**EAT SMART, EAT HEALTHY
WITH THE ULTIMATE REFERENCE GUIDE
FOR TODAY'S HEALTH-CONSCIOUS CONSUMER**

Are you serious about good eating? Are you counting carbs? Boosting protein? Restricting salt? Whatever your nutritional needs, it's essential that you have the most up-to-date, comprehensive nutritional information available. Whether you're under a doctor's supervision or just trying to maintain a healthy lifestyle, you're in good hands with Corinne T. Netzer, the bestselling expert who sets the standard against which all others are measured with the latest, most accurate nutritional information available.

Now you can make *informed* choices among the foods you love best. With Corinne T. Netzer's help, you can find essential food counts quickly and easily in one indispensable guide. . . . Keep a copy in the kitchen . . . take it to the office . . . carry it with you on trips—it's the best and most authoritative dietary reference available—the one book you can't afford to miss!

THOUSANDS MORE LISTINGS THAN EVER BEFORE!

**THE COMPLETE BOOK
OF FOOD COUNTS
6TH EDITION**

CORINNE T. NETZER

Sixth Edition

THE
COMPLETE
BOOK
OF
FOOD COUNTS

Corinne T. Netzer

A DELL BOOK

Published by
Dell Publishing
a division of
Random House, Inc.
New York, New York

ISBN: 0-440-22564-7

Manufactured in the United States of America

Published simultaneously in Canada

January 2003

10 9 8 7 6 5

OPM

For
Pat Ladew

Introduction

The sixth edition of *The Complete Book of Food Counts* is the largest compilation of essential food data in this format. It contains data (calories, protein, carbohydrates, fat, cholesterol, sodium, and fiber) for basic generic foods, brand-name foods, and restaurant chains. Whether you are interested in dieting or nutrition—or both—you will find this book unique and invaluable as a reference.

Since this book is alphabetized, you should have no difficulty finding whatever you wish to look up. There are, however, times when you may have to look in more than one place. If you are searching for a particular food and cannot find it immediately, look for it under a category, such as cakes, puddings, cookies, soups. Wherever sensible, I have cross-referenced listings, but the pressure of space has made it impossible to do that for every item.

Compare only foods listed in similar measures. This rule particularly applies to the confusion between measures by capacity and measures by weight. Eight ounces is not necessarily equivalent to eight fluid ounces or one cup. Eight ounces is a measure of how much something weighs; one cup is a measure of how much space it occupies. For instance, a cup of lightweight food, such as puffed rice or popcorn, weighs about one ounce, and eight ounces of the same product would fill many cups. Naturally, you can convert a similar unit of measure into a smaller or larger amount. The following table may be useful in making such conversions.

Equivalents by Capacity
(all measures level)
1 quart = 4 cups
1 cup = 8 fluid ounces
= ½ pint
= 16 tablespoons
2 tablespoons = 1 fluid ounce
1 tablespoon = 3 teaspoons

Equivalents by Weight
1 pound = 16 ounces
3.57 ounces = 100 grams
1 ounce = 28.35 grams

All the material contained in *The Complete Book of Food Counts* is based on information from the United States government, from producers and processors of brand-name foods, and from food chains. The data contained herein is the most complete and accurate information available as this book goes to press. Please bear in mind that seasonal and regional differences can affect the nutritional value of foods. Also, the food industry often changes recipes and sizes and may discontinue products or add new ones. In the future I will revise and update this book to keep you completely informed.

Good luck and good dieting.

Corinne T. Netzer

ABBREVIATIONS AND SYMBOLS

cal.	calories
carbo.	carbohydrates
chol.	cholesterol
cont.	container
diam.	diameter
fl.	fluid
gms	grams
"	inch
<	less than
lb(s).	pound(s)
mgs.	milligrams
n.a.	not available
oz.	ounce
pc(s).	piece(s)
pkg.	package
pkt.	packet
prot.	protein
sod.	sodium
sq.	square
tbsp.	tablespoon
tsp.	teaspoon
tr.	trace
w/	with
*	prepared according to basic package directions, except as noted

---

Note: Brand-name foods and restaurants listed in italics denote registered trademarks.

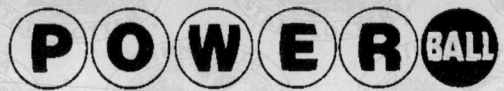

POWERBALL

PROGRESSIVE PRINT-N-PLAY
INSTANT FUN WITH A
PROGRESSIVE JACKPOT!
HAVE YOU PLAYED TODAY?

091-048325633-1263-32

POWER PLAY NO

001 02 04 13 15 59 PB 06Q6

SAT FEB 25 12
$2.00
02/25/12 09:13:50
091-048325633-1263-32
T02357620   R00235762
018424

FOR WINNING NUMBERS, PLEASE

VISIT YOUR LOTTERY RETAILER,
OR VISIT WWW.MNLOTTERY.COM,
OR CALL 651-634-1111.

PHONE NO. _____

For your protection, we encourage you to always sign your ticket whenever presenting for payment or having it checked to determine winning status.

To claim your prize: Complete information above and sign. Prize amounts of less than $600 may be paid at any Lottery Retailer provided funds are available. Prize amounts of $600 or more require a claim form, which can be obtained from our website at www.mnlottery.com or by contacting the Lottery. All Lottery Offices will pay prizes up to $30,000, or the player may submit the ticket for payment by mail. Complete the ticket back, sign, and mail the ticket with a claim form to MINNESOTA STATE LOTTERY, P.O. BOX 131000, ROSEVILLE, MN 55113. Prizes over $30,000 must be claimed, in person, at Lottery Headquarters at 2645 Long Lake Road, Roseville, Minnesota.

Important: Tickets are bearer instruments until signed. All tickets, transactions, and winners are subject to the rules of the Minnesota State Lottery. Tickets are VOID if torn, altered, illegible, or incomplete. The Lottery is not responsible for lost or stolen tickets.   Website: www.mnlottery.com PH: 651-635-8273

RMF REV. 02/08 Part# MN1000-01

GAMBLING PROBLEM? Call 1-800-333-HOPE Not a winning numbers line.	CARE FOR TICKETS:	
		Do not deface / Do not iron / Avoid heat / Keep dry

AC-
SERIES

850730256

SIGNATURE _____

NAME _____

ADDRESS _____

CITY _____ STATE _____ ZIP _____

PHONE NO. _____

For your protection, we encourage you to always sign your ticket whenever presenting for payment or having it checked to determine winning status.

To claim your prize: Complete information above and sign. Prize amounts of less than $600 may be paid at any Lottery Retailer provided funds are available. Prize amounts of $600 or more require a claim form, which can be obtained from our website at www.mnlottery.com or by contacting the Lottery. All Lottery Offices will pay prizes up to $30,000, or the player may submit the ticket for payment by mail. Complete the ticket back, sign, and mail the ticket with a claim form to MINNESOTA STATE LOTTERY, P.O. BOX 131000, ROSEVILLE, MN 55113. Prizes over $30,000 must be claimed, in person, at Lottery Headquarters at 2645 Long Lake Road, Roseville, Minnesota.

Important: Tickets are bearer instruments until signed. All tickets, transactions, and winners are subject to the rules of the Minnesota State Lottery. Tickets are VOID if torn, altered, illegible, or incomplete. The Lottery is not responsible for lost or stolen tickets.   Website: www.mnlottery.com PH: 651-635-8273

RMF REV. 02/08 Part# MN1000-01

GAMBLING PROBLEM? Call 1-800-333-HOPE Not a winning numbers line.	CARE FOR TICKETS:	
		Do not deface / Do not iron / Avoid heat / Keep dry

AC-
SERIES

850730257

SIGNATURE _____

NAME _____

THE
COMPLETE
BOOK
OF
FOOD COUNTS

A

Food and Measure	cal.	prot. (gms)	carbo. (gms)	fat (gms)	chol. (mgs)	sod. (mgs)	fiber (gms)
Abalone, meat only,							
raw, 4 oz.	119	19.4	6.8	.9	96	341	0
Abruzzese sausage							
(*Boar's Head*), 1 oz.	100	8.0	<1.0	8.0	15	540	0
Acerola, fresh:							
10 fruits	15	.2	3.7	.1	0	3	.5
peeled, 1 cup	31	.4	7.5	.3	0	7	1.1
Acerola juice, fresh,							
8 fl. oz.	56	1.0	11.6	.7	0	7	.7
Acorn squash:							
raw:							
(*Frieda's*), ¾ cup,							
3 oz.	35	1.0	9.0	0	0	0	2.0
4" squash, 15.2 oz.	172	3.5	44.9	.4	0	13	6.6
cubed, 1 cup	56	1.1	14.6	.1	0	4	2.1
baked, cubed, ½ cup	57	1.1	14.9	.1	0	4	4.5
boiled, mashed, ½ cup	42	.8	10.8	.1	0	4	3.2
Adobo sauce (*Doña Maria*), 2 tbsp. . . .	230	2.0	10.0	15.0	0	370	2.0
Adobo seasoning							
(*Goya*), ¼ tsp	0	0	0	0	0	360	0
Adzuki beans:							
dry (*Arrowhead Mills*),							
¼ cup	160	11.0	29.0	.5	0	0	6.0
boiled, ½ cup	147	8.7	28.5	.1	0	9	8.4
Adzuki beans, canned,							
(*Eden* Aduki), ½ cup	110	7.0	19.0	0	0	10	5.0
Aioli, see "Mayonnaise"							
Alfalfa sprouts, 1 cup:							
(*Jonathan's*)	25	3.0	3.0	.5	0	5	2.0
w/dill sprouts (*Jonathan's*)	30	3.0	4.0	.5	0	15	2.0
w/garlic (*Jonathan's*) .	27	3.0	4.0	.5	0	5	2.0
w/onion (*Jonathan's*) .	25	3.0	3.0	.5	0	5	2.0

Food and Measure	cal.	prot. (gms)	carbo. (gms)	fat (gms)	chol. (mgs)	sod. (mgs)	fiber (gms)
Alfalfa sprouts *(cont.)*							
w/radish sprouts							
(*Jonathan's*)	30	3.0	3.0	1.5	0	5	2.0
Alfredo sauce, can or							
jar, ¼ cup, except							
as noted:							
(*Classico* Di Roma) . .	110	2.0	3.0	10.0	50	480	0
(*Five Brothers*							
Creamy)	110	2.0	3.0	10.0	35	420	0
(*Progresso*), ½ cup . .	200	8.0	7.0	15.0	50	850	1.0
(*Watkins* Pasta Top-							
per), 2 tbsp.	30	1.0	3.0	1.5	5	270	0
cheese, see "Cheese							
sauce, cooking"							
garlic (*Five Brothers*) .	100	2.0	3.0	10.0	30	360	0
garlic, roasted (*Clas-*							
sico Di Sorrento) . .	110	2.0	3.0	10.0	50	460	0
mushroom:							
(*Five Brothers*)	80	2.0	3.0	7.0	25	380	0
(*Francesco Rinaldi*)	60	2.0	3.0	4.0	10	480	0
(*Healthy Choice*) . .	45	3.0	3.0	3.0	<5	430	0
tomato, see "Pasta							
sauce"							
Alfredo sauce, refrig-							
erated, ¼ cup:							
(*Buitoni*)	130	4.0	7.0	10.0	35	420	0
(*Buitoni* Light)	80	4.0	5.0	5.0	15	350	0
(*Di Giorno*)	180	3.0	3.0	18.0	25	560	0
(*Di Giorno* Reduced							
Fat)	130	5.0	10.0	8.0	35	580	0
Alfredo sauce mix:							
(*Knorr* Pasta Sauces),							
2 tbsp.	60	2.0	7.0	3.0	5	760	0
(*McCormick*), 1 cup*	90	3.0	4.0	6.0	0	860	0
Allspice, 1 tsp.	5	.1	1.4	.2	0	1	.4
Almond, shelled:							
(*Fisher*), 1 oz.	170	7.0	6.0	14.0	0	0	3.0
(*Setton Farm*), 3 tbsp.,							
1.1 oz.	130	6.0	4.0	9.0	0	0	3.0
whole, natural:							
(*Blue Diamond*),							
3 tbsp.	180	6.0	6.0	15.0	0	0	4.0
(*House of Bazzini*),							
1 oz.	170	6.0	6.0	14.0	0	0	4.0

Food and Measure	cal.	prot. (gms)	carbo. (gms)	fat (gms)	chol. (mgs)	sod. (mgs)	fiber (gms)
(*Sonoma* Organic), ¼ cup, 1.1 oz.	180	6.0	6.0	15.0	0	0	4.0
dried:							
1 oz.	167	5.7	5.8	14.8	0	3	3.1
slivered, 1 cup	795	26.9	27.5	70.5	0	15	14.7
dry-roasted, salted, 1 oz.	167	4.6	6.9	14.7	0	221	3.9
lightly salted (*Blue Diamond*), 3 tbsp.	180	6.0	4.0	17.0	0	110	3.0
oil-roasted, salted:							
(*Blue Diamond* 6 oz.), 3 tbsp. . .	180	6.0	4.0	17.0	0	110	3.0
(*Blue Diamond* 4.5 oz.), 3 tbsp.	190	7.0	4.0	17.0	0	110	3.0
salted, 1 oz.	176	5.8	4.5	16.4	0	221	3.2
sliced:							
(*Bazzini's Nut Club*), 1 oz.	170	6.0	6.0	14.0	0	0	4.0
blanched (*Blue Diamond*), ⅓ cup . .	200	7.0	6.0	17.0	0	0	4.0
slivered (*Planters*), 2-oz. pkg.	340	6.0	11.0	31.0	0	0	6.0
slivered, blanched:							
(*Bazzini's Nut Club*), 1 oz.	170	6.0	5.0	14.0	0	2	3.0
(*Blue Diamond*), ¼ cup	200	7.0	6.0	16.0	0	0	4.0
toasted:							
1 oz.	167	5.8	6.5	14.4	0	3	3.2
sliced (*Blue Diamond*), ⅓ cup . .	200	7.0	7.0	17.0	0	0	4.0
barbecue:							
(*Blue Diamond* 6 oz.) 3 tbsp. . .	170	6.0	5.0	15.0	0	250	4.0
(*Blue Diamond* 4.5 oz.), 3 tbsp.	180	7.0	5.0	16.0	0	260	4.0
frosted, slivered (*Blue Diamond* Fabs), 1-oz. pkg. . .	150	4.0	12.0	10.0	0	70	2.0
green onion, slivered:							
(*Blue Diamond*), ¼ cup	210	6.0	7.0	18.0	0	240	3.0
(*Blue Diamond* Gorbs), 3 tbsp. .	180	5.0	6.0	15.0	0	200	3.0

Food and Measure	cal.	prot. (gms)	carbo. (gms)	fat (gms)	chol. (mgs)	sod. (mgs)	fiber (gms)
Almond *(cont.)*							
honey-roasted:							
(*Blue Diamond*							
8 oz.), 3 tbsp. . . .	170	5.0	8.0	14.0	0	35	2.0
(*Blue Diamond*							
4.5 oz.), 3 tbsp.	180	5.0	8.0	15.0	0	40	3.0
1 oz.	168	5.2	7.9	14.2	0	37	3.9
smoke flavor, 3 tbsp.:							
(*Blue Diamond*							
Smokehouse							
8 / 40 oz.)	180	6.0	4.0	16.0	0	170	2.0
(*Blue Diamond*							
Smokehouse							
4.5 oz.)	180	6.0	5.0	17.0	0	180	3.0
smoked (*Planters*),							
1 oz.	170	4.0	6.0	15.0	0	200	3.0
Almond butter (*Arrow-*							
head Mills), 2 tbsp.	210	5.0	7.0	20.0	0	0	2.0
Almond meal, 1 oz.	116	11.2	8.2	5.2	0	2	n.a.
Almond paste, see							
"Pastry filling"							
Almond syrup (*Trader*							
Vic's Orgeat),							
2 tbsp.	100	0	25.0	0	0	15	0
Amaranth, whole-grain,							
1 oz.	106	4.1	18.8	1.8	0	6	4.3
Amaranth flakes, see							
"Cereal, ready-to-							
eat"							
Amaranth flour (*Arrow-*							
head Mills), ¼ cup	110	4.0	19.0	1.5	0	0	2.0
Amaranth leaves,							
½ cup:							
raw, trimmed	4	.3	.6	<.1	0	3	n.a.
boiled, drained	14	1.4	1.0	.1	0	14	n.a.
Amaranth seeds							
(*Arrowhead Mills*),							
¼ cup	170	7.0	29.0	2.0	0	0	3.0
Amaretto syrup							
(*Ferrara*), 2 oz. . . .	130	0	32.0	0	0	12	0
Anasazi beans, dry							
(*Arrowhead Mills*),							
¼ cup	150	10.0	27.0	.5	0	0	9.0
Anchovy, fresh, Eu-							

Food and Measure	cal.	prot. (gms)	carbo. (gms)	fat (gms)	chol. (mgs)	sod. (mgs)	fiber (gms)
ropean, meat only, raw, 1 oz.	37	5.8	0	1.4	17	29	0
Anchovy, canned, in olive oil:							
(Bumble Bee), 6 pcs.	25	4.0	0	1.5	15	750	0
(Crown Prince Natural), 9 pcs.	35	4.0	0	2.5	15	1050	0
(Granadaisa), 9 pcs.	35	4.0	0	2.5	15	1050	0
drained, 1 oz.	60	8.2	0	2.8	24	1040	0
5 medium, .7 oz. ...	42	5.8	.0	1.9	3	734	0
Anchovy paste (Reese's), 1 tbsp.	30	2.0	0	2.5	55	940	0
Andouille sausage, see "Sausage"							
Angel-hair pasta: dry, see "Pasta"							
refrigerated:							
(Buitoni), 1¼ cups	230	9.0	43.0	2.5	85	20	2.0
(Di Giorno), 2 oz.	160	6.0	31.0	1.5	0	115	2.0
Angel-hair pasta dish, mix, 1 cup*:							
w/garlic and butter (Pasta Roni)	260	8.0	40.0	8.0	5	760	2.0
w/herbs (Pasta Roni)	320	9.0	42.0	13.0	5	820	2.0
w/lemon and butter (Pasta Roni)	360	9.0	48.0	15.0	0	1270	2.0
w/Parmesan (Pasta Roni)	320	9.0	38.0	14.0	5	880	2.0
primavera (Pasta Roni)	330	9.0	38.0	16.0	5	990	2.0
tomato, spicy (Near East)	240	8.0	41.0	6.0	0	630	3.0
tomato Parmesan (Pasta Roni)	280	10.0	40.0	9.0	10	920	2.0
Angle-hair pasta entree, frozen, 1 pkg.:							
(Lean Cuisine Everyday Favorites), 10 oz. .	240	9.0	43.0	4.0	5	690	4.0
w/chunky tomato, meat sauce (Budget Gourmet), 8 oz. ..	240	8.0	39.0	5.0	10	450	3.0
Anise seed, 1 tsp. ..	7	.4	1.1	.3	0	<1	.3
Antelope, meat only, roasted, 4 oz.	170	33.4	0	3.0	143	51	0

Food and Measure	cal.	prot. (gms)	carbo. (gms)	fat (gms)	chol. (mgs)	sod. (mgs)	fiber (gms)
Appaloosa beans, dry, (*Frieda's*), ½ cup ..	120	7.0	22.0	0	0	0	9.0
Apple, fresh:							
raw, w/peel:							
(*Dole*), 1 medium	80	0	22.0	0	0	0	5.0
(*Frieda's* Lady),							
5 oz.	80	0	21.0	.5	0	0	3.0
·2¾" apple	81	.3	21.1	.5	0	1	3.7
sliced, ½ cup	32	.1	8.4	.2	0	0	3.0
raw, peeled:							
2¾" apple	72	.2	19.0	.4	0	<1	2.4
sliced, ½ cup	31	.1	8.2	.2	0	0	1.0
cooked, peeled, sliced,							
boiled, ½ cup	45	.2	11.7	.3	0	1	2.0
Apple, can or jar:							
cinnamon (*Del Monte Fruitrageous*),							
4 oz.	80	0	19.0	0	0	10	<1.0
pie, spiced, in sauce							
(*Del Monte Fruit Pleasures*), ½ cup	70	0	18.0	0	0	10	<1.0
sweetened, sliced,							
drained, ½ cup ...	68	.2	17.0	<.1	0	3	1.7
Apple, coated, candy or caramel (*Tastee*),							
3-oz. apple	160	3.0	26.0	5.0	0	20	4.0
Apple, dried (see also "Apple snack"):							
(*Sonoma* Organic),							
11 rings, 1.4 oz. ..	110	0	29.0	0	0	0	4.0
(*Sunsweet*), ¼ cup,							
1.4 oz.	110	<1.0	27.0	0	0	270	3.0
dehydrated:							
(*AlpineAire*), 1 oz.	100	0	26.0	0	0	150	2.0
½ cup	104	.4	28.1	.2	0	74	7.4
flakes, unsulfured							
(*AlpineAire*), 1 oz.	110	0	26.0	0	0	95	1.0
sulfured:							
1 ring	16	.1	4.2	0	0	6	4.2
½ cup	104	.4	28.3	.1	0	75	7.5
Apple, escalloped, see "Apple dish"							
Apple, frozen, un-heated, ½ cup	42	0	10.7	0	0	3	1.6

Food and Measure	cal.	prot. (gms)	carbo. (gms)	fat (gms)	chol. (mgs)	sod. (mgs)	fiber (gms)
Apple butter, 1 tbsp.:							
(*Eden* Organic)	20	0	6.0	0	0	0	0
(*Kraft*)	25	0	6.0	0	0	0	0
(*Lost Acres*)	35	0	9.0	0	0	0	0
(*Lucky Leaf/*							
Musselman's)	30	0	8.0	0	0	0	0
(*Smucker's* Cider) . . .	45	0	11.0	0	0	10	0
(*Tap'n Apple*)	20	0	5.0	0	0	0	<1.0
Apple chips, see							
"Apple snack"							
Apple cider, see							
"Apple drink" and							
"Apple Juice"							
Apple cider, alcoholic							
(*Hard Core* Crisp),							
12 fl. oz.	190	1.0	19.0	0	0	15	0
Apple cinnamon syrup							
(*Knott's Berry Farm*							
Light), ¼ cup	100	0	25.0	0	0	15	0
Apple dip, 2 tbsp.:							
caramel:							
(*Marzetti*)	150	1.0	23.0	6.0	4	90	0
(*Marzetti* Fat Free)	120	1.0	27.0	0	0	120	0
peanut butter caramel							
(*Marzetti*)	130	3.0	16.0	7.0	0	160	1.0
Apple dish, frozen:							
cinnamon (*Boston*							
Market), ½ cup . . .	260	0	53.0	5.0	0	10	2.0
escalloped (*Stouffer's*							
Side Dish), 6 oz. . .	210	1.0	43.0	4.0	0	40	3.0
Apple drink, 8 fl. oz.,							
except as noted:							
(*Libby's* Nectar),							
11.5-fl.-oz. can . . .	200	0	49.0	0	0	10	0
(*Musselman's* Little							
Brown Jug Cider) . .	120	0	31.0	0	0	25	0
sparkling (*Lucky Leaf/*							
Musselman's Cider)	150	0	36.0	0	0	20	0
Apple drink blends,							
8 fl. oz., except as							
noted:							
cranberry (*Tropicana*),							
11.5 fl. oz.	200	0	49.0	0	0	45	0

Food and Measure	cal.	prot. (gms)	carbo. (gms)	fat (gms)	chol. (mgs)	sod. (mgs)	fiber (gms)
Apple drink blends *(cont.)*							
raspberry blackberry (*Tropicana Twister*)	120	0	31.0	0	0	20	0
herbal cider (*Turkey Hill*)	100	0	24.0	0	0	10	0
raspberry blackberry (*Tropicana Twister*), 11.5 fl. oz.	180	0	45.0	0	0	30	0
Apple dumpling, frozen (*Pepperidge Farm*), 3-oz. pc. . .	250	3.0	33.0	11.0	0	180	1.0
Apple fritters, frozen (*Mrs. Paul's*), 2 pcs.	240	3.0	33.0	11.0	<5	570	1.0
Apple juice, 8 fl. oz., except as noted:							
(*After the Fall* Organic)	90	0	22.0	0	0	20	0
(*Apple Time*)	120	0	31.0	0	0	25	0
(*Dole*)	110	<1.0	27.0	0	0	10	0
(*Dole*), 10 fl. oz.	140	1.0	34.0	0	0	15	0
(*Dole*), 11.5 fl. oz. . ,	160	<1.0	39.0	0	0	15	0
(*Edon* Organic)	80	0	23.0	0	0	0	0
(*Langers* Cider/ Harvest)	120	0	28.0	0	0	0	0
(*Lincoln*)	120	0	31.0	0	0	25	0
(*Lucky Leaf/ Musselman's*)	120	0	31.0	0	0	25	0
(*Lucky Leaf* 100%) . .	120	0	31.0	0	0	20	0
(*Martinelli's* Juice/ Cider)	140	1.0	35.0	0	0	0	0
(*Martinelli's* Sparkling), 10 fl. oz.	180	1.0	43.0	0	0	0	1.0
(*Mott's* Natural)	110	0	27.0	0	0	25	0
(*Mott's* from Concentrate)	120	0	29.0	0	0	10	0
(*Nantucket Nectars* Cider/Pressed)	100	0	25.0	0	0	10	<1.0
(*R. W. Knudsen* Aseptic Organic)	110	0	28.0	0	0	5	0
(*R. W. Knudsen* Natural/ Gravenstein Organic/ Cider & Spice)	120	<1.0	30.0	0	0	25	0
(*Santa Cruz Organic*)	120	<1.0	30.0	0	0	25	0
(*Season's Best*)	110	1.0	27.0	0	0	10	0

Food and Measure	cal.	prot. (gms)	carbo. (gms)	fat (gms)	chol. (mgs)	sod. (mgs	fiber (gms)
(*Season's Best*), 10 fl. oz.	140	1.0	34.0	0	0	15	0
(*Season's Best*), 11.5 fl. oz.	160	0	40.0	0	0	30	0
(*Season's Best* Calcium/ Vitamin C), 10 fl. oz.	140	<1.0	35.0	0	0	30	0
(*Snapple*)	120	0	30.0	0	0	10	0
(*Speas Farm* Juice/ Cider)	120	0	31.0	0	0	25	0
(*Ziegler's* Cider)	120	0	30.0	0	0	25	0
cider, sparkling:							
(*Heinke's*)	120	1.0	30.0	0	0	25	0
(*R. W. Knudsen*) ..	110	0	28.0	0	0	5	0
frozen* (*Cascadian Farm*)	120	0	30.0	0	0	15	0
Apple juice blends, 8 fl. oz.:							
all blends:							
(*Martinelli's*)	110	0	27.0	0	0	4	0
except apricot (*R. W. Knudsen*)	120	<1.0	30.0	0	0	25	0
apricot (*R. W. Knudsen*)	120	<1.0	30.0	0	0	35	0
cranberry (*R. W. Knudsen* Aseptic) .	110	1.0	29.0	0	0	25	0
grape (*Juicy Juice*) ..	120	0	29.0	0	0	10	0
Apple pastry (see also specific listings):							
puffs (*Entenmann's*), 3-oz. pc.	270	2.0	37.0	13.0	0	230	1.0
strudel (*Entenmann's*), ¼ pastry	340	3.0	50.0	15.0	0	240	2.0
Apple snack:							
(*Weight Watchers*), 1 pkg.	50	0	13.0	0	0	125	2.0
w/caramel (*Sonoma* Apple-Teasers), 10 rings, 1.4 oz. ..	110	0	25.0	0	0	15	3.0
chips:							
(*Tastee*), 1 oz.	130	0	22.0	6.0	0	10	2.0
(*Weight Watchers*), 1 pkg.	70	0	18.0	0	0	125	3.0

Food and Measure	cal.	prot. (gms)	carbo. (gms)	fat (gms)	chol. (mgs)	sod. (mgs)	fiber (gms)
Apple snack, chips *(cont.)*							
all flavors except pink lady (*Seneca*), 1 oz.	140	0	20.0	7.0	0	15	2.0
pink lady (*Seneca*), 1 oz.	160	0	20.0	9.0	0	15	4.0
Applesauce, ½ cup, except as noted:							
(*Lucky Leaf* Chunky) .	90	0	22.0	0	0	10	2.0
(*Lucky Leaf* 4-Pack), 6 oz.	120	0	30.0	0	0	10	3.0
(*Lucky Leaf/ Musselman's* 6-Pack), 4 oz.	80	0	20.0	0	0	10	2.0
(*Mott's* Original)	110	0	27.0	0	0	0	1.0
(*Mott's* Original), 4-oz. cont.	90	0	22.0	0	0	0	1.0
(*Musselman's*)	90	0	22.0	0	0	10	2.0
(*Musselman's* Chunky)	100	0	25.0	0	0	10	2.0
(*Musselman's* Chunky 6-Pack), 4 oz.	80	0	21.0	0	0	10	2.0
(*Musselman's* Premium), 4 oz.	90	0	22.0	0	0	10	2.0
(*S&W*)	90	0	21.0	0	0	5	1.0
cinnamon:							
(*Apple Time*)	100	0	25.0	0	0	10	2.0
(*Apple Time* Original Unsweetened), 4 oz.	50	0	12.0	0	0	10	2.0
(*Lucky Leaf/ Musselman's*) . .	100	0	25.0	0	0	10	2.0
(*Lucky Leaf/ Musselman's* 6-Pack), 4 oz. . .	80	0	21.0	0	0	10	2.0
(*Mott's*), 4-oz. cont.	100	0	26.0	0	0	0	1.0
(*Musselman's* 4-Pack), 6 oz. . .	130	0	31.0	0	0	10	3.0
unsweetened/natural:							
(*Apple Time* Original)	50	0	13.0	0	0	10	2.0
(*Eden* Organic) . . .	50	0	15.0	0	0	15	2.0
(*Langers*)	50	0	13.0	0	0	5	2.0

Food and Measure	cal.	prot. (gms)	carbo. (gms)	fat (gms)	chol. (mgs)	sod. (mgs)	fiber (gms)
(*Lucky Leaf* Old Fashioned/ *Musselman's*) ..	50	0	13.0	0	0	20	2.0
(*Lucky Leaf* Old Fashioned/ *Musselman's* 4-Pack), 6 oz. ...	70	0	18.0	0	0	25	3.0
(*Lucky Leaf* Old Fashioned/ *Musselman's* 6-Pack), 4 oz. ...	50	0	12.0	0	0	20	2.0
(*Mott's*), 3.9-oz. cont.	50	0	12.0	0	0	0	1.0
(*Santa Cruz Organic* Gravenstein) ...	45	<1.0	15.0	0	0	5	2.0
(*S&W*)	50	0	13.0	0	0	5	2.0
Applesauce blends, 4-oz. cont., except as noted:							
all fruits:							
(*Santa Cruz Organic*), ½ cup	45	<1.0	15.0	0	0	5	2.0
except strawberry and strawberry-banana (*Mott's Fruitsations*) ...	90	0	23.0	0	0	0	1.0
berry, mixed (*Mott's*)	90	0	22.0	0	0	0	1.0
mixed fruit (*Mott's Rugrats*)	90	0	22.0	0	0	0	1.0
strawberry:							
(*Mott's*)	80	0	22.0	0	0	10	1.0
(*Mott's Fruitsa-tions*)	90	0	23.0	0	0	10	1.0
strawberry-banana (*Mott's Fruitsa-tions*)	90	0	23.0	0	0	5	1.0
watermelon (*Mott's Rugrats*)	100	0	23.0	0	0	0	1.0
Apricot, fresh:							
(*Dole*), 3 medium, 4 oz.	60	0	11.0	1.0	0	0	1.0
3 medium, 12 per lb.	51	1.5	11.8	.4	0	1	2.5
pitted, ½ cup:							
halves	37	1.1	8.6	.3	0	1	1.9
sliced	40	1.2	9.2	.3	0	2	2.0

Food and Measure	cal.	prot. (gms)	carbo. (gms)	fat (gms)	chol. (mgs)	sod. (mgs)	fiber (gms)
Apricot, can or jar,							
½ cup, halves,							
except as noted:							
(*Del Monte* Lite)	60	0	16.0	0	0	10	1.0
in juice:							
(*Libby's*)	80	1.0	21.0	0	0	10	1.0
w/liquid	59	.8	15.1	<.1	0	5	2.0
in light syrup:							
(*Del Monte Orchard*							
Select)	80	0	21.0	0	0	10	1.0
almond flavored							
(*Del Monte*)	90	0	22.0	0	0	10	1.0
almond flavored							
(*S&W* Sun)	90	<1.0	22.0	0	0	25	1.0
w/liquid	80	.7	20.9	<.1	0	5	2.0
in heavy syrup:							
(*Del Monte*)	100	0	26.0	0	0	10	1.0
w/liquid	107	.7	27.7	.1	0	5	2.1
whole, peeled							
(*S&W*)	120	<1.0	29.0	0	0	10	1.0
Apricot, dried:							
(*Setton Farm*), 5 pcs.	90	1.0	22.0	0	0	10	2.0
(*Sonoma* Organic),							
10 pcs., 1.4 oz. ...	130	2.0	31.0	0	0	0	3.0
(*Sun•Maid Fast*							
Fruits), ¼ cup,							
1.4 oz.	110	1.0	25.0	0	0	0	2.0
(*Sunsweet*), 1.4 oz.,							
about 5 pcs.	100	1.0	26.0	0	0	30	3.0
(*Sunsweet Fruitlings*),							
⅓ cup, 1.4 oz.	110	1.0	29.0	0	0	30	3.0
dehydrated, ½ cup ..	190	2.9	49.3	.4	0	15	n.a.
sulfured, ½ cup	155	2.4	40.1	.3	0	7	5.9
sun-dried (*Sunsweet*							
California), 1.4 oz.,							
about 5 pcs.	100	1.0	24.0	0	0	0	4.0
Apricot, frozen,							
sweetened,							
½ cup	119	.9	30.4	.1	0	5	2.1
Apricot butter (*Lost*							
Acres), 1 tbsp. ...	45	0	11.0	0	0	10	0
Apricot juice, blend							
(*Ceres*), 5.25 fl. oz.	87	0	21.0	0	0	n.a.	0

Food and Measure	cal.	prot. (gms)	carbo. (gms)	fat (gms)	chol. (mgs)	sod. (mgs)	fiber (gms)
Apricot nectar:							
(*Goya*), 6 fl. oz.	120	0	29.0	0	0	30	0
(*Goya*), 8 fl. oz.	130	1.0	31.0	0	0	15	0
(*Libby's*), 5.5 fl. oz. . .	100	<1.0	24.0	0	0	5	0
(*Libby's*), 8 fl. oz. . . .	150	<1.0	36.0	0	0	10	0
(*Libby's*), 11.5 fl. oz. . .	210	1.0	24.0	0	0	10	0
(*R. W. Knudsen/Santa Cruz Organic*), 8 fl. oz.	120	<1.0	30.0	0	0	35	0
(*S&W*), 11.5 fl. oz. . .	210	2.0	53.0	0	0	20	1.0
Apricot sauce, sweet and spicy (*Susan Elaine's*), 2 tbsp. . . .	60	0	15.0	0	0	10	0
Apricot syrup, ¼ cup:							
(*Knott's Berry Farm*)	210	0	52.0	0	0	30	0
(*Smucker's*)	210	0	52.0	0	0	0	0
Arame, see "Seaweed"							
Arby's, 1 serving:							
breakfast items:							
biscuit w/bacon . . .	360	9.0	27.0	24.0	10	1000	1.0
biscuit w/butter . . .	280	5.0	27.0	17.0	0	780	.5
biscuit w/ham	330	12.0	28.0	20.0	30	1610	1.0
biscuit w/sausage	460	12.0	28.0	33.0	25	1130	1.0
croissant w/bacon	340	10.0	28.0	23.0	30	520	1.0
croissant w/ham . .	310	13.0	29.0	19.0	50	1130	0
croissant w/sausage	440	13.0	29.0	32.0	45	600	0
sourdough w/bacon	420	16.0	66.0	10.0	10	960	3.0
sourdough w/ham .	390	19.0	67.0	6.0	30	1570	2.0
sourdough w/sausage	520	19.0	67.0	19.0	25	1040	2.0
add egg	110	5.0	2.0	9.0	175	170	0
add Swiss cheese .	45	3.0	0	3.0	10	220	0
French *Toastix,* no syrup	370	7.0	48.0	17.0	0	440	4.0
syrup, .5 oz.	130	0	32.0	0	0	45	0
sandwiches:							
roast beef:							
Arby's melt	340	16.0	36.0	15.0	70	890	2.0
Arby-Q	360	16.0	40.0	14.0	70	1530	2.0
beef 'n cheddar	480	23.0	43.0	24.0	90	1240	2.0
Big Montana . . .	630	47.0	41.0	32.0	155	2080	3.0
giant	480	32.0	41.0	23.0	110	1440	3.0
junior	310	16.0	34.0	13.0	70	740	2.0
regular	350	21.0	34.0	16.0	85	950	2.0
super	470	22.0	47.0	23.0	85	1130	3.0

Food and Measure	cal.	prot. (gms)	carbo. (gms)	fat (gms)	chol. (mgs)	sod. (mgs)	fiber (gms)
Arby's, sandwiches *(cont.)*							
chicken:							
bacon 'n Swiss	610	31.0	49.0	33.0	110	1550	2.0
breast fillet	540	24.0	47.0	30.0	90	1160	2.0
cordon bleu	630	34.0	47.0	35.0	120	1820	2.0
grilled deluxe ...	450	29.0	37.0	22.0	110	1050	2.0
roast, club	520	29.0	38.0	28.0	115	1440	2.0
hot ham 'n Swiss ..	340	23.0	35.0	13.0	90	1450	1.0
sub:							
French dip	440	28.0	42.0	18.0	100	1680	2.0
hot ham 'n Swiss	530	29.0	45.0	27.0	110	1860	3.0
Italian	780	29.0	49.0	53.0	120	2440	3.0
Philly beef 'n							
Swiss	700	36.0	46.0	42.0	130	1940	4.0
roast beef	760	35.0	47.0	48.0	130	2230	3.0
turkey	630	26.0	51.0	37.0	100	2170	2.0
Market Fresh:							
grilled chicken							
supreme	610	41.0	39.0	34.0	155	1860	2.0
roast beef/Swiss	810	37.0	73.0	42.0	130	1780	5.0
roast ham/Swiss	730	36.0	74.0	34.0	125	2180	5.0
roast chicken							
Caesar	820	43.0	75.0	38.0	140	2160	5.0
roast turkey ranch							
and bacon	880	48.0	74.0	44.0	155	2320	5.0
roast turkey/							
Swiss	760	43.0	75.0	33.0	130	1920	5.0
ultimate BLT ...	820	24.0	72.0	49.0	110	1480	5.0
light deluxe:							
grilled chicken ..	280	29.0	30.0	5.0	55	1170	3.0
roast chicken ...	260	23.0	33.0	5.0	40	1010	3.0
roast turkey	260	23.0	33.0	5.0	40	980	3.0
salad, no dressing:							
chicken, roast	160	20.0	15.0	2.5	40	700	6.0
chicken, grilled ...	210	30.0	14.0	4.5	65	800	6.0
garden	70	4.0	14.0	1.0	0	45	6.0
side	25	2.0	5.0	0	0	20	2.0
Market Fresh:							
Caesar	90	7.0	8.0	4.0	10	170	3.0
Caesar, chicken	230	33.0	8.0	8.0	80	920	3.0
Caesar side	45	4.0	4.0	2.0	5	95	2.0
chicken finger ..	570	30.0	39.0	34.0	65	1300	3.0
turkey club	350	33.0	9.0	21.0	90	920	3.0

Food and Measure	cal.	prot. (gms)	carbo. (gms)	fat (gms)	chol. (mgs)	sod. (mgs)	fiber (gms)
sides:							
chicken fingers:							
4-pack	640	31.0	42.0	38.0	70	1590	0
snack	580	19.0	55.0	32.0	35	1450	3.0
fries, curly:							
cheddar	460	6.0	54.0	24.0	5	1290	4.0
large	620	8.0	78.0	30.0	0	1540	7.0
medium	400	5.0	50.0	20.0	0	990	4.0
small	310	4.0	39.0	15.0	0	770	3.0
fries, home style:							
large	560	6.0	79.0	24.0	0	1070	6.0
medium	370	4.0	53.0	16.0	0	710	4.0
small	300	3.0	42.0	13.0	0	570	3.0
Jalapeño Bites	330	7.0	30.0	21.0	40	670	2.0
mozzarella sticks ..	470	18.0	34.0	29.0	60	1330	2.0
onion petals	410	4.0	43.0	24.0	0	300	2.0
potato, baked:							
broccoli/cheddar	540	12.0	71.0	24.0	50	680	7.0
butter/sour cream	500	8.0	65.0	24.0	55	170	6.0
deluxe	650	20.0	67.0	34.0	90	750	6.0
potato cakes, 2 ...	250	2.0	26.0	16.0	0	490	3.0
dressings, 2 oz.:							
BBQ vinaigrette ...	140	0	9.0	11.0	0	660	0
bleu cheese	300	2.0	3.0	31.0	45	580	0
buttermilk ranch ..	360	1.0	2.0	39.0	5	490	0
buttermilk ranch,							
reduced cal.	60	1.0	13.0	0	0	750	1.0
Caesar	310	1.0	1.0	34.0	60	470	0
honey French	290	0	18.0	24.0	0	410	<1.0
Italian, reduced cal.	25	0	3.0	1.0	0	1030	<1.0
Italian Parmesan ..	240	1.0	4.0	24.0	0	950	0
Thousand Island ..	290	1.0	9.0	28.0	35	480	0
sauces/condiments:							
Arby's Sauce, ½ oz.	15	0	4.0	0	0	180	0
au jus, 3 oz.	5	.3	.9	0	0	386	0
BBQ sauce, 1 oz.	40	0	10.0	0	0	350	0
Bronco Berry Sauce,							
1.5 oz.	90	0	23.0	0	0	35	0
croutons:							
cheese/garlic ...	100	2.5	10.0	6.3	n.a.	138	0
seasoned	30	1.0	5.0	1.0	0	70	1.0
honey mustard							
sauce, 1 oz. ...	130	0	5.0	12.0	10	160	0
Horsey Sauce, ½ oz.	60	0	3.0	5.0	5	150	0

Food and Measure	cal.	prot. (gms)	carbo. (gms)	fat (gms)	chol. (mgs)	sod. (mgs)	fiber (gms)
Arby's, sauces/condiments *(cont.)*							
ketchup pkt.	10	0	2.0	0	0	100	0
marinara sauce,							
1.5 oz.	35	1.0	4.0	1.0	0	260	1.0
mayo pkt.	90	0	0	10.0	10	65	0
mayo, light, pkt. ..	20	0	1.0	1.5	0	110	0
mustard pkt.	5	0	0	0	0	60	0
Tangy Southwest							
Sauce, 1.5 oz. ..	250	0	3.0	26.0	30	290	0
desserts/shakes:							
apple turnover	420	4.0	65.0	16.0	0	230	2.0
cherry turnover ...	410	4.0	63.0	16.0	0	250	1.0
hot chocolate	110	2.0	23.0	1.0	0	120	0
shake, 14 oz.:							
chocolate	480	10.0	84.0	16.0	45	370	0
jamocha	470	10.0	82.0	15.0	45	390	0
strawberry	500	11.0	87.0	13.0	15	340	0
vanilla	470	10.0	83.0	15.0	45	360	0
Arrowhead:							
raw, 1 medium corm,							
2⅝"	12	.6	2.4	<.1	0	3	.<1.0
boiled, drained,							
1 medium corm,							
.4 oz.	9	.5	1.9	<.1	0	2	<1.0
Arrowroot, raw, sliced,							
½ cup	36	2.5	8.0	.1	0	16	.8
Arrowroot flour, 1 cup	457	.4	112.8	.1	0	2	4.4
Artichoke, globe, fresh:							
raw:							
(*Dole*), 1 medium,							
2 oz. edible	25	2.0	6.0	0	0	70	3.0
4.5-oz. choke	60	4.2	13.5	.2	0	120	6.9
5.7-oz. choke	76	5.3	17.0	.2	0	152	8.9
boiled, 4.2 oz.	60	4.2	13.4	.2	0	114	6.5
hearts, boiled, drained,							
½ cup	42	2.9	9.4	.1	0	80	4.5
Artichoke, canned:							
(*Progresso*), 1 pc.,							
2.9 oz.	30	2.0	6.0	0	0	240	1.0
bottoms (*Gourmet*							
Award), 3 pcs. ...	18	2.0	3.0	0	0	488	2.0
hearts:							
(*Pompeian*), ½ cup	35	2.0	6.0	0	0	420	4.0

Food and Measure	cal.	prot. (gms)	carbo. (gms)	fat (gms)	chol. (mgs)	sod. (mgs	fiber (gms)
(*Reese*), 4.5 oz., 4 quarters	50	3.0	9.0	0	0	380	2.0
marinated, see "Artichoke appetizer"							
Artichoke, frozen:							
bottoms (*Bonduelle*), 3 oz.	25	2.0	4.0	0	0	70	2.0
hearts:							
(*Birds Eye* Deluxe), ½ cup	40	3.0	8.0	0	0	45	6.0
9-oz. pkg.	96	6.7	19.8	1.1	0	120	9.9
quartered (*Bonduelle*), 3 oz. ...	35	2.0	7.0	0	0	70	2.0
Artichoke, Jerusalem, see "Jerusalem artichoke"							
Artichoke appetizer, marinated:							
(*Pompeian*), 1 oz. ...	25	.5	2.0	.5	0	90	.5
(*Progresso*), 2 pcs., 1.1 oz.	50	0	2.0	5.0	0	110	0
grilled (*Antica Cucuma Mediteranea*), 1 oz.	40	1.0	2.0	3.0	0	180	0
quarters (*S&W*), 2 pcs., 1 oz.	20	0	2.0	2.0	0	80	1.0
salad (*Reese*), ⅓ cup .	150	1.0	7.0	14.0	0	270	<1.0
Artichoke dip (*Victoria*), 2 tbsp.	30	0	2.0	2.0	0	310	1.0
Artichoke paste (*Cucina Aromatica*), 1 oz.	155	.2	3.5	15.0	<5	440	2.8
Artichoke sauce (*Italia In Talola*), 2 tbsp. .	110	0	2.0	12.0	0	360	<1.0
Arugula, fresh:							
10 leaves	5	.5	.7	.1	0	5	.3
½ cup	3	.3	.4	<.1	0	<1	.2
Asparagus, fresh: raw, trimmed:							
(*Dole*), 5 spears ...	25	2.0	4.0	0	0	0	2.0
4 small spears, 1.8 oz.	14	1.3	2.6	.1	0	1	1.2
purple (*Frieda's*), 3 oz.	20	3.0	4.0	0	0	0	1.0

Food and Measure	cal.	prot. (gms)	carbo. (gms)	fat (gms)	chol. (mgs)	sod. (mgs)	fiber (gms)
Asparagus, raw, trimmed *(cont.)*							
white (*Frieda's*),							
⅔ cup, 3 oz. . . .	20	2.0	4.0	0	0	0	2.0
boiled, 4 spears,							
½"-diam. base	14	1.6	2.5	.2	0	7	1.3
boiled, drained, cuts,							
½ cup	22	2.3	3.8	.3	0	10	1.9
Asparagus, can							
or jar:							
all styles (*Del Monte*)							
½ cup	20	2.0	3.0	0	0	420	1.0
spears:							
(*Green Giant*), 4.5 oz.,							
about 5 pcs. . . .	20	2.0	3.0	0	0	400	1.0
(*Reese* White), ⅓							
of 15-oz. can . . .	20	2.0	4.0	0	0	550	1.0
pickled (*Hogue*							
Farms), 3 pcs.,							
1.1 oz.	10	1.0	1.0	0	0	75	0
blend (*S&W*), 6 pcs.	15	2.0	4.0	0	0	260	1.0
cuts, ½ cup:							
(*Bush's Best*)	25	3.0	2.0	0	0	380	1.0
(*Green Giant*)	20	2.0	3.0	0	0	420	1.0
(*Green Giant* 50%							
Less Sodium) . .	20	2.0	3.0	0	0	210	1.0
(*Libby's*)	20	2.0	3.0	0	0	290	2.0
drained, ½ cup	23	2.6	3.0	.8	0	350	2.0
Asparagus, freeze-							
dried, diced							
(*AlpineAire*), ½ cup	35	4.0	4.0	0	0	0	1.0
Asparagus, frozen:							
boiled, drained, 1 cup	50	5.3	8.8	.8	0	7	2.9
spears:							
(*Birds Eye* Deluxe),							
3 oz.	20	3.0	4.0	0	0	5	1.0
(*Seabrook Farms*),							
7 pcs., 3 oz. . . .	20	3.0	3.0	0	0	5	2.0
boiled, 4 pcs.	17	1.8	2.9	.3	0	2	1.2
cuts:							
(*Birds Eye* Deluxe),							
½ cup	25	3.0	4.0	0	0	5	2.0
(*Green Giant*),							
⅔ cup	20	2.0	3.0	0	0	90	2.0

Food and Measure	cal.	prot. (gms)	carbo. (gms)	fat (gms)	chol. (mgs)	sod. (mgs)	fiber (gms)
stir-fry blend (*Birds Eye*), 2 cups frozen	90	5.0	16.0	.5	0	35	3.0
Asparagus bean, see "Winged bean"							
Atemoya (*Frieda's*), 3-oz. fruit	80	2.0	20.0	0	0	10	4.0
Au jus gravy, ¼ cup:							
(*Franco-American*)	10	<1.0	2.0	.5	<5	310	0
(*Heinz* Bistro)	20	1.0	1.0	1.0	0	360	0
Au jus gravy mix, 1 tsp.:							
(*Knorr* Classics)	10	0	2.0	0	0	310	0
(*Lawry's*)	10	0	2.0	0	0	390	0
(*McCormick*)	5	0	1.0	0	0	310	0
Aubergine, see "Eggplant"							
***Auntie Anne's*:**							
pretzel, 1 pc.:							
almond	350	9.0	72.0	1.5	0	390	2.0
almond w/butter . .	400	9.0	72.0	8.0	20	400	2.0
cinnamon sugar . . .	350	9.0	74.0	2.0	0	410	2.0
cinnamon sugar w/butter	450	8.0	83.0	9.0	25	430	3.0
garlic	320	9.0	66.0	1.0	0	830	2.0
garlic w/butter	350	9.0	68.0	4.5	10	850	2.0
Glazin' Raisin	470	11.0	104.0	.5	0	460	3.0
Glazin' Raisin w/ butter	510	11.0	107.0	4.0	10	480	4.0
jalapeño	270	8.0	58.0	1.0	0	780	2.0
jalapeño w/butter . .	310	8.0	59.0	4.5	10	940	2.0
original	340	10.0	72.0	1.0	0	900	3.0
original w/butter . .	370	10.0	72.0	4.0	10	930	3.0
Parmesan herb . . .	390	11.0	74.0	5.0	10	780	4.0
Parmesan herb w/butter	440	10.0	72.0	13.0	30	660	9.0
sesame	350	11.0	63.0	6.0	0	840	3.0
sesame w/butter . .	410	12.0	64.0	12.0	15	860	7.0
sour cream/onion	310	9.0	66.0	1.0	0	920	2.0
sour cream/onion w/butter	340	9.0	66.0	5.0	10	930	2.0
whole wheat	350	11.0	72.0	1.5	0	1100	7.0
whole wheat w/butter	370	11.0	72.0	4.5	10	1120	7.0

Food and Measure	cal.	prot. (gms)	carbo. (gms)	fat (gms)	chol. (mgs)	sod. (mgs)	fiber (gms)
Auntie Anne's (cont.)							
dipping sauce, 1.25 oz., except as noted:							
caramel, 1.5 oz. . .	135	1.0	27.0	3.0	5	110	0
cheese sauce	100	3.0	4.0	8.0	10	510	0
chocolate flavored	130	1.0	24.0	4.0	2	65	1.0
cream cheese, light	70	3.0	1.0	6.0	25	140	0
cream cheese, strawberry	110	2.0	4.0	10.0	35	105	0
hot salsa cheese . .	100	2.0	4.0	8.0	10	550	0
marinara sauce . . .	10	0	4.0	0	0	180	0
mustard, sweet . . .	60	<1.0	8.0	1.0	40	120	0
Auntie Anne's							
lemonade, 22 fl. oz.	180	0	43.0	0	0	0	0
Dutch Ice, 14 fl. oz.:							
cherry, wild	210	0	48.0	0	0	25	0
kiwi-banana	190	0	44.0	0	0	30	0
lemonade	315	0	77.0	0	0	0	0
mocha	400	0	74.0	10.0	0	100	0
orange creme	280	0	64.0	0	0	35	0
pina colada	220	0	53.0	0	0	15	0
raspberry, blue . . .	165	0	36.0	0	0	20	0
strawberry	220	0	50.0	0	0	40	0
Dutch Ice, 20 fl. oz.:							
cherry, wild	300	0	68.0	0	0	35	0
kiwi-banana	270	0	63.0	0	0	40	0
lemonade	455	0	110.0	0	0	0	0
mocha	570	0	105.0	15.0	0	150	0
orange creme	400	0	92.0	0	0	50	0
piña colada	535	0	125.0	0	0	50	0
raspberry, blue . . .	230	0	55.0	0	0	30	0
strawberry	315	0	72.0	0	0	60	0
Australian blue squash (*Frieda's*), ¾ cup, 3 oz.	30	1.0	7.0	0	0	0	1.0
Avocado:							
(*Frieda's* Cocktail), 1.4-oz. pc.	60	1.0	3.0	6.0	0	0	2.0
all varieties:							
cubed, ½ cup	121	1.5	18.1	11.5	0	15	7.5
pureed, ½ cup	185	2.3	8.5	17.6	0	12	5.8
California:							
pulp from 1 medium, 6.1 oz.	306	3.7	12.0	30.0	0	21	8.5

Food and Measure	cal.	prot. (gms)	carbo. (gms)	fat (gms)	chol. (mgs)	sod. (mgs)	fiber (gms)
pureed, ½ cup	204	2.4	8.0	19.9	0	14	5.6
Florida, pureed, ½ cup	129	1.8	10.2	10.2	0	6	6.1
Avocado dip, see "Guacamole"							

B

Food and Measure	cal.	prot. (gms)	carbo. (gms)	fat (gms)	chol. (mgs)	sod. (mgs)	fiber (gms)
Baba ghanoush, see "Eggplant appetizer"							
Bacon, cooked, 2 slices, except as noted:							
(*Armour*)	90	5.0	0	7.0	15	340	0
(*Black Label*)	80	5.0	0	7.0	15	330	0
(*Boar's Head* Domestic)	70	4.0	0	6.0	10	190	0
(*Boar's Head* Imported)	60	4.0	0	5.0	10	190	0
(*Hormel* Fully Cooked), 2½ slices	70	5.0	0	5.0	20	290	0
(*Hormel* Microwave)	80	5.0	0	7.0	15	340	0
(*Jones Dairy Farm* Country Carved) . .	90	4.0	0	8.0	15	350	0
(*Old Smokehouse*) . . .	80	5.0	0	7.0	15	280	0
(*Oscar Mayer*)	70	4.0	0	6.0	15	290	0
(*Oscar Mayer* Center Cut)	50	4.0	0	4.0	15	270	0
(*Oscar Mayer* Ready-to-Serve), 3 slices	70	5.0	0	5.0	15	220	0
(*Plumrose*)	80	5.0	0	7.0	15	320	0
(*Range Brand*)	110	7.0	0	9.0	20	460	0
(*Red Label*)	80	5.0	0	7.0	15	330	0
(*Rock River*)	80	3.0	0	8.0	15	350	0
(*Thorn Apple Valley*)	80	4.0	0	7.0	10	240	0
(*Tobin's First Prize* Hardwood)	100	4.0	0	9.0	10	300	0
thick cut, 1 slice:							
(*Jones Dairy Farm* Country Carved)	70	3.0	0	6.0	15	290	0
(*Oscar Mayer*)	60	4.0	0	5.0	10	250	0
turkey, see "Turkey bacon"							

Food and Measure	cal.	prot. (gms)	carbo. (gms)	fat (gms)	chol. (mgs)	sod. (mgs	fiber (gms)
Bacon, Canadian:							
(*Boar's Head*), 2 oz.	70	12.0	1.0	2.0	35	570	0
(*Hormel*), 2 oz.	70	10.0	0	3.0	30	640	0
(*Hormel Pillow Pack*),							
2 oz.	80	10.0	2.0	3.5	30	900	0
(*Jones Dairy Farm*							
Lean Choice),							
3 slices, 2.8 oz. ..	70	11.0	0	3.0	30	460	0
(*Oscar Mayer*), 1 oz.	30	5.0	0	1.0	15	380	0
unheated, 2 oz.	89	11.7	1.9	4.0	28	799	0
Bacon, Irish, back							
(*Dawn Irish Gold*),							
2 slices, 2 oz.	140	10.0	1.0	10.0	30	570	0
Bacon, Italian, .5 oz.:							
(*Boar's Head*) ......:	50	2.0	0	4.5	10	180	0
(*Daniele* Pancetta) ...	50	2.0	0	4.5	10	230	0
"Bacon," vegetarian,							
frozen, 2 slices,							
except as noted:							
(*Morningstar Farms*							
Breakfast Strips) ..	60	2.0	2.0	4.5	0	220	<1.0
(*Worthington*							
Stripples)	60	2.0	2.0	4.5	0	220	<1.0
Canadian (*Yves*), 2 oz.	80	17.0	1.0	.5	0	480	1.0
Bacon bits, 1 tbsp.:							
(*Hormel*)	30	3.0	0	1.5	5	250	0
(*Oscar Mayer*)	25	3.0	0	1.5	5	220	0
chips (*Hormel* Crispy)	45	.5	0	2.5	10	170	0
pieces (*Hormel*)	25	3.0	0	1.5	10	180	0
pieces (*Oscar Mayer*							
Smoke Flavor)	25	3.0	0	.5	5	180	0
"Bacon" bits,							
imitation, 1½ tbsp.:							
(*Bac'n Pieces*)	30	3.0	2.0	1.5	0	220	0
chips/bits (*Bac*Os*) ..	30	3.0	2.0	1.5	0	120	0
Bacon dip, 2 tbsp.:							
cheddar (*Kraft Dips*)	60	1.0	3.0	5.0	<5	180	0
horseradish (*Heluva*							
Good)	60	1.0	2.0	5.0	20	190	0
ranch, see "Ranch dip"							
Bacon dip mix, 1 tsp.:							
cheddar (*Watkins*) ...	10	0	2.0	0	0	140	0
horseradish (*Watkins*)	10	1.0	1.0	0	0	90	0

Food and Measure	cal.	prot. (gms)	carbo. (gms)	fat (gms)	chol. (mgs)	sod. (mgs)	fiber (gms)
Bagel, 1 pc., except as noted:							
plain:							
(*Awrey's*), 2 oz. . . .	150	6.0	31.0	0	0	320	2.0
(*Awrey's*), 2.6 oz.	190	8.0	40.0	.5	0	430	3.0
(*Awrey's*), 4 oz. . . .	270	10.0	58.0	1.0	0	620	4.0
(*Thomas'* New York Style), 3.7 oz. . .	280	10.0	56.0	1.5	0	530	2.0
mini (*Awrey's*), .9 oz.	70	3.0	16.0	0	0	170	1.0
plain, onion, poppy, or sesame seed, 2 oz.	157	6.0	30.4	.9	0	304	1.3
blueberry:							
(*Awrey's*), 4 oz. . . .	280	10.0	61.0	1.0	0	580	4.0
(*Thomas'* New York Style), 3.7 oz. . .	300	10.0	59.0	2.0	0	470	3.0
cinnamon raisin:							
(*Awrey's*), 2 oz. . . .	150	6.0	32.0	0	0	310	3.0
(*Awrey's*), 2.6 oz.	190	8.0	42.0	.5	0	410	4.0
(*Awrey's*), 4 oz. . . .	280	10.0	61.0	1.0	0	580	4.0
cinnamon swirl (*Thomas'* New York Style), 3.7 oz.	300	10.0	57.0	3.0	0	490	4.0
cranberry orange (*Thomas'* Gourmet), ½ pc., 2 oz.	150	5.0	31.0	.5	0	250	2.0
egg, 2 oz.	158	6.0	30.2	1.2	14	288	1.3
multigrain (*Thomas'* New York Style), 3.7 oz.	280	11.0	55.0	2.0	0	460	4.0
oat bran, 2 oz.	145	6.1	30.4	.7	0	289	2.1
onion (*Thomas'* New York Style), 3.7 oz.	280	11.0	54.0	1.5	0	510	3.0
sesame (*Thomas'* New York Style), 3.7 oz.	300	11.0	55.0	3.5	0	530	32.0
whole wheat (*Thomas'* New York Style), 3.7 oz.	280	13.0	57.0	2.0	0	450	10.0
wildberry blueberry (*Thomas'* Gourmet), ½ pc., 2 oz.	170	5.0	33.0	1.0	0	270	2.0
Bagel, frozen, 1 pc., except as noted:							

Food and Measure	cal.	prot. (gms)	carbo. (gms)	fat (gms)	chol. (mgs)	sod. (mgs	fiber (gms)
plain:							
(*Lender's*)	150	6.0	30.0	.5	0	320	1.0
(*Lender's* Bagelette), 2 pcs.	140	5.0	27.0	.5	0	290	1.0
(*Lender's Big 'n Crusty*)	250	9.0	52.0	1.0	0	540	1.0
(*Sara Lee*)	210	8.0	43.0	.5	0	500	2.0
blueberry:							
(*Lender's Big 'n Crusty*)	250	9.0	51.0	1.0	0	440	2.0
(*Sara Lee*)	210	8.0	41.0	1.0	0	570	2.0
swirl (*Lender's*) ...	160	5.0	32.0	.5	0	260	1.0
chocolate chip swirl							
(*Lender's*)	160	6.0	33.0	1.0	<5	240	2.0
cinnamon raisin:							
(*Lender's*)	160	5.0	32.0	1.0	0	240	1.0
(*Lender's Big 'n Crusty*)	260	8.0	52.0	2.5	0	390	2.0
(*Sara Lee*)	220	8.0	45.0	1.0	0	320	3.0
cinnamon swirl							
(*Lender's*)	150	5.0	32.0	.5	0	270	1.0
egg:							
(*Lender's*)	160	6.0	30.0	1.0	15	320	1.0
(*Lender's Big 'n Crusty*)	260	9.0	52.0	1.5	30	510	1.0
(*Sara Lee*)	210	7.0	44.0	.5	0	460	2.0
garlic (*Lender's*)	150	6.0	29.0	1.0	0	280	2.0
honey wheat (*Lender's Big 'n Crusty*)	230	8.0	49.0	.5	0	410	2.0
oat bran (*Sara Lee*) ..	210	8.0	42.0	1.0	0	570	3.0
onion:							
(*Lender's*)	150	5.0	30.0	1.0	0	300	1.0
(*Lender's Big 'n Crusty*)	250	9.0	52.0	1.0	0	520	2.0
(*Sara Lee*)	210	7.0	44.0	0	0	540	2.0
poppy seed:							
(*Lender's*)	150	6.0	30.0	1.0	0	290	2.0
(*Sara Lee*)	210	8.0	41.0	1.0	0	570	2.0
pumpernickel							
(*Lender's*)	150	5.0	31.0	1.0	0	340	1.0
rye (*Lender's*)	150	5.0	30.0	1.0	0	320	2.0
sesame seed:							
(*Lender's*)	150	6.0	29.0	1.5	0	290	1.0

Food and Measure	cal.	prot. (gms)	carbo. (gms)	fat (gms)	chol. (mgs)	sod. (mgs)	fiber (gms)
Bagel, frozen, sesame seed *(cont.)*							
(*Sara Lee*)	210	8.0	42.0	1.5	0	530	2.0
soft (*Lender's*)	210	6.0	37.0	.5	10	330	2.0
strawberry swirl							
(*Lender's*)	160	5.0	33.0	.5	0	240	2.0
Bagel chips:							
plain (*Burns & Ricker*),							
3 pcs., 1 oz.	130	3.0	19.0	4.5	0	70	1.0
cinnamon raisin							
(*Burns & Ricker*),							
3 pcs., 1 oz.	130	3.0	20.0	4.5	0	105	1.0
garlic (*Burns & Ricker*),							
3 pcs., 1 oz.	130	4.0	20.0	4.5	0	250	1.0
rice (*Hain*), .4-oz. pc.:							
butter sesame	45	1.0	9.0	.5	0	100	0
cinnamon raisin . . .	50	1.0	10.0	1.0	0	10	0
everything	50	1.0	10.0	1.0	0	120	1.0
onion poppy	45	1.0	9.0	1.0	0	100	0
sea salt (*Burns &*							
Ricker), 3 pcs.,							
1 oz.	130	4.0	20.0	4.5	0	170	1.0
sesame (*Burns &*							
Ricker), 3 pcs.,							
1 oz.	130	4.0	19.0	4.0	0	200	1.0
Bagel sandwich, see							
"Toaster bagel,							
muffin, and pastry"							
Bagel spread mix:							
apple-cinnamon							
(*Watkins*),1 tsp. . . .	20	0	5.0	0	0	0	0
onion-dill (*Watkins*),							
1 tsp.	10	0	3.0	0	0	300	0
strawberry cream							
(*Watkins*), 1½ tsp.	25	0	7.0	0	0	0	0
Baked beans, ½ cup:							
(*Allens*)	150	6.0	29.0	1.0	0	350	8.0
(*B&M* Original)	170	7.0	30.0	2.0	<5	380	6.0
(*Bush's Best* Bold &							
Spicy)	120	6.0	24.0	.5	0	550	5.0
(*Bush's Best* Boston							
Recipe)	170	6.0	32.0	1.5	0	440	6.0
(*Bush's Best* Country							
Style)	170	7.0	33.0	1.0	0	680	7.0

Food and Measure	cal.	prot. (gms)	carbo. (gms)	fat (gms)	chol. (mgs)	sod. (mgs)	fiber (gms)
(*Bush's Best* Homestyle)	150	6.0	28.0	1.5	5	480	8.0
(*Bush's Best* Original)	150	7.0	29.0	1.0	0	550	7.0
(*Campbell's* New England Style)	160	5.0	29.0	2.5	<5	410	6.0
(*Campbell's* Old Fashioned)	180	5.0	32.0	3.0	5	460	6.0
(*Eden* Organic)	150	8.0	27.0	0	0	130	7.0
(*Greene's Farm*)	150	6.0	32.0	.5	0	540	7.0
w/bacon:							
(*S&W*)	140	5.0	29.0	.5	0	510	6.0
and onion (*B&M*) .	190	8.0	36.0	2.0	<5	450	8.0
w/bacon/brown sugar flavor (*Campbell's* Old Fashioned) ...	160	5.0	29.0	3.0	<5	460	6.0
barbecue:							
(*Bush's Best*)	160	6.0	32.0	1.0	0	510	6.0
(*S&W* Country) ...	140	6.0	28.0	.5	0	510	6.0
(*S&W* Ranch)	140	6.0	25.0	1.5	0	640	8.0
chili, see "Chili beans"							
w/franks, see "Beans and franks"							
honey mustard (*S&W*)	140	6.0	28.0	.5	0	600	6.0
maple:							
(*B&M*)	150	6.0	28.0	1.0	0	340	6.0
cured (*Bush's Best*)	150	7.0	28.0	1.0	0	620	7.0
sugar (*S&W*)	150	7.0	29.0	0	0	640	6.0
w/onion (*Bush's Best*)	150	7.0	26.0	1.5	0	500	6.0
w/pork:							
(*Campbell's*)	110	5.0	20.0	1.0	<5	360	5.0
(*Showboat*)	120	6.0	22.0	1.5	5	550	6.0
(*Trappey's/Wagon Master*)	110	5.0	21.0	1.0	0	710	7.0
peas (*East Texas Fair* Peas 'n Pork)	110	6.0	19.0	1.5	0	540	5.0
tomato sauce (*Campbell's*) ...	130	5.0	24.0	2.0	5	420	6.0
vegetarian:							
(*Bearitos* Fat Free Original)	130	6.0	26.0	0	0	360	3.0
(*B&M*)	150	6.0	28.0	1.0	0	340	6.0
(*Bush's Best*)	130	5.0	24.0	0	0	550	6.0
(*Heinz*)	140	6.0	27.0	.5	0	480	5.0
black (*Bearitos*) ...	110	6.0	22.0	0	0	360	3.0

Food and Measure	cal.	prot. (gms)	carbo. (gms)	fat (gms)	chol. (mgs)	sod. (mgs)	fiber (gms)
Baking mix (see also "Biscuit mix"):							
(*Arrowhead Mills*), ¼ cup	140	5.0	30.0	.5	0	320	2.0
(*Bisquick*), ⅓ cup	160	3.0	25.0	6.0	0	490	1.0
(*Bisquick* Reduced Fat), ⅓ cup	140	3.0	27.0	3.0	0	500	<1.0
(*Hodgson Mill* InstaBake), ⅓ cup	150	4.0	25.0	5.0	0	540	3.0
sweet (*Bisquick*), ⅓ cup	170	1.0	31.0	4.0	0	260	0
wheat free (*Arrowhead Mills*), ¼ cup	120	2.0	27.0	.5	0	300	1.0
Baking powder:							
(*Calumet*), ⅛ tsp.	0	0	0	0	0	60	0
(*Featherweight* Sodium Free), ¼ tsp.	0	0	0	0	0	0	0
(*Watkins*), ¼ tsp.	0	0	0	0	U	150	0
Baking soda, ½ tsp.	0	0	0	0	0	630	0
Baklava, frozen: (*Apollo/Athens*), 4½ pcs., 4.4 oz.	540	7.0	62.0	31.0	5	230	2.0
Balsam pear, ½ cup, except as noted:							
(*Frieda's* Bittermelon), 1 cup, 3 oz.	15	1.0	3.0	0	0	0	2.0
leafy-tips:							
raw	7	1.3	.8	.2	0	3	.6
boiled, drained	10	1.0	2.0	.1	0	4	.6
pods, ½" pcs.:							
raw	8	.5	1.7	.1	0	3	1.3
boiled, drained	12	.5	2.7	.1	0	4	1.2
Bamboo shoots, fresh, slices, ½ cup:							
raw	21	2.0	4.0	.2	0	3	.7
boiled, drained	8	.9	1.2	.1	0	3	<1.0
Bamboo shoots, canned, ½ cup:							
(*La Choy*)	10	<1.0	2.0	0	0	10	<1.0
drained	13	1.1	2.1	.3	0	5	2.0
Banana (see also "Plantain"), fresh:							
(*Dole*), 1 medium, 4.4 oz.	110	1.0	29.0	0	0	0	4.0

Food and Measure	cal.	prot. (gms)	carbo. (gms)	fat (gms)	chol. (mgs)	sod. (mgs)	fiber (gms)
(*Frieda's* Baby Nino/ Burro/Ice Cream), 3-oz. fruit	80	1.0	20.0	0	0	0	1.0
(*Frieda's* Red), 5 oz. . .	130	1.0	33.0	.5	0	0	2.0
8¾" banana	105	1.2	26.7	.6	0	1	2.7
sliced, ½ cup	69	.8	17.6	.4	0	1	1.8
mashed, ½ cup	104	1.2	26.4	.5	0	1	2.7
red, 7¼" long	118	1.6	30.7	.3	0	1	n.a.
Banana, dried:							
(*AlpineAire*), 2 oz. . . .	50	1.0	12.0	0	0	0	1.0
(*Frieda's*), 1.2-oz. pc.	30	0	8.0	0	0	0	1.0
dehydrated, ¼ cup . . .	87	1.0	22.1	.5	0	1	1.9
Banana drink blends:							
(*After the Fall Banana Casablanca*), 8 fl. oz.	100	1.0	19.0	0	0	10	0
(*Libby's* Nectar), 11.5-fl.-oz. can . . .	190	0	47.0	0	0	35	0
Banana milk drink, see "Milk, flavored"							
Banana squash (*Frieda's*), ¾ cup, 3 oz.	30	1.0	7.0	0	0	0	1.0
Banana-strawberry juice (*R. W. Knudsen*), 8 fl. oz.	120	<1.0	30.0	0	0	25	0
Barbecue beans, see "Baked beans"							
Barbecue sauce (see also "Grilling sauce"), 2 tbsp.:							
(*Bull's Eye* Original) . .	60	0	13.0	0	0	330	0
(*D. L. Jardine's* 5-Star)	40	0	10.0	0	0	270	0
(*Honeycup*)	50	1.0	11.0	.5	0	140	0
(*Hunt's* Original)	50	<1.0	13.0	0	0	290	<1.0
(*KC Masterpiece*)	60	<1.0	15.0	0	0	230	0
(*Kraft* Char-Grill)	60	0	13.0	0	0	450	0
(*Kraft* Original)	40	0	11.0	0	0	420	0
(*Kraft* Steakhouse Style)	50	0	12.0	0	0	360	0
(*Kraft* Thick 'N Spicy Original)	50	0	12.0	0	0	430	0
(*Lea & Perrins*)	50	1.0	13.0	0	0	125	0
(*Maull's*)	40	0	10.0	0	0	320	0
(*Maull's* Sweet-N-Mild)	60	0	12.0	0	0	280	0

Food and Measure	cal.	prot. (gms)	carbo. (gms)	fat (gms)	chol. (mgs)	sod. (mgs)	fiber (gms)
Barbecue sauce *(cont.)*							
(*Maull's* Sweet-N-Smoky)	60	0	13.0	0	0	300	0
(*Mrs. Renfro's*)	35	<1.0	8.0	0	0	220	0
(*Silver Dollar City*) ...	40	0	11.0	0	0	400	0
(*Silver Dollar City* Ozark Recipe)	50	0	14.0	0	0	330	0
(*Sweet Baby Ray's*)	70	0	17.0	0	0	290	0
(*Sylvia's* Original) ...	40	0	9.0	0	0	290	1.0
(*Texas Best* Original Rib Style)	50	0	11.0	0	0	390	0
all varieties (*Muir Glen* Grill Chef)	40	0	8.0	0	0	265	<1.0
beer (*Maull's*)	45	0	9.0	0	0	310	0
brown sugar:							
(*Kraft*)	60	0	15.0	0	0	350	0
Spicy (*Bull's Eye*) ..	70	0	16.0	0	0	300	0
Cajun:							
(*Texas Best*)	50	0	12.0	0	0	360	0
Spicy (*Kraft Thick 'N Spicy*)	45	0	12.0	0	0	430	0
garlic, roasted (*Kraft*)	50	0	12.0	0	0	360	0
hickory smoke:							
(*Bull's Eye* Smokehouse) ..	60	0	13.0	0	0	340	0
(*Kraft*)	40	0	9.0	0	0	420	0
(*Kraft Thick 'N Spicy*)	50	0	12.0	0	0	450	0
bacon (*Kraft Thick 'N Spicy*)	60	0	13.0	1.0	0	570	0
bacon, smoky (*Bull's Head*) ..	60	<1.0	13.0	0	0	330	0
brown sugar (*Hunt's*)	70	0	17.0	0	0	380	<1.0
hot (*Kraft*)	40	0	9.0	0	0	370	0
molasses (*Kraft*) ..	70	0	16.0	0	0	350	0
w/onion bits (*Kraft*)	45	0	11.0	0	0	360	0
sweet (*Bull's Eye*)	60	<1.0	15.0	0	0	370	0
honey:							
(*KC Masterpiece* Steakhouse)	60	1.0	14.0	0	0	250	0
(*Kraft*)	50	0	13.0	0	0	360	0
(*Kraft Thick 'N Spicy*)	60	0	13.0	0	0	340	0
(*Sweet Baby Ray's*)	70	0	16.0	0	0	300	0

Food and Measure	cal.	prot. (gms)	carbo. (gms)	fat (gms)	chol. (mgs)	sod. (mgs)	fiber (gms)
hickory smoke							
(*Kraft*)	60	0	14.0	0	0	370	<1.0
smoke (*Bull's Eye*)	50	0	11.0	0	0	310	0
spicy (*Kraft*)	60	0	14.0	0	0	360	0
spicy (*Bull's Eye*) ..	50	0	12.0	0	0	310	0
teriyaki (*KC Master-*							
piece)	60	0	14.0	0	0	610	0
honey garlic:							
(*Bull's Eye*)	60	0	14.0	0	0	310	0
(*Kraft*)	50	0	12.0	0	0	350	0
honey mustard:							
(*Kraft*)	60	0	13.0	0	0	300	0
(*Kraft Thick 'N*							
Spicy)	60	0	14.0	0	0	310	0
(*Hunt's*)	45	0	11.0	0	0	390	<1.0
Dijon (*KC Master-*							
piece)	60	0	10.0	1.0	0	570	0
hot:							
(*D. L. Jardine's*							
Killer Hot)	35	0	6.0	1.5	0	400	0
(*Kraft*)	40	0	9.0	0	0	500	0
spicy (*Bull's Eye*) ..	60	0	13.0	0	0	390	0
jalapeño (*Maull's*) ...	50	0	12.0	0	0	300	0
Jamaican (*Helen's*							
Tropical Exotics) ..	60	1.0	12.0	1.5	0	610	1.0
Kansas City style:							
(*Kraft*)	50	0	11.0	0	0	310	0
(*Kraft Thick 'N*							
Spicy)	60	0	14.0	0	0	310	<1.0
(*Maull's*)	60	0	15.0	0	0	320	0
Korean style (*Sun*							
Luck)	45	<1.0	7.0	1.5	0	550	0
mesquite:							
(*Bull's Eye* Texas)	60	0	13.0	0	0	380	0
(*D. L. Jardine's*) ...	35	0	6.0	1.5	0	380	0
(*Kraft*)	40	0	9.0	0	0	420	0
(*Kraft Thick 'N*							
Spicy)	50	0	12.0	0	0	430	0
(*Texas Best*)	50	0	11.0	0	0	350	0
molasses (*Kraft*)	70	0	16.0	0	0	390	0
mustard (*D. L. Jardine's*							
Chick'n-Lik'n)	40	0	10.0	0	0	270	0
w/onion bits:							
(*Kraft*)	50	0	11.0	0	0	360	0

Food and Measure	cal.	prot. (gms)	carbo. (gms)	fat (gms)	chol. (mgs)	sod. (mgs)	fiber (gms)
Barbecue sauce, w/onion bits *(cont.)*							
(*Maull's*)	45	0	9.0	0	0	310	0
pecan, Texas (*D. L. Jardine's*)	35	0	7.0	1.5	0	330	0
smoke, triple (*Kraft*)	50	0	12.0	0	0	430	0
smoky (*Maull's*)	40	0	10.0	0	0	310	0
Southwest sweet chile (*Kraft*)	50	0	11.0	0	0	380	0
spicy (*KC Masterpiece*)	60	0	14.0	0	0	380	0
teriyaki (*Kraft*)	50	0	12.0	0	0	310	0
tropical, and marinade (*World Harbors Maui Mountain*) . . .	50	0	11.0	0	0	270	0
Barbecue sauce concentrate, 2 tsp.:							
(*Watkins* Original) . . .	30	0	5.0	1.0	0	300	0
honey (*Watkins*)	30	0	5.0	1.0	0	290	0
mesquite (*Watkins*) . .	30	0	5.0	1.0	0	300	0
Barbecue seasoning:							
(*McCormick*), ¼ tsp.	0	0	0	0	0	230	0
hickory (*Wyler's Shakers*), 1 tsp. . .	10	0	2.0	0	0	420	0
Barley, pearled:							
dry:							
(*Arrowhead Mills*), ¼ cup	170	5.0	37.0	.5	0	0	6.0
(*Jack Rabbit*), ¼ cup	100	3.0	24.0	0	0	0	5.0
(*Quaker* Scotch Quick), ⅓ cup . .	170	5.0	37.0	1.0	0	0	5.0
(*Quaker* Scotch Regular), ¼ cup	170	5.0	37.0	1.0	0	0	5.0
1 cup	704	19.8	155.5	2.3	0	18	31.2
cooked, 1 cup	193	3.6	44.3	.7	0	5	6.0
Barley flakes (*Arrowhead Mills*), ⅓ cup	110	4.0	28.0	1.0	0	0	5.0
Barley flour (*Arrowhead Mills*), ¼ cup	93	3.0	19.0	.5	0	0	3.0
Barley malt syrup, see "Malt syrup"							
Barley sauce (*Westbrae Natural Mellow*), 1 tsp. . . .	10	0	1.0	0	0	100	0

Food and Measure	cal.	prot. (gms)	carbo. (gms)	fat (gms)	chol. (mgs)	sod. (mgs	fiber (gms)
Basella, see "Vine spinach"							
Basil, fresh:							
1 oz.	8	.7	1.2	.2	0	0	.3
5 medium leaves	1	.1	.1	<.1	0	0	.1
chopped, 2 tbsp. . . .	1	.1	.2	<.1	0	0	.2
Basil, dried:							
ground, 1 tbsp.	11	.7	2.7	.2	0	2	.5
ground, 1 tsp.	4	.2	.9	.1	0	<1	.2
Bass (see also "Sea Bass"), meat only:							
freshwater, 4 oz.:							
raw	129	21.4	0	4.2	77	79	0
baked, broiled, or microwaved	166	27.4	0	5.4	99	102	0
striped, 4 oz.:							
raw	110	20.1	0	2.7	91	78	0
baked, broiled, or microwaved	141	25.8	0	3.4	117	100	0
Batter and seasoning mix (see also specific listings):							
all purpose (*Don's Chuck Wagon*), ¼ cup	100	4.0	20.0	0	0	580	1.0
all varieties (*Watkins*), 1½ tbsp.	50	1.0	11.0	0	0	620	1.0
Bay leaf, dried, crumbled, 1 tsp. . .	5	.1	.3	.1	0	<1	<1.0
Bean casserole, dried, five bean (*Alpine-Aire*), 12 oz.	300	16.0	47.0	5.0	n.a.	760	15.0
Bean dip, 2 tbsp.:							
(*Fritos*)	40	2.0	5.0	1.0	0	170	1.0
(*Marie's*)	140	.5	2.0	14.0	10	160	.5
black bean, spicy or mild (*Guiltless Gourmet*)	30	2.0	5.0	0	0	100	1.0
hot (*Fritos*)	40	2.0	5.0	1.0	0	210	1.0
pinto (*Bearitos*)	25	1.0	5.0	0	0	150	1.0
Bean dishes, see specific bean listings							

Food and Measure	cal.	prot. (gms)	carbo. (gms)	fat (gms)	chol. (mgs)	sod. (mgs)	fiber (gms)
Bean loaf, frozen, 9–bean (*Natural Touch*), 1" slice ...	160	8.0	13.0	8.0	<5	350	5.0
Bean salad, ½ cup: (*S&W* Deli Style)	90	4.0	17.0	0	0	670	6.0
marinated:							
dill (*S&W*)	50	2.0	14.0	0	0	560	3.0
mixed bean (*S&W*)	90	4.0	19.0	0	0	620	6.0
3–bean:							
(*Green Giant*)	90	3.0	20.0	0	0	490	4.0
(*Hanover*), ⅓ cup	100	2.0	22.0	.5	0	120	3.0
Bean sauce, spicy brown (*House of Tsang*), 1 tsp.	15	0	3.0	0	0	130	0
Bean sprouts, fresh, see specific listings							
Bean sprouts, canned (*La Choy*), ⅔ cup	15	1.0	3.0	0	0	50	<1.0
Bean-carrot blend, frozen, baby (*Birds Eye*), 3 oz.	30	1.0	5.0	0	0	25	2.0
Beans, see specific listings							
Beans, baked, see "Baked beans"							
Beans, mixed, dried, soup (*Jack Rabbit*), ¼ cup	80	8.0	23.0	0	0	80	13.0
Beans, mixed, canned (*Westbrae Natural* Salad Beans), ½ cup	90	6.0	1.0	0	0	140	5.0
Beans, snap or string, see "Green bean"							
Beans and franks:							
(*Hormel*), 7.5-oz. can	290	11.0	34.0	12.0	50	1310	6.0
(*Kid's Kitchen* Wieners), 1 cup ...	310	13.0	37.0	13.0	45	760	8.0
(*Van Camp's Beanee Weenee* Original), 7.75-oz. can	230	14.0	29.0	9.0	30	910	7.0
baked flavor (*Van Camp's Beanee Weenee*), 7.75-oz. can	340	16.0	48.0	12.0	30	1300	7.0

Food and Measure	cal.	prot. (gms)	carbo. (gms)	fat (gms)	chol. (mgs)	sod. (mgs)	fiber (gms)
Beans and rice, see "Rice dishes, mix"							
Bear, meat only, simmered, 4 oz. ..	294	36.8	0	15.2	111	81	0
Béarnaise sauce, in jars (*Maille* Dipping), 2 tbsp.	140	0	2.7	14.0	3	300	0
Béarnaise sauce mix (*Knorr*), 1 tsp. ...	10	0	2.0	0	0	110	0
Beaver, meat only, roasted, 4 oz.	240	39.5	0	7.9	133	67	0
Beechnuts, dried, shelled, 1 oz.	164	1.8	9.5	14.2	0	11	n.a.
Beef, choice grade, meat only[1], 4 oz.:							
brisket, whole:							
braised, lean w/fat	437	26.6	0	35.8	107	69	0
braised, lean only	274	33.7	0	14.5	105	79	0
chuck, arm pot roast:							
braised, lean w/fat	395	30.6	0	29.2	112	67	0
braised, lean only	255	37.4	0	10.5	115	75	0
chuck, blade roast:							
braised, lean w/fat	412	29.7	0	31.5	117	73	0
braised, lean only	298	35.2	0	16.3	120	81	0
flank steak[2]:							
braised, lean only .	269	31.8	0	14.7	81	82	0
broiled, lean only ..	256	30.0	0	14.2	77	92	0
ground, raw:							
extra lean	265	21.1	0	19.3	78	75	0
lean	298	20.0	0	23.4	85	78	0
regular	351	18.8	0	30.0	96	77	0
ground, broiled, medium:							
extra lean	290	28.8	0	18.5	95	79	0
lean	308	28.0	0	20.9	99	87	0
regular	328	27.3	0	23.5	102	94	0
porterhouse steak:							
broiled, lean w/fat	346	28.2	0	25.1	94	69	0
broiled, lean only ..	247	31.9	0	12.2	91	75	0

1. *Retail cuts trimmed to ¼" fat, except as noted.*
2. *Trimmed to 0" fat.*

Food and Measure	cal.	prot. (gms)	carbo. (gms)	fat (gms)	chol. (mgs)	sod. (mgs)	fiber (gms)
Beef *(cont.)*							
rib, whole:							
roasted, lean w/fat	426	25.1	0	35.4	96	71	0
roasted, lean only	276	30.9	0	15.9	91	82	0
rib, large end (ribs 6–9):							
roasted, lean w/fat	434	25.3	0	36.2	96	71	0
roasted, lean only	284	31.2	0	16.7	92	83	0
rib, small end (ribs 10–12):							
broiled, lean w/fat	376	26.7	0	31.3	95	70	0
broiled, lean only ..	264	31.8	0	14.3	91	78	0
round, bottom:							
braised, lean w/fat	322	32.5	0	20.3	109	57	0
braised, lean only	249	35.8	0	10.7	109	58	0
round, eye of:							
roasted, lean w/fat	273	30.2	0	16.0	82	67	0
roasted, lean only	198	32.9	0	6.5	78	70	0
round, full cut:							
broiled, loan w/fat	272	31.0	0	15.4	91	69	0
broiled, lean only ..	217	33.1	0	8.3	88	73	0
round, tip:							
roasted, lean w/fat	280	30.1	0	16.9	94	70	0
roasted, lean only	213	32.6	0	8.3	92	74	0
round, top:							
broiled, lean w/fat	254	34.2	0	12.0	96	68	0
broiled, lean only ..	214	35.9	0	6.7	95	69	0
fried, lean w/fat ...	314	36.7	0	17.4	110	77	0
fried, lean only	257	39.8	0	9.7	110	81	0
shank, crosscuts:							
braised, lean w/fat	298	34.8	0	16.6	91	69	0
braised, lean only	228	38.2	0	7.2	88	73	0
short ribs:							
braised, lean w/fat	534	24.5	0	47.6	107	57	0
braised, lean only	335	34.9	0	20.6	105	66	0
sirloin, top:							
broiled, lean w/fat	305	31.3	0	19.0	102	70	0
broiled, lean only ..	229	34.4	0	9.1	101	75	0
fried, lean w/fat ...	370	31.9	0	25.9	111	79	0
fried, lean only	270	36.8	0	12.4	112	87	0
T–bone steak:							
broiled, lean w/fat	338	28.3	0	24.0	94	69	0
broiled, lean only ..	243	31.9	0	11.8	91	75	0

Food and Measure	cal.	prot. (gms)	carbo. (gms)	fat (gms)	chol. (mgs)	sod. (mgs	fiber (gms)
tenderloin:							
broiled, lean w/fat	345	28.4	0	24.8	98	67	0
broiled, lean only ..	252	32.0	0	12.7	95	71	0
top loin:							
broiled, lean w/fat	338	28.8	0	23.8	90	71	0
broiled, lean only ..	243	32.5	0	11.5	86	77	0
Beef, canned, see "Beef entree, can or pkg." and specific listings							
Beef, corned (see also "Beef lunch meat"), cooked:							
(*Boar's Head* Brisket), 2.4 oz.	180	16.0	0	13.0	50	550	0
(*Boar's Head* Brisket First Cut), 2.5 oz.	130	17.0	0	7.0	30	590	0
(*Mosey's*), 4 oz.	200	14.0	1.0	15.0	55	1180	0
(*Nathan's*), 4 oz.	160	14.0	1.0	11.0	60	1310	0
(*Swift Premium*), 4 oz.	160	16.0	2.0	10.0	50	1100	0
brisket, 4 oz.	285	20.6	.5	21.5	111	1286	0
Beef, corned, canned, 2 oz.:							
(*Delta*)	120	13.0	0	8.0	50	500	0
(*Hormel*)	120	15.0	0	7.0	50	490	0
(*Libby's*)	120	15.0	0	7.0	50	490	0
hash, see "Beef hash"							
Beef, dried:							
(*Armour*), 1.1 oz. ...	60	8.0	2.0	1.5	25	1370	0
(*Hormel*), 1 oz.	45	8.0	0	1.0	20	1010	0
(*Hormel* Can), 1 oz. .	50	8.0	1.0	1.5	25	1190	0
cured, 1 oz.	47	8.3	.4	1.1	n.a.	984	0
freeze-dried (*Alpine-Aire*), ½ oz.	60	11.0	0	2.0	35	180	0
Beef, refrigerated, cooked:							
roast, au jus (*Always Tender*), 5 oz.	200	28.0	3.0	9.0	75	450	0
seasoned strips: (*Tyson Time Trimmers*), 3 oz.	140	20.0	1.0	6.0	55	420	0

Food and Measure	cal.	prot. (gms)	carbo. (gms)	fat (gms)	chol. (mgs)	sod. (mgs)	fiber (gms)
Beef, refrigerated *(cont.)*							
steak, grilled (*Louis Rich Carving Board*), 3 oz. . .	110	18.0	<1.0	4.0	65	800	0
sirloin, filet of, 4 oz.:							
peppercorn (*Always Tender*)	160	18.0	2.0	4.0	50	570	0
teriyaki (*Always Tender*)	170	19.0	4.0	3.5	50	580	0
tips, w/gravy (*Always Tender*), ½ cup . . .	150	20.0	5.0	6.0	55	760	1.0
"Beef," vegetarian (see also "Burger, vegetarian" and "Vegetarian dishes"), frozen:							
corned "beef":							
roll (*Worthington*), ⅜" slice, 1.9 oz.	130	9.0	4.0	9.0	0	510	2.0
sliced (*Worthington*), 4 slices, 2 oz. . .	140	10.0	5.0	9.0	0	520	2.0
grounds (*Quorn*), ⅔ cup, 3 oz.	80	13.0	5.0	2.5	0	220	4.0
smoked (*Worthington*), 6 slices, 2 oz.	120	11.0	6.0	6.0	0	730	3.0
Beef dinner, frozen, 1 pkg.:							
chicken fried steak (*Banquet Extra Helping*), 16 oz. . .	820	29.0	63.0	50.0	60	2260	6.0
mesquite w/barbecue sauce (*Healthy Choice*), 11 oz. . . .	320	21.0	38.0	9.0	55	490	5.0
oven roasted (*Healthy Choice*), 10.15 oz. . .	280	18.0	35.0	8.0	50	600	4.0
patty, charbroiled (*Healthy Choice*), 11 oz.	310	16.0	40.0	9.0	45	550	4.0
pot roast:							
(*Swanson Hungry-Man*), 18.5 oz. .	390	20.0	59.0	8.0	40	1500	7.0
(*Swanson Traditional Favorites*), 14 oz.	320	19.0	44.0	8.0	35	1200	4.0

Food and Measure	cal.	prot. (gms)	carbo. (gms)	fat (gms)	chol. (mgs)	sod. (mgs)	fiber (gms)
Yankee (*Banquet Extra Helping*), 14.5 oz.	410	25.0	33.0	20.0	70	1680	3.0
Yankee (*Healthy Choice*), 11 oz. .	330	20.0	41.0	9.0	40	600	8.0
Yankee (*Stouffer's* HomeStyle), 16 oz.	360	20.0	48.0	10.0	45	1620	8.0
roast, w/gravy (*Swanson Traditional Favorites*), 10.5 oz.	370	19.0	40.0	15.0	40	700	6.0
Salisbury steak: (*Banquet Extra Helping*), 16.5 oz.	740	27.0	37.0	54.0	130	2200	7.0
(*Healthy Choice*), 11.5 oz.	330	18.0	48.0	7.0	50	470	6.0
(*Stouffer's* Home-Style), 16 oz. ..	550	28.0	49.0	27.0	60	1360	5.0
(*Swanson Hungry-Man*), 16.25 oz.	610	30.0	45.0	34.0	95	1710	5.0
sirloin, chopped (*Swanson Traditional Favorites*), 14.75 oz.	490	27.0	49.0	20.0	70	1240	10.0
sirloin tips (*Swanson Hungry-Man*), 15.75 oz.	440	25.0	49.0	16.0	55	960	6.0
steak, country fried (*Stouffer's* Home-Style), 16 oz.	560	22.0	61.0	25	50	1750	7.0
Stroganoff (*Healthy Choice*), 11 oz. ...	330	22.0	40.0	9.0	60	600	7.0
tips, portobello (*Healthy Choice*), 11.25 oz.	310	23.0	34.0	9.0	40	600	7.0
Beef entree, can or pkg., 1 cup, except as noted:							
hash, see "Beef hash"							
pot roast (*Dinty Moore American Classics*), 1 bowl	200	24.0	19.0	3.0	45	730	2.0

Food and Measure	cal.	prot. (gms)	carbo. (gms)	fat (gms)	chol. (mgs)	sod. (mgs)	fiber (gms)
Beef entree, can or pkg. *(cont.)*							
roast:							
w/gravy (*Hormel*), ½ cup	150	25.0	3.0	4.0	75	640	0
w/potatoes (*Dinty Moore American Classics*), 1 bowl	240	24.0	24.0	5.0	45	870	2.0
Salisbury steak (*Dinty Moore American Classics*), 1 bowl ..	320	21.0	28.0	15.0	40	1380	3.0
stew:							
(*Castleberry*)	340	10.0	16.0	26.0	50	900	3.0
(*Dinty Moore* Can)	180	10.0	18.0	8.0	30	920	2.0
(*Dinty Moore* Can), 7.5-oz. can	190	11.0	15.0	10.0	30	840	2.0
(*Dinty Moore* Microwave Cup)	160	8.0	16.0	7.0	30	900	2.0
(*Dinty Moore American Classics*), 1 bowl	250	15.0	22.0	11.0	45	1170	2.0
(*Hormel* Microcup)	150	10.0	14.0	6.0	25	890	2.0
burger (*Dinty Moore* Microwave Cup)	240	12.0	19.0	13.0	40	930	3.0
Beef entree, dried, 1 serving:							
barbecue, and turkey w/beans (*AlpineAire*)	370	23.0	61.0	3.0	40	770	8.0
rotini (*AlpineAire*) ...	360	22.0	59.0	3.5	40	560	2.0
stew, hearty:							
(*Mountain House Double/Four*) ...	200	13.0	31.0	2.0	25	1190	4.0
(*Mountain House Single*)	280	18.0	44.0	3.5	35	1690	5.0
Stroganoff:							
(*AlpineAire*)	310	20.0	37.0	9.0	55	950	1.0
(*Mountain House Double/Four*) ...	320	14.0	37.0	13.0	20	1050	2.0
(*Mountain House Single*)	390	17.0	46.0	16.0	25	1320	2.0
tamale pie (*AlpineAire Western*)	380	23.0	50.0	10.0	55	1050	7.0
teriyaki (*Mountain House*)	330	14.0	54.0	6.0	20	1170	2.0

Food and Measure	cal.	prot. (gms)	carbo. (gms)	fat (gms)	chol. (mgs)	sod. (mgs	fiber (gms)
vegetable stew (*Alpine-Aire*)	220	16.0	30	3.5	n.a.	800	5.0
Beef entree, frozen (see also "beef, refrigerated"), 1 pkg., except as noted:							
barbecue sauce, rice and beans (*Healthy Choice* Duo), 8.5 oz.	250	19.0	34.0	4.0	35	600	2.0
and broccoli:							
(*Healthy Choice* Bowl), 10.5 oz.	300	17.0	41.0	8.0	35	600	1.0
(*Stouffer's Skillet Sensations*), ½ of 25-oz. pkg.	320	17.0	51.0	5.0	30	1250	3.0
Hunan (*Lean Cuisine Everyday Favorites*), 8.5 oz.	240	11.0	40.0	3.5	20	690	2.0
Burgundy, w/garlic mashed potato (*Michelina's*), 8.5 oz.	300	19.0	21.0	14.0	35	1020	2.0
chipped, creamed:							
(*Banquet* Hot Sandwich Toppers), 4-oz. bag	120	7.0	8.0	6.0	25	700	0
(*Freezer Queen* Cook-in-Pouch), 4 oz.	100	6.0	8.0	5.0	15	360	1.0
(*Stouffer's*), ½ of 11-oz. pkg.	160	10.0	8.0	10.0	35	620	0
chunky, and tomato (*Stouffer's* Home-Style), 10 oz.	280	18.0	35.0	8.0	45	1360	4.0
cured, cream sauce (*Michelina's*), 8 oz.	420	17.0	40.0	20.0	60	770	0
enchilada, see "Enchilada entree"							
fajita (*Uncle Ben's* Bowl), 12 oz.	360	26.0	48.0	7.0	50	1260	6.0
home-style:							
(*Lean Cuisine Hearty Portions*), 14.25 oz.	350	23.0	44.0	9.0	30	1160	9.0

Food and Measure	cal.	prot. (gms)	carbo. (gms)	fat (gms)	chol. (mgs)	sod. (mgs)	fiber (gms)
Beef entree, frozen, home-style *(cont.)*							
(*Stouffer's Skillet Sensations*), ½ of 25-oz. pkg.	350	19.0	41.0	12.0	30	1340	7.0
nacho bake (*Ortega*), ¼ of 36-oz. pkg. . . .	400	19.0	36.0	20.0	30	1510	3.0
w/noodles, see "Noodle entree, frozen"							
Oriental:							
(*Budget Gourmet*), 8 oz.	200	10.0	32.0	3.5	10	1160	2.0
(*Lean Cuisine Cafe Classics*), 9.25 oz.	210	14.0	30.0	3.5	25	530	2.0
and peppers (*Yu Sing*), 8 oz.	290	10.0	44.0	7.0	15	1200	2.0
patty:							
onion gravy and (*Freezer Queen* Family), 1 patty w/gravy	260	13.0	12.0	17.0	55	1010	3.0
w/vegetables (*Banquet*), 9.5 oz.	310	11.0	22.0	20.0	40	1090	2.0
Western style (*Banquet*), 9.5 oz.	360	14.0	28.0	21.0	40	1400	3.0
patty, charbroiled:							
gravy and (*Freezer Queen* Meal), 9.5 oz.	270	17.0	15.0	16.0	25	900	6.0
gravy and (*Morton*), 9 oz.	310	10.0	26.0	18.0	30	1210	5.0
mushroom gravy (*Banquet* Family), 1 patty w/gravy	250	11.0	6.0	20.0	35	750	2.0
mushroom gravy and (*Freezer Queen* Family), 1 patty w/gravy	180	9.0	6.0	12.0	25	610	3.0
pepper steak:							
(*Marie Callender's Skillet Meal*), ½ of 24-oz. pkg.	320	18.0	39.0	12.0	40	1380	6.0
(*Michelina's*), 8 oz.	260	11.0	44.0	4.5	20	910	2.0

Food and Measure	cal.	prot. (gms)	carbo. (gms)	fat (gms)	chol. (mgs)	sod. (mgs)	fiber (gms)
(*Michelina's*), 8.5 oz.	280	12.0	46.0	4.0	20	1040	2.0
green (*Stouffer's* HomeStyle), 10.5 oz.	270	21.0	33.0	6.0	40	760	2.0
w/rice (*Budget Gourmet*), 8.5 oz.	230	10.0	35.0	6.0	20	840	2.0
peppercorn:							
(*Lean Cuisine Cafe Classics*), 8.75 oz.	260	16.0	32.0	7.0	25	690	4.0
sirloin (*Michelina's*), 8.5 oz.	290	13.0	33.0	13.0	55	1160	2.0
and peppers, w/rice:							
(*Freezer Queen Deluxe Family*), 1 cup	230	14.0	38.0	2.5	25	780	1.0
(*Freezer Queen Home-style*), 8.5 oz.	210	14.0	35.0	1.5	20	710	1.0
pie/pot pie:							
(*Banquet*), 7 oz. ...	400	9.0	38.0	23.0	30	1000	1.0
(*Marie Callender's*), 9.5 oz.	630	19.0	58.0	36.0	25	700	3.0
(*Marie Callender's* 16.5 oz.), 1 cup	550	16.0	50.0	32.0	20	610	3.0
(*Swanson*), 7 oz.	420	13.0	42.0	22.0	25	730	2.0
(*Swanson Potato-Topped*), 12 oz.	480	20.0	42.0	26.0	50	1240	13.0
portobello (*Lean Cuisine Cafe Classics*), 9 oz.	220	14.0	24.0	7.0	35	590	2.0
pot roast:							
(*Country Skillet*), ¼ of 32-oz. pkg.	200	15.0	23.0	5.0	95	980	2.0
(*Freezer Queen Meal*), 9.25 oz.	140	9.0	20.0	2.5	15	560	5.0
(*Freezer Queen Deluxe Family*), 1 cup	170	22.0	18.0	3.5	50	470	3.0
(*Lean Cuisine Cafe Classics*), 9 oz.	190	15.0	19.0	6.0	30	690	3.0
(*Marie Callender's Skillet Meal*), ½ of 22-oz. pkg.	330	22.0	300	13.0	75	1200	3.0

Food and Measure	cal.	prot. (gms)	carbo. (gms)	fat (gms)	chol. (mgs)	sod. (mgs)	fiber (gms)
Beef entree, frozen, pot roast *(cont.)*							
(*Michelina's*), 10 oz.	270	17.0	35.0	5.0	10	890	4.0
country style (*Marie Callender's* Bowl), 11.85 oz.	250	18.0	35.0	4.0	40	1050	5.0
old-fashioned (*Marie Callender's*), 15 oz.	500	50.0	56.0	17.0	115	1460	3.0
and potatoes (*Stouffer's* Home-Style), 8⅞ oz. ..	260	15.0	30.0	9.0	30	790	4.0
Yankee (*Banquet*), 9.4 oz.	210	15.0	21.0	8.0	40	1050	3.0
Yankee (*Stouffer's Oven Sensations*), ½ of 24-oz. pkg.	320	18.0	41.0	9.0	40	1130	3.0
and rice, fiesta (*Lean Cuisine Skillet Sensations*), ½ of 24-oz. pkg.	300	19.0	48.0	3.5	25	760	6.0
w/roast potato and peppers (*Stouffer's Oven Sensations*), ½ of 24-oz. pkg. ..	300	17.0	44.0	6.0	25	830	7.0
roast/roasted:							
(*Lean Cuisine Cafe Classics*), 9.25 oz.	260	18.0	28.0	8.0	50	590	4.0
(*Marie Callender's*), 14.5 oz.	390	24.0	30.0	19.0	70	1240	11.0
sirloin (*Michelina's* Supreme), 8 oz.	240	11.0	34.0	6.0	50	920	2.0
sirloin (*Michelina's* Supreme), 8.5 oz.	270	13.0	33.0	9.0	50	900	2.0
Salisbury steak:							
(*Banquet*), 9.5 oz.	380	12.0	28.0	24.0	60	1140	3.0
(*Freezer Queen* Meal), 9.5 oz. ..	280	14.0	21.0	15.0	40	900	6.0
(*Lean Cuisine Cafe Classics*), 9.5 oz.	290	25.0	26.0	9.0	45	690	3.0
(*Lean Cuisine Hearty Portions*), 15.5 oz.	300	22.0	40.0	6.0	40	890	8.0

Food and Measure	cal.	prot. (gms)	carbo. (gms)	fat (gms)	chol. (mgs)	sod. (mgs	fiber (gms)
(*Marie Callender's*), 10 oz.	320	21.0	31.0	13.0	85	1420	4.0
(*Stouffer's* Home-Style), 9⅝ oz. .	360	24.0	27.0	17.0	65	1160	1.0
brown gravy and (*Banquet* Family), 1 patty w/gravy	240	9.0	7.0	20.0	40	900	1.0
and gravy (*Marie Callender's*), 14 oz.	550	30.0	51.0	25.0	85	1680	6.0
and gravy (*Master Choice*), 1 pc. w/gravy	380	24.0	39.0	26.0	95	1090	<1.0
and gravy (*Michelina's* Family), ¼ of 32-oz. pkg. ..	320	13.0	23.0	21.0	50	1290	2.0
and gravy, w/macaroni and cheese (*Freezer Queen* Family Buffet), ¼ pkg.	430	20.0	42.0	20.0	40	1990	2.0
and gravy, w/mashed potato (*Michelina's*), 8 oz.	330	14.0	21.0	21.0	55	1360	2.0
and gravy, w/ whipped potato (*Freezer Queen* Homestyle), 8.5 oz.	300	18.0	26.0	14.0	30	840	5.0
gravy and (*Banquet* Hot Sandwich Toppers), 5-oz. bag	210	9.0	8.0	16.0	25	790	2.0
gravy and (*Freezer Queen* Cook-in-Pouch), 5 oz. ..	150	8.0	8.0	10.0	20	680	2.0
gravy and (*Freezer Queen* Family), 1 patty w/gravy	160	9.0	6.0	11.0	20	810	3.0
gravy and (*Morton*), 9 oz.	310	7.0	24.0	20.0	30	1100	3.0
and red skin mashed potato (*Healthy Choice* Duo), 8 oz.	210	17.0	23.0	6.0	35	600	3.0

Food and Measure	cal.	prot. (gms)	carbo. (gms)	fat (gms)	chol. (mgs)	sod. (mgs)	fiber (gms)
Beef entree, frozen, Salisbury steak (cont.)							
w/shells and cheese (*Michelina's*), 10.5 oz.	450	24.0	33.0	25.0	60	1730	2.0
sliced:							
(*Banquet*), 9 oz. ...	270	26.0	17.0	10.0	70	740	4.0
brown gravy and (*Banquet* Family), 2 slices w/gravy	140	13.0	5.0	8.0	40	850	<1.0
sliced, gravy and:							
(*Banquet* Hot Sandwich Toppers), 4 oz.	70	8.0	5.0	2.0	25	440	0
(*Freezer Queen* Cook-in-Pouch), 4 oz.	60	9.0	5.0	1.0	20	400	<1.0
(*Freezer Queen* Deluxe Family), ⅔ cup	80	11.0	6.0	1.5	35	690	0
w/mashed potato (*Freezer Queen* Family Buffet*), ¼ pkg.	220	13.0	32.0	5.0	35	1110	5.0
w/mashed potato, carrots (*Freezer Queen*), 9 oz. ...	140	14.0	17.0	2.0	25	840	3.0
steak, chicken-fried:							
(*Banquet*), 10 oz.	420	15.0	39.0	23.0	35	1200	4.0
and gravy (*Marie Callender's*), 15 oz.	650	20.0	58.0	37.0	50	2260	7.0
steak, Philly (*Healthy Choice* Bread Stuffs), 6.1 oz.	310	17.0	50.0	5.0	20	600	3.0
steak, sirloin, and garlic potato (*Birds Eye Steak Voila!*), 1 cup* ...	240	13.0	26.0	9.0	25	650	3.0
stew, hearty (*Banquet* Family), 1 cup	170	10.0	18.0	7.0	30	1120	4.0
stir-fry (*Contessa*), 1¾ cups	190	13.0	28.0	3.0	20	820	4.0

Food and Measure	cal.	prot. (gms)	carbo. (gms)	fat (gms)	chol. (mgs)	sod. (mgs)	fiber (gms)
Stroganoff:							
(*Budget Gourmet*), 8 oz.	240	13.0	32.0	6.0	20	690	3.0
(*Marie Callender's*), 13 oz.	510	32.0	59.0	16.0	70	1140	4.0
(*Marie Callender's* Skillet Meal), ½ of 22-oz. pkg. . .	340	21.0	31.0	15.0	70	1290	2.0
(*Marie Callender's* Skillet Meal), ¼ of 35-oz. pkg. . .	270	17.0	25.0	12.0	60	1020	1.0
(*Stouffer's* Home-Style), 9.75 oz.	370	21.0	32.0	17.0	65	950	3.0
(*Stouffer's Skillet Sensations*), ¼ of 40-oz. pkg.	340	19.0	38.0	12.0	35	1090	4.0
taco olé (*Uncle Ben's Mini Bowl*), 8 oz.	350	15.0	42.0	15.0	40	1160	3.0
teriyaki:							
(*Healthy Choice Medley*), 9.5 oz.	330	19.0	48.0	7.0	40	600	7.0
(*Lean Cuisine Skillet Sensations*), ½ of 24-oz. pkg. . .	320	16.0	52.0	5.0	20	860	4.0
w/rice (*Yu Sing*), 8 oz.	270	10.0	58.0	2.5	10	1140	2.0
tips:							
sirloin and mushroom rice (*Healthy Choice* Duo), 8 oz.	270	20.0	35.0	6.0	35	600	4.0
in mushroom sauce (*Marie Callender's*), 13.6 oz.	430	25.0	39.0	19.0	50	1620	6.0
Southern (*Lean Cuisine Cafe Classics*), 8.75 oz.	270	16.0	37.0	6.0	35	690	4.0
spiral pasta and (*Healthy Choice Medley*), 9.5 oz.	300	20.0	40.0	7.0	40	600	4.0
w/vegetables:							
(*Lean Cuisine Cafe Classics*), 9 oz.	200	13.0	31.0	3.0	25	610	4.0

Food and Measure	cal.	prot. (gms)	carbo. (gms)	fat (gms)	chol. (mgs)	sod. (mgs)	fiber (gms)
Beef entree, frozen, w/vegetables *(cont.)*							
savory (*Lean Cuisine Skillet Sensations*), ½ of 24-oz. pkg. ...	290	18.0	38.0	7.0	35	760	9.0
Beef entree mix (see also "Hamburger entree mix"), Stroganoff (*Lipton Sizzle & Stir*), ⅙ box	160	5.0	28.0	3.0	10	720	1.0
Beef gravy, ¼ cup:							
(*Boston Market*)	30	2.0	3.0	1.0	5	340	0
(*Franco-American*) ...	25	1.0	3.0	1.0	<5	340	0
(*Franco-American* Fat Free)	20	1.0	3.0	0	<5	290	0
(*Franco-American Slow Roast*)	25	1.0	3.0	.5	<5	310	0
(*Heinz Fat Free Savory*)	20	2.0	3.0	0	<5	350	0
Beef gravy mix, herb (*McCormick*), ¼ cup*	30	1.0	3.0	1.0	0	290	0
Beef hash, corned, (*Jones Dairy Farm*), 2 oz.	100	6.0	5.0	6.0	20	290	0
Beef hash, canned, 1 cup, except as noted:							
corned:							
(*Armour*)	440	19.0	23.0	30.0	100	840	2.0
(*Broadcast*)	420	17.0	33.0	24.0	55	1230	6.0
(*Broadcast*), 7.5 oz.	350	15.0	28.0	20.0	45	1030	5.0
(*Libby's*)	420	17.0	33.0	24.0	55	1230	6.0
(*Libby's Morning Classics*)	360	12.0	33.0	20.0	30	1390	2.0
(*Mary Kitchen*) ...	390	21.0	22.0	24.0	80	1000	2.0
(*Mary Kitchen*), 7.5 oz.	370	19.0	19.0	24.0	75	950	1.0
(*Mary Kitchen 50% Less Fat*)	280	19.0	25.0	12.0	65	1070	3.0
(*Stagg*)	450	23.0	29.0	26.0	90	1250	2.0
roast (*Mary Kitchen*)	390	21.0	22.0	24.0	70	790	2.0
Beef hash, dried, roast (*AlpineAire* All American), 2 oz. ..	220	18.0	28.0	4.5	50	920	3.0

Food and Measure	cal.	prot. (gms)	carbo. (gms)	fat (gms)	chol. (mgs)	sod. (mgs)	fiber (gms)
Beef jerky, see "Sausage stick"							
Beef lunch meat (see also "Bologna," etc.), 2 oz., except as noted:							
(*Carl Buddig* 6 oz.) ..	75	10.0	1.0	4.0	40	790	0
cooked, seasoned							
(*Briar Street Market*)	50	9.0	1.0	1.5	20	440	0
corned:							
(*Black Bear* Brisket)	90	9.0	2.0	5.0	35	550	0
(*Boar's Head* Brisket)	120	11.0	0	8.0	40	590	0
(*Boar's Head* Brisket First Cut)	80	12.0	0	3.5	40	460	0
(*Boar's Head* Cap-Off Top Round)	80	14.0	0	2.5	30	360	0
(*Boar's Head Custom Cut* Round)	80	12.0	0	3.0	30	510	0
(*Briar Street Market*)	60	9.0	1.0	2.0	30	640	0
(*Carl Buddig* 6 oz.) .	75	10.0	1.0	4.0	40	740	0
(*Healthy Choice*) ..	60	10.0	0	1.5	30	430	0
(*Healthy Deli*)	80	11.0	2.0	3.0	30	480	0
(*Sara Lee*), 2 slices, 1.6 oz.	45	7.0	0	2.0	25	520	0
eye round:							
pepper seasoned (*Boar's Head*) ..	90	14.0	0	3.0	40	130	0
oven roasted (*Boar's Head* Deluxe) ...	80	14.0	0	2.5	30	120	0
flame roasted:							
medium (*Sara Lee*)	70	13.0	1.0	2.0	30	240	0
rare (*Sara Lee*) ...	80	13.0	1.0	2.5	35	210	0
London broil (*Healthy Deli*)	70	11.0	2.0	2.5	25	300	0
peppered (*Sara Lee*)	70	12.0	1.0	2.0	25	310	0
roast:							
(*Alpine Lace*)	70	13.0	1.0	1.5	40	200	0
(*Briar Street Market*)	60	10.0	1.0	1.5	25	410	0
(*Healthy Choice*) ..	60	10.0	2.0	1.5	25	480	0
(*Healthy Choice* Deli Traditions), 1-oz. slice	30	5.0	1.0	1.0	10	240	0
(*Healthy Choice* Whole Muscle), 2 slices, 1.5 oz.	50	8.0	1.0	1.0	20	450	0

Food and Measure	cal.	prot. (gms)	carbo. (gms)	fat (gms)	chol. (mgs)	sod. (mgs)	fiber (gms)
Beef lunch meat, roast *(cont.)*							
(*Sara Lee*), 2 slices, 1.6 oz.	50	9.0	0	1.5	25	260	0
Cajun (*Boar's Head*)	80	14.0	0	2.0	35	200	0
garlic herb (*Healthy Choice Savory Selections*), 6 slices, 1.9 oz.	60	10.0	1.0	1.5	25	470	0
Italian style (*Healthy Choice*)	60	11.0	1.0	1.5	25	480	0
Italian style (*Healthy Deli*)	70	11.0	1.0	1.5	30	320	0
Italian style braciole, seasoned (*Boar's Head*)	80	12.0	2.0	2.0	40	350	0
medium (*Healthy Choice*)	70	10.0	1.0	1.5	25	480	0
top round, medium (*Sara Lee*)	80	13.0	1.0	2.5	35	210	0
top round, seasoned (*Healthy Deli*) ..	70	12.0	0	2.0	30	320	0
well done (*Healthy Deli*)	70	12.0	0	2.0	30	320	0
round (*Boar's Head Custom Cut* No Salt)	90	14.0	0	3.0	35	40	0
top round:							
(*Boar's Head* Cap-Off No Salt)	70	14.0	0	2.0	30	40	0
(*Boar's Head* Deluxe Low Sodium Half) ...	80	15.0	<1.0	2.5	30	80	0
(*Boar's Head* Deluxe Low Sodium Whole)	90	14.0	0	3.0	30	80	0
oven roasted (*Boar's Head* No Salt) ..	90	14.0	0	3.0	30	40	0
seasoned filet (*Boar's Head*) ..	80	14.0	0	2.5	40	105	0
Beef pie, see "Beef entree, frozen"							
Beef pocket (see also "Beef sandwich"),							

Food and Measure	cal.	prot. (gms)	carbo. (gms)	fat (gms)	chol. (mgs)	sod. (mgs)	fiber (gms)
frozen, 4.5-oz. pc., except as noted:							
barbecue (*Hot Pockets*)	340	10.0	47.0	12.0	15	740	2.0
and cheddar (*Hot Pockets*)	350	12.0	44.0	14.0	45	660	2.0
cheeseburger:							
(*Hot Pockets*)	330	14.0	41.0	13.0	35	570	2.0
(*Lean Pockets*) ...	300	13.0	43.0	7.0	25	570	2.0
fajita (*Hot Pockets*) ..	330	12.0	37.0	14.0	40	650	2.0
jalapeño steak (*Hot Pockets*)	330	11.0	40.0	14.0	45	640	2.0
Philly steak/cheese:							
(*Croissant Pockets*)	350	12.0	40.0	16.0	45	630	2.0
(*Deli Stuffs*)	340	13.0	43.0	13.0	40	560	3.0
(*Lean Pockets*) ...	280	12.0	42.0	7.0	25	520	3.0
potato topped (*Mrs. Patterson's Aussie Pie*), 5.5 oz.	340	14.0	33.0	16.0	50	840	2.0
Beef sandwich, frozen, 1 pc., except as noted:							
barbecued (*Hormel Quick Meal*)	370	15.0	38.0	17.0	45	560	1.0
cheeseburger:							
(*Hormel Quick Meal*)	400	19.0	36.0	20.0	55	600	1.0
(*White Castle*), 2 pcs.	310	15.0	28.0	17.0	30	480	6.0
bacon (*Hormel Quick Meal*)	420	22.0	34.0	22.0	65	800	1.0
(*Kid's Kitchen*), 2 pcs.	400	18.0	44.0	16.0	60	600	1.0
hamburger:							
(*Hormel Quick Meal*)	350	17.0	34.0	16.0	45	400	1.0
(*White Castle*), 2 pcs.	270	12.0	28.0	14.0	20	270	5.0
patty, w/cheese (*Kid Cuisine*), 8.5 oz. ..	450	14.0	59.0	17.0	30	650	4.0
Beef sausage, see "Sausage"							

Food and Measure	cal.	prot. (gms)	carbo. (gms)	fat (gms)	chol. (mgs)	sod. (mgs)	fiber (gms)
Beef seasoning mix:							
pot roast (*McCormick Bag'n Season*), ⅛ pkg.	10	0	1.0	0	0	390	0
stew:							
(*Adolph's Meal Makers*), 1 tbsp.	10	0	3.0	0	0	700	0
(*Knorr Recipe Classics* Goulash), 1⅓ tbsp.	40	<1.0	6.0	1.5	0	530	0
(*Lawry's*), 1 tsp. ...	10	<1.0	2.0	0	0	370	0
(*McCormick Bag'n Season*), ⅛ pkg.	15	1.0	1.0	0	0	670	0
Stroganoff:							
(*Lawry's*), 1 tbsp.	20	0	5.0	0	0	500	0
(*McCormick*), ⅛ pkg.	15	0	3.0	0	0	350	0
Swiss steak (*McCormick Bag'n Season*), ⅛ pkg. ...	15	0	2.0	0	0	430	0
Beef spread, roast (*Underwood*), ¼ cup	140	9.0	0	11.0	45	390	0
Beef stew, see "Beef entree"							
Beef stew base, see "Soup base, mix"							
Beef-tomato drink, see "Tomato-beef drink"							
Beefalo, meat only, roasted, 4 oz.	213	34.8	0	7.2	66	93	0
Beer, 12 fl. oz.:							
regular	146	.9	13.2	0	0	19	0
light	100	.7	4.8	0	0	10	0
Beet, fresh:							
raw:							
(*Frieda's*), 3 oz. ...	35	1.0	8.0	0	0	65	2.0
2 medium, 2" diam.	70	2.6	15.6	.3	0	126	4.6
trimmed, sliced, ½ cup	29	1.1	6.5	.1	0	53	1.9
boiled, drained:							
2 medium, 2" diam.	44	1.7	10.0	.2	0	77	1.7
sliced, ½ cup	38	1.4	8.5	.2	0	65	1.4

Food and Measure	cal.	prot. (gms)	carbo. (gms)	fat (gms)	chol. (mgs)	sod. (mgs	fiber (gms)
Beet, canned, ½ cup, except as noted:							
whole or sliced:							
(*Aunt Nellie's*)	35	<1.0	8.0	0	0	240	2.0
(*Del Monte*)	35	1.0	8.0	0	0	290	2.0
(*Libby's*)	35	<1.0	8.0	0	0	240	2.0
(*S&W*)	30	1.0	7.0	0	0	230	1.0
(*Veg-All*)	40	<1.0	8.0	0	0	300	1.0
w/liquid	36	1.0	8.3	.1	0	324	1.4
sliced, w/ or w/out onion (*Aunt Nellie's/Lohmann/ Libby's*), 4 slices, 1 oz.	20	0	4.0	0	0	55	0
Harvard:							
(*Aunt Nellie's/ Lohmann*), ⅓ cup, ...	60	0	14.0	0	0	270	2.0
(*Greenwood* Sweet & Tangy)	100	1.0	27.0	0	0	370	1.0
(*Libby's*), ⅓ cup ..	60	0	14.0	0	0	270	2.0
w/liquid	89	1.0	22.4	.1	0	199	1.0
pickled:							
whole, 2 pcs.:							
(*Aunt Nellie's/ Lohmann*) ...	20	0	5.0	0	0	65	<1.0
tiny (*Libby's*) ...	20	0	5.0	0	0	65	<1.0
whole or sliced:							
(*Greenwood* Sweet & Tangy), 1 oz.	25	0	6.0	0	0	100	0
(*S&W*), 1 oz. ..	15	0	4.0	0	0	50	1.0
crinkle (*Del Monte*)	80	1.0	19.0	0	0	380	2.0
w/liquid	74	.9	18.5	.1	0	300	3.0
raspberry flavor, julienne or crinkle (*Aunt Nellie*), 1 oz.	20	0	5.0	0	0	100	0
Beet greens, ½ cup:							
raw, 1" pcs.	4	.4	.8	<.1	0	38	.7
boiled, drained, 1" pcs.	20	1.9	3.9	.1	0	173	2.1
Berliner, pork and beef, 1 oz.	65	4.3	.7	4.9	13	368	0

Food and Measure	cal.	prot. (gms)	carbo. (gms)	fat (gms)	chol. (mgs)	sod. (mgs)	fiber (gms)
Berries, mixed, frozen:							
(*Cascadian Farm Harvest Berries*),							
1 cup	65	1.0	16.0	1.0	0	0	5.0
(*Tree of Life* Organic),							
¾ cup	60	0	16.0	0	0	0	3.0
in syrup (*Big Valley's Burst o' Berries/ Flavorland Berry Bonanza*), ⅔ cup . .	160	<1.0	38.0	0	0	0	1.0
Berry drink blends:							
(*Kool-Aid Bursts*), 6.75 fl. oz.	90	0	23.0	0	0	35	0
(*Tang Berry Panic*), 6.75 fl. oz.	100	0	25.0	0	0	30	0
(*Tang Berry Panic*), 8 fl. oz.	120	0	32.0	0	0	35	0
black and blue (*WhipperSnapple*), 10 fl. oz.	160	0	40.0	0	0	60	0
blue (*Kool-Aid Bursts*), 6.75 fl. oz.	100	0	24.0	0	0	30	0
red (*Capri Sun All Natural*), 6.75 fl. oz.	100	0	25.0	0	0	20	0
punch, 8 fl. oz.:							
(*Tropicana*)	130	0	32.0	0	0	15	0
frozen* (*Minute Maid*)	110	0	31.0	0	0	5	0
Berry juice blends, 8 fl. oz.:							
(*After the Fall* Oregon)	100	0	25.0	0	0	25	0
(*Juicy Juice*)	130	1.0	30.0	0	0	10	0
(*Santa Cruz Organic* Nectar)	120	<1.0	30.0	0	0	25	0
Berry-cherry drink mix* (*Kool-Aid Blastin' Berry Cherry*), 8 fl. oz. . .	70	0	17.0	0	0	0	0
Biryani paste, see "Curry paste"							
Biscuit, 2-oz. pc.:							
buttermilk (*Awrey's*)	200	4.0	31.0	7.0	0	510	2.0
plain or buttermilk . . .	206	3.5	27.5	9.4	<1	596	.7

Food and Measure	cal.	prot. (gms)	carbo. (gms)	fat (gms)	chol. (mgs)	sod. (mgs	fiber (gms)
Biscuit, refrigerated,							
1 pc., except as noted:							
(*Big Country Butter*							
Tastin')	100	2.0	13.0	4.0	0	360	0
(*Grands!* Extra Rich) .	220	4.0	25.0	11.0	0	570	<1.0
(*Grands!* HomeStyle) .	180	4.0	24.0	8.0	0	600	<1.0
(*Grands! Butter Tastin'*)	180	4.0	23.0	9.0	0	600	<1.0
(*Pillsbury Butter Tastin'*)	180	4.0	21.0	9.0	0	570	<1.0
(*Pillsbury* Country),							
3 pcs.	150	4.0	29.0	2.0	0	540	<1.0
buttermilk:							
(*Big Country* Fluffy)	100	2.0	14.0	4.0	0	360	0
(*Grands!*)	190	4.0	24.0	9.0	0	600	<1.0
(*Pillsbury*), 3 pcs.	150	4.0	29.0	2.0	0	540	<1.0
(*Hungry Jack*)	100	2.0	14.0	4.5	0	360	0
(*Pillsbury* Home-							
style)	190	4.0	22.0	9.0	0	580	<1.0
(*Pillsbury* Tender							
Layer), 3 pcs. ..	160	4.0	22.0	4.5	0	520	<1.0
flaky (*Hungry Jack*)	100	2.0	14.0	4.5	0	360	0
cheddar garlic (*Pills-							
bury Home Baked							
Classics*)	190	6.0	19.0	10.0	10	710	<1.0
cinnamon and sugar							
(*Hungry Jack*)	110	2.0	17.0	4.0	0	280	<1.0
corn, golden (*Grands!*)	190	4.0	28.0	7.0	0	610	<1.0
flaky:							
(*Grands!*)	200	4.0	25.0	9.0	0	580	<1.0
(*Hungry Jack*)	100	2.0	14.0	4.5	0	360	0
honey butter (*Hungry*							
Jack)	110	2.0	17.0	4.0	0	280	0
Southern style:							
(*Big Country*)	100	2.0	14.0	4.0	0	360	0
(*Grands!*)	190	4.0	23.0	9.0	0	600	<1.0
(*Pillsbury* Home-							
style)	180	4.0	21.0	9.0	0	570	<1.0
wheat, golden (*Grands!*							
Reduced Fat)	190	4.0	27.0	7.0	0	600	2.0
Biscuit mix, dry							
(*Arrowhead Mills*),							
¼ cup	120	5.0	23.0	1.0	0	200	3.0
Bison, meat only,							
roasted, 4 oz.	162	32.3	0	2.7	93	65	0

Food and Measure	cal.	prot. (gms)	carbo. (gms)	fat (gms)	chol. (mgs)	sod. (mgs)	fiber (gms)
Bitter melon, see "Balsam pear"							
Black bean, dried:							
dry (*Frieda's*), ⅓ cup	120	8.0	20.0	0	0	240	11.0
boiled, ½ cup	113	7.6	20.4	.5	0	1	7.5
turtle:							
dry (*Arrowhead*							
Mills), ¼ cup . . .	150	10.0	28.0	.5	0	10	9.0
boiled, ½ cup	120	7.5	22.4	.3	0	3	4.9
Black bean, canned, ½ cup:							
(*Allens*)	100	6.0	20.0	1.5	0	310	8.0
(*Bush's Best*)	100	7.0	20.0	.5	0	470	7.0
(*Eden* Organic)	100	7.0	18.0	0	0	15	6.0
(*Progresso*)	110	7.0	17.0	1.0	0	400	7.0
(*S&W*)	70	5.0	17.0	0	0	480	6.0
(*S&W* 50% Salt)	70	5.0	17.0	0	0	260	6.0
(*Westbrae Natural*) . .	90	6.0	16.0	0	0	140	4.0
w/ginger and lemon							
(*Eden* Organic) . . .	120	7.0	21.0	0	0	200	7.0
seasoned:							
(*S&W* Caribbean) . .	100	6.0	18.0	0	0	540	7.0
(*S&W* San Antonio)	90	6.0	20.0	.5	0	670	6.0
(*S&W* Santa Fe) . . .	90	6.0	21.0	1.0	0	680	6.0
(*Trappey's*)	120	7.0	20.0	1.5	0	410	7.0
turtle (*Hain* Organic)	100	7.0	17.0	1.0	0	140	7.0
Black bean, dehydrated (*Alpine-Aire*), 1 oz.	100	6.0	18.0	.5	0	0	9.0
Black bean sauce, 1 tbsp.:							
(*Ka•Me*)	20	1.0	3.0	.5	0	280	0
chili (*Heaven and Earth*)	30	1.0	4.0	1.5	0	400	0
garlic, spicy (*Annie Chun's*)	50	1.0	6.0	4.0	0	440	0
Blackberry, fresh, ½ cup	37	.5	9.2	.3	0	tr.	3.6
Blackberry, canned:							
(*Allens*), ⅔ cup	60	2.0	13.0	.5	0	20	9.0
in light syrup (*Oregon*), ½ cup	120	1.0	29.0	0	0	10	6.0
in syrup, ½ cup	118	1.7	29.6	.2	0	3	4.4

Food and Measure	cal.	prot. (gms)	carbo. (gms)	fat (gms)	chol. (mgs)	sod. (mgs)	fiber (gms)
Blackberry, frozen:							
(*Cascadian Farm*),							
1 cup	80	1.0	20.0	.5	0	10	3.0
unsweetened, ½ cup	49	.9	11.8	.3	0	1	3.8
Blackberry syrup							
(*Smucker's*), ¼ cup	210	0	52.0	0	0	0	0
Black-eyed peas:							
fresh, see "Cowpeas"							
mature, dry:							
(*Frieda's*), ⅓ cup,							
3 oz.	130	8.0	21.0	1.0	0	250	11.0
(*Jack Rabbit*),							
¼ cup	90	9.0	23.0	0	0	25	10.0
mature, boiled,							
½ cup	100	6.7	17.9	.5	0	3	5.6
Black-eyed peas,							
canned, ½ cup:							
(*Eden* Organic)	90	6.0	16.0	1.0	0	25	4.0
fresh shell:							
(*Allens/East Texas*							
Fair/Dorman) ...	120	7.0	21.0	1.0	0	350	6.0
(*Bush's Best*)	110	7.0	18.0	1.0	0	500	5.0
w/snaps (*Allens/*							
East Texas Fair)	120	8.0	20.0	1.0	0	420	5.0
w/snaps (*Bush's*							
Best)	110	7.0	17.0	.5	0	550	5.0
w/jalapeño							
(*Trappey's*)	120	7.0	20.0	1.0	0	580	5.0
mature:							
(*Allens*)	110	7.0	18.0	1.0	0	275	4.0
(*Bush's Best*)	100	5.0	19.0	0	0	410	4.0
(*Showboat*)	100	5.0	19.0	0	0	410	4.0
w/bacon (*Allens/*							
Sunshine)	120	7.0	20.0	1.5	0	390	5.0
w/bacon (*Bush's*							
Best)	110	6.0	18.0	1.0	5	630	5.0
w/bacon (*Trappey's*)	120	7.0	19.0	2.0	0	350	5.0
w/bacon and							
jalapeño (*Bush's*							
Best)	120	6.0	16.0	2.5	5	660	5.0
w/bacon and							
jalapeño							
(*Trappey's*)	110	6.0	19.0	2.0	0	470	5.0

Food and Measure	cal.	prot. (gms)	carbo. (gms)	fat (gms)	chol. (mgs)	sod. (mgs)	fiber (gms)
Black-eyed peas, canned, mature *(cont.)*							
seasoned *(Glory Foods)*	120	7.0	20.0	1.0	0	530	5.0
Black-eyed peas, frozen, ½ cup:							
(Birds Eye Southern)	110	7.0	21.0	.5	0	10	4.0
boiled, drained	112	7.2	20.2	.6	0	5	4.3
Blimpie, 1 serving:							
6" cold sub:							
Blimpie Best	410	39.0	47.0	13.0	50	1480	4.0
cheese trio/wheat . .	490	26.0	48.0	23.0	55	1110	5.0
cheese trio/white . .	490	25.0	48.0	23.0	55	1130	3.0
club/wheat	370	23.0	48.0	11.0	30	1180	5.0
club/white	370	23.0	48.0	10.0	30	1200	4.0
ham, salami, provolone/wheat	450	24.0	47.0	20.0	55	1350	5.0
ham, salami, provolone/white	480	24.0	49.0	20.0	55	1370	3.0
ham and Swiss/ wheat	400	26.0	46.0	14.0	50	1040	5.0
ham and Swiss/ white	410	25.0	48.0	14.0	50	1050	3.0
roast beef/wheat . .	390	37.0	45.0	8.0	65	1380	5.0
roast beef/white . . .	390	37.0	47.0	7.0	65	1370	3.0
tuna/wheat	650	18.0	49.0	45.0	55	860	5.0
tuna/white	660	18.0	51.0	44.0	55	880	3.0
turkey/wheat	330	19.0	48.0	7.0	0	1190	5.0
turkey/white	330	19.0	48.0	6.0	0	1200	3.0
6" hot sub:							
beef melt, smoky cheddar	380	23.0	42.0	12.0	50	1200	1.0
Chik Max/wheat . . .	495	25.8	69.3	12.8	0	1370	4.0
Chik Max/white . . .	483	33.6	69.9	11.6	0	1293	4.0
Grille Max/wheat . .	425	18.8	71.3	7.3	5	900	5.0
Grille Max/white . . .	413	18.1	71.9	6.1	5	823	5.0
grilled chicken	400	28.0	52.0	9.0	30	950	2.0
Italian meatball . . .	500	23.0	52.0	22.0	25	970	2.0
Mexi Max/wheat . .	405	25.0	65.0	5.8	0	1080	5.0
Mexi Max/white . .	393	25.0	66.0	4.6	0	1003	5.0
roast turkey cordon bleu	430	29.0	43.0	14.0	60	1180	1.0
steak and cheese . .	550	27.0	51.0	26.0	70	1080	2.0
Vegi Max/wheat . . .	415	24.0	60.0	7.8	30	1050	5.0
Vegi Max/white . . .	403	24.0	61.0	7.0	30	980	5.0

Food and Measure	cal.	prot. (gms)	carbo. (gms)	fat (gms)	chol. (mgs)	sod. (mgs)	fiber (gms)
wraps:							
chicken Caesar ...	610	26.0	56.0	31.0	35	1770	3.0
Italian, zesty	530	24.0	59.0	22.0	45	1850	3.0
Southwestern	590	28.0	56.0	28.0	75	1990	3.0
sides and salads w/out dressing:							
antipasto salad ...	200	19.0	9.0	11.0	50	950	3.0
chef salad	150	17.0	8.0	6.0	40	600	3.0
chili w/cheese and beef	240	14.0	27.0	8.0	40	1060	10.0
club salad	130	14.0	7.0	6.0	30	450	3.0
coleslaw, ½ cup ..	180	1.0	13.0	13.0	<5	230	1.0
green salad, tossed	35	2.0	7.0	.5	0	20	3.0
ham and Swiss salad	170	16.0	7.0	8.0	40	500	3.0
macaroni salad, ⅔ cup	360	4.0	25.0	25.0	10	660	1.0
pasta, Italian, supreme salad ..	180	3.0	20.0	7.0	0	840	1.0
potato salad, ⅔ cup	270	2.0	19.0	19.0	10	560	1.0
potato salad, mustard, ⅔ cup	160	2.0	21.0	5.0	5	660	1.0
roast beef salad ...	120	19.0	8.0	2.5	25	480	3.0
tuna salad	130	22.0	7.0	1.5	45	400	3.0
turkey salad	90	15.0	8.0	.5	25	580	3.0
dressing, 1 fl. oz.:							
Blimpie	120	1.0	16.0	8.0	0	570	<1.0
Blimpie Special Sub	70	0	0	7.0	0	0	0
blue cheese	220	2.0	2.0	24.0	40	440	0
buttermilk ranch ..	270	0	1.0	29.0	5	360	0
buttermilk ranch, light	90	1.0	10.0	1.0	0	350	0
honey French	240	0	16.0	20.0	0	350	0
Italian, fat free	20	0	5.0	0	0	670	0
Italian, light	20	0	3.0	1.0	0	810	0
Thousand Island ..	210	0	7.0	21.0	25	360	0
sauces:							
guacamole, 1 oz.	194	1.8	7.4	17.5	<1	468	1.4
mayonnaise, 1 tbsp.	100	0	1.0	11.0	10	60	0
soup, 1 cup:							
chicken noodle ...	140	8.0	20.0	3.0	30	1190	2.0
chicken w/white and wild rice	230	10.0	21.0	12.0	30	1210	2.0

Food and Measure	cal.	prot. (gms)	carbo. (gms)	fat (gms)	chol. (mgs)	sod. (mgs)	fiber (gms)
Blimpie, soup *(cont.)*							
potato, cream of ...	190	5.0	24.0	9.0	<5	860	3.0
Blimpie potato chips:							
regular	210	3.0	25.0	11.0	0	190	2.0
cheddar/sour cream	210	3.0	25.0	11.0	<5	220	1.0
jalapeño	210	2.0	25.0	11.0	0	250	2.0
Lea & Perrins:							
barbecue	210	3.0	25.0	10.0	0	270	2.0
sour cream/onion	210	2.0	25.0	11.0	<5	250	1.0
zesty	210	3.0	25.0	3.0	<5	220	2.0
bread:							
6" sub roll:							
marbled rye	246	9.5	47.3	2.5	0	586	2.3
wheat	235	9.0	40.5	4.0	0	475	3.5
white	240	8.5	43.0	3.5	0	490	3.5
wrap, spinach herb	308	7.8	49.0	7.8	0	781	1.7
wrap, traditional ...	301	7.8	47.9	7.6	0	761	1.6
wrap, veggie	240	8.4	43.5	8.4	0	503	1.5
cookie:							
chocolate chunk ..	201	2.0	26.0	10.0	15	201	1.0
macadamia white							
chunk	210	2.0	26.0	10.0	20	140	1.0
oatmeal raisin	191	6.0	27.0	6.0	15	201	1.0
peanut butter	221	4.0	27.0	12.0	15	201	1.0
sugar	330	3.0	24.2	17.0	30	290	0
baked goods:							
brownie, fudge ...	243	2.6	33.6	10.8	20	168	n.a.
cinnamon roll	631	9.0	90.0	25.0	0	692	0
muffin:							
banana nut	472	8.0	55.0	23.0	55	442	n.a.
blueberry	412	7.0	55.0	18.0	55	452	n.a.
bran/raisin	442	7.0	64.0	18.0	20	502	n.a.
Blintz, frozen:							
apple (*Empire* Kosher),							
2 pcs.	220	6.0	36.0	5.5	<5	260	5.0
blueberry (*Empire*							
Kosher), 2 pcs. ...	190	4.0	36.0	7.0	10	260	2.0
cheese:							
(*Empire* Kosher),							
2 pcs.	200	11.0	29.0	6.0	20	310	3.0
(*Ratner's*), 1 pc. ..	90	7.0	15.0	.5	20	15	<1.0
cherry (*Empire* Kosher),							
2 pcs.	200	5.0	36.0	4.0	10	280	3.0

Food and Measure	cal.	prot. (gms)	carbo. (gms)	fat (gms)	chol. (mgs)	sod. (mgs)	fiber (gms)
potato:							
(*Empire* Kosher),							
2 pcs.	190	6.0	32.0	6.0	10	530	3.0
(*Ratner's*), 1 pc. ..	110	3.0	17.0	3.0	15	130	1.0
Blintz, nondairy, frozen, 1 pc.:							
apple, blueberry, or cherry and "cheese" (*Tofutti* Pillows),							
2.25 oz.	70	2.0	2.0	5.0	0	290	0
"cheese" (*Tofutti* Mintz's), 2 oz.	90	3.0	2.0	4.0	0	170	2.0
Blood sausage, 1 oz.	107	4.1	.4	9.8	34	n.a.	0
Bloody Mary mixer, 8 fl. oz., except as noted:							
(*D. L. Jardine's* Red Snapper), 3 oz. ...	25	1.0	5.0	0	0	680	0
(*Mr & Mrs T*)	40	1.0	9.0	0	0	1440	0
spicy:							
(*Mr & Mrs T* Rich & Spicy)	50	1.0	11.0	0	0	970	0
(*Trader Vic's*), 4 fl. oz.	20	1.0	6.0	0	0	690	0
Blue squash, see "Australian blue squash"							
Blueberry, fresh, ½ cup	41	.5	10.2	.3	0	5	2.0
Blueberry, can or jar:							
(*S&W*), ⅓ cup	70	0	16.0	0	0	0	6.0
in light syrup (*Oregon*), ½ cup	110	<1.0	26.0	0	0	5	2.0
in heavy syrup, ½ cup	113	.8	28.2	.4	0	4	1.9
Blueberry, dried:							
(*Frieda's*), ¼ cup ...	140	1.0	33.0	0	0	0	4.0
(*Sonoma*), ¼ cup ...	140	1.0	33.0	0	0	0	5.0
freeze-dried (*Alpine-Aire*), .5 oz.	60	1.0	17.0	1.0	0	0	0
Blueberry, frozen:							
(*Big Valley*), ⅔ cup ..	70	<1.0	12.0	0	0	0	4.0
(*Cascadian Farm*), 1 cup	90	1.0	22.0	.5	0	10	2.0

Food and Measure	cal.	prot. (gms)	carbo. (gms)	fat (gms)	chol. (mgs)	sod. (mgs)	fiber (gms)
Blueberry, frozen *(cont.)*							
(*Tree of Life* Organic),							
1 cup	80	1.0	20.0	0	0	0	2.0
unsweetened, ½ cup	40	3.3	9.4	.5	0	1	2.1
sweetened, ½ cup . . .	94	.5	25.2	.2	0	2	2.4
Blueberry juice blend							
(*After the Fall* Maine							
Coast), 8 fl. oz. . . .	90	0	25.0	0	0	20	0
Blueberry syrup,							
¼ cup:							
(*Estee*)	80	0	20.0	0	0	70	0
(*Maple Grove Farms*)	210	0	52.0	0	0	0	0
(*Smucker's*)	210	0	52.0	0	0	0	0
Bluefish, meat only:							
raw, 4 oz.	141	22.7	0	4.8	67	68	0
baked, broiled, or							
microwaved, 4 oz.	180	29.1	0	6.2	86	87	0
Boar, wild, meat only,							
roasted, 4 oz.	181	32.1	0	5.0	87	68	0
Bocconcini pasta dish,							
mix, four cheese							
Parmesano (*Land O*							
Lakes), 2.5 oz. . . .	280	10.0	43.0	8.0	10	770	2.0
Bockwurst, raw, 1 oz.	87	3.8	.1	7.8	17	313	0
Bok choy, see							
"Cabbage, Chinese"							
Bologna (see also							
"Ham bologna," etc.),							
2 oz., except as noted:							
(*Black Bear* German)	160	7.0	1.0	14.0	30	450	0
(*Boar's Head*)	150	7.0	<1.0	13.0	35	530	0
(*Boar's Head* Lebanon)	100	11.0	3.0	5.0	40	680	0
(*Johnsonville* Ring							
Original)	170	7.0	1.0	15.0	35	460	0
(*Oscar Mayer*), 1-oz.							
slice	90	5.0	<1.0	8.0	30	300	0
(*Oscar Mayer*),							
2 slices, .7 oz. . . .	160	5.0	2.0	14.0	45	500	0
(*Oscar Mayer*),							
3 slices, 2.6 oz. . .	250	8.0	3.0	23.0	75	800	0
(*Oscar Mayer* Fat							
Free), 1 oz.	20	3.0	2.0	0	10	250	0
(*Oscar Mayer* Light),							
1-oz. slice	60	3.0	2.0	4.0	20	300	0

Food and Measure	cal.	prot. (gms)	carbo. (gms)	fat (gms)	chol. (mgs)	sod. (mgs)	fiber (gms)
(*Oscar Mayer/Oscar Mayer* Thick Cut) ..	190	6.0	2.0	17.0	55	610	0
beef:							
(*Boar's Head*)	150	7.0	0	13.0	35	520	0
(*Hebrew National*), 4 slices, 2 oz. ..	90	8.0	1.0	5.0	20	440	0
(*Johnsonville* Ring)	170	7.0	1.0	15.0	35	460	0
(*Oscar Mayer*), 1-oz. slice	90	3.0	<1.0	8.0	20	310	0
(*Oscar Mayer*), 1.4-oz. slice	130	5.0	<1.0	12.0	30	450	0
(*Oscar Mayer*), 1.5-oz. slice	140	5.0	<1.0	13.0	30	480	0
(*Oscar Mayer*), 2 slices, 1.7 oz.	150	5.0	<1.0	14.0	35	520	0
(*Oscar Mayer* Light), 1-oz. slice	60	3.0	2.0	4.0	15	310	0
garlic:							
(*Boar's Head*)	150	7.0	1.0	13.0	35	530	0
(*Oscar Mayer*), 1.4-oz. slice	130	4.0	1.0	12.0	40	420	0
ring (*Oscar Mayer* Wisconsin)	180	6.0	2.0	16.0	35	460	0
"Bologna," vegetarian, frozen:							
(*Worthington Bolono*), 3 slices, 3 oz.	80	10.0	2.0	3.5	0	720	2.0
(*Yves* Deli Slices), 2.2 oz.	70	15.0	2.0	0	0	460	0
Boniato, raw (*Frieda's*), 3 oz.	100	1.0	24.0	0	0	10	3.0
Bonito, meat only, raw, 4 oz.	146	29.3	.5	2.3	n.a.	50	0
Borage:							
raw, 1" pcs., ½ cup ..	9	.8	1.4	.3	0	35	<1.0
boiled, drained, 4 oz.	28	2.4	4.0	.9	0	98	<2.0
Boston Market, 1 serving:							
entrees:							
chicken:							
½ w/skin	590	70.0	4.0	33.0	280	1010	0
dark, ¼ w/skin ..	320	30.0	2.0	21.0	155	500	0
dark, ¼ w/out skin	190	22.0	1.0	10.0	115	440	0

Food and Measure	cal.	prot. (gms)	carbo. (gms)	fat (gms)	chol. (mgs)	sod. (mgs)	fiber (gms)
Boston Market, entrees, chicken (cont.)							
white, ¼ w/skin, wing	280	40.0	2.0	12.0	135	510	0
white, ¼ w/out skin, wing ...	170	33.0	2.0	4.0	85	480	0
pot pie	780	32.0	61.0	46.0	135	1480	4.0
salad, chunky, ¾ cup	370	28.0	3.0	27.0	120	800	1.0
ham, honey glaze, lean, 5 oz.	210	25.0	9.0	9.0	75	1490	0
meat loaf, w/brown gravy, 7 oz.	390	30.0	19.0	22.0	120	1040	1.0
meat loaf, w/tomato sauce, 8 oz. ...	370	30.0	22.0	18.0	120	1170	2.0
turkey breast, rotisserie, 5 oz.	170	36.0	1.0	1.0	100	850	0
sandwiches, 1 pc.:							
chicken, w/cheese and sauce	750	41.0	72.0	33.0	135	1860	5.0
chicken, no cheese or sauce	430	34.0	62.0	4.5	65	910	4.0
chicken, BBQ	540	30.0	84.0	9.0	75	1690	3.0
chicken salad	680	39.0	63.0	30.0	120	1360	4.0
ham, w/cheese and sauce	750	38.0	72.0	34.0	100	130	5.0
ham, no cheese or sauce	440	25.0	66.0	8.0	45	1450	4.0
meat loaf, w/cheese	860	46.0	95.0	33.0	165	2270	6.0
meat loaf, no cheese	690	40.0	86.0	21.0	120	1610	6.0
turkey, w/cheese and sauce	710	45.0	68.0	28.0	110	1390	4.0
turkey, no cheese or sauce	400	45.0	61.0	3.5	60	1070	4.0
turkey, open face ..	500	37.0	61.0	12.0	80	2170	3.0
turkey club	650	39.0	64.0	26.0	105	1590	4.0
sides, hot, ¾ cup, except as noted:							
apples, cinnamon	250	0	56.0	4.5	0	45	3.0
baked beans	270	8.0	48.0	5.0	0	540	12.0
black beans and rice, 1 cup	300	8.0	45.0	10.0	0	1050	5.0
broccoli rice casserole	240	5.0	26.0	12.0	40	800	2.0

Food and Measure	cal.	prot. (gms)	carbo. (gms)	fat (gms)	chol. (mgs)	sod. (mgs	fiber (gms)
butternut squash . .	160	2.0	25.0	6.0	15	580	3.0
carrots, glazed	280	1.0	35.0	15.0	0	80	4.0
chicken gravy, 1 oz.	15	0	2.0	1.0	0	170	0
corn, kernel	180	5.0	30.0	4.0	0	170	2.0
green bean casse- role	130	2.0	10.0	9.0	20	440	2.0
green beans	80	1.0	5.0	6.0	0	200	3.0
macaroni and cheese	280	13.0	32.0	11.0	30	830	1.0
potato, mashed, ⅔ cup	210	3.0	24.0	9.0	25	570	1.0
potato, mashed, and gravy	230	4.0	26.0	10.0	25	740	1.0
potatoes, new	130	3.0	25.0	2.5	0	150	2.0
red beans and rice, 1 cup	260	8.0	45.0	5.0	5	1050	4.0
rice pilaf, ⅔ cup . .	180	5.0	32.0	5.0	0	600	2.0
spinach, creamed .	260	9.0	11.0	20.0	55	740	2.0
squash casserole . .	330	7.0	20.0	24.0	70	1110	3.0
stuffing, savory . . .	310	6.0	44.0	12.0	0	1140	3.0
sweet potato casserole	280	3.0	39.0	18.0	10	190	2.0
vegetables, steamed, ⅔ cup	35	2.0	7.0	.5	0	35	3.0
sides, cold, ¾ cup:							
coleslaw	300	2.0	30.0	19.0	20	540	3.0
cranberry relish . . .	370	2.0	84.0	5.0	0	5	5.0
cucumber salad . . .	90	1.0	5.0	8.0	0	640	1.0
fruit salad	70	1.0	15.0	.5	0	10	1.0
potato salad	340	2.0	30.0	24.0	30	870	2.0
tortellini salad	380	14.0	29.0	24.0	90	530	2.0
salad, Caesar:							
entree	670	18.0	24.0	57.0	40	1480	3.0
w/out dressing	230	16.0	14.0	12.0	20	500	3.0
side	268	7.0	10.0	23.0	16	592	1.0
soup, 1 cup:							
chicken noodle . . .	130	11.0	12.0	4.5	40	1310	2.0
chicken tortilla	220	10.0	19.0	11.0	35	1410	2.0
baked goods:							
apple pie, double crust	440	3.0	53.0	25.0	0	190	2.0
apple pie, Dutch . . .	380	4.0	58.0	18.0	15	115	<1.0
brownie, 1 pc. . . .	450	6.0	47.0	27.0	80	190	3.0

Food and Measure	cal.	prot. (gms)	carbo. (gms)	fat (gms)	chol. (mgs)	sod. (mgs)	fiber (gms)
Boston Market, baked goods *(cont.)*							
chocolate chip							
cookie, 1 pc. . . .	340	4.0	48.0	17.0	25	240	1.0
corn bread, 1 loaf	200	3.0	33.0	6.0	25	390	1.0
Bouillon (see also "Bouillon concentrate"):							
beef:							
(*Herb-Ox*), 1 cube	5	0	<1.0	0	0	900	0
(*Herb-Ox* Instant), 1 tsp. or pkt. . . .	5	0	<1.0	0	0	1020	0
(*Herb-Ox* Instant Low Sodium), 1 pkt.	10	0	2.0	0	0	5	0
(*Knorr*), ½ cube . .	15	<1.0	1.0	1.0	0	830	0
(*Maggie* Instant), 1 tsp.	5	0	0	0	0	570	0
(*MBT/Wyler's*), 1 pkt.	15	1.0	2.0	0	0	780	0
(*MBT/Wyler's* Very Low Sodium), 1 pkt.	15	<1.0	3.0	0	0	5	0
(*Weight Watchers*), ⅛ pkg.	10	0	2.0	0	0	800	0
(*Wyler's*), 1 cube . .	5	0	1.0	0	0	920	0
(*Wyler's*), 1 tsp.	5	0	1.0	0	0	810	0
(*Wyler's* Reduced Sodium), 1 cube	5	0	1.0	0	0	610	0
(*Wyler's* Sodium Free), 1 tsp.	10	0	2.0	0	0	0	0
(*Wyler's Shakers* Bouillon/ Seasoning), 1 tsp.	5	0	1.0	0	0	630	0
(*Wyler's Shakers* Bouillon/Seasoning Reduced Sodium), 1 tsp.	10	0	2.0	0	0	420	0
beef and French onion (*Wyler's Shakers* Bouillon/Seasoning), 1 tsp.	5	0	1.0	0	0	650	0
chicken:							
(*Doña Maria*), 1 tsp.	10	0	0	.5	0	930	0

Food and Measure	cal.	prot. (gms)	carbo. (gms)	fat (gms)	chol. (mgs)	sod. (mgs)	fiber (gms)
(*Herb-Ox/Herb-Ox* Instant), 1 cube, 1 tsp., or 1 pkt.	5	0	<1.0	0	0	1100	0
(*Herb-Ox* Instant Low Sodium), 1 pkt.	10	0	2.0	0	0	5	0
(*Knorr*), ½ cube ..	20	<1.0	<1.0	1.5	0	1270	0
(*Maggi* Instant), 1 tsp.	5	0	1.0	0	0	640	0
(*MBT/Wyler's*), 1 pkt.	15	<1.0	2.0	0	0	860	0
(*MBT/Wyler's* Very Low Sodium), 1 pkt.	15	0	3.0	0	0	10	0
(*Weight Watchers*), ⅛ pkg.	10	0	2.0	0	0	830	0
(*Wyler's*), 1 cube ..	5	0	1.0	0	0	920	0
(*Wyler's*), 1 tsp.	5	0	0	0	0	810	0
(*Wyler's* Reduced Sodium), 1 tsp.	5	0	1.0	0	0	610	0
(*Wyler's Shakers* Bouillon/Seasoning Reduced Sodium), 1 tsp.	10	0	2.0	0	0	420	0
garlic and herb (*Wyler's Shakers* Bouillon/Seasoning), 1 tsp.	5	0	1.0	0	0	650	0
w/parsley (*Wyler's Shakers* Bouillon/ Seasoning), 1 tsp.	5	0	1.0	0	0	630	0
tomato (*Doña Maria*), 1 tsp.	10	0	1.0	.5	0	640	0
fish (*Knorr*), ½ cube	10	<1.0	0	1.0	0	980	0
ham (*Knorr*), ½ cube	15	0	<1.0	1.0	0	1030	0
Italian, zesty (*Wyler's Shakers* Bouillon/ Seasoning), 1 tsp.	10	0	2.0	0	0	630	0
vegetable:							
(*Knorr* Vegetarian), ½ cube	15	<1.0	1.0	1.0	0	830	0
(*Morga*), ½ cube ..	22	.5	1.3	1.6	0	300	0
(*Maggi* Vegetarian), 1 cube	5	0	1.0	0	0	820	0

Food and Measure	cal.	prot. (gms)	carbo. (gms)	fat (gms)	chol. (mgs)	sod. (mgs)	fiber (gms)
Bouillon concentrate, liquid, 2 tsp.:							
beef:							
(*Bovril*)	10	<1.0	1.0	0	0	930	0
(*Knorr*).	15	2.0	1.0	0	0	850	0
chicken:							
(*Bovril*)	15	<1.0	2.0	.5	0	880	0
(*Knorr*)	5	<1.0	<1.0	0	0	740	0
Bourguignonne seasoning mix (*Knorr*), 1 tbsp.	35	<1.0	6.0	1.0	0	410	0
Bow-tie pasta, see "Pasta, dry"							
Bow-tie pasta dish, mix:							
w/chicken flavor vegetable sauce (*Knorr* Side Dish), ⅓ cup	110	4.0	20.0	1.5	0	400	1.0
w/herb sauce, savory (*Knorr* Side Dish), ⅔ cup	260	12.0	47.0	2.0	<5	790	6.0
and red lentil (*Marrakesh Express*), 1 cup*	220	12.0	39.0	2.0	35	370	5.0
Bow-tie pasta entree, frozen, w/chicken (*Lean Cuisine Cafe Classics*), 9.5 oz.	220	15.0	32.0	4.0	40	690	5.0
Boysenberry, fresh, see "Blackberry"							
Boysenberry, canned, in light syrup (*Oregon*), ½ cup . .	120	<1.0	27.0	0	0	10	3.0
Boysenberry, frozen, unsweetened, ½ cup	33	.7	8.1	.1	0	1	2.6
Boysenberry nectar (*R. W. Knudsen*), 8 fl. oz.	130	<1.0	33.0	0	0	35	0
Boysenberry syrup (*Smucker's*), ¼ cup	210	0	52.0	0	0	0	0
Brains, 4 oz.:							
beef, fried	222	14.3	0	18.0	2262	179	0

Food and Measure	cal.	prot. (gms)	carbo. (gms)	fat (gms)	chol. (mgs)	sod. (mgs)	fiber (gms)
lamb, fried	310	19.2	0	25.2	2840	178	0
pork, braised	156	13.8	0	10.8	2894	103	0
veal, fried	242	16.4	0	19.0	2404	200	0
Bran, see "Cereal" and specific grains							
Bratwurst, 1 link, except as noted:							
(*Black Bear*), 3.2 oz.	240	11.0	0	22.0	40	670	0
(*Black Bear* Hungarian Brand), 3.2 oz. . . .	230	11.0	0	21.0	40	650	0
(*Boar's Head*), 4 oz. .	300	19.0	0	25.0	75	650	0
(*Johnsonville* Cooked), 2.7 oz.	240	9.0	2.0	22.0	50	760	0
(*Johnsonville* Fresh), 3.4 oz.	250	12.0	1.0	22.0	65	960	0
(*Johnsonville* Stadium Style), 2.7 oz.	240	9.0	2.0	22.0	50	760	0
beef (*Johnsonville*), 2.7 oz.	240	9.0	2.0	21.0	60	640	0
bites (*Johnsonville*), 6 links, 2 oz.	200	7.0	1.0	18.0	40	530	0
chicken (*Bilinski's* Bratwurst), 2 oz. . .	70	11.0	2.0	2.0	25	280	0
fresh, grilled, 3 oz.: (*Johnsonville/ Johnsonville* Beer 'n Bratwurst) . .	290	14.0	1.0	25.0	65	800	0
cheddar (*Johnson- ville*)	300	15.0	2.0	25.0	65	800	0
honey and garlic (*Johnsonville*) . .	280	13.0	5.0	22.0	60	700	0
hot 'n spicy (*John- sonville*)	290	14.0	2.0	25.0	60	760	0
roasted garlic or onion (*Johnson- ville*)	290	14.0	1.0	25.0	65	800	0
smoked: (*Johnsonville*), 2.78 oz.	240	9.0	2.0	21.0	60	640	0
(*Johnsonville* Light), 2.3 oz.	140	10.0	3.0	9.0	35	640	0
"Bratwurst," vege- tarian, frozen (*Boca*), 2.5-oz. link	130	12.0	6.0	7.0	0	870	1.0

Food and Measure	cal.	prot. (gms)	carbo. (gms)	fat (gms)	chol. (mgs)	sod. (mgs)	fiber (gms)
Bratwurst burger, grilled (*Johnsonville*), 2.5 oz.	240	11.0	1.0	21.0	55	660	0
Braunschweiger (see also "Liverwurst"):							
chub, 2 oz.:							
(*Jones Dairy Farm Light*)	100	10.0	1.0	6.0	140	500	0
(*Jones Dairy Farm Original 8 oz.*) . .	160	8.0	1.0	14.0	115	520	0
(*Jones Dairy Farm Original 16 oz.*)	150	9.0	1.0	12.0	130	520	0
w/bacon, 20% (*Jones Dairy Farm*)	150	9.0	1.0	12.0	120	560	0
w/onion (*Jones Dairy Farm*)	160	8.0	2.0	13.0	110	560	0
chunk, 2 oz.:							
(*Jones Dairy Farm Light*)	90	10.0	1.0	5.0	125	430	0
(*Jones Dairy Farm Original*)	180	8.0	1.0	16.0	110	460	0
sliced:							
(*Jones Dairy Farm 8 oz.*), 2 slices . .	150	6.0	1.0	13.0	90	370	0
(*Jones Dairy Farm 12 oz.*), 1 slice . .	110	5.0	1.0	10.0	70	280	0
(*Oscar Mayer*), 1 oz.	100	4.0	1.0	9.0	50	320	0
spread (*Oscar Mayer*), 2 oz.	190	8.0	1.0	17.0	90	630	0
Brazil nuts, shelled, 8 medium or 6 large, 1 oz.	186	4.1	3.6	18.8	0	<1	1.6
Bread, 1 slice, except as noted:							
(*Arnold Health Nut*) . .	110	5.0	20.0	2.0	0	220	2.0
banana swirl (*Pepperidge Farm*) . .	90	2.0	15.0	2.0	0	100	<1.0
bran (*Arnold Bran'nola*)	110	4.0	20.0	1.5	0	170	3.0
buttermilk:							
(*Pepperidge Farm Farmhouse*)	110	4.0	22.0	1.0	0	210	1.0
(*Pillsbury*)	90	3.0	15.0	1.5	0	150	<1.0
bran (*Shiloh Farms*) . .	80	4.0	16.0	1.0	0	135	2.0

Food and Measure	cal.	prot. (gms)	carbo. (gms)	fat (gms)	chol. (mgs)	sod. (mgs)	fiber (gms)
cheddar, white, garlic (*Great Harvest*) ...	130	5.0	18.0	4.5	15	360	0
cinnamon swirl (*Pepperidge Farm*)	140	4.0	25.0	3.5	0	170	1.0
flatbread, onion (*Kontos*), ½ loaf ..	120	7.0	15.0	3.5	0	160	1.0
focaccia, sprouted, 5-grain (*Shiloh Farms*), 4-oz. pc.	360	11.0	52.0	16.0	0	130	10.0
French toast swirl:							
brown sugar cinnamon (*Pepperidge Farm*)	140	4.0	25.0	3.5	0	170	1.0
maple syrup cinnamon (*Pepperidge Farm*)	130	4.0	25.0	2.5	0	180	<1.0
honey wheat, see "wheat, honey," below							
Italian:							
(*Pepperidge Farm*)	90	3.0	15.0	1.5	0	180	<1.0
(*Pepperidge Farm* Light)	45	2.0	9.0	0	0	90	1.0
(*Rhodes*)	130	5.0	23.0	2.0	0	280	1.0
(*Wonder* Light), 2 slices	80	4.0	19.0	1.0	0	230	5.0
(*Wonder* Seeded) ..	70	2.0	13.0	1.0	0	180	.0
kamut (*Shiloh Farms* Egyptian Wheat)	90	6.0	18.0	1.0	0	115	3.0
multigrain:							
(*LifeWorks*), 2 slices	170	9.0	27.0	2.5	0	330	3.0
7-grain (*Healthy Choice*)	80	4.0	18.0	1.0	0	170	4.0
7-grain (*Pepperidge Farm* Light)	45	2.0	9.0	0	0	95	<1.0
7-grain (*Pepperidge Farm Farmhouse* Harvest)	110	4.0	20.0	1.5	0	190	2.0
9-grain (*Cobblestone Mill* Hearty)	120	5.0	23.0	2.0	0	250	2.0
9-grain (*Great Harvest*)	110	4.0	23.0	.5	0	250	3.0

Food and Measure	cal.	prot. (gms)	carbo. (gms)	fat (gms)	chol. (mgs)	sod. (mgs)	fiber (gms)
Bread, multigrain *(cont.)*							
9-grain *(Pepperidge Farm* Natural Whole Grain) . . .	90	4.0	15.0	1.0	0	140	3.0
12-grain *(Arnold)* .	110	4.0	30.0	1.5	0	190	3.0
soft *(Healthy Choice)*	60	3.0	12.0	.5	0	120	2.0
multigrain, sprouted:							
(Shiloh Farms Firehouse), 2 oz. . .	160	9.0	29.0	2.0	0	200	5.0
(Shiloh Farms Sandwich)	80	4.0	17.0	.5	0	100	3.0
5-grain *(Shiloh Farms)*	90	5.0	19.0	.5	0	110	4.0
5-grain *(Shiloh Farms* Hearth) . .	130	7.0	28.0	1.0	0	150	5.0
5-grain sourdough *(Shiloh Farms)* . .	140	7.0	28.0	1.5	0	170	4.0
7-grain *(Shiloh Farms* No Salt) . .	90	5.0	19.0	.5	0	0	3.0
7-grain *(Shiloh Farms)*	90	5.0	19.0	.5	0	130	3.0
10-grain *(Shiloh Farms)*, 2 slices .	140	9.0	26.0	1.5	0	120	5.0
oat, country *(Pepperidge Farm* Hearty Slices)	110	5.0	19.0	1.5	0	180	2.0
oat bran:							
(Arnold), 2 slices . .	170	8.0	30.0	3.0	0	340	4.0
(Shiloh Farms)	90	5.0	18.0	1.0	0	130	3.0
oatmeal:							
(Pepperidge Farm)	60	2.0	11.0	1.0	0	160	1.0
(Pepperidge Farm Light)	45	2.0	9.0	0	0	90	<1.0
pita, 2-oz. pc.:							
white *(Sahara)*	160	5.0	32.0	1.5	0	350	2.0
whole wheat *(Sahara)*	140	6.0	27.0	1.5	0	310	5.0
potato:							
(Home Pride)	70	2.0	13.0	1.0	0	130	0
(Martin's)	100	4.0	14.0	1.5	0	115	1.0
(Stroehmann Dutch Country)	90	3.0	18.0	1.0	0	170	<1.0
golden *(Pepperidge Farm Farmhouse)*	110	3.0	21.0	1.0	0	220	1.0

Food and Measure	cal.	prot. (gms)	carbo. (gms)	fat (gms)	chol. (mgs)	sod. (mgs)	fiber (gms)
pumpernickel:							
(*Arnold*)	80	3.0	15.0	1.0	0	200	<1.0
(*Cobblestone Mill* German Classic), 2 slices	160	6.0	32.0	1.5	0	420	2.0
(*Rubschlager* Cocktail), 3 slices	80	3.0	14.0	1.0	0	180	2.0
(*Rubschlager* Danish/West- phalian)	70	2.0	14.0	.5	0	135	2.0
dark (*Pepperidge Farm* Party), 5 slices	130	5.0	24.0	1.5	0	290	3.0
raisin:							
(*Monk's*)	70	2.0	14.0	1.0	0	95	2.0
whole wheat (*Shiloh Farms*), 2 slices	140	7.0	30.0	1.0	0	160	3.0
raisin cinnamon:							
(*Great Harvest*) ...	100	3.0	24.0	0	0	280	3.0
swirl (*Pepperidge Farm*)	80	3.0	14.0	1.5	0	105	1.0
swirl (*Sun•Maid*) ..	80	2.0	16.0	1.5	0	95	1.0
rye:							
(*Arnold* Real Jewish Melba Thin), 2 slices	110	3.0	21.0	1.5	0	300	1.0
(*Arnold* Real Jewish Seeds/Seedless)	80	3.0	15.0	1.5	0	220	<1.0
(*Cobblestone Mill* New York Jewish Classic), 2 slices	160	6.0	31.0	2.0	0	480	2.0
(*Friehofer's* Seeded/ Seedless)	90	3.0	15.0	1.5	0	220	<1.0
(*Levy's* Real Jewish Seeds/Seedless)	90	3.0	16.0	1.5	0	230	<1.0
(*Monk's*)	60	2.0	12.0	0	0	115	2.0
(*Pepperidge Farm* Deli Seedless) ..	80	3.0	15.0	1.0	0	210	1.0
(*Pepperidge Farm* Jewish Party), 5 slices	120	4.0	25.0	1.0	0	430	3.0
dill (*Arnold* Real Jewish)	80	2.0	15.0	1.0	0	180	<1.0
soft (*Beefsteak*) ...	70	2.0	14.0	1.0	0	200	0

Food and Measure	cal.	prot. (gms)	carbo. (gms)	fat (gms)	chol. (mgs)	sod. (mgs)	fiber (gms)
Bread (cont.)							
soft (*Beefsteak* Light), 2 slices ..	80	5.0	17.0	1.0	0	260	5.0
rye/pumpernickel:							
marble (*Arnold*) ...	80	3.0	15.0	1.0	0	210	<1.0
swirl (*Pepperidge Farm* Deli Swirl)	80	3.0	15.0	1.0	0	220	1.0
sesame wheat:							
(*Pepperidge Farm* Hearty Slices) ..	110	4.0	19.0	2.0	0	190	2.0
(*Pepperidge Farm* Farmhouse)	110	4.0	19.0	2.0	0	190	2.0
sourdough:							
(*Cobblestone Mill* San Francisco Classic), 2 slices	160	6.0	32.0	1.5	0	370	2.0
(*Rubschlager* Cocktail), 3 slices	80	3.0	14.0	1.0	0	180	2.0
spelt (*Shiloh Farms*)	100	4.0	21.0	1.0	0	140	2.0
stone-ground (*Home Pride*)	70	3.0	13.0	1.0	0	140	1.0
sunflower:							
(*Great Harvest*) ...	110	4.0	21.0	2.0	0	270	3.0
and bran (*Monk's*)	60	3.0	11.0	1.5	0	90	2.0
whole wheat (*Shiloh Farms*), 2 slices	160	2.0	23.0	4.5	5	250	4.0
wheat:							
(*Arnold* Country) ..	100	4.0	19.0	1.5	0	190	1.0
(*Home Pride*)	80	2.0	14.0	1.0	0	190	0
(*Nature's Own* Light), 2 slices	80	5.0	19.0	1.0	0	200	5.0
(*Pan Wonder* De Trigo), 2 slices ..	110	4.0	20.0	1.5	0	240	2.0
(*Pepperidge Farm* Very Thin), 3 slices	120	4.0	21.0	2.0	0	220	3.0
(*Pillsbury*)	80	3.0	15.0	1.0	0	115	1.0
(*Rhodes*)	130	6.0	24.0	2.0	0	280	2.0
(*Shiloh Farms* Butter Hearth)	150	6.0	28.0	1.5	<5	100	<1.0
(*Shiloh Farms* Home-style), 2 slices ..	160	7.0	29.0	1.5	<5	115	<1.0
(*Wonder* Light), 2 slices	80	5.0	18.0	.5	0	240	5.0

Food and Measure	cal.	prot. (gms)	carbo. (gms)	fat (gms)	chol. (mgs)	sod. (mgs	fiber (gms)
stone-ground (*Pepperidge Farm* 100%)	70	3.0	11.0	1.0	0	95	2.0
wheat, honey:							
(*Nature's Own*) ...	60	3.0	12.0	.5	0	125	1.0
(*Nature's Own Light*), 2 slices	80	5.0	19.0	1.0	0	200	5.0
soft (*Healthy Choice*)	60	3.0	12.0	.5	0	120	2.0
wheat berry (*Arnold*)	110	4.0	21.0	1.0	0	220	2.0
wheat berry (*Cobblestone Mill* Hearty)	110	4.0	23.0	1.0	0	220	2.0
wheat berry (*Home Pride*)	70	2.0	14.0	1.0	0	140	1.0
whole (*Great Harvest*)	100	3.0	23.0	0	0	290	3.0
wheat, whole:							
(*Arnold* 100%)	90	5.0	18.0	1.0	0	190	3.0
(*Arnold Brick Oven* 100%), 2 slices	130	6.0	22.0	3.0	0	200	4.0
(*Cobblestone Mill* 100% Hearty) ..	100	5.0	21.0	1.5	0	240	3.0
(*Monk's* 100%) ...	60	3.0	10.0	1.0	0	10	2.0
(*Nature's Own* 100%)	50	4.0	10.0	1.0	0	115	3.0
(*Nature's Own* 100% Sugar Free)	50	3.0	11.0	1.0	0	110	2.0
(*Shiloh Farms*), 2 slices	140	7.0	26.0	1.5	0	260	4.0
(*Shiloh Farms* No Salt), 2 slices ...	140	7.0	26.0	1.5	0	0	3.0
stone-ground (*Arnold* 100%) ..	70	3.0	12.0	.5	0	135	2.0
stone-ground (*Wonder* 100%)	80	3.0	13.0	1.5	0	190	2.0
whole grain (*Pepperidge Farm* German)	90	4.0	15.0	1.0	0	140	3.0
wheat and rye (*Shiloh Farms* Zesty), 2 slices	140	9.0	26.0	2.0	0	160	5.0
white:							
(*Arnold* Country) ..	110	3.0	20.0	1.5	0	240	<1.0
(*Arnold Brick Oven*), 2 slices	130	4.0	25.0	2.0	0	250	<1.0

Food and Measure	cal.	prot. (gms)	carbo. (gms)	fat (gms)	chol. (mgs)	sod. (mgs)	fiber (gms)
Bread, white *(cont.)*							
(*Arnold Brick Oven*							
Big Slice)	90	3.0	17.0	1.5	0	170	<1.0
(*Great Harvest*) . . .	100	3.0	22.0	0	0	410	<1.0
(*Monk's*)	60	3.0	12.0	1.0	0	130	2.0
(*Nature's Own*							
Butterbread) . . .	60	3.0	12.0	.5	0	140	1.0
(*Nature's Own* Light							
Premium),							
2 slices	80	5.0	19.0	1.0	0	190	5.0
(*Pepperidge Farm*							
Original)	70	2.0	13.0	1.5	0	135	0
(*Pepperidge Farm*							
Sandwich),							
2 slices	130	4.0	23.0	2.5	0	260	<1.0
(*Pepperidge Farm*							
Toasting)	90	3.0	16.0	1.0	0	200	0
(*Pepperidge Farm*							
Very Thin),							
3 slices	120	4.0	24.0	1.0	0	250	1.0
(*Pepperidge Farm*							
Farmhouse							
Hearty)	110	5.0	20.0	1.5	<5	260	<1.0
(*Pillsbury*)	80	3.0	15.0	1.0	0	170	1.0
(*Rhodes*)	140	5.0	17.0	2.0	0	280	2.0
(*Wonder* Light),							
2 slices	80	4.0	19.0	.5	0	260	5.0
(*Wonder* Giant),							
2 slices	120	3.0	23.0	1.5	0	250	1.0
(*Wonder* Small),							
2 slices	110	3.0	20.0	1.5	0	230	1.0
honey (*Pillsbury*) . .	80	3.0	15.0	1.0	0	140	<1.0
whole grain (*Healthy*							
Choice 100%)	80	3.0	18.0	1.0	0	170	3.0
Bread, brown, canned							
(*B&M*), ½" slice . .	130	3.0	29.0	.5	0	390	2.0
Bread, frozen:							
corn bread (*Boston*							
Market), 2.25-oz.							
mini loaf	210	3.0	33.0	6.0	15	280	4.0
buttermilk (*Pillsbury*),							
1-oz. slice	90	3.0	15.0	1.5	0	150	0

Food and Measure	cal.	prot. (gms)	carbo. (gms)	fat (gms)	chol. (mgs)	sod. (mgs)	fiber (gms)
French, crusty (*Pillsbury* Tube), ⅛ loaf	150	5.0	27.0	2.0	0	370	<1.0
garlic:							
(*Marie Callender's* Original), 1 pc. .	190	4.0	23.0	8.0	<5	330	2.0
(*New York*), 2 slices, 1", 2 oz.	190	4.0	28.0	7.0	0	390	1.0
(*New York* Reduced Fat), 2 slices, 1", 2 oz.	160	4.0	29.0	3.0	0	340	1.0
(*Pepperidge Farm*), 2 slices, ½"	170	5.0	15.0	10.0	30	270	1.0
Parmesan (*Pepperidge Farm*), 2 slices, ½"	170	6.0	20.0	7.0	10	280	2.0
Parmesan/Romano (*Marie Callender's*), 1 pc.	200	5.0	23.0	10.0	5	430	2.0
toast, Texas, 1 slice:							
garlic (*New York*), 1.4 oz.	170	2.0	16.0	10.0	0	260	1.0
garlic, w/cheese (*New York*), 1.7 oz.	180	4.0	17.0	11.0	5	350	1.0
garlic, Parmesan (*New York*), 1.7 oz.	190	6.0	19.0	11.0	5	380	1.0
garlic, pizza (*New York*), 1.8 oz. ..	160	5.0	18.0	7.0	5	410	1.0
mozzarella/Monterey Jack (*Pepperidge Farm*), 1.6 oz. ..	160	5.0	20.0	7.0	<5	250	<1.0
Parmesan (*Pepperidge Farm*), 1.4 oz.	160	4.0	14.0	9.0	20	250	<1.0
wheat (*Pillsbury*), 1-oz. slice	80	3.0	15.0	10	0	115	1.0
white, honey (*Pillsbury*), 1-oz. slice	80	3.0	15.0	1.0	0	140	0
Bread, mix (see also "Bread mix, sweet"):							
cheese herb (*Hodgson Mill* European), ¼ cup	130	5.0	21.0	2.0	0	250	<1.0

Food and Measure	cal.	prot. (gms)	carbo. (gms)	fat (gms)	chol. (mgs)	sod. (mgs)	fiber (gms)
Bread mix *(cont.)*							
French (*Eagle Mills* Country), 1/9 loaf*	160	6.0	29.0	2.0	0	310	1.0
Italian (*Eagle Mills* Classic), 1/9 loaf* ..	160	6.0	29.0	2.0	0	310	1.0
multigrain:							
(*Arrowhead Mills*), 1/3 cup	160	7.0	31.0	1.0	0	200	3.0
(*Eagle Mills* Hearty), 1/11 loaf*	150	5.0	28.0	2.0	0	290	2.0
9 (*Hodgson Mill*), 1/4 cup	130	5.0	22.0	2.0	0	150	2.0
oat, honey (*Eagle Mills*), 1/11 loaf*	150	5.0	28.0	2.5	0	290	1.0
potato (*Hodgson Mill* Wholesome), 1/4 cup	120	5.0	23.0	0	0	170	<1.0
rye:							
(*Arrowhead Mills*), 1/3 cup	160	5.0	33.0	.5	0	190	3.0
(*Eagle Mills* Old World), 1/11 loaf*	150	6.0	26.0	2.5	0	290	2.0
caraway (*Hodgson Mill*), 1/4 cup ...	120	5.0	22.0	2.0	0	190	3.0
sourdough (*Eagle Mills* San Francisco), 1/9 loaf*	160	6.0	29.0	2.0	0	310	1.0
spelt (*Arrowhead Mills*), 1/3 cup	150	6.0	31.0	1.0	0	190	5.0
wheat:							
cracked (*Pillsbury* Bread Machine), 1/12 pkg.	130	4.0	25.0	2.0	0	260	1.0
whole (*Arrowhead Mills*), 1/3 cup ...	150	7.0	31.0	1.0	0	190	5.0
whole (*Eagle Mills* Harvest), 1/11 loaf*	140	5.0	28.0	2.0	0	330	3.0
whole, honey (*Hodgson Mill*), 1/4 cup	120	5.0	22.0	2.0	0	160	3.0
white:							
(*Arrowhead Mills*), 1/3 cup	150	4.0	31.0	.5	0	170	2.0

Food and Measure	cal.	prot. (gms)	carbo. (gms)	fat (gms)	chol. (mgs)	sod. (mgs)	fiber (gms)
(*Eagle Mills* Home-style), ⅑ loaf*	160	5.0	30.0	3.0	0	310	1.0
(*Hodgson Mill*), ¼ cup	120	5.0	22.0	2.0	0	170	3.0
(*Pillsbury* Bread Machine Country), 1/12 pkg.	130	4.0	25.0	2.0	0	250	<1.0
Bread mix, sweet, dry, except as noted:							
apple walnut, no icing (*Eagle Mills*), ¼ cup	150	4.0	24.0	3.5	0	230	1.0
banana:							
(*Betty Crocker* Quick), ½ loaf*	170	3.0	25.0	7.0	35	200	0
(*Pillsbury* Quick Bread/Muffin), 1/14 pkg.	110	2.0	23.0	1.0	0	160	<1.0
chocolate, no icing (*Eagle Mills* Nugget), ¼ cup	150	4.0	26.0	3.5	5	160	1.0
chocolate chip swirl (*Pillsbury* Bread/Muffin), 1/14 pkg.	150	1.0	27.0	4.5	0	135	<1.0
cinnamon, no icing (*Eagle Mills* Sunrise), ¼ cup	150	4.0	26.0	3.0	0	170	2.0
cinnamon streusel (*Betty Crocker* Quick), 1/14 loaf*	180	2.0	28.0	7.0	30	160	0
corn bread, see "Corn bread mix"							
cranberry orange (*Betty Crocker* Quick), 1/12 loaf*	180	3.0	29.0	6.0	35	180	0
date (*Pillsbury* Bread/Muffin), 1/14 pkg.	130	2.0	28.0	1.5	0	130	1.0
fruit, no icing (*Eagle Mills* Harvest), ¼ cup	140	4.0	26.0	2.5	0	270	1.0
gingerbread (*Hodgson Mill*), ¼ cup	110	2.0	24.0	0	0	260	2.0

Food and Measure	cal.	prot. (gms)	carbo. (gms)	fat (gms)	chol. (mgs)	sod. (mgs)	fiber (gms)
Bread mix, sweet *(cont.)*							
lemon poppy seed:							
(*Betty Crocker*							
Quick), 1/12 loaf* .	170	3.0	25.0	7.0	35	200	0
(*Pillsbury* Bread/							
Muffin), 1/14 pkg.	130	2.0	25.0	2.5	0	135	<1.0
no icing (*Eagle Mills*),							
1/4 cup	140	4.0	25.0	3.0	5	190	1.0
Bread crumbs, 1/4 cup							
or 1 oz.:							
(*Old Bay* Dip & Crisp)	110	3.0	15.0	2.0	0	800	1.0
all purpose (*Golden*							
Dipt Fry Easy)	120	2.0	20.0	1.0	0	750	1.0
plain (*Progresso*)	110	4.0	19.0	1.5	0	210	1.0
garlic and herb							
(*Progresso*)	100	4.0	18.0	1.5	0	530	1.0
Italian:							
(*Contadina*)	100	3.0	19.0	1.5	0	720	1.0
(*Progresso*)	110	4.0	20.0	1.5	0	430	1.0
Parmesan (*Progresso*)	110	4.0	19.0	1.5	0	870	1.0
Bread cubes, see							
"Stuffing"							
Bread dough, sweet							
(*Rhodes*), 1/9 loaf,							
1.8 oz.	145	5.0	24.0	3.0	10	260	1.00
Bread stick:							
(*Stella D'oro* Fat Free),							
1 pc.	70	2.0	15.0	0	0	150	1.0
(*Stella D'oro* Original),							
1 pc.	40	1.0	7.0	1.0	0	40	0
(*Stella D'oro* Sodium							
Free), 1 pc.	45	1.0	7.0	1.0	0	0	0
garlic (*Stella D'oro*							
Traditional), 2 pcs.	70	2.0	14.0	0	0	150	1.0
onion:							
(*Stella D'oro*), 1 pc.	40	1.0	6.0	1.0	0	35	0
(*Toufayan*), 2 pcs.	55	2.0	11.0	.5	0	90	1.0
pepper, cracked (*Stella*							
D'oro Snack Stix),							
4 pcs.	70	2.0	11.0	22.0	0	290	<1.0
potato onion (*Stella*							
D'oro Snack Stix),							
4 pcs.	70	2.0	11.0	2.0	0	300	0

Food and Measure	cal.	prot. (gms)	carbo. (gms)	fat (gms)	chol. (mgs)	sod. (mgs)	fiber (gms)
salted (*Stella D'oro* Snack Stix), 4 pcs.	70	2.0	11.0	2.0	0	290	<1.0
sesame:							
(*Stella D'oro*), 1 pc.	50	1.0	7.0	2.5	0	45	1.0
(*Stella D'oro* Low-fat), 2 pcs.	70	2.0	14.0	1.0	0	90	1.0
(*Toufayan*), 2 pcs.	55	2.0	8.0	1.0	0	85	1.0
Bread stick, frozen or refrigerated:							
(*Pillsbury*), 2 pcs. ..	140	4.0	25.0	2.5	0	370	<1.0
corn bread twists (*Pillsbury*), 1 pc. .	130	3.0	17.0	6.0	0	340	0
garlic (*Pepperidge Farm*), 1 pc.	180	4.0	29.0	5.0	0	320	1.0
garlic w/herbs (*Pillsbury*), 2 pcs.	180	4.0	25.0	7.0	0	580	<1.0
garlic Parmesan (*New York*), 1 pc.	180	4.0	29.0	5.0	0	320	1.0
Parmesan (*Pillsbury*), 2 pcs.	180	4.0	25.0	7.0	0	580	<1.0
Breadfruit, raw, ½ cup	113	1.2	29.8	.3	0	2	5.4
Breadfruit seeds:							
boiled, shelled, 1 oz. .	48	1.5	9.1	.7	0	n.a.	n.a.
roasted, shelled, 1 oz.	59	1.8	11.4	.8	0	8	1.7
Breadnut tree seeds, dried, 1 oz.	104	2.4	22.5	.5	0	15	4.2
Breakfast dish, see specific listings							
Breakfast sandwich (see also "Burrito, breakfast" and "Toaster bagel, muffin, and pastry"), 1 pc.:							
biscuit, sausage, egg: (*Hormel Quick Meals*), 4.5 oz.	390	12.0	31.0	24.0	120	830	1.0
cheese (*Great Starts*), 5.5 oz.	460	16.0	37.0	28.0	115	1060	3.0
croissant, sausage, egg, cheese (*Great Starts*), 5 oz.	470	17.0	27.0	33.0	100	840	1.0

Food and Measure	cal.	prot. (gms)	carbo. (gms)	fat (gms)	chol. (mgs)	sod. (mgs)	fiber (gms)
Breakfast sandwich *(cont.)*							
muffin, egg:							
Canadian bacon, cheese (*Great Starts*), 4.1 oz.	290	14.0	25.0	15.0	95	750	2.0
Canadian bacon, cheese (*Great Starts* Lite), 4.2 oz.	230	14.0	29.0	6.0	30	720	2.0
cheese (*Hormel Quick Meals*), 4.5 oz.	260	17.0	29.0	8.0	90	980	0
muffin, vegetarian:							
patty (*Morningstar Farms Scramblers*)	240	22.0	32.0	2.5	5	700	5.0
patty, cheese (*Morningstar Scramblers*)	280	28.0	35.0	3.0	10	1000	5.0
pocket, egg/cheese:							
bacon (*Hot Pockets*)	170	5.0	17.0	9.0	45	260	1.0
sausage (*Croissant Pockets*)	340	11.0	38.0	16.0	80	480	2.0
sausage (*Hot Pockets*)	180	5.0	16.0	10.0	35	260	1.0
Broad bean, fresh:							
raw, ½ cup	40	3.1	6.4	.4	0	28	2.3
boiled, drained, 4 oz.	64	5.4	11.5	.6	0	47	<3.0
Broad beans, mature (see also "Habas"):							
raw (*Frieda's* Fava), ¾ cup, 3 oz.	290	22.0	50.0	1.5	0	10	n.a.
boiled, ½ cup	93	6.5	16.7	.3	0	4	4.6
Broad beans, mature, canned, ½ cup:							
(*Progresso* Fava)	110	6.0	20.0	.5	0	250	5.0
w/liquid	91	7.0	15.9	.3	0	580	4.7
Broccoli, fresh:							
raw:							
(*Dole*), 5.2-oz. stalk	45	5.0	8.0	.5	0	55	5.0
(*Mann's Broccoli Wokly*), 4 oz. . .	30	2.0	7.0	0	0	30	3.0
8.7-oz. stalk	42	4.5	7.9	.5	0	40	4.5
chopped, ½ cup . .	12	1.3	2.3	.2	0	12	1.3

Food and Measure	cal.	prot. (gms)	carbo. (gms)	fat (gms)	chol. (mgs)	sod. (mgs)	fiber (gms)
raw, baby (*Mann's Broccolini*), 2.9 oz., about 8 stalks	35	3.0	6.0	0	0	25	1.0
boiled, drained:							
1 stalk, 6.3 oz. ...	51	5.4	9.1	.6	0	46	5.2
chopped, ½ cup ..	22	2.3	3.9	.2	0	20	2.3
Broccoli, Chinese, see "Kale, Chinese"							
Broccoli, dried (*AlpineAire*), .25 oz.	25	2.0	4.0	0	0	20	2.0
Broccoli, frozen, 1 cup, except as noted:							
spears:							
(*Birds Eye*), 3 oz.	25	3.0	4.0	0	0	20	2.0
10-oz. pkg.	84	8.7	15.2	1.0	0	49	8.5
spears or chopped, boiled, drained	52	5.7	9.8	.2	0	44	5.5
florets:							
(*Birds Eye* Baby/ Deluxe), 3 oz. ...	25	3.0	5.0	0	0	35	2.0
(*Green Giant*), 1⅓ cups	25	2.0	4.0	0	0	20	2.0
(*Seabrook Farms*)	25	2.0	4.0	0	0	20	2.0
cuts:							
(*Birds Eye*), ½ cup	25	2.0	5.0	0	0	30	3.0
(*Cascadian Farm*), ½ cup	24	3.0	4.0	0	0	20	3.0
(*Green Giant*)	25	2.0	4.0	0	0	20	0
(*Tree of Life*), 1 cup	25	2.0	4.0	0	0	20	2.0
chopped:							
(*Birds Eye*), ⅓ cup	25	2.0	5.0	0	0	15	2.0
(*Green Giant*), ¾ cup	25	2.0	4.0	0	0	20	2.0
10-oz. pkg.	75	8.0	13.6	.8	0	68	8.5
in cheese sauce:							
(*Birds Eye*), 4 oz.	70	3.0	7.0	4.0	5	500	2.0
(*Green Giant*), ⅔ cup	80	3.0	9.0	3.0	<5	570	2.0
cheddar (*Cascadian Farm*), ½ cup ...	60	5.0	7.0	2.5	5	290	3.0

Food and Measure	cal.	prot. (gms)	carbo. (gms)	fat (gms)	chol. (mgs)	sod. (mgs)	fiber (gms)
Broccoli combinations, fresh, 4 oz.:							
carrots:							
(*Mann's*)	35	2.0	7.0	0	0	35	3.0
red cabbage (*Mann's* Cole Slaw)	35	1.0	6.0	0	0	65	3.0
snap peas, celery (*Mann's Broccoli Wokly* Stir Fry) . .	35	2.0	7.0	0	0	40	3.0
cauliflower, red cabbage (*Mann's* Rainbow Salad)	30	1.0	6.0	0	0	60	3.0
Broccoli combinations, frozen:							
baby, blend (*Birds Eye*), ¾ cup	70	4.0	8.0	1.5	0	30	3.0
carrots:							
cauliflower (*Green Giant Select*), ⅔ cup	25	2.0	4.0	0	0	30	2.0
water chestnuts (*Birds Eye*), ½ cup	30	2.0	7.0	0	0	30	3.0
water chestnuts (*Green Giant Select*), ⅔ cup .	25	1.0	5.0	0	0	30	2.0
cauliflower (*Birds Eye*), ½ cup	20	2.0	4.0	0	0	20	2.0
cauliflower, carrots:							
(*Birds Eye*), ½ cup .	25	2.0	5.0	0	0	30	2.0
(*McKenzie's* Garden Fresh), ½ cup . .	25	2.0	4.0	0	0	25	2.0
in cheese sauce (*Birds Eye*), ½ cup	70	3.0	7.0	4.0	5	460	2.0
in cheese sauce (*Green Giant*), ⅔ cup	80	3.0	9.0	3.0	<5	560	2.0
cauliflower, red pepper (*Birds Eye*), ½ cup	20	2.0	5.0	0	0	20	2.0
corn, red peppers (*Birds Eye*), ½ cup	50	3.0	12.0	0	0	15	3.0

Food and Measure	cal.	prot. (gms)	carbo. (gms)	fat (gms)	chol. (mgs)	sod. (mgs	fiber (gms)
red pepper, onion, mushrooms (*Birds Eye*), ½ cup	25	2.0	5.0	0	0	20	2.0
stir-fry (*Birds Eye*), 1 cup	30	2.0	5.0	0	0	30	2.0
Broccoli dish, frozen:							
au gratin (*Stouffer's Family Style Favorites*), ½ cup	100	5.0	8.0	5.0	10	370	2.0
in cheese sauce (*Freezer Queen Family Side Dish*), ⅔ cup	80	2.0	12.0	1.5	<5	370	12.0
pancake (*Dr. Praeger's*) 1.3-oz. cake	70	2.0	8.5	3.0	15	150	1.0
and pasta, cauliflower, carrots, in cheese sauce (*Freezer Queen Family Side Dish*), ⅔ cup	120	3.0	14.0	2.0	<5	310	3.0
pot pie (*Amy's*), 7.5 oz.	430	11.0	46.0	22.0	45	630	4.0
soufflé (*Melrose*), ⅓ cup	80	4.0	9.0	3.0	45	260	2.0
Broccoli rabe, fresh:							
(*Andy Boy*), ⅛ bunch	30	3.0	3.0	0	0	45	2.0
(*Frieda's* Rapini, 3 oz.	25	3.0	4.0	0	0	25	0
Broccoli rabe, frozen (*Seabrook Farms*), 1 cup	25	2.0	4.0	0	0	35	2.0
Broccoli sprouts (*Jonathan's*), 1 cup	35	2.0	5.0	.5	0	25	4.0
Broccoli-cheese pocket, frozen, 1 pc.:							
(*Amy's*), 4.5 oz.	270	8.0	37.0	10.0	15	560	3.0
croissant (*Sara Lee*), 3.7 oz.	280	11.0	30.0	13.0	30	430	2.0
Broiling sauce, see "Grilling sauce" and specific listings							
Brown gravy, in jar, w/onions (*Franco-American*), ¼ cup	25	0	4.0	1.0	<5	340	0

Food and Measure	cal.	prot. (gms)	carbo. (gms)	fat (gms)	chol. (mgs)	sod. (mgs)	fiber (gms)
Brown gravy mix:							
(*Bistro*), 2 tsp.	15	0	4.0	0	0	460	0
(*Knorr* Classic), 2 tsp.	20	<1.0	3.0	.5	0	420	0
(*Hain*), 2 tsp.	15	<1.0	3.0	0	0	270	0
(*Lawry's*), 2 tsp.	20	0	4.0	0	0	370	0
(*Loma Linda Gravy Quik/Natural Touch*), ¼ cup*..........	20	<1.0	4.0	0	0	360	0
(*McCormick*), ¼ cup*	20	0	3.0	.5	0	340	0
onion, see "Lyonnaise gravy mix"							
Brownie:							
chocolate, 1 pc.:							
(*Awrey's* Decadent)	220	2.0	31.0	11.0	30	110	1.0
chunk (*Entenmann's* Ultimate)	320	3.0	41.0	17.0	45	190	2.0
peanut (*Awrey's* Sensation)	230	3.0	27.0	13.0	30	135	1.0
fudge:							
(*Entenmann's*), ½ pc., 1.5 oz.	200	3.0	24.0	11.0	40	55	2.0
nut (*Awrey's*), 1 pc.	210	2.0	28.0	11.0	25	100	2.0
mini:							
(*Entenmann's Little Bites*), 3 pcs., 2.2 oz.	300	3.0	36.0	16.0	45	200	1.0
(*Hostess* Bites), 3 pcs., 1.3 oz. ..	170	2.0	21.0	9.0	30	80	1.0
Brownie, refrigerated ¹⁄₁₂ pkg.:							
chocolate bar (*Nestlé* Tollhouse)	180	2.0	26.0	7.0	15	160	2.0
walnut (*Nestlé* Tollhouse)	170	2.0	23.0	9.0	20	125	<1.0
Brownie mix, 1 pc.*, except as noted:							
(*Arrowhead Mills*) ...	110	2.0	27.0	0	0	100	2.0
(*Arrowhead Mills* Fat Free)	120	2.0	28.0	0	0	110	2.0
(*Duncan Hines* Turtle Chocolate Lover's)	150	1.0	20.0	8.0	15	95	0
caramel swirl (*Pillsbury* Thick 'n Fudgy), ¹⁄₁₄ pkg.	120	1.0	23.0	2.5	0	95	<1.0

Food and Measure	cal.	prot. (gms)	carbo. (gms)	fat (gms)	chol. (mgs)	sod. (mgs)	fiber (gms)
cheesecake swirl (*Pillsbury* Thick 'n Fudgy), 1/18 pkg. ..	110	<1.0	19.0	3.0	0	80	<1.0
chocolate:							
chunk (*Betty Crocker* Supreme)	180	2.0	25.0	9.0	20	95	0
chunk (*Duncan Hines* Chocolate Lover's)	160	2.0	23.0	7.0	15	100	0
chunk (*Pillsbury* Thick 'n Fudgy), 1/16 pkg.	120	1.0	22.0	3.5	0	85	<1.0
dark, fudge (*Betty Crocker* Supreme)	170	2.0	24.0	7.0	20	110	0
dark, fudge, w/chunks (*Duncan Hines*)	150	1.0	20.0	8.0	15	95	0
dark, w/*Hershey's* syrup (*Betty Crocker* Supreme)	170	2.0	25.0	7.0	20	110	0
double (*Pillsbury* Thick 'n Fudgy), 1/6 pkg.	120	1.0	23.0	2.5	0	90	<1.0
German (*Betty Crocker* Supreme)	200	2.0	29.0	8.0	20	130	1.0
walnut (*Duncan Hines* Chocolate Lover's)	160	2.0	20.0	9.0	15	95	1.0
frosted (*Betty Crocker* Supreme)	210	2.0	30.0	9.0	20	135	1.0
fudge:							
(*Betty Crocker* Original Supreme)	160	2.0	27.0	6.0	20	110	0
(*Betty Crocker* Pouch)	190	2.0	27.0	8.0	25	125	1.0
(*Betty Crocker* Supreme)	190	2.0	30.0	7.0	20	130	1.0
(*Betty Crocker* Supreme Family)	170	2.0	24.0	7.0	20	105	0
(*Betty Crocker* Supreme Family No Cholesterol)	140	2.0	24.0	4.0	0	105	0
("*Jiffy*"), 1/5 cup ..	150	1.0	28.0	4.0	0	150	<1.0
(*Pillsbury* Rich and Moist), 1/20 pkg.	120	1.0	23.0	2.5	0	75	<1.0

Food and Measure	cal.	prot. (gms)	carbo. (gms)	fat (gms)	chol. (mgs)	sod. (mgs)	fiber (gms)
Brownie mix, fudge *(cont.)*							
(*Sweet Rewards* Low Fat)	130	2.0	27.0	2.5	0	115	1.0
(*Sweet Rewards* Reduced Fat) ...	140	2.0	27.0	3.5	20	110	0
chewy (*Duncan Hines* Family) ...	170	2.0	25.0	8.0	25	110	1.0
chewy (*Duncan Hines* Family Snack Size)	170	2.0	24.0	7.0	20	125	0
double (*Duncan Hines* Chocolate Lover's)	170	2.0	28.0	6.0	25	115	1.0
hot (*Betty Crocker* Supreme)	170	2.0	23.0	8.0	20	110	0
hot, swirl (*Pillsbury* Thick 'n Fudgy), 1/14 pkg.	130	1.0	23.0	3.5	0	90	<1.0
rich (*Pillsbury* Ready to Bake!), 1/12 pkg.	180	2.0	25.0	8.0	0	105	<1.0
peanut butter chunk (*Betty Crocker* w/*Reese's Pieces*)	180	3.0	23.0	9.0	20	105	0
turtle (*Betty Crocker*)	170	2.0	23.0	8.0	20	100	0
walnut:							
(*Betty Crocker* Supreme)	180	2.0	22.0	9.0	20	95	0
(*Pillsbury* Thick 'n Fudgy), 1/12 pkg.	150	2.0	24.0	5.0	0	105	<1.0
white chunk (*Pillsbury* Thick 'n Fudgy), 1/16 pkg.	120	1.0	21.0	4.0	0	90	<1.0
wheat free (*Arrowhead Mills*)	120	3.0	26.0	2.0	0	110	2.0
Browning sauce:							
(*GravyMaster*), 1/4 tsp.	0	0	<1.0	0	0	30	0
(*Kitchen Bouquet*), 1 tsp.	15	0	3.0	0	0	10	0
Bruegger's Bagels:							
bagels, 1 pc.:							
plain	300	12.0	61.0	2.0	0	540	4.0
blueberry	330	11.0	68.0	2.0	0	530	4.0
chocolate chip	310	11.0	69.0	4.5	0	500	4.0
cinnamon raisin ...	320	11.0	68.0	2.0	0	510	4.0

Food and Measure	cal.	prot. (gms)	carbo. (gms)	fat (gms)	chol. (mgs)	sod. (mgs	fiber (gms)
cinnamon sugar . . .	340	12.0	71.0	2.0	0	540	6.0
cranberry orange . .	330	11.0	68.0	2.0	0	510	4.0
everything	310	12.0	62.0	2.0	0	710	4.0
garlic	310	12.0	62.0	2.0	0	540	4.0
honey grain	330	13.0	64.0	3.0	0	500	5.0
jalapeño	310	12.0	63.0	2.0	0	550	4.0
onion	310	12.0	62.0	2.0	0	540	4.0
poppy	310	12.0	61.0	2.5	0	540	4.0
pumpernickel	320	12.0	64.0	2.5	0	600	5.0
rosemary olive oil .	350	11.0	62.0	6.0	0	530	4.0
salt	300	12.0	61.0	2.0	0	1540	4.0
sesame	320	12.0	61.0	2.0	0	540	4.0
sun-dried tomato . .	310	12.0	64.0	2.0	0	630	4.0
cream cheese, 2 tbsp.:							
plain	90	2.0	4.0	8.0	25	85	0
plain, light	70	2.0	3.0	4.5	15	90	0
bacon scallion	100	2.0	4.0	8.0	30	105	0
chive	100	2.0	2.0	9.0	30	90	0
herb garlic, light . .	70	4.0	3.0	4.5	15	85	0
honey walnut	110	2.0	5.0	8.0	25	85	0
jalapeño	100	2.0	3.0	9.0	30	100	0
olive pimiento	100	2.0	2.0	9.0	30	90	0
smoked salmon . . .	100	2.0	2.0	9.0	25	105	0
strawberry, light . .	70	4.0	4.0	4.0	15	85	0
veggie, garden	90	2.0	3.0	8.0	25	95	0
veggie, garden, light	60	4.0	2.0	4.0	15	75	0
wildberry	100	2.0	4.0	9.0	25	85	0
bagel sandwich, 1 pc.:							
egg/cheese	480	22.0	66.0	15.0	190	840	4.0
egg/cheese/bacon .	560	26.0	66.0	22.0	200	1070	4.0
egg/cheese/ham . .	520	28.0	66.0	17.0	205	1350	4.0
egg/cheese/sausage	680	33.0	66.0	33.0	235	1570	4.0
chicken fajita	500	28.0	74.0	12.0	85	970	5.0
chicken salad, mayo	460	24.0	67.0	12.0	55	820	4.0
garden veggie	390	17.0	70.0	6.0	15	580	5.0
ham, honey mustard	440	24.0	77.0	4.5	30	1440	4.0
Leonardo da Veggie	460	19.0	69.0	11.0	40	740	4.0
smoked salmon . . .	470	26.0	66.0	12.0	55	590	4.0
turkey, herb	530	28.0	73.0	14.0	55	1180	4.0
turkey, w/mayo . . .	480	25.0	65.0	14.0	35	1220	4.0
turkey, Santa Fe . . .	480	29.0	71.0	10.0	55	1630	4.0
salmon/spreads:							
hummus, 2 tbsp.	60	2.0	4.0	3.5	0	85	2.0

Food and Measure	cal.	prot. (gms)	carbo. (gms)	fat (gms)	chol. (mgs)	sod. (mgs)	fiber (gms)
Bruegger's Bagels, salmon/spreads *(cont.)*							
smoked salmon, 2 oz.	90	15.0	<1.0	3.0	30	840	0
tuna salad, 2.5 oz.	180	8.0	6.0	14.0	20	440	0
dessert, 1 serving:							
blondie	370	5.0	42.0	23.0	25	220	2.0
Bruegger Bar	420	6.0	47.0	24.0	15	240	3.0
cappuccino bar	420	5.0	45.0	25.0	60	125	1.0
chocolate chunk brownie	330	4.0	39.0	19.0	55	150	2.0
lemon bar	350	4.0	39.0	20.0	85	260	0
mint brownie	300	3.0	34.0	17.0	40	95	0
oatmeal cranberry mountain	380	6.0	44.0	22.0	55	240	3.0
pecan chocolate chunk	350	4.0	32.0	24.0	80	160	1.0
raspberry sammies	300	3.0	41.0	14.0	35	115	1.0
Bruscetta, frozen, pesto, mozzarella, tomato (*Cedarlane*), 1.25-oz. pc.	100	3.0	10.0	5.0	5	190	.5
Brussels sprouts, fresh:							
raw:							
(*Dole*), 4 pcs., 3 oz.	40	2.0	6.0	.5	0	25	3.0
½ cup	19	1.5	3.9	.1	0	11	1.8
boiled, .7-oz. pc.	8	.5	1.8	.1	0	4	.9
boiled, drained, ½ cup	30	2.0	6.8	.4	0	17	3.4
Brussels sprouts, frozen:							
(*Birds Eye* Deluxe), 11 pcs.	35	3.0	7.0	0	0	15	3.0
boiled, drained, ½ cup	33	2.8	6.5	.3	0	18	1.4
in butter sauce (*Green Giant*), ⅔ cup	60	3.0	9.0	1.5	<5	270	4.0
Brussels sprouts combinations, frozen, w/cauliflower, carrots (*Birds Eye*), ½ cup	30	2.0	7.0	0	0	20	3.0
Buckwheat:							
whole grain, 1 oz.	97	3.8	20.3	1.0	0	<1	2.8
whole grain, 1 cup	584	22.5	121.6	5.8	0	1	17.0

Food and Measure	cal.	prot. (gms)	carbo. (gms)	fat (gms)	chol. (mgs)	sod. (mgs)	fiber (gms)
Buckwheat flour:							
(*Arrowhead Mills*),							
¼ cup	100	4.0	21.0	1.0	0	0	3.0
(*Hodgson Mill*),							
⅓ cup	160	7.0	33.0	1.0	0	10	2.0
1 cup	402	15.1	84.7	3.7	0	n.a.	12.0
Buckwheat groats:							
dry, ¼ cup:							
brown (*Arrowhead*							
Mills)	140	5.0	30.0	1.0	0	0	3.0
whole (*Wolff's*) . . .	150	5.0	32.0	1.0	0	10	2.0
roasted:							
(*Wolff's* Kasha),							
¼ cup	170	6.0	35.0	1.0	0	10	2.0
dry, 1 oz.	98	3.3	21.2	.8	0	3	n.a.
cooked, 1 cup	182	6.7	39.5	1.2	0	8	n.a.
Buffalo wing sauce,							
2 tbsp.:							
hot:							
(*Nance's* Chicken							
Wing)	15	2.0	3.0	0	0	650	0
(*World Harbors*							
After Glow)	30	0	7.0	0	0	390	0
mild (*Nance's* Chicken							
Wing)	20	0	4.0	0	0	630	0
Buffalo wing season-							
ing (*McCormick*							
Bag'n Season),							
⅙ pkg.	30	0	5.0	0	0	710	0
Bulgur:							
dry:							
(*Arrowhead Mills*),							
¼ cup	150	5.0	33.0	.5	0	0	4.0
1 cup	479	17.2	106.2	1.9	0	23	25.6
w/soy grits (*Hodgson*							
Mill), ¼ cup	120	6.0	24.0	1.0	0	0	1.0
cooked, 1 cup	152	5.6	33.8	.4	0	9	8.2
salad, see "Tabouli"							
Bulgur dish mix, see							
"Tabouli salad mix"							
and "Wheat pilaf							
mix"							
Bun, see "Roll"							

Food and Measure	cal.	prot. (gms)	carbo. (gms)	fat (gms)	chol. (mgs)	sod. (mgs)	fiber (gms)
Bun, sweet, 1 pc.:							
cheese (*Entenmann's*)	300	6.0	37.0	15.0	55	300	1.0
cinnamon:							
(*Entenmann's Light*)	170	3.0	33.0	3.0	0	260	2.0
(*Hostess* Sweet							
Roll)	210	3.0	34.0	7.0	10	190	0
iced (*Rhodes*)	265	4.0	44.0	8.0	5	260	1.0
no icing (*Rhodes*)	220	4.0	37.0	6.0	0	240	1.0
swirl (*Entenmann's*)	320	5.0	44.0	14.0	50	290	2.0
honey glazed (*Hostess*)	320	4.0	34.0	19.0	15	210	1.0
honey iced (*Drake's*)	420	5.0	44.0	25.0	0	270	1.0
orange:							
iced (*Rhodes*)	285	4.0	49.0	9.0	5	270	1.0
no icing (*Rhodes*)	240	4.0	42.0	7.0	0	250	1.0
sticky (*Entenmann's*)	260	4.0	39.0	10.0	40	240	1.0
Bun, sweet, frozen or refrigerated, 1 pc.:							
caramel, sticky							
(*Pillsbury*)	170	2.0	24.0	7.0	0	330	<1.0
cinnamon, w/icing:							
(*Grands!*)	330	5.0	52.0	11.0	0	670	1.0
(*Pillsbury Home Baked Classics*)	340	6.0	55.0	11.0	0	560	1.0
(*Pillsbury* Reduced Fat)	140	2.0	24.0	3.5	0	340	<1.0
(*Pillsbury* Tube) . . .	150	2.0	23.0	5.0	0	350	<1.0
cream cheese (*Grands!*)	330	5.0	52.0	11.0	<5	660	1.0
cream cheese (*Pillsbury*)	150	2.0	23.0	6.0	0	350	<1.0
orange flavor, w/icing (*Pillsbury*)	170	2.0	25.0	7.0	0	340	<1.0
Burbot, meat only:							
raw, 4 oz.	102	21.9	0	.9	68	110	0
baked, broiled, or microwaved, 4 oz.	130	28.1	0	1.2	87	141	0
Burdock root:							
(*Frieda's* Gobo Root), ¾ cup, 3 oz.	60	1.0	15.0	0	0	0	3.0
raw, 7.3-oz. pc.	112	1.3	13.6	.1	0	4	5.1
raw, pieces, ½ cup . .	43	.9	10.3	.1	0	3	1.9
boiled, 1" pcs., ½ cup	55	1.3	13.2	.1	0	3	1.1

Food and Measure	cal.	prot. (gms)	carbo. (gms)	fat (gms)	chol. (mgs)	sod. (mgs	fiber (gms)
Burger, see "Beef sandwich"							
Burger, vegetarian:							
canned:							
(*Loma Linda Redi-Burger*), ⅝" slice	120	18.0	7.0	2.5	0	450	4.0
(*Loma Linda Vege-Burger*), ¼ cup	70	11.0	2.0	1.5	0	115	2.0
(*Worthington*), ¼ cup	60	9.0	2.0	2.0	0	270	1.0
frozen, crumbles:							
(*Boca*), ½ cup	80	12.0	7.0	.5	0	380	4.0
(*Morningstar Farms* Burger Style Recipe), ⅔ cup	80	10.0	4.0	2.5	0	210	2.0
(*Morningstar Farms* Ground Meatless), ½ cup	60	10.0	4.0	0	0	260	2.0
(*Morningstar Farms* Harvest Burgers), ½ cup	70	12.0	5.0	0	0	200	3.0
(*Worthington Gran Burger*), 3 tbsp.	60	10.0	3.0	.5	0	410	2.0
frozen patties, see "Burger patty, vegetarian, frozen"							
mix, dry:							
(*Loma Linda Patty Mix*), ⅓ cup	90	14.0	7.0	1.0	0	480	5.0
(*Loma Linda Vita-Burger*), ¼ cup chunks or 3 tbsp. granules	70	10.0	6.0	1.0	0	350	3.0
Burger patty, vegetarian, frozen, 1 pc., 2.5 oz., except as noted:							
(*Boca* Vegan)	90	13.0	6.0	1.0	0	350	4.0
(*Harmony Farms* Soy)	110	12.0	7.0	3.0	0	230	4.0
(*Morningstar Farms* Quarter Prime), 3.4 oz.	140	24.0	6.0	2.0	0	370	3.0

Food and Measure	cal.	prot. (gms)	carbo. (gms)	fat (gms)	chol. (mgs)	sod. (mgs)	fiber (gms)
Burger patty, vegetarian, frozen *(cont.)*							
(*Morningstar Farms Better'n Burgers*) ..	100	13.0	6.0	2.0	0	310	3.0
(*Morningstar Farms Garden Grille*)	120	6.0	18.0	2.5	<5	280	4.0
(*Morningstar Farms Grillers*), 2.25 oz.	140	15.0	5.0	6.0	0	260	2.0
(*Morningstar Farms Grillers* Prime) ...	170	16.0	5.0	9.0	0	390	2.0
(*Morningstar Farms Hard Rock Café*), 3 oz.	170	6.0	18.0	8.0	0	340	3.0
(*Morningstar Farms Harvest Burgers Original*), 3.2 oz. ..	140	18.0	8.0	4.0	0	390	5.0
(*Natural Touch Okara Pattie*), 2.25 oz. ..	120	12.0	6.0	5.0	0	300	3.0
(*Natural Touch Hard Rock Café*), 3 oz.	170	6.0	18.0	8.0	0	340	3.0
(*Natural Touch Vegan Burger*), 2.75 oz.	70	11.0	6.0	0	0	370	3.0
(*Tofutti Quit Beef'n*) ..	140	18.0	8.0	4.0	0	370	5.0
(*Yves*), 3 oz.	119	16.0	9.0	2.0	0	480	4.0
(*Yves* Veggie Chick'n), 3 oz.	120	17.0	6.0	3.0	0	390	3.0
all American:							
(*Amy's*)	170	19.0	19.0	3.0	0	370	5.0
(*Boca*)	110	14.0	6.0	3.5	<5	370	4.0
black bean, spicy:							
(*Morningstar Farms*), 2.75 oz.	150	11.0	16.0	4.5	0	470	5.0
(*Morningstar Farms Refrigerated*), 3.3 oz.	120	9.0	19.0	1.0	0	560	5.0
(*Natural Touch*), 2.75 oz.	110	11.0	15.0	1.0	0	330	5.0
black bean and mushroom (*Yves*), 3 oz.	100	12.0	13.0	0	0	450	7.0
Bombay (*Dr. Praeger's*), 2.8 oz.	100	8.0	9.5	3.3	0	190	4.0
California:							
(*Amy's*)	130	6.0	19.0	5.0	0	390	5.0
(*Dr. Praeger's*), 2.8 oz.	100	8.0	9.5	3.3	0	190	4.0

Food and Measure	cal.	prot. (gms)	carbo. (gms)	fat (gms)	chol. (mgs)	sod. (mgs)	fiber (gms)
w/cheese (*Dr. Praeger's Royale*), 3 oz.	120	9.0	11.5	4.0	5	258	2.0
w/"cheese" (*Tofutti Quit Beef'n*)	180	9.0	8.0	6.0	0	340	5.0
Chicago (*Amy's*)	160	11.0	20.0	5.0	5	390	4.0
garlic:							
(*Harmony Farms Soy*)	110	12.0	10.0	3.0	0	240	3.0
roasted (*Boca*)	100	14.0	7.0	2.0	<5	400	5.0
garden vegetable:							
(*Morningstar Farms*), 2.4 oz.	100	10.0	9.0	2.5	0	350	4.0
(*Morningstar Farms Refrigerated*), 3.5 oz.	150	17.0	13.0	3.5	0	520	6.0
(*Natural Touch Garden Veggie Patties*), 2.4 oz.	100	10.0	8.0	2.5	0	280	3.0
(*Yves*), 3 oz.	90	11.0	11.0	0	0	470	7.0
grilled vegetable (*Boca*)	80	13.0	6.0	1.0	0	350	5.0
Italian (*Morningstar Farms Harvest Burger*), 3.2 oz. ..	140	17.0	8.0	4.5	0	370	5.0
mushroom (*Harmony Farms Soy*)	110	11.0	9.0	3.0	0	320	3.0
onion:							
(*Harmony Farms Soy*)	90	10.0	7.0	3.0	0	230	3.0
roasted (*Boca*)	90	13.0	8.0	1.0	0	460	5.0
oven roasted (*Morningstar Farms*), 2.4 oz.	120	12.0	9.0	4.0	0	470	3.0
pizza, tomato basil (*Morningstar Farms*), 2.4 oz.	130	11.0	7.0	6.0	10	320	3.0
salsa (*Boca*)	90	13.0	8.0	1.0	<5	380	5.0
Southwestern (*Morningstar Farms Harvest Burgers*), 3.2 oz.	140	16.0	9.0	4.0	0	370	5.0
Texas (*Amy's*)	130	12.0	15.0	2.5	0	270	3.0
Thai (*Natural Touch*), 2.4 oz.	100	10.0	7.0	3.5	0	380	3.0

Food and Measure	cal.	prot. (gms)	carbo. (gms)	fat (gms)	chol. (mgs)	sod. (mgs)	fiber (gms)
Burger King, 1 serving:							
breakfast dishes:							
Cini-minis, w/out icing, 4 rolls ...	440	6.0	51.0	23.0	25	710	1.0
Croissan'wich, egg, cheese	320	12.0	24.0	19.0	185	730	<1.0
Croissan'wich, sausage, cheese	420	14.0	23.0	31.0	45	840	<1.0
Croissan'wich, sausage, egg, cheese	520	19.0	24.0	39.0	210	1090	1.0
Egg'wich, Canadian bacon, egg	380	15.0	35.0	19.0	125	680	3.0
Egg'wich, Canadian bacon, egg, cheese	420	18.0	36.0	23.0	140	900	3.0
Egg'wich, egg, cheese	410	15.0	36.0	23.0	130	760	3.0
french toast sticks, 5 pcs.	390	6.0	46.0	20.0	0	440	2.0
hash brown rounds	440	6.0	51.0	23.0	0	710	1.0
syrup	80	0	21.0	0	0	20	0
vanilla icing, 1 oz.	110	0	20.0	3.0	0	40	0
whipped blend *Land O Lakes* ...	25	0	0	3.5	0	30	0
burgers/sandwiches:							
bacon double cheeseburger ...	580	35.0	32.0	34.0	110	1240	2.0
BK Homestyle Griller	480	26.0	35.0	27.0	75	760	2.0
BK ¼ Lb. Burger	490	26.0	50.0	21.0	60	950	3.0
BK Smokehouse Cheddar Griller ..	720	39.0	32.0	48.0	125	1240	2.0
BK Veggie Burger	330	14.0	45.0	10.0	0	770	4.0
BK Veggie Burger, w/out mayo	290	14.0	40.0	7.0	0	690	4.0
cheeseburger	360	19.0	31.0	17.0	50	790	2.0
cheeseburger, double	540	32.0	32.0	31.0	100	1050	2.0
Double Whopper ..	1060	59.0	52.0	69.0	185	1100	4.0
Double Whopper, w/out mayo	900	59.0	52.0	51.0	175	980	4.0
Double Whopper w/cheese	1150	64.0	53.0	76.0	210	1530	4.0

Food and Measure	cal.	prot. (gms)	carbo. (gms)	fat (gms)	chol. (mgs)	sod. (mgs)	fiber (gms)
Double Whopper							
w/cheese, w/out							
mayo	990	64.0	53.0	59.0	195	1410	4.0
hamburger	310	17.0	31.0	13.0	40	580	2.0
hamburger, double .	450	28.0	31.0	24.0	75	620	2.0
King Supreme	550	30.0	32.0	34.0	100	790	2.0
Whopper	760	35.0	52.0	46.0	100	1000	4.0
Whopper, w/out							
mayo	600	34.0	52.0	28.0	85	870	4.0
Whopper w/cheese	850	39.0	53.0	53.0	120	1430	4.0
Whopper w/cheese,							
w/out mayo	690	39.0	53.0	36.0	110	1310	4.0
Whopper Jr.	390	17.0	32.0	22.0	45	570	2.0
Whopper Jr., w/out							
mayo	310	17.0	31.0	13.0	40	510	2.0
Whopper Jr.							
w/cheese	440	19.0	32.0	26.0	55	790	2.0
Whopper Jr.							
w/cheese, w/out							
mayo	360	19.0	32.0	17.0	50	730	2.0
sandwiches:							
BK Big Fish	710	24.0	66.0	39.0	50	1160	4.0
chicken, specialty	560	25.0	52.0	28.0	60	1270	3.0
chicken, specialty,							
w/out mayo	460	25.0	52.0	17.0	55	1190	3.0
Chicken Whopper	580	39.0	48.0	26.0	75	1370	3.0
Chicken Whopper,							
w/out mayo	420	38.0	47.0	9.0	60	1250	3.0
Chicken Whopper Jr.	350	26.0	30.0	14.0	45	900	2.0
Chicken Whopper Jr.,							
w/out mayo	270	25.0	30.0	6.0	40	840	2.0
sandwich condiments:							
ketchup, ½ oz. . . .	15	0	4.0	0	0	180	0
tartar sauce, ½ oz.	70	0	0	8.0	5	100	0
Chicken Tenders:							
4 pcs.	170	11.0	10.0	9.0	25	420	0
5 pcs.	220	14.0	13.0	12.0	30	530	<1.0
6 pcs.	250	16.0	15.0	14.0	35	630	<1.0
8 pcs.	340	22.0	20.0	19.0	50	840	<1.0
dipping sauce, 1 oz.:							
barbecue	35	0	9.0	0	0	400	0
honey flavored	90	0	23.0	0	0	0	0
honey mustard . . .	90	0	9.0	6.0	10	150	0
marinara	20	0	5.0	0	0	280	0

Food and Measure	cal.	prot. (gms)	carbo. (gms)	fat (gms)	chol. (mgs)	sod. (mgs)	fiber (gms)
Burger King, dipping sauce *(cont.)*							
ranch, .9 oz.	120	1.0	1.0	13.0	5	85	0
sweet and sour ...	40	0	10.0	0	0	65	0
sides:							
fries, salted:							
king	600	7.0	76.0	30.0	0	1070	7.0
king, no salt added	600	7.0	76.0	30.0	0	620	7.0
large	500	6.0	63.0	25.0	0	880	5.0
large, no salt added	500	6.0	63.0	25.0	0	510	5.0
medium	360	4.0	46.0	18.0	0	640	4.0
medium, no salt added	360	4.0	46.0	18.0	0	380	4.0
small	230	3.0	29.0	11.0	0	410	2.0
small, no salt added	230	3.0	29.0	11.0	0	240	2.0
onion rings:							
king	550	8.0	70.0	27.0	5	800	5.0
largo	480	7.0	60.0	23.0	0	690	5.0
medium	320	4.0	40.0	16.0	0	460	3.0
small	180	2.0	22.0	9.0	0	260	2.0
salad, no dressing or croutons:							
chicken Caesar ...	160	25.0	5.0	6.0	40	730	3.0
garden	25	1.0	5.0	0	0	15	2.0
shakes:							
vanilla, medium ...	720	15.0	73.0	41.0	125	280	1.0
vanilla, small	560	11.0	56.0	32.0	95	220	1.0
syrup added:							
chocolate, medium	790	15.0	89.0	42.0	125	380	2.0
chocolate, small	620	12.0	72.0	32.0	95	310	2.0
strawberry, medium	780	15.0	88.0	41.0	125	300	1.0
strawberry, small	620	11.0	71.0	32.0	95	230	1.0
dessert:							
cookies	440	4.0	57.0	21.0	15	390	2.0
Dutch apple pie ...	340	2.0	52.0	14.0	1	470	1.0
Hershey's sundae pie	310	3.0	33.0	18.0	10	135	<1.0
hot fudge brownie royale	440	6.0	62.0	19.0	50	250	6.0

Food and Measure	cal.	prot. (gms)	carbo. (gms)	fat (gms)	chol. (mgs)	sod. (mgs)	fiber (gms)
Burrito, frozen, 1 pc.:							
(*El Monterey Family Classic* Supreme), 5 oz.	290	13.0	37.0	10.0	30	370	1.0
bean, black, vegetable (*Amy's*), 6 oz.	320	9.0	54.0	8.0	0	540	4.0
bean/cheese:							
(*Amy's*), 6 oz.	280	10.0	43.0	8.0	10	540	6.0
(*El Monterey*), 4 oz.	230	8.0	35.0	7.0	5	460	3.0
(*El Monterey*), 5 oz.	290	10.0	44.0	9.0	10	270	4.0
(*El Monterey*), 8 oz.	470	16.0	70.0	14.0	15	420	7.0
(*El Monterey*), 10 oz.	590	18.0	87.0	17.0	20	530	9.0
(*El Monterey* Reduced Fat), 4 oz.	210	8.0	35.0	3.5	0	180	3.0
(*Las Campanas*), 4 oz.	270	10.0	41.0	7.0	3	480	6.0
(*Patio*), 5 oz.	300	9.0	46.0	9.0	15	690	4.0
bean/rice (*Amy's*), 6 oz.	270	9.0	48.0	6.0	0	550	5.0
bean/rice/cheese (*Cedarlane* Low Fat), 6 oz.	260	13.0	48.0	1.0	0	490	7.0
beef, red hot (*Las Campanas*), 4 oz.	300	9.0	39.0	12.0	10	520	6.0
beef/bean:							
(*El Monterey*), 4 oz.	290	8.0	34.0	14.0	15	460	3.0
(*El Monterey*), 5 oz.	420	10.0	44.0	21.0	30	320	4.0
(*El Monterey*), 8 oz.	580	17.0	68.0	27.0	30	930	7.0
(*El Monterey*), 10 oz.	730	21.0	85.0	34.0	40	1160	9.0
(*El Monterey* Reduced Fat), 4 oz.	260	9.0	34.0	9.0	15	190	3.0
(*Las Campanas*), 4 oz.	310	10.0	39.0	12.0	10	500	5.0
hot (*Patio*), 5 oz. . .	320	10.0	43.0	12.0	25	840	4.0
hot, red chili peppers (*Patio*), 5 oz. . . .	320	10.0	42.0	12.0	20	850	4.0
medium (*Patio*), 5 oz.	310	10.0	45.0	10.0	20	860	4.0
mild (*Patio*), 5 oz.	330	10.0	45.0	12.0	20	890	4.0
spicy, red hot (*El Monterey*), 5 oz.	370	11.0	43.0	17.0	20	330	4.0

Food and Measure	cal.	prot. (gms)	carbo. (gms)	fat (gms)	chol. (mgs)	sod. (mgs)	fiber (gms)
Burrito, frozen, beef/bean *(cont.)*							
spicy, red hot (*El Monterey*), 8 oz.	600	17.0	69.0	28.0	30	520	7.0
spicy, red hot (*El Monterey*), 10 oz.	750	21.0	86.0	35.0	40	650	9.0
beef/bean, green chili:							
(*El Monterey*), 4 oz.	290	8.0	34.0	14.0	15	340	3.0
(*El Monterey*), 5 oz.	370	10.0	42.0	17.0	20	490	4.0
(*El Monterey*), 8 oz.	580	16.0	68.0	27.0	30	540	6.0
(*El Monterey*), 10 oz.	730	20.0	85.0	34.0	40	680	8.0
(*Las Campanas*), 4 oz.	300	10.0	39.0	12.0	10	480	5.0
beef/bean, red chili:							
(*El Monterey*), 4 oz.	280	8.0	33.0	13.0	15	450	3.0
(*El Monterey*), 5 oz.	350	10.0	42.0	16.0	20	650	4.0
(*El Monterey*), 8 oz.	560	17.0	66.0	25.0	30	1030	6.0
(*El Monterey*), 10 oz.	700	21.0	83.0	31.0	40	1290	8.0
chicken:							
(*El Monterey*), 4 oz.	210	5.0	32.0	6.0	0	420	1.0
(*El Monterey Family Classic* Ultimate), 5 oz.	290	12.0	40.0	9.0	20	920	2.0
(*Las Campanas*), 4 oz.	200	7.0	36.0	3.0	10	530	2.0
(*Patio*), 5 oz.	290	11.0	44.0	8.0	20	740	2.0
fajita (*El Monterey Family Classic*), 5 oz.	250	10.0	40.0	6.0	15	430	2.0
steak fajita (*El Monterey Family Classic*), 5 oz.	250	10.0	40.0	6.0	15	430	2.0
vegetable, roasted, and cheese (*Cedarlane*), 6 oz.	550	14.0	48.0	8.0	15	590	3.0
Burrito, breakfast, frozen, 1 pc.:							
(*Amy's*), 6 oz.	210	9.0	38.0	6.0	0	540	5.0
bacon (*Great Starts*), 3.5 oz.	250	10.0	27.0	11.0	90	540	1.0
egg, bacon, cheese, salsa (*El Monterey Family Classics*), 4.5 oz.	270	12.0	33.0	12.0	110	760	1.0

Food and Measure	cal.	prot. (gms)	carbo. (gms)	fat (gms)	chol. (mgs)	sod. (mgs)	fiber (gms)
sausage:							
(*El Monterey Family Classics*), 4.5 oz.	290	8.0	31.0	14.0	55	660	1.0
(*Great Starts*), 3.5 oz.	240	9.0	24.0	12.0	90	500	1.0
Burrito dinner, frozen, con queso (*Patio*), 10-oz. pkg.	490	12.0	60.0	22.0	20	1420	10.0
Burrito entree, frozen, 1 pkg.:							
bean and cheese (*Michelina's*), 8.5 oz.	400	12.0	55.0	15.0	25	1110	4.0
spicy hot (*Patio*), 11 oz.	390	10.0	58.0	13.0	15	1520	5.0
Burrito entree kit:							
(*Chi-Chi's*), 2 shells and seasoning	300	7.0	52.0	7.0	0	1180	2.0
(*Old El Paso*), 1 shell, 2 tsp. seasoning, 3 tbsp. salsa	150	3.0	26.0	4.0	0	790	1.0
(*Old El Paso*), w/beef*	270	14.0	27.0	12.0	40	840	1.0
Burrito seasoning mix:							
(*Chi-Chi's* Fiesta), ¼ pkg.	40	0	6.0	1.0	0	520	1.0
(*Lawry's*), 1 tbsp. ...	30	1.0	6.0	0	0	700	0
(*McCormick*) ⅙ pkg.	25	0	5.0	.5	0	500	0
Butter:							
(*Land O Lakes Ultra Creamy* Unsalted), 1 tbsp.	110	0	0	12.0	30	0	0
(*Land O Lakes Ultra Creamy* Salted), 1 tbsp.	110	0	0	12.0	30	85	0
regular, unsalted:							
(*Land O Lakes*), 1 tbsp.	100	0	0	11.0	30	0	0
1 stick or 4 oz. ...	813	1.0	0	92.0	248	12	0
1 tbsp.	100	.1	0	11.4	31	1	0
1 tsp.	34	<.1	0	3.8	10	<1	0
regular, salted:							
(*Land O Lakes*), 1 tbsp.	100	0	0	11.0	30	85	0
1 stick or 4 oz. ...	813	1.0	0	92.0	248	937	0

Food and Measure	cal.	prot. (gms)	carbo. (gms)	fat (gms)	chol. (mgs)	sod. (mgs)	fiber (gms)
Butter, regular, salted *(cont.)*							
1 tbsp.	100	.1	0	11.4	31	115	0
1 tsp.	34	<.1	0	3.8	10	39	0
whipped, unsalted:							
(*Land O Lakes*),							
1 tbsp.	70	0	0	7.0	20	0	0
½ cup or 1 stick . .	542	.6	<.1	61.3	165	8	0
1 tbsp.	67	.1	tr.	7.6	20	1	0
1 tsp.	23	tr.	tr.	2.6	7	<1	0
whipped, salted:							
(*Land O Lakes*),							
1 tbsp.	70	0	0	7.0	20	50	0
½ cup or 1 stick . .	542	.6	<.1	61.3	165	625	0
1 tbsp.	67	.1	tr.	7.6	20	78	0
1 tsp.	23	tr.	tr.	2.6	7	26	0
light, 1 tbsp.:							
salted (*Land O Lakes*)	50	<1.0	0	6.0	20	70	0
unsalted (*Land O Lakes*)	50	<1.0	0	6.0	20	0	0
whipped, salted (*Land O Lakes*) .	35	0	0	3.5	10	45	0
Butter, flavored, 1 tbsp.:							
garlic (*Land O Lakes*)	100	0	0	11.0	20	95	0
honey:							
(*Land O Lakes*) . . .	90	0	4.0	8.0	15	35	0
plain or cinnamon (*Downey's*)	60	0	11.0	1.0	<5	10	0
Butter beans, see "Lima beans"							
Butter flavor seasoning, 1 tsp.:							
(*Molly McButter*) . . .	5	0	1.0	0	0	180	0
garlic-herb (*Molly McButter*)	5	0	1.0	0	0	125	0
Butter oil, see "Oil"							
Butter salt:							
(*Watkins*), ¼ tsp. . . .	0	0	0	0	0	400	0
(*McCormick*), ¼ tsp. .	0	0	0	0	0	310	0
Butterbur, fresh:							
raw, .2-oz. stalk	1	<.1	.2	<.1	0	<1	<1.0
boiled, drained, 4 oz.	9	.3	2.4	<.1	0	5	n.a.

Food and Measure	cal.	prot. (gms)	carbo. (gms)	fat (gms)	chol. (mgs)	sod. (mgs)	fiber (gms)
Butterbur, canned, chopped, ½ cup	2	.1	.2	.1	0	3	n.a.
Buttercup squash (*Frieda's*), ¾ cup, 3 oz.	30	1.0	7.0	0	0	0	1.0
Butterfish, meat only:							
raw, 4 oz.	166	19.6	0	9.1	74	100	0
baked, broiled, or microwaved, 4 oz.	212	25.1	0	11.7	94	129	0
Buttermilk, see "Milk"							
Butternut, dried:							
in shell, 1 lb.	750	30.5	14.8	69.8	0	1	5.8
shelled, 1 oz.	174	7.1	3.4	16.2	0	<1	1.3
Butternut squash:							
(*Frieda's*), ¾ cup, 3 oz.	30	1.0	7.0	0	0	0	1.0
raw, cubed, ½ cup	32	.7	8.1	.1	0	3	1.1
baked, cubed, ½ cup	41	.9	10.7	.1	0	4	2.9
Butternut squash, frozen:							
12-oz. pkg.	192	6.0	49.0	.3	0	8	4.4
boiled, drained, mashed, ½ cup	47	1.5	12.1	.1	0	2	n.a.
Butterscotch baking chips, 1 tbsp.							
(*Hershey's*)	80	<1.0	10.0	4.0	0	10	0
(*Nestlé*)	80	0	9.0	4.0	0	15	0
Butterscotch syrup (*Smucker's* Sundae Syrup), 2 tbsp.	100	1.0	25.0	0	0	110	0
Butterscotch topping, 2 tbsp.:							
(*Kraft*)	130	<1.0	28.0	1.5	<5	150	0
(*Mrs. Richardson's*)	130	1.0	29.0	.5	0	220	0
(*Smucker's*)	130	0	31.0	0	0	110	<1.0
caramel:							
(*Mrs. Richardson's*)	130	2.0	28.0	1.5	5	70	0
(*Smucker's* Special Recipe)	130	1.0	30.0	1.0	<5	70	<1.0

C

Food and Measure	cal.	prot. (gms)	carbo. (gms)	fat (gms)	chol. (mgs)	sod. (mgs)	fiber (gms)
Cabbage:							
raw:							
5¾" head, 2½ lbs.	228	13.1	49.3	2.4	0	164	20.9
shredded, ½ cup ..	9	.5	1.9	.1	0	6	.8
boiled, drained,							
shredded, ½ cup ..	17	.8	3.4	.3	0	6	2.1
Cabbage, Chinese,							
½ cup, except as							
noted:							
bok choy:							
(*Frieda's*), 1 cup,							
3 oz.	10	1.0	2.0	0	0	55	1.0
(*Frieda's* Baby),							
⅔ cup, 3 oz. . . .	10	1.0	2.0	0	0	35	1.0
raw, whole, 1 lb. ..	52	6.0	8.7	.8	0	257	4.0
raw, shredded	5	.5	.8	.1	0	23	.4
boiled, drained,							
shredded	10	1.3	1.5	.1	0	29	1.4
pe-tsai:							
raw, whole, 1 lb. ..	68	5.1	13.6	.8	0	38	4.2
raw, shredded	6	.5	1.2	.1	0	3	.4
boiled, drained,							
shredded	8	.9	1.4	.1	0	6	1.0
Cabbage, dehydrated,							
diced (*AlpineAire*),							
.7 oz.	70	3.0	13.0	.5	0	40	5.0
Cabbage, marinated,							
see "Kimchee"							
Cabbage, mustard							
(*Frieda's* Gai Choy),							
1 cup, 3 oz.	20	2.0	4.0	0	0	20	2.0
Cabbage, napa							
(*Frieda's*), 1 cup,							
3 oz.	15	1.0	3.0	0	0	10	1.0

Food and Measure	cal.	prot. (gms)	carbo. (gms)	fat (gms)	chol. (mgs)	sod. (mgs)	fiber (gms)
Cabbage, red, fresh:							
raw:							
whole, 1 lb.	100	5.0	22.2	.9	0	38	7.3
shredded (*Dole* Classic), 3 oz. . .	25	1.0	5.0	0	0	10	2.0
shredded (*Fresh Express*), 1 cup	20	1.0	4.0	0	0	30	1.0
shredded, ½ cup . .	10	.5	2.1	.1	0	4	.7
boiled, drained, shredded, ½ cup . .	16	.8	3.5	.2	0	6	1.5
Cabbage, red, can or jar, sweet/sour:							
(*Aunt Nellie's/ Lohmann*), 2 tbsp.	20	0	5.0	0	0	90	0
(*Greenwood*), ½ cup	100	1.0	24.0	0	0	380	0
Cabbage, savoy:							
raw:							
(*Frieda's Salad Savoy*), 3 oz. . .	25	2.0	5.0	0	0	25	3.0
whole, 1 lb.	100	7.3	22.1	.4	0	102	11.2
shredded, ½ cup . .	10	.7	2.1	<.1	0	10	1.1
boiled, drained, shredded, ½ cup . .	18	1.3	4.0	.1	0	17	n.a.
Cabbage, Tuscan (*Frieda's*), ⅔ cup, 3 oz.	20	1.0	2.0	0	0	15	2.0
Cabbage entree, frozen, stuffed (*Lean Cuisine Everyday Favorites*), 9.5 oz.	210	9.0	25.0	8.0	20	590	5.0
Cactus pads, fresh:							
raw:							
(*Frieda's*), 3 oz. . . .	20	1.0	4.0	0	0	5	1.0
sliced, 1 cup	14	1.1	2.9	.1	0	19	2.0
cooked:							
1 cup	22	2.0	4.9	.1	0	30	3.0
1 pad	4	.4	1.0	<.1	0	6	.6
Cactus pads, canned:							
(*Doña Maria* Nopalitos), 2 tbsp.	5	0	1.0	0	0	500	0
(*La Costeña* Nopalitos), 1 cup	20	0	4.0	0	0	2580	2.0

Food and Measure	cal.	prot. (gms)	carbo. (gms)	fat (gms)	chol. (mgs)	sod. (mgs)	fiber (gms)
Cactus pads, canned *(cont.)*							
in escabeche (*Royal Crown* Nopalitos), ⅔ cup	5	0	1.0	0	0	690	2.0
sliced, 2 tbsp.:							
(*Doña Maria* Nopalitos)	5	0	1.0	0	0	560	0
(*Embasa* Nopalitos)	5	0	1.0	0	0	830	2.0
Cactus pear, see "Prickly pear"							
Cajun seasoning (*McCormick*), ¼ tsp.	0	0	0	0	0	135	0
Cake, ⅛ cake, except as noted:							
almond topped (*Entenmann's*)	180	4.0	23.0	8.0	25	120	<1.0
apple, crumb (*Entenmann's* Orchard Delight)	260	3.0	40.0	10.0	15	140	1.0
banana:							
chocolate chip (*Awrey's* Marquise), 1/16 cake	310	2.0	39.0	17.0	30	200	<1.0
crunch (*Entenmann's*)	220	2.0	32.0	10.0	40	280	<1.0
iced (*Entenmann's*)	290	2.0	40.0	15.0	45	230	1.0
loaf (*Entenmann's Light*)	140	2.0	33.0	0	0	260	<1.0
sheet (*Awrey's*), 1/24 cake	350	3.0	40.0	20.0	55	290	<1.0
Black Forest (*Awrey's*), 1/12 cake	370	2.0	42.0	22.0	40	310	1.0
blueberry crumb (*Entenmann's* Orchard Delight)	250	2.0	38.0	10.0	20	190	1.0
butter, ⅙ cake:							
(*Entenmann's Deluxe Desserts Sunshine*)	320	4.0	44.0	14.0	100	370	<1.0
loaf (*Entenmann's*)	210	5.0	30.0	9.0	75	270	<1.0
carrot, iced:							
cream cheese							

Food and Measure	cal.	prot. (gms)	carbo. (gms)	fat (gms)	chol. (mgs)	sod. (mgs)	fiber (gms)
(*Awrey's* Layer), 1/16 cake	390	4.0	48.0	21.0	35	240	1.0
sheet (*Awrey's* Supreme), 1/24 cake	400	5.0	50.0	21.0	45	280	1.0
cheesecake, see "Cheesecake"							
cherry cordial (*Awrey's* Marquise), 1/16 cake	250	2.0	29.0	15.0	20	180	<1.0
chocolate:							
(*Awrey's* Marquise Killer), 1/16 cake	280	2.0	41.0	13.0	25	190	1.0
blackout (*Entenmann's Deluxe Desserts*), 1/9 cake	240	2.0	35.0	11.0	40	190	2.0
chip crumb (*Entenmann's Deluxe Desserts*), 1/9 cake	390	3.0	48.0	21.0	40	190	1.0
creme filled (*Entenmann's*)	300	2.0	42.0	15.0	15	240	2.0
crunch (*Entenmann's*), 1/9 cake	300	3.0	46.0	12.0	25	360	1.0
double, butter cream (*Awrey's* 3-Layer), 1/16 cake	330	3.0	47.0	16.0	35	330	2.0
double, butter cream (*Awrey's* 2-Layer), 1/16 cake	250	3.0	38.0	11.0	35	290	1.0
double, sheet (*Awrey's*), 1/24 cake	320	4.0	45.0	15.0	45	320	2.0
double, torte (*Awrey's* 8"), 1/12 cake	340	3.0	53.0	15.0	40	340	2.0
fudge (*Entenmann's*)	260	2.0	39.0	12.0	15	230	2.0
German, butter cream (*Awrey's* 3-Layer), 1/16 cake	370	4.0	45.0	20.0	80	270	<1.0
German, sheet (*Awrey's*), 1/24 cake	320	4.0	40.0	18.0	95	330	1.0

Food and Measure	cal.	prot. (gms)	carbo. (gms)	fat (gms)	chol. (mgs)	sod. (mgs)	fiber (gms)
Cake, chocolate *(cont.)*							
peanut (*Awrey's Marquise Fantasy*), 1/16 cake	330	6.0	38.0	19.0	25	270	<1.0
tropical (*Awrey's Marquise*), 1/16 cake	230	3.0	34.0	11.0	25	210	<1.0
white iced, butter cream (*Awrey's 2-Layer*), 1/16 cake	270	3.0	35.0	15.0	40	330	1.0
chocolate layers, no icing (*Awrey's*), 1/16 cake	300	5.0	45	12.0	75	500	2.0
coffee cake:							
(*Awrey's Long John*), 1/12 cake	180	3.0	25.0	8.0	2	170	0
butter (*Entenmann's French*)	210	2.0	28.0	10.0	55	220	<1.0
cheese (*Entenmann's*)	160	3.0	21.0	7.0	25	140	<1.0
cheese, cherry (*Entenmann's Light*), 1/9 cake	140	3.0	31.0	0	0	220	1.0
coconut, butter cream:							
sheet (*Awrey's*), 1/24 cake	380	3.0	41.0	23.0	45	390	0
yellow (*Awrey's 3-Layer*), 1/16 cake	390	3.0	46.0	23.0	45	360	0
crumb cake:							
(*Entenmann's Light Delight*), 1/9 cake	210	3.0	36.0	6.0	0	200	1.0
(*Entenmann's Ultimate*), 1/10 cake	250	2.0	33.0	13.0	15	260	<1.0
Danish, pecan (*Entenmann's Ultimate*)	250	3.0	22.0	17.0	30	160	2.0
Danish ring (*Entenmann's*), 1/5 cake	250	4.0	27.0	14.0	30	200	<1.0
Danish twist:							
cheese (*Entenmann's*)	230	3.0	28.0	12.0	30	200	<1.0
cinnamon apple (*Entenmann's Light*)	140	2.0	34.0	0	0	160	1.0

Food and Measure	cal.	prot. (gms)	carbo. (gms)	fat (gms)	chol. (mgs)	sod. (mgs	fiber (gms)
lemon (*Entenmann's Light*)	130	2.0	30.0	0	0	200	1.0
raspberry (*Entenmann's* Light)	140	2.0	32.0	0	0	190	1.0
devil's food, iced (*Entenmann's*)	280	2.0	38.0	14.0	15	260	<1.0
(*Entenmann's* Metropolitan), 1/8 cake	340	3.0	46.0	16.0	45	270	<1.0
espresso, French (*Awrey's* Marquise), 1/16 cake	330	2.0	30.0	23.0	30	200	<1.0
fruit (*Claxton*), 1/12 cake	420	6.0	72.0	12.0	35	100	8.0
golden, fudge iced (*Entenmann's*), 1/8 cake	340	3.0	48.0	16.0	50	260	1.0
loaf (*Entenmann's* Old Fashioned)	200	2.0	27.0	9.0	40	200	<1.0
lemon:							
(*Awrey's* Marquise), 1/16 cake	270	2.0	33.0	14.0	45	210	0
butter cream (*Awrey's* 3-Layer), 1/16 cake	340	2.0	38.0	20.0	45	310	0
coconut (*Entenmann's*), 1/8 cake	380	3.0	44.0	22.0	50	300	<1.0
crunch (*Entenmann's*), 1/9 cake	320	3.0	48.0	13.0	50	280	<1.0
marble loaf (*Entenmann's* Ali Butter)	190	2.0	26.0	8.0	55	250	<1.0
Neapolitan torte (*Awrey's*), 1/12 cake	360	3.0	41.0	21.0	45	330	0
orange:							
butter cream (*Awrey's* 3-Layer), 1/16 cake	340	2.0	43.0	20.0	40	300	0
sheet (*Awrey's* Frosty), 1/24 cake	350	3.0	42.0	19.0	40	300	0
peach, Georgia (*Awrey's* Marquise), 1/16 cake	260	2.0	34.0	14.0	30	220	0
pineapple loaf (*Entenmann's*)	220	3.0	30.0	11.0	45	210	0

Food and Measure	cal.	prot. (gms)	carbo. (gms)	fat (gms)	chol. (mgs)	sod. (mgs)	fiber (gms)
Cake *(cont.)*							
pound:							
(*Hostess*), ⅙ cake .	260	4.0	39.0	9.0	15	320	1.0
pumpkin, spice, or cranberry orange (*Capitol*), ¼ cake	250	3.0	39.0	10.0	35	350	<1.0
raisin loaf (*Entenmann's*)	220	3.0	33.0	8.0	45	200	1.0
raspberries and cream (*Awrey's* Marquise), 1/16 cake	260	2.0	34.0	14.0	25	210	0
raspberry:							
(*Awrey's* Marquise Extrodinaire), 1/16 cake	370	2.0	48.0	20.0	45	240	1.0
nut (*Awrey's* Marquise), 1/16 cake	290	3.0	35.0	16.0	30	200	0
red velvet (*Awrey's* Marquise), 1/16 cake	310	3.0	34.0	19.0	30	230	<1.0
rocky road (*Entenmann's*)	260	3.0	39.0	12.0	15	220	2.0
sour cream loaf (*Entenmann's*)	220	2.0	24.0	12.0	50	150	1.0
sponge, no icing, sheet (*Awrey's*), 1/24 cake	180	3.0	28.0	7.0	40	320	0
strawberry torte (*Awrey's* Supreme), 1/12 cake	270	2.0	39.0	12.0	40	290	<1.0
white layers, no icing (*Awrey's*), 1/16 cake	320	5.0	47.0	12.0	80	490	0
yellow:							
white iced, sheet (*Awrey's*), 1/24 cake	370	3.0	40.0	22.0	45	400	0
yellow iced (*Awrey's* Layer), 1/16 cake	300	2.0	35.0	17.0	45	320	0
Cake, frozen, ⅛ cake, except as noted:							
cappuccino (*Manzoni*), ⅕ cake	260	2.0	30.0	15.0	25	50	0
carrot, iced:							
(*Oregon Farms*), ⅙ cake	300	3.0	37.0	16.0	30	360	1.0

Food and Measure	cal.	prot. (gms)	carbo. (gms)	fat (gms)	chol. (mgs)	sod. (mgs)	fiber (gms)
layer (*Pepperidge Farm*), 1/9 cake ..	320	3.0	32.0	20.0	30	190	1.0
cheesecake, see "Cheesecake, frozen"							
chocolate layer:							
(*Pepperidge Farm Decadence*)	300	3.0	32.0	18.0	25	150	1.0
double (*Sara Lee*)	260	3.0	33.0	13.0	10	230	2.0
fudge (*Pepperidge Farm*)	250	3.0	31.0	11.0	30	160	1.0
German (*Sara Lee*)	280	3.0	35.0	14.0	15	250	1.0
chocolate mousse (*Manzoni*), 1/5 cake	270	4.0	40.0	11.0	30	70	<2.0
coconut, layer:							
(*Pepperidge Farm*)	250	2.0	35.0	11.0	25	115	<1.0
(*Sara Lee*)	260	2.0	33.0	14.0	15	210	1.0
coffee cake, 1/8 cake, except as noted:							
butter streusel (*Sara Lee*)	220	4.0	25.0	12.0	35	240	<1.0
cheese (*Sara Lee* Reduced Fat) ...	180	3.0	28.0	6.0	20	230	0
crumb (*Sara Lee*) ..	220	3.0	32.0	9.0	15	210	<1.0
pecan (*Sara Lee*) ..	230	4.0	24.0	12.0	25	170	<1.0
raspberry (*Sara Lee*)	220	3.0	27.0	8.0	15	220	<1.0
corn, see "Corn cake"							
fudge stripe, layer (*Pepperidge Farm*)	250	2.0	31.0	13.0	25	140	1.0
golden, layer, fudge:							
(*Pepperidge Farm*)	250	2.0	33.0	12.0	35	120	<1.0
(*Sara Lee*)	260	2.0	34.0	13.0	15	200	1.0
pound, 1/4 cake:							
(*Sara Lee* Butter) ..	320	4.0	38.0	16.0	85	280	<1.0
(*Sara Lee* Reduced Fat)	280	4.0	42.0	11.0	65	350	<1.0
chocolate swirl (*Sara Lee*)	330	5.0	42.0	16.0	75	350	<1.0
strawberry swirl (*Sara Lee*)	290	4.0	44.0	11.0	60	140	<1.0
strawberry:							
layer, stripe (*Pepperidge Farm*)	250	2.0	32.0	12.0	15	110	<1.0

Food and Measure	cal.	prot. (gms)	carbo. (gms)	fat (gms)	chol. (mgs)	sod. (mgs)	fiber (gms)
Cake, frozen, strawberry *(cont.)*							
shortcake layer *(Sara Lee)*	180	2.0	27.0	7.0	15	140	<1.0
tiramisu *(Manzoni)*, ⅕ cake	230	2.0	30.0	11.0	55	70	0
vanilla layer *(Sara Lee)*	260	2.0	32.0	14.0	15	210	0
Cake, mix, 1/12 cake*, except as noted:							
angel food:							
(Duncan Hines Moist Deluxe) ..	190	3.0	34.0	6.0	0	300	0
(Pillsbury)	140	3.0	31.0	0	0	340	0
(SuperMoist Traditional)	130	3.0	30.0	0	0	150	0
(SuperMoist Easy Pouch), ¼ pkg.	170	3.0	37.0	0	0	330	0
chocolate swirl *(SuperMoist)* ...	150	3.0	34.0	0	0	310	0
confetti *(SuperMoist)*	150	3.0	34.0	0	0	320	0
white *(SuperMoist* One Step)	140	3.0	32.0	0	0	320	0
banana *(Duncan Hines Moist Deluxe Supreme)*	250	3.0	36.0	11.0	55	290	0
brownie, w/mini kisses *(Betty Crocker Stir 'n Bake)*, ⅙ pkg. ..	220	2.0	36.0	7.0	0	160	1.0
butter pecan *(SuperMoist)*	240	3.0	35.0	10.0	55	280	0
butterscotch *(Duncan Hines* Moist Deluxe)	250	3.0	36.0	11.0	55	290	0
caramel *(Duncan Hines* Moist Deluxe)	250	3.0	36.0	11.0	55	290	0
carrot:							
(SuperMoist), 1/10 cake*	320	4.0	42.0	15.0	65	360	0
cream cheese *(Betty Crocker Stir 'n Bake)*, ⅙ pkg. ..	250	2.0	46.0	7.0	0	300	0
cheesecake, see "Cheesecake mix"							
cherry chip *(SuperMoist)*, 1/10 cake* ..	300	4.0	41.0	13.0	65	340	0

Food and Measure	cal.	prot. (gms)	carbo. (gms)	fat (gms)	chol. (mgs)	sod. (mgs)	fiber (gms)
cherry, wild, vanilla (*Duncan Hines* Moist Deluxe)	250	3.0	36.0	11.0	55	290	0
chocolate:							
(*Estee*), 1/5 cake* ..	190	2.0	36.0	4.0	0	240	1.0
(*Pillsbury Moist Supreme*), 1/12 pkg.	180	2.0	34.0	4.5	0	320	<1.0
butter recipe (*Pillsbury Moist Supreme*), 1/12 pkg.	180	2.0	33.0	4.0	0	330	1.0
butter recipe (*SuperMoist*)	250	4.0	35.0	11.0	75	420	1.0
chip (*SuperMoist*)	250	3.0	35.0	11.0	55	270	0
dark (*Pillsbury Moist Supreme*), 1/12 pkg.	180	2.0	34.0	4.0	0	320	1.0
dark, fudge (*Duncan Hines* Moist Deluxe)	290	4.0	34.0	15.0	55	360	1.0
fudge (*SuperMoist*)	270	3.0	35.0	12.0	55	340	1.0
fudge, creamy swirls (*SuperMoist*), 1/9 cake*	210	3.0	32.0	8.0	50	250	1.0
German (*Duncan Hines* Moist Deluxe)	240	3.0	32.0	12.0	55	430	1.0
German (*SuperMoist*)	270	3.0	36.0	13.0	55	330	0
milk (*SuperMoist*)	240	4.0	34.0	10.0	55	300	1.0
mocha (*Duncan Hines* Moist Deluxe)	290	4.0	34.0	15.0	55	360	1.0
swirl, double (*SuperMoist*)	270	4.0	35.0	13.0	55	330	1.0
Swiss (*Duncan Hines* Moist Deluxe)	290	4.0	34.0	15.0	55	360	1.0
coffee cake:							
(*Aunt Jemima* Easy), 1/8 pkg.	160	2.0	27.0	5.0	0	240	<1.0

Food and Measure	cal.	prot. (gms)	carbo. (gms)	fat (gms)	chol. (mgs)	sod. (mgs)	fiber (gms)
Cake, mix, coffee cake *(cont.)*							
cinnamon (*Betty Crocker Stir 'n Bake* Streusel), ⅙ pkg.	200	2.0	36.0	6.0	10	220	0
cinnamon (*Pillsbury* Streusel), 1/16 pkg.	190	1.0	36.0	5.0	0	200	0
chocolate chip (*Pillsbury* Streusel), 1/16 pkg.	210	2.0	38.0	6.0	0	200	<1.0
devil's food:							
(*Duncan Hines* Moist Deluxe) ..	290	4.0	34.0	15.0	55	360	1.0
("*Jiffy*"), ⅕ cake*	220	3.0	40.0	5.0	0	520	1.0
(*Pillsbury Moist Supreme*), 1/12 pkg.	180	2.0	33.0	4.0	0	330	2.0
(*SuperMoist*)	270	3.0	35.0	13.0	55	340	1.0
(*Sweet Rewards*) ..	200	4.0	36.0	5.0	55	380	1.0
chocolate frosting (*Betty Crocker Stir 'n Bake*), ⅙ pkg.	240	2.0	43.0	7.0	0	270	1.0
fudge:							
butter (*Duncan Hines* Moist Deluxe), 1/10 cake*	320	3.0	40.0	17.0	80	300	2.0
marble (*Duncan Hines* Moist Deluxe)	250	3.0	36.0	11.0	55	290	0
marble (*SuperMoist*), 1/10 cake*	290	4.0	43.0	12.0	65	330	0
gingerbread (*Betty Crocker* Cake/Cookie Mix), ⅛ cake*	230	3.0	39.0	6.0	25	350	0
golden, butter recipe (*Duncan Hines* Moist Deluxe)	320	3.0	42.0	16.0	80	190	2.0
lemon:							
(*Duncan Hines* Moist Deluxe Supreme)	250	3.0	36.0	11.0	55	290	0
(*Pillsbury Moist Supreme*), 1/12 pkg.	170	1.0	35.0	3.0	0	270	0

Food and Measure	cal.	prot. (gms)	carbo. (gms)	fat (gms)	chol. (mgs)	sod. (mgs)	fiber (gms)
(*SuperMoist*)	240	3.0	36.0	10.0	55	290	0
marble (*Manischewitz*), ¼ cup	230	2.0	48.0	4.0	0	710	2.0
orange (*Duncan Hines* Moist Deluxe Supreme)	250	3.0	36.0	11.0	55	290	0
party swirl (*Super-Moist*)	250	3.0	35.0	11.0	55	280	0
pineapple: (*Duncan Hines* Moist Deluxe Supreme)	250	3.0	36.0	11.0	55	290	0
(*SuperMoist*)	250	3.0	35.0	10.0	55	290	0
upside down (*Betty Crocker*), ⅛ cake*	400	3.0	64.0	14.0	35	330	0
pound, ⅛ cake*: (*Betty Crocker*) . . .	260	4.0	45.0	8.0	55	210	0
(*Betty Crocker* No Cholesterol)	250	4.0	45.0	7.0	0	220	0
rainbow chip (*Super-Moist*), ⅒ cake* . .	300	4.0	41.0	13.0	65	340	0
red velvet (*Duncan Hines* Moist Deluxe)	240	3.0	33.0	11.0	55	280	1.0
sour cream white (*SuperMoist*), ⅒ cake*	280	3.0	41.0	12.0	65	370	0
spice: (*Duncan Hines* Moist Deluxe) . .	250	3.0	36.0	11.0	55	290	0
(*SuperMoist*)	240	3.0	35.0	10.0	55	290	0
strawberry: (*Duncan Hines* Moist Deluxe Supreme)	250	3.0	36.0	11.0	55	290	0
(*Pillsbury Moist Supreme*), ½ pkg.	180	1.0	35.0	4.0	0	270	<1.0
(*SuperMoist*)	250	3.0	35.0	10.0	55	280	0
vanilla, French: (*Duncan Hines* Moist Deluxe) . .	250	3.0	36.0	11.0	55	290	0
(*Pillsbury Moist Supreme*), ½ pkg.	180	2.0	34.0	4.0	0	270	<1.0

Food and Measure	cal.	prot. (gms)	carbo. (gms)	fat (gms)	chol. (mgs)	sod. (mgs)	fiber (gms)
Cake, mix, vanilla, French *(cont.)*							
(*SuperMoist*), 1/12 pkg.	170	1.0	35.0	3.0	0	270	0
(*SuperMoist*)	240	3.0	35.0	10.0	55	290	0
vanilla, golden (*SuperMoist*)	240	3.0	35.0	10.0	55	290	0
white:							
(*Estee*), 1/5 cake*	200	2.0	38.0	4.0	0	170	<1.0
(*"Jiffy"*), 1/5 cake*	210	2.0	41.0	4.5	0	320	<1.0
(*Pillsbury Moist Supreme*), 1/12 pkg.	180	2.0	34.0	4.0	0	270	<1.0
(*SuperMoist*)	230	3.0	34.0	10.0	0	300	0
(*SuperMoist* Richer Recipe)	250	3.0	34.0	11.0	55	300	0
(*Sweet Rewards*)	190	3.0	36.0	4.0	0	310	0
yellow:							
(*Duncan Hines* Moist Deluxe)	250	3.0	36.0	11.0	55	290	0
(*"Jiffy"* Golden), 1/5 pkg.	210	2.0	41.0	4.5	0	340	<1.0
(*Pillsbury Moist Supreme*), 1/12 pkg.	180	1.0	35.0	3.5	0	290	0
(*SuperMoist*)	250	3.0	35.0	10.0	55	290	0
(*Sweet Rewards*)	200	3.0	37.0	4.5	55	300	0
butter recipe (*SuperMoist*)	260	3.0	36.0	11.0	75	370	0
chocolate frosting (*Betty Crocker Stir 'n Bake*), 1/6 pkg.	240	2.0	43.0	7.0	10	240	<1.0
w/fudge, creamy swirls (*SuperMoist*), 1/9 cake*	210	3.0	32.0	8.0	50	230	0
Cake, snack (see also specific listings), 1 pc., except as noted:							
Boston creme (*Drake's*), 1.5 oz.	180	1.0	25.0	8.0	0	110	1.0
butter loaf slice (*Entenmann's*), 3 oz.	330	4.0	47.0	14.0	110	420	<1.0

Food and Measure	cal.	prot. (gms)	carbo. (gms)	fat (gms)	chol. (mgs)	sod. (mgs)	fiber (gms)
cheese puffs:							
(Entenmann's), 3 oz.	330	5.0	30.0	21.0	30	310	<1.0
guava (Entenmann's), 2.8 oz.	290	4.0	33.0	17.0	15	250	1.0
cherry (Mr. Kipling Bakewells), 1.4-oz. pc.	170	2.0	23.0	7.0	5	55	<1.0
chocolate:							
(Devil Dogs), 1.6 oz.	180	2.0	26.0	7.0	0	150	1.0
(Funny Bones), 2 pcs., 2.5 oz. ..	300	4.0	41.0	13.0	0	220	4.0
(Hostess Ding Dongs), 2 pcs., 2.8 oz.	360	3.0	47.0	18.0	5	210	2.0
(Hostess Ho-Ho's), 2 pcs., 2 oz.	250	2.0	34.0	12.0	20	150	1.0
(Hostess Suzy Q's), 2 oz.	230	2.0	35.0	9.0	10	270	1.0
(Ring Dings), 2 pcs., 2.7 oz.	340	2.0	43.0	18.0	0	220	2.0
(Yodels), 2 pcs., 2.2 oz.	290	2.0	34.0	16.0	0	160	1.0
chocolate marshmallow or banana (Salerno Scooter Pie), 1.2-oz. pc.	140	1.0	23.0	5.0	0	80	0
coconut, crème filled (Drake's Mini Coco Bites), 4 pcs., 2.5 oz.	320	3.0	36.0	19.0	10	200	2.0
coffee cake:							
(Drake's), 1.2-oz. pc.	140	1.0	20.0	6.0	5	100	0
(Drake's), 2.25-oz. pc. ...	270	3.0	39.0	12.0	10	180	1.0
(Little Debbie), 3.4 oz.	370	4.0	64.0	11.0	15	320	1.0
crumb (Hostess), 1.1-oz. pc.	140	1.0	19.0	6.0	10	110	0
crumb cake:							
(Entenmann's), 3 oz.	360	4.0	50.0	16.0	85	350	1.0
(Hostess Light), 1 oz.	90	1.0	19.0	.5	0	100	0
cupcake:							
cream filled (Entenmann's Light), 2 oz.	160	1.0	39.0	0	0	150	1.0

Food and Measure	cal.	prot. (gms)	carbo. (gms)	fat (gms)	chol. (mgs)	sod. (mgs)	fiber (gms)
Cake, snack, cupcake (cont.)							
creme filled, golden (*Sunny Doodles*), 2 pcs., 2 oz. . . .	220	2.0	33.0	8.0	5	180	1.0
creme filled (*Little Debbie*), 1.7 oz.	210	1.0	29.0	10.0	0	110	0
orange (*Hostess*), 1.5-oz. pc.	160	1.0	27.0	5.0	10	150	0
cupcake, chocolate:							
(*Hostess*), 1.8 oz.	180	2.0	30.0	6.0	5	290	1.0
(*Hostess* Lowfat), 1.6 oz.	140	2.0	29.0	1.5	0	190	1.0
creme-filled (*Entenmann's* Light), 2 oz.	160	1.0	39.0	0	0	160	1.0
creme-filled (*Hostess*), 1.8-oz. pc.	180	2.0	30.0	6.0	5	290	1.0
creme-filled (*Yankee Doodles*), 3 pcs., 3 oz.	320	4.0	49.0	12.0	0	310	2.0
cream-filled, mini (*Yankee Doodles*), 4 pcs., 1.8 oz. . . .	190	2.0	30.0	7.0	0	180	1.0
devil's food, creme filled, 1 pc.:							
(*Little Debbie* Cremes*), 1.7 oz.	190	1.0	29.0	8.0	0	170	0
(*Twinkies*), 1.6 oz.	170	1.0	27.0	6.0	0	220	0
fudge rounds (*Little Debbie*), 2 oz.	240	2.0	38.0	9.0	<5	125	1.0
golden, cream filled:							
(*Twinkies*), 1.5-oz. pc.	150	1.0	25.0	5.0	15	200	0
(*Twinkies* Lowfat), 1.5-oz. pc.	130	1.0	27.0	1.5	10	190	0
marble (*Entenmann's*), 3 oz.	320	4.0	45.0	14.0	105	400	<1.0
pecan spin wheels:							
(*Aunt Fanny's*), 1 oz.	100	1.0	16.0	4.0	0	80	0
(*Drake's*), 1 oz. . . .	100	1.0	16.0	4.0	0	70	<1.0
pound:							
(*Awrey's* Golden), 2.6 oz.	250	4.0	37.0	10.0	45	270	<1.0

Food and Measure	cal.	prot. (gms)	carbo. (gms)	fat (gms)	chol. (mgs)	sod. (mgs)	fiber (gms)
(*Drake's*), 2 pcs., 2.3 oz.	250	4.0	32.0	11.0	25	380	0
raspberry sponge (*Mr. Kipling*), 2 pcs., 2.3 oz.	260	3.0	33.0	2.0	15	190	<1.0
Cake, snack, mix (see also "Cookie mix" and specific listings), 1 pc.*:							
chocolate bar (*Betty Crocker Hershey*) .	150	1.0	21.0	6.0	15	110	0
chocolate peanut butter bar (*Betty Crocker Supreme*)	190	3.0	26.0	9.0	20	190	0
date bar (*Betty Crocker*)	150	1.0	23.0	6.0	0	90	1.0
lemon bar (*Betty Crocker Sunkist*) ..	140	2.0	24.0	4.5	40	90	0
Calabaza (*Frieda's*), ½ cup, 3 oz.	10	1.0	2.0	0	0	0	1.0
Calamari, see "Squid"							
Calamari dish, frozen:							
breaded (*Contessa*), 2 oz. or 13 pcs., w/2 tbsp. sauce ...	170	5.0	16.0	9.0	65	520	0
crisps, breaded (*Acadian Gourmet*), 12 pcs., 3.1 oz. ...	230	9.0	19.0	13.0	100	580	2.0
Calves' liver, see "Liver"							
Camote, see "Boniato"							
Camouflage melon (*Frieda's*), 1 cup, 5 oz.	50	1.0	13.0	0	0	15	1.0
Candy:							
almond, Jordan:							
(*Blue Diamond*), 13 pcs., 1.4 oz.	190	4.0	28.0	7.0	0	0	1.0
(*House of Bazzini*), 1 oz.	180	3.0	30.0	6.0	0	0	1.0
almond, chocolate coated:							
(*Chocolate World*), 11 pcs., 1.3 oz.	210	4.0	18.0	14.0	5	30	2.0
(*Ferrara Pan*), 14 pcs., 1.4 oz.	210	4.0	17.0	16.0	2	30	1.0
(*Lindt*), 1.4 oz. ...	220	5.0	16.0	17.0	5	25	0

Food and Measure	cal.	prot. (gms)	carbo. (gms)	fat (gms)	chol. (mgs)	sod. (mgs)	fiber (gms)
Candy (cont.)							
almond bar:							
(*Mars*), 1.8-oz. bar	240	3.0	32.0	12.0	5	70	2.0
(*Mars* Fun Size),							
2 bars	190	3.0	24.0	10.0	5	65	1.0
(*Pot of Gold*),							
2.75-oz. bar	450	10.0	36.0	30.0	10	50	3.0
(*Baby Ruth*),							
2.1-oz. bar	270	4.0	36.0	13.0	0	130	2.0
(*Baby Ruth* Fun Size),							
1-oz. bar	130	2.0	17.0	6.0	0	60	<1.0
(*Bittyfinger*), 2 bars ..	170	2.0	27.0	7.0	0	75	<1.0
(*Buncha Crunch*),							
1.4-oz. bag	200	2.0	26.0	10.0	10	60	<1.0
butter rum, 2 pcs.:							
(*LifeSavers*)	20	0	5.0	0	0	0	0
(*Nips*)	60	0	11.0	1.5	0	40	0
(*Butterfinger*),							
2.1-oz. bar	270	3.0	44.0	11.0	0	120	1.0
(*Butterfinger* Fun Size),							
.75-oz. bar	100	2.0	15.0	4.0	0	40	0
(*Butterfinger BB's*),							
1.7-oz. bag	220	2.0	34.0	9.0	0	85	1.0
(*Butterfinger Treasures*),							
3 pcs., 1.2 oz.	180	2.0	23.0	9.0	5	40	<1.0
butterscotch:							
(*Estee* No Sugar),							
2 pcs.	25	0	12.0	0	0	50	0
(*Hershey's Taste-tations*), 3 pcs.,							
6 oz.	60	0	12.0	1.5	<5	85	0
(*Land O Lakes*),							
3 pcs., .6 oz. ...	70	0	17.0	0	0	35	0
(*Candy Bar Factory*),							
3-oz. pkg.	440	8.0	47.0	24.0	10	160	3.0
candy cane (*Spangler*),							
.5-oz. pc.	55	0	14.0	0	0	0	0
candy corn, 1 oz. ...	110	0	27.0	0	0	40	0
caramel:							
(*Hershey's* Classic),							
6 pcs., 1.3 oz. ...	160	1.0	27.0	5.0	5	90	0
(*Hershey's Taste-tations*), 3 pcs.,							
.6 oz.	60	0	12.0	1.5	<5	85	0

Food and Measure	cal.	prot. (gms)	carbo. (gms)	fat (gms)	chol. (mgs)	sod. (mgs)	fiber (gms)
(*Nips*), 2 pcs.	60	0	11.0	1.5	0	40	0
(*Treasures*), 3 pcs., 1.2 oz.	170	1.0	22.0	9.0	5	60	<1.0
(*Werther's Original*), 3 pcs., .5 oz. ...	60	0	13.0	1.0	<5	60	0
chocolate coated (*Milk Duds*), 1.8-oz. box	240	2.0	37.0	9.0	0	100	0
chocolate coated (*Pom Poms*), 1.6 oz.	200	1.0	35.0	6.0	<5	70	2.0
chocolate coated (*Rolo*), 1.9-oz. pkg.	260	3.0	36.0	11.0	10	110	0
chocolate filled (*Hershey's*), 6 pcs., 1.3 oz.	160	1.0	26.0	6.0	<5	65	0
vanilla and chocolate (*Estee*), 5 pcs.	115	1.0	26.0	5.0	0	65	0
caramel cookie bar: (*Twix*), 2 pcs., 2 oz.	280	3.0	37.0	14.0	5	115	1.0
(*Twix* Fun Size), 1 pc.	80	1.0	10.0	4.0	0	30	0
(*Twix* Miniatures), 3 pcs., 1.1 oz. ..	150	1.0	19.0	7.0	0	60	0
caramel fudge bar (*Hershey's Sweet Escapes*), .7-oz. bar	70	<1.0	13.0	2.0	0	50	0
caramel peanut butter bar (*Hershey's Sweet Escapes*), .7-oz. bar	80	1.0	13.0	2.5	0	70	0
cherries, w/chocolate: bing, dried, 5 pcs., 1.4 oz.	190	2.0	26.0	9.0	<5	25	3.0
dark (*Cella*), 2 pcs.	110	<1.0	18.0	4.0	0	10	1.0
milk (*Cella*), 2 pcs.	110	<1.0	18.0	4.0	0	15	2.0
thins (*Andes* Jubilee), 8 pcs.	200	2.0	22.0	13.0	0	15	<1.0
chocolate, bittersweet: (*Lindt* Excellence), 4 pcs., 1.4 oz. ..	220	3.0	13.0	17.0	0	12	2.0
(*Lindt* Surfin), 5 pcs., 1.3 oz.	200	2.0	19.0	12.5	0	5	0

Food and Measure	cal.	prot. (gms)	carbo. (gms)	fat (gms)	chol. (mgs)	sod. (mgs)	fiber (gms)
Candy, chocolate, bittersweet *(cont.)*							
hazelnut (*Lindt*), 12 pcs., 1.4 oz.	230	3.0	16.0	17.0	<5	5	3.0
chocolate, candy coated:							
(*M&M's*), 1.7-oz. pkg.	240	2.0	34.0	10.0	5	30	1.0
(*M&M's* Fun Size), 1 pkg.	100	1.0	15.0	4.5	5	15	1.0
(*M&M's Minis*), 1.08-oz. tube . . .	150	1.0	21.0	7.0	5	20	1.0
almond (*M&M's*), 1.3-oz. pkg.	200	3.0	21.0	11.0	5	15	2.0
crispy (*M&M's*), 1.5-oz. pkg. . . .	200	2.0	31.0	8.0	5	60	1.0
crispy (*M&M's* Fun Size), 3 pkgs. . .	200	2.0	30.0	8.0	5	60	1.0
dolce de leche (*M&M's* Single), 1 pkg.	250	3.0	31.0	13.0	5	40	0
peanut (*M&M's*), 1.74-oz. pkg. . .	250	5.0	30.0	13.0	5	25	2.0
peanut (*M&M's* Fun Size), 1 pkg. . . .	110	2.0	13.0	5.0	0	10	1.0
peanut butter (*M&M's*), 1.63-oz. pkg.	240	5.0	26.0	14.0	5	100	2.0
chocolate, dark:							
(*Dove*), 1.3-oz. bar	200	2.0	22.0	12.0	5	0	2.0
(*Dove* Miniatures), 7 pcs.	220	2.0	26.0	14.0	5	0	2.0
(*Estee* Bar), 7 sqs.	200	2.0	23.0	14.0	10	10	0
(*Hershey's Special Dark*), 1.45-oz. bar	220	2.0	24.0	13.0	<5	0	3.0
(*Hershey's Special Dark* Miniatures), 5 pcs., 1.5 oz. . .	230	2.0	25.0	14.0	<5	0	3.0
(*Lindt* Thins), 15 pcs., 1.5 oz.	260	2.0	20.0	19.0	0	5	0
almond (*Hershey's Nuggets*), 4 pcs., 1.3 oz.	220	3.0	19.0	15.0	<5	0	3.0

Food and Measure	cal.	prot. (gms)	carbo. (gms)	fat (gms)	chol. (mgs)	sod. (mgs	fiber (gms)
mint filled (*Ghirardelli*), 3 pcs., 1.5 oz. . .	200	1.0	29.0	11.0	0	0	1.0
chocolate, hard, plain or mint:							
(*Hershey's Taste-tations*), 3 pcs.	60	0	12.0	1.5	<5	30	0
(*Nips*), 2 pcs.	60	0	11.0	.5	0	40	0
(*Nips* Parfait), 2 pcs.	60	0	10.0	2.0	0	30	0
chocolate, milk:							
(*Cadbury*), 9 blocks, 1.4 oz.	220	3.0	24.0	12.0	10	45	<1.0
(*Dove*), 1.3-oz. bar	200	2.0	22.0	12.0	5	25	1.0
(*Dove Promises*), 5 pcs., 1.4 oz. . .	220	2.0	24.0	13.0	5	25	1.0
(*Estee* Bar), 7 sqs.	230	4.0	17.0	17.0	20	65	0
(*Hershey's*), 1.5-oz. bar	230	3.0	25.0	13.0	10	40	1.0
(*Hershey's Hugs*), 9 pcs., 1.4 oz. . .	220	3.0	23.0	13.0	10	35	0
(*Hershey's Kiss* Giant), ⅕ pkg., 1.4 oz.	210	3.0	23.0	12.0	10	35	1.0
(*Hershey's Kisses*), 1.5-oz. pkg. . . .	230	3.0	24.0	13.0	10	35	1.0
(*Hershey's Kisses* Extra Creamy), 9 pcs., .4 oz. . . .	220	3.0	24.0	12.0	10	40	1.0
(*Hershey's Nuggets*), 4 pcs., 1.4 oz. . .	210	3.0	23.0	12.0	10	35	1.0
(*Hershey's Sym-phony*), 1.5-oz. bar	230	4.0	24.0	13.0	10	40	<1.0
(*Lindt* Excellence), 12 pcs., 1.4 oz.	210	2.0	21.0	13.0	0	0	3.0
(*Lindt* Fairy Tales), 14 pcs., 1.4 oz.	210	3.0	22.0	12.0	5	60	0
(*Lindt* Milk Truffle Bar), 5 pcs., 1.5 oz.	260	2.0	17.0	21.0	5	35	0
(*Lindt* Mocca), 12 pcs., 1.4 oz. .	220	2.0	22.0	13.0	10	45	1.0

Food and Measure	cal.	prot. (gms)	carbo. (gms)	fat (gms)	chol. (mgs)	sod. (mgs)	fiber (gms)
Candy, chocolate, milk *(cont.)*							
(*Lindt* Swiss Classic Milk), 12 pcs., 1.4 oz.	210	3.0	23.0	12.0	5	75	1.0
(*Lindt* Swiss Milk Gold), 5 pcs., 1.3 oz.	200	3.0	21.0	11.5	5	60	0
(*Lindt* Thins), 15 pcs., 1.5 oz.	230	2.0	22.0	15.0	5	35	0
(*Nestlé*), 1.45-oz. bar	220	2.0	26.0	13.0	10	25	<1.0
almond (*Cadbury* Roast), 9 blocks, 1.4 oz.	220	4.0	21.0	13.0	10	80	1.0
almond (*Hershey's*), 1.45-oz. bar	230	5.0	20.0	14.0	5	35	1.0
almond (*Hershey's Bites*), 17 pcs., 1.4 oz.	220	4.0	20.0	14.0	5	30	1.0
almond (*Hershey's Kisses*), 9 pcs., 1.4 oz.	230	4.0	21.0	14.0	10	30	1.0
almond (*Hershey's Nuggets*), 4 pcs., 1.3 oz.	210	4.0	20.0	13.0	5	30	1.0
almond (*Lindt* Alba), 5 pcs., 1.5 oz. ..	240	3.0	20.0	16.0	5	45	1.0
almond (*Lindt* Swiss), 12 pcs., 1.4 oz.	220	4.0	18.0	14.0	5	50	1.0
almond toffee (*Hershey's Symphony*), 1.5-oz. bar	230	4.0	22.0	14.0	10	50	1.0
caramel (*Caramello*), 1.23-oz. bar ...	170	2.0	22.0	8.0	10	45	0
caramel (*Ghirardelli*), 3 pcs. 1.5 oz. ..	210	2.0	25.0	12.0	10	60	<1.0
caramel (*Lindt*), 5 pcs., 1.5 oz. ..	210	2.0	23.0	11.0	8	45	.5
chocolate filled (*Ghirardelli*), 3 pcs., 1.5 oz. ..	210	2.0	25.0	13.0	5	25	<1.0

Food and Measure	cal.	prot. (gms)	carbo. (gms)	fat (gms)	chol. (mgs)	sod. (mgs)	fiber (gms)
cookies and mint (*Hershey's*), 1.5-oz. bar	230	3.0	27.0	12.0	10	80	1.0
crisps (*Cadbury's Krisp*), 9 blocks, 1.4 oz.	200	3.0	25.0	10.0	10	80	<1.0
crisps (*Estee* Bar), 7 sqs.	370	7.0	29.0	26.0	30	110	0
crisps (*Krackel*), 1.45-oz. bar ...	220	3.0	26.0	11.0	<5	80	<1.0
crisps (*Nestlé Crunch*), 1.55-oz. bar ...	230	2.0	29.0	12.0	10	65	<1.0
crisps (*Nestlé Crunch* Fun Size), 4 bars	200	2.0	26.0	10.0	10	60	<1.0
eggs, candy coated (*Hershey*), 1.5-oz. pkg. ...	220	3.0	30.0	10.0	5	30	<1.0
fruit and nuts (*Cadbury*), 9 blocks, 1.4 oz.	210	3.0	24.0	11.0	5	45	1.0
fruit and nuts (*Chunky*), 1.4-oz. bar	210	3.0	24.0	11.0	5	20	1.0
fruit and nuts (*Estee* Bar), 7 sqs.	220	4.0	18.0	16.0	20	65	0
hazelnut (*Lindt* Swiss), 5 pcs., 1.3 oz.	210	3.0	19.0	14.0	<5	60	1.0
hazelnut (*Lindt* Swiss), 12 pcs., 1.4 oz.	230	3.0	19.0	16.0	<5	60	1.0
hazelnut w/raisins (*Lindt*), 5 pcs., 1.3 oz.	210	3.0	21.0	12.0	<5	40	1.0
orange filled (*Ghirardelli*), 3 pcs., 1.5 oz.	210	2.0	25.0	13.0	5	30	<1.0
peanut (*Mr. Goodbar*), 1.7-oz. bar	270	5.0	25.0	17.0	<5	20	2.0
pistachio (*Lindt*), 5 pcs., 1.5 oz. ..	250	3.0	20.0	17.0	<5	55	1.0

Food and Measure	cal.	prot. (gms)	carbo. (gms)	fat (gms)	chol. (mgs)	sod. (mgs)	fiber (gms)
Candy, chocolate, milk *(cont.)*							
raisins and almonds (*Hershey's Nuggets*), 4 pcs., 1.4 oz.	190	3.0	23.0	10.0	5	30	1.0
raisins, hazelnuts, almonds (*Lindt*), 12 pcs., 1.4 oz.	200	3.0	22.0	12.0	<5	45	1.0
toffee and almonds (*Hershey's Nuggets*), 4 pcs., 1.3 oz.	210	4.0	20.0	13.0	10	45	1.0
chocolate, white:							
(*Lindt* White Lindor Truffle), 7 pcs., 1.4 oz.	240	2.0	17.0	19.0	5	25	0
(*Lindt* Swiss), 4 pcs., 1.3 oz.	220	2.0	19.0	15.5	5	45	0
(*Lindt* Swiss), 12 pcs., 1.4 oz	230	3.0	22.0	14.0	5	45	0
cookies (*Hershey's Cookies 'n' Creme*), 1.5-oz. bar	220	4.0	25.0	12.0	5	95	0
cookies (*Hershey's Cookies 'n' Creme Bites*), 18 pcs., 1.4 oz.	210	4.0	23.0	11.0	<5	85	0
cookies (*Hershey's Cookies 'n' Creme Nuggets*), 4 pcs., 1.3 oz.	190	3.0	21.0	10.0	5	80	0
crisps (*Nestlé White Crunch*), 1.4-oz. bar	220	3.0	23.0	13.0	10	70	0
chocolate twists:							
(*I. M. Good*), 3 pcs., .6 oz.	120	1.0	27.0	5.0	0	90	0
(*Twizzlers*), 3 pcs., 1.5 oz.	150	1.0	32.0	1.5	0	95	<1.0
chocolate wafer bar (*Lindt*), 5 pcs., 1.5 oz.	220	3.0	24.0	14.0	5	25	<1.0

Food and Measure	cal.	prot. (gms)	carbo. (gms)	fat (gms)	chol. (mgs)	sod. (mgs	fiber (gms)
coconut, chocolate coated:							
(*Mounds*), 1.9-oz. pkg.	250	2.0	31.0	13.0	0	80	3.0
almond (*Almond Joy*), 1.7-oz. bar	240	2.0	29.0	13.0	0	70	2.0
almond (*Almond Joy Bites*), 18 pcs., 1.4 oz.	220	2.0	22.0	14.0	<5	15	1.0
white (*Lindt Excellence*), 4 pcs., 1.4 oz.	240	2.0	19.0	17.0	5	50	1.0
coffee (*Nips*), 2 pcs.	50	0	10.0	1.5	0	40	0
cotton candy (*Fluffy Stuff*), ½ bag, 1.6 oz.	180	0	44.0	0	0	0	0
creme de menthe, chocolate thin (*Andes*), 8 pcs. . . .	200	2.0	22.0	13.0	0	15	<1.0
fruit flavor:							
(*Charms Sour Balls*), 1 pc.	20	0	5.0	0	0	0	0
(*Charms Squares*), 2 pcs.	25	0	6.0	0	0	0	0
(*Chuckles*), 4 pcs., 1.6 oz.	150	0	37.0	0	0	15	0
(*Estee* Assorted No Sugar), 5 pcs. . . .	30	0	16.0	0	0	0	0
(*LifeSavers*), 2 pcs.	20	0	5.0	0	0	0	0
(*LifeSavers* Large), 4 pcs.	60	0	16.0	0	0	0	0
(*LifeSavers Delites*), 5 pcs.	30	0	15.0	0	0	0	0
(*Skittles* Original), 1.5 oz.	170	0	39.0	2.0	0	5	0
(*Skittles* Original Single), 2.2-oz. bag	240	0	54.0	2.5	0	10	0
(*Skittles Sours* Original Single), 1 bag	200	0	44.0	2.0	0	5	0
(*Starburst* Hard), 3 pcs., .5 oz. . . .	50	0	13.0	0	0	25	0

Food and Measure	cal.	prot. (gms)	carbo. (gms)	fat (gms)	chol. (mgs)	sod. (mgs)	fiber (gms)
Candy, fruit flavor *(cont.)*							
(*Tootsie Flavor Roll*),							
6 pcs., 1.4 oz.	170	0	35.0	3.0	0	25	0
(*Twizzlers Twist-n-*							
Fill), 1-oz. pc.	90	<1.0	21.0	.5	0	110	0
all flavors, except							
cherry (*Pull 'n'*							
Peel), 1.2-oz. pc.	110	1.0	26.0	0	0	80	0
cherry (*Nibs*),							
27 pcs., 1.4 oz.	140	1.0	31.0	1.0	0	85	0
cherry (*Pull 'n' Peel*),							
3 pcs., 1.3 oz.	120	1.0	27.0	0	0	85	0
cherry (*Switzer*							
Bites), 18 pcs.,							
1.4 oz.	140	1.0	31.0	1.0	0	120	<1.0
and creme (*Creme*							
Savers), 3 pcs.	60	<1.0	11.0	1.5	0	35	0
citrus sour slices							
(*Estee*), 9 pcs.	60	0	30.0	0	0	50	0
hard (*Jolly Rancher*),							
3 pcs., .6 oz.	70	0	17.0	0	0	10	0
strawberry twists							
(*Twizzlers*),							
1.7-oz. pkg.	170	1.0	38.0	.5	0	125	0
twists (*Starburst*							
Single),							
2-oz. pkg.	200	0	45.0	2.0	0	25	0
tropical (*Estee* No							
Sugar), 5 pcs.	30	0	16.0	0	0	0	0
tropical or wild							
cherry (*Skittles*							
Single), 1 bag	240	0	54.0	2.5	0	10	0
fruit flavor, chews:							
(*Chewmongus*),							
.6-oz. pc.	60	0	15.0	.5	0	0	0
(*Jolly Rancher*),							
2 oz.	210	0	48.0	0	0	0	0
(*LifeSavers Fruit*							
Chews), 11 pcs.	150	0	36.0	1.5	0	45	0
(*Starburst*), 2.1-oz.							
pkg.	240	0	48.0	5.0	0	0	0
fruit flavor, gummed:							
(*Amazin' Fruit*),							
1.5-oz. bag	140	2.0	32.0	0	0	50	0

Food and Measure	cal.	prot. (gms)	carbo. (gms)	fat (gms)	chol. (mgs)	sod. (mgs)	fiber (gms)
(*Dots* Original/Tropical/Wild Berry), 12 pcs., 1.5 oz.	150	0	37.0	0	0	20	0
(*Gummi Bears*), 1.4-oz. pkg. . . .	110	4.0	24.0	0	0	170	0
(*Gummi Jujubes*), 45 pcs., 1.4 oz.	110	4.0	24.0	0	0	170	0
(*Gummi Savers*), 10 pcs.	130	1.0	30.0	0	0	0	0
(*Jolly Rancher* Gummis), 1.7-oz. pkg.	150	2.0	36.0	0	0	0	0
(*Jolly Rancher Jolly Jellies* Sweet n' Fruity), 1.3-oz. pkg.	110	<1.0	28.0	0	0	45	0
(*Jujubes*), 1.5-oz. box	130	0	32.0	0	0	120	0
(*Jujyfruits*), 2.1-oz. box	200	0	51.0	0	0	45	0
(*Jujyfruits* Soft), 15 pcs., 1.4 oz.	130	0	32.0	0	0	170	0
(*LifeSavers* Fruit Slices), 9 pcs., 1.4 oz.	140	0	36.0	0	0	10	0
(*Sour Dudes*), 2-oz. bag	190	0	48.0	0	0	40	0
apple rings (*Estee*), 5 pcs.	70	0	28.0	0	0	5	0
gum, chewing:							
(*Doublemint/Juicy Fruit/Big Red/ Winterfresh/ Wrigley's Spearmint*), 1 pc. . . .	10	0	2.0	0	0	0	0
(*Eclipse*), 2 pcs. . .	5	0	2.0	0	0	0	0
(*Eggums*), 2 pcs. . .	10	0	3.0	0	0	0	0
(*Extra* Sugar Free), 1 pc.	5	0	2.0	0	0	0	0
(*Freedent*), 1 pc. .	10	0	2.0	0	0	0	0
(*Rainblo*), 1 pc. . .	15	0	4.0	0	0	0	0
(*Rainblo Jumblo*), 1 pc.	45	0	11.0	0	0	0	0
(*Rainblo Mega Eggs*), 1 pc. . . .	200	0	51.0	0	0	10	0

Food and Measure	cal.	prot. (gms)	carbo. (gms)	fat (gms)	chol. (mgs)	sod. (mgs)	fiber (gms)
Candy *(cont.)*							
hard, see "fruit flavor," above and specific flavors							
hazelnuts, chocolate coated (*Lindt*), 1.4 oz.	220	4.0	17.0	17.0	5	25	2.0
honey (*Bit-O-Honey*), 1.7-oz. bar	190	1.0	40.0	.5	0	125	0
(*Hot Dollars* Soft), 15 pcs., 1.4 oz. . . .	130	0	32.0	0	0	20	0
jelly beans, 1.4 oz.:							
(*Jolly Rancher Jolly Beans*), 25 pcs.	130	0	33.0	0	0	30	0
(*LifeSavers*), 32 pcs.	150	0	37.0	0	0	0	0
(*Smucker's*), 25 pcs.	150	0	37.0	0	0	0	0
(*Starburst*), ¼ cup	150	0	38.0	0	0	15	0
licorice:							
(*Crows/Mason Dots*), 12 pcs., 1.5 oz.	150	0	37.0	0	0	20	0
(*Diamond*), 10 pcs., 1.4 oz.	120	0	31.0	0	0	105	0
(*Nibs*), 22 pcs. . . .	140	1.0	31.0	1.0	0	220	0
(*Switzer Bites*), 18 pcs., 1.4 oz.	130	1.0	31.0	.5	0	210	<1.0
(*Twizzlers*), 3 pcs., 1.23 oz.	120	1.0	27.0	.5	0	180	0
(*Twizzlers* Bites), 16 pcs., 1.4 oz.	130	1.0	30.0	1.0	0	210	0
jelly beans (*Jelly Belly*), 35 pcs., 1.4 oz.	140	0	37.0	0	0	10	0
twists (*Twizzlers*), 2.5-oz. pkg. . . .	240	3.0	55.0	1.0	0	350	0
licorice, candy coated:							
(*Good & Fruity*), 1.75-oz. box . . .	180	0	45.0	0	0	30	0
(*Good & Plenty*), 1.75-oz. box . . .	170	<1.0	43.0	0	0	120	0
lollipop, all flavors, 1 pop:							
(*Candy Cane Pops*)	60	0	16.0	0	0	10	0
(*Caramel Apple Pops*)	70	0	17.0	.5	0	20	0

Food and Measure	cal.	prot. (gms)	carbo. (gms)	fat (gms)	chol. (mgs)	sod. (mgs	fiber (gms)
(*Charms*), 1 flat or 3 mini, .5 oz.	60	0	14.0	0	0	0	0
(*Charms Blow Pop* Regular)	70	0	17.0	0	0	0	0
(*Charms Blow Pop* Super)	150	0	36.0	.5	0	0	<1.0
(*Charms Sweet/Sour Pop* Regular)	70	0	18.0	0	0	0	0
(*Charms Way-2-Sour Blow Pop* Regular)	70	0	17.0	0	0	0	0
(*Dum-Dums*), .2 oz.	20	0	5.0	0	0	0	0
(*Fruit Smoothie Pops*)	60	0	16.0	0	0	5	0
(*Hot Chocolate Pops*)	70	0	17.0	.5	0	45	0
(*Jolly Rancher*)	60	0	16.0	0	0	10	0
(*Starburst* Chew Pop)	50	0	13.0	0	0	5	0
(*Sugar Daddy* Large)	200	1.0	43.0	2.5	<5	100	0
(*Sugar Daddy* Junior), 3 pops	160	<1.0	34.0	2.0	<5	80	0
(*Tootsie Pops*), .6 oz.	60	0	16.0	0	0	10	0
malted milk balls:							
(*Whoppers*), 18 pcs., 1.44 oz.	190	1.0	31.0	7.0	0	135	<1.0
(*Whoppers*), .75-oz. pouch	150	<1.0	16.0	3.5	0	70	0
(*Whoppers* Eggs), 6 pcs., 1.3 oz.	180	1.0	27.0	7.0	0	95	0
(*Whoppers* Mini Eggs), 1.7-oz. pkg.	230	2.0	36.0	9.0	0	125	<1.0
marshmallow:							
(*Kraft Jet-Puffed*), 5 pcs.	110	<1.0	27.0	0	0	40	0
egg, chocolate coated (*Hershey's*), .9-oz. pc.	100	1.0	17.0	3.5	<5	15	0
peanut (*Spangler*), 6 pcs.	163	0	41.0	0	0	0	0
(*Mexican Hats*), 10 pcs., 1.4 oz.	120	0	30.0	0	0	210	0
(*Milky Way*), 2-oz. bar	270	2.0	41.0	10.0	5	95	1.0

Food and Measure	cal.	prot. (gms)	carbo. (gms)	fat (gms)	chol. (mgs)	sod. (mgs)	fiber (gms)
Candy *(cont.)*							
(*Milky Way* Fun Size), 2 bars	180	2.0	28.0	7.0	5	65	0
(*Milky Way* Lite), 1.57-oz. bar	170	2.0	34.0	5.0	5	75	0
(*Milky Way* Lite Miniatures), 5 pcs.	150	1.0	29.0	4.5	5	65	0
(*Milky Way* Midnight), 1.76-oz. bar	220	1.0	36.0	8.0	5	85	1.0
(*Milky Way* Midnight Fun Size), 2 bars . .	170	1.0	28.0	7.0	5	65	1.0
(*Milky Way* Midnight Miniatures), 5 pcs.	180	1.0	29.0	7.0	5	70	1.0
(*Milky Way* Miniatures), 5 pcs.	190	2.0	30.0	7.0	5	70	0
mint:							
(*Junior* Chews), 26 pcs., 1.4 oz. .	150	0	33.0	1.0	0	130	0
(*LifeSavers*), 2 pcs.	20	0	5.0	0	0	0	0
(*LifeSavers* Large), 4 pcs.	60	0	16.0	0	0	0	0
assorted (*Estee* No Sugar), 5 pcs. . .	30	0	16.0	0	0	0	0
jelly filled (*Richardson's* After Dinner), 15 pcs., 1.5 oz.	170	0	40.0	0	0	0	0
peppermint (*Hershey's Tastetations*), 3 pcs., .6 oz.	60	0	15.0	0	0	15	0
mint, chocolate coated:							
(*After Eight* Thins), 8 pcs., 1.5 oz. . .	170	<1.0	31.0	5.0	0	0	<1.0
(*Andes* Mint Parfait), 8 pcs.	210	2.0	22.0	13.0	0	20	0
(*Andes* Mint Patties), 3 pcs., 1.5 oz. . .	180	0	38.0	3.0	0	5	0
(*Junior Mints*), 16 pcs., 1.4 oz.	160	1.0	34.0	2.5	0	5	<1.0
(*York* Bites), 15 pcs., 1.4 oz.	150	<1.0	31.0	3.0	0	20	<1.0
(*York* Peppermint Pattie), 1.4-oz. pkg.	160	<1.0	32.0	3.0	0	10	<1.0

Food and Measure	cal.	prot. (gms)	carbo. (gms)	fat (gms)	chol. (mgs)	sod. (mgs)	fiber (gms)
peppermint swirl (*Estee*), 3 pcs. .	30	0	14.0	0	0	0	0
(*Nestlé Mocha Crunch*), 1.3-oz. bar	200	2.0	21.0	12.0	10	65	0
(*Nestlé Turtles*), 2 pcs.	160	2.0	20.0	9.0	<5	40	<1.0
nonpareils (*Sno Caps*), 2.3-oz. box	300	2.0	48.0	13.0	0	0	3.0
(*NutRageous*), 1.9-oz. bar	290	6.0	29.0	17.0	0	75	2.0
nougat, w/chocolate:							
chocolate (*Charleston Chew*), 1.9 oz.	230	3.0	40.0	6.0	0	50	1.0
strawberry (*Charleston Chew*), 1.9 oz.	230	1.0	42.0	6.0	0	60	<1.0
vanilla (*Charleston Chew*), 1.9 oz. .	230	2.0	40.0	7.0	0	50	1.0
vanilla, mini (*Charleston Chew*), 13 pcs., 1.4 oz.	180	1.0	30.0	6.0	0	35	0
(*Oh Henry!*), .9-oz. bar	120	2.0	16.0	5.0	<5	60	0
(*100 Grand*), 1.5-oz. pkg.	190	1.0	30.0	8.0	5	75	<1.0
pecan caramel cluster (*Pot of Gold*), 2 oz.	310	4.0	31.0	19.0	10	85	1.0
peanut, butter toffee:							
(*Fisher*), 1 oz. . . .	130	3.0	17.0	6.0	0	150	1.0
(*Old Dominion*), 1 oz.	140	4.0	16.0	7.0	0	20	2.0
(*Smithfield Tavern*), 2 tbsp., 1 oz. . .	180	6.0	7.0	14.0	0	140	2.0
peanut, chocolate coated:							
(*Goobers*), 1.38-oz. bag	210	4.0	20.0	13.0	5	15	1.0
dark (*Setton Farm*), ¼ cup, 1.6 oz.	230	7.0	15.0	20.0	0	20	2.0
milk (*Setton Farm*), ¼ cup, 1.6 oz.	240	7.0	18.0	18.0	<5	20	2.0
peanut bar:							
(*PayDay*), 1.8-oz. bar	260	6.0	29.0	13.0	0	210	2.0
(*Planters*), 1.6 oz. . .	230	6.0	22.0	14.0	0	70	2.0
peanut brittle (*Estee*), ⅓ box	160	3.0	28.0	9.0	10	115	1.0

Food and Measure	cal.	prot. (gms)	carbo. (gms)	fat (gms)	chol. (mgs)	sod. (mgs)	fiber (gms)
Candy (cont.)							
peanut butter, chocolate:							
(*5th Avenue*), 2 oz.	280	5.0	38.0	12.0	<5	95	1.0
(*Reese's* Crunchy Cookie Cups), .6-oz. pkg.	90	1.0	10.0	5.0	0	45	<1.0
(*Reese's* Crunchy Cookie Cups Miniatures), 5 pcs., 1.4 oz.	200	3.0	23.0	11.0	<5	105	1.0
(*Reese's* Cup), 1.2-oz. pkg. . . .	180	3.0	19.0	10.0	0	105	1.0
(*Reese's* Cup Miniatures), 1.6-oz. pkg. . . .	250	4.0	26.0	14.0	<5	130	2.0
(*Reese's Bites*), 16 pcs., 1.4 oz. .	210	4.0	22.0	12.0	<5	70	1.0
(*Treasures*), 4 pcs., 1.5 oz.	240	3.0	22.0	16.0	5	80	1.0
candy coated (*Reese's Pieces*), 1.6-oz. pkg. . . .	230	6.0	26.0	11.0	0	90	1.0
crunchy, bar (*Hershey's Sweet Escapes*), .7-oz. bar	90	2.0	13.0	3.0	0	40	0
egg (*Reese's*), 1.2 oz.	180	4.0	19.0	10.0	0	145	1.0
peanut butter cookie (*Twix*), 2 pcs., 1.8 oz.	280	4.0	28.0	17.0	5	120	2.0
peanut butter parfait (*Nips*), 2 pcs. . . .	60	<1.0	10.0	2.0	0	45	0
(*Pot of Gold* All Nuts), 1.5 oz.	240	4.0	22.0	15.0	<5	40	1.0
praline, chocolate (*Lindt*), 3 pcs., 1.3 oz.	200	2.0	18.0	14.0	5	40	0
pretzel, chocolate:							
(*Estee*), 7 pcs. . . .	130	2.0	19.0	6.0	0	270	<1.0
milk (*Flipz*), 1 oz.	130	1.0	19.0	6.0	<5	90	<1.0
white fudge (*Flipz*), 1 oz.	140	2.0	19.0	6.0	0	95	0

Food and Measure	cal.	prot. (gms)	carbo. (gms)	fat (gms)	chol. (mgs)	sod. (mgs)	fiber (gms)
raisins, chocolate coated:							
(*Estee*), 1.4 cup ...	180	3.0	27.0	6.0	<5	45	1.0
(*Lindt*), 1.5 oz. ...	190	2.0	25.0	10.0	5	20	2.0
(*Raisinets*), 1.58-oz. bag	190	2.0	31.0	8.0	<5	15	1.0
(*Setton Farm*), 2 tbsp.	100	1.0	18.0	4.0	<5	15	1.0
(*Red Hot Dollars*), 15 pcs., 1.4 oz. ..	140	0	34.0	0	0	0	0
(*Robin Eggs*), 8 pcs., 1.4 oz.	180	1.0	31.0	6.0	0	70	0
(*Robin Eggs Mini*), 1.8-oz. box	230	1.0	40.0	7.0	0	115	<1.0
(*Snickers*), 2-oz. bar .	280	4.0	35.0	14.0	5	140	1.0
(*Snickers* Fun Size), 2 bars	190	3.0	24.0	10.0	5	100	1.0
(*Snickers* Miniature), 4 pcs.	170	3.0	22.0	9.0	5	90	1.0
(*Snickers Crunchier*), 1.56-oz. bar or 3 fun-size bars	230	4.0	25.0	13.0	5	140	1.0
soy nuts, chocolate dipped (*Tofutti* Totally Nuts), 1 oz.	190	1.0	30.0	7.0	0	100	<1.0
(*Spree/SweeTarts*), 8 pcs., .5 oz.	60	0	14.0	0	0	0	0
(*Spree/SweeTarts* Mini Chewy), .5 oz.	60	0	13.0	0	0	0	0
strawberry, see "fruit flavor," above							
(*Sugar Babies*), 30 pcs., 1.6 oz. ..	180	<1.0	39.0	2.0	0	70	0
(*3 Musketeers*), 2.1-oz. bar	260	2.0	46.0	8.0	5	110	1.0
(*3 Musketeers* Fun Size), 2 bars	140	1.0	26.0	4.5	5	60	0
(*3 Musketeers* Miniatures), 7 pcs.	170	1.0	32.0	5.0	5	80	1.0
toffee:							
(*Estee*), 5 pcs. ...	30	0	16.0	0	0	0	0
(*Heath* Bar), 1.4 oz.	210	1.0	24.0	12.0	10	135	<1.0
(*Heath* Bits), 1 tbsp.	80	<1.0	9.0	4.5	<5	60	0

Food and Measure	cal.	prot. (gms)	carbo. (gms)	fat (gms)	chol. (mgs)	sod. (mgs)	fiber (gms)
Candy, toffee *(cont.)*							
(Heath Bites),							
15 pcs., 1.4 oz. . .	210	1.0	25.0	12.0	5	100	<1.0
(Heath Bits O'							
Brickle), 1 tbsp.	80	<1.0	9.0	5.0	5	80	0
(Skor), 1.4-oz. bar	210	2.0	23.0	12.0	20	110	0
crunch, chocolate							
thin *(Andes),*							
8 pcs.	200	2.0	24.0	11.0	0	45	0
(Tootsie Roll Midgees),							
6 pcs., 1.4 oz.	160	<1.0	33.0	3.0	0	40	<1.0
(Tootsie Roll Snack Bar),							
2 bars, 1 oz.	110	<1.0	23.0	2.0	0	30	<1.0
(Top Secret), 2.2-oz.							
bar	320	6.0	35.0	17.0	0	30	2.0
truffles, chocolate:							
(Godiva), 1.5 oz. . .	220	2.0	24.0	13.0	10	15	0
(Pot of Gold Shells),							
1.5 oz.	210	2.0	26.0	11.0	5	25	1.0
amaretto, hazelnut,							
milk, mint, or orange							
(Lindt Lindor),							
.42-oz. ball	70	1.0	5.0	6.0	0	5	0
dark *(Lindt* Lindor),							
.42-oz. ball	70	1.0	5.0	6.0	0	0	0
peanut butter *(Lindt*							
Lindor), .42-oz.							
ball	70	1.0	5.0	6.0	0	20	0
white *(Lindt* Lindor)	80	1.0	5.0	6.0	0	10	0
vanilla almond café							
(Nips), 2 pcs.	50	0	10.0	1.0	0	40	0
wafer, chocolate, triple							
(Hershey's Sweet							
Escapes), .7-oz. bar	80	<1.0	13.0	2.5	0	30	0
wafer, w/chocolate:							
(Kit Kat), 4-pc. bar,							
1.5 oz.	220	3.0	27.0	11.0	<5	25	<1.0
(Kit Kat Chunky),							
1.9-oz. bar	290	3.0	35.0	15.0	<5	35	1.0
(Kit Kat Bites),							
15 pcs., 1.4 oz.	200	3.0	25.0	10.0	<5	25	<1.0
(Whatchamacallit),							
1.7-oz. bar	240	4.0	30.0	11.0	5	140	<1.0

Food and Measure	cal.	prot. (gms)	carbo. (gms)	fat (gms)	chol. (mgs)	sod. (mgs)	fiber (gms)
(*White Rabbit*), 8 pcs., 1.4 oz.	160	2.0	32.0	2.5	6	52	0
(*Wonderball*), 1-oz. pc.	140	1.0	21.0	6.0	<5	10	0
(*Wunderbeans*), 1.5-oz. box	150	0	37.0	0	0	10	0
(*Zagut*), 1.7-oz. bar ..	230	3.0	31.0	10.0	0	85	2.0
(*Zero*), 1.8-oz. bar ...	230	3.0	36.0	8.0	0	110	<1.0
Cane syrup, 1 tbsp.	52	0	13.4	0	0	<1	0
Cannellini beans, see "Kidney beans"							
Cannelloni dinner, frozen (*Amy's*), 9-oz. pkg.	330	16.0	34.0	12.0	35	390	6.0
Cannelloni entree, frozen, 1 pkg.:							
(*Lean Cuisine Everyday Favorites*), 9⅛ oz.	220	21.0	27.0	2.0	15	550	3.0
ricotta (*Wolfgang Puck's*), 12 oz. ...	420	20.0	37.0	21.0	80	610	13.0
Cannoli shell (*Ferrara*), .5-oz. shell	80	1.0	8.0	4.0	0	0	0
Cantaloupe:							
(*Dole*), ¼ medium ...	50	1.0	12.0	0	0	25	1.0
½ of 5" melon	94	2.3	22.3	.7	0	23	2.1
cubed, 1 cup	56	1.4	13.4	.5	0	14	1.3
Caper berries (*Haddon House*), ½ oz.	0	0	1.0	0	0	410	
Capers, 1 tbsp.:							
(*Crosse & Blackwell*)	5	0	1.0	0	0	350	0
(*Italica*)	0	0	<1.0	0	0	460	0
Capicola, see "Ham lunch meat"							
Capon, see "Chicken"							
Caponata, see "Eggplant appetizer"							
Cappuccino, see "Coffee, iced" and "Coffee, flavored, mix"							
Carambola:							
(*Frieda's* Starfruit), 5 oz.	45	1.0	11.0	0	0	0	4.0
1 medium, 4.7 oz. ..	42	.7	9.9	.4	0	2	3.4
sliced, ½ cup	18	.3	1.0	.2	0	1	1.5

Food and Measure	cal.	prot. (gms)	carbo. (gms)	fat (gms)	chol. (mgs)	sod. (mgs)	fiber (gms)
Carambola, dried (*Frieda's* Starfruit), ⅓ cup, 1.4 oz. ...	120	2.0	29.0	0	0	5	10.0
Caramel dip, see "Apple dip"							
Caramel syrup (*Smucker's* Sundae Syrup), 2 tbsp. ...	100	1.0	2.0	0	0	110	0
Caramel topping, 2 tbsp.:							
(*Hershey's Chocolate Shoppe*)	100	0	25.0	0	0	95	0
(*Kraft*)	120	2.0	28.0	0	0	90	0
(*Mrs. Richardson's*) ..	130	1.0	31.0	0	0	75	0
(*Smucker's*)	130	1.0	31.0	0	0	110	<1.0
(*Smucker's* Microwave)	110	0	28.0	0	0	122	0
(*Smucker's Magic Shell*)	220	2.0	13.0	18.0	5	30	0
(*Smucker's Plate Scrapers*)	100	1.0	25.0	0	0	105	0
butterscotch, see "Butterscotch topping"							
hot (*Smucker's*)	120	1.0	29.0	3.0	0	60	0
Caraway seed, 1 tsp.	7	.4	1.1	.3	0	<1	<1.0
Carbonara sauce mix (*Knorr* Pasta Sauces), 2 tbsp.	70	4.0	5.0	3.5	10	880	0
Cardamom, ground:							
1 tsp.	6	.2	1.4	.1	0	<1	.5
1 tbsp.	18	.6	4.0	.4	0	1	1.6
Cardoon:							
raw:							
(*Frieda's*), 1 cup, 3 oz.	15	1.0	4.0	0	0	140	1.0
shredded, ½ cup ..	18	.6	4.4	.1	0	151	1.4
boiled, drained, 4 oz.	25	.9	6.0	.1	0	200	n.a.
Caribbean spice rub (*Watkins*), ¼ tsp.	0	0	0	0	0	0	0
Caribou, meat only, roasted, 4 oz.	189	33.8	0	5.0	123	68	0
Carissa:							
1 medium, .8 oz. ...	12	.1	2.7	.3	0	1	n.a.

Food and Measure	cal.	prot. (gms)	carbo. (gms)	fat (gms)	chol. (mgs)	sod. (mgs)	fiber (gms)
sliced, ½ cup	46	.4	10.2	1.0	0	2	n.a.
Carl's Jr., 1 serving:							
breakfast items:							
bacon, 2 strips ...	45	3.0	0	4.0	10	150	0
burrito	550	29.0	36.0	32.0	495	980	1.0
eggs, scrambled ..	180	13.0	1.0	14.0	455	110	0
English muffin w/margarine ...	210	5.0	28.0	9.0	0	300	2.0
French Toast Dips, w/out syrup	370	6.0	42.0	20.0	0	430	1.0
sausage, 1 patty ..	190	7.0	2.0	18.0	40	480	0
sourdough	410	26.0	33.0	20.0	275	930	1.0
Sunrise Sandwich, no bacon or sausage	360	13.0	28.0	21.0	245	470	<1.0
quesadilla	370	15.0	38.0	17.0	240	910	1.0
sandwiches:							
Carl's bacon Swiss crispy chicken ..	760	31.0	72.0	38.0	90	1550	3.0
Carl's Catch Fish ..	530	16.0	55.0	28.0	80	1030	2.0
Carl's Famous Star .	590	24.0	50.0	32.0	70	910	3.0
Carl's ranch crispy chicken	660	24.0	71.0	31.0	70	1180	3.0
Carl's western bacon crispy chicken ..	760	31.0	91.0	28.0	80	1900	3.0
Charbroiled BBQ Chicken	290	25.0	41.0	3.5	60	840	2.0
Charbroiled BBQ Club	470	31.0	37.0	23.0	95	1110	2.0
Charbroiled Santa Fe Chicken	540	28.0	37.0	31.0	95	1210	2.0
charbroiled sirloin steak	550	30.0	52.0	24.0	80	1080	2.0
double sourdough bacon cheese-burger	880	50.0	37.0	59.0	165	1010	2.0
Double Western Bacon Cheese-burger	920	51.0	65.0	50.0	155	1770	3.0
Famous Bacon Cheeseburger ..	700	31.0	51.0	41.0	95	1310	3.0
hamburger	280	14.0	36.0	9.0	35	480	1.0
sourdough bacon cheeseburger ...	640	30.0	37.0	41.0	95	690	2.0

Food and Measure	cal.	prot. (gms)	carbo. (gms)	fat (gms)	chol. (mgs)	sod. (mgs)	fiber (gms)
Carls' Jr., sandwiches (cont.)							
sourdough ranch cheeseburger ...	720	33.0	43.0	46.0	95	800	3.0
Southwest spicy chicken	620	18.0	48.0	41.0	65	1640	2.0
spicy chicken	480	14.0	47.0	26.0	40	1220	2.0
Super Star	790	41.0	51.0	47.0	130	980	3.0
Western Bacon Cheeseburger ..	660	31.0	64.0	30.0	85	1410	3.0
sandwich cheese:							
American, large ...	60	3.0	1.0	5.0	15	260	0
American, small ...	50	3.0	1.0	4.0	10	200	0
Swiss style	50	4.0	0	4.0	15	230	0
side dishes:							
chicken stars, 6 pcs.	260	13.0	14.0	16.0	40	480	<1.0
CrissCut Fries	410	5.0	43.0	24.0	0	950	4.0
french fries:							
large	620	10.0	80.0	29.0	0	380	6.0
medium	460	7.0	59.0	22.0	0	280	5.0
small	290	5.0	37.0	14.0	0	180	3.0
hash brown nuggets	330	3.0	32.0	21.0	0	470	2.0
onion rings	430	7.0	53.0	22.0	0	700	3.0
zucchini	320	6.0	31.0	19.0	0	860	2.0
potatoes:							
plain, no margarine	290	6.0	68.0	0	0	20	6.0
bacon/cheese	640	21.0	75.0	29.0	40	1660	6.0
broccoli/cheese ...	530	11.0	76.0	21.0	15	940	6.0
sour cream/chives	430	7.0	70.0	14.0	10	180	6.0
salads:							
Charbroiled Chicken Salad-to-Go	200	25.0	12.0	7.0	75	440	4.0
Garden Salad-to-Go	50	3.0	4.0	2.5	10	60	2.0
salad dressings, 2 oz.:							
blue cheese	320	2.0	1.0	35.0	25	370	0
French, fat free ...	60	0	16.0	0	0	680	<1.0
house	220	1.0	3.0	22.0	25	450	0
Italian, fat free	15	0	4.0	0	0	770	0
Thousand Island ..	230	<1.0	5.0	23.0	20	420	0
breads/sauces:							
bread sticks	35	1.0	7.0	.5	0	60	<1.0
croutons	30	1.0	5.0	1.0	0	105	0
BBQ sauce	50	1.0	11.0	0	0	270	0
jelly or jam	40	0	9.0	0	0	15	0
honey sauce	90	0	22.0	0	0	0	0

Food and Measure	cal.	prot. (gms)	carbo. (gms)	fat (gms)	chol. (mgs)	sod. (mgs)	fiber (gms)
mustard sauce	50	0	11.0	0	0	210	0
salsa	10	0	2.0	0	0	160	0
sweet 'n' sour sauce	50	0	12.0	0	0	80	0
table syrup	90	0	21.0	0	0	0	0
bakery/desserts:							
blueberry muffin ..	340	5.0	49.0	14.0	40	340	1.0
bran raisin muffin	370	6.0	61.0	14.0	45	410	6.0
cheese Danish	400	5.0	49.0	23.0	15	390	1.0
chocolate cake	300	3.0	46.0	12.0	30	350	1.0
chocolate chip cookie	350	3.0	46.0	18.0	20	330	1.0
strawberry swirl cheesecake	290	6.0	30.0	17.0	55	230	0
shakes:							
chocolate, regular	770	21.0	140.0	15.0	65	520	<1.0
chocolate, small ...	530	14.0	96.0	10.0	45	350	0
strawberry, regular	750	20.0	133.0	15.0	65	490	0
strawberry, small ..	510	14.0	91.0	10.0	45	330	0
vanilla, regular	700	22.0	115.0	16.0	70	530	0
vanilla, small	470	15.0	78.0	11.0	50	350	0
Carnival squash (*Frieda's*), ¾ cup, 3 oz.	30	1.0	7.0	0	0	0	1.0
Carob drink mix, powder, 3 tsp. ...	45	.2	11.2	tr.	0	12	<1.0
Carob flour, 1 cup ...	395	4.8	91.6	.7	0	36	41.0
Carp, meat only:							
raw, 4 oz.	144	20.2	0	6.4	75	58	0
baked, broiled, or microwaved, 4 oz.	184	25.9	0	8.1	95	71	0
Carrot, fresh:							
raw:							
(*Dole*), 7" long, 1¼" diam.	35	1.0	8.0	0	0	40	2.0
(*Frieda's Gold*), ⅔ cup, 3 oz. ...	35	1.0	9.0	0	0	30	3.0
whole, 7½" long, 2.8 oz.	31	.7	7.3	.1	0	25	2.2
crinkle cut (*Mann's*), 3 oz.	35	1.0	9.0	0	0	30	3.0
shredded (*Dole*), 3 oz.	40	1.0	9.0	0	0	45	2.0
shredded (*Fresh Express*), 1 cup	45	1.0	10.0	0	0	55	3.0

Food and Measure	cal.	prot. (gms)	carbo. (gms)	fat (gms)	chol. (mgs)	sod. (mgs)	fiber (gms)
Carrot, fresh, raw *(cont.)*							
shredded, ½ cup ..	24	.6	5.6	.1	0	19	1.7
raw, baby:							
(*Grimmway*), 3 oz.	38	1.0	9.0	0	0	30	2.0
(*Mann's*), 3 oz. ...	38	1.0	9.0	0	0	44	2.0
1 medium,							
2¾" long	4	.1	.8	.1	0	3	.2
peeled mini (*Dole*),							
3 oz.	40	1.0	9.0	0	0	45	2.0
boiled, drained, sliced,							
½ cup	35	.9	8.2	.1	0	52	2.6
Carrot, can or jar,							
½ cup:							
whole, baby:							
(*Bonduelle*)	21	0	4.0	0	0	370	1.0
(*Greenleaf*)	21	0	4.0	0	0	370	1.0
(*Reese*)	15	<1.0	3.0	0	0	410	1.0
whole, sliced, or							
julienne (*S&W*) ...	30	1.0	5.0	0	0	390	2.0
sliced:							
(*Allens/Crest Top*)	35	0	8.0	0	0	40	3.0
(*Del Monte*)	35	0	8.0	0	0	300	3.0
(*Libby's*)	25	<1.0	6.0	0	0	270	2.0
(*Veg-All*)	30	0	5.0	0	0	320	2.0
w/liquid	28	.8	6.2	.2	0	297	1.1
drained	17	.5	4.0	.1	0	176	1.1
Carrot, dehydrated,							
(*AlpineAire*), .75 oz.	80	2.0	17.0	0	0	55	2.0
Carrot, frozen:							
baby:							
(*Birds Eye*), ½ cup	40	1.0	9.0	0	0	45	2.0
(*John Cope's*), 3 oz.	35	1.0	6.0	0	0	45	2.0
bell, small (*Bonduelle*							
Parisian), 3 oz. ...	35	0	8.0	0	0	45	2.0
honey glazed:							
(*Green Giant*), 1 cup	90	1.0	13.0	3.5	0	180	2.0
baby (*Cascadian*							
Farm), 1 cup ...	60	1.0	14.0	0	0	160	3.0
sliced:							
(*Birds Eye*), ½ cup	35	1.0	9.0	0	0	45	3.0
(*John Cope's*),							
⅔ cup	35	1.0	6.0	0	0	45	2.0

Food and Measure	cal.	prot. (gms)	carbo. (gms)	fat (gms)	chol. (mgs)	sod. (mgs)	fiber (gms)
boiled, drained, ½ cup	26	.9	6.0	.1	0	43	2.6
Carrot chips (*Hain*), 22 pcs., 1.1 oz. . . .	160	2.0	18.0	9.0	0	170	2.0
Carrot drink blend (*Santa Cruz Organic Super Carrot Zest*), 8 fl. oz.	130	1.0	30.0	0	0	30	0
Carrot juice (*Hollywood*), 8 fl. oz. . . .	120	2.0	27.0	1.0	0	250	1.0
Carrot juice blends:							
(*AriZona* Crazy Berry), 8 fl. oz.	110	.5	26.0	0	0	25	.6
(*AriZona* Crazy Cocktail), 8 fl. oz.	110	.5	27.0	0	0	25	.6
(*Ceres*), 5.25 fl. oz. . . .	87	0	21.0	0	0	n.a.	0
Casaba:							
¹⁄₁₀ of 7¾" melon	43	1.5	10.2	.2	0	20	1.3
cubed, 1 cup	44	1.5	10.5	.2	0	10	1.4
Cashew, 1 oz., except as noted:							
(*Bazzini's Nut Club* Salted), ¼ cup	200	5.0	8.0	16.0	0	45	2.0
(*Bazzini's Nut Club* Unsalted), ¼ cup . .	200	5.0	8.0	16.0	0	5	2.0
(*Fisher* Jumbo)	170	5.0	8.0	15.0	0	140	1.0
(*Frito-Lay* Salted)	180	5.0	7.0	15.0	0	190	1.0
(*Planters* Fancy)	170	5.0	8.0	14.0	0	120	1.0
(*Planters* Halves)	170	6.0	7.0	14.0	0	55	1.0
(*Planters* Halves w/Pieces)	170	6.0	7.0	14.0	0	120	1.0
(*Planters* Salted)	160	n.a.	8.0	14.0	0	160	1.0
raw, whole, ¼ cup:							
(*Bazzini's Nut Club*)	180	5.0	8.0	4.0	0	0	3.0
(*Blue Diamond*) . . .	190	5.0	9.0	15.0	0	0	3.0
dry-roasted:							
18 medium, 1 oz. . . .	163	4.4	9.3	13.2	0	4	.9
whole or halves, 1 cup	787	21.0	44.8	63.5	0	21	4.1
oil-roasted:							
18 medium, 1 oz. . . .	163	4.6	8.1	13.7	0	5	1.1
whole (*Blue Diamond*), ¼ cup . .	210	6.0	10.0	17.0	0	240	1.0

Food and Measure	cal.	prot. (gms)	carbo. (gms)	fat (gms)	chol. (mgs)	sod. (mgs)	fiber (gms)
Cashew, oil-roasted *(cont.)*							
whole or halves,							
1 cup	748	21.0	37.1	62.7	0	22	4.9
honey-roasted							
(*Planters*), 2-oz. pkg.	310	n.a.	23.0	24.0	0	170	3.0
roasted, 1.2 oz.:							
(*Setton Farm*)	200	5.0	10.0	16.0	0	40	1.0
(*Setton Farm*							
Unsalted)	200	5.0	10.0	16.0	0	0	1.0
Cashew butter (*Arrow-*							
head Mills), 2 tbsp.	160	5.0	8.0	14.0	0	0	1.0
Cassava (see also							
"Yuca root"), raw:							
14.4-oz. root	653	5.6	155.2	1.1	0	57	7.3
1 cup	330	2.8	78.4	.6	0	29	3.7
Catfish, channel, 4 oz.:							
farmed, meat only:							
raw	153	17.7	0	8.6	15	60	0
baked, broiled, or							
microwaved . . .	172	21.2	0	9.1	73	91	0
wild, meat only:							
raw, 4 oz.	108	18.6	0	3.2	66	49	0
baked, broiled, or							
microwaved · · ·	119	20.9	0	3.2	82	57	0
Catjang, boiled,							
½ cup	100	7.0	17.5	.6	0	16	3.1
Cauliflower, fresh:							
raw:							
(*Dole*), ⅙ medium							
head, 3.5 oz. . . .	25	2.0	5.0	0	0	30	5.0
florets (*Mann's*							
Cauliettes), 4 oz.	30	2.0	6.0	0	0	35	3.0
florets, 3 pcs.	14	1.1	2.9	.1	0	17	1.4
1" pcs., ½ cup	13	1.0	2.6	.1	0	15	1.3
boiled, drained, 1" pcs.,							
½ cup	14	1.1	2.6	.3	0	9	1.7
green:							
raw, ⅕ head	28	2.7	5.7	.3	0	22	3.0
raw, 1" pcs., ½ cup . .	16	1.5	3.0	.2	0	12	1.6
boiled, drained,							
1" pcs., ½ cup	20	1.9	3.9	.2	0	14	2.0
Cauliflower, frozen:							
(*Birds Eye*), ½ cup . .	20	2.0	4.0	0	0	15	2.0

Food and Measure	cal.	prot. (gms)	carbo. (gms)	fat (gms)	chol. (mgs)	sod. (mgs)	fiber (gms)
florets (*Green Giant*), 1 cup	20	2.0	3.0	0	0	25	2.0
boiled, drained, 1" pcs., ½ cup	17	1.5	3.4	.2	0	16	2.0
in cheese sauce (*Green Giant*), ½ cup	60	2.0	7.0	2.5	<5	510	1.0
Cauliflower combinations, frozen, nuggets, w/carrots and snow pea pods (*Birds Eye*), ½ cup	30	2.0	6.0	0	0	25	2.0
Cavatelli pasta dish, frozen, w/cheese (*Celentano*), 1 cup	400	14.0	77.0	1.5	15	10	4.0
Cavatelli pasta dish, mix, 1 cup*:							
butter and herb (*Lipton* Pasta & Sauce) . . .	270	7.0	40.0	9.5	5	830	2.0
roasted garlic chicken (*Lipton* Pasta & Sauce)	260	7.0	40.0	8.5	5	850	<1.0
Cavatappi pasta dish, mix, sun-dried tomato/basil pesto (*Land O Lakes*), 2.5 oz.	260	8.0	47.0	4.5	0	1040	2.0
Caviar (see also "Roe"), 1 tbsp., except as noted:							
black or red	40	3.9	.6	2.9	94	240	0
carp roe (*Krinos* Tarama)	20	3.0		.5	50	700	0
lumpfish, black, red, or gold (*Romanoff*)	15	1.0	0	1.0	50	380	0
salmon (*Romanoff*) . .	35	3.0	0	1.5	55	310	0
sturgeon, granular (*Romanoff* Beluga/ Osetra/Sevruga), 1 oz.	74	9.5	.9	4.3	n.a.	624	0
whitefish, black or gold (*Romanoff*)	25	1.0	1.0	1.5	45	300	0
Caviar spread, see "Taramosalata"							
Cayenne, see "Pepper"							

Food and Measure	cal.	prot. (gms)	carbo. (gms)	fat (gms)	chol. (mgs)	sod. (mgs)	fiber (gms)
Ceci, see "Garbanzo beans"							
Celeriac, fresh, raw:							
(*Frieda's* Celery Root),							
¾ cup, 3 oz.	35	1.0	8.0	0	0	85	2.0
trimmed, 4 oz.	44	1.7	10.4	.3	0	113	2.0
trimmed, ½ cup	31	1.2	7.2	.2	0	78	1.4
Celery:							
raw:							
(*Dole*), 2 stalks . . .	20	1.0	2.0	0	0	100	2.0
7½"-stalk, 1.6 oz. .	6	.3	1.5	.1	0	35	.7
diced, ½ cup	10	.5	2.2	.1	0	52	1.0
boiled, drained, diced,							
½ cup	13	.6	3.0	.1	0	68	1.2
Celery, Chinese							
(*Frieda's* Kun Choy),							
1 cup, 3 oz.	15	1.0	3.0	0	0	75	1.0
Celery, dehydrated,							
(*AlpineAire*), .3 oz.	25	1.0	5.0	0	0	125	1.0
Celery, dried, flake/							
seed (*Tone's*), 1 tsp.	9	.1	.9	.5	0	4	.3
Celery root, see							
"Celeriac"							
Celery salt:							
(*Tone's*), 1 tsp.	6	.3	.6	.4	0	1584	.2
(*McCormick*), ¼ tsp.	0	0	0	0	0	250	0
(*Watkins*), ¼ tsp. . . .	0	0	0	0	0	270	0
Cellophane noodles,							
see "Noodle, Asian"							
Celtus, raw, trimmed:							
1 oz.	6	.2	1.0	.1	0	3	.3
.3-oz. leaf	1	<.1	.3	0	0	1	.1
Cereal, ready-to-eat							
(see also specific							
grains), 1 cup,							
except as noted:							
amaranth flakes:							
(*Arrowhead Mills*)	128	3.0	23.0	1.0	0	0	2.0
(*Health Valley*),							
¾ cup	100	3.0	24.0	0	0	90	4.0
(*Boo Berry*)	120	1.0	27.0	1.0	0	210	0
bran:							
(*Kellogg's All-Bran*							
Original), ½ cup .	80	4.0	23.0	1.0	0	80	10.0

Food and Measure	cal.	prot. (gms)	carbo. (gms)	fat (gms)	chol. (mgs)	sod. (mgs)	fiber (gms)
(*Kellogg's All-Bran Bran Buds*), ⅓ cup	80	2.0	24.0	.5	0	200	13.0
(*Multi-Bran Chex*)	200	4.0	49.0	1.5	0	380	8.0
(*Post 100% Bran*), ⅓ cup	80	4.0	22.0	1.0	0	125	9.0
apple/cinnamon (*Health Valley Organic*), ¾ cup .	160	5.0	41.0	0	0	10	7.0
extra fiber (*Kellogg's All-Bran*), ½ cup	50	3.0	20.0	1.0	0	120	13.0
flakes (*Arrowhead Mills*)	90	4.0	18.0	1.0	0	80	5.0
flakes (*Hearty Start*), ¾ cup	90	3.0	23.0	.5	0	230	5.0
flakes (*Kellogg's Complete*), ¾ cup	90	3.0	23.0	.5	0	210	5.0
flakes (*Post Premium*), ¾ cup ..	100	3.0	24.0	.5	0	210	5.0
flakes, w/flax (*New Morning*)	110	4.0	21.0	1.0	0	5	5.0
bran, raisin:							
(*Arrowhead Mills*)	190	6.0	41.0	1.5	0	300	10.0
(*Erewhon*)	170	5.0	40.0	1.0	0	100	6.0
(*General Mills Para su Familia*), 1⅓ cups	170	5.0	41.0	1.5	0	320	6.0
(*General Mills Raisin Nut Bran*), ¾ cup	200	4.0	41.0	4.0	0	250	4.0
(*Gold Medal*), 1⅓ cups	170	5.0	41.0	1.5	0	320	6.0
(*Health Valley*), ¾ cup	160	5.0	40.0	0	0	10	6.0
(*Kellogg's*)	190	5.0	45.0	1.5	0	350	8.0
(*Kellogg's Raisin Bran Crunch*) ...	190	3.0	45.0	1.0	0	210	4.0
(*Malt-O-Meal*)	200	6.0	47.0	1.5	0	390	8.0
(*Post*)	190	4.0	46.0	1.0	0	360	8.0
(*Skinner's*)	170	6.0	41.0	1.0	0	85	7.0
(*Total*)	170	4.0	41.0	1.0	0	240	5.0
(*Wheaties*)	180	4.0	44.0	1.0	0	250	5.0
cinnamon cluster (*Post*)	220	4.0	48.0	3.0	0	250	7.0
flakes (*Health Valley*), 1¼ cups	190	5.0	47.0	0	0	90	6.0

Food and Measure	cal.	prot. (gms)	carbo. (gms)	fat (gms)	chol. (mgs)	sod. (mgs)	fiber (gms)
Cereal, ready-to-eat, bran, raisin *(cont.)*							
w/flax (*New Morning*)	90	3.0	22.0	.5	0	60	6.0
buckwheat flakes, maple (*Arrowhead Mills*)	160	4.0	35.0	1.0	0	210	3.0
corn:							
(*Barbara's Puffins*), ¾ cup	90	2.0	23.0	1.0	0	190	5.0
(*Barbara's Puffins Organic Eco Bag*)	100	2.0	25.0	1.0	0	210	6.0
(*Cocoa Puffs*)	120	1.0	26.0	1.0	0	170	0
(*Corn Bursts*)	120	1.0	29.0	0	0	120	0
(*Corn Chex*)	110	2.0	26.0	0	0	280	0
(*Cornfetti*), ¾ cup	110	2.0	24.0	1.0	0	130	<1.0
(*Ginseng Crunch*), ¾ cup	110	2.0	22.0	2.0	0	60	3.0
(*Health Valley CrunchEms*), 1¼ cups	110	2.0	27.0	0	0	160	2.0
(*Kellogg's Corn Pops*)	120	1.0	28.0	0	0	120	0
(*Kellogg's Crispix*) .	110	2.0	25.0	0	0	210	<1.0
cinnamon (*Barbara's Puffins*), 1¼ cups	100	2.0	26.0	1.0	0	150	6.0
cinnamon (*Kellogg's Crispix*), ¾ cup	120	1.0	26.0	1.0	0	180	<1.0
maple (*Arrowhead Mills*)	190	5.0	43.0	3.0	0	140	6.0
puffed (*Arrowhead Mills*)	60	2.0	11.0	.5	0	0	0
puffed (*Health Valley*)	110	2.0	26.0	0	0	5	2.0
cornflakes:							
(*Arrowhead Mills*)	130	3.0	30.0	0	0	65	2.0
(*Country*)	110	2.0	26.0	0	0	270	0
(*Erewhon*), 1¼ cups	210	5.0	45.0	2.5	0	100	3.0
(*Kellogg's Corn Flakes*)	100	2.0	24.0	0	0	200	1.0
(*Kellogg's Cocoa Frosted Flakes*), ¾ cup	120	1.0	28.0	0	0	170	0

Food and Measure	cal.	prot. (gms)	carbo. (gms)	fat (gms)	chol. (mgs)	sod. (mgs)	fiber (gms)
(*Kellogg's Frosted Flakes*), ¾ cup ...	120	1.0	28.0	0	0	150	1.0
(*Kellogg's Honey Crunch Corn Flakes*), ¾ cup ..	120	2.0	26.0	1.0	0	210	1.0
(*Malt-O-Meal*)	110	2.0	26.0	0	0	320	1.0
(*Post Toasties*) ...	100	2.0	24.0	0	0	260	1.0
(*Total*), 1⅓ cups ..	110	2.0	24.0	0	0	210	0
blue (*Health Valley Organic*), ¾ cup	100	3.0	24.0	0	0	10	4.0
w/flax (*New Morning*)	120	2.0	26.0	1.0	0	60	1.0
juice sweetened (*Barbara's*)	110	2.0	26.0	0	0	130	2.0
frosted (*General Mills Para Su Familia*), ¾ cup	110	1.0	26.0	0	0	250	0
frosted (*Malt-O-Meal*), ¾ cup ...	120	1.0	28.0	0	0	200	1.0
honey frosted (*New Morning*)	120	2.0	25.0	1.0	0	60	1.0
corn and amaranth (*Erewhon Aztec*) ..	110	2.0	26.0	0	0	70	1.0
flax, golden (*Health Valley*), ½ cup	190	6.0	38.0	3.0	0	30	6.0
granola:							
(*Kellogg's Lowfat*), ½ cup	190	4.0	39.0	3.0	0	120	3.0
all varieties (*Health Valley*), ⅔ cup .	190	5.0	42.0	2.0	0	90	6.0
clusters, w/honey (*Oatiola*), ¾ cup .	200	5.0	42.0	2.0	0	60	3.0
fruit (*Nature Valley Lowfat*), ⅔ cup .	210	4.0	44.0	2.5	0	210	3.0
oats and honey (*Quaker 100% Natural*), ½ cup .	220	5.0	31.0	9.0	0	20	3.5
oats, honey, raisins (*Quaker 100% Natural*), ½ cup .	225	5.0	34.0	9.0	0	25	3.5
w/raisins (*Kellogg's Lowfat*), ⅔ cup .	220	5.0	48.0	3.0	0	150	3.0
w/raisins (*Quaker 100% Natural*), ⅔ cup .	210	5.0	44.0	3.0	0	130	3.0

Food and Measure	cal.	prot. (gms)	carbo. (gms)	fat (gms)	chol. (mgs)	sod. (mgs)	fiber (gms)
Cereal, ready-to-eat, granola *(cont.)*							
kamut:							
(*Kamutios*)	120	5.0	23.0	1.0	0	90	1.0
flakes (*Arrowhead Mills*)	110	4.0	25.0	1.0	0	75	3.0
flakes (*Erewhon*), ⅔ cup	110	5.0	25.0	0	0	75	4.0
puffed (*Arrowhead Mills*)	50	2.0	11.0	0	0	0	1.0
millet, puffed (*Arrowhead Mills*)	60	2.0	12.0	.5	0	0	0
multigrain (see also "granola," above):							
(*Apple Jacks*)	130	1.0	30.0	.5	0	150	1.0
(*Apple Zings*)	130	1.0	30.0	1.0	0	150	1.0
(*Barbara's* Organic Fruity Punch) ...	110	2.0	26.0	.5	0	120	0
(*Barbara's* Organic SoyEssence), ¾ cup	100	3.0	25.0	.5	0	115	5.0
(*Barbara's* Shredded Spoonfuls), ¾ cup	120	5.0	23.0	1.5	0	200	4.0
(*Barbara's* Grain-Shop*), ⅔ cup ..	90	3.0	24.0	1.0	0	110	8.0
(*Basic 4*)	200	4.0	42.0	3.0	0	320	3.0
(*Berry Berry Kix*), ¾ cup	120	1.0	26.0	1.5	0	180	0
(*Berry Colossal Crunch*), ¾ cup	120	1.0	26.0	1.5	0	210	1.0
(*Cinnamon Toast Crunch*), ¾ cup	130	1.0	24.0	3.5	0	210	1.0
(*Cinni-Mini Crunch*), ¾ cup	130	1.0	24.0	3.5	0	210	1.0
(*Coco-Roos*), ¾ cup	120	1.0	27.0	1.0	0	190	0
(*Cocoa Dyna-Bites*), ¾ cup	120	1.0	26.0	1.0	0	160	0
(*Colossal Crunch*), ¾ cup	120	1.0	26.0	1.5	0	230	1.0
(*Cookie Crisp*)	120	1.0	26.0	1.0	0	180	0
(*Country Inn Specialties Green Gables Inn*), ½ cup	210	4.0	37.0	6.0	0	160	4.0

Food and Measure	cal.	prot. (gms)	carbo. (gms)	fat (gms)	chol. (mgs)	sod. (mgs)	fiber (gms)
(*Country Inn Specialties Greyfield Inn*), ¾ cup	210	3.0	38.0	6.0	0	220	3.0
(*Country Inn Specialties Inn at Ormsby Hill*)	220	4.0	49.0	2.0	0	300	3.0
(*Erewhon Apple Stroodles*), ¾ cup	110	3.0	25.0	.5	0	15	1.0
(*Erewhon Banana-O's*), ¾ cup	110	2.0	26.0	0	0	15	2.0
(*Fiber One*), ½ cup	60	2.0	24.0	1.0	0	130	14.0
(*French Toast Crunch*), ¾ cup	120	1.0	26.0	1.0	0	180	0
(*Frosted Mini-Spooners*)	190	5.0	45.0	1.0	0	0	6.0
(*Froot Loops*)	120	1.0	28.0	1.0	0	150	1.0
(*Fruity Dyno-Bites*), ¾ cup	100	<1.0	24.0	.5	0	160	0
(*General Mills* Cinnamon Grahams), ¾ cup	120	1.0	26.0	1.0	0	240	1.0
(*GinkgOs*)	120	4.0	21.0	1.0	0	60	2.0
(*Golden Crisp*), ¾ cup	110	1.0	25.0	0	0	40	0
(*Golden Grahams*), ¾ cup	120	1.0	25.0	1.0	0	270	1.0
(*Golden Puffs*), ¾ cup	100	2.0	25.0	0	0	40	<1.0
(*Grape-Nuts*), ½ cup	210	6.0	47.0	1.0	0	340	5.0
(*Grape-Nuts O's*) ..	120	3.0	28.0	0	0	160	2.0
(*Harmony*), 1¼ cups	200	5.0	44.0	1.0	0	350	2.0
(*Honey Buzzers*), 1⅓ cups	110	1.0	26.0	.5	0	220	<1.0
(*Honey Graham Crunch*), ¾ cup	120	1.0	25.0	1.0	0	270	1.0
(*Honey Nut Chex*), ¾ cup	120	1.0	26.0	.5	0	220	0
(*Honey Nut Clusters*)	210	4.0	46.0	2.5	0	270	3.0
(*Honeycomb*), 1⅓ cups	110	2.0	26.0	.5	0	220	<1.0
(*Kaboom*), 1¼ cups	120	2.0	24.0	1.0	0	290	1.0

Food and Measure	cal.	prot. (gms)	carbo. (gms)	fat (gms)	chol. (mgs)	sod. (mgs)	fiber (gms)
Cereal, ready-to-eat, multigrain *(cont.)*							
(*Kashi* Medley), ½ cup	100	3.0	20.0	1.0	0	50	2.0
(*Kashi* Pilaf), ½ cup	170	6.0	30.0	3.0	0	15	6.0
(*Kellogg's Froot Loops*)	120	1.0	28.0	1.0	0	150	1.0
(*Kashi GoLean*), ¾ cup	120	8.0	28.0	1.0	0	35	10.0
(*Kashi GoLean Crunch*)	190	9.0	36.0	3.0	0	95	8.0
(*Kashi Good Friends*), ¾ cup	90	3.0	24.0	1.0	0	70	8.0
(*Kellogg's Marsh-mallow Blasted Froot Loops*)	120	1.0	27.0	.5	0	105	0
(*Kellogg's Müeslix*), ⅔ cup	200	5.0	40.0	3.0	0	170	4.0
(*Kellogg's Product 19*)	100	2.0	25.0	0	0	210	1.0
(*Kellogg's Smart Set*)	180	3.0	43.0	.5	0	280	2.0
(*Kellogg's Special K Plus*)	210	4.0	47.0	2.0	0	250	3.0
(*Kix*), 1⅓ cups	120	2.0	26.0	.5	0	270	1.0
(*Multi-Grain Cheerios*)	110	3.0	24.0	1.0	0	200	3.0
(*Pebbles* Cinna-Crunch), 1¼ cups	130	1.0	27.0	1.5	0	90	<1.0
(*Post Waffle Crisp*)	130	2.0	24.0	2.5	0	115	<1.0
(*Quaker Life*), ¾ cup	120	3.0	25.0	1.5	0	165	2.0
(*Sunrise Organic*), ¾ cup	110	2.0	26.0	.5 —	0	190	1.0
(*Team Cheerios*)	120	2.0	25.0	1.0	0	210	2.0
(*Tootie Fruities*)	120	2.0	28.0	1.0	0	150	1.0
(*Total* Whole Grain), ¾ cup	110	2.0	23.0	1.0	0	190	3.0
(*Trix*)	120	1.0	27.0	1.0	0	190	1.0
(*Uncle Sam*)	190	7.0	38.0	5.0	0	135	10.0
(*Wafflers*), ⅔ cup	110	2.0	26.0	1.0	0	65	2.0
(*Wheaties Energy Crunch*)	210	6.0	42.0	3.0	0	310	4.0

Food and Measure	cal.	prot. (gms)	carbo. (gms)	fat (gms)	chol. (mgs)	sod. (mgs	fiber (gms)
almond crunch w/raisins (*Kellogg's Healthy Choice*)	210	5.0	45.0	2.5	0	230	5.0
apple pie (*Kashi Pillows*), ¾ cup	200	3.0	46.0	1.0	0	25	2.0
banana nut (*Health Valley Crunches & Flakes*), ¾ cup	200	5.0	41.0	3.0	0	30	4.0
banana nut (*Post Banana Nut Crunch*)	240	5.0	44.0	6.0	0	230	5.0
banana nut (*Post Selects Banana Nut Crunch*)	240	5.0	44.0	6.0	0	230	5.0
blueberry (*Post Selects Blueberry Morning*), 1¼ cups	230	4.0	48.0	3.5	0	240	2.0
brown sugar and oat (*Total*), ¾ cup ..	110	2.0	23.0	.5	0	210	0
brown sugar squares (*Kellogg's Healthy Choice*)	190	5.0	44.0	1.0	0	210	5.0
chocolate (*Kashi Pillows*), ¾ cup .	200	3.0	45.0	1.0	0	50	2.0
cinnamon (*Wafflers*), ⅔ cup	110	2.0	26.0	1.0	0	65	2.0
cocoa (*Barbara's Crunch Stars*) ..	110	2.0	26.0	.5	0	140	1.0
cocoa (*Pebbles*), ¾ cup	120	1.0	25.0	1.0	0	180	0
cranberry almond (*Post Selects Cranberry Almond Crunch*)	210	4.0	44.0	3.0	0	200	3.0
cranberry crunch (*Health Valley*), ¾ cup	190	4.0	38.0	3.0	0	140	3.0
dates, raisins, walnuts (*Fruit & Fibre*)	190	4.0	42.0	3.0	0	240	6.0
flakes (*Arrowhead Mills*)	140	3.0	29.0	1.5	0	130	3.0

Food and Measure	cal.	prot. (gms)	carbo. (gms)	fat (gms)	chol. (mgs)	sod. (mgs)	fiber (gms)
Cereal, ready-to-eat, multigrain (cont.)							
flakes (*Grape-Nuts*), ¾ cup	110	3.0	24.0	1.0	0	120	3.0
flakes (*Health Valley Organic Fiber 7*), ¾ cup	100	3.0	24.0	0	0	90	4.0
flakes (*Health Valley Organic Healthy Fiber*), ¾ cup . . .	100	3.0	23.0	0	0	15	4.0
w/fruit, nuts (*Kellogg's Just Right*)	220	4.0	49.0	2.0	0	280	3.0
fruit juice sweet (*Fruit-e-o's*)	120	2.0	25.0	1.0	0	60	2.0
honey (*Barbara's Crunch Stars*) . .	110	2.0	26.0	0	0	50	2.0
honey (*Health Valley Crunches & Flakes*), ¾ cup	130	3.0	31.0	0	0	35	4.0
honey (*Health Valley Fiber 7*), ¾ cup .	110	3.0	27.0	0	0	90	4.0
maple (*Wafflers*), ⅔ cup	110	2.0	26.0	1.0	0	65	2.0
peaches, raisins, almonds (*Fruit & Fibre*)	190	4.0	42.0	2.5	0	260	7.0
pecans (*Post Selects Great Grains*), ½ cup	220	5.0	38.0	6.0	0	200	4.0
puffed (*Kashi*)	70	3.0	13.0	<1.0	0	0	2.0
puffed, honey (*Kashi*)	120	3.0	25.0	1.0	0	6—	2.0
raisins, dates, pecans (*Post Selects Great Grains*), ½ cup	200	4.0	39.0	4.5	0	135	4.0
raspberry (*Health Valley Rhapsody*), ¾ cup	200	5.0	41.0	3.0	0	100	4.0
strawberry crisp (*Kashi Pillows*), ¾ cup	200	3.0	46.0	1.0	0	25	2.0
vanilla nut (*Wafflers*), ⅔ cup	110	2.0	26.0	1.0	0	65	2.0

Food and Measure	cal.	prot. (gms)	carbo. (gms)	fat (gms)	chol. (mgs)	sod. (mgs)	fiber (gms)
oat bran:							
(*Health Valley Oat Bran O's*), ¾ cup	100	3.0	23.0	0	0	90	3.0
(*Kellogg's Cracklin' Oat Bran*), ¾ cup	200	4.0	35.0	7.0	0	140	5.0
(*Quaker*), 1¼ cups	210	7.0	43.0	3.0	0	210	6.0
almond crunch (*Health Valley*), ½ cup	200	6.0	34.0	3.0	0	90	5.0
oat bran flakes:							
(*Arrowhead Mills*)	140	6.0	24.0	2.5	0	80	4.0
(*Health Valley Organic*), ¾ cup	100	3.0	24.0	0	0	90	4.0
(*Kellogg's Complete*), ¾ cup	110	3.0	23.0	1.0	0	210	4.0
(*New Morning*)	110	4.0	21.0	1.0	0	60	5.0
w/raisins (*Health Valley*), ¾ cup ..	110	3.0	26.0	0	0	90	4.0
oats/oatmeal:							
(*Alpha-Bits*)	130	3.0	27.0	1.5	0	210	1.0
(*Arrowhead Mills Nature O's*)	130	4.0	24.0	2.0	0	5	3.0
(*Barbara's Breakfast O's*)	120	5.0	22.0	2.0	0	115	3.0
(*Cheerios*)	110	3.0	22.0	2.0	0	280	3.0
(*Frosted Cheerios*) .	120	2.0	26.0	1.0	0	210	1.0
(*Frosted Toasty O's*)	110	2.0	25.0	1.0	0	210	2.0
(*Honey Bunches of Oats*), ¾ cup ...	120	2.0	25.0	1.5	0	180	2.0
(*Honey Nut Cheerios*)	120	3.0	24.0	1.5	0	270	2.0
(*Honey Nut Toasty O's*)	110	3.0	24.0	1.0	0	270	2.0
(*Kashi Heart to Heart*), ¾ cup ..	110	4.0	25.0	1.5	0	90	5.0
(*Oatios Original*)	120	4.0	21.0	1.0	0	60	2.0
(*Post Oreo O's*), ¾ cup	110	1.0	21.0	2.5	0	110	<1.0
(*Quaker Oatmeal Squares*)	210	6.0	44.0	3.0	0	270	4.5
(*Quaker Toasted*) ..	110	4.0	23.0	1.5	0	285	2.0
(*Quaker Toasted Oatmeal Original*)	190	5.0	39.0	2.5	0	220	4.0
(*Toasty O's*)	110	4.0	22.0	2.0	0	280	3.0

Cereal, ready-to-eat, oats/oatmeal *(cont.)*

Food and Measure	cal.	prot. (gms)	carbo. (gms)	fat (gms)	chol. (mgs)	sod. (mgs)	fiber (gms)
w/almond (*Honey Bunches of Oats*), ¾ cup	130	3.0	24.0	2.5	0	170	2.0
w/almond (*Oatmeal Crisp*)	220	5.0	42.0	4.5	0	240	4.0
apple (*Health Valley Crunch O's*), ¾ cup	120	3.0	25.0	1.0	0	90	3.0
apple cinnamon (*Barbara's* Toasted O's), ¾ cup	110	3.0	24.0	1.0	0	90	2.0
apple cinnamon (*Cheerios*), ¾ cup	120	2.0	25.0	1.5	0	120	1.0
apple cinnamon (*Oatios*)	90	2.0	21.0	1.5	0	60	5.0
apple cinnamon (*Oatmeal Crisp*)	210	5.0	45.0	2.0	0	250	4.0
apple cinnamon (*Toasty O's*), ¾ cup	120	2.0	25.0	1.5	0	160	1.0
blueberry (*Oatiola*)	200	5.0	41.0	1.5	0	60	4.0
cinnamon (*Mother's* Oat Crunch)	230	6.0	50.0	3.0	0	250	5.0
cinnamon (*Quaker* Oatmeal Squares)	230	6.0	47.0	2.5	0	265	5.0
cinnamon (*Quaker Life*), ¾ cup	120	3.0	25.0	1.0	0	145	2.0
flakes (*Mother's Harvest*), ¾ cup	110	3.0	24.0	1.0	0	205	2.0
flakes, apple almond (*Mother's Harvest*), ¾ cup	115	3.0	24.0	2.0	0	175	2.5
honey (*Health Valley Crunch O's*), ¾ cup	120	3.0	26.0	0	0	90	3.0
honey (*Mother's Round-ups*), ¾ cup	105	2.0	24.0	1.0	0	175	1.0
honey almond (*Oatios*)	100	3.0	22.0	1.0	0	60	3.0

Food and Measure	cal.	prot. (gms)	carbo. (gms)	fat (gms)	chol. (mgs)	sod. (mgs)	fiber (gms)
honey nut (*Barbara's* Toasty O's), ¾ cup	120	3.0	23.0	2.0	0	90	2.0
honey nut (*Health Valley* Organic O's), ¾ cup	120	3.0	24.0	1.5	0	130	4.0
honey nut (*Quaker* Toasted Oatmeal)	190	4.0	40.0	3.0	0	185	3.5
marshmallow (*Alpha-Bits*)	110	2.0	25.0	1.0	0	210	1.0
marshmallow (*Lucky Charms*)	120	2.0	25.0	1.0	0	210	1.0
raisin (*Oatmeal Crisp*)	210	5.0	44.0	2.0	0	220	4.0
shredded (*Barbara's* Bite Size), 1¼ cups	220	6.0	46.0	2.5	0	260	6.0
shredded (*Barbara's* Organic Eco Bag), 1¼ cups	210	8.0	41.0	3.0	0	240	5.0
sweetened (*Arrowhead Mills* Nature O's)	160	8.0	31.0	2.5	0	110	3.0
vanilla almond, shredded (*Barbara's*)	220	7.0	42.0	3.0	0	210	4.3
rice:							
(*Health Valley* CrunchEms*), 1¼ cups	110	2.0	26.0	0	0	150	2.0
(*Kellogg's Cocoa Krispies*), ¾ cup	120	1.0	27.0	1.0	0	190	1.0
(*Kellogg's Razzle Dazzle Rice Krispies*), ¾ cup	110	1.0	25.0	0	0	170	0
(*Kellogg's Rice Krispies*), 1¼ cups	120	2.0	29.0	0	0	320	0
(*Kellogg's Rice Krispies Treats*), ¾ cup	120	1.0	26.0	1.5	0	190	0
(*Kellogg's Special K*)	110	6.0	23.0	0	0	220	<1.0
(*Rice Chex*), 1¼ cups	120	2.0	27.0	0	0	290	0
crispy (*Malt-O-Meal*), 1¼ cups	130	2.0	29.0	0	0	320	0

Food and Measure	cal.	prot. (gms)	carbo. (gms)	fat (gms)	chol. (mgs)	sod. (mgs)	fiber (gms)
Cereal, ready-to-eat, rice *(cont.)*							
flakes (*Arrowhead Mills*)	80	3.0	19.0	1.0	0	210	2.0
puffed (*Arrowhead Mills*)	60	2.0	13.0	.5	0	0	0
puffed (*Malt-O-Meal*)	60	1.0	13.0	0	0	20	0
puffed (*Quaker*), . .	55	1.0	12.0	0	0	0	0
rice, brown:							
(*Barbara's Rice Crisps*)	120	2.0	25.0	1.0	0	125	1.0
(*Erewhon Rice Twice*), ¾ cup . .	120	2.0	26.0	0	0	60	0
crispy (*Erewhon The Original*)	110	2.0	25.0	0	0	180	1.0
crispy (*Erewhon The Original No Salt*)	110	2.0	25.0	0	0	10	1.0
crispy (*New Morning*)	110	2.0	23.0	1.0	0	5	1.0
crispy, frosted (*New Morning* Cocoa) .	210	6.0	45.0	1.5	0	60	6.0
soy, ½ cup:							
(*Health Valley*) . . .	180	12.0	31.0	2.0	0	230	4.0
apple cinnamon or honey nut (*Health Valley*)	180	11.0	31.0	2.0	0	230	3.0
spelt flakes (*Arrowhead Mills*)	100	4.0	23.0	.5	0	100	4.0
wheat:							
(*Barbara's* Organic Crispy Wheats), ¾ cup	110	3.0	25.0	.5	0	190	3.0
(*Erewhon* Fruit 'n Wheat), ¾ cup . .	170	5.0	39.0	1.5	0	105	5.0
(*Frosted Wheaties*), ¾ cup	110	1.0	27.0	0	0	200	0
(*Kellogg's Honey Frosted Mini-Wheats* Bite-Size), 24 pcs.	200	6.0	48.0	1.0	0	5	6.0
(*Kellogg's Mini-Wheats* Frosted Bite-Size), 24 pcs.	200	6.0	48.0	1.0	0	5	6.0

Food and Measure	cal.	prot. (gms)	carbo. (gms)	fat (gms)	chol. (mgs)	sod. (mgs)	fiber (gms)
(*Kellogg's Mini-Wheats* Frosted Original), 5 pcs.	180	5.0	41.0	1.0	0	5	5.0
(*Wheat Chex*)	180	5.0	40.0	1.0	0	420	5.0
(*Wheaties*)	110	3.0	24.0	1.0	0	220	3.0
apple cinnamon (*Kellogg's Mini-Wheats*), ¾ cup .	180	4.0	44.0	1.0	0	170	5.0
blueberry (*Kellogg's Mini-Wheats*), ¾ cup	180	4.0	43.0	1.0	0	180	5.0
bran, see "bran," above							
flakes (*Arrowhead Mills*)	160	5.0	37.0	.5	0	200	6.0
flakes (*Erewhon*) ..	180	6.0	42.0	1.0	0	135	6.0
germ, see "Wheat germ"							
raisins (*Kellogg's Mini-Wheats*), ¾ cup	180	5.0	42.0	1.0	0	5	5.0
strawberry (*Kellogg's Mini-Wheats*), ¾ cup	170	4.0	40.0	1.0	0	15	5.0
wheat, puffed:							
(*Arrowhead Mills*)	60	2.0	13.0	.5	0	0	1.0
(*Kellogg's Smacks*), ¾ cup	100	2.0	24.0	.5	0	50	1.0
(*Malt-O-Meal*)	50	2.0	11.0	0	0	60	1.0
(*Quaker*), 1¼ cup	55	2.5	11.0	0	0	0	1.5
wheat, shredded:							
(*Arrowhead Mills*)	180	5.0	41.0	.5	0	0	6.0
(*Barbara's*), 2 pcs.	140	4.0	31.0	1.0	0	0	5.0
(*Post Honey Nut Shredded Wheat Spoon Size*)	200	5.0	43.0	1.5	0	70	4.0
(*Post The Original Shredded Wheat Spoon Size*)	170	6.0	40.0	1.0	0	0	6.0
(*Quaker*), 3 pcs. ..	220	7.0	50.0	1.0	0	0	7.0
w/bran (*Post The Original Shredded Wheat 'N Bran Spoon Size*), 1¼ cups	200	7.0	48.0	1.0	0	0	8.0

Food and Measure	cal.	prot. (gms)	carbo. (gms)	fat (gms)	chol. (mgs)	sod. (mgs)	fiber (gms)
Cereal, ready-to-eat, wheat, shredded *(cont.)*							
frosted (*Post Spoon Size*)	180	4.0	43.0	1.0	0	5	5.0
sweetened (*Arrowhead Mills*)	200	5.0	44.0	1.0	0	0	6.0
Cereal, cooking/hot							
(see also specific grains), dry, 1 pkt., except as noted:							
barley:							
(*Arrowhead Mills Bits O Barley*), ⅓ cup	140	5.0	33.0	1.0	0	0	6.0
(*Erewhon Barley Plus*), ¼ cup ...	170	5.0	37.0	1.0	0	0	4.0
buckwheat, cream of (*Wolff's*), ⅓ cup ..	90	1.0	21.0	0	0	0	0
couscous:							
apple cinnamon (*Marrakesh Express Cocorico*)	260	8.0	55.0	0	0	90	2.0
banana (*Marrakesh Express Cocorico*)	280	8.0	54.0	4.0	0	40	3.0
blueberry (*Marrakesh Express Cocorico*)	270	9.0	54.0	2.0	0	40	3.0
peach (*Marrakesh Express Cocorico*)	280	7.0	59.0	1.0	5	35	0
strawberry (*Marrakesh Express Cocorico*)	250	9.0	50.0	2.0	0	40	3.0
farina, see "wheat," below							
grits, see "Corn grits"							
multigrain:							
(*Country Choice Naturals*), ½ cup	130	5.0	29.0	1.5	0	0	5.0
(*Health Valley Terrific 10 Grain!*)	220	12.0	41.0	2.5	0	210	5.0
(*Quaker*), ½ cup ..	130	5.0	29.0	1.0	0	0	5.0
4 grain plus flax (*Arrowhead Mills*), ¼ cup	150	6.0	28.0	2.0	0	0	6.0
5 grain (*AlpineAire*)	230	7.0	48.0	1.5	0	500	6.0

Food and Measure	cal.	prot. (gms)	carbo. (gms)	fat (gms)	chol. (mgs)	sod. (mgs)	fiber (gms)
5 grain, fruit-nut (*AlpineAire*)	250	8.0	47.0	3.5	0	190	6.0
7 grain (*Arrowhead Mills*), ⅓ cup ...	140	6.0	25.0	1.5	0	0	5.0
7 grain, wheat free (*Arrowhead Mills*), ¼ cup	120	4.0	25.0	1.5	0	0	2.0
apple cinnamon (*Health Valley* Cup)	210	9.0	41.0	2.0	0	230	4.0
apple cranberry cobbler (*Cream of Wheat*)	140	3.0	32.0	1.0	0	130	3.0
apple spice (*Kashi Go*), ½ cup	270	7.0	56.0	3.0	0	0	6.0
banana almond (*Kashi Go*), ½ cup	280	7.0	57.0	3.5	0	5	6.0
banana nut (*Health Valley* Cup)	240	10.0	45.0	3.0	0	240	4.0
banana nut bread (*Harvest Morning*)	150	3.0	32.0	1.5	0	210	3.0
berry tart (*Kashi Go*), ½ cup	260	7.0	55.0	3.0	0	5	6.0
blueberry (*Kashi Go Bliss*), ½ cup ...	250	7.0	55.0	3.0	0	5	6.0
blueberry muffin (*Harvest Morning*)	140	2.0	31.0	1.0	0	170	2.0
cherry vanilla (*Kashi Go*), ½ cup	260	7.0	54.0	3.0	0	15	6.0
maple (*Health Valley* Cup)	240	9.0	47.0	2.0	0	290	4.0
peach (*Kashi Go Just Peachy*), ½ cup	260	7.0	54.0	3.0	0	0	6.0
raspberry Danish (*Harvest Morning*)	140	2.0	32.0	1.5	0	115	3.0
oat bran:							
(*Hodgson Mill*), ¼ cup	120	6.0	23.0	3.0	0	3	6.0
(*Quaker*), ½ cup ..	150	7.0	25.0	3.0	0	0	6.0

Food and Measure	cal.	prot. (gms)	carbo. (gms)	fat (gms)	chol. (mgs)	sod. (mgs)	fiber (gms)
Cereal, ready-to-eat, oat bran *(cont.)*							
flakes (*Kellogg's Complete*), ¾ cup	110	3.0	23.0	1.0	0	210	4.0
w/toasted wheat germ (*Erewhon*), ⅓ cup	170	10.0	31.0	2.5	0	0	5.0
oats/oatmeal:							
(*Arrowhead Mills* Instant Oatmeal)	110	4.0	20.0	2.0	0	0	3.0
(*Arrowhead Mills* Steel Cut Oats), ¼ cup	170	6.0	29.0	3.0	0	0	5.0
(*Country Choice Naturals* Regular/ Quick), ½ cup ..	150	5.0	27.0	3.0	0	0	4.0
(*Crystal Wedding Oats*), ½ cup ...	150	5.0	27.0	3.0	0	0	4.0
(*H-O* Instant), ½ cup	150	5.0	27.0	3.0	0	0	4.0
(*H-O* Regular)	110	4.0	18.0	2.5	0	220	3.0
(*H-O* Quick), ½ cup	150	5.0	27.0	3.0	0	0	4.0
(*Maypo* Instant), ½ cup	210	7.0	37.0	2.5	0	110	3.0
(*Quaker* Instant Oatmeal)	100	4.0	19.0	2.0	0	80	3.0
(*Quaker* Old Fashioned/Quick Oats), ½ cup ...	150	5.0	27.0	3.0	0	0	4.0
(*Quaker Sun Country* Fortified Quick Oats), ½ cup ...	150	5.0	27.0	3.0	0	0	4.0
w/added oat bran (*Erewhon* Instant Oatmeal)	130	6.0	25.0	2.5	0	0	4.0
apple, baked (*Quaker* Instant Oatmeal)	150	3.0	31.0	2.0	0	230	3.0
apple, baked (*Quaker Express* Instant Oatmeal Cup)	200	4.0	42.0	2.5	0	320	4.0

Food and Measure	cal.	prot. (gms)	carbo. (gms)	fat (gms)	chol. (mgs)	sod. (mgs)	fiber (gms)
apple cinnamon:							
(*Country Choice Naturals*)	140	4.0	25.0	2.0	0	25	3.0
(*Erewhon* Instant Oatmeal)	130	5.0	24.0	2.0	0	100	3.0
(*Health Valley* Cup Amazing Apple)	210	9.0	41.0	2.0	0	230	4.0
(*H-O*)	130	3.0	26.0	2.0	0	100	3.0
(*Malt-O-Meal* Big Bowl)	190	4.0	41.0	2.0	0	260	5.0
(*Quaker* Instant Oatmeal)	130	3.0	27.0	1.5	0	170	3.0
apple raisin (*Erewhon* Instant Oatmeal)	140	5.0	26.0	2.0	0	100	3.0
banana nut (*Health Valley* Cup Banana Gone Nuts)	240	10.0	45.0	3.0	0	240	4.0
brown sugar, golden (*Quaker* Instant Oatmeal)	165	5.0	33.0	2.0	0	315	3.0
brown sugar, golden (*Quaker Express* Instant Oatmeal Cup)	200	5.0	42.0	2.5	0	290	3.0
cinnamon, raisin, almond (*Arrowhead Mills* Instant) ...	130	5.0	24.0	2.0	0	0	2.0
cinnamon and brown sugar (*H-O*)	160	4.0	32.0	2.0	0	220	3.0
cinnamon roll (*Quaker* Instant Oatmeal)	160	4.0	33.0	2.0	0	240	3.0
cinnamon roll (*Quaker Express* Instant Oatmeal Cup) ...	200	5.0	41.0	2.5	0	250	4.0
cinnamon spice (*Malt-O-Meal* Big Bowl)	200	6.0	54.0	3.0	0	360	5.0
cinnamon spice (*Quaker* Instant Oatmeal)	170	4.0	35.0	2.0	0	250	3.0
honey nut (*Quaker* Instant Oatmeal)	170	4.0	31.0	3.5	0	240	3.0
maple (*Maypo* Vermont), ⅓ cup	180	6.0	33.0	2.0	0	80	3.0

Food and Measure	cal.	prot. (gms)	carbo. (gms)	fat (gms)	chol. (mgs)	sod. (mgs)	fiber (gms)
Cereal, ready-to-eat, oats/oatmeal *(cont.)*							
maple, apple, spice (*Arrowhead Mills* Instant)	130	4.0	25.0	2.0	0	40	2.0
maple brown sugar:							
(*H-O*)	160	4.0	32.0	2.0	0	220	3.0
(*Malt-O-Meal* Big Bowl)	230	6.0	49.0	2.0	0	360	5.0
(*Quaker* Instant Oatmeal)	160	4.0	32.0	2.0	0	260	3.0
maple spice (*Erewhon* Instant Oatmeal)	130	5.0	25.0	2.0	0	100	3.0
maple syrup (*Country Choice Naturals*)	170	5.0	29.0	3.0	0	0	3.0
peach (*Quaker Express* Instant Oatmeal Cup) .	200	4.0	42.0	2.5	0	280	4.0
peaches and cream (*Quaker* Instant Oatmeal)	140	3.0	27.0	2.5	0	190	2.0
raisin, date, walnut (*Erewhon* Instant Oatmeal)	130	4.0	24.0	2.5	0	40	3.0
raisin, date, walnut (*Quaker* Instant Oatmeal)	140	3.0	27.0	2.5	0	240	2.0
raisin spice (*Quaker* Instant Oatmeal)	150	3.0	33.0	2.0	0	240	3.0
strawberries and cream (*Quaker* Instant Oatmeal)	140	3.0	27.0	2.5	0	190	2.0
sweet and mellow (*H-O*)	150	4.0	30.0	2.0	0	200	3.0
vanilla, French (*Quaker* Instant Oatmeal)	160	4.0	33.0	2.0	0	250	3.0
rice:							
(*Arrowhead Mills Rice & Shine*), ¼ cup	150	3.0	32.0	1.0	0	0	2.0
(*Cream of Rice*), ¼ cup	170	4.0	38.0	0	0	0	0

Food and Measure	cal.	prot. (gms)	carbo. (gms)	fat (gms)	chol. (mgs)	sod. (mgs)	fiber (gms)
(*Lundberg* Organic Hot 'n Creamy), ⅓ cup	190	4.0	43.0	2.0	0	0	3.0
almond, sweet (*Lundberg* Hot 'n Creamy), ⅓ cup	200	3.0	40.0	3.5	0	0	4.0
brown (*Erewhon* Cream), ¼ cup . .	170	5.0	36.0	1.0	0	30	1.0
cinnamon raisin (*Lundberg* Hot 'n Creamy), ⅓ cup	190	3.0	42.0	1.5	0	0	4.0
wheat:							
(*Arrowhead Mills Bear Mush*), ¼ cup	160	5.0	33.0	1.0	0	0	2.0
(*Cream of Wheat* Instant Original)	100	4.0	21.0	0	0	170	1.0
(*Cream of Wheat* 24 Pack)	120	5.0	25.0	0	0	0	1.0
(*Cream of Wheat* 12 Pack)	120	5.0	25.0	0	0	90	1.0
(*H-O Cream Farina* Quick), 3 tbsp.	120	3.0	26.0	0	0	0	3.0
(*Malt-O-Meal* Original), 3 tbsp.	120	5.0	26.0	.5	0	0	1.0
(*Wheatena*), ⅓ cup	160	5.0	33.0	1.0	0	0	5.0
apple cinnamon (*Malt-O-Meal*), 3 tbsp.	120	3.0	28.0	0	0	0	1.0
baked apple cinnamon (*Cream of Wheat*)	130	4.0	30.0	0	0	210	1.0
brown sugar cinnamon (*Cream of Wheat*)	130	4.0	29.0	0	0	220	1.0
chocolate (*Malt-O-Meal*), 3 tbsp. . .	120	4.0	26.0	.5	0	0	1.0
cracked (*Arrowhead Mills*), ¼ cup . . .	140	5.0	29.0	.5	0	0	6.0
cracked (*Hodgson Mill*), ¼ cup . . .	110	4.0	26.0	1.0	0	0	8.0
farina (*Cream of Wheat*), 3 tbsp.	120	5.0	25.0	0	0	90	0

Food and Measure	cal.	prot. (gms)	carbo. (gms)	fat (gms)	chol. (mgs)	sod. (mgs)	fiber (gms)
Cereal, ready-to-eat, wheat *(cont.)*							
farina (*H-O* Cream), 3 tbsp.	120	3.0	26.0	0	0	0	1.0
farina (*Malt-O-Meal*), 3 tbsp.	120	4.0	26.0	0	0	0	1.0
farina (*Quaker* Creamy Wheat), ¼ cup	150	5.0	35.0	.5	0	0	1.0
maple brown sugar (*Cream of Wheat*)	130	5.0	30.0	0	0	140	0
maple brown sugar (*Malt-O-Meal*), 3 tbsp.	120	3.0	28.0	0	0	0	1.0
Cereal, freeze-dried, granola, 1 serving:							
(*AlpineAire* Fat Free)	180	4.0	38.0	1.0	0	50	5.0
almond (*AlpineAire*) . .	300	9.0	41.0	11.0	0	0	5.0
w/milk:							
(*Mountain House*)	250	8.0	36.0	9.0	0	55	4.0
blueberry honey (*AlpineAire*)	340	15.0	65.0	2.0	n.a.	190	7.0
honey apple (*Alpine-Aire*)	280	14.0	53.0	1.5	n.a.	200	7.0
strawberry honey (*AlpineAire*)	340	18.0	65.0	2.0	n.a.	190	7.0
Cereal crumbs, see "Cornflake crumbs"							
Cereal bar, see "Granola/cereal bar"							
Cervelat, see "Summer sausage"							
Chayote:							
raw:							
(*Frieda's*), ⅔ cup, 3 oz.	20	1.0	5.0	0	0	0	3.0
1 medium, 7.2 oz.	49	1.8	11.0	.6	0	8	6.1
1" pcs., ½ cup	16	.6	3.6	.2	0	3	2.0
boiled, drained, 1" pcs., ½ cup . .	19	.5	4.1	.4	0	1	2.3
Cheese (see also "Cheese Food" and "Cheese Spread"), 1 oz., except as noted:							

Food and Measure	cal.	prot. (gms)	carbo. (gms)	fat (gms)	chol. (mgs)	sod. (mgs)	fiber (gms)
American, processed:							
(*Alpine Lace* Reduced Fat)	80	6.0	2.0	6.0	20	200	0
(*Boar's Head* Loaf)	100	6.0	1.0	9.0	25	380	0
(*Boar's Head* Slice), ⅔ oz.	70	4.0	1.0	6.0	15	260	0
(*Boar's Head* Slice), 2 slices, 1 oz.	110	5.0	1.0	9.0	20	380	0
(*Chedasharp*), ...	110	6	<1.0	9.0	30	400	0
(*Chedasharp* Slice), 2 slices, 1 oz. .:.	100	5	<1.0	9.0	30	460	0
(*Healthy Choice* Slice), ¾-oz. slice	40	5.0	2.0	1.0	5	200	0
(*Kraft Deli Deluxe*)	100	6.0	1.0	9.0	30	400	0
(*Kraft Deli Deluxe* Singles), ⅔ oz.	70	4.0	<1.0	6.0	15	310	0
(*Kraft Deli Deluxe* Singles), ¾ oz.	80	4.0	<1.0	7.0	20	340	0
(*Kraft Deli Deluxe* Singles)	110	5.0	<1.0	9.0	30	450	0
(*Land O Lakes*), ¾-oz. slice	70	4.0	2.0	5.0	15	330	0
(*Land O Lakes* Golden Velvet) ..	80	5.0	2.0	6.0	20	380	0
(*Land O Lakes* Light)	70	7.0	1.0	4.0	0	360	0
(*Land O Lakes* Loaf)	110	5.0	1.0	9.0	26	430	0
(*Sara Lee*)	110	6.0	0	9.0	30	350	0
(*Sara Lee* Slice), ¾-oz. slice	80	5.0	0	7.0	15	280	0
(*Sargento* Deli), ⅔-oz. slice	70	4.0	<1.0	6.0	20	240	0
sharp (*Land O Lakes*)	110	6.0	<1.0	9.0	30	380	0
blend, three cheese, shredded (*Kraft*), ¼ cup	110	8.0	<1.0	8.0	25	400	0
blue:							
(*Flora Danica* Danish)	110	6.0	0	9.0	15	330	0
creamy (*Boar's Head*)	90	6.0	0	8.0	30	360	0
brick (*Land O Lakes*)	100	7.0	<1.0	8.0	30	160	0
Brie	95	5.9	.1	7.9	20	229	0

Food and Measure	cal.	prot. (gms)	carbo. (gms)	fat (gms)	chol. (mgs)	sod. (mgs)	fiber (gms)
Cheese *(cont.)*							
Brie, creamy *(Saga)* ..	110	5.0	0	9.0	13.0	200	0
butterkase *(Boar's Head)*	100	6.0	0	9.0	30	180	0
Camembert	85	5.6	.1	6.9	20	239	0
(Chedarella)	100	7.0	0	8.0	25	200	0
(Chedasharp)	110	6.0	<1.0	9.0	30	400	0
cheddar:							
(Alpine Lace Reduced Fat)*	70	8.0	1.0	4.5	15	170	0
(Boar's Head Canadian)*	110	7.0	0	10.0	35	170	0
(Boar's Head Vermont)	110	7.0	0	10.0	30	170	0
(Cracker Barrel) ...	120	6.0	0	10.0	30	180	0
(Cracker Barrel Reduced Fat) ...	90	7.0	<1.0	6.0	20	240	0
(Kraft)	120	6.0	0	10.0	30	180	0
(Land O Lakes) ...	110	7.0	<1.0	9.0	30	180	0
(Land O Lakes Processed)	110	6.0	<1.0	9.0	30	360	0
(Sara Lee)	110	7.0	1.0	9.0	30	180	0
(Sara Lee Slice), ¾-oz. slice	90	5.0	0	7.0	20	140	0
aged or medium *(Sargento* Deli), ¾-oz. slice	80	5.0	0	7.0	20	130	0
extra sharp *(Cabot Hunter's Vermont)*	110	7.0	1.0	9.0	30	180	0
extra sharp *(Heluva Good New York State)*	110	7.0	1.0	9.0	30	180	0
mild *(Kraft Marbled)*	110	7.0	<1.0	9.0	30	180	0
mild or sharp *(Kraft Reduced Fat)* ...	90	7.0	<1.0	6.0	20	240	0
mild or sharp, cubed *(Kraft)*, 8 pcs., 1.1 oz.	130	7.0	0	11.0	30	210	0
sharp *(Boar's Head Slicing)*	110	7.0	<1.0	9.0	30	190	0
sharp *(Cracker Barrel Marbled)*	120	6.0	0	10.0	30	180	0
sharp *(Cracker Barrel* Vermont)*	110	7.0	<1.0	9.0	30	180	0

Food and Measure	cal.	prot. (gms)	carbo. (gms)	fat (gms)	chol. (mgs)	sod. (mgs)	fiber (gms)
sharp (*Healthy Choice* Slice), ¾-oz. slice	40	5.0	2.0	1.0	<5	220	0
sharp, white (*Cracker Barrel* Vermont) .	110	7.0	<1.0	9.0	30	180	0
(*Heluva* Good)	110	7.0	1.0	9.0	30	180	0
cheddar, shredded, ¼ cup:							
(*Kraft*)	110	6.0	1.0	9.0	25	180	0
double (*Sargento* Chef Style)	110	7.0	1.0	9.0	30	180	0
mild (*Sargento* Light)	70	8.0	<1.0	4.5	10	200	0
mild or sharp (*Kraft* Reduced Fat) . . .	80	7.0	<1.0	6.0	20	230	0
mild or sharp (*Sargento* Chef Style/Fancy)	110	7.0	1.0	9.0	30	180	0
cheddar blend (*Kraft* Classic Melts), ¼ cup	110	6.0	1.0	9.0	20	290	0
cheddar/Monterey Jack:							
(*Kraft Marbled*) . . .	110	7.0	<1.0	9.0	30	190	0
cubed (*Kraft*), 8 pcs., 1.1 oz.	120	7.0	0	10.0	30	210	0
diced or shredded (*Sargento*), ¼ cup	110	7.0	1.0	9.0	30	180	0
shredded (*Kraft*), ¼ cup	110	6.0	1.0	9.0	25	190	0
shredded (*Kraft* Mexican Style), ¼ cup	110	6.0	<1.0	9.0	25	190	0
shredded, w/jalapeño (*Kraft* Mexican style), ¼ cup . . .	110	6.0	1.0	9.0	25	190	0
Cheshire	110	6.6	1.4	8.7	29	198	0
Colby:							
(*Boar's Head*)	110	7.0	<1.0	9.0	30	170	0
(*Kraft*)	110	7.0	<1.0	9.0	30	180	0
(*Kraft* Reduced Fat)	80	7.0	0	6.0	20	220	0
(*Land O Lakes*) . . .	110	7.0	<1.0	9.0	30	160	0
(*Sara Lee*)	110	7.0	1.0	9.0	30	170	0

Food and Measure	cal.	prot. (gms)	carbo. (gms)	fat (gms)	chol. (mgs)	sod. (mgs)	fiber (gms)
Cheese, Colby *(cont.)*							
(*Sara Lee* Slice),							
¾-oz. slice	110	7.0	<1.0	9.0	30	170	0
(*Sargento* Deli),							
¾ -oz. slice	80	5.0	<1.0	7.0	20	130	0
Colby Jack:							
(*Heluva* Good)	110	7.0	1.0	9.0	30	170	0
(*Land O Lakes*) . . .	110	6.0	<1.0	9.0	30	180	0
(*Sara Lee*)	100	7.0	0	8.0	30	170	0
(*Sara Lee* Slice),							
1-oz. slice	100	7.0	0	8.0	30	170	0
Colby Jack, shredded,							
¼ cup or 1 oz.:							
(*Kraft*)	100	6.0	1.0	8.0	25	190	0
(*Kraft* Reduced Fat)	80	7.0	<1.0	6.0	15	190	0
(*Sargento* Fancy) . .	110	6.0	<1.0	9.0	25	190	0
Colby/Monterey Jack:							
(*Kraft*)	110	7.0	<1.0	9.0	30	180	0
cubed (*Kraft*), 4 pcs.,							
1 oz.	110	7.0	0	9.0	30	180	0
cubed (*Kraft*							
Marbled), 8 pcs.,							
1.1 oz.	120	8.0	<1.0	10.0	30	210	0
cottage, 4%, ½ cup:							
(*Breakstone*)	120	13.0	5.0	5.0	25	420	0
(*Crowley*)	120	14.0	5.0	5.0	25	450	0
(*Darigold* Large							
Curd)	130	14.0	5.0	5.0	25	490	0
(*Darigold* Small							
Curd)	120	14.0	5.0	5.0	25	470	0
(*Friendship*)	110	12.0	4.0	5.0	25	430	0
(*Friendship* California							
Style)	110	15.0	3.0	5.0	20	380	0
(*Hood*)	110	13.0	5.0	4.5	25	390	0
(*Knudsen* Large							
Curd)	120	14.0	3.0	5.0	25	360	0
(*Knudsen* Small							
Curd)	120	13.0	5.0	5.0	25	430	0
chive (*Darigold*) . .	120	13.0	5.0	5.0	25	470	0
pineapple (*Darigold*)	150	11.0	17.0	4.0	20	410	0
pineapple (*Friend-*							
ship)	140	12.0	14.0	4.0	15	300	0
pineapple (*Hood*)	130	10.0	15.0	3.5	15	290	0

Food and Measure	cal.	prot. (gms)	carbo. (gms)	fat (gms)	chol. (mgs)	sod. (mgs)	fiber (gms)
cottage, 2%:							
(*Breakstone's* Large Curd), 4-oz. cont.	90	13.0	4.0	3.0	15	380	0
(*Breakstone's* Large Curd), ½ cup . . .	90	13.0	5.0	2.5	15	400	0
(*Breakstone's* Small Curd), 4-oz. cont.	90	13.0	4.0	2.0	15	380	0
(*Breakstone's* Small Curd), ½ cup . . .	90	14.0	5.0	2.5	15	400	0
(*Darigold*), ½ cup .	100	14.0	5.0	2.5	15	470	0
(*Friendship* Pot Style), ½ cup . . .	90	15.0	3.0	2.5	10	400	0
cottage, 2%, 5.5 oz.:							
apple cinnamon (*Knudsen Cottage Doubles*)	140	14.0	17.0	2.5	15	400	0
blueberry (*Breakstone's/Knudsen Cottage Doubles*)	150	14.0	17.0	2.5	15	400	<1.0
peach or pineapple (*Breakstone's/ Knudsen Cottage Doubles*)	140	14.0	16.0	2.5	15	400	0
raspberry (*Knudsen Cottage Doubles*)	150	14.0	19.0	2.5	15	400	<1.0
strawberry (*Breakstone's/Knudsen Cottage Doubles*)	150	14.0	18.0	2.5	15	400	0
cottage, 1.5%:							
peach (*Knudsen*), 4-oz. cont.	110	10.0	13.0	1.5	10	320	0
pineapple (*Knudsen*), 4-oz. cont.	110	10.0	12.0	1.5	10	320	0
pineapple (*Knudsen*), ½ cup	120	11.0	14.0	2.0	10	360	0
strawberry (*Knudsen*), 4-oz. cont.	110	10.0	13.0	1.5	10	310	0
tropical fruit (*Knudsen*), 4-oz. cont.	110	10.0	13.0	1.5	10	330	0
cottage, 1%, ½ cup:							
(*Crowley*)	90	14.0	6.0	1.5	15	480	0
(*Friendship* Lowfat)	90	16.0	3.0	1.0	5	360	0

Food and Measure	cal.	prot. (gms)	carbo. (gms)	fat (gms)	chol. (mgs)	sod. (mgs)	fiber (gms)
Cheese, cottage, 1% *(cont.)*							
(*Friendship* Lowfat No Salt)	90	16.0	4.0	1.0	5	50	0
(*Hood* Low Fat) . . .	80	13.0	6.0	1.0	10	380	0
(*Light 'n' Lively*) . .	80	12.0	5.0	1.5	10	380	0
pineapple (*Friendship* Lowfat) . . .	120	12.0	16.0	1.0	5	290	0
cottage, nonfat, ½ cup:							
(*Breakstone's Free*)	80	13.0	7.0	0	10	430	0
(*Crowley*)	90	14.0	7.0	0	5	470	0
(*Darigold*)	90	15.0	6.0	0	5	460	0
(*Friendship*)	80	15.0	4.0	0	<5	380	0
(*Hood*)	80	13.0	7.0	0	5	320	0
(*Knudsen Free*) . . .	80	13.0	7.0	0	5	420	0
(*Light 'n' Lively Free*)	80	13.0	7.0	0	10	450	0
peach (*Friendship*)	110	12.0	15.0	0	<5	300	0
pineapple (*Friendship*)	110	12.0	16.0	0	<5	300	0
cream cheese, 2 tbsp., except as noted:							
(*Boar's Head*)	100	2.0	2.0	10.0	30	100	0
(*Friendship*)	100	2.0	1.0	10.0	35	120	0
(*Philadelphia*), 1 oz.	100	2.0	<1.0	10.0	30	90	0
(*Philadelphia* Light)	60	3.0	2.0	4.5	15	150	0
(*Philadelphia Free*) .	30	5.0	1.0	0	<5	200	0
(*Philadelphia Free*), 1-oz. pouch. . . .	25	5.0	1.0	0	<5	170	0
blueberry (*Philadelphia* Light)	70	2.0	6.0	4.0	15	120	0
blueberry (*Philadelphia*), 1 oz.	60	2.0	5.0	3.5	15	105	0
cheesecake (*Philadelphia*)	100	1.0	4.0	8.0	35	105	0
chive and onion (*Philadelphia*), 1 oz.	90	1.0	1.0	8.0	35	135	0
chive and onion (*Philadelphia* Light)	60	3.0	2.0	4.5	15	180	0
chive and onion or garden vegetable (*Philadelphia*) . .	90	2.0	1.0	9.0	35	150	0

Food and Measure	cal.	prot. (gms)	carbo. (gms)	fat (gms)	chol. (mgs)	sod. (mgs)	fiber (gms)
garden vegetable or roasted garlic (*Philadelphia* Light)	60	3.0	3.0	4.5	15	180	0
honey nut (*Philadelphia*)	100	1.0	4.0	8.0	30	100	0
jalapeño (*Philadelphia* Light)	60	3.0	2.0	4.5	15	200	0
pineapple or strawberry (*Philadelphia*)	90	1.0	4.0	8.0	30	100	0
raspberry (*Philadelphia* Light)	70	2.0	6.0	4.0	15	120	0
salmon (*Philadelphia*)	90	2.0	1.0	8.0	35	210	0
soft (*Friendship*) ..	100	2.0	1.0	10.0	35	120	0
soft (*Philadelphia*)	100	2.0	1.0	9.0	35	120	0
strawberry (*Philadelphia* Light) ..	70	2.0	6.0	4.0	15	120	0
strawberry (*Philadelphia* Free) ...	40	4.0	6.0	0	<5	190	0
whipped (*Philadelphia*)	70	1.0	<1.0	7.0	25	85	0
whipped, chive or salmon (*Philadelphia*)	60	2.0	1.0	6.0	20	130	0
Edam:							
(*Boar's Head*)	90	7.0	0	7.0	20	280	0
1 oz.	90	7.0	0	7.0	25	280	0
farmer:							
(*Friendship*)	50	5.0	0	2.5	10	120	0
(*Friendship* No Salt)	50	5.0	0	1.5	10	10	0
feta:							
(*Alpine Lace* Reduced Fat) ...	50	6.0	1.0	3.0	10	370	0
(*Athenos* Mild)	80	5.0	<1.0	6.0	20	190	0
(*Athenos* Traditional)	80	5.0	<1.0	6.0	20	320	0
(*Athenos* Traditional Reduced Fat) ...	60	6.0	<1.0	4.0	10	390	0
(*Boar's Head*)	60	5.0	1.0	4.0	10	370	0
(*Krinos*)	90	5.0	0	8.0	24	430	0
in brine (*Athenos* Traditional), ¼ cup	80	5.0	1.0	6.0	20	330	<1.0

Food and Measure	cal.	prot. (gms)	carbo. (gms)	fat (gms)	chol. (mgs)	sod. (mgs)	fiber (gms)
Cheese, feta *(cont.)*							
basil-tomato							
(*Athenos*)	80	5.0	<1.0	6.0	20	220	0
garlic-herb							
(*Athenos*)	80	5.0	1.0	6.0	20	340	<1.0
peppercorn							
(*Athenos*)	80	5.0	<1.0	6.0	20	330	0
sun-dried tomato-basil (*Alpine Lace Reduced Fat*) ...	50	5.0	1.0	3.0	10	370	0
feta, crumbled, ¼ cup:							
(*Athenos* Mild)	80	5.0	1.0	6.0	20	340	<1.0
(*Athenos* Traditional)	80	5.0	1.0	6.0	20	330	<1.0
(*Athenos* Traditional Reduced Fat) ...	60	6.0	1.0	4.0	10	400	<1.0
basil-tomato (*Athenos* 4 oz.)	90	6.0	2.0	7.0	25	360	<1.0
basil-tomato (*Athenos* Reduced Fat)	60	6.0	<1.0	4.0	10	400	0
garlic-herb (*Athenos*)	90	6.0	1.0	7.0	20	380	<1.0
fontina:							
(*Boar's Head*)	110	6.0	0	10.0	30	170	0
(*Classica*)	110	7.0	<1.0	8.5	25	160	0
garlic herb (*Kraft Parm Plus!*), 2 tsp.	15	<1.0	2.0	.5	0	90	0
(*Gjetost*)	130	3.0	11.0	9.0	30	90	0
Gloucester, double (*Boar's Head*)	110	7.0	0	10.0	35	200	0
goat:							
(*Laura Chenel Select* Chèvre)	80	4.0	1.0	7.0	25	120	0
(*Snofrisk*)	70	2.0	2.0	8.0	15	170	0
hard type	128	8.7	.6	10.1	30	98	0
mild (*Chavrie*), 1.1 oz.	50	3.0	1.0	4.0	20	120	0
semisoft type	103	6.1	.7	8.5	22	146	0
soft type	76	5.3	.3	6.0	13	104	0
w/basil, roasted garlic (*Chavrie*), 1.1 oz.	50	3.0	1.0	4.0	20	150	0
garlic herb or four peppers (*Mont-chevrê*)	70	4.0	1.0	6.0	20	130	0

Food and Measure	cal.	prot. (gms)	carbo. (gms)	fat (gms)	chol. (mgs)	sod. (mgs)	fiber (gms)
gorgonzola:							
(*Galbani* Dolcelatte)	93	5.0	<1.0	8.0	22	234	0
(*Stella*)	100	6.0	<1.0	9.0	25	390	0
Gouda (*Boar's Head*)	110	6.0	0	9.0	30	280	0
Gruyère:							
(*Boar's Head*)	120	8.0	0	9.0	35	230	0
1 oz.	117	8.5	.1	9.2	31	95	0
hickory smoked							
(*Boar's Head*) . .	100	7.0	0	8.0	20	360	0
havarti:							
(*Sara Lee*)	120	5.0	0	10.0	25	150	0
cream, all varieties							
(*Boar's Head*) . .	110	6.0	0	10.0	35	210	0
hoop (*Friendship*) . . .	20	5.0	0	0	0	10	0
Italian blend, shredded:							
fine (*Kraft Hearty*),							
¼ cup	90	6.0	2.0	7.0	20	210	0
garlic (*Kraft*),							
¼ cup	90	6.0	2.0	6.0	20	220	0
garlic (*Sargento*),							
¼ cup	100	7.0	1.0	7.0	20	170	0
4 cheese (*Maggio* Fancy)	90	7.0	<1.0	6.0	20	190	<1.0
4 cheese (*Sargento* Light), ¼ cup . . .	70	8.0	1.0	3.5	10	210	0
6 cheese (*Sargento*), ¼ cup	90	7.0	0	7.0	20	200	0
jalapeño:							
(*Alpine Lace* Reduced Fat) . . .	80	6.0	2.0	6.0	20	260	0
Jack (*Land O Lakes*)	100	5.0	<1.0	8.0	25	460	0
(*Jarlsberg*)	100	7.0	0	8.0	20	180	0
(*Jarlsberg Lite*)	70	9.0	0	3.5	10	130	0
Kasseri (*Krinos*), 1½" cube, 1.2 oz.	100	8.0	1.0	7.0	18	240	0
(*The Laughing Cow*):							
Babybel	90	7.0	0	7.0	10	230	0
Bonbel	100	6.0	0	8.0	25	230	0
Cheezbits, 6 pcs.	70	4.0	2.0	6.0	20	330	0
mini, 1 pc.:							
Babybel Light . . .	45	6.0	0	3.0	5	180	0
Babybel/Bonbel	70	5.0	0	6.0	15	170	0
wedge, 1 pc.:							
original	50	2.0	1.0	4.0	15	280	0

Food and Measure	cal.	prot. (gms)	carbo. (gms)	fat (gms)	chol. (mgs)	sod. (mgs)	fiber (gms)
Cheese, *The Laughing Cow*, wedge *(cont.)*							
light	30	3.0	1.0	2.0	10	260	0
light, flavored . .	35	3.0	1.0	2.0	10	270	0
Limburger (*Knirps*) . .	80	7.0	0	6.0	20	200	0
mascarpone:							
(*Bel Gioioso*)	124	2.0	.5	13.0	36	16	0
tiramisu flavor (*Bel Gioioso*)	130	2.0	3.0	13.0	35	15	0
Mexican, shredded, 4 cheese, ¼ cup:							
(*Kraft*)	110	6.0	1.0	9.0	25	190	0
(*Maggio* Fancy) . . .	110	6.0	1.0	9.0	25	200	0
(*Sargento*)	110	6.0	<1.0	9.0	25	200	0
(*Sargento* Light) . .	70	8.0	<1.0	4.5	10	200	0
Monterey Jack:							
(*Boar's Head*)	100	6.0	0	9.0	25	170	0
(*Kraft*)	110	6.0	0	9.0	30	190	0
(*Kraft* Reduced Fat)	80	7.0	<1.0	6.0	20	240	0
(*Land O Lakes*) . . .	110	6.0	<1.0	9.0	30	160	0
(*Sara Lee*)	100	7.0	0	8.0	30	170	0
(*Sara Lee* Slice), ¾-oz. slice	80	5.0	0	7.0	20	135	0
(*Sargento* Slice), ¾-oz. slice	80	5.0	0	6.0	20	135	0
hot pepper (*Land O Lakes*)	110	6.0	<1.0	8.0	30	140	0
jalapeño (*Heluva Good*)	100	7.0	0	8.0	25	180	0
jalapeño (*Kraft*) . . .	110	7.0	<1.0	9.0	30	190	0
jalapeño (*Sara Lee* Slice), ¾-oz. slice	80	5.0	0	6.0	20	125	0
Monterey Jack, shredded, ¼ cup:							
(*Kraft*)	100	6.0	1.0	8.0	25	190	0
(*Sargento* Fancy) . .	110	7.0	0	9.0	30	190	0
mozzarella:							
(*Alpine Lace* Reduced Fat) . . .	70	8.0	1.0	3.0	10	200	0
(*Boar's Head*)	90	6.0	<1.0	7.0	25	140	0
(*Land O Lakes*) . . .	80	7.0	<1.0	6.0	15	190	0
(*Sara Lee* Slice), ¾-oz. slice	60	6.0	<1.0	4.0	10	130	0

Food and Measure	cal.	prot. (gms)	carbo. (gms)	fat (gms)	chol. (mgs)	sod. (mgs)	fiber (gms)
(*Sargento* Deli 8 oz.), ¾-oz. slice	60	5.0	1.0	4.0	10	140	0
(*Sargento* Deli 12 oz.), ¾-oz. slice	60	5.0	1.0	4.0	15	140	0
(*Sargento* Deli Light), .8-oz. slice	60	7.0	<1.0	3.0	10	170	0
whole milk (*Maggio*)	80	6.0	1.0	6.0	25	180	0
part skim (*Kraft*) ..	80	8.0	<1.0	5.0	15	200	0
part skim (*Maggio*)	80	7.0	<1.0	6.0	20	220	0
part skim (*Sara Lee*)	80	8.0	1.0	5.0	15	170	0
mozzarella, shredded, ¼ cup:							
(*Kraft* Reduced Fat)	70	8.0	<1.0	4.0	15	190	0
(*Sargento* Chef Style/Fancy)	80	7.0	1.0	6.0	15	190	0
(*Sargento* Light)	70	8.0	<1.0	3.5	10	200	0
whole milk (*Kraft*)	90	6.0	1.0	6.0	20	200	0
whole milk (*Sargento* Chef Style)	100	7.0	0	8.0	25	190	0
part skim (*Kraft*) ..	80	6.0	1.0	5.0	20	220	0
part skim (*Maggio*)	80	8.0	1.0	5.0	15	170	0
mozzarella/Parmesan, shredded (*Kraft* Italian Style), ¼ cup	90	6.0	1.0	7.0	20	220	0
Muenster:							
(*Alpine Lace* Reduced Sodium)	110	7.0	1.0	9.0	25	85	0
(*Boar's Head*)	100	6.0	0	8.0	25	180	0
(*Boar's Head* Low Sodium)	100	6.0	0	8.0	20	75	0
(*Land O Lakes*) ...	100	6.0	0	8.0	25	190	0
(*Sara Lee*)	100	6.0	0	8.0	25	190	0
(*Sara Lee* Slice), ¾-oz. slice	60	5.0	0	7.0	20	150	0
(*Sargento* Deli), ¾-oz. slice	80	5.0	0	6.0	20	135	0
nacho/taco blend, shredded (*Sargento*), ¼ cup	110	6.0	1.0	9.0	25	240	0
Neufchâtel:							
(*Boar's Head*), 2 tbsp.	70	2.0	2.0	6.0	20	190	0

Food and Measure	cal.	prot. (gms)	carbo. (gms)	fat (gms)	chol. (mgs)	sod. (mgs)	fiber (gms)
Cheese, Neufchâtel *(cont.)*							
(*Philadelphia*)	70	3.0	<1.0	6.0	20	120	0
(*Nokkelost*)	100	7.0	2.0	8.0	20	135	0
Parmesan, grated:							
(*Boar's Head*),							
1 tbsp.	20	1.0	1.0	1.0	5	55	0
(*Kraft*), 2 tsp.	20	2.0	0	1.5	<5	75	0
(*Kraft*), .2-oz. pkg.	25	2.0	0	2.0	5	100	0
(*Kraft* Reduced Fat),							
2 tsp.	20	<1.0	2.0	1.0	<5	75	0
(*Land O Lakes*),							
1 tbsp.	20	2.0	0	1.5	<5	60	0
(*Maggio*), 1 tbsp.	25	1.0	1.0	1.5	5	90	0
Parmesan, shredded:							
(*Kraft*), ¼ cup	110	9.0	1.0	8.0	25	410	0
(*Maggio*), 1 tbsp.	20	2.0	0	1.0	0	35	0
(*Sargento* Fancy),							
¼ cup	110	9.0	1.0	7.0	25	300	0
(*Sargento* Fancy),							
2 tsp.	20	2.0	0	1.5	<5	55	0
Parmesan style (*Kraft* Reduced Fat Topping), 2 tsp.	20	<1.0	2.0	1.0	<5	75	0
Parmesan/mozzarella/ Romano, shredded (*Sargento Angel Hair* Blend), ¼ cup	100	8.0	1.0	7.0	20	280	0
Parmesan/Romano:							
grated (*Kraft*), 2 tsp.	20	2.0	0	1.5	<5	85	0
shredded (*Sargento*), ¼ cup	110	9.0	1.0	7.0	25	340	0
pepper, red, zesty (*Kraft Parm Plus!*), 2 tsp.	15	<1.0	2.0	.5	0	90	0
pepper Jack blend (*Sargento*), ¼ cup	110	6.0	<1.0	9.0	25	180	0
pimiento, processed (*Kraft* Deluxe)	100	6.0	<1.0	8.0	25	430	0
pizza blend, shredded, ¼ cup:							
(*Maggio* Fancy) ...	100	7.0	1.0	7.0	20	180	0
(*Sargento Pizza Double Cheese*)	90	7.0	1.0	6.0	20	190	0

Food and Measure	cal.	prot. (gms)	carbo. (gms)	fat (gms)	chol. (mgs)	sod. (mgs)	fiber (gms)
cheddar/mozzarella (Kraft)	100	6.0	<1.0	8.0	25	200	0
four cheese (Kraft)	90	6.0	1.0	7.0	20	230	0
mozzarella/smoke provolone (Kraft)	90	6.0	1.0	7.0	20	210	0
Port du Salut	100	6.7	.2	8.0	35	151	0
provolone:							
(Alpine Lace Reduced Fat) . . .	70	9.0	1.0	5.0	15	120	0
(Boar's Head Lower Sodium)	100	7.0	1.0	8.0	20	140	0
(Boar's Head Picante/ Sharp)	100	7.0	1.0	8.0	25	250	0
(Land O Lakes) . . .	100	7.0	<1.0	8.0	20	240	0
(Sara Lee)	100	7.0	1.0	8.0	30	60	0
(Sara Lee Slice), ¾-oz. slice	80	6.0	0	6.0	15	190	0
(Sargento Deli), ⅔-oz. slice	70	5.0	0	5.0	15	125	0
(Sargento Deli Light), ⅔-oz. slice	45	5.0	<1.0	2.5	5	125	0
ricotta, ¼ cup:							
whole milk (Break- stone's)	110	7.0	2.0	8.0	25	65	0
whole milk (Maggio)	100	6.0	3.0	7.0	25	150	1.0
whole milk	108	7.0	1.9	8.0	32	52	0
part skim (Maggio)	80	4.0	3.0	5.0	20	150	1.0
nonfat (Maggio) . . .	50	7.0	3.0	0	5	170	0
Romano, grated:							
(Boar's Head Pecorino), 1 tbsp.	20	1.0	1.0	1.5	5	95	0
(Kraft), 2 tsp.	25	2.0	0	1.5	5	90	0
(Maggio), 1 tbsp.	25	1.0	2.0	1.5	0	85	0
Romano, shredded (Maggio), 1 tbsp.	20	1.0	0	1.5	0	100	0
Roquefort	105	6.1	.6	8.7	26	513	0
Stilchester (Anco) . . .	110	7.0	0	10.0	30	170	0
string (Maggio)	80	8.0	<1.0	5.0	15	170	0
Swiss:							
(Alpine Lace Reduced Fat) . . .	90	8.0	1.0	6.0	20	35	0
(Boar's Head Gold Label Imported)	110	8.0	<1.0	8.0	20	65	0
(Boar's Head Lacy)	90	9.0	0	6.0	15	35	0

Food and Measure	cal.	prot. (gms)	carbo. (gms)	fat (gms)	chol. (mgs)	sod. (mgs)	fiber (gms)
Cheese, Swiss (cont.)							
(*Boar's Head* Natural)	100	8.0	<1.0	8.0	25	60	0
(*Boar's Head* Natural No Salt)	110	8.0	<1.0	8.0	25	10	0
(*Kraft*)	110	8.0	0	9.0	30	50	0
(*Land O Lakes*) . . .	110	8.0	<1.0	8.0	25	75	0
(*Sara Lee*)	110	8.0	1.0	8.0	30	60	0 ·
(*Sara Lee* Slice), ¾-oz. slice	80	6.0	0	6.0	20	45	0
(*Sargento* Deli) . . .	110	8.0	1.0	8.0	25	60	0
(*Sargento* Deli), ⅔-oz. slice	70	5.0	<1.0	5.0	20	40	0
(*Sargento* Deli Light), .8-oz. slice	70	8.0	<1.0	3.5	15	40	0
aged (*Sargento* Deli), ⅔-oz. slice	70	5.0	0	5.0	20	40	0
Swiss, baby:							
(*Boar's Head*)	110	7.0	<1.0	9.0	25	135	0
(*Cracker Barrel*) . . .	110	7.0	0	9.0	25	110	0
(*Land O Lakes*) . . .	110	8.0	<1.0	8.0	25	75	0
(*Sara Lee*)	110	7.0	1.0	9.0	25	125	0
(*Sara Lee* Slice), ¾-oz. slice	90	6.0	0	6.0	15	160	0
Swiss, processed:							
(*Kraft*)	90	6.0	0	7.0	25	340	0
(*Kraft* Deluxe Singles), ¾ oz. .	70	5.0	0	5.0	20	310	0
(*Kraft* Deluxe Singles).	90	7.0	<1.0	7.0	25	410	0
Swiss, shredded, ¼ cup:							
(*Kraft*)	110	7.0	1.0	8.0	25	60	0
(*Sargento*)	110	8.0	<1.0	8.0	25	60	0
Swiss/American, processed (*Land O Lakes*)	100	6.0	<1.0	8.0	25	380	0
taco blend, shredded, ¼ cup:							
(*Kraft* Mexican Style)	110	6.0	2.0	9.0	25	230	0
(*Sargento*)	110	6.0	1.0	9.0	25	220	0
Wisconsin (*Cracker Barrel* Aged Reserve)	110	7.0	<1.0	9.0	30	180	0

Food and Measure	cal.	prot. (gms)	carbo. (gms)	fat (gms)	chol. (mgs)	sod. (mgs)	fiber (gms)
"Cheese," substitute and nondairy:							
(*Smart Beat* Lactose Free), ⅔-oz. slice	25	4.0	3.0	0	0	180	0
American, slices:							
(*Smart Beat*), ⅔ oz.	25	4.0	3.0	0	0	180	0
(*Tofutti*), ⅔-oz. slice	70	2.0	2.0	5.0	0	290	0
(*Yves* The Good Slice), .7 oz. ...	35	4.0	0	2.0	0	290	0
cheddar:							
(*Yves* The Good Slice), .7 oz. ...	35	4.0	1.0	2.0	0	280	1.0
creamy (*Smart Balance*), ⅔-oz. slice	40	4.0	2.0	2.0	<5	290	0
mellow (*Smart Beat*), ⅔-oz. slice	25	4.0	3.0	0	0	180	0
sharp (*Smart Beat*), ⅔-oz. slice	25	4.0	3.0	0	0	220	0
shredded (*Tofutti Better Than Cheddar*), 1 oz.	70	2.0	2.0	5.0	0	290	0
cream cheese, 1 oz.:							
all varieties (*Tofutti Better Than Cream Cheese*)	80	1.0	1.0	8.0	0	135	0
plain or herb and chive (*Tofutti Better Than Cream Cheese Low Fat*)	40	1.0	2.0	4.0	0	135	0
garlic, roasted (*Tofutti*), ⅔-oz. slice	70	2.0	2.0	5.0	0	290	0
jalapeño Jack (*Yves* The Good Slice), .7 oz.	35	4.0	0	2.0	0	250	0
mozzarella:							
(*Tofutti*), ⅔-oz. slice	70	2.0	2.0	5.0	0	290	0
(*Yves* The Good Slice), .7 oz. ...	30	4.0	0	2.0	0	270	0
mozzarella, shredded (*Smart Balance*), 1 oz.	80	7.0	0	5.0	0	120	0

Food and Measure	cal.	prot. (gms)	carbo. (gms)	fat (gms)	chol. (mgs)	sod. (mgs)	fiber (gms)
"Cheese" substitute and nondairy *(cont.)*							
Swiss (*Yves* The Good Slice), .7 oz.	35	4.0	1.0	2.0	0	260	0
Cheese appetizer (see also "Cheese sticks"), frozen, three cheese (*Apollo/Athens* Tiropita), 4½ pcs., 4.4 oz.	540	7.0	62.0	31.0	5	230	2.0
Cheese dip, 2 oz., except as noted:							
(*Cheez Whiz*)	90	3.0	4.0	7.0	15	490	0
blue (*Marzetti* Veggie Dip)	180	1.0	1.0	19.0	20	220	0
cheddar:							
mild (*Fritos*)	60	1.0	3.0	4.0	5	330	0
mild (*Snyder's*), 1 oz.	80	3.0	3.0	6.0	10	420	0
mild (*Utz*)	45	2.0	2.0	3.0	5	250	0
jalapeño (*Fritos*) . .	50	1.0	4.0	4.0	5	300	0
jalapeño (*Utz*)	30	0	2.0	2.5	0	250	0
chili (*Fritos*)	45	1.0	3.0	3.0	<5	310	0
cream cheese, see "Fruit dip"							
nacho:							
beef (*Ortega*)	60	4.0	4.0	3.5	10	290	0
chicken (*Ortega*) . .	45	3.0	3.0	2.5	5	200	0
salsa:							
(*Chi-Chi's*)	90	3.0	4.0	7.0	15	480	0
(*Old El Paso*)	40	<1.0	3.0	3.0	<5	300	0
(*Tostitos*), 4 tbsp. . .	80	2.0	10.0	5.0	<10	560	<2.0
medium (*Cheez Whiz*)	90	3.0	4.0	7.0	15	500	0
Cheese food (see also "Cheese" and "Cheese products"):							
American:							
(*Kraft* Singles Reduced Fat), ⅔ oz.	45	4.0	1.0	3.0	10	260	0
(*Kraft* Singles Reduced Fat), ¾ oz.	50	4.0	1.0	3.0	10	280	0
(*Velveeta*), 1 oz . . .	90	5.0	2.0	7.0	25	380	0
Cheddar, ¾ oz.:							
(*Kraft* Singles)	70	4.0	2.0	5.0	20	260	0

Food and Measure	cal.	prot. (gms)	carbo. (gms)	fat (gms)	chol. (mgs)	sod. (mgs	fiber (gms)
(*Kraft* Singles Reduced Fat)	50	4.0	1.0	3.0	10	290	0
w/garlic or jalapeño (*Kraft*), 1 oz. ...	90	5.0	2.0	7.0	20	370	0
Italian seasoning (*Land O Lakes*), 1 oz.	90	5.0	2.0	7.0	20	420	0
jalapeño (*Land O Lakes*), 1 oz. ...	90	5.0	2.0	6.0	20	390	0
Mexican style, w/jalapeño (*Kraft* Singles), ¾ oz.	70	4.0	2.0	5.0	20	270	0
Monterey (*Kraft* Singles), ¾ oz.	70	4.0	2.0	5.0	20	280	0
onion (*Land O Lakes*), 1 oz. ...	90	5.0	2.0	7.0	20	450	0
pepperoni (*Land O Lakes*), 1 oz. ...	90	6.0	1.0	7.0	25	430	0
pimiento (*Kraft* Singles), ¾ oz.	70	4.0	2.0	5.0	20	260	0
salami (*Land O Lakes*), 1 oz. ...	90	5.0	2.0	7.0	30	420	0
Swiss (*Kraft* Singles), ¾ oz.	70	4.0	2.0	5.0	20	290	0
Cheese powder (*AlpineAire*), 1 oz. .	170	11.0	0	14.0	n.a.	560	0
Cheese product (see also "Cheese food"), ¾-oz. slice, except as noted:							
(*Velveeta*), 1 oz.	80	5.0	3.0	6.0	25	400	0
(*Velveeta* Slice)	60	3.0	1.0	4.5	20	270	0
(*Velveeta Light* Reduced Fat), 1 oz. ..	60	5.0	3.0	3.0	15	450	0
American: (*Kraft Free* Singles)	30	5.0	2.0	0	<5	270	0
white (*Kraft Free* Singles)	30	5.0	3.0	0	<5	300	0
cheddar, sharp (*Kraft Free* Singles)	30	5.0	2.0	0	<5	280	0
w/jalapeño (*Velveeta*), 1 oz.	80	5.0	3.0	6.0	25	380	0

Food and Measure	cal.	prot. (gms)	carbo. (gms)	fat (gms)	chol. (mgs)	sod. (mgs)	fiber (gms)
Cheese product *(cont.)*							
mozzarella (*Kraft Free* Singles)	30	5.0	2.0	0	<5	270	0
Swiss (*Kraft Free* Singles)	30	5.0	2.0	0	<5	260	0
Cheese puffs, see "Cake, snack"							
Cheese salt (*Watkins*), ¼ tsp.	0	0	0	0	0	310	0
Cheese sandwich dinner, frozen, grilled (*Swanson Fun Feast*), 6.5-oz. pkg.	530	12.0	54.0	29.0	30	810	5.0
Cheese sauce, 2 tbsp.:							
(*Cheez Whiz*)	90	3.0	3.0	7.0	10	560	0
(*Cheez Whiz* Pasteurized	90	3.0	4.0	7.0	15	490	0
(*Cheez Whiz* Squeezable)	90	2.0	4.0	8.0	15	540	0
Romano (*Watkins* Pasta Topper)	30	1.0	4.0	1.0	5	260	0
Cheese sauce, cooking, in jars, ¼ cup:							
Alfredo:							
(*Ragú Cheese Creations!* Classic)	110	1.0	3.0	10.0	25	340	0
(*Ragú Cheese Creations* Light)	80	2.0	3.0	6.0	25	460	0
four cheese (*Five Brothers*)	120	2.0	2.0	12.0	25	300	0
four cheese (*Healthy Choice*)	45	2.0	3.0	3.0	<5	480	0
Parmesan, light (*Ragú Cheese Creations!*)	80	2.0	3.0	6.0	25	440	0
cheddar, double (*Ragú Cheese Creations!*)	100	2.0	3.0	9.0	25	490	0
garlic:							
creamy (*Five Brothers*)	100	2.0	3.0	10.0	30	360	0
roasted, and Parmesan (*Ragú Cheese Creations!*)	110	2.0	3.0	10.0	20	340	0

Food and Measure	cal.	prot. (gms)	carbo. (gms)	fat (gms)	chol. (mgs)	sod. (mgs)	fiber (gms)
Parmesan and:							
mozzarella (*Ragú Cheese Creations!*)	60	6.0	3.0	4.5	25	430	0
Romano (*Ragú Cheese Creations!*)	60	2.0	3.0	4.5	25	430	0
Cheese sauce, cooking, refrigerated, four (*Di Giorno*), ¼ cup ...	160	4.0	2.0	15.0	30	450	0
Cheese sauce mix, creamy cheddar (*Knorr Pasta Sauces*), 2 tbsp.	60	1.0	7.0	3.0	10	580	0
Cheese spread (see also "Cheese," and "Cheese Product"), 2 tbsp., except as noted:							
(*Cheez Whiz*)	90	5.0	2.0	7.0	25	510	0
(*Velveeta*), 1 oz.	80	4.0	3.0	6.0	20	430	0
American (*Easy Cheese*)	100	6.0	2.0	7.0	25	400	0
w/bacon (*Kraft*).	90	5.0	<1.0	8.0	25	570	0
blue cheese (*Kraft Roka*)	80	3.0	2.0	7.0	30	290	0
cheddar:							
(*Easy Cheese* Baseball)	90	4.0	3.0	7.0	25	410	0
sharp (*Easy Cheese*)	100	6.0	3.0	7.0	25	440	0
cheddar and bacon (*Easy Cheese*)	100	6.0	3.0	7.0	25	410	0
feta:							
(*Athenos*)	80	3.0	<1.0	7.0	20	190	0
w/garlic and chives (*Cypress*), 1 oz.	110	4.0	0	10.0	20	210	0
sun-dried tomato-basil (*Athenos*)	80	3.0	<1.0	7.0	20	180	<1.0
Limburger (*Mohawk Valley*)	80	5.0	0	7.0	25	470	0
olive and pimiento (*Kraft*)	80	2.0	3.0	7.0	25	200	0
pimiento (*Kraft*)	80	2.0	3.0	6.0	25	140	0
pineapple (*Kraft*)	70	2.0	4.0	5.0	25	100	0

Food and Measure	cal.	prot. (gms)	carbo. (gms)	fat (gms)	chol. (mgs)	sod. (mgs)	fiber (gms)
Cheese spread *(cont.)*							
sharp (*Kraft Old English*)	90	5.0	<1.0	8.0	25	520	0
Cheese sticks, frozen, breaded:							
(*Master Choice*), 1 pc.	140	5.0	9.0	9.0	10	460	<1.0
mozzarella, 2 pcs.:							
(*Giorgio*)	120	4.0	10.0	7.0	15	300	0
w/sauce (*Farm Rich Dippers*)	180	8.0	16.0	10.0	0	480	<1.0
Cheese topping, see "Nacho topping"							
Cheeseburger, see "Beef sandwich"							
Cheesecake:							
(*Best Little Baker*), 3-oz. cont.	180	4.0	18.0	10.0	75	110	0
pineapple filled (*Entenmann's*), ⅕ cont.	350	7.0	37.0	10.0	85	300	<1.0
strawberry (*Jell-O*), 3.5-oz. cake	150	2.0	25.0	4.5	5	120	0
Cheesecake, frozen, ¼ cake, except as noted:							
(*Baby Watson* New York's) . . .	260	4.0	19.0	18.0	65	150	<1.0
(*Mrs. Smith's* Original), ⅙ cake	520	9.0	44.0	35.0	140	350	1.0
(*Mrs. Smith's Nestlé Butterfinger*), ⅙ cake	550	9.0	54.0	34.0	115	340	2.0
(*Sara Lee* Original) . .	350	7.0	39.0	18.0	50	320	1.0
(*Sara Lee* 25% Reduced Fat)	310	9.0	40.0	13.0	70	310	2.0
cherry (*Sara Lee*)	350	6.0	55.0	12.0	35	310	2.0
chocolate (*Mrs. Smith's*), ⅙ cake . .	550	8.0	50.0	37.0	120	320	2.0
chocolate chip (*Sara Lee*)	410	8.0	47.0	21.0	65	300	2.0
chocolate mousse (*Sara Lee*), ⅕ cake	400	5.0	37.0	25.0	30	190	2.0
French (*Sara Lee*), ⅙ cake	350	5.0	24.0	21.0	20	280	1.0

Food and Measure	cal.	prot. (gms)	carbo. (gms)	fat (gms)	chol. (mgs)	sod. (mgs)	fiber (gms)
strawberry:							
cream (*Sara Lee*) . .	330	6.0	49.0	12.0	40	310	2.0
French (*Sara Lee*), ⅙ cake	320	4.0	43.0	14.0	20	230	1.0
streusel (*Mrs. Smith's*), ⅙ cake	530	7.0	54.0	32.0	85	300	1.0
Cheesecake bar, 1pc.:							
(*Philadelphia* Classic)	190	2.0	17.0	12.0	20	80	0
chocolate (*Philadelphia* Decadence) . .	200	2.0	19.0	12.0	20	85	<1.0
strawberry or white chocolate raspberry (*Philadelphia*)	180	2.0	19.0	10.0	20	75	0
Cheesecake mix*:							
(*Betty Crocker* Original), ⅛ cake	400	6.0	32.0	27.0	100	380	0
(*Jell-O* No Bake Homestyle), ⅙ cake	370	5.0	51.0	18.0	35	550	<1.0
cherry or strawberry (*Jell-O* No Bake), ⅑ cake	300	3.0	47.0	12.0	25	370	<1.0
chocolate chip (*Betty Crocker*), ⅛ cake .	410	6.0	34.0	28.0	100	360	1.0
strawberry swirl, ⅛ cake:							
(*Betty Crocker*) . . .	380	6.0	33.0	25.0	95	360	0
(*Jell-O* No Bake Reduced Fat) . .	250	5.0	45.0	6.0	15	380	0
Cherimoya (see also "Custard apple"):							
(*Frieda's*), 5 oz.	120	2.0	34.0	.5	0	0	3.0
1 medium, 1.9 lb. . . .	515	7.1	131.3	2.2	0	n.a.	13.1
Cherry, fresh:							
(*Dole*), 1 cup, approx. 21 cherries	90	2.0	22.0	.5	0	0	3.0
sour, red, ½ cup:							
w/pits	26	.5	6.3	.2	0	2	.6
red, pitted	39	.8	9.4	.2	0	3	.9
sweet, w/pits, ½ cup .	52	.9	12.0	.7	0	1	1.7
sweet, 10 medium . .	49	.8	11.3	.7	0	<1	1.6
Cherry, canned, ½ cup:							
sour, pitted:							
in water	44	1.0	10.9	.1	0	9	1.3

Food and Measure	cal.	prot. (gms)	carbo. (gms)	fat (gms)	chol. (mgs)	sod. (mgs)	fiber (gms)
Cherry, canned, sour, pitted *(cont.)*							
in light syrup	95	.9	24.3	.1	0	9	1.0
in heavy syrup	116	.9	29.8	.1	0	9	1.0
sweet, w/liquid:							
in water	57	1.0	14.6	.2	0	1	1.9
in juice	68	1.1	17.3	<.1	0	4	1.9
in light syrup	84	.8	21.8	.2	0	4	1.9
sweet, dark, in heavy syrup *(Oregon)* . . .	100	<1.0	24.0	0	0	5	1.0
sweet, pitted, in heavy syrup:							
bing or Royal Anne *(Oregon)*	110	1.0	26.0	0	0	10	1.0
dark *(Del Monte)* . .	100	<1.0	24.0	0	0	10	<1.0
dark *(S&W)*	140	1.0	34.0	0	0	10	1.0
Cherry, candied, red or green:							
(Seneca Glacé), 6 pcs., 1.1 oz. . .	90	0	23.0	0	0	25	0
(S&W Glacé), 5 pcs., 1.1 oz.	80	0	20.0	0	0	20	0
w/pineapple, 2 tbsp.: *(Paradise/White Swan)*	110	0	29.0	0	0	25	1.0
(Seneca Glacé)	100	0	24.0	0	0	20	0
Cherry, dried: bing, ¼ cup, 1.4 oz.:							
(Frieda's)	120	2.0	26.0	0	0	5	3.0
(Sonoma)	140	1.0	34.0	0	0	0	2.0
sweet-tart *(Sonoma)*, ¼ cup, 1.4 oz. . . .	140	1.0	33.0	0	0	0	2.0
tart *(Frieda's)*, ⅓ cup, 1.4 oz.	150	2.0	33.0	0	0	0	2.0
Cherry, frozen: dark sweet:							
(Big Valley), ¾ cup	90	1.0	20.0	0	0	0	3.0
(Cascadian Farm), 1 cup	72	1.0	17.0	1.0	0	0	2.0
unsweetened, ½ cup	36	7.1	8.5	.3	0	1	1.2
sweetened, ½ cup . . .	116	1.5	29.0	.2	0	1	2.7
Cherry, maraschino, red or green, 1 pc.:							
(Haddon House)	10	0	2.0	0	0	0	0
(S&W)	10	0	3.0	0	0	0	0

Food and Measure	cal.	prot. (gms)	carbo. (gms)	fat (gms)	chol. (mgs)	sod. (mgs)	fiber (gms)
large (*Aunt Nellie's*) ..	10	0	3.0	0	0	0	0
small (*Aunt Nellie's*) ..	10	0	2.0	0	0	0	0
Cherry, West Indian, see "Acerola"							
Cherry drink:							
(*Kool-Aid Bursts*), 6.75 fl. oz.	90	0	23.0	0	0	40	0
(*R. W. Knudsen* Cider), 8 fl. oz.	120	1.0	31.0	0	0	35	0
(*Santa Cruz Organic* Nectar), 8 fl. oz. ..	110	<1.0	26.0	0	0	20	0
(*Tang Cherry Craze*), 8 fl. oz.	100	0	27.0	0	0	30	0
black, concentrate* (*R. W. Knudsen*), 8 fl. oz.	130	1.0	31.0	0	0	15	0
wild (*Capri Sun All Natural*), 6.75-fl. oz.	110	0	30.0	0	0	20	0
Cherry drink mix*, 8 fl. oz.:							
(*Kool-Aid* Sugar Sweetened)	60	0	16.0	0	0	0	0
freeze (*Kool-Aid Slushies*)	140	0	35.0	0	0	80	2.0
Cherry juice, 8 fl. oz., except as noted:							
(*Eden* Organic)	140	1.0	33.0	1.0	0	30	0
(*Juicy Juice*)	130	0	30.0	0	0	10	0
(*Juicy Juice*), 12 fl. oz.	190	0	45.0	0	0	15	0
black (*R. W. Knudsen*)	180	2.0	43.0	0	0	40	0
Cherry juice blends, 8 fl. oz.:							
(*After the Fall* Very Cherry)	100	0	26.0	0	0	20	0
black, concentrate* (*R. W. Knudsen*) ..	130	1.0	31.0	0	0	15	0
cider (*R. W. Knudsen*)	130	<1.0	33.0	0	0	35	0
frozen* (*Cascadian Farm* Mountain) ...	120	0	30.0	0	0	9	0
Cherry syrup, mara-schino (*Trader Vic's*), 1 fl. oz.	90	0	23.0	0	0	15	0

Food and Measure	cal.	prot. (gms)	carbo. (gms)	fat (gms)	chol. (mgs)	sod. (mgs)	fiber (gms)
Cherry-berry, dried (*Sunsweet Fruitlings*), 1.4 oz., ⅓ cup	130	1.0	31.0	0	0	0	3.0
Chervil, dried, 1 tsp.	1	.1	.3	<.1	0	<1	.1
Chestnut, Chinese, shelled, 1 oz.:							
dried	103	1.9	22.7	.5	0	2	<1.0
boiled or steamed ...	44	.8	9.6	.2	0	1	<1.0
roasted	68	1.3	14.9	.3	0	1	<1.0
Chestnut, European: raw:							
in shell, 1 lb.	714	8.1	152.8	7.6	0	9	27.2
shelled, w/peel, 1 cup, 13 pcs. ..	308	3.5	66.0	3.3	0	4	11.7
dried, peeled, 1 oz. ...	105	1.4	23.3	1.1	0	11	<2.0
boiled, 1 oz.	37	.8	7.9	.4	0	8	<1.0
roasted, peeled:							
1 oz.	70	.9	15.0	.6	0	1	3.3
1 cup, 17 kernels ..	350	4.3	75.7	3.2	0	3	16.7
Chestnuts, European, in jars (*Minerve*), 4 whole, 1.1 oz. ...	50	1.0	12.0	0	0	0	2.0
Chicken, fresh, 4 oz., except as noted:							
broiler-fryer, roasted:							
w/skin, ½ chicken, 10.5 oz. (15.8 oz. w/bone)	715	81.6	0	40.7	263	244	0
w/skin	271	31.0	0	15.4	100	93	0
meat only	215	32.8	0	8.4	101	98	0
meat only, chopped or diced, 1 cup	266	40.5	0	10.4	125	120	0
skin only, 1 oz.	129	5.8	0	11.5	24	18	0
dark meat only	232	31.0	0	11.0	105	105	0
light meat only	196	35.1	0	5.1	96	87	0
breast, w/skin, ½ breast, 3½ oz. (8.5 oz. w/bone)	193	29.2	0	7.6	83	69	0
drumstick, w/skin, 1.8 oz. (2.9 oz. w/bone)	112	14.1	0	5.8	48	47	0
leg, w/skin (5.7 oz. w/bone)	265	29.6	0	15.4	105	99	0

Food and Measure	cal.	prot. (gms)	carbo. (gms)	fat (gms)	chol. (mgs)	sod. (mgs)	fiber (gms)
thigh, w/skin, 2.2 oz. (2.9 oz. w/bone)	153	15.5	0	9.6	58	52	0
wing, w/skin, 1.2 oz. (2.3 oz. w/bone)	99	9.1	0	6.6	29	28	0
capon, roasted, w/skin:							
½ capon, 1.4 lbs. (2 lbs. w/bone)	1457	184.5	0	74.2	549	313	0
w/skin	260	32.8	0	13.2	98	56	0
ground, see "Chicken, ground"							
roaster, roasted:							
w/skin, ½ chicken, 1 lb. (1.5 lbs. w/bone)	1071	115.0	0	64.3	365	349	0
meat w/skin	253	27.2	0	15.2	86	83	0
stewing, stewed:							
w/skin, ½ chicken, 9.2 oz. (13½ oz. w/bone)	744	70.2	0	49.2	205	190	0
meat w/skin	323	30.5	0	21.4	90	83	0
meat only	269	34.5	0	13.5	94	88	0
meat only, chopped or diced, 1 cup	332	42.6	0	16.6	117	109	0
Chicken, canned:							
chunk, 2 oz.:							
(*Hormel*)	70	11.0	0	2.5	35	250	0
(*Swanson*)	70	11.0	<1.0	2.0	35	230	<1.0
breast:							
(*Hormel*)	60	13.0	0	1.0	30	290	0
(*Hormel* No Salt) . .	60	12.0	0	1.0	30	35	0
(*Swanson*)	60	11.0	1.0	1.0	25	230	0
Chicken, freeze-dried, cooked, diced (*AlpineAire*), ½ oz.	60	13.0	0	.5	35	15	0
Chicken, frozen or refrigerated, raw, 4 oz., except as noted:							
whole:							
(*Tyson* Young/ Cut-up)	250	19.0	0	19.0	65	70	0
roaster (*Tyson Fresh Sunday Best/ Tyson* Young) . .	220	20.0	0	15.0	80	75	0

Food and Measure	cal.	prot. (gms)	carbo. (gms)	fat (gms)	chol. (mgs)	sod. (mgs)	fiber (gms)
Chicken, frozen or refrigerated, raw *(cont.)*							
whole, rotisserie:							
all flavors, except honey, dark (*Perdue*)	240	15.0	1.0	20.0	105	340	0
all flavors, except honey, white (*Perdue*)	170	19.0	1.0	10.0	80	370	0
honey, dark (*Perdue*)	240	15.0	2.0	20.0	95	360	0
honey, white (*Perdue*)	170	20.0	2.0	10.0	85	360	0
whole, toasted garlic:							
dark (*Perdue*)	260	16.0	1.0	21.0	100	440	0
white (*Perdue*)	180	20.0	1.0	10.0	90	440	0
breast:							
whole (*Tyson*)	190	21.0	1.0	12.0	80	40	0
half (*Tyson Individually Fresh Frozen*), 5.2-oz. pc.	220	29.0	0	12.0	100	260	0
split (*Tyson*)	190	21.0	1.0	12.0	80	40	0
split, broth basted (*Tyson Tasty-basted*)	210	20.0	0	14.0	50	270	0
split, skinless (*Tyson*)	130	25.0	0	3.0	75	70	0
quarters (*Tyson*) . .	250	19.0	0	19.0	65	70	0
breast, boneless, skinless:							
(*Perdue Individually Frozen*), 5.9 oz. .	160	35.0	0	1.5	100	310	0
(*Perdue Fit 'n Easy*)	110	26.0	0	1.0	75	45	0
(*Perdue Oven Stuffer*)	130	27.0	0	2.0	75	45	0
(*Tyson*)	140	25.0	0	4.0	65	40	0
(*Tyson Individually Fresh Frozen*), 4.7-oz. pc.	160	28.0	0	5.0	75	140	0
fillet (*Tyson Thin & Fancy*)	120	28.0	0	1.0	60	30	0
thin sliced (*Perdue Fit 'n Easy*), 2.8 oz.	80	18.0	0	1.5	50	35	0
breast, boneless, skinless, seasoned:							

Food and Measure	cal.	prot. (gms)	carbo. (gms)	fat (gms)	chol. (mgs)	sod. (mgs	fiber (gms)
barbecue, mesquite (*Chicken By George*)	130	21.0	5.0	3.0	60	700	0
broth basted, split (*Tyson* Tasty-basted)	110	21.0	0	3.0	45	190	0
Cajun (*Chicken By George*)	130	21.0	3.0	4.0	60	700	0
Caribbean grill (*Chicken By George*)	150	22.0	8.0	4.0	60	550	0
chili lime (*Tyson* Tastybasted) ...	100	22.0	2.0	1.0	40	570	0
fajita (*Tyson* Tasty-basted)	110	21.0	4.0	.5	35	450	0
garlic herb (*Perdue*)	110	22.0	3.0	1.0	60	740	0
Italian (*Perdue*) ...	110	22.0	3.0	1.0	60	740	0
Italian (*Tyson* Tasty-basted)	100	22.0	2.0	5.0	55	800	0
Italian blue cheese (*Chicken By George*)	130	20.0	2.0	5.0	60	790	0
lemon herb (*Chicken By George*)	120	20.0	3.0	3.0	60	800	0
lemon herb (*Tyson* Tastybasted) ...	100	22.0	2.0	1.0	45	490	0
lemon oregano (*Chicken By George*)	130	20.0	3.0	4.0	50	600	0
lemon pepper (*Perdue*)	110	22.0	3.0	1.0	60	740	0
mustard dill (*Chicken By George*)	140	20.0	2.0	5.0	65	650	0
roasted (*Chicken By George*)	110	21.0	0	3.0	55	500	0
rosemary, garlic, thyme (*Perdue*), 3.5 oz.	100	20.0	1.0	1.5	60	830	0
teriyaki (*Chicken By George*)	130	21.0	6.0	3.0	55	530	0
teriyaki (*Perdue*) ..	110	22.0	3.0	1.0	60	680	0

Food and Measure	cal.	prot. (gms)	carbo. (gms)	fat (gms)	chol. (mgs)	sod. (mgs)	fiber (gms)
Chicken, frozen or refrigerated, raw, breast, boneless, skinless *(cont.)*							
teriyaki, (*Tyson* Tastybasted) ...	120	21.0	8.0	1.0	45	670	0
tomato herb (*Perdue*), 3.5 oz.	100	20.0	1.0	1.5	60	750	0
tomato herb basil (*Chicken By George*)	140	20.0	5.0	5.0	60	630	0
cut-up:							
(*Tyson* Pick of the Chix)	210	20.0	1.0	14.0	100	55	0
skinless (*Tyson* Pick of the Chix)	150	22.0	0	7.0	80	15	0
drumsticks:							
(*Tyson*)	150	21.0	0	7.0	115	85	0
(*Tyson Individually Fresh Frozen*), 2 pcs.	140	17.0	0	7.0	90	280	0
broth basted (*Tyson* Tastybasted) ...	120	18.0	0	6.0	80	320	0
skinless (*Tyson*) ..	130	21.0	0	5.0	110	95	0
breast, skinless, split broth basted (*Tyson* Tastybasted)	130	22.0	0	5.0	50	310	0
gizzards and hearts (*Tyson*)	90	20.0	0	1.0	235	65	0
leg, whole (*Tyson*) ...	230	19.0	1.0	17.0	115	70	0
leg quarters:							
(*Tyson*)	230	19.0	1.0	17.0	115	70	0
honey barbecue (*Tyson* Tastybasted)	210	15.0	3.0	16.0	70	470	0
salsa (*Tyson* Tastybasted)	240	16.0	4.0	18.0	75	280	0
strips, seasoned:							
Parmesan garlic (*Perdue Simply Sauté*)	110	22.0	3.0	1.5	65	800	0
savory (*Perdue Simply Sauté Classic*)	110	23.0	2.0	1.0	65	600	0
spicy (*Perdue Simply Sauté Fiesta*)	160	18.0	4.0	8.0	85	710	0

Food and Measure	cal.	prot. (gms)	carbo. (gms)	fat (gms)	chol. (mgs)	sod. (mgs)	fiber (gms)
stuffed, 5.9-oz. pc.:							
w/broccoli, cheese (*Tyson*)	320	20.0	23.0	16.0	50	870	3.0
cordon bleu (*Tyson*)	350	25.0	24.0	17.0	55	1320	3.0
Kiev (*Tyson*)	460	20.0	24.0	32.0	115	980	2.0
w/wild rice, mushrooms (*Tyson*)	300	23.0	25.0	12.0	50	860	1.0
tenderloin:							
(*Perdue* Individually Frozen)	110	24.0	0	1.5	65	160	0
(*Perdue Fit 'n Easy*)	120	27.0	0	1.0	70	45	0
(*Tyson Individually Fresh Frozen*), 4 pcs., 4.6 oz. ...	110	25.0	0	1.0	55	220	0
tenders:							
breast (*Tyson*)	110	26.0	0	5.0	55	40	0
broth basted (*Tyson* Tastybasted) ...	100	22.0	0	.5	50	230	0
honey barbecue (*Tyson* Tastybasted)	120	21.0	7.0	1.5	40	570	0
thigh:							
(*Perdue* Individually Frozen), 6.2-oz. pc.	260	29.0	0	16.0	140	270	0
(*Tyson*)	250	17.0	0	20.0	100	80	0
(*Tyson Individually Fresh Frozen*), 4.9-oz. pc.	380	17.0	0	34.0	110	350	0
broth basted (*Tyson* Tastybasted) ...	270	16.0	0	23.0	80	240	0
thigh, boneless, skinless:							
cutlets (*Tyson*)	160	19.0	0	10.0	90	75	0
fajita (*Tyson* Tastybasted)	150	16.0	2.0	8.0	75	600	0
salsa (*Tyson* Tastybasted)	140	17.0	5.0	6.0	60	710	0
teriyaki (*Tyson* Tastybasted) ...	150	17.0	7.0	6.0	65	910	0
thigh, skinless (*Tyson*)	210	19.0	0	15.0	95	75	0
wing:							
(*Tyson/Tyson* Jumbo Pack)	250	18.0	1.0	20.0	125	60	0

Food and Measure	cal.	prot. (gms)	carbo. (gms)	fat (gms)	chol. (mgs)	sod. (mgs)	fiber (gms)
Chicken, frozen or refrigerated, raw *(cont.)*							
(*Tyson Individually Fresh Frozen*), 4 pcs., 4.2 oz. . . .	240	20.0	0	18.0	95	220	0
broth basted (*Tyson Tastybasted*) . . .	230	17.0	0	18.0	80	260	0
Chicken, frozen or refrigerated, cooked (see also "Chicken entree, frozen"), 3 oz., except as noted:							
whole:							
(*Tyson*), 3 oz.	160	16.0	1.0	11.0	75	490	0
dark (*Perdue*)	210	17.0	0	16.0	110	55	0
dark (*Perdue Oven Stuffer*)	210	18.0	0	15.0	100	60	0
white (*Perdue*)	170	21.0	0	10.0	85	45	0
white (*Perdue Oven Stuffer*)	170	21.0	0	9.0	80	50	0
whole, barbecue (*Empire* Kosher), 5 oz.	280	31.0	1.0	17.0	110	480	
whole, garlic toasted:							
dark (*Perdue*)	190	16.0	1.0	14.0	100	330	0
white (*Perdue*)	160	19.0	1.0	9.0	75	320	0
whole, rotisserie:							
all flavors, except honey, dark (*Perdue*)	180	15.0	0	13.0	100	260	0
all flavors, except honey, white (*Perdue*)	140	17.0	0	7.0	75	260	0
honey, dark (*Perdue*)	200	12.0	1.0	16.0	80	300	0
honey, white (*Perdue*)	140	16.0	1.0	8.0	80	300	0
barbecue, smoky (*Wampler*), 1 cup .	430	42.0	31.0	15.0	140	1020	1.0
bites:							
(*Country Skillet*), 10 pcs.	280	14.0	16.0	17.0	25	610	1.0
(*Country Skillet Value Pack*), 5 pcs.	270	12.0	18.0	16.0	20	720	1.0

Food and Measure	cal.	prot. (gms)	carbo. (gms)	fat (gms)	chol. (mgs)	sod. (mgs	fiber (gms)
breast, whole:							
(*Perdue*)	160	21.0	0	9.0	80	45	0
(*Perdue Oven*							
Stuffer)	150	21.0	0	8.0	70	40	0
breast, split:							
(*Perdue*), 6.8 oz. ..	370	48.0	0	20.0	180	100	0
(*Tyson*), 5.1-oz. pc.	260	34.0	1.0	13.0	110	670	0
skinless (*Perdue*),							
5.8 oz.	250	46.0	0	7.0	150	95	0
breast, quarters							
(*Perdue*)	170	20.0	0	10.0	80	50	0
breast, boneless,							
skinless:							
(*Perdue Individually*							
Frozen), 4.2 oz.	140	32.0	0	1.5	90	280	0
(*Perdue Fit 'n Easy*)	110	25.0	0	1.0	70	30	0
(*Perdue Oven*							
Stuffer)	120	25.0	0	1.5	70	30	0
(*Tyson*), 3.7-oz. pc.	130	26.0	1.0	2.5	70	580	0
diced (*Tyson*)	110	22.0	1.0	1.5	55	510	0
diced (*Tyson Time*							
Trimmers)	90	20.0	0	1.0	45	240	0
shredded (*Tyson*) ..	110	21.0	2.0	1.5	55	350	0
tenderloin (*Perdue*							
Individually							
Frozen)	100	23.0	0	1.0	55	100	0
tenderloin (*Perdue*							
Fit 'n Easy)	100	24.0	0	.5	60	30	0
thin sliced (*Perdue*							
Fit 'n Easy), 2 oz.	80	16.0	0	1.0	45	20	0
breast, barbecue fried							
(*Empire* Kosher) ..	170	21.0	3.0	8.0	45	440	<1.0
breast, boneless,							
seasoned:							
garlic herb (*Perdue*)	90	18.0	3.0	1.0	50	620	0
lemon pepper or							
Italian (*Perdue*)	90	18.0	3.0	1.0	50	610	0
lemon pepper							
(*Perdue Short*							
Cuts), ½ cup ...	100	19.0	1.0	2.5	60	490	0
honey roasted							
(*Perdue Short*							
Cuts), ½ cup ...	100	18.0	2.0	2.0	45	450	0

Food and Measure	cal.	prot. (gms)	carbo. (gms)	fat (gms)	chol. (mgs)	sod. (mgs)	fiber (gms)
Chicken, frozen or refrigerated, cooked, breast, boneless *(cont.)*							
Italian (*Perdue Short Cuts*), ½ cup . . .	100	19.0	0	2.5	60	380	0
roasted (*Perdue Short Cuts Original*), ½ cup	90	19.0	1.0	2.0	50	500	0
rosemary garlic thyme (*Perdue*)	90	20.0	1.0	1.5	60	820	0
Southwestern (*Perdue Short Cuts*), ½ cup . . .	100	18.0	1.0	2.5	60	410	0
teriyaki (*Perdue*) . .	90	18.0	3.0	1.0	50	560	0
tomato herb (*Perdue*)	90	20.0	1.0	1.5	60	740	0
breast fillet, breaded (*Tyson*), 2.8-oz. pc.	150	15.0	8.0	6.0	35	330	1.0
cacciatore (*Wampler*), 1 cup	260	30.0	10.0	9.0	90	600	2.0
cutlets, breaded:							
(*Perdue*), 3.5 oz. . .	220	15.0	15.0	11.0	55	600	0
(*Perdue* Low Fat) . .	110	14.0	12.0	1.0	35	730	0
Italian (*Perdue* Low Fat)	120	15.0	11.0	2.0	40	690	0
drum and thigh, fried (*Empire* Kosher) . .	240	16.0	7.0	16.0	80	260	2.0
drumsticks:							
barbecue, honey (*Tyson* Family Pack), 3.1-oz. pc.	150	17.0	5.0	7.0	85	470	2.0
barbecue, hot (*Tyson*), 2 pcs., 3.5 oz.	160	22.0	3.0	7.0	100	620	1.0
roasted (*Perdue*), 2.2 oz.	110	14.0	0	6.0	80	65	0
roasted (*Perdue Oven Stuffer*), 3.6 oz.	190	22.0	0	11.0	120	100	0
roasted (*Tyson* Multi-Serve), 2 pcs., 3.8 oz. . .	220	27.0	1.0	12.0	50	580	0
roasted (*Tyson* Single Serve), 3 pcs., 5.8 oz. . .	330	40.0	1.0	18.0	225	870	0

Food and Measure	cal.	prot. (gms)	carbo. (gms)	fat (gms)	chol. (mgs)	sod. (mgs	fiber (gms)
fajita (*Wampler*), 1 cup	210	23.0	13.0	7.0	70	1350	2.0
fillet, battered and breaded (*Empire Kosher*), 4 oz.	240	21.0	13.0	11.0	30	380	2.0
fried, bone-in:							
(*Banquet* Original)	280	14.0	15.0	18.0	65	630	1.0
(*Country Skillet*) ..	270	14.0	13.0	18.0	65	620	1.0
country (*Banquet*)	270	14.0	13.0	18.0	65	620	1.0
cut (*Empire* Kosher)	200	15.0	8.0	12.0	75	240	0
honey barbecue, skinless (*Banquet*)	230	18.0	9.0	13.0	55	480	2.0
hot/spicy (*Banquet*)	260	14.0	13.0	18.0	65	730	1.0
skinless (*Banquet*)	220	18.0	7.0	13.0	65	480	2.0
Southern (*Banquet*)	280	14.0	15.0	18.0	65	700	1.0
leg:							
whole, roasted (*Perdue*), 5.6 oz.	370	33.0	0	27.0	200	105	0
quarters (*Perdue*)	220	17.0	0	17.0	105	55	0
nuggets:							
(*Banquet* Fun), 4 pcs.	220	11.0	10.0	24.0	45	540	<1.0
(*Banquet* Original), 6 pcs.	270	11.0	13.0	19.0	40	540	1.0
(*Country Skillet*), 5 pcs.	270	12.0	18.0	16.0	20	720	1.0
(*Perdue*), 5 pcs. ..	210	15.0	15.0	11.0	50	580	0
(*Perdue* Individually Frozen), 5 pcs.	250	11.0	15.0	16.0	40	720	1.0
(*Tyson*), 6 pcs. ...	280	11.0	14.0	20.0	50	490	2.0
(*Tyson* Family Pack), 6 pcs.	240	14.0	11.0	16.0	30	410	1.0
breast (*Banquet*), 7 pcs.	280	11.0	13.0	20.0	40	500	1.0
breast (*Perdue* Golden Brown), 5 pcs.	240	11.0	14.0	15.0	35	530	0
breast (*Tyson*), 6 pcs.	220	13.0	11.0	14.0	40	480	0
w/cheese (*Perdue*), 5 pcs.	230	15.0	15.0	13.0	55	670	0
mozzarella (*Banquet*), 6 pcs.	280	9.0	19.0	18.0	40	630	1.0
Southern (*Banquet*), 6 pcs.	260	12.0	15.0	17.0	35	550	1.0

Food and Measure	cal.	prot. (gms)	carbo. (gms)	fat (gms)	chol. (mgs)	sod. (mgs)	fiber (gms)
Chicken, frozen or refrigerated, cooked, nuggets (cont.)							
Southern (*Tyson*), 6 pcs.	260	11.0	11.0	9.0	40	540	1.0
Southern fried (*Country Skillet*), 5 pcs.	270	11.0	17.0	18.0	20	550	1.0
patty, 1 pc.:							
(*Banquet* Original)	190	7.0	10.0	14.0	30	440	1.0
(*Country Skillet*) ..	190	9.0	12.0	11.0	20	490	1.0
(*Tyson*), 2.6-oz. pc.	180	10.0	12.0	11.0	25	300	1.0
(*Tyson* Family Pack)	210	12.0	9.0	14.0	25	360	1.0
(*Tyson Thick 'n Crispy*)	220	10.0	10.0	15.0	40	370	1.0
Southern (*Banquet*)	190	8.0	10.0	13.0	25	420	<1.0
Southern fried (*Country Skillet*)	190	9.0	12.0	12.0	20	440	1.0
patty, breast, 1 pc.:							
baked (*Banquet* Fat Free)	100	9.0	15.0	0	20	400	<1.0
grilled (*Banquet*) ..	110	15.0	3.0	4.5	35	490	1.0
grilled, hickory barbecue (*Banquet*)	150	13.0	3.0	9.0	40	440	0
Southern (*Tyson*)	180	11.0	8.0	12.0	30	360	0
popcorn:							
(*Banquet*), 11 pcs.	190	8.0	22.0	8.0	20	510	1.0
(*Tyson Bites* Family Pack), 6 pcs. ..	210	14.0	17.0	9.0	25	650	2.0
shredded, barbecue (*Tyson*), ¼ cup ...	90	7.0	11.0	5.0	30	280	0
strips:							
Buffalo (*Tyson* Family Pack), 2 pcs., 3 oz. ...	190	12.0	17.0	9.0	20	1050	1.0
crispy (*Tyson* Family Pack), 2 pcs., 2.5 oz.	160	13.0	10.0	7.0	25	410	1.0
Parmesan garlic (*Perdue Simply Sauté*)	100	20.0	2.0	1.5	55	710	0
savory (*Perdue Simply Sauté Classic*)	90	19.0	1.0	1.0	55	500	0

Food and Measure	cal.	prot. (gms)	carbo. (gms)	fat (gms)	chol. (mgs)	sod. (mgs)	fiber (gms)
spicy (*Perdue Simply Sauté Fiesta*)	140	16.0	3.0	7.0	75	630	0
strips, breast:							
(*Tyson Time Trimmers*)	90	20.0	0	1.0	45	240	0
Southwestern (*Tyson Time Trimmers*)	110	18.0	2.0	3.0	40	400	0
strips, breast, breaded:							
(*Perdue Kick'N Chicken* Original)	120	14.0	14.0	1.0	35	750	0
barbecue (*Perdue Kick'N Chicken*)	120	12.0	16.0	1.0	30	720	0
hot and spicy (*Perdue Kick'N Chicken*)	110	12.0	13.0	1.0	30	930	0
sweet and sour (*Wampler*), 1 cup	250	20.0	35.0	4.0	55	510	1.0
tenderloin, breaded:							
(*Perdue*)	140	15.0	13.0	2.5	35	480	0
(*Perdue* Individually Frozen)	200	15.0	13.0	10.0	300	510	0
(*Tyson*), 2 pcs., 3 oz.	180	12.0	15.0	8.0	25	440	1.0
Southern (*Tyson*), 2 pcs., 3.5 oz. . .	210	15.0	14.0	11.0	30	480	1.0
spicy (*Tyson*), 2 pcs.	200	14.0	16.0	9.0	25	790	0
tenders:							
(*Banquet* Original), 3 pcs.	250	12.0	15.0	16.0	40	480	<1.0
(*Tyson* Family Pack), 5 pcs., 3 oz. . .	240	14.0	11.0	16.0	30	410	1.0
breast (*Banquet* Fat Free), 3 pcs. . . .	120	13.0	16.0	0	30	480	1.0
breast (*Country Skillet*), 3 pcs. .	240	11.0	16.0	14.0	25	450	1.0
breast, baked (*Butterball*), 3 pcs.	170	14.0	15.0	6.0	35	410	1.0
breast, breaded (*Tyson*), 5 pcs., 3 oz.	230	12.0	11.0	15.0	35	290	1.0
breast, Buffalo (*Banquet*), 5 pcs.	230	12.0	16.0	13.0	30	560	0

Food and Measure	cal.	prot. (gms)	carbo. (gms)	fat (gms)	chol. (mgs)	sod. (mgs)	fiber (gms)
Chicken, frozen or refrigerated, cooked, tenders *(cont.)*							
breast, honey battered (*Tyson*), 5 pcs., 3 oz. . . .	220	12.0	9.0	15.0	45	380	1.0
grilled, hickory smoked (*Butterball*), 4 pcs. w/sauce	160	17.0	12.0	5.0	50	570	1.0
grilled, Oriental (*Butterball*), 4 pcs. w/sauce . .	160	17.0	12.0	5.0	45	560	1.0
Southern (*Banquet*), 3 pcs.	260	12.0	16.0	16.0	40	460	1.0
thigh, roasted, 1 pc.:							
(*Perdue*), 3.2 oz. . .	240	17.0	0	19.0	115	65	0
(*Tyson* Single Serve), 3.6 oz.	270	22.0	1.0	19.0	40	490	0
wings:							
(*Banquet* Firehouse Big), 2 pcs.	190	14.0	1.0	14.0	75	700	0
(*Banquet* Smokehouse Big), 2 pcs.	200	14.0	4.0	14.0	70	300	0
(*Tyson* Tabasco), 3 pcs., 2.7 oz. . .	170	17.0	1.0	10.0	100	330	1.0
barbecue (*Master Choice*), 3 pcs., 3 oz.	220	13.0	6.0	16.0	45	580	0
barbecue (*Tyson*), 3 pcs., 3.2 oz. . .	200	19.0	2.0	13.0	110	330	0
barbecue, honey (*Banquet*), 4 pcs.	260	15.0	11.0	18.0	55	440	0
barbecue, honey (*Tyson*), 5 pcs., 3 oz.	210	19.0	4.0	12.0	120	540	1.0
hot and spicy (*Banquet*), 4 pcs.	220	15.0	6.0	15.0	70	310	0
hot and spicy (*Perdue* Individually Frozen) . . .	180	16.0	1.0	12.0	95	430	0
hot and spicy (*Tyson*), 4 pcs., 3.4 oz.	220	20.0	1.0	15.0	110	560	0

Food and Measure	cal.	prot. (gms)	carbo. (gms)	fat (gms)	chol. (mgs)	sod. (mgs)	fiber (gms)
hot and spicy (*Tyson* Party Pack), 4 pcs., 3.2 oz.	190	18.0	2.0	12.0	100	900	0
roasted (*Perdue*), 2 pcs., 3.2 oz. . .	210	19.0	0	15.0	115	75	0
teriyaki (*Tyson*), 4 pcs., 3.4 oz. . .	190	21.0	2.0	12.0	120	210	2.0
wingettes, roasted:							
(*Perdue*), 3 pcs. . .	210	19.0	0	15.0	110	70	0
(*Perdue Oven Stuffer*), 3 pcs., 3.4 oz.	220	21.0	0	15.0	120	80	0
Chicken, ground							
raw, 4 oz.:							
(*Perdue Fit 'n Easy*)	180	19.0	0	12.0	135	75	0
(*Shady Brook Farms*)	180	23.0	0	10.0	95	90	0
(*Tyson*)	150	18.0	0	9.0	75	65	0
(*Wampler*)	220	22.0	0	14.0	90	85	0
breast (*Perdue Fit 'n Easy*)	100	24.0	0	.5	65	75	0
cooked, 3 oz.:							
(*Perdue Fit 'n Easy*)	170	18.0	0	11.0	125	50	0
(*Tyson Crumbles*) .	110	16.0	1.0	5.0	70	510	0
breast (*Perdue Fit 'n Easy*)	80	19.0	0	.5	55	65	0
"Chicken," vegetarian:							
canned:							
diced (*Worthington Chik*), ¼ cup . . .	50	9.0	2.0	0	0	220	1.0
fried (*Worthington FriChik*), 2 pcs.	140	12.0	3.0	8.0	0	350	1.0
fried (*Worthington FriChik Lowfat*), 2 pcs.	80	10.0	2.0	3.0	0	430	1.0
fried, w/gravy (*Loma Linda Chik'n*), 2 pcs.	160	12.0	4.0	10.0	0	440	2.0
sliced (*Worthington Chik*), 3 slices . .	80	15.0	3.0	.5	0	360	2.0
frozen/refrigerated:							
(*Morningstar Farms Chik Patties*), 1 pc.	150	9.0	15.0	6.0	0	490	2.0

Food and Measure	cal.	prot. (gms)	carbo. (gms)	fat (gms)	chol. (mgs)	sod. (mgs)	fiber (gms)
"Chicken," vegetarian, frozen/refrigerated *(cont.)*							
(*Morningstar Farms Chik Nuggets*), 4 pcs.	160	13.0	17.0	4.0	0	670	5.0
(*Worthington ChicKetts*), 2 slices, ⅜" ...	120	13.0	2.0	7.0	0	390	2.0
Buffalo wings (*Morningstar Farms*), 5 pcs.	200	12.0	18.0	9.0	0	630	3.0
chunk (*Veggie Master Vege*), ¼ pkg.	124	7.9	7.6	6.8	0	256	6.7
cutlets (*Quorn*), 3.5-oz. pc.	200	10.0	20.0	8.0	0	610	4.0
diced (*Worthington Meatless*), ¼ cup	60	11.0	3.0	0	0	260	<1.0
drumstick (*Worthington ChickStiks*), 1.7-oz pc.	100	10.0	4.0	6.0	0	300	2.0
nuggets (*Boca Chik'n*), 4 pcs. .	190	16.0	16.0	7.0	0	570	2.0
nuggets (*Loma Linda Chik-Nuggets*), 5 pcs.	240	12.0	13.0	16.0	0	710	5.0
nuggets (*Morningstar Farms*), 4 pcs.	180	13.0	17.0	6.0	0	590	5.0
nuggets (*Morningstar Farms Chik Nuggets*), 4 pcs.	160	13.0	17.0	4.0	0	670	5.0
nuggets (*Quorn*), 3–5 pcs., 3 oz.	180	8.0	18.0	8.0	0	650	3.0
nuggets (*Veggie Master Vege*), ¼ pkg.	126	6.0	2.8	6.5	0	116	2.8
patty (*Boca Chik'n*), 1 pc.	150	13.0	12.0	6.0	<5	470	2.0
patty (*Quorn*), 1 pc.	160	8.0	12.0	7.0	0	525	3.0
patty (*Worthington Crispy Chik Patties*), 1 pc. ..	150	10.0	15.0	6.0	0	400	1.0

Food and Measure	cal.	prot. (gms)	carbo. (gms)	fat (gms)	chol. (mgs)	sod. (mgs)	fiber (gms)
roll (*Worthington Meatless*), ⅜" slice	90	9.0	2.0	4.5	0	240	<1.0
slices (*Worthington Meatless*), 2 slices, 2 oz.	80	9.0	1.0	4.5	0	370	<1.0
tenders (*Quorn*), 1 cup	90	12.0	8.0	2.0	0	350	3.0
mix (*Loma Linda* Supreme), ⅓ cup	90	15.0	6.0	1.0	0	720	4.0
Chicken Dijon seasoning (*Knorr Recipe Classics*), 1 tbsp.	30	0	5.0	1.0	0	430	0
Chicken dinner, frozen, 1 pkg.:							
baked (*Stouffer's* HomeStyle), 14 oz.	410	30.0	55.0	8.0	60	560	4.0
boneless:							
w/herb gravy (*Swanson Traditional Favorites*), 11 oz.	320	18.0	46.0	7.0	40	1020	3.0
white meat (*Swanson Hungry-Man*), 13.75 oz.	660	34.0	73.0	26.0	60	1740	5.0
breaded, country (*Healthy Choice*), 10.25 oz.	350	16.0	51.0	9.0	45	480	5.0
breast, stir-fry (*Healthy Choice*), 11.9 oz.	360	19.0	57.0	6.0	25	600	5.0
broccoli Alfredo (*Healthy Choice*), 11.5 oz.	300	25.0	34.0	7.0	50	530	2.0
Dijon (*Healthy Choice*), 11 oz.	310	22.0	40.0	7.0	50	600	5.0
fettuccine (*Stouffer's* HomeStyle), 16.75 oz.	640	39.0	67.0	24.0	40	1610	4.0
fried:							
(*Banquet Extra Helping*), 14.7 oz.	910	34.0	70.0	55.0	160	2400	5.0
(*Swanson*), 11.5 oz.	600	24.0	58.0	31.0	70	1360	5.0
(*Swanson Fun Feast*), 10 oz. edible	590	14.0	64.0	31.0	55	1100	4.0

Food and Measure	cal.	prot. (gms)	carbo. (gms)	fat (gms)	chol. (mgs)	sod. (mgs)	fiber (gms)
Chicken dinner, frozen, fried *(cont.)*							
(*Swanson Traditional Favorites* Classic), 10.5 oz. edible	600	24.0	58.0	31.0	70	1360	5.0
boneless white meat (*Banquet Extra Helpings*), 13 oz.	720	22.0	41.0	52.0	80	1970	7.0
boneless white meat (*Swanson Traditional Favorites*), 11 oz.	430	23.0	49.0	16.0	40	1010	5.0
herb, country (*Healthy Choice*), 11.35 oz.	280	17.0	40.0	6.0	30	600	6.0
honey glazed (*Healthy Choice*), 11 oz. ...	320	20.0	48.0	6.0	35	600	4.0
mesquite, barbecue (*Healthy Choice*), 10.5 oz.	320	21.0	38.0	9.0	55	490	5.0
nuggets:							
(*Swanson Fun Feast*), 9 oz. ...	850	16.0	59.0	32.0	35	1010	4.0
(*Swanson Traditional Favorites*), 11 oz.	670	23.0	71.0	28.0	40	1030	6.0
parmigiana (*Healthy Choice*), 11 oz. ...	320	20.0	40.0	9.0	20	600	6.0
roast:							
boneless, w/herb gravy (*Swanson Hungry-Man*), 15.25 oz.	540	35.0	65.0	15.0	40	1550	7.0
breast (*Healthy Choice*), 11 oz.	230	20.0	23.0	7.0	50	470	6.0
sesame, breast (*Healthy Choice*), 10.8 oz.	360	19.0	54.0	7.0	20	600	4.0
sweet/sour (*Healthy Choice*), 11 oz. ...	350	20.0	53.0	7.0	45	360	5.0
teriyaki (*Healthy Choice*), 11 oz. ...	270	18.0	37.0	6.0	45	600	3.0
Chicken entree, can or pkg., 1 cup, except as noted:							
à la king (*Swanson*), 10.5-oz. can	340	17.0	16.0	23.0	70	1260	2.0

Food and Measure	cal.	prot. (gms)	carbo. (gms)	fat (gms)	chol. (mgs)	sod. (mgs	fiber (gms)
chow mein (*La Choy*)	80	8.0	6.0	3.5	20	1190	3.0
and dumpling:							
(*Dinty Moore*), 7.5 oz.	200	15.0	21.0	6.0	35	890	1.0
(*Dinty Moore* Microwave Cup)	200	15.0	21.0	6.0	35	890	1.0
stew (*Dinty Moore*)	260	13.0	30.0	10.0	45	1100	3.0
and noodles (*Dinty Moore American Classics*), 1 bowl ..	270	19.0	28.0	8.0	75	1280	2.0
noodles and, see "Noodle entree, can or pkg."							
w/potatoes (*Dinty Moore American Classics*), 1 bowl ..	240	20.0	25.0	4.0	35	990	2.0
stew (*Dinty Moore*) ..	220	12.0	16.0	11.0	40	980	2.0
Chicken entree, dried, 1 serving:							
(*AlpineAire* Kung Fu)	360	16.0	68.0	2.5	25	890	3.0
(*AlpineAire* Sierra) ...	330	21.0	53.0	3.0	25	670	2.0
(*AlpineAire* Summer)	330	23.0	38.0	10.0	50	650	1.0
à la king and noodles (*Mountain House*)	390	25.0	42.0	14.0	85	990	3.0
almond (*AlpineAire*) ..	380	24.0	53.0	8.0	20	780	5.0
brown rice, w/vegetables (*AlpineAire*)	330	20.0	55.0	3.0	30	1300	8.0
gumbo (*AlpineAire*) ..	520	21.0	102.0	2.5	35	1420	17.0
lemon herb (*AlpineAire*)	260	18.0	44.0	1.5	n.a.	440	4.0
noodles and (*Mountain House*)	270	12.0	44.0	5.0	45	1420	2.0
Oriental style, and vegetables (*Mountain House*)	300	16.0	44.0	6.0	20	1070	8.0
pasta Parmesan (*AlpineAire*)	300	25.0	39.0	5.0	n.a.	650	4.0
peach and pecan (*AlpineAire*)	380	18.0	54.0	10.0	35	590	3.0
Polynesian (*Mountain House*)	270	12.0	44.0	5.0	30	1020	1.0
primavera (*AlpineAire*)	260	16.0	44.0	2.5	25	660	2.0

Food and Measure	cal.	prot. (gms)	carbo. (gms)	fat (gms)	chol. (mgs)	sod. (mgs)	fiber (gms)
Chicken entree, dried *(cont.)*							
rice and:							
(*Mountain House Double/Four*) ...	400	11.0	59.0	14.0	25	1470	2.0
(*Mountain House Single*)	510	14.0	74.0	17.0	35	1840	3.0
rice, Mexican, and							
(*Mountain House*)	300	16.0	46.0	6.0	35	1220	6.0
rotelle (*AlpineAire*) ...	350	23.0	44.0	10.0	60	870	1.0
stew (*Mountain House*)	300	22.0	34.0	12.0	50	1180	4.0
teriyaki (*Mountain House*)	280	12.0	49.0	3.5	30	1020	3.0
Chicken entree, frozen (see also "Chicken, frozen or refrigerated, cooked"), 1 pkg., except as noted:							
à la king:							
(*Freezer Queen Cook-in-Pouch*), 4 oz	60	8.0	5.0	1.5	20	530	3.0
(*Michelina's*), 8 oz.	280	14.0	39.0	8.0	70	770	2.0
(*Stouffer's*), 11.5 oz.	370	21.0	47.0	11.0	45	1300	2.0
à l'orange (*Lean Cuisine Cafe Classics*), 9 oz. ...	230	20.0	33.0	1.5	40	300	2.0
Alfredo:							
(*Birds Eye Chicken Voila!*), 1 cup* .	230	15.0	26.0	8.0	20	660	2.0
(*Green Giant Complete Skillet Meal!*), ¼ pkg.	290	20.0	37.0	7.0	40	920	2.0
(*Lean Cuisine Skillet Sensations*), ¼ of 40-oz. pkg. ..	280	20.0	36.0	6.0	30	590	3.0
(*Stouffer's Skillet Sensations*), ½ of 25-oz. pkg. ..	450	26.0	51.0	16.0	40	910	5.0
(*Marie Callender's Skillet Meal*), ½ of 23-oz. pkg. ..	500	25.0	32.0	30.0	80	1230	7.0
(*Marie Callender's Skillet Meal*), ¼ of 37-oz. pkg. ..	400	20.0	26.0	25.0	65	990	6.0

Food and Measure	cal.	prot. (gms)	carbo. (gms)	fat (gms)	chol. (mgs)	sod. (mgs)	fiber (gms)
broccoli (*Banquet* Family), 1 cup ..	250	11.0	22.0	13.0	60	740	3.0
and almonds, w/rice (*Yu Sing*), 9 oz. ..	300	12.0	49.0	6.0	20	1220	2.0
bake, country (*Healthy Choice* Bowl), 11 oz.	260	20.0	28.0	7.0	60	600	4.0
baked:							
(*Lean Cuisine Cafe Classics*), 8⅝ oz.	240	17.0	33.0	4.5	30	690	3.0
and cheddar rice (*Stouffer's Oven Sensations*), ½ of 24-oz. pkg. ..	390	21.0	50.0	12.0	40	1220	7.0
w/sour cream–chive mashed potato (*Healthy Choice* Duo), 8.5 oz.	210	18.0	24.0	4.5	40	600	3.0
barbecue:							
(*Banquet*), 9.9 oz.	330	16.0	37.0	13.0	50	1210	2.0
honey, w/rice (*Michelina's*), 8.5 oz.	290	9.0	56.0	3.0	15	910	2.0
sauce (*Lean Cuisine Hearty Portions*), 13⅞ oz.	370	20.0	60.0	6.0	40	840	6.0
w/basil cream sauce (*Lean Cuisine Cafe Classics*), 8.5 oz.	290	19.0	37.0	7.0	35	630	0
and biscuits (*Freezer Queen* Deluxe Family), 1 cup	200	13.0	28.0	4.0	35	710	4.0
breast:							
baked (*Stouffer's* HomeStyle), 8⅞ oz.	260	22.0	18.0	11.0	65	680	3.0
in barbecue sauce (*Stouffer's* Home-Style), 10 oz. ..	500	17.0	44.0	25.0	65	1320	2.0
cheesy rice and (*Marie Callender's*), 10 oz.	370	23.0	34.0	17.0	60	1280	7.0

Food and Measure	cal.	prot. (gms)	carbo. (gms)	fat (gms)	chol. (mgs)	sod. (mgs)	fiber (gms)
Chicken entree, frozen, breast *(cont.)*							
lemon sauce, pasta, green beans (*Mamma Rita's*), ½ of 18-oz. pkg.	240	23.0	25.0	8.0	50	150	3.0
w/mushroom gravy (*Stouffer's* Home-Style), 10 oz. . .	350	23.0	27.0	17.0	60	940	2.0
oven roasted (*Boston Market* Home Style), 6 oz.	180	23.0	0	7.0	105	800	0
strips, breaded (*Marie Callender's*), 8.75 oz.	500	29.0	42.0	24.0	70	1410	5.0
strips, breaded, w/macaroni and cheese (*Healthy Choice* Duo), 8 oz.	270	22.0	34.0	5.0	40	600	1.0
and vegetables (*Healthy Choice* Medley), 11.5 oz.	230	18.0	29.0	5.0	25	550	6.0
and broccoli:							
(*Healthy Choice* Bread Stuffs), 6.1 oz.	310	17.0	50.0	4.0	25	600	2.0
bake (*Stouffer's* Family Style Favorites), ⅕ of 40-oz. pkg.	330	19.0	26.0	17.0	50	1040	2.0
w/cheese and rice, creamy (*Banquet* Family), 1 cup . .	280	14.0	25.0	14.0	45	980	2.0
cacciatore (*Mamma Rita's*), ½ of 18-oz. pkg.	290	30.0	19.0	11.0	70	360	3.0
carbonara:							
(*Healthy Choice* Medley), 9 oz. . .	310	23.0	39.0	7.0	40	600	2.0
(*Lean Cuisine Cafe Classics*), 9 oz.	280	17.0	36.0	7.0	30	690	4.0
cheddar cheese and, bake (*Stouffer's*), 11.5 oz.	450	25.0	41.0	21.0	50	1230	3.0

Food and Measure	cal.	prot. (gms)	carbo. (gms)	fat (gms)	chol. (mgs)	sod. (mgs	fiber (gms)
cheese, three:							
(*Birds Eye Chicken Voila!*), 1 cup*	220	14.0	24.0	8.0	20	570	1.0
(*Lean Cuisine Skillet Sensations*), ½ of 24-oz. pkg.	370	26.0	45.0	10.0	50	820	3.0
chow mein:							
(*Contessa*), 1¾ cups	320	6.0	55.0	2.5	25	1060	3.0
(*Lean Cuisine Everyday Favorites*), 9 oz.	240	14.0	37.0	3.5	35	590	3.0
(*Yu Sing*), 8.75 oz.	270	8.0	43.0	6.0	15	1210	2.0
cordon bleu (*Marie Callender's*), 13 oz.	610	33.0	58.0	28.0	75	1920	6.0
creamed (*Stouffer's*), 6.5 oz.	250	17.0	11.0	15.0	50	720	0
croquettes, gravy and (*Freezer Queen* Family), 1 patty w/gravy	160	8.0	14.0	8.0	10	600	2.0
and dumplings:							
(*Marie Callender's*), 14 oz.	390	17.0	34.0	20.0	130	1650	4.0
(*Stouffer's* Home-Style), 10 oz.	340	21.0	35.0	13.0	65	1320	3.0
country style (*Banquet* Family), 1 cup	290	12.0	30.0	14.0	40	1270	2.0
enchilada, see "Enchilada"							
fettuccine:							
(*Lean Cuisine Everyday Favorites*), 9.25 oz.	270	21.0	33.0	6.0	40	690	3.0
(*Lean Cuisine Hearty Portions*), 13⅝ oz.	400	31.0	49.0	9.0	50	980	4.0
(*Stouffer's* Home-Style), 10.5 oz.	350	22.0	34.0	14.0	40	1050	2.0
Alfredo (*Healthy Choice* Medley), 8.5 oz.	280	25.0	30.0	7.0	35	600	4.0

Food and Measure	cal.	prot. (gms)	carbo. (gms)	fat (gms)	chol. (mgs)	sod. (mgs)	fiber (gms)
Chicken entree, frozen, fettuccine (cont.)							
Alfredo (*Uncle Ben's Pasta Bowl*), 12 oz.	350	27.0	47.0	7.0	40	1160	2.0
Florentine:							
(*Lean Cuisine Hearty Portions*), 13.25 oz.	380	25.0	53.0	7.0	45	890	6.0
baked (*Lean Cuisine Everyday Favorites*), 8 oz.	220	13.0	32.0	4.5	25	640	3.0
fingers:							
(*Banquet*), 7.1 oz.	570	18.0	57.0	30.0	60	1010	2.0
barbecue sauce (*Freezer Queen Meal*), 9 oz.	350	16.0	39.0	14.0	30	920	6.0
fried:							
(*Banquet* Original), 9 oz.	470	21.0	35.0	27.0	90	1500	2.0
(*Kid Cuisine*), 10.1 oz.	440	16.0	47.0	21.0	50	850	5.0
(*Morton*), 9 oz.	470	20.0	30.0	30.0	90	1100	3.0
boneless white meat (*Banquet*), 8.25 oz.	490	14.0	49.0	27.0	65	1150	2.0
breast (*Stouffer's HomeStyle*), 8⅞ oz.	350	16.0	34.0	17.0	55	980	3.0
country, and gravy (*Marie Callender's*), 16 oz.	620	24.0	63.0	30.0	75	2300	6.0
country, w/gravy and mashed potato (*Marie Callender's Family*), 1 patty w/gravy, ½ cup potato	240	17.0	39.0	27.0	60	1890	2.0
garlic:							
(*Lean Cuisine Skillet Sensations*), ½ of 24-oz. pkg.	340	20.0	56.0	4.5	20	730	4.0
and pasta (*Tyson Meal Kit*), 1 cup*	190	14.0	23.0	5.0	15	380	0

Food and Measure	cal.	prot. (gms)	carbo. (gms)	fat (gms)	chol. (mgs)	sod. (mgs)	fiber (gms)
w/rice (*Yu Sing*), 8 oz.	240	8.0	42.0	3.0	10	1010	2.0
zesty (*Birds Eye Chicken Voila!*), 1 cup*	270	15.0	28.0	11.0	25	550	1.0
glazed:							
(*Lean Cuisine Cafe Classics*), 8.5 oz.	240	22.0	25.0	6.0	55	480	0
(*Lean Cuisine Hearty Portions*), 13 oz.	360	29.0	43.0	8.0	70	590	2.0
(*Michelina's*), 8 oz.	250	10.0	43.0	4.0	15	810	2.0
breast (*Marie Callender's*), 10 oz.	340	21.0	35.0	13.0	30	930	5.0
country, breast (*Healthy Choice Medley*), 8.5 oz.	250	19.0	31.0	5.0	30	600	3.0
orange (*Budget Gourmet*), 8 oz.	270	11.0	46.0	4.5	20	650	1.0
w/rice (*Michelina's*), 9.5 oz.	310	21.0	49.0	6.0	40	710	2.0
grilled:							
(*Lean Cuisine Cafe Classics*), 9⅜ oz.	250	22.0	29.0	5.0	40	690	3.0
Alfredo, w/broccoli (*Michelina's*), 10 oz.	410	22.0	36.0	19.0	85	990	2.0
breast (*Marie Callender's*), 10 oz.	300	15.0	33.0	12.0	35	950	5.0
breast, and pasta (*Healthy Choice Duo*), 9 oz.	240	21.0	26.0	6.0	40	600	4.0
breast, and rice w/mushroom sauce (*Marie Callender's* Bowl), 12 oz.	370	23.0	51.0	8.0	55	1210	4.0
fiesta (*Lean Cuisine Cafe Classics*), 8.5 oz.	260	15.0	40.0	4.5	35	520	3.0
w/mashed potato (*Healthy Choice Duo/Medley*), 8.5 oz.	200	21.0	19.0	6.0	40	600	4.0

Food and Measure	cal.	prot. (gms)	carbo. (gms)	fat (gms)	chol. (mgs)	sod. (mgs)	fiber (gms)
Chicken entree, frozen, grilled *(cont.)*							
and mashed potato (*Marie Callender's*), 10 oz.	340	24.0	20.0	18.0	90	1090	1.0
in mushroom sauce (*Marie Callender's*), 14 oz.	480	33.0	54.0	15.0	65	1030	7.0
and penne pasta (*Lean Cuisine Hearty Portions*), 14 oz.	360	26.0	47.0	7.0	40	870	5.0
salsa, w/rice (*Birds Eye Chicken Voila!*), 1 cup* .	240	14.0	35.0	5.0	25	1180	3.0
Sonoma (*Healthy Choice Medley*), 9 oz.	230	18.0	30.0	4.0	45	530	3.0
Southwestern (*Marie Callender's*), 14 oz.	410	34.0	43.0	11.0	80	2020	6.0
herb:							
(*Marie Callender's Skillet Meal*), ½ of 24-oz. pkg.	290	22.0	42.0	4.0	35	1030	5.0
garden (*Birds Eye Chicken Voila!*), 1 cup*	310	16.0	28.0	15.0	40	540	2.0
and roast potato (*Lean Cuisine Skillet Sensations*), ½ of 24-oz. pkg.	260	16.0	40.0	4.5	25	890	5.0
herb roasted:							
(*Lean Cuisine Cafe Classics*), 8 oz.	200	17.0	24.0	3.5	35	690	3.0
and mashed potato (*Marie Callender's*), 14 oz.	580	42.0	26.0	34.0	205	2100	7.0
home style:							
(*Country Skillet*), ¼ of 32-oz. pkg.	170	10.0	25.0	4.0	20	880	2.0
(*Stouffer's Skillet Sensations*), ½ of 25-oz. pkg. ..	390	22.0	47.0	13.0	50	1040	7.0

Food and Measure	cal.	prot. (gms)	carbo. (gms)	fat (gms)	chol. (mgs)	sod. (mgs)	fiber (gms)
and pasta (*Healthy Choice* Solo), 9 oz.	270	21.0	32.0	6.0	35	570	5.0
honey mustard (*Lean Cuisine Cafe Classics*), 8 oz.	270	19.0	40.0	3.5	35	690	1.0
honey roasted:							
(*Lean Cuisine Cafe Classics*), 8.5 oz.	270	13.0	41.0	6.0	25	690	5.0
(*Marie Callender's*), 14 oz.	440	45.0	27.0	17.0	140	1170	7.0
lemon herb (*Marie Callender's* Bowl), 12.4 oz.	420	23.0	54.0	12.0	70	1610	3.0
lo mein:							
(*Green Giant Complete Skillet Meal!*), ¼ pkg.	250	16.0	30.0	7.0	40	710	3.0
(*Yu Sing*), 8.5 oz.	220	13.0	34.0	2.5	20	1060	3.0
mandarin:							
(*Budget Gourmet*), 8.5 oz.	240	8.0	38.0	6.0	15	780	2.0
(*Healthy Choice* Medley), 10 oz.	280	20.0	43.0	3.5	35	520	4.0
(*Lean Cuisine Everyday Favorites*), 9 oz.	240	14.0	36.0	4.0	25	610	2.0
marsala, w/garlic mashed potato (*Michelina's*), 8.5 oz.	280	20.0	22.0	14.0	60	1110	2.0
Mediterranean (*Lean Cuisine Cafe Classics*), 10.5 oz.	260	17.0	38.0	4.0	20	690	4.0
Monterey, creamy (*Ortega Skillet*), ½ of 23-oz. pkg.	430	20.0	48.0	17.0	50	1210	8.0
nacho (*Ortega Skillet Supreme*), ½ of 23-oz. pkg.	380	20.0	49.0	11.0	50	1810	8.0
and noodles:							
(*Budget Gourmet*), 8.5 oz.	370	14.0	31.0	21.0	90	760	2.0
chunky (*Marie Callender's*), 10 oz.	430	18.0	33.0	25.0	70	1030	4.0

Food and Measure	cal.	prot. (gms)	carbo. (gms)	fat (gms)	chol. (mgs)	sod. (mgs)	fiber (gms)
Chicken entree, frozen, and noodles *(cont.)*							
creamy (*Green Giant Complete Skillet Meals!*), ¼ pkg.	320	21.0	45.0	6.0	35	1310	3.0
escalloped (*Stouffer's*), 10 oz.	460	18.0	36.0	27.0	60	1170	4.0
escalloped (*Stouffer's Family Style Favorites*), ⅕ of 40-oz. pkg.	370	15.0	25.0	23.0	45	1130	2.0
honey ginger (*Uncle Ben's* Noodle Bowl), 12 oz. . .	430	25.0	69.0	5.0	85	1700	3.0
nuggets:							
(*Banquet*), 6.75 oz.	430	16.0	38.0	21.0	35	860	3.0
(*Freezer Queen Family*), 6 pcs., 3 oz.	250	12.0	16.0	15.0	25	960	2.0
(*Freezer Queen Meal*), 6 oz. . . .	250	11.0	27.0	17.0	20	1010	3.0
(*Kid Cuisine*), 9.1 oz.	500	18.0	50.0	25.0	45	1070	3.0
(*Morton*), 7 oz. . . .	340	12.0	31.0	19.0	30	470	2.0
w/macaroni and cheese (*Freezer Queen Family Buffet*), ¼ pkg.	460	19.0	43.0	24.0	40	1710	3.0
olé (*Healthy Choice Solo*), 9 oz.	270	16.0	42.0	4.0	20	600	5.0
Oriental:							
(*Healthy Choice Medley*), 8.5 oz.	240	21.0	28.0	5.0	35	600	7.0
(*Lean Cuisine Skillet Sensations*), ½ of 24-oz. pkg. . .	270	16.0	44.0	3.0	25	890	5.0
(*Stouffer's*), 10⅝ oz.	250	12.0	38.0	5.0	25	1130	3.0
glazed (*Lean Cuisine Hearty Portions*), 14 oz.	370	21.0	66.0	2.0	35	850	4.0
and pasta (*Tyson Meal Kit*), 1 cup*	180	14.0	19.0	5.0	15	380	0
pappardelle (*Wolfgang Puck's*), 12 oz. . . .	430	23.0	48.0	17.0	105	730	3.0

Food and Measure	cal.	prot. (gms)	carbo. (gms)	fat (gms)	chol. (mgs)	sod. (mgs)	fiber (gms)
Parmesan (*Lean Cuisine Cafe Classics*), 10⅞ oz.	300	21.0	41.0	6.0	35	690	5.0
parmigiana:							
(*Banquet*), 9.5 oz.	320	10.0	29.0	18.0	50	900	3.0
(*Marie Callender's*), 16 oz.	660	30.0	63.0	32.0	50	920	5.0
(*Michelina's* Parmigiano), 10 oz. . .	410	20.0	48.0	15.0	35	960	3.0
(*Stouffer's* Home-Style), 12 oz. . .	460	24.0	54.0	16.0	45	1060	5.0
(*Wolfgang Puck's*), 12 oz.	540	29.0	58.0	21.0	95	910	4.0
pasta:							
cheese, three (*Tyson* Meal Kit), 1 cup*	190	14.0	23.0	2.0	15	570	0
cheesy (*Green Giant Complete Skillet Meal!*), ¼ pkg.	300	19.0	39.0	7.0	40	970	3.0
garlic (*Green Giant Complete Skillet Meal!*), ¼ pkg.	250	16.0	30.0	7.0	40	710	3.0
primavera (*Banquet*), 9.5 oz.	320	11.0	40.0	12.0	25	840	6.0
vegetable and, bake (*Stouffer's*), 12 oz.	380	24.0	46.0	11.0	55	1200	4.0
patty:							
(*Freezer Queen* Meal), 7.5 oz. . .	360	16.0	36.0	17.0	30	880	5.0
breaded (*Morton*), 6.75 oz.	340	10.0	24.0	22.0	35	840	3.0
in peanut sauce (*Lean Cuisine Cafe Classics*), 9 oz.	260	20.0	32.0	6.0	30	690	4.0
penne and, bake (*Stouffer's*), 11.5 oz.	350	21.0	37.0	13.0	45	1140	4.0
pesto:							
(*Birds Eye Chicken Voila!*), 1 cup* .	240	15.0	24.0	9.0	25	690	1.0
w/penne (*Michelina's*), 8 oz.	250	13.0	36.0	6.0	25	540	2.0
piccata:							
(*Healthy Choice* Medley), 9 oz. . .	270	17.0	40.0	5.0	30	600	2.0

Food and Measure	cal.	prot. (gms)	carbo. (gms)	fat (gms)	chol. (mgs)	sod. (mgs)	fiber (gms)
Chicken entree, frozen, piccata *(cont.)*							
(*Lean Cuisine Cafe Classics*), 9 oz.	300	14.0	41.0	9.0	30	690	2.0
(*Michelina's*), 9 oz.	340	14.0	41.0	12.0	45	1250	1.0
pie/pot pie:							
(*Banquet*), 7 oz. . .	380	10.0	36.0	22.0	40	950	1.0
(*Lean Cuisine Everyday Favorites*), 9.5 oz.	300	19.0	38.0	8.0	30	580	5.0
(*Marie Callender's*), 9.5 oz.	680	14.0	53.0	43.0	20	1100	3.0
(*Marie Callender's* 16.5 oz.), 1 cup	540	12.0	44.0	35.0	15	1040	2.0
(*Stouffer's*), 10 oz.	730	21.0	61.0	44.0	55	1060	3.0
(*Stouffer's*), ½ of 16-oz. pie	590	17.0	53.0	34.0	55	890	2.0
(*Swanson*), 7 oz.	410	10.0	43.0	22.0	25	780	2.0
(*Swanson Potato-Topped*), 12 oz.	440	15.0	40.0	23.0	50	1250	6.0
au gratin (*Marie Callender's* 16.5 oz.), 1 cup . .	580	15.0	46.0	37.0	25	970	<1.0
broccoli (*Banquet*), 7 oz.	350	10.0	32.0	20.0	35	830	2.0
broccoli (*Marie Callender's*), 9.5 oz.	670	16.0	54.0	43.0	25	1000	4.0
broccoli (*Marie Callender's* 16.5 oz.), 1 cup	620	14.0	41.0	45.0	25	960	3.0
broccoli, w/cheddar-potato (*Swanson Potato-Topped*), 12 oz.	450	15.0	48.0	22.0	55	1310	11.0
white meat, deep dish (*Swanson Hungry-Man*), 1 cup	520	14.0	52.0	29.0	40	890	3.0
and potato casserole, home style (*Marie Callender's* Bowl), 12.05 oz.	310	22.0	30.0	12.0	55	990	4.0

Food and Measure	cal.	prot. (gms)	carbo. (gms)	fat (gms)	chol. (mgs)	sod. (mgs)	fiber (gms)
primavera:							
(*Lean Cuisine Skillet Sensations*), ½ of 24-oz. pkg. . .	300	16.0	51.0	4.0	25	890	5.0
w/spirals (*Michelina's*), 8 oz. . . .	250	14.0	35.0	6.0	30	760	2.0
and rice:							
w/broccoli and cheese (*Marie Callender's* Skillet Meal), ½ of 25-oz. pkg.	410	30.0	40.0	14.0	70	1400	7.0
savory (*Stouffer's Skillet Sensations*), ¼ of 40-oz. pkg.	300	14.0	51.0	35.0	30	1270	3.0
rice, fried:							
(*Contessa*), 1¾ cups	260	17.0	49.0	3.5	100	680	4.0
(*Michelina's* Family), 1 cup	270	9.0	46.0	4.5	15	690	2.0
(*Tyson* Meal Kit), ½ pkg., 2½ cups	480	24.0	74.0	10.0	80	1510	3.0
(*Yu Sing*), 8 oz. . .	360	14.0	58.0	7.0	25	950	2.0
and egg rolls (*Banquet*), 8.5 oz.	330	12.0	51.0	9.0	60	1270	5.0
roast/roasted:							
(*Lean Cuisine Everyday Favorites*), 8⅛ oz.	250	15.0	32.0	7.0	25	620	3.0
(*Lean Cuisine Hearty Portions*), 12.5 oz.	330	23.0	49.0	5.0	40	740	4.0
garlic (*Stouffer's Oven Sensations*), ½ of 24-oz. pkg.	320	15.0	39.0	11.0	25	1720	7.0
herb (*Michelina's*), 10 oz.	270	21.0	33.0	5.0	50	810	3.0
red pepper (*Healthy Choice* Bowl), 9.5 oz.	340	20.0	50.0	7.0	50	600	4.0
and vegetables (*Marie Callender's* Skillet Meal), ½ of 25-oz. pkg. . .	300	21.0	30.0	10.0	50	1200	4.0

Food and Measure	cal.	prot. (gms)	carbo. (gms)	fat (gms)	chol. (mgs)	sod. (mgs)	fiber (gms)
Chicken entree, frozen, roast/roasted *(cont.)*							
and vegetables (*Marie Callender's* Skillet Meal), ¼ of 40-oz. pkg.	240	16.0	24.0	8.0	40	960	3.0
sesame (*Healthy Choice* Medley), 9 oz.	240	13.0	35.0	6.0	25	600	4.0
sliced, gravy and (*Freezer Queen* Cook-in-Pouch), 4 oz.	60	6.0	4.0	2.5	15	620	1.0
Sorrentino, w/linguine (*Michelina's*), 8.5 oz.	320	17.0	38.0	9.0	45	1000	2.0
and spinach pasta wrap (*Wolfgang Puck's*), 12 oz. . . .	460	22.0	68.0	11.0	100	540	6.0
stir-fry:							
(*Contessa*), 1¾ cups	180	13.0	28.0	1.5	25	1270	4.0
(*Tyson* Meal Kit), ½ pkg., 2¾ cups	430	21.0	73.0	4.5	45	700	5.0
w/stuffing and gravy (*Stouffer's Oven Sensations*), ½ of 21-oz. pkg.	380	18.0	48.0	13.0	55	1930	5.0
sweet and sour:							
(*Green Giant Complete Skillet Meal!*), ¼ pkg.	320	14.0	52.0	1.5	25	550	3.0
(*Marie Callender's*), 14 oz.	570	23.0	86.0	15.0	40	700	7.0
w/rice (*Healthy Choice* Bowl), 12 oz.	380	21.0	66.0	3.5	45	600	5.0
w/rice (*Freezer Queen* Homestyle), 8.5 oz.	280	15.0	51.0	2.0	25	710	2.0
w/rice (*Michelina's* Family), 1 cup . .	280	9.0	5.0	2.5	15	710	1.0
w/rice (*Yu Sing*), 8.5 oz.	340	11.0	68.0	3.5	20	880	1.0
teriyaki:							
(*Birds Eye Chicken Voila!*), 1 cup* .	240	13.0	26.0	9.0	25	700	2.0

Food and Measure	cal.	prot. (gms)	carbo. (gms)	fat (gms)	chol. (mgs)	sod. (mgs)	fiber (gms)
(*Green Giant Complete Skillet Meal!*), ¼ pkg.	250	15.0	45.0	1.5	25	810	3.0
(*Marie Callender's*), 10 oz.	310	17.0	46.0	7.0	25	930	4.0
(*Marie Callender's* Bowl), 12 oz.	400	26.0	66.0	4.0	45	1440	6.0
(*Marie Callender's* Skillet Meal), ½ of 24-oz. pkg.	270	18.0	38.0	5.0	45	1100	2.0
(*Stouffer's Skillet Sensations*), ½ of 25-oz. pkg.	320	15.0	58.0	3.0	30	1440	3.0
w/rice (*Healthy Choice* Bowl), 10.5 oz.	300	19.0	45.0	5.0	50	600	4.0
w/rice (*Michelina's*), 8.5 oz.	290	10.0	65.0	2.5	15	1230	1.0
tetrazzini (*Michelina's*), 8 oz.	320	14.0	35.0	12.0	35	690	2.0
and tomatoes, fire-roasted (*Michelina's*), 8 oz.	240	9.0	35.0	7.0	15	640	2.0
and vegetables: (*Lean Cuisine Cafe Classics*), 10.5 oz.	250	18.0	33.0	5.0	30	690	3.0
grilled (*Stouffer's Skillet Sensations*), ½ of 25-oz. pkg.	400	21.0	45.0	15.0	30	1240	3.0
herb, country (*Cascadian Farm Veggie & Chicken Bowl*), 8.5 oz.	240	14.0	38.0	3.0	25	630	2.0
w/noodles (*Freezer Queen Homestyle*), 8 oz.	170	12.0	27.0	2.0	15	530	4.0
orange Dijon (*Cascadian Farm Veggie & Chicken Bowl*), 8.5 oz.	240	12.0	42.0	3.0	35	360	3.0
rice (*Uncle Ben's* Bowl), 12 oz.	360	21.0	56.0	5.0	25	1020	3.0

Food and Measure	cal.	prot. (gms)	carbo. (gms)	fat (gms)	chol. (mgs)	sod. (mgs)	fiber (gms)
Chicken entree, frozen, and vegetables *(cont.)*							
rice bake (*Stouffer's Family Style Favorites* Grandmas), ¼ of 36-oz. pkg.	360	19.0	36.0	15.0	70	1040	2.0
stir-fry (*Michelina's*), 8 oz.	200	9.0	29.0	5.0	15	900	3.0
teriyaki (*Cascadian Farm* Veggie & Chicken Bowl), 8.5 oz.	240	12.0	38.0	4.0	35	670	2.0
Thai (*Cascadian Farm* Veggie & Chicken Bowl), 8.5 oz.	260	10.0	42.0	6.0	35	370	2.0
in wine sauce (*Lean Cuisine Cafe Classics*), 8⅛ oz.	220	20.0	23.0	5.0	45	690	2.0
Chicken entree mix, 1 cup*, except as noted:							
Alfredo, three cheese *Lipton Sizzle & Stir*), ⅙ box, 2 oz.	220	6.0	27.0	9.0	10	890	1.0
au gratin bake (*Stove Top Oven Classics*), ⅙ box	200	5.0	33.0	5.0	10	840	2.0
cheddar, mild, and shells (*Lipton Sizzle & Stir*), ⅙ box, 2 oz.	190	6.0	29.0	6.0	15	850	<1.0
cheddar and broccoli (*Chicken Helper*) ..	310	27.0	28.0	9.0	60	760	<1.0
cheddar and mozzarella (*Chicken Helper Oven Favorites*), 8.4 oz.*	320	23.0	34.0	11.0	50	750	<1.0
cheese, four (*Chicken Helper*)	310	24.0	27.0	12.0	55	790	0
cheesy chicken bake (*Stove Top Oven Classics*), ⅙ box ..	230	6.0	40.0	5.0	10	890	1.0

Food and Measure	cal.	prot. (gms)	carbo. (gms)	fat (gms)	chol. (mgs)	sod. (mgs)	fiber (gms)
chicken biscuit bake (*Chicken Helper Oven Favorites*), 8.3 oz.*	290	22.0	35.0	7.0	50	830	2.0
chicken fried rice (*Chicken Helper*)	260	23.0	22.0	8.0	120	660	1.0
chicken herb rice (*Chicken Helper*)	260	24.0	24.0	7.0	55	440	1.0
chicken and mashed potatoes (*Chicken Helper*)	250	20.0	24.0	9.0	50	790	1.0
chicken Parmesan pasta: (*Chicken Helper*)	290	25.0	30.0	8.0	55	850	1.0
bake (*Stove Top Oven Classics*), ⅙ box	210	8.0	38.0	3.5	<5	960	2.0
chicken and stuffing (*Chicken Helper*)	290	25.0	28.0	9.0	60	830	1.0
creamy chicken and rice (*Chicken Helper Oven Favorites*), 8 oz.*	290	20.0	30.0	10.0	45	680	0
creamy roasted garlic (*Chicken Helper*)	290	27.0	29.0	8.0	60	720	1.0
fajita rice (*Chicken Helper*)	250	24.0	28.0	5.0	55	820	1.0
fettucine Alfredo (*Chicken Helper*)	290	26.0	28.0	8.0	60	830	1.0
garlic, w/pasta: (*Campbell's Supper Bakes*), ⅙ pkg.	230	11.0	44.0	1.0	<5	780	2.0
(*Campbell's Supper Bakes*), ⅙ pkg.*	370	33.0	44.0	7.0	75	870	2.0
herb, w/rice: (*Campbell's Supper Bakes*), ⅙ pkg.	190	5.0	40.0	1.0	<5	790	1.0
(*Campbell's Supper Bakes*), ⅙ pkg.*	330	27.0	40.0	7.0	70	880	1.0
herbed, savory, and bow ties (*Lipton Sizzle & Stir*), ⅙ box, 2 oz.	170	5.0	28.0	4.0	5	840	1.0
honey mustard bake (*Kraft Classics*), ⅙ box	220	6.0	43.0	2.5	0	910	2.0

Food and Measure	cal.	prot. (gms)	carbo. (gms)	fat (gms)	chol. (mgs)	sod. (mgs)	fiber (gms)
Chicken entree mix *(cont.)*							
lemon, w/herb rice:							
(*Campbell's* Supper Bakes), ⅙ pkg.	200	4.0	43.0	1.0	<5	790	2.0
(*Campbell's* Supper Bakes), ⅙ pkg.*	340	26.0	43.0	7.0	70	880	2.0
lemon garlic and rice (*Lipton Sizzle & Stir*), ⅙ box, 2 oz.	180	2.0	33.0	3.5	5	960	1.0
potatoes, mashed, and gravy bake (*Stove Top Oven Classics*), ⅙ box	120	3.0	24.0	2.0	<5	540	2.0
potatoes au gratin (*Chicken Helper Oven Favorites*), 8.1 oz.*	270	20.0	29.0	9.0	45	910	2.0
roast chicken, traditional, bake (*Stove Top Oven Classics*), ⅙ box	190	6.0	35.0	3.0	0	890	2.0
Southwestern (*Chicken Helper*)	240	23.0	27.0	5.0	55	810	1.0
stuffing, home style, and gravy (*Chicken Helper Oven Favorites*), 7.8 oz.*	310	21.0	32.0	11.0	50	980	1.0
sweet and sour (*Lipton Sizzle & Stir*), 2.5 oz.	220	4.0	46.0	2.5	0	700	1.0
teriyaki stir-fry, and rice (*Lipton Sizzle & Stir*), ⅙ box, 2 oz.	200	4.0	34.0	4.5	5	880	<1.0
Chicken fat:							
1 oz.	178	1.1	0	19.3	16	9	0
rendered (*Empire Kosher*), 1 tbsp. . .	120	0	<1.0	13.0	10	0	0
Chicken frankfurter, see "Frankfurter"							
Chicken giblets, simmered:							
4 oz.	178	29.3	1.1	5.4	446	66	0
chopped, 1 cup	228	37.5	1.4	6.9	570	85	0

Food and Measure	cal.	prot. (gms)	carbo. (gms)	fat (gms)	chol. (mgs)	sod. (mgs)	fiber (gms)
Chicken gravy, can or jar, ¼ cup:							
(*Boston Market*)	30	1.0	3.0	1.5	5	340	0
(*Franco-American*) ...	25	<1.0	3.0	3.0	<5	290	<1.0
(*Franco-American* Fat Free)	15	<1.0	3.0	0	<1	310	0
(*Franco-American Slow Roast*)	20	1.0	3.0	.5	<5	240	0
(*Heinz* Fat Free)	20	2.0	3.0	0	<5	350	0
giblet (*Franco-American*)	20	1.0	3.0	2.0	10	310	0
Chicken gravy mix, ¼ cup*:							
(*Lawry's*)	25	0	4.0	1.0	0	290	0
(*McCormick*)	20	0	4.0	0	0	330	0
roasted (*Knorr*)	30	2.0	3.0	1.0	5	310	0
roasted, and herb (*McCormick*)	25	0	3.0	1.0	0	260	0
vegetarian:							
(*Hain*)	25	<1.0	6.0	0	0	360	0
(*Loma Linda Gravy Quik/Natural Touch*)	20	1.0	3.0	0	0	440	0
Chicken lunch meat, breast, 2 oz., except as noted:							
(*Carl Buddig* 6 oz.) ..	85	10.0	1.0	5.0	30	530	0
(*Healthy Choice* Skinless)	50	9.0	1.0	1.0	20	470	0
(*Louis Rich*), 2 slices, 1.6 oz.	45	9.0	<1.0	.5	25	480	0
(*Wampler* Gourmet) ..	60	10.0	2.0	1.5	30	450	0
(*Wampler* Premium) .	90	8.0	2.0	5.0	30	540	0
barbecue:							
(*Black Bear*)	70	11.0	1.0	1.5	30	450	0
(*Boar's Head Bar B Q Sauce Basted*)	60	11.0	3.0	.5	30	490	0
browned (*Healthy Choice*)	60	11.0	1.0	1.0	25	400	0
grilled (*Louis Rich Carving Board*), 6 slices, 1.6 oz. ..	45	9.0	1.0	.5	25	480	0
oil browned (*Wampler*)	60	11.0	1.0	1.0	30	370	0

Food and Measure	cal.	prot. (gms)	carbo. (gms)	fat (gms)	chol. (mgs)	sod. (mgs)	fiber (gms)
Chicken lunch meat *(cont.)*							
oven roasted:							
(*Boar's Head* Golden Oven)	50	11.0	1.0	.5	30	430	0
(*Butterball*), 5 slices, 1.9 oz.	50	10.0	3.0	0	25	480	0
(*Carl Buddig*), 2.5-oz. pkg. ...	110	12.0	1.0	7.0	40	680	0
(*Carl Buddig* Premium), 2.5-oz. pkg. ...	60	12.0	1.0	1.0	30	630	0
(*Healthy Choice*), 1-oz. slice	25	5.0	2.0	0	5	240	0
(*Healthy Choice* 10 oz.), 1-oz. slice	35	5.0	2.0	1.0	10	240	0
(*Healthy Choice* Deli), 1-oz. slice .	30	6.0	1.0	0	10	240	0
(*Healthy Choice Deli Traditions*), 6 slices, 1.8 oz.	60	9.0	3.0	1.5	25	470	0
(*Louis Rich*), 1 oz.	40	5.0	<1.0	2.0	15	330	0
(*Louis Rich* Fat Free), 3 slices, 1.8 oz.	45	10.0	<1.0	0	20	640	0
(*Louis Rich* Fat Free), 4 slices, 2 oz. ..	50	11.0	<1.0	0	25	700	0
(*Sara Lee*)	50	11.0	1.0	.5	20	470	0
(*Sara Lee*), 3 slices, 1.8 oz.	50	10.0	1.0	.5	20	430	0
(*The Turkey Store*) .	50	10.0	0	1.5	20	420	0
honey (*Carl Buddig*), 2.5-oz. pkg. ...	70	12.0	3.0	1.0	30	640	0
rotisserie flavor (*Sara Lee*)	50	10.0	1.0	1.0	25	470	0
slow roasted (*Shady Brook Farms*)	60	12.0	1.0	.5	30	400	0
smoked:							
(*Healthy Choice*), 1-oz. slice	30	5.0	2.0	1.0	15	240	0
(*Healthy Choice Deli Traditions*), 6 slices, 1.9 oz.	60	10.0	3.0	1.5	25	470	0
mesquite (*Healthy Choice*)	60	11.0	1.0	1.0	30	440	0

Food and Measure	cal.	prot. (gms)	carbo. (gms)	fat (gms)	chol. (mgs)	sod. (mgs)	fiber (gms)
Chicken pie, frozen, see "Chicken entree, frozen"							
Chicken pie, refrigerated, 1 cup:							
(*Mrs. Budd's* Fancy Vegetable)	310	12.0	30.0	16.0	35	900	2.0
(*Mrs. Budd's* Original)	330	11.0	32.0	17.0	35	890	1.0
Chicken pocket (see also "Chicken sandwich"), frozen, 4.5-oz. pc., except as noted:							
(*Mrs. Paterson's* Aussie Pie), 5.5 oz.	460	12.0	45.0	25.0	90	770	2.0
(*Mrs. Paterson's* Aussie Pie Low Fat), 5.5 oz.	380	13.0	44.0	17.0	35	800	1.0
broccoli (*Lean Pockets* Supreme)	280	10.0	42.0	7.0	30	570	2.0
broccoli and cheddar:							
(*Croissant Pockets*)	320	10.0	41.0	13.0	35	430	2.0
(*Hot Pockets*)	310	12.0	40.0	11.0	40	460	2.0
fajita:							
(*Lean Pockets*) . . .	260	11.0	39.0	7.0	35	600	2.0
potato topped (*Mrs. Paterson's Aussie Pie*), 5.5 oz. . . .	350	17.0	33.0	17.0	55	760	2.0
Italian melt (*Croissant Pockets*)	380	11.0	37.0	20.0	20	690	2.0
Parmesan (*Lean Pockets*)	300	13.0	44.0	7.0	35	450	2.0
Chicken and rice seasoning (*A Taste of Thai*), ¼ pkt. . .	15	0	3.0	0	0	740	0
Chicken salad, ⅓ cup:							
(*Wampler*)	200	9.0	9.0	14.0	30	420	1.0
(*Wampler* Lowfat) . . .	90	8.0	9.0	1.5	20	440	0
Chicken sandwich, frozen, 1 pc.:							
breaded (*Hormel Quick Meal*)	340	15.0	40.0	13.0	35	520	1.0
grilled (*Hormel Quick Meal*)	310	19.0	36.0	10.0	55	580	1.0

Food and Measure	cal.	prot. (gms)	carbo. (gms)	fat (gms)	chol. (mgs)	sod. (mgs)	fiber (gms)
Chicken sauce, cooking (see also specific listings), ½ cup, except as noted:							
cacciatore (*Chicken Tonight*)	70	2.0	10.0	1.5	0	530	2.0
Dijon (*Lawry's* Weekday Gourmet), 2 tbsp.	40	<1.0	5.0	2.0	0	370	0
French, country (*Chicken Tonight*)	120	<1.0	6.0	10.0	15	860	1.0
honey mustard, light (*Chicken Tonight*)	60	1.0	13.0	.5	0	420	3.0
mushroom, creamy (*Chicken Tonight*)	80	<1.0	5.0	6.0	10	750	1.0
orange (*Lawry's* Weekday Gourmet), 2 tbsp.	30	0	6.0	1.0	0	300	0
wing, see "Buffalo wing sauce"							
Chicken sauce mix (see also specific listings), ¼ pkg.:							
cheese, three (*McCormick*)	45	1.0	2.0	3.0	0	470	0
herb:							
country (*McCormick*) ...	40	1.0	4.0	2.0	0	470	0
lemon (*McCormick*)	30	0	5.0	0	0	410	0
teriyaki (*McCormick*)	40	1.0	5.0	1.0	0	520	0
Chicken sausage, see "Sausage"							
Chicken seasoning, dry, ¼ tsp.:							
(*McCormick* Original)	0	0	0	0	0	130	0
Montreal (*McCormick Grill Mates*)	0	0	0	0	0	60	0
Montreal, garlic, roasted (*McCormick Grill Mates*)	0	0	0	0	0	170	0
herb (*McCormick*) ...	0	0	0	0	0	85	0
mesquite (*McCormick*)	0	0	0	0	0	70	0
rotisserie (*McCormick*)	0	0	0	0	0	130	0

Food and Measure	cal.	prot. (gms)	carbo. (gms)	fat (gms)	chol. (mgs)	sod. (mgs)	fiber (gms)
Chicken seasoning and coating mix, ⅛ pkg., except as noted:							
(*Don's Chuck Wagon* Baking Mix), ¼ cup	95	3.0	21.0	0	0	850	1.0
(*McCormick* Season 'n Fry)	35	0	6.0	0	0	760	0
(*McCormick Bag'n Season*), ⅙ pkg. . .	20	0	3.0	0	0	460	0
(*Shake 'n Bake* Original)	40	1.0	7.0	1.0	0	220	0
barbecue (*Shake 'n Bake Glazes*)	45	0	9.0	1.0	0	410	0
Buffalo wings (*Shake 'n Bake Glazes*), ⅒ pkg.	40	0	8.0	1.0	0	300	0
country style (*McCormick Bag'n Season*), ⅙ pkg. . .	25	0	3.0	1.0	0	880	0
home style flour recipe (*Oven Fry*) .	40	<1.0	7.0	1.0	0	470	0
honey, tangy (*Shake 'n Bake Glazes*) . . .	45	0	9.0	1.0	0	300	0
Italian herb (*McCormick Bag'n Season*)	15	0	2.0	0	0	480	0
nuggets, crispy (*Shake 'n Bake*), ⅙ pkg.	50	1.0	9.0	1.0	0	360	0
Oriental (*McCormick Bag'n Season*), ⅙ pkg.	25	0	4.0	0	0	550	0
Southwest style (*McCormick Bag'n Season*), ⅙ pkg. . .	25	0	3.0	.5	0	490	0
stir-fry (*McCormick*), ⅙ pkg.	20	0	4.0	0	0	520	0
Chicken spread (*Underwood*), ¼ cup	140	10.0	2.0	10.0	30	400	0
Chick-fil-A, 1 serving:							
chicken soup, hearty breast of, 1 cup . . .	100	9.0	13.0	1.5	20	940	1.0

Food and Measure	cal.	prot. (gms)	carbo. (gms)	fat (gms)	chol. (mgs)	sod. (mgs)	fiber (gms)
Chick-fil-A (cont.)							
chicken dishes:							
char-grilled chicken garden salad . . .	180	23.0	8.0	6.0	70	730	3.0
Chick-fil-A chicken Caesar salad . . .	240	31.0	6.0	10.0	85	1170	2.0
Chick-fil-A Chickin Strips, 4 pcs.	250	25.0	12.0	11.0	70	570	0
Chick-fil-A nuggets, 8-pack	260	26.0	12.0	12.0	70	1090	<1.0
Chick-n-Strips salad	340	30.0	19.0	16.0	85	680	3.0
Chick-fil-A sandwich:							
char-grilled, club . .	360	30.0	31.0	13.0	80	1370	2.0
char-grilled, regular	280	25.0	29.0	7.0	60	1000	1.0
chicken salad	350	20.0	32.0	15.0	65	880	5.0
regular	410	28.0	38.0	16.0	60	1300	1.0
chicken cool wraps:							
Caesar	460	38.0	51.0	11.0	85	1540	3.0
char-grilled	390	31.0	53.0	7.0	70	1120	3.0
spicy	390	31.0	51.0	7.0	70	1150	3.0
side items, small:							
carrot-raisin salad .	130	1.0	22.0	5.0	0	90	2.0
Chick-fil-A Waffle Potato Fries	280	3.0	37.0	14.0	15	105	5.0
coleslaw	210	1.0	14.0	17.0	20	180	2.0
side salad	80	5.0	6.0	5.0	15	110	2.0
sauces:							
barbecue	45	0	11.0	0	0	180	0
Dijon honey mustard	50	0	2.0	5.0	5	65	0
honey mustard . . .	45	0	10.0	0	0	150	0
Polynesian	110	0	13.0	6.0	0	210	0
dressings:							
basil vinaigrette . . .	210	0	4.0	21.0	0	160	0
blue cheese	190	1.0	2.0	20.0	20	370	0
buttermilk ranch . . .	190	1.0	2.0	20.0	10	330	0
Caesar	200	1.0	1.0	21.0	45	300	0
Dijon honey mustard, fat free	60	0	14.0	0	0	200	0
Italian, light	20	0	3.0	.5	0	640	0
spicy	210	0	2.0	22.0	10	170	0
Thousand Island . .	170	0	6.0	16.0	10	300	0
Truett's special house	150	0	7.0	13.0	5	290	0
desserts:							
brownie, fudge nut	330	4.0	45.0	15.0	20	210	2.0

Food and Measure	cal.	prot. (gms)	carbo. (gms)	fat (gms)	chol. (mgs)	sod. (mgs)	fiber (gms)
cheese cake, slice	340	6.0	30.0	21.0	90	270	2.0
Icedream, small cone	160	4.0	28.0	4.0	15	80	0
lemon pie, slice ...	320	7.0	51.0	10.0	110	220	3.0
Chickpeas, see "Garbanzo beans"							
Chicory, witloof:							
(*Frieda's* Belgium Endive), 2 cups, 3 oz.	15	1.0	3.0	0	0	20	3.0
5–7" head, 1.9 oz.	9	.5	2.1	.1	0	1	1.6
½ cup	8	.4	1.8	<.1	0	1	1.4
Chicory greens:							
trimmed, 1 oz.	7	.5	1.3	.1	0	13	1.1
chopped, ½ cup	21	1.5	4.2	.3	0	41	3.6
Chicory root:							
1 medium, 2.6 oz. ..	44	.8	10.5	.1	0	30	n.a.
1" pcs., ½ cup	33	.6	7.9	.1	0	23	n.a.
Chili, can or pkg. (see also "Chili starter"), 1 cup, except as noted:							
w/beans:							
(*Broadcast*)	350	20.0	36.0	15.0	50	1030	11.0
(*Castleberry*)	350	14.0	26.0	21.0	45	1090	8.0
(*Hormel*)	270	16.0	34.0	7.0	30	1220	7.0
(*Hormel*), 7.5-oz. can	230	14.0	29.0	6.0	30	1070	6.0
(*Hormel* Chunky) ..	270	18.0	34.0	7.0	35	1240	7.0
(*Hormel* Microcup)	220	15.0	27.0	6.0	30	1050	6.0
(*Stagg* Classic) ...	330	17.0	28.0	17.0	45	820	5.0
(*Stagg* Chili Laredo)	320	18.0	27.0	15.0	45	1150	6.0
(*Stagg* Chunkero)	300	16.0	26.0	15.0	45	830	5.0
(*Stagg* Country) ..	320	15.0	29.0	16.0	45	1130	5.0
(*Stagg* Dynamite Hot)	330	18.0	30.0	16.0	50	870	6.0
(*Stagg* Silverado) ..	230	18.0	33.0	3.0	45	880	6.0
(*Stagg* Steak House)	330	18.0	16.0	21.0	65	1060	2.0
hot (*Hormel*)	270	16.0	34.0	7.0	30	1220	7.0
hot (*Hormel*), 7.5 oz.	230	14.0	29.0	6.0	30	1070	6.0
hot (*Hormel* Micro- cup)	220	15.0	27.0	6.0	30	1050	6.0
w/out beans:							
(*Hormel*)	210	16.0	17.0	9.0	40	970	3.0

Food and Measure	cal.	prot. (gms)	carbo. (gms)	fat (gms)	chol. (mgs)	sod. (mgs)	fiber (gms)
Chili, can or pkg. w/out beans *(cont.)*							
(*Hormel* Microcup)	190	14.0	15.0	8.0	30	800	2.0
(*Stagg Double Barrel Beef*)	340	18.0	19.0	22.0	65	1250	2.0
hot (*Hormel*)	210	16.0	17.0	9.0	40	970	3.0
chicken:							
w/beans (*Greene's Farm*)	230	21.0	29.0	3.5	50	800	9.0
w/beans (*Stagg Ranch House*) ..	290	19.0	32.0	9.0	50	810	6.0
w/out beans (*Stagg Chicken Grande*)	250	18.0	17.0	12.0	75	1030	2.0
w/macaroni:							
(*Chef Boyardee* Chili Mac), ½ of 15-oz. can	260	10.0	30.0	11.0	30	1480	3.0
(*Hormel* Microcup Chili Mac)	200	11.0	17.0	9.0	25	980	2.0
turkey:							
w/beans (*Stagg Turkey Ranchero*)	240	22.0	31.0	3.0	35	880	6.0
w/beans (*Health Valley* 99% Fat Free)	220	16.0	34.0	3.0	30	480	8.0
w/beans (*Hormel*)	210	17.0	26.0	3.0	45	1200	5.0
w/out beans (*Hormel*)	190	24.0	17.0	3.0	75	1250	3.0
vegetable/vegetarian:							
(*Bearitos* Lowfat Premium Original)	200	12.0	36.0	2.0	0	500	9.0
(*Greene's Farm*) ...	170	11.0	33.0	1.0	0	650	10.0
(*Hormel*)	200	12.0	38.0	1.0	0	780	7.0
(*Natural Touch*) ...	170	18.0	21.0	1.0	0	870	11.0
(*Stagg Vegetable Garden*)	200	10.0	37.0	1.0	0	870	7.0
(*Worthington*)	290	19.0	21.0	15.0	0	1130	9.0
(*Worthington* Lowfat)	170	18.0	21.0	1.0	0	870	11.0
black bean (*Bearitos* Lowfat Premium)	160	10.0	29.0	1.5	0	510	8.0
black bean or 3 bean (*Health Valley* 99% Fat Free) ..	160	13.0	28.0	1.0	0	320	12.0

Food and Measure	cal.	prot. (gms)	carbo. (gms)	fat (gms)	chol. (mgs)	sod. (mgs)	fiber (gms)
burrito or enchilada flavor (*Health Valley* 99% Fat Free)	160	14.0	30.0	1.0	0	390	12.0
fajita flavor (*Health Valley* 99% Fat Free)	160	14.0	30.0	1.0	0	390	11.0
lentil (*Health Valley*)	160	15.0	28.0	1.0	0	390	11.0
lentil (*Health Valley* No Salt)	160	14.0	30.0	1.0	0	65	11.0
medium (*Amy's*) . .	190	8.0	26.0	6.0	0	590	7.0
medium, w/vegetables (*Amy's*) . .	190	7.0	29.0	6.0	0	590	8.0
mild or spicy (*Health Valley*)	160	14.0	30.0	1.0	0	390	11.0
mild or spicy (*Health Valley* No Salt) . .	160	14.0	30.0	1.0	0	65	11.0
spicy (*Amy's*)	190	8.0	26.0	6.0	0	590	7.0
spicy (*Bearitos* Low Fat Premium) . . .	200	12.0	36.0	2.0	0	500	9.0
Chili, frozen or refrigerated (see also "Chili entree, frozen"):							
turkey, w/beans (*Wampler*), 1 cup .	250	23.0	22.0	7.0	75	1840	4.0
vegetarian:							
(*Tabatchnick*), 7.5 oz.	210	12.0	28.0	6.0	0	530	10.0
(*Yves*), 10.5-oz. pkg.	230	21.0	37.0	1.0	0	850	14.0
Chili, mix, dry, ¾ cup:							
black bean (*Taste Adventure*)	240	17.0	43.0	1.5	0	490	11.0
five bean (*Taste Adventure*)	260	19.0	45.0	1.5	0	490	14.0
red bean (*Taste Adventure*)	240	17.0	43.0	1.5	0	480	12.0
Chili beans (see also "Chili starter" and "Mexican beans"), canned, ½ cup:							
(*Blue Boy*)	120	6.0	22.0	0	0	450	6.0
(*Bush's Best*)	120	6.0	20.0	1.0	0	480	6.0
(*Eden* Organic)	130	9.0	21.0	0	0	250	7.0

Food and Measure	cal.	prot. (gms)	carbo. (gms)	fat (gms)	chol. (mgs)	sod. (mgs)	fiber (gms)
Chili beans *(cont.)*							
(Joan of Arc)	110	6.0	20.0	1.0	0	490	5.0
(S&W)	110	7.0	23.0	1.0	0	470	6.0
(Westbrae Natural) . .	90	6.0	15.0	0	0	140	5.0
chipotle *(S&W)*	90	7.0	21.0	0	0	570	6.0
hot *(Bush's Best)* . . .	120	6.0	20.0	1.0	0	480	6.0
spicy *(Eden* Pintos) . .	125	6.0	24.0	0	0	195	7.0
Chili dinner, frozen, w/corn bread *(Amy's)*, 10.5-oz. pkg.	320	11.0	59.0	6.0	10	780	8.0
Chili dip (see also "Salsa"), chunky *(La Victoria)*, 2 tbsp.	10	0	2.0	0	0	140	0
Chili entree, dried, 1 serving:							
(AlpineAire Mountain)	300	23.0	48.0	3.0	0	1280	13.0
w/beef: *(AlpineAire* Black Bart)	320	29.0	39.0	4.5	65	1430	10.0
macaroni *(Mountain House)*	300	15.0	39.0	9.0	20	800	4.0
turkey *(AlpineAire)* . . .	350	33.0	43.0	5.0	n.a.	890	12.0
Chili entree, frozen, 1 pkg., except as noted:							
bean, three *(Lean Cuisine Everyday Favorites)*, 10 oz.	250	10.0	39.0	6.0	10	590	10.0
w/beans *(Stouffer's)*, 8.75 oz.	290	19.0	29.0	11.0	45	1000	6.0
w/beans and rice *(Healthy Choice* Bowl Homestyle), 11 oz.	380	24.0	59.0	6.0	45	600	9.0
black bean, w/rice *(Michelina's)*, 10 oz.	400	13.0	76.0	5.0	0	510	10.0
and corn bread *(Marie Callender's)*, 16 oz.	560	27.0	67.0	21.0	60	2110	7.0
w/macaroni *(Michelina's* Chili-Mac), 8 oz.	290	14.0	38.0	9.0	25	850	3.0
Chili pepper, see "Pepper, chili"							

Food and Measure	cal.	prot. (gms)	carbo. (gms)	fat (gms)	chol. (mgs)	sod. (mgs)	fiber (gms)
Chili pepper paste, see "Thai sauce"							
Chili powder:							
(*McCormick*), ¼ tsp.	0	0	0	0	0	20	0
1 tbsp.	24	.9	4.1	1.3	0	76	2.6
1 tsp.	8	.3	1.4	.4	0	26	.9
Chili relish, hot, Indian (*Patak's* Chile), 1 tbsp.	50	<1.0	0	5.0	0	510	0
Chili sauce, black bean, see "Black bean sauce"							
Chili sauce, hot, see "Hot sauce" and "Thai sauce"							
Chili sauce, tomato:							
(*Bennetts*), 1 tbsp. . .	15	0	4.0	0	0	125	0
(*Del Monte*), 1 tbsp. . .	20	0	5.0	0	0	480	0
(*Heinz*), 1 tbsp.	15	0	4.0	0	0	230	0
(*Nance's*), 2 tbsp. . . .	25	0	5.0	0	0	150	0
(*Red Gold*), 1 tbsp. .	20	0	5.0	0	0	180	0
Chili seasoning mix:							
(*Adolph's Meal Makers*), 1 tbsp. . .	30	<1.0	5.0	1.0	0	270	0
(*Bearitos*), 4 tsp.	30	1.0	5.0	.5	0	620	0
(*Hain*), 1⅓ tsp.	40	1.0	7.0	1.0	0	410	2.0
(*Lawry's*), 1 tbsp. . . .	25	<1.0	5.0	1.0	0	460	0
(*McCormick Original*), ½ pkg.	30	1.0	5.0	.5	0	310	0
(*Shotgun Willie's* Texas), 3 tbsp.	50	2.0	8.0	0	0	180	0
(*Tempo*), 1½ tbsp. . .	45	1.0	10.0	.5	0	820	0
hot (*McCormick*), ¼ pkg.	35	1.0	4.0	1.0	0	340	0
mild (*McCormick*), ¼ pkg.	30	1.0	5.0	0	0	400	0
Chili starter, canned, ½ cup, except as noted:							
(*Bush's Chili Magic* Traditional)	110	5.0	19.0	1.0	0	890	5.0
(*Bush's Chili Magic* Traditional), 1 cup*	220	22.0	15.0	8.0	55	770	3.0
(*S&W* Chili Makins) . .	80	6.0	19.0	0	0	750	6.0

Food and Measure	cal.	prot. (gms)	carbo. (gms)	fat (gms)	chol. (mgs)	sod. (mgs)	fiber (gms)
Chili starter *(cont.)*							
(*S&W* Chili Makins							
Homestyle)	80	7.0	19.0	0	0	630	6.0
black bean (*S&W* Chili							
Makins)	80	6.0	19.0	0	0	750	6.0
Louisiana:							
(*Bush's Chili Magic*)	110	4.0	21.0	1.5	0	1070	5.0
(*Bush's Chili Magic*),							
1 cup*	220	22.0	16.0	7.0	60	820	3.0
Mexican:							
(*Bush's Chili Magic*)	120	5.0	22.0	1.5	0	1030	4.0
(*Bush's Chili Magic*),							
1 cup*	230	24.0	15.0	9.0	55	860	4.0
Texas:							
(*Bush's Chili Magic*)	120	5.0	20.0	2.0	0	1130	5.0
(*Bush's Chili Magic*),							
1 cup*	230	22.0	15.0	9.0	55	880	4.0
Chimichanga, frozen:							
beef and bean (*El							
Monterey*), 4 oz. ...	310	8.0	34.0	15.0	15	480	3.0
beef and cheese (*El							
Monterey Family							
Classic*), 5 oz.	310	14.0	35.0	13.0	35	340	1.0
chicken and cheese							
(*El Monterey Family							
Classic*), 5 oz.	320	13.0	38.0	13.0	25	350	2.0
Chipotle sauce (*La							
Morena*), 2 tbsp. ...	25	<1.0	6.0	0	0	680	0
Chitterlings, pork,							
simmered, 4 oz. ...	344	11.6	0	32.6	162	44	0
Chives:							
fresh:							
1 oz.	9	.9	1.2	.2	0	1	.9
chopped, 1 tbsp. ...	1	.1	.1	<.1	0	<1	.1
freeze-dried:							
¼ cup	2	.2	.5	<.1	0	24	<1.0
1 tbsp.	1	<.1	.1	<.1	0	6	<1.0
Chocolate, see "Candy"							
Chocolate, baking,							
½ oz. or 1 tbsp.,							
except as noted:							
(*Nestlé Choco Bake*)	80	1.0	4.0	8.0	0	0	2.0
bar:							
(*German's*), 2 sqs.	70	<1.0	8.0	3.5	0	0	<1.0

Food and Measure	cal.	prot. (gms)	carbo. (gms)	fat (gms)	chol. (mgs)	sod. (mgs)	fiber (gms)
bittersweet (*Baker's*)	70	<1.0	7.0	6.0	0	0	1.0
semisweet (*Baker's*)	70	<1.0	8.0	4.5	0	0	1.0
semisweet (*Hershey's*)	70	<1.0	9.0	4.0	0	0	0
semisweet (*Nestlé*)	70	<1.0	9.0	4.0	0	0	<1.0
unsweetened (*Baker's*)	70	2.0	4.0	7.0	0	0	2.0
unsweetened (*Hershey's*)	90	2.0	4.0	7.0	0	0	2.0
unsweetened (*Nestlé*)	80	2.0	5.0	7.0	0	0	3.0
white (*Baker's*)	80	1.0	8.0	4.5	<5	15	0
white (*Hershey's*) . .	80	1.0	9.0	4.0	0	30	0
white (*Nestlé*)	80	1.0	8.0	5.0	<5	15	0
bits, mini (*M&M's*), 1 tbsp.	70	1.0	10.0	3.5	5	10	0
chips or morsels:							
milk (*Baker's*)	70	<1.0	9.0	3.5	0	15	0
milk (*Hershey's*) . .	80	1.0	9.0	4.5	<5	10	0
milk (*Hershey's* Bake Shoppe Reduced Fat) . . .	60	<1.0	11.0	3.5	0	0	0
milk (*Nestlé*)	70	<1.0	9.0	4.0	<5	0	0
mint (*Nestlé*)	70	<1.0	9.0	4.0	0	0	<1.0
semisweet (*Baker's* Flavored)	70	0	10.0	3.5	0	15	0
semisweet (*Baker's* Real)	60	<1.0	10.0	3.5	0	10	<1.0
semisweet (*Hershey's*)	80	<1.0	10.0	4.0	0	0	0
semisweet (*Nestlé/ Nestlé* Mini)	70	<1.0	9.0	4.0	0	0	<1.0
semisweet, mint or raspberry (*Hershey's*)	80	<1.0	10.0	4.0	0	0	0
white (*Hershey's*) . .	80	1.0	9.0	4.0	0	30	0
white (*Nestlé*)	80	<1.0	9.0	4.0	0	20	0
chunks:							
(*Nestlé*)	70	1.0	8.0	4.0	0	0	1.0
white (*Baker's*)	80	<1.0	9.0	5.0	<5	15	0
milk chocolate, mini (*Hershey's Kisses*), 11 pcs., .5 oz.	80	1.0	9.0	4.5	<5	15	0

Food and Measure	cal.	prot. (gms)	carbo. (gms)	fat (gms)	chol. (mgs)	sod. (mgs)	fiber (gms)
Chocolate, baking *(cont.)*							
sprinkles, see "Chocolate sprinkles"							
Chocolate dip, see "Fruit dip"							
Chocolate drink:							
(*Hershey's*), 1 box . . .	130	2.0	28.0	1.0	0	200	0
(*Yoo-Hoo*), 8 fl oz. . .	130	2.0	29.0	1.0	0	180	0
(*Yoo-Hoo*), 9 fl. oz. . .	150	2.0	33.0	1.0	0	200	0
(*Yoo-Hoo* Lite), 9 fl. oz.	70	2.0	15.0	1.0	0	190	0
Chocolate drink mix, 2 tbsp.:							
(*Nesquik*)	90	1.0	19.0	.5	0	30	1.0
(*Nesquik* No Sugar) . .	40	1.0	7.0	1.0	0	45	2.0
Chocolate milk, see "Milk, flavored"							
Chocolate shake (*Hershey's*), 7 fl. oz.	230	6.0	41.0	4.5	20	290	1.0
Chocolate sprinkles:							
candy coated (*Hershey's*), 1 tbsp.	70	<1.0	10.0	3.0	<5	10	0
mint (*Hershey's York Chocolate Shoppe*), 2 tbsp.	170	1.0	21.0	9.0	0	0	0
Chocolate syrup, 2 tbsp., except as noted:							
(*Fox's U-Bet*)	120	1.0	29.0	0	0	35	0
(*Hershey's*), 2-oz. pouch	150	1.0	36.0	.5	0	35	1.0
(*Hershey's* Lite)	50	0	12.0	0	0	35	<1.0
(*Hershey's Chocolate Shoppe* Apple Pie a la Mode Fat Free) . .	100	0	25.0	0	0	90	<1.0
(*Hershey's Special Dark*)	110	<1.0	26.0	0	0	35	0
(*Nesquik*)	100	1.0	23.0	.5	0	30	<1.0
(*Smucker's* Sundae) .	110	1.0	26.0	0	0	20	0
cherries jubilee sundae (*Hershey's Chocolate Shoppe*)	110	<1.0	26.0	0	0	20	<1.0
flavored (*Estee*)	15	<1.0	5.0	0	0	40	0
malt (*Hershey's*), 2-oz. pouch	140	<1.0	36.0	0	0	100	<1.0

Food and Measure	cal.	prot. (gms)	carbo. (gms)	fat (gms)	chol. (mgs)	sod. (mgs)	fiber (gms)
mint (*Hershey's Chocolate Shoppe*)	110	<1.0	26.0	0	0	25	<1.0
Chocolate topping, 2 tbsp.:							
(*Hershey's Shell*)	230	1.0	16.0	18.0	0	15	1.0
(*Kraft*)	110	2.0	26.0	0	0	30	1.0
(*Smucker's Magic Shell*)	210	1.0	16.0	17.0	0	20	1.0
(*Smucker's Plate Scrapers*)	100	1.0	23.0	1.0	0	20	1.0
crisps (*Hershey's Krackel Shell*)	190	<1.0	14.0	17.0	0	25	<1.0
dark (*Dove*)	140	<1.0	22.0	5.0	0	80	1.0
fudge:							
(*Hershey's*)	130	2.0	19.0	5.0	5	40	<1.0
(*Hershey's Shell*) ..	190	1.0	15.0	14.0	0	55	2.0
(*Mrs. Richardson's Chocolate Lovers*)	130	1.0	20.0	6.0	0	40	<1.0
(*Smucker's*)	130	0	28.0	1.5	0	60	1.0
(*Smucker's Magic Shell*)	200	1.0	19.0	14.0	0	50	1.0
double (*Hershey's*)	120	2.0	24.0	2.0	<5	75	<1.0
hot (*Hershey's*) ...	130	2.0	20.0	4.5	<5	180	<1.0
hot (*Hershey's Chocolate Shoppe* Fat Free)	100	1.0	23.0	0	0	135	1.0
hot (*Kraft*)	140	1.0	24.0	4.5	0	100	<1.0
hot (*Mrs. Richardson's*)	140	1.0	19.0	7.0	0	75	0
hot (*Mrs. Richardson's* Fat Free) ..	100	1.0	25.0	0	0	80	<1.0
hot (*Mrs. Richardson's Singles*), 1 pouch	180	1.0	25.0	9.0	0	105	1.0
hot (*Smucker's*) ...	140	2.0	24.0	4.0	0	60	1.0
hot (*Smucker's Light*)	90	2.0	23.0	0	0	95	2.0
hot (*Smucker's Microwave*)	130	2.0	24.0	2.5	0	50	<1.0
hot (*Smucker's Microwave Fat Free*)	110	2.0	26.0	0	0	70	<1.0

Food and Measure	cal.	prot. (gms)	carbo. (gms)	fat (gms)	chol. (mgs)	sod. (mgs)	fiber (gms)
Chocolate topping, fudge *(cont.)*							
hot (*Smucker's* Special Recipe)	140	2.0	22.0	4.0	0	70	<1.0
milk (*Dove*)	130	2.0	21.0	4.0	0	75	1.0
toffee, see "Toffee topping"							
white (*Smucker's Plate Scrapers*)	110	0	22.0	2.5	0	65	0
Chorizo, see "Sausage"							
Chow chow pickle:							
(*Crosse & Blackwell*), 1 tbsp.	10	0	1.0	0	0	105	<1.0
hot or mild (*Mrs. Renfro's*), 1 tbsp. .	10	0	3.0	0	0	45	0
relish (*Stubb's*), ½ cup	70	2.0	13.0	1.0	0	600	2.0
Chrysanthemum garland, 1" pcs.:							
raw, ½ cup	2	.2	.5	<.1	0	7	.4
boiled, drained, ½ cup	10	.8	2.2	.1	0	27	1.2
Church's Chicken:							
chicken, 1 pc.:							
breast, 2.8 oz. . . .	200	19.0	4.3	12.4	65	510	0
leg, 2 oz.	140	12.7	2.4	9.1	45	160	0
Tender Strip, 1.1 oz.	80	6.0	4.5	4.0	15	140	.5
thigh, 2.8 oz.	230	16.2	5.3	16.2	80	520	0
wing, 3.1 oz.	250	18.5	7.7	16.1	60	540	0
sides:							
biscuit, 2.1 oz. . . .	250	2.2	25.6	16.4	<5	640	1.0
coleslaw, 3 oz. . . .	92	4.2	8.4	5.5	0	230	2.0
corn on cob, 5.7 oz.	139	4.4	23.5	3.2	0	15	9.0
french fries, 2.7 oz.	210	3.3	28.5	10.5	0	60	2.0
jalapeño bombers, 5 oz.	300	10.0	36.0	12.0	35	1210	4.0
macaroni and cheese, 3.6 oz.	140	5.0	15.0	7.0	10	460	<1.0
okra, fried, 2.8 oz.	210	2.7	19.1	16.1	0	520	4.0
potatoes w/gravy, 3.7 oz.	90	1.2	14.0	3.3	0	520	1.0
rice, Cajun, 3.1 oz.	130	1.3	15.6	7.0	5	260	<1.0
apple pie, 3.1 oz. . . .	280	2.3	40.5	12.3	<5	340	1.0
Churro, cinnamon:							
(*Bearitos*), ½ cup	150	1.0	20.0	7.0	0	<1	0

Food and Measure	cal.	prot. (gms)	carbo. (gms)	fat (gms)	chol. (mgs)	sod. (mgs)	fiber (gms)
Chutney, 1 tbsp., except as noted:							
(*Trader Vic's* Calcutta), 2 tbsp.	44	.5	11.0	0	0	270	0
apple curry (*Crosse & Blackwell*)	25	0	7.0	0	0	20	0
cranberry:							
(*Crosse & Blackwell*)	40	0	10.0	0	0	0	0
(*Susan Elaine's*), 2 tbsp.	80	0	21.0	0	0	10	0
ginger pineapple (*Neera's*)	31	0	7.0	0	0	54	0
mango:							
(*Bombay Brand* Major Grey's), 2 tbsp.	110	0	25.0	0	0	210	0
(*Crosse & Blackwell* Major Grey's) . . .	60	0	14.0	0	0	170	0
(*Neera's*)	20	0	5.0	0	0	26	0
(*Patak's*)	50	<1.0	12.0	.5	0	240	0
ginger (*Bombay Brand*), 2 tbsp.	90	0	23.0	0	0	25	1.0
ginger (*Patak's* Major Grey)	50	0	12.0	.5	0	90	0
hot (*Crosse & Blackwell*)	60	0	14.0	0	0	170	0
hot (*Patak's*)	60	0	12.0	.5	0	70	0
lime (*Patak's*)	50	0	12.0	0	0	240	0
sweet, mild (*Patak's*)	60	0	13.0	0	0	70	0
peach (*Neera's*)	22	0	6.0	0	0	30	0
pear cardamom (*Neera's*)	30	0	7.0	0	0	23	0
tomato:							
(*Neera's*)	22	0	5.0	1.0	0	23	0
dried (*Sonoma*) . . .	35	0	9.0	0	0	0	0
mint (*Neera's*)	22	0	5.0	2.0	0	54	0
vegetable (*Neera's*) . .	21	0	2.0	2.0	0	49	0
Cilantro, see "Coriander"							
Cinnamon, ground, 1 tsp.	6	.1	2.1	.1	0	1	1.4
Cinnamon baking chips (*Hershey's*), 1 tbsp.	80	1.0	9.0	4.0	0	35	0

Food and Measure	cal.	prot. (gms)	carbo. (gms)	fat (gms)	chol. (mgs)	sod. (mgs)	fiber (gms)
Cisco, meat only:							
raw, 4 oz.	112	21.5	0	2.2	57	62	0
smoked, 4 oz.	201	18.6	0	13.5	36	545	0
Citron, candied, diced:							
(*Seneca* Glacé), 2 tbsp.	70	0	18.0	0	0	25	<1.0
(*S&W* Glacé), 39 pcs.,							
1.1 oz.	90	0	23.0	0	0	25	1.0
Citronella root, see							
"Lemon grass"							
Citrus drink, 8 fl. oz.,							
except as noted:							
(*Capri Sun Citrus*							
Cooler), 6.75 fl. oz.	90	0	23.0	0	0	20	0
frozen*	114	.7	28.5	0	0	7	0
punch:							
(*Minute Maid*)	120	0	32.0	0	0	25	0
(*Tropicana*)	140	0	36.0	0	0	15	0
tangy (*Sunny Delight*)	120	0	29.0	0	0	190	0
Citrus pepper blend							
(*McCormick*),							
¼ tsp.	0	0	0	0	0	30	0
Clam, meat only:							
raw:							
4 oz.	84	14.5	2.9	1.1	39	64	0
9 large or 20 small,							
6.3 oz.	133	23.0	4.6	1.8	60	100	0
boiled, poached, or							
steamed, 4 oz. . . .	168	29.0	5.8	2.2	76	127	0
Clam, canned, 2 oz. or							
¼ cup, except as							
noted:							
whole:							
baby (*Bumble Bee*)	50	9.0	2.0	1.0	40	270	0
baby (*Chicken of the*							
Sea)	30	6.0	1.0	0	10	290	0
baby (*Crown Prince*							
Natural), ⅓ cup	50	8.0	1.0	1.0	25	70	0
baby, boiled (*Crown*							
Prince), ⅓ cup . .	50	8.0	2.0	1.5	40	260	0
small (*3 Diamonds*)	45	9.0	1.0	.5	25	290	0
chopped:							
ocean (*Chinco-*							
teague)	30	6.0	1.0	0	10	290	0

Food and Measure	cal.	prot. (gms)	carbo. (gms)	fat (gms)	chol. (mgs)	sod. (mgs)	fiber (gms)
sea, Eastern (*Chincoteague*)	25	6.0	0	0	15	260	0
chopped or minced:							
(*Chicken of the Sea*)	30	5.0	2.0	0	12	370	0
(*Doxsee*)	25	4.0	2.0	0	10	320	0
(*Neptune* Fancy Atlantic Surf) ...	20	4.0	1.0	0	10	320	0
(*Neptune* Atlantic Ocean)	30	5.0	2.0	0	5	430	0
minced (*Progresso*) ..	25	4.0	2.0	0	10	250	0
smoked, baby (*Reese*), ⅓ cup	120	9.0	3.0	9.0	30	130	0
Clam chowder, see "Soup"							
Clam dish, frozen:							
casino (*Matlaw's*), 2 pcs., 1.3 oz.	60	3.0	7.0	3.0	0	260	1.0
fried:							
(*Chincoteague*), 3 oz.	265	6.0	24.0	16.0	5	527	1.0
(*Gorton's*), 3 oz. ..	250	8.0	20.0	15.0	10	310	0
(*Mrs. Paul's/Van de Kamp's*), 18 pcs., 3 oz.	250	9.0	26.0	12.0	20	560	1.0
crisps (*Acadian Gourmet*), 22 pcs., 3.1 oz.	310	9.0	27.0	18.0	10	1130	2.0
on half shell (*Chincoteague*), 2 pcs. ...	20	4.0	1.0	0	10	15	0
Oreganata (*Matlaw's*), 2 pcs., 1.2 oz.	90	3.0	7.0	6.0	0	180	1.0
stuffed:							
(*Chincoteague*), 1 pc.	130	7.0	9.0	7.0	15	180	0
(*Morning Catch*), 2 pcs.	180	8.0	21.0	8.0	0	730	3.0
(*Matlaw's* Box), 2 pcs., 3.7 oz.	180	8.0	21.0	8.0	0	730	3.0
(*Matlaw's* Tray), 2.7-oz. pc.	130	6.0	13.0	6.0	0	530	2.0
Clam juice, 8 fl. oz., except as noted:							
(*Crown Prince*), 1 tbsp.	5	1.0	0	0	0	100	0

Food and Measure	cal.	prot. (gms)	carbo. (gms)	fat (gms)	chol. (mgs)	sod. (mgs)	fiber (gms)
Clam juice *(cont.)*							
ocean (*Chincoteague*)	10	2.0	1.0	0	0	1490	0
sea (*Chincoteague*) ..	15	1.0	0	0	0	590	0
and tomato, see							
"Tomato-clam drink"							
Clam sauce, canned:							
red, ½ cup:							
(*Crown Prince*) ...	60	3.0	5.0	3.0	10	250	<1.0
(*Olde Cape Cod*) ..	100	5.0	12.0	3.0	0	160	0
(*Progresso*)	60	4.0	8.0	1.0	10	350	1.0
(*Rienzi*)	70	4.0	7.0	2.5	0	490	2.0
white, ½ cup:							
(*Bookbinder's*)	300	4.0	4.0	30.0	0	860	<1.0
(*Chincoteague*) ...	120	4.0	9.0	8.0	10	490	0
(*Crown Prince*) ...	90	5.0	3.0	6.0	15	430	<1.0
(*Olde Cape Cod*) ..	100	6.0	6.0	6.0	15	340	0
(*Progresso*)	140	7.0	5.0	10.0	15	510	0
(*Progresso* Authen-							
tic)	150	9.0	5.0	10.0	20	710	0
creamy (*Progresso*)	110	5.0	8.0	6.0	10	440	0
Clover sprouts (*Jona-*							
than's), 1 cup	25	3.0	3.0	.5	0	5	2.0
Cloves, ground:							
1 tbsp.	21	.4	4.0	1.3	0	16	<1.0
1 tsp.	7	.1	1.3	.4	0	5	.2
Cobbler, frozen:							
apple:							
(*Marie Callender's*),							
¼ of 17-oz. pkg.	370	2.0	45.0	20.0	0	170	2.0
(*Mrs. Smith's*), ⅛							
of 32-oz. pkg. ..	270	2.0	43.0	10.0	0	250	2.0
(*Mrs. Smith's*), 1/18							
of 79-oz. pkg. ..	280	2.0	42.0	12.0	0	260	2.0
berry (*Marie Cal-*							
lender's), ¼ of							
17-oz. pkg.	370	3.0	41.0	21.0	<5	220	1.0
blackberry:							
(*Mrs. Smith's*), ⅛							
of 32-oz. pkg. ..	260	2.0	43.0	10.0	0	250	2.0
(*Mrs. Smith's*), 1/18							
of 79-oz. pkg. ..	270	3.0	41.0	12.0	0	260	3.0
cherry:							
(*Marie Callender's*),							
¼ of 17-oz. pkg.	380	3.0	50.0	19.0	5	240	0

Food and Measure	cal.	prot. (gms)	carbo. (gms)	fat (gms)	chol. (mgs)	sod. (mgs	fiber (gms)
(*Mrs. Smith's*), ⅛ of 32-oz.	280	2.0	46.0	10.0	0	250	<1.0
(*Mrs. Smith's*), ⅟₁₈ of 79-oz. pkg. ..	300	3.0	47.0	12.0	0	260	<1.0
peach:							
(*Marie Callender's*), ¼ of 17-oz. pkg.	360	3.0	47.0	18.0	0	240	0
(*Mrs. Smith's*), ⅟₁₈ of 79-oz. pkg. ..	270	3.0	40.0	12.0	0	260	1.0
Cocktail sauce, see "Seafood sauce"							
Cocoa, 1 tbsp., except as noted:							
(*Ghirardelli*)	35	2.0	5.0	3.0	0	0	3.0
(*Hershey's/ Hershey's* European Style)	20	1.0	3.0	.5	0	0	1.0
(*Hershey's* Breakfast)	30	1.0	3.0	1.5	0	0	1.0
(*Nestlé* Baking)	15	1.0	3.0	.5	0	0	1.0
(*Watkins*), 1 tsp.	20	1.0	3.0	.5	0	0	1.0
Cocoa mix, 1 pkt., except as noted:							
(*Baker's*), 3 tbsp. ...	150	2.0	29.0	3.0	<5	170	<1.0
(*Hershey's* Classic) ..	120	1.0	24.0	2.0	5	110	1.0
(*Hershey's* Goodnight Hug)	150	2.0	27.0	4.0	5	140	0
chocolate:							
(*Country Choice Naturals* Royal)	100	2.0	24.0	0	0	150	<1.0
(*Land O Lakes* Supreme)	160	4.0	25.0	5.0	0	180	0
almond (*Hershey's* Hot Cocoa Collection)	150	3.0	27.0	3.0	0	150	1.0
amaretto (*Land O Lakes*)	160	3.0	24.0	5.0	0	135	0
caramel (*Land O Lakes*)	160	4.0	25.0	5.0	0	180	0
cherry, black (*Land O Lakes*)	150	3.0	24.0	5.0	0	150	1.0
cinnamon (*Land O Lakes*)	160	4.0	25.0	5.0	0	220	0

Food and Measure	cal.	prot. (gms)	carbo. (gms)	fat (gms)	chol. (mgs)	sod. (mgs)	fiber (gms)
Cocoa mix, chocolate *(cont.)*							
cinnamon spice, Irish mint, or orange cream (*Country Choice Naturals*)	100	3.0	24.0	0	0	160	<1.0
dark (*Carnation Homemade Classics*), 1⅔ tbsp.	90	1.0	21.0	1.0	0	70	1.0
double (*Carnation Meltdown*)	150	2.0	29.0	3.0	0	150	1.0
Dutch (*Hershey's Hot Cocoa Collection*)	160	1.0	27.0	5.0	0	180	1.0
Dutch (*Hershey's Hot Cocoa Collection* Fat Free) ...	50	2.0	10.0	0	0	160	<1.0
hazelnut (*Land O Lakes*)	160	4.0	25.0	5.0	0	220	0
Irish creme (*Land O Lakes*)	160	4.0	25.0	5.0	0	180	0
milk (*Carnation*) ...	120	2.0	23.0	2.0	0	190	<1.0
milk (*Carnation Homemade Classics*), 1⅔ tbsp.	90	<1.0	23.0	.5	0	55	1.0
milk (*Hershey's Goodnight Kiss*)	150	2.0	27.0	3.5	0	160	<1.0
mint (*Hershey's Hot Cocoa Collection*)	150	3.0	27.0	3.0	0	140	1.0
mint (*Land O Lakes*)	160	4.0	25.0	5.0	0	220	0
mocha (*Land O Lakes*)	160	3.0	24.0	5.0	0	135	0
raspberry (*Hershey's Hot Cocoa Collection*)	150	3.0	27.0	3.0	0	135	1.0
raspberry (*Land O Lakes*)	160	4.0	25.0	5.0	0	180	0
rich (*Carnation*) ...	120	<1.0	23.0	3.0	0	180	<1.0
rich (*Carnation* Fat Free)	25	1.0	5.0	0	0	125	<1.0
rich (*Carnation* No Sugar)	50	2.0	10.0	0	0	190	<1.0

Food and Measure	cal.	prot. (gms)	carbo. (gms)	fat (gms)	chol. (mgs)	sod. (mgs	fiber (gms)
Irish creme:							
(*Hershey's Hot*							
Cocoa Collection)	150	3.0	27.0	3.0	0	140	1.0
(*Watkins*), 1 oz.,							
about 3 tbsp. . .	110	2.0	25.0	1.5	2	170	0
w/marshmallows:							
(*Carnation* Fat Free)	40	2.0	8.0	0	0	125	<1.0
(*Carnation Marsh-*							
mallow Madness)	180	<1.0	36.0	4.0	0	250	<1.0
(*Hershey's* Classic)	120	1.0	24.0	2.0	5	100	1.0
chocolate, rich							
(*Carnation*)	120	<1.0	23.0	.5	0	170	<1.0
chocolate, rich							
(*Carnation* Fat							
Free)	40	1.0	8.0	0	0	130	<1.0
chocolate, rich							
(*Carnation* No							
Sugar)	50	4.0	9.0	.5	0	170	<1.0
s'mores (*Carnation*)	130	0	25.0	3.5	0	160	<1.0
vanilla, French:							
(*Carnation*)	120	1.0	22.0	3.0	0	150	<1.0
(*Hershey's Hot*							
Cocoa Collection)	140	2.0	28.0	2.5	0	150	0
(*Hershey's Hot*							
Cocoa Collection							
Fat Free)	50	2.0	11.0	0	0	150	<1.0
(*Land O Lakes*) . . .	160	4.0	25.0	5.0	0	220	0
(*Watkins*), 1 oz.,							
about 3 tbsp. . .	110	1.0	23.0	1.5	2	120	1.0
Cocoa-coffee mix							
(*Trader Vic's Kafe-*							
La-Te), 2 rounded							
tsp., ½ oz.	50	0	13.0	0	0	30	0
Coconut, fresh, shelled:							
(*Frieda's* White/Young),							
¼ cup, 1.4 oz. . . .	140	1.0	6.0	13.0	0	10	4.0
1 oz.	100	.9	4.3	9.5	0	6	2.6
shredded or grated							
(*Dole*), 1 cup not							
packed	283	3.0	12.0	27.0	0	16	7.0
shredded or grated,							
1 cup not packed . .	283	2.7	12.2	26.8	0	16	7.2

Food and Measure	cal.	prot. (gms)	carbo. (gms)	fat (gms)	chol. (mgs)	sod. (mgs)	fiber (gms)
Coconut, can or pkg.:							
dried, toasted, 1 oz.	168	1.5	12.6	13.4	0	11	1.0
flaked, 2 tbsp.:							
(*Baker's Angel Flake* Bag)	70	<1.0	6.0	5.0	0	45	1.0
(*Baker's Angel Flake* Can).	70	<1.0	6.0	6.0	0	0	1.0
(*Baker's* Premium Shred)	60	0	5.0	4.5	0	35	<1.0
flaked, sweetened, ⅓ cup	117	.8	11.8	7.9	0	63	1.1
Coconut cream:							
(*Goya* Coco Cream of Coconut), 2 tbsp.	140	0	22.0	5.0	0	15	0
1 tbsp.	36	.5	1.6	3.4	0	10	.4
Coconut milk:							
(*Goya*), 1 tbsp.	50	1.0	1.0	5.0	0	5	0
(*A Taste of Thai*), ¼ cup	110	1.0	2.0	11.0	0	15	0
(*A Taste of Thai* Lite), ⅓ cup	45	1.0	3.0	4.0	0	20	0
Coconut nectar (*R. W. Knudsen*), 8 fl. oz.	140	1.0	26.0	5.0	0	55	2.0
Coconut water (*Goya*), 12 fl. oz.	150	2.0	31.0	2.5	0	85	10.0
Cod, meat only:							
Atlantic, 4 oz.:							
raw	93	20.2	0	.8	49	62	0
baked, broiled, or microwaved ...	119	25.9	0	1.0	62	88	0
Pacific, 4 oz.:							
raw	93	20.3	0	.7	42	81	0
baked, broiled, or microwaved ...	119	26.0	0	.9	53	103	0
Cod, canned:							
Atlantic, w/liquid, 4 oz.	119	25.8	0	1.0	62	247	0
in biscayan sauce (*Goya*), ¼ cup	100	7.0	1.0	8.0	30	450	0
Cod, dried, Atlantic, salted, 1 oz.	81	17.6	0	.7	42	1968	0
Cod entree, frozen:							
au gratin (*Oven Poppers*), 5-oz. pc. ...	220	24.0	5.0	11.0	75	450	1.0

Food and Measure	cal.	prot. (gms)	carbo. (gms)	fat (gms)	chol. (mgs)	sod. (mgs)	fiber (gms)
fillets, breaded, 1 pc.:							
(*Mrs. Paul's*)	260	15.0	17.0	14.0	35	350	0
(*Van de Kamp's* Premium)	220	14.0	19.0	10.0	35	410	0
stuffed w/broccoli, cheese (*Oven Poppers*), 5-oz. pc. ...	150	20.0	4.0	6.0	55	330	1.0
Cod liver oil, see "Oil"							
Coffee:							
brewed, 6 fl. oz.	4	.1	.8	0	0	4	0
instant, regular, 1 rounded tsp. ...	4	.2	.7	tr.	0	1	0
Coffee, flavored, mix, 1 pkt., except as noted:							
amaretto (*Bigelow* Classic)	90	0	11.0	4.0	0	90	0
café français (*General Foods International Coffees*), 2 tbsp. ...	90	<1.0	11.0	5.0	0	135	<1.0
café Vienna:							
(*General Foods International Coffees*), 2 tbsp.	100	<1.0	17.0	3.5	0	170	<1.0
(*General Foods International Coffees* Fat/Sugar Free), 1⅓ tbsp.	25	0	5.0	0	0	75	0
cappuccino:							
(*Land O Lakes* Suprema)	130	4.0	23.0	3.0	0	125	0
amaretto (*General Foods International Coffees*) ..	90	<1.0	17.0	2.5	0	50	0
amaretto (*Nescafé* Frothé), 3 tbsp.	80	1.0	16.0	1.5	0	95	0
amaretto Italia (*Land O Lakes*)	130	4.0	23.0	3.0	0	140	0
café mocha (*General Foods International Coffees*)	100	1.0	18.0	2.5	0	45	0

Food and Measure	cal.	prot. (gms)	carbo. (gms)	fat (gms)	chol. (mgs)	sod. (mgs)	fiber (gms)
Coffee, flavored, mix, cappuccino (cont.)							
café mocha, decaf (General Foods International Coffees)	100	1.0	18.0	2.5	0	45	0
caramel (Nescafé Frothé), 3 tbsp.	80	1.0	16.0	1.0	0	95	0
crème caramel (General Foods International Coffees)	100	<1.0	20.0	2.0	0	50	0
Irish cream (General Foods International Coffees) . .	90	<1.0	17.0	2.5	0	50	0
Italian (General Foods International Coffees), 2 tbsp.	80	<1.0	15.0	2.5	0	70	0
iced, all flavors (Land O Lakes)	60	1.0	14.0	0	0	0	0
latte (Nescafé Frothé), 3 tbsp.	90	1.0	14.0	3.0	0	70	0
orange (General Foods International Coffees), 2 tbsp.	100	<1.0	17.0	3.0	0	150	<1.0
Suisse mocha (Land O Lakes)	130	3.0	23.0	3.0	0	95	1.0
vanilla, French (General Foods International Coffees)	90	<1.0	18.0	2.0	0	50	0
vanilla, French (Land O Lakes)	130	4.0	23.0	3.0	0	132	0
vanilla, French (Nescafé Frothé), 3 tbsp.	80	1.0	15.0	2.0	0	80	0
vanilla, French, decaf (General Foods International Coffees) . .	90	<1.0	17.0	2.5	0	50	0
cappuccino, iced: chocolate (General Foods International Coffees Coolers)	60	0	16.0	0	0	0	<1.0

Food and Measure	cal.	prot. (gms)	carbo. (gms)	fat (gms)	chol. (mgs)	sod. (mgs)	fiber (gms)
hazelnut (General Foods International Coffees Coolers)	60	0	14.0	0	0	0	<1.0
vanilla, French (General Foods International Coffees Coolers) ...	60	0	15.0	0	0	0	0
chocolate, Swiss white (General Foods International Coffees), 2 tbsp. ...	110	<1.0	18.0	4.5	0	50	0
chocolate café, Viennese (General Foods International Coffees), 2 tbsp. ...	80	0	15.0	2.0	0	40	0
chocolate chocolate or chocolate mint (Bigelow)	90	0	11.0	4.0	0	100	0
chocolate mocha: (Nescafé Frothé Regular/Decaf), 3 tbsp.	80	1.0	16.0	1.5	0	75	0
hazel, mint, or raspberry (Nescafé Frothé), 3 tbsp.	80	1.0	16.0	1.5	0	100	0
English toffee (General Foods International Coffees), 2 tbsp. ...	100	0	18.0	3.0	0	60	0
hazelnut: (Bigelow)	90	0	11.0	4.0	0	90	0
Belgian café (General Foods International Coffees), 1⅓ tbsp.	70	<1.0	12.0	2.0	0	60	0
Irish creme (Bigelow)	90	0	12.0	3.0	0	90	0
Kahlúa café (General Foods International Coffees), 2 tbsp. ...	80	<1.0	14.0	3.0	0	80	<1.0
raspberry (Bigelow Supreme)	90	0	13.0	3.0	0	100	0
Suisse mocha: (General Foods International Coffees), 2 tbsp.	80	<1.0	14.0	3.0	0	60	<1.0

Food and Measure	cal.	prot. (gms)	carbo. (gms)	fat (gms)	chol. (mgs)	sod. (mgs)	fiber (gms)
Coffee, flavored, mix, Suisse mocha *(cont.)*							
(*General Foods International Coffees* Fat/Sugar Free), 1⅓ tbsp.	25	0	5.0	0	0	35	<1.0
decaf (*General Foods International Coffees*), 2 tbsp.	80	<1.0	14.0	3.5	0	50	<1.0
vanilla, French:							
(*Bigelow*)	80	0	12.0	3.0	0	100	0
(*General Foods International Coffees*), 2 tbsp. . .	100	<1.0	15.0	4.0	0	85	0
(*General Foods International Coffees* Fat/Sugar Free), 1⅓ tbsp.	25	0	5.0	0	0	65	0
Coffee, iced, 8 fl. oz., except as noted:							
café latte (*Blue Luna Café*)	130	3.0	24.0	2.0	7	90	0
café mocha (*Blue Luna Café* Lite)	70	3.0	10.0	2.0	7	90	0
cappuccino, all flavors (*Frappuccino*), 9.5 fl.oz.	190	6.0	39.0	3.0	12	110	0
latte supreme (*AriZona*)	110	3.0	21.0	2.0	6	95	.7
mocha latte (*AriZona*)	110	4.0	21.0	2.0	5	95	.7
Coffee, iced, mix, see "Coffee, flavored, mix"							
Coffee creamer, see "Creamer"							
Coffee liqueur, 1 fl. oz.:							
53 proof	117	<.1	16.3	.1	0	3	0
w/cream, 34 proof . . .	102	.9	6.5	4.9	0	29	0
Coffee substitute, cereal grain, 1 tsp., except as noted:							
(*Natural Touch* Kaffree Roma)	10	0	2.0	0	0	0	0
(*Postum*)	10	0	3.0	0	0	0	0

Food and Measure	cal.	prot. (gms)	carbo. (gms)	fat (gms)	chol. (mgs)	sod. (mgs)	fiber (gms)
Cold cuts, see "Lunch meat" and specific listings							
Coleslaw:							
(*Blue Ridge Farms*), ½ cup	130	1.0	20.0	4.5	5	470	2.0
(*Chef's Express*), 4 oz.	190	1.0	15.0	15.0	10	310	2.0
Coleslaw blend, see "Salad blend" and "Salad kit"							
Coleslaw dressing, see "Salad dressing"							
Coleslaw seasoning:							
(*McCormick Produce Partners*), ⅒ pkg.	10	0	2.0	0	0	340	0
(*Watkins*), ½ tsp. ...	5	0	1.0	0	0	190	0
Collard greens, fresh:							
raw, 1 oz.	9	.4	2.0	.1	0	6	1.0
raw, chopped, ½ cup	6	.3	1.3	<.1	0	4	.7
boiled, drained, chopped, ½ cup ..	17	.9	3.9	.1	0	10	1.3
Collard greens, canned, ½ cup:							
(*Allens/Sunshine*) ...	30	1.0	5.0	.5	0	20	3.0
chopped (*Bush's Best*)	30	2.0	4.0	0	0	410	2.0
seasoned:							
(*Glory Foods*)	50	3.0	7.0	1.0	0	470	3.0
(*Sylvia's*)	45	1.0	8.0	1.0	0	475	3.0
Collard greens, frozen, chopped:							
(*Birds Eye* Southern), 1 cup	30	2.0	2.0	0	0	20	2.0
(*Seabrook Farms*), ½ cup	30	2.0	2.0	0	0	20	2.0
boiled, drained, ½ cup	31	2.5	6.1	.4	0	42	n.a.
Collins drink mix (*Bar-Tender's*), 1 pouch	70	0	16.0	0	0	30	0
Cookie (see also "Cake, snack" and specific listings):							
almond:							
(*Frieda's*), 2 pcs., 1 oz.	170	2.0	19.0	10.0	0	75	0

Food and Measure	cal.	prot. (gms)	carbo. (gms)	fat (gms)	chol. (mgs)	sod. (mgs)	fiber (gms)
Cookie, almond *(cont.)*							
(*Grandma's* Bites), 11 pcs., 1 oz. .	260	3.0	42.0	9.0	0	280	1.0
(*Stella D'oro* Breakfast Treats), .8-oz. pc.	100	1.0	16.0	3.0	10	80	<1.0
(*Stella D'oro* Chinese Dessert), 1.2-oz. pc.	170	2.0	21.0	9.0	5	90	<1.0
butter (*Jules Destrooper*), 11 pcs., 1.1 oz.	127	2.0	24.0	3.0	6	182	0
fudge dipped (*Stella D'oro*), 1 pc. . . .	120	3.0	18.0	4.0	5	35	1.0
toast (*Stella D'oro*), 2 pcs., 1 oz.	110	2.0	21.0	2.5	30	85	1.0
animal:							
(*Ernie's*), 1 box . . .	250	4.0	41.0	9.0	0	290	1.0
(*Hain*), 9 pcs., 1 oz.	110	2.0	16.0	2.0	0	80	0
(*Nabisco Barnum's Animalc*), 10 pcs., 1.1 oz.	140	2.0	23.0	4.0	0	150	0
chocolate chip (*Barbara's Snackimals*), 8 pcs., 1.1 oz.	120	2.0	18.0	5.0	0	85	1.0
chocolate chip (*Keebler*), 7 pcs., 1 oz.	130	2.0	22.0	4.5	0	120	0
frosted (*Keebler*), 6 pcs., 1 oz. . . .	130	1.0	18.0	6.0	0	65	0
iced (*Keebler*), 6 pcs., 1.1 oz.	150	2.0	24.0	5.0	0	110	0
oatmeal (*Barbara's Snackimals* Wheat Free), 8 pcs., 1.1 oz.	120	2.0	19.0	5.0	0	75	2.0
sprinkled (*Keebler*), 6 pcs., 1.1 oz. . .	150	2.0	24.0	4.5	0	105	0
vanilla (*Barbara's*), 8 pcs., 1 oz. . . .	130	2.0	20.0	5.0	0	105	1.0
vanilla (*Barbara's Snackimals*), 8 pcs., 1.1 oz. . .	120	2.0	19.0	4.5	0	55	1.0

Food and Measure	cal.	prot. (gms)	carbo. (gms)	fat (gms)	chol. (mgs)	sod. (mgs)	fiber (gms)
anisette:							
(*Stella D'oro* Sponge), 2 pcs., 1 oz.	90	2.0	19.0	1.0	40	80	<1.0
(*Stella D'oro* Toast), 3 pcs., 1.2 oz.	130	2.0	27.0	1.0	35	150	<1.0
apple cinnamon:							
(*Newtons Cobblers*), .75-oz. pc.	70	1.0	17.0	0	0	40	<1.0
filled (*Barbara's* Whole Wheat), .7-oz. pc.	60	1.0	14.0	0	0	20	2.0
apple filled (*Newtons*), 2 pcs., 1 oz.	90	1.0	21.0	0	0	65	<1.0
apple raisin (*Health Valley* Jumbo), .9-oz. pc.	80	2.0	19.0	0	0	90	3.0
apple spice (*Health Valley* Fat Free), 3 pcs., 1.2 oz.	100	2.0	24.0	0	0	90	3.0
apricot (*Health Valley* Delight), 3 pcs., 1.2 oz.	100	2.0	24.0	0	0	90	3.0
apricot raspberry (*Pepperidge Farm* Verona), 3 pcs., 1.1 oz.	140	2.0	22.0	6.0	5	110	<1.0
arrowroot:							
(*Nabisco*), 1.2-oz. pc.	20	0	4.0	.5	0	15	0
(*Peek Freans*), 5 pcs., 1.4 oz.	180	3.0	31.0	5.0	0	215	1.0
(*Bahlsen* Afrika), 8 pcs., 1.1 oz.	170	2.0	17.0	10.0	5	20	2.0
(*Bahlsen* Nuss Dessert), 3 pcs., 1.1 oz.	180	2.0	17.0	11.0	10	60	0
banana sandwich, chocolate filled (*Delicious Chiquita Banana Ramas*), 2 pcs., .9 oz.	120	1.0	17.0	5.0	0	55	<1.0
banana split wafer (*Estee*), 5 pcs.	155	1.0	22.0	8.5	0	10	0

Food and Measure	cal.	prot. (gms)	carbo. (gms)	fat (gms)	chol. (mgs)	sod. (mgs)	fiber (gms)
Cookie *(cont.)*							
biscotti:							
(*Almondina* Choconut), 4 pcs., 1.1 oz	140	4.0	20.0	6.0	0	15	3.0
all varieties (*Health Valley* Low Fat), 2 pcs., 1.1 oz. . .	120	3.0	23.0	3.0	0	50	3.0
almond (*Stella D'oro*) .8-oz. pc.	100	2.0	15.0	3.0	10	55	0
cashew (*Stella D'oro*), .7-oz. pc.	110	1.0	13.0	6.0	5	50	0
chocolate, chocolate dipped (*Nonnis* Decadent), 1.2-oz. pc	130	2.0	19.0	5.0	25	65	1.0
chocolate chunk (*Stella D'oro*), .8-oz. pc.	90	2.0	16.0	2.5	10	60	0
chocolate dipped (*Nonni's* Cioccolati), 1.28-oz. pc. . . .	130	2.0	19.0	6.0	25	70	1.0
hazelnut (*Stella D'oro*), .8-oz. pc.	100	2.0	15.0	3.5	10	60	0
vanilla, French (*Stella D'oro*), .8-oz. pc.	90	2.0	16.0	2.5	10	65	0
vanilla, French, fudge dipped (*Stella D'oro*), 1 pc.	120	3.0	18.0	4.0	10	55	0
blueberry filled:							
(*Barbara's* Traditional), .7-oz. pc.	60	1.0	14.0	1.0	0	25	1.0
(*Health Valley* Cobbler Bites), 2 pcs., .9 oz.	100	2.0	21.0	1.5	0	40	1.0
butter:							
(*Bahlsen* Leaves), 7 pcs., 1 oz. . . .	140	2.0	19.0	7.0	15	50	<1.0
(*Bahlsen* Leibniz), 6 pcs., 1.1 oz. . .	130	2.0	23.0	3.5	10	125	1.0

Food and Measure	cal.	prot. (gms)	carbo. (gms)	fat (gms)	chol. (mgs)	sod. (mgs)	fiber (gms)
(*Demitasse* Minis Petit Beurre), 10 pcs., 1 oz.	110	2.0	22.0	2.0	<5	100	0
(*Keebler*), 5 pcs., 1.1 oz.	150	2.0	22.0	6.0	0	170	<1.0
(*Peek Freans* Petit Beurre), 6 pcs., 1.4 oz.	180	2.5	31.0	5.0	<5	165	1.0
(*Pepperidge Farm* Chessman), 3 pcs., .9 oz.	120	2.0	18.0	5.0	20	80	<1.0
chocolate top (*Carr's*), 2 pcs., 1 oz.	150	2.0	19.0	7.0	0	40	2.0
fudge filled (*E. L. Fudge*), 2 pcs., .9 oz.	120	1.0	17.0	6.0	<5	70	<1.0
waffle (*Jules Destrooper*), 2 pcs., .9 oz.	130	2.0	16.0	6.0	35	90	0
cappuccino:							
crisp (*Murray* Sugar Free), 4 pcs., 1.1 oz.	150	2.0	23.0	5.0	0	85	<1.0
sandwich (*Café Cremes*), 2 pcs.	160	1.0	22.0	8.0	0	130	0
caramel (*SnackWell's* Delights), .6-oz. pc.	70	1.0	13.0	2.0	0	35	0
chocolate:							
(*Bahlsen* Leibniz), 4 pcs., 1 oz.	140	2.0	18.0	7.0	5	60	1.0
(*Pizzelle*), 5 pcs., 1.1 oz.	150	3.0	20.0	6.0	15	20	0
(*Stella D'oro*), 2 pcs., 1 oz.	130	2.0	19.0	6.0	5	55	1.0
(*Stella D'oro* Breakfast Treat), .8-oz. pc.	100	2.0	15.0	3.5	10	70	<1.0
(*Stella D'oro* Margherite), 2 pcs., 1.1 oz.	140	2.0	22.0	5.0	15	90	<1.0
crisps (*SnackWell's* Bite Size), 18 pcs., 1 oz.	130	1.0	25.0	2.5	0	180	1.0

Food and Measure	cal.	prot. (gms)	carbo. (gms)	fat (gms)	chol. (mgs)	sod. (mgs)	fiber (gms)
Cookie, chocolate *(cont.)*							
double Dutch (*Barbara's* Crisp), .6-oz. pc.	80	1.0	10.0	4.0	5	60	1.0
milk (*Carr's Imperials*), 2 pcs., 1 oz.	150	2.0	18.0	7.0	<5	50	1.0
top, w/nuts (*Pepperidge Farm Geneva*), 3 pcs., 1.1 oz.	160	2.0	19.0	9.0	0	95	1.0
wafer (*Estee*), 5 pcs.	150	1.0	19.0	9.0	0	10	0
wafer (*Nabisco Famous*), 5 pcs., 1.2 oz.	140	2.0	24.0	4.0	<5	230	1.0
wafer (*Nilla*), 8 pcs., 1.1 oz.	110	1.0	23.0	2.0	0	120	0
chocolate almond (*Pepperidge Farm Dessert Bliss*), 3 pcs., 1.1 oz.	170	2.0	22.0	8.0	<5	75	1.0
chocolate chip/chunk:							
(*Barbara's* Crisp), .6-oz. pc.	80	1.0	10.0	4.0	5	60	1.0
(*Chips Ahoy!*), 3 pcs., 1.1 oz. . .	160	2.0	21.0	8.0	0	105	1.0
(*Chips Ahoy! Chewy*) 3 pcs., 1.3 oz.	170	2.0	24.0	8.0	0	125	<1.0
(*Chips Ahoy! Chunky*), .6-oz. pc.	80	1.0	10.0	4.0	5	35	0
(*Chips Ahoy! Mini*), 5 pcs., 1.1 oz. . .	150	2.0	20.0	7.0	0	95	<1.0
(*Chips Ahoy! Reduced Fat*), 3 pcs., 1.1 oz.	140	2.0	22.0	5.0	0	10	<1.0
(*Entenmann's* Soft), 3 pcs., 1.1 oz. . .	150	1.0	20.0	7.0	10	60	<1.0
(*Entenmann's* Soft Chocolatey), .7-oz. pc.	100	1.0	31.0	5.0	10	60	<1.0

Food and Measure	cal.	prot. (gms)	carbo. (gms)	fat (gms)	chol. (mgs)	sod. (mgs	fiber (gms)
(*Entenmann's* Soft Chocolatey Light), 2 pcs., 1.1 oz. . .	120	1.0	21.0	3.5	0	85	1.0
(*Entenmann's* Soft Chunk), 1.8-oz. pc.	240	2.0	31.0	12.0	20	170	<1.0
(*Estee*), 4 pcs., 1 oz.	150	2.0	21.0	7.0	0	35	<1.0
(*Famous Amos*), 4 pcs., 1 oz. . . .	130	<2.0	18.0	6.0	0	90	0
(*Famous Amos* Belgian), 4 pcs., 1 oz.	150	2.0	20.0	7.0	<5	90	<1.0
(*Famous Amos* Big Chunk), 1-oz. pc.	140	2.0	19.0	7.0	<5	110	<1.0
(*Grandma's* Home-style), 1.4-oz. pc.	200	2.0	28.0	9.0	15	125	1.0
(*Grandma's* Rich N'Chewy), 1 pkg.	270	2.0	39.0	12.0	10	130	1.0
(*Grandma's* Bites), 12 pcs., 1 oz. .	280	3.0	38.0	12.0	15	200	1.0
(*Health Valley* Healthy Chips), 3 pcs., 1.2 oz. . .	100	2.0	24.0	0	0	90	3.0
(*Keebler Chips Deluxe*), ½-oz. pc.	80	1.0	9.0	4.5	0	60	0
(*Keebler Chips Deluxe* Chocolate Lovers'), .6-oz. pc.	90	1.0	11.0	5.0	5	80	0
(*Keebler Chips Deluxe* Mini), 4 pcs., 1 oz. . . .	150	2.0	19.0	8.0	<5	90	<1.0
(*Keebler Cookie Stix*), 4 pcs., 1 oz.	130	2.0	19.0	5.0	5	100	<1
(*Keebler Soft Batch*), .6-oz. pc.	80	<1.0	10.0	3.5	0	70	<1.0
(*Pepperidge Farm Chesapeake*), .9-oz. pc.	140	2.0	15.0	8.0	10	80	0
(*Pepperidge Farm Montauk*), .9-oz. pc.	130	1.0	17.0	7.0	10	90	0
(*Pepperidge Farm Nantucket*), 1-oz. pc.	140	2.0	18.0	7.0	10	80	1.0

Food and Measure	cal.	prot. (gms)	carbo. (gms)	fat (gms)	chol. (mgs)	sod. (mgs)	fiber (gms)
Cookie, chocolate chip/chunk *(cont.)*							
(*Pepperidge Farm Tahoe*), .9-oz. pc.	140	2.0	15.0	8.0	10	90	0
(*SnackWell's* Bite Size), 13 pcs., 1 oz.	130	2.0	22.0	4.0	0	160	<1.0
(*Tofutti*), 1 pc.	139	1.0	19.0	6.0	0	79	1.0
(*Weight Watchers*), 2 pcs., 1.1 oz.	140	2.0	22.0	5.0	0	90	1.0
(*Westbrae Natural*), .9-oz. pc.	110	1.0	18.0	4.0	10	125	1.0
w/cashews (*Famous Amos* Big Chunk), 1-oz. pc.	140	2.0	18.0	7.0	<5	110	<1.0
chocolate (*Westbrae Natural*), .9-oz. pc.	90	1.0	18.0	3.0	5	85	1.0
coconut (*Keebler Chips Deluxe*), .6-oz. pc.	80	1.0	10.0	5.0	0	45	<1.0
crisps (*SnackWell's* Bite Size), 18 pcs.	150	1.0	27.0	4.0	0	180	1.0
crispy (*Entenmann's Little Bites*), 8 pcs., 1.8 oz.	240	2.0	33.0	12.0	0	120	1.0
double (*Entenmann's Soft*), .7-oz. pc.	100	1.0	14.0	5.0	10	65	<1.0
double (*Health Valley Healthy Chips* Fat Free), 3 pcs., 1.2 oz.	100	3.0	24.0	0	0	90	3.0
double (*SnackWell's*), 13 pcs., 1.1 oz.	130	2.0	22.0	4.0	0	190	1.0
fudge (*Chips Ahoy!*), 3 pcs., 1.1 oz.	160	2.0	23.0	7.0	<5	150	1.0
fudge (*Grandma's* Homestyle), 1.4-oz. pc.	190	2.0	28.0	7.0	10	80	1.0
fudge (*Grandma's* Mini), 1.4 oz.	190	2.0	28.0	7.0	10	80	1.0
w/macadamias (*Famous Amos* Big Chunk), 1-oz. pc.	150	2.0	18.0	8.0	<5	110	<1.0

Food and Measure	cal.	prot. (gms)	carbo. (gms)	fat (gms)	chol. (mgs)	sod. (mgs	fiber (gms)
milk (*Entenmann's*), .7-oz. pc.	100	1.0	13.0	5.0	10	60	<1.0
w/pecans (*Chips Ahoy! Mini*), 5 pcs., 1.1 oz.	150	2.0	19.0	9.0	0	105	<1.0
w/pecans (*Famous Amos*), 4 pcs., 1 oz.	140	<2.0	17.0	7.0	0	90	<1.0
w/pecan (*Westbrae Natural*), .9-oz. pc.	110	1.0	18.0	5.0	5	110	1.0
w/peanut butter cups (*Keebler Chips Deluxe*), .6-oz. pc.	80	1.0	9.0	4.5	0	45	0
rainbow (*Keebler Chips Deluxe*), .6-oz. pc.	80	1.0	10.0	4.0	0	45	<1.0
rainbow (*Keebler Chips Deluxe Mini*), 4 pcs., 1 oz.	150	2.0	19.0	8.0	<5	100	<1.0
soft, chewy (*Keebler Chips Deluxe*), .6-oz. pc.	80	1.0	11.0	3.5	5	60	0
toffee (*Famous Amos*), 4 pcs., 1 oz.	130	<1.0	18.0	6.0	0	115	0
walnut (*Country Choice Naturals*), .8-oz. pc.	100	1.0	15.0	3.5	5	65	<1.0
walnut (*Westbrae Natural*), .9-oz. pc.	110	1.0	17.0	5.0	10	130	0
walnut, crunch (*Keebler Chips Deluxe*), .6-oz. pc.	90	1.0	9.0	6.0	0	60	<1.0
white, w/macadamias (*Entenmann's Soft*), .7-oz. pc.	100	1.0	12.0	6.0	10	65	<1.0
chocolate mint (*Anna's*), 6 pcs., 1 oz.	135	2.0	18.0	6.0	0	80	<1.0
chocolate mocha (*Pepperidge Farm Salzburg*), 2 pcs., 1 oz.	150	2.0	21.0	6.0	0	65	1.0

Food and Measure	cal.	prot. (gms)	carbo. (gms)	fat (gms)	chol. (mgs)	sod. (mgs)	fiber (gms)
Cookie *(cont.)*							
chocolate sandwich:							
(*Estee*), 3 pcs., 1.1 oz.	160	2.0	24.0	6.0	0	60	1.0
(*Hydrox*), 3 pcs., 1.1 oz.	150	2.0	21.0	7.0	0	125	1.0
(*Murray* Sugar Free), 3 pcs., 1 oz.	120	2.0	19.0	6.0	0	90	<1.0
(*Oreo*), 3 pcs., 1.2 oz.	160	1.0	23.0	7.0	0	220	1.0
(*Oreo* Mini), 9 pcs., 1 oz.	140	1.0	21.0	6.0	0	150	1.0
(*Oreo* Reduced Fat), 3 pcs., 1.2 oz.	130	1.0	25.0	3.5	0	190	1.0
(*Oreo Double Stuff*), 2 pcs., 1 oz.	140	1.0	19.0	7.0	0	150	<1.0
(*Pepperidge Farm Bordeaux*), 4 pcs., 1 oz.	130	2.0	19.0	5.0	10	95	<1.0
(*Pepperidge Farm Brussels*), 3 pcs., 1.1 oz.	150	2.0	20.0	7.0	5	80	1.0
(*Pepperidge Farm Milano Endless Chocolate*), 3 pcs., 1.2 oz.	180	2.0	21.0	10.0	<5	85	1.0
(*Pepperidge Farm Milano*), 3 pcs., 1.2 oz.	180	2.0	21.0	10.0	10	80	<1.0
(*SnackWell's*), 2 pcs., .9 oz.	110	1.0	20.0	3.0	0	210	<1.0
creme filled (*Droxies*), 3 pcs., 1.1 oz.	140	2.0	21.0	6.0	0	95	<1.0
double (*Pepperidge Farm Milano*), 2 pcs., 1 oz.	140	2.0	17.0	8.0	10	70	<1.0
fudge covered (*Oreo*), .75-oz. pc.	110	2.0	14.0	6.0	0	75	1.0
milk (*Pepperidge Farm Milano*), 3 pcs., 1.2 oz.	170	2.0	21.0	9.0	10	110	<1.0

Food and Measure	cal.	prot. (gms)	carbo. (gms)	fat (gms)	chol. (mgs)	sod. (mgs)	fiber (gms)
mint or orange (*Pepperidge Farm Milano*), 2 pcs., .9 oz.	130	1.0	16.0	7.0	<5	65	<1.0
raspberry (*Pepperidge Farm Milano*), 2 pcs., .9 oz.	130	1.0	16.0	7.0	<5	40	<1.0
chocolate stick:							
hazelnut filled (*Pepperidge Farm Pirouette*), 2 pcs., .9 oz.	130	1.0	19.0	6.0	10	60	<1.0
milk, wafer (*Larzaroni* Cannoli), 4 pcs., 1.1 oz.	150	1.0	23.0	6.0	0	55	0
cinnamon (*Stella D'oro* Viennese), 1-oz. pc.	100	2.0	17.0	2.5	10	65	0
coconut:							
(*Demitasse* Minis), 10 pcs., 1 oz.	120	2.0	21.0	3.0	0	70	0
(*Estee*), 4 pcs., 1 oz.	140	2.0	19.0	6.0	0	25	<1.0
(*Estee* Smart Treats), 3 pcs., 1 oz.	110	2.0	22.0	3.5	0	110	1.0
(*Lazzaroni* Samba), 5 pcs., 1.1 oz.	160	3.0	14.0	10.0	0	150	2.0
(*Miss Meringue*), 4 pcs., 1.25 oz.	110	1.0	23.0	2.0	0	20	1.0
almond (*Barbara's Nature's Choice* Dipped), 1.1-oz. bar	120	2.0	20.0	4.5	0	10	1.0
creme (*SnackWell's*), 2 pcs., 1 oz.	110	<1.0	19.0	4.0	0	80	1.0
coffee creme sandwich (*Peek Freans*), 2 pcs., 1.1 oz.	150	1.0	21.0	7.0	0	70	0
coffee mocha wafer stick (*Lazzaroni* Cannoli), 4 pcs., 1.1 oz.	150	2.0	22.0	6.0	0	85	0

Food and Measure	cal.	prot. (gms)	carbo. (gms)	fat (gms)	chol. (mgs)	sod. (mgs)	fiber (gms)
Cookie (cont.)							
creme sandwich:							
(*Peek Freans* Tropical Cremes), 2 pcs.	130	2.0	20.0	5.0	0	15	0
(*SnackWell's*), 1.7-oz. pkg.	210	2.0	38.0	5.0	0	240	0
(*Cuetara* Maria), 5 pcs., 1 oz.	110	2.0	20.0	2.5	0	65	0
Danish (*Keebler* Wedding), 4 pcs., 1 oz	120	1.0	20.0	5.0	0	80	<1.0
date (*Health Valley* Delight Fat Free), 3 pcs., 1.2 oz.	100	2.0	24.0	0	0	90	3.0
(*Delicious Heath*), 3 pcs., 1.3 oz.	170	1.0	21.0	10.0	15	125	0
(*Delicious Nestlé Butterfinger*), 3 pcs., 1 oz.	130	2.0	18.0	6.0	5	125	<1.0
devil's food:							
(*SnackWell's*), 1.1-oz. pkg.	90	1.0	22.0	0	0	55	<1.0
(*SnackWell's* Golden), .6-oz. pc.	50	1.0	11.0	.5	0	25	0
(*SnackWell's* Fat Free), .6-oz. pc.	50	1.0	12.0	0	0	30	0
egg biscuit:							
(*Stella D'oro* Jumbo), 2 pcs., .8 oz.	90	2.0	18.0	1.0	30	60	<1.0
vanilla (*Stella D'oro* Roman), 1.2-oz. pc.	140	2.0	21.0	5.0	20	125	<1.0
espresso bean (*Barbara's Nature's Choice* Dipped), 1.1-oz. bar	120	2.0	22.0	3.0	0	10	1.0
fig filled/bar:							
(*Barbara's* Traditional), .7-oz. pc.	60	1.0	14.0	1.0	0	25	1.0
(*Barbara's* Wheat Free), .7-oz. pc.	60	<1.0	15.0	0	0	20	1.0
(*Barbara's* Whole Wheat), .7-oz. pc.	60	<1.0	16.0	0	0	20	2.0

Food and Measure	cal.	prot. (gms)	carbo. (gms)	fat (gms)	chol. (mgs)	sod. (mgs)	fiber (gms)
(*Estee*), 2 pcs., 1 oz.	100	1.0	23.0	1.0	0	20	3.0
(*Fig Newton*), 2 pcs., 1.1 oz.	110	1.0	22.0	2.5	0	115	1.0
(*Fig Newton* Fat Free), 2 pcs., 1 oz.	90	1.0	20.0	0	0	110	1.0
(*Health Valley Cobbler Bites*), 2 pcs., .9 oz.	100	2.0	21.0	1.5	0	40	1.0
(*Tofutti*), 2 pcs. ..	100	1.0	21.0	2.0	0	35	1.0
fortune (*Frieda's*), 4 pcs., 1 oz.	120	2.0	23.0	1.0	5	65	1.0
fruit, Hawaiian (*Health Valley*), 3 pcs., 1.2 oz.	100	2.0	24.0	0	0	90	3.0
fruit filled (*Bahlsen Deloba*), 4 pcs., 1 oz.	120	2.0	19.0	5.0	0	80	1.0
fudge:							
(*Estee*) 4 pcs., 1 oz.	150	2.0	19.0	7.0	0	45	1.0
(*Grandma's* Mini), 9 pcs., 1 oz.	150	2.0	21.0	7.0	0	180	1.0
(*Stella D'oro* Swiss), 2 pcs., 1 oz.	130	1.0	16.0	7.0	5	55	0
brownie, double (*Country Choice Naturals*), .8-oz. pc.	80	1.0	14.0	3.0	5	35	1.0
double, and caramel (*Fudge Shoppe*), 2 pcs., 1.1 oz. ..	140	1.0	20.0	7.0	0	65	<1.0
double, chewy (*Murray* Sugar Free), 3 pcs., 1.2 oz.	140	2.0	23.0	6.0	0	110	2.0
mint (*Fudge Shoppe* Grasshoppers), 4 pcs., 1 oz.	150	2.0	19.0	7.0	0	85	<1.0
sticks (*Fudge Shoppe*), 3 pcs., 1 oz.	150	1.0	19.0	8.0	0	55	0
striped (*Fudge Shoppe*), 3 pcs., 1.1 oz.	160	<1.0	21.0	8.0	0	140	<1.0

Food and Measure	cal.	prot. (gms)	carbo. (gms)	fat (gms)	chol. (mgs)	sod. (mgs)	fiber (gms)
Cookie, fudge *(cont.)*							
striped (*Fudge Shoppe* Reduced Fat), 3 pcs., 1 oz.	140	1.0	21.0	5.0	0	100	<1.0
fudge sandwich:							
(*E. L. Fudge*), 2 pcs., .9 oz.	120	2.0	17.0	6.0	0	70	<1.0
vanilla (*Grandma's*), 3 pcs., 1 oz. . . .	120	1.0	21.0	4.0	0	130	<1.0
ginger (*Country Choice Naturals*), .8-oz. pc.	90	1.0	17.0	2.0	5	80	<1.0
ginger lemon creme sandwich (*Carr's*), 2 pcs., 1 oz.	140	1.0	19.0	7.0	<5	105	<1.0
ginger snaps:							
(*Murray* Sugar Free), 6 pcs., 1 oz. . . .	110	2.0	21.0	4.0	0	100	<1.0
(*Nabisco*), 4 pcs., 1 oz.	120	1.0	22.0	2.5	0	230	<1.0
(*Sunchine*), 5 pcs., 1.2 oz.	150	2.0	24.0	6.0	0	120	0
(*Westbrae Natural*), 3 pcs., 1 oz. . . .	130	2.0	18.0	6.0	0	60	2.0
graham cracker:							
(*Cinnamon Crisp*), 8 pcs., 1.1 oz. . .	130	2.0	24.0	3.0	0	230	1.0
(*Cinnamon Crisps Low Fat Grahams*), 8 pcs., 1 oz.	110	2.0	23.0	1.5	0	160	1.0
(*Estee* Old Fashioned), 2 pcs.	90	3.0	17.0	2.0	0	115	2.0
(*Graham Selects* Original), 8 pcs., 1 oz.	130	2.0	23.0	3.0	0	135	<1.0
(*Honey Maid*), 8 pcs., 1 oz.	120	2.0	22.0	3.0	0	180	1.0
(*Honey Maid* Low Fat), 8 pcs., 1 oz.	110	2.0	23.0	1.5	0	200	<1.0
(*Nabisco*), 4 pcs., 1 oz.	120	2.0	22.0	3.0	0	180	1.0
amaranth (*Health Valley* Original), 6 pcs., 1 oz. . . .	120	3.0	22.0	3.0	0	80	3.0

Food and Measure	cal.	prot. (gms)	carbo. (gms)	fat (gms)	chol. (mgs)	sod. (mgs)	fiber (gms)
cinnamon (*Hain*), 2 pcs., 1 oz. ...	80	2.0	12.0	3.0	0	115	0
cinnamon (*Honey Maid* Low Fat), 8 pcs., 1 oz.	110	2.0	23.0	1.5	0	170	<1.0
cinnamon (*New Morning*), 2 pcs., 1.1 oz.	100	2.0	20.0	2.0	0	125	1.0
cinnamon (*New Morning* Mini Bites), 15 pcs., 1.1 oz.	120	2.0	24.0	2.5	0	135	1.0
cinnamon (*Snackin' Grahams* Bite Size), 21 pcs., 1 oz.	130	2.0	23.0	3.0	0	210	1.0
cinnamon or honey (*Teddy Grahams*), 24 pcs., 1.1 oz. ..	130	2.0	23.0	4.0	0	150	<1.0
ginger (*New Morning*), 2 pcs., 1.1 oz. ..	140	2.0	26.0	4.5	0	180	1.0
honey (*Blue's Clues*), 24 pcs., 1.1 oz. .	130	2.0	23.0	4.0	0	150	<1.0
honey (*Hain*), 2 pcs., 1 oz.	80	2.0	12.0	3.0	0	115	0
honey (*Keebler*), 8 pcs., 1.1 oz. ..	140	2.0	23.0	4.5	0	170	0
honey (*Keebler Low Fat Grahams*), 9 pcs., 1.1 oz. ..	120	2.0	25.0	1.5	0	210	1.0
honey (*New Morning*), 2 pcs., 1.1 oz.	110	2.0	21.0	2.0	0	135	1.0
honey (*New Morning* Mini Bites), 15 pcs., 1.1 oz. .	120	2.0	24.0	2.5	0	135	1.0
honey, animal (*Hain*), 15 pcs., 1 oz. ..	80	2.0	12.0	3.0	0	115	0
lemon (*New Morning* Mini Bites), 15 pcs., 1.1 oz.	120	2.0	23.0	2.5	0	130	1.0
oat bran (*Health Valley*), 6 pcs., 1 oz.	120	3.0	22.0	3.0	0	80	3.0

Food and Measure	cal.	prot. (gms)	carbo. (gms)	fat (gms)	chol. (mgs)	sod. (mgs)	fiber (gms)
Cookie, graham cracker (cont.)							
oatmeal crunch (*Honey Maid*), 8 pcs., 1 oz. . . .	130	2.0	23.0	2.5	0	150	1.0
peanut butter, animal (*Hain*), 15 pcs., 1.1 oz.	140	4.0	20.0	5.0	0	140	1.0
vanilla, French (*Hain*), 2 pcs., 1.1 oz.	100	2.0	16.0	3.0	0	120	1.0
graham, chocolate:							
(*Dizzy Grizzlies*), 8 pcs., 1.1 oz. . .	150	1.0	24.0	5.0	0	110	<1.0
(*Graham Selects*), 8 pcs., 1.1 oz. . .	130	2.0	23.0	4.0	0	115	0
(*Hain*), 2 pcs., 1.1 oz.	120	3.0	21.0	3.0	0	120	1.0
(*Honey Maid*), 8 pcs., 1 oz. . . .	120	2.0	22.0	3.0	0	170	1.0
(*New Morning*), 2 pcs., 1.1 oz. . .	120	3.0	21.0	3.0	0	120	1.0
(*Teddy Grahams* Snacks), 24 pcs., 1.1 oz.	130	2.0	22.0	4.5	0	170	1.0
animal (*Hain*), 15 pcs., 1.1 oz.	120	3.0	21.0	3.0	0	120	1.0
milk chocolate (*Fliptz*), 9 pcs., 1 oz.	130	1.0	19.0	6.0	<5	90	<1.0
chip (*Teddy Grahams*), 24 pcs., 1.1 oz.	140	2.0	22.0	4.5	0	150	1.0
graham, fudge coated:							
(*Fudge Favorites*), 3 pcs., 1.1 oz. . .	140	1.0	18.0	7.0	0	125	<1.0
(*Fudge Shoppe Deluxe*), 3 pcs., .9 oz.	140	1.0	19.0	7.0	0	105	<1.0
(*Fudge Shoppe Deluxe* Reduced Fat), 3 pcs., .9 oz.	120	1.0	19.0	5.0	0	130	0
white (*Fliptz*), 8 pcs., 1 oz.	140	2.0	19.0	6.0	0	95	0

Food and Measure	cal.	prot. (gms)	carbo. (gms)	fat (gms)	chol. (mgs)	sod. (mgs)	fiber (gms)
graham, vanilla frosted (*Dizzy Grizzlies*), 8 pcs., 1.1 oz.	150	1.0	24.0	6.0	0	105	<1.0
hazelnut (*Bahlsen Kipferl*), 4 pcs., 1 oz.	150	2.0	16.0	9.0	5	10	0
holiday (*Stella D'oro Trinkets*), 4 pcs., 1.1 oz.	160	2.0	20.0	8.0	10	125	<1.0
honey almond (*Westbrae Natural*), .9-oz. pc.	110	1.0	17.0	4.0	10	135	1.0
kichel (*Manischewitz*), 4 pcs., .5 oz.	70	2.0	8.0	4.0	105	45	1.0
lemon:							
(*Country Choice Naturals*), .8-oz. pc.	90	1.0	17.0	2.0	5	75	<1.0
(*Estee* Smart Treats), 3 pcs., 1 oz. . . .	110	2.0	22.0	3.0	0	90	1.0
(*Miss Meringue*), 4 pcs., 1.25 oz. .	100	1.0	24.0	0	0	20	0
creme wafer (*Estee*), 5 pcs.	150	1.0	22.0	8.0	0	10	0
crisp (*Murray* Sugar Free), 4 pcs., 1.1 oz.	140	2.0	22.0	4.5	0	90	<1.0
w/hazelnuts (*Lazzaroni* Limonelli), 5 pcs., 1 oz. . . .	140	2.0	16.0	8.0	5	30	2.0
nut (*Pepperidge Farm*), 3 pcs., 1.1 oz.	170	2.0	19.0	8.0	15	60	2.0
snaps (*Westbrae Natural*), 3 pcs., 1.1 oz.	140	2.0	20.0	6.0	0	60	2.0
thins (*Estee*), 4 pcs., 1 oz.	140	2.0	19.0	6.0	0	25	<1.0
yogurt (*Barbara's Nature's Choice* Dipped), 1.1-oz. bar	120	2.0	22.0	3.5	0	10	1.0
lemon or lime (*Pepperidge Farm Spritzers*), 5 pcs., 1.1 oz.	140	1.0	21.0	7.0	<5	60	0

Food and Measure	cal.	prot. (gms)	carbo. (gms)	fat (gms)	chol. (mgs)	sod. (mgs)	fiber (gms)
Cookie *(cont.)*							
lemon sandwich:							
(*Murray Sugar Free*), 3 pcs., 1 oz. . . .	120	1.0	20.0	6.0	0	115	1.0
(*SnackWell's*), 3 pcs.	140	1.0	23.0	6.0	0	150	0
(*Vienna Fingers*), 2 pcs., 1 oz. . . .	140	2.0	21.0	6.0	0	90	0
lime (*Peek Freans Calypso*), 2 pcs. . .	130	1.0	20.0	5.0	0	15	0
marshmallow, choco-late coated:							
(*Mallomars*), 2 pcs., .9 oz.	120	1.0	17.0	5.0	0	35	<1.0
(*Peek Freans Dream Puffs*), 2 pcs., .9 oz.	110	<1.0	18.0	4.0	0	50	0
(*Pinwheels*), 1 pc.	130	<1.0	21.0	5.0	0	35	<1.0
mint, fudge coated (*Mystic Mint*), .6-oz. pc.	90	0	11.0	4.5	0	65	0
mint creme (*Snack-Well's*), 2 pcs., .9 oz.	110	1.0	19.0	3.5	0	70	<1.0
molasses:							
(*Grandma's* Home-style), 1.4-oz. pc.	160	2.0	29.0	4.0	<5	230	<1.0
crisps (*Pepperidge Farm*), 5 pcs., 1.1 oz.	150	2.0	20.0	6.0	0	140	<1.0
oatmeal:							
(*Barbara's* Crisp), .6-oz. pc.	70	1.0	11.0	3.0	5	65	1.0
(*Keebler* Country Style), 2 pcs., .8 oz.	120	2.0	17.0	5.0	0	115	<1.0
(*Murray Sugar Free*), 3 pcs., 1.1 oz. . .	140	2.0	20.0	7.0	0	170	<1.0
(*Nabisco* Family Favorites), .6-oz. pc.	80	1.0	12.0	3.0	0	65	0
chocolate chip (*Country Choice Naturals*), .8-oz. pc.	100	1.0	15.0	4.0	5	65	<1.0

Food and Measure	cal.	prot. (gms)	carbo. (gms)	fat (gms)	chol. (mgs)	sod. (mgs	fiber (gms)
chocolate chip (*Health Valley*), .8-oz. pc.	100	2.0	14.0	4.0	0	50	1.0
chocolate chip, w/walnuts (*Famous Amos*), 4 pcs., 1 oz. ...	140	<2.0	16.0	7.0	0	120	<1.0
iced (*Nabisco* Family Favorites), .6-oz. pc.	80	1.0	12.0	3.0	0	55	0
peanut crunch (*Health Valley*), .8-oz. pc.	100	2.0	14.0	4.0	0	60	1.0
snaps (*Westbrae Natural*), 3 pcs., 1.1 oz.	140	2.0	20.0	6.0	0	70	2.0
oatmeal raisin: (*Country Choice Naturals*), .8-oz. pc.	100	1.0	13.0	4.0	5	65	<1.0
(*Entenmann's* Soft Light), 2 pcs., 1.1 oz.	100	2.0	23.0	0	0	135	2.0
(*Estee*), 4 pcs., 1 oz.	130	2.0	19.0	5.0	0	25	1.0
(*Famous Amos*), 4 pcs., 1 oz. ...	130	<2.0	20.0	6.0	5	135	<1.0
(*Grandma's* Home-style), 1.4-oz. pc.	180	2.0	30.0	6.0	10	240	1.0
(*Health Valley*), .8-oz. pc.	90	2.0	14.0	3.5	0	50	1.0
(*Health Valley* Fat Free), 3 pcs., 1.2 oz.	100	2.0	24.0	0	0	80	3.0
(*Tofutti*), 1 pc. ...	118	2.0	20.0	4.0	0	75	2.0
(*Weight Watchers*), 2 pcs., 1.1 oz. ..	120	2.0	22.0	2.0	0	90	1.0
(*Westbrae Natural*), .9-oz. pc.	100	2.0	18.0	2.0	5	110	1.0
soft (*Pepperidge Farm*), .9-oz. pc.	110	1.0	17.0	4.0	15	60	1.0
orange (*Pepperidge Farm Spritzers*), 5 pcs., 1.1 oz.	140	1.0	21.0	7.0	<5	55	0

Food and Measure	cal.	prot. (gms)	carbo. (gms)	fat (gms)	chol. (mgs)	sod. (mgs)	fiber (gms)
Cookie *(cont.)*							
pastry puffs, cappuccino chocolate (*Ferrara*), 5 pcs., 1.1 oz.	150	1.0	18.0	7.0	0	200	0
peach-apricot (*Newtons Cobblers*), .75-oz. pc.	70	1.0	17.0	0	0	55	0
peanut, roasted (*Barbara's Nature's Choice* Dipped), 1.1-oz. bar	130	3.0	20.0	4.5	0	50	1.0
peanut butter:							
(*Country Choice Naturals*), .8-oz. pc.	80	1.0	11.0	5.0	10	75	<1.0
(*Grandma's* Homestyle), 1.4-oz. pc.	200	4.0	24.0	10.0	10	200	1.0
(*Grandma's* Mini), 9 pcs., 1 oz. ...	150	2.0	21.0	7.0	0	140	1.0
(*Hain* Cookie Jar Bits), 17 pcs., .5 oz.	60	1.0	12.0	1.0	0	105	0
(*Murray* Sugar Free), 3 pcs., 1 oz. ...	150	3.0	18.0	7.0	<5	160	1.0
(*Tofutti*), 1 pc. ...	137	3.0	18.0	7.0	0	108	1.0
chip (*SnackWell's* Bite Size), 13 pcs., 1 oz.	120	3.0	20.0	4.0	0	210	<1.0
creme wafer (*Estee*), 5 pcs.	150	1.0	22.0	8.0	0	40	0
fudge (*Fudge Shoppe* Sticks), 3 pcs., 1 oz.	150	2.0	18.0	8.0	0	60	<1.0
nut (*Westbrae Natural*), .9-oz. pc.	110	2.0	17.0	3.5	5	110	0
peanut butter sandwich:							
(*E. L. Fudge*), 2 pcs., .9 oz.	120	2.0	16.0	6.0	0	150	<1.0
(*Estee*), 3 pcs., 1.1 oz.	160	4.0	22.0	7.0	0	55	1.0
(*Grandma's*), 5 pcs., 1 oz.	210	3.0	28.0	10.0	0	200	1.0
(*Nutter Butter*), 1.4-oz. pkg. ...	260	4.0	36.0	11.0	5	210	2.0

Food and Measure	cal.	prot. (gms)	carbo. (gms)	fat (gms)	chol. (mgs)	sod. (mgs)	fiber (gms)
(*Nutter Butter* Bite Size), 10 pcs. ...	150	3.0	20.0	6.0	0	125	1.0
chocolate (*Nutter Butter*), 2 pcs., 1 oz.	130	2.0	19.0	5.0	0	130	1.0
patties (*Nutter Butter*), 5 pcs. .	160	3.0	17.0	9.0	0	80	1.0
(*Peek Freans* Nice), 4 pcs., 1.2 oz.	160	2.0	25.0	6.0	0	100	1.0
pfeffernusse:							
(*Archway*), 2 pcs., 1 oz.	100	1.0	23.0	1.0	5	90	1.0
(*Stella D'oro*), 3 pcs., 1 oz.	120	1.0	21.0	3.0	15	55	0
pralines and creme (*Pepperidge Farm Dessert Bliss*), 3 pcs., 1.1 oz.	160	2.0	23.0	7.0	5	95	<1.0
rainbow:							
(*Beigel's*), 1.2-oz. pc.	120	2.0	15.0	6.0	5	15	1.0
(*Keebler Cookie Stix*), 5 pcs., 1.2 oz.	150	2.0	23.0	6.0	5	110	<1.0
raspberry:							
(*Health Valley* Fat Free Jumbo), .9-oz. pc.	80	2.0	19.0	0	0	90	3.0
filled (*Barbara's* Fat/ Wheat Free), .7-oz. pc.	60	1.0	15.0	0	0	25	1.0
filled (*Newtons* Fat Free), 2 pcs., 1 oz.	90	1.0	21.0	0	0	100	<1.0
vanilla (*Westbrae Natural*), .9-oz. pc.	110	1.0	17.0	4.0	10	135	0
rocky road (*Country Choice Naturals*), .8-oz. pc.	90	1.0	13.0	4.0	5	30	1.0
sandwich, 1.1 oz.:							
(*Estee*), 3 pcs. ...	160	2.0	24.0	6.0	0	45	1.0
assorted (*Pepperidge Farm Crème Magnifique*), 2 pcs.	150	2.0	21.0	7.0	5	60	1.0
sesame (*Stella D'oro* Regina), 3 pcs., 1.1 oz.	150	2.0	210	6.0	10	85	1.0

Food and Measure	cal.	prot. (gms)	carbo. (gms)	fat (gms)	chol. (mgs)	sod. (mgs)	fiber (gms)
Cookie *(cont.)*							
shortbread:							
(*Barbara's* Traditional							
Crisp), .6-oz. pc.	80	1.0	10.0	4.0	10	40	1.0
(*Estee*), 4 pcs., 1 oz.	130	2.0	22.0	4.0	0	150	<1.0
(*Lorna Doone*),							
4 pcs., 1 oz. . . .	140	2.0	19.0	7.0	5	130	<1.0
(*Murray* Sugar Free),							
8 pcs., 1 oz. . . .	120	2.0	20.0	4.5	0	115	1.0
(*Simply Sandies*),							
.6-oz. pc.	80	1.0	9.0	4.5	10	70	0
(*SnackWell's*), 3 pcs.	130	1.0	21.0	5.0	5	150	<1.0
(*Westbrae Natural*							
Original), 3 pcs.,							
1.1 oz.	130	1.0	19.0	5.0	15	80	1.0
almond (*Crookes &*							
Hanson English),							
.9-oz. pc.	120	1.0	13.0	8.0	20	70	0
almond (*Sandies*),							
.6-oz. pc.	80	1.0	9.0	5.0	5	50	0
chocolate (*Westbrae*							
Natural), 4 pcs.,							
1.1 oz	140	2.0	18.0	7.0	15	105	2.0
fudge striped (*Fudge*							
Favorites), 3 pcs.,							
1.1 oz.	160	2.0	21.0	8.0	0	150	<1.0
fudge striped,							
covered (*Fudge*							
Shoppe Mini),							
14 pcs., 1.1 oz. . .	150	1.0	20.0	7.0	0	110	<1.0
pecan (*Pecanz*),							
.6-oz. pc.	90	3.0	9.0	5.0	<5	50	0
pecan (*Sandies*),							
.6-oz. pc.	80	<1.0	9.0	5.0	<5	75	<1.0
pecan (*Sandies* Mini),							
4 pcs., 1.1 oz. . .	160	2.0	17.0	10.0	<5	100	<1.0
pecan (*Sandies*							
Reduced Fat),							
.6-oz. pc.	80	<1.0	11.0	3.0	0	60	0
s'mores (*Hain* Cookie							
Jar Bits), 17 pcs.,							
.5 oz.	60	1.0	12.0	0	0	20	0
(*Social Tea*), 6 pcs.,							
1 oz.	120	2.0	22.0	3.5	5	115	<1.0

Food and Measure	cal.	prot. (gms)	carbo. (gms)	fat (gms)	chol. (mgs)	sod. (mgs)	fiber (gms)
(*Stella D'oro Angel Wings*), 2 pcs., .9 oz.	140	2.0	13.0	9.0	<5	80	<1.0
(*Stella D'oro Angelica Goodies*), .8-oz. pc.	100	2.0	15.0	4.0	15	45	0
(*Stella D'oro Anginetti*), 4 pcs., 1.1 oz.	140	2.0	23.0	4.0	40	10	<1.0
(*Stella D'oro* Continental Collection), 1 oz.	130	3.0	20.0	2.5	5	55	0
(*Stella D'oro Lady Stella* Assortment), 3 pcs., 1 oz.	130	1.0	19.0	5.0	5	55	0
(*Stella D'oro Margherite* Combination), 2 pcs., 1.1 oz.	140	2.0	22.0	6.0	10	75	<1.0
(*Stella D'oro Royal Nuggets*), 1.1 oz. .	140	11.0	9.0	6.0	60	150	<1.0
strawberry (*Miss Meringue*), 4 pcs., 1.25 oz.	100	1.0	24.0	0	0	20	0
strawberry filled:							
(*Health Valley Cobbler Bites*), 2 pcs., .9 oz.	100	2.0	21.0	1.5	0	40	1.0
(*Newtons*), 2 pcs., 1 oz.	90	1.0	21.0	0	0	95	0
strawberry-kiwi (*Tropical Newtons*), 2 pcs., 1 oz.	90	1.0	19.0	1.5	0	55	0
sugar:							
(*Grandma's* Bites), 12 pcs., 1 oz. . .	280	3.0	38.0	13.0	5	180	1.0
(*Pepperidge Farm*), 3 pcs., 1.1 oz. ...	140	2.0	20.0	6.0	15	90	<1.0
sugar wafer:							
(*Biscos*), 8 pcs., 1 oz.	140	<1.0	21.0	6.0	0	40	0
(*Keebler*), 3 pcs., .9 oz.	130	1.0	19.0	6.0	0	20	0
chocolate (*Keebler*), 3 pcs., .9 oz. ...	140	1.0	18.0	7.0	0	30	<1.0
lemon (*Keebler*), 3 pcs., .9 oz. ...	130	1.0	19.0	6.0	0	20	0

Food and Measure	cal.	prot. (gms)	carbo. (gms)	fat (gms)	chol. (mgs)	sod. (mgs)	fiber (gms)
Cookie, sugar wafer *(cont.)*							
lemon (*Murray* Sugar Free), 6 pcs., 1.1 oz.	150	1.0	21.0	8.0	0	40	2.0
peanut butter (*Keebler*), 4 pcs., 1.1 oz.	160	3.0	18.0	9.0	0	80	<1.0
strawberry (*Murray* Sugar Free), 6 pcs., 1.1 oz.	150	1.0	21.0	8.0	0	45	1.0
vanilla (*Murray* Sugar Free), 6 pcs., 1.1 oz.	160	1.0	21.0	9.0	0	35	1.0
vanilla:							
(*Grandma's* Mini), 9 pcs., 1 oz. ...	150	2.0	22.0	7.0	<5	85	<1.0
thins (*Estee*), 4 pcs.	140	2.0	19.0	6.0	0	25	<1.0
wafer (*Estee*), 5 pcs.	150	1.0	21.0	8.0	0	10	0
wafer (*Keebler Golden*), 8 pcs., 1.1 oz.	150	1.0	20.0	7.0	0	120	<1.0
wafer (*Keebler Golden* Reduced Fat), 8 pcs., 1.1 oz.	130	2.0	25.0	3.5	0	140	<1.0
wafer (*Murray* Sugar Free), 9 pcs., 1.1 oz.	120	2.0	23.0	4.0	0	85	<1.0
wafer (*Nilla*), 8 pcs., 1.1 oz.	140	1.0	21.0	6.0	5	115	0
wafer (*Nilla* Reduced Fat), 8 pcs., 1 oz.	120	1.0	24.0	2.0	0	105	0
wafer, rainbow (*Keebler*), 8 pcs., 1.1 oz.	130	1.0	20.0	5.0	0	125	0
vanilla sandwich:							
(*Café Cremes*), 2 pcs.	160	1.0	22.0	7.0	0	130	0
(*Cameo*), 2 pcs., 1 oz.	130	1.0	21.0	5.0	0	105	0
(*Cameo*), 1.9-oz. pkg.	250	2.0	40.0	9.0	0	200	1.0
(*Estee*), 3 pcs., 1.1 oz.	160	2.0	25.0	5.0	0	35	<1.0

Food and Measure	cal.	prot. (gms)	carbo. (gms)	fat (gms)	chol. (mgs)	sod. (mgs	fiber (gms)
(*Grandma's*), 5 pcs., 1 oz.	210	2.0	30.0	10.0	5	125	<1.0
(*Murray* Sugar Free), 3 pcs., 1 oz. ...	120	1.0	21.0	5.0	0	65	2.0
(*Vienna Fingers*), 2 pcs., 1 oz. ...	140	2.0	21.0	6.0	0	105	<1.0
(*Vienna Fingers* Reduced Fat), 2 pcs., 1 oz.	130	1.0	22.0	4.5	0	105	<1.0
vanilla fudge sandwich (*Café Cremes*), 2 pcs.	200	1.0	27.0	10.0	0	140	1.0
vanilla-strawberry wafer (*Estee*), 5 pcs. ...	150	1.0	22.0	8.0	0	10	0
Cookie, mix*, 2 pcs., except as noted:							
chocolate chip:							
(*Arrowhead Mills*), 1 pc.	80	1.0	16.0	1.5	0	110	0
(*Betty Crocker*)	160	2.0	22.0	8.0	10	105	0
(*Duncan Hines*) ...	170	2.0	22.0	8.0	10	100	0
(*Pillsbury*), 2 small or 1 large	140	1.0	21.0	6.0	<5	140	<1.0
wheat free (*Arrowhead Mills*), 1 pc.	80	1.0	16.0	1.5	0	105	<1.0
chocolate chunk:							
(*Pillsbury*), 2 small or 1 large	140	1.0	21.0	6.0	<5	140	<1.0
double (*Betty Crocker*)	150	2.0	21.0	6.0	10	100	0
chocolate peanut butter (*Betty Crocker*)	150	3.0	20.0	7.0	10	120	0
oatmeal:							
(*Betty Crocker*) ...	150	2.0	22.0	6.0	10	105	<1.0
chocolate chip (*Betty Crocker*)	150	2.0	21.0	7.0	10	135	0
raisin (*Arrowhead Mills*), 1 pc. ...	70	1.0	16.0	0	0	110	1.0
peanut butter:							
(*Betty Crocker*) ...	160	3.0	20.0	8.0	10	135	0
(*Duncan Hines*) ...	140	2.0	16.0	8.0	10	120	0
sugar:							
(*Betty Crocker*) ...	160	2.0	22.0	8.0	10	115	0

Food and Measure	cal.	prot. (gms)	carbo. (gms)	fat (gms)	chol. (mgs)	sod. (mgs)	fiber (gms)
Cookie mix, sugar *(cont.)*							
golden (*Duncan Hines*)	150	1.0	21.0	7.0	20	90	0
white chunk:							
(*Betty Crocker*) . . .	160	2.0	22.0	8.0	10	110	0
(*Pillsbury*), 2 small or 1 large	150	1.0	21.0	7.0	<5	150	<1.0
Cookie, frozen, ruga- lach (*Tofutti*), .75-oz. pc.	130	10.0	14.0	8.0	0	65	0
Cookie, refrigerated, 1 oz., except as noted:							
(*Pillsbury M&M's*) . . .	130	1.0	18.0	6.0	<5	75	<1.0
chocolate chip:							
(*Nestlé Toll House/ Nestlé Toll House Big Batch*), 2 tbsp., 1 pc.*	140	2.0	20.0	6.0	10	100	0
(*Nestlé Toll House Reduced Fat*), 2 tbsp., 1 pc.* . .	130	2.0	23.0	3.5	5	130	1.0
(*Pillsbury*)	140	1.0	17.0	7.0	<5	90	<1.0
(*Pillsbury* Dough) .	110	1.0	17.0	2.0	<5	75	<1.0
(*Pillsbury* Ready to Bake!)	120	1.0	15.0	6.0	<5	80	<1.0
(*Pillsbury* Reduced Fat)	110	1.0	18.0	2.0	<5	85	<1.0
bar (*Nestlé Toll House*), 1 pc.* . .	110	1.0	16.0	5.0	10	90	1.0
oatmeal (*Pillsbury*)	120	1.0	16.0	6.0	<5	95	<1.0
peanut butter (*Nestlé Toll House*), 2 tbsp., 1 pc.*	150	3.0	19.0	7.0	10	110	0
walnut (*Nestlé Toll House*), 2 tbsp., 1 pc.*	110	1.0	14.0	6.0	10	115	0
walnut (*Pillsbury*) .	130	1.0	16.0	7.0	5	90	<1.0
walnut (*Pillsbury* Ready to Bake!), 1 pc.	120	1.0	14.0	7.0	5	80	<1.0
and white fudge (*Nestlé Toll House*), 2 tbsp., 1 pc.* . .	150	2.0	21.0	6.0	10	110	1.0

Food and Measure	cal.	prot. (gms)	carbo. (gms)	fat (gms)	chol. (mgs)	sod. (mgs)	fiber (gms)
chocolate chip and chunk, double (*Pillsbury*)	140	1.0	17.0	7.0	5	85	<1.0
chocolate chunk:							
(*Nestlé Toll House*), 2 tbsp., 1 pc.* . .	150	2.0	22.0	6.0	10	110	1.0
(*Pillsbury*)	140	1.0	17.0	7.0	5	85	<1.0
white (*Pillsbury*) . .	130	1.0	17.0	6.0	5	100	0
gingerbread (*Pillsbury*), 2 slices, ¼"	140	1.0	18.0	7.0	15	105	0
peanut butter (*Pillsbury*)	130	2.0	16.0	6.0	5	130	0
sugar:							
(*Pillsbury*)	130	1.0	19.0	5.0	10	115	0
(*Pillsbury* Ready to Bake!), 1 pc. . . .	110	1.0	14.0	6.0	10	100	0
bar (*Nestlé Toll House*), 1 pc.* . .	110	1.0	15.0	5.0	10	80	<1.0
Cookie crumbs:							
(*Oreo Crunchies*), 2 tbsp.	50	0	8.0	2.5	0	60	0
chocolate (*Oreo*), 2 tbsp.	90	0	13.0	4.0	0	85	<1.0
graham cracker:							
(*Honey Maid*), 2½ tbsp.	70	1.0	12.0	1.5	0	100	0
(*Keebler*), 3 tbsp. . .	80	2.0	13.0	2.0	0	150	<1.0
Cookie pie crust, see "Pie crust"							
Cookie topping, 2 tbsp.:							
dough crunch (*Smucker's Magic Shell*)	210	1.0	16.0	16.0	0	15	0
(*Hershey's* Cookies 'n' Creme)	180	2.0	14.0	13.0	0	50	0
Coquito nuts (*Frieda's*), 11 pcs., 1 oz.	110	21.0	5.0	10.0	0	5	3.0
Coriander, fresh, ¼ cup	1	.1	.1	<.1	0	1	.1
Coriander, dried:							
(*Watkins* cilantro), ¼ tsp.	0	0	0	0	0	0	0
leaf, 1 tsp.	2	.1	.3	<.1	0	1	.1
seed, 1 tsp.	5	.2	1.0	.3	0	1	.5

Food and Measure	cal.	prot. (gms)	carbo. (gms)	fat (gms)	chol. (mgs)	sod. (mgs)	fiber (gms)
Corkscrew pasta, see "Pasta"							
Corkscrew pasta dish mix, 1 cup*:							
four-cheese sauce (*Pasta Roni*)	390	12.0	49.0	17.0	10	950	2.0
garlic sauce, creamy (*Pasta Roni*)	350	9.0	40.0	17.0	5	950	2.0
Corn, fresh:							
baby, .28-oz. ear	9	.3	2.0	.1	0	1	.2
golden or white raw, 5-oz. ear	123	4.6	27.2	1.7	0	21	3.9
kernels, boiled, drained, ½ cup .	89	2.7	20.6	1.1	0	14	2.3
white, boiled, drained, 2.72-oz. ear	83	2.6	19.3	1.0	0	13	2.1
Corn, canned, ½ cup, except as noted:							
kernel, golden:							
(*Blue Boy*)	90	2.0	19.0	.5	0	290	2.0
(*Del Monte*)	90	2.0	18.0	1.0	0	360	3.0
(*Del Monte* Supersweet No Salt) . .	60	2.0	11.0	1.0	0	10	3.0
(*Del Monte* Supersweet No Sugar)	60	2.0	11.0	1.0	0	360	3.0
(*Del Monte* Supersweet Vac Pack)	70	2.0	13.0	1.0	0	270	3.0
(*Del Monte* Supersweet Vac Pack No Salt)	70	2.0	13.0	1.0	0	10	3.0
(*Green Giant*)	80	2.0	18.0	.5	0	360	2.0
(*Green Giant* 50% Less Sodium) . .	80	1.0	17.0	0	0	180	1.0
(*Green Giant Niblets*), ⅓ cup	70	2.0	15.0	0	0	230.	2.0
(*Green Giant Niblets* Extra Sweet), ⅓ cup	50	2.0	10.0	.5	0	200	2.0
(*Green Giant Niblets* No Salt), ⅓ cup	60	2.0	13.0	0	0	0	2.0
(*Greene's Farm* Garden)	60	2.0	15.0	.5	0	170	2.0
(*Hain*)	90	2.0	14.0	1.0	0	340	2.0
(*Libby's*)	90	2.0	19.0	.5	0	290	2.0

Food and Measure	cal.	prot. (gms)	carbo. (gms)	fat (gms)	chol. (mgs)	sod. (mgs)	fiber (gms)
(*Libby's* No Salt) ..	80	2.0	16.0	.5	0	40	<1.0
(*Libby's* Vac Pack) .	80	2.0	17.0	0	0	210	1.0
(*S&W* Sweet & Crispy), ⅓ cup .	70	2.0	12.0	1.5	0	170	2.0
(*Veg-All*)	80	2.0	16.0	1.0	0	340	2.0
kernel, gold/white:							
(*Del Monte* Supersweet)	80	2.0	18.0	.5	0	360	2.0
(*Green Giant* Super Sweet), ⅓ cup ..	50	1.0	11.0	0	0	200	1.0
kernel, white:							
(*Del Monte*)	60	2.0	11.0	1.0	0	360	3.0
(*Green Giant* Shoepeg), ⅓ cup	80	2.0	16.0	.5	0	220	1.0
kernel, w/peppers:							
(*Del Monte* Fiesta Supersweet) ...	50	2.0	12.0	1.0	0	310	2.0
(*Green Giant* Mexicorn*), ⅓ cup ...	60	2.0	14.0	0	0	250	1.0
cream style, golden:							
(*Blue Boy*)	90	2.0	20.0	0	0	360	2.0
(*Del Monte*)	90	2.0	20.0	.5	0	360	2.0
(*Del Monte* No Salt)	90	2.0	20.0	.5	0	10	2.0
(*Del Monte* Supersweet)	60	1.0	14.0	.5	0	360	2.0
(*Del Monte* Supersweet No Salt) ..	60	1.0	14.0	.5	0	10	2.0
(*Green Giant*)	80	2.0	17.0	.5	0	410	2.0
(*Libby's*)	90	2.0	20.0	0	0	360	2.0
(*S&W*)	60	1.0	14.0	.5	0	360	2.0
(*Veg-All*)	100	2.0	21.0	1.0	0	280	2.0
cream style, white							
(*Del Monte*)	100	2.0	21.0	1.0	0	360	2.0
Corn, frozen:							
on cob, 1 ear, except as noted:							
(*Birds Eye* 4 Pack) .	140	5.0	34.0	1.5	0	20	2.0
(*Birds Eye* 8/12 Pack Little Ears)	80	3.0	18.0	1.0	0	10	1.0
(*Cascadian Farm*), 2 ears	120	4.0	28.0	1.0	0	5	3.0
(*Green Giant Niblets*)	150	4.0	32.0	1.0	0	10	3.0
(*John Cope's* 3–5")	140	5.0	34.0	1.5	0	20	2.0

Food and Measure	cal.	prot. (gms)	carbo. (gms)	fat (gms)	chol. (mgs)	sod. (mgs)	fiber (gms)
Corn, frozen, on the cob *(cont.)*							
(*John Cope's* Mini 2–3")	80	3.0	18.0	1.0	0	10	1.0
(*John Cope's* Super Sweet 5")	120	4.0	22.0	1.5	0	5	5.0
white (*John Cope's* Silver Queen 5")	150	4.0	31.0	1.5	0	5	3.0
kernel, golden:							
(*Birds Eye*), ⅓ cup	70	3.0	17.0	.5	0	0	2.0
(*Birds Eye* 10 oz. Box), ⅓ cup	60	2.0	14.0	1.0	0	0	2.0
(*Cascadian Farm*), ¾ cup	90	3.0	21.0	1.0	0	0	5.0
(*Green Giant Niblets*), ⅔ cup	80	3.0	17.0	.5	0	60	3.0
(*Green Giant Niblets* Extra Sweet), ⅔ cup	70	2.0	13.0	1.0	0	0	2.0
(*John Cope's*), ⅔ cup	80	3.0	15.0	1.0	0	0	2.0
(*John Cope's* Shoe-peg), ⅔ cup ...	80	3.0	19.0	1.0	0	10	1.0
(*John Cope's* Super Sweet), ⅓ cup ..	80	2.0	17.0	.5	0	0	1.0
(*Seabrook Farms*), ⅔ cup	80	3.0	19.0	1.0	0	10	1.0
(*Tree of Life* Organic), ⅔ cup	80	3.0	19.0	1.0	0	10	1.0
kernel, gold/white:							
(*Birds Eye*), ½ cup .	60	2.0	11.0	1.0	0	330	2.0
(*Green Giant*), ¾ cup	70	2.0	14.0	1.0	0	0	2.0
kernel, white:							
(*Green Giant* Shoe-peg), ¾ cup	100	3.0	20.0	1.0	0	0	3.0
(*John Cope's* Super Sweet), ⅓ cup ..	80	2.0	17.0	.5	0	0	1.0
(*McKenzie's*), ½ cup	80	3.0	19.0	1.0	0	10	1.0
baby (*Birds Eye*), ⅔ cup	110	3.0	22.0	1.0	0	10	3.0
cream style:							
white (*John Cope's* Sweet 'n Creamy), ⅓ cup	100	3.0	17.0	2.5	<5	120	1.0

Food and Measure	cal.	prot. (gms)	carbo. (gms)	fat (gms)	chol. (mgs)	sod. (mgs)	fiber (gms)
in butter sauce:							
(*Cascadian Farm*), ½ cup	100	3.0	19.0	3.0	5	310	2.0
(*Green Giant Niblets*), ⅔ cup	110	3.0	22.0	1.5	<5	340	2.0
Corn, dried:							
(*John Cope's*), ¼ cup	130	2.0	15.0	1.0	0	0	1.0
freeze-dried, ½ cup:							
(*AlpineAire*)	90	3.0	16.0	1.5	0	0	3.0
(*Mountain House*)	90	3.0	16.0	1.5	0	0	2.0
Corn, whole-grain:							
1 oz.	103	2.7	21.1	1.3	0	10	n.a.
1 cup	605	15.6	123.3	7.9	0	58	n.a.
Corn blend, frozen, baby, and bean (*Birds Eye*), 3 oz.	60	3.0	12.0	.5	0	10	2.0
Corn bran, crude, 1 cup	170	6.4	65.1	.7	0	5	64.3
Corn bread, see "Bread, frozen"							
Corn bread mix, dry, ¼ cup, except as noted:							
(*Arrowhead Mills*)	120	5.0	24.0	1.0	0	270	4.0
(*Aunt Jemima* Easy), ⅛ pkg.	145	2.0	24.0	4.5	0	440	1.0
(*Hodgson Mill* Cornbread/Muffin)	130	4.0	28.0	.5	0	240	3.0
(*Glory Foods*)	140	2.0	24.0	3.5	0	440	1.0
jalapeño (*Hodgson Mill*)	100	4.0	21.0	.5	0	310	1.0
sweet cake:							
(*Chi-Chi's* Cake), ½ cup	100	1.0	22.0	.5	0	120	0
(*El Torito*), ⅛ pkt.	100	1.0	22.0	.5	0	120	0
(*Kentucky Kernel*)	120	2.0	24.0	1.5	0	310	0
Corn cake, frozen (*El Torito*), ⅓ cup	180	2.0	33.0	4.0	10	340	1.0
Corn chips/crisps (see also "Snack chips"), 1 oz., except as noted:							
(*Bachman*), 1.1 oz.	150	2.0	20.0	7.0	0	125	2.0
(*Baked Bugles*), 1.1 oz.	130	2.0	23.0	3.5	0	380	0

Food and Measure	cal.	prot. (gms)	carbo. (gms)	fat (gms)	chol. (mgs)	sod. (mgs)	fiber (gms)
Corn chips/crisps *(cont.)*							
(*Bugles*), 1.1 oz.	160	1.0	18.0	9.0	0	310	<1.0
(*Corn Nuts* Original),							
⅓ cup	120	1.0	20.0	4.5	0	180	2.0
(*Fritos*)	160	2.0	15.0	10.0	0	170	1.0
(*Fritos* King Size)	160	2.0	16.0	10.0	0	150	1.0
(*Fritos* Scoops)	160	2.0	16.0	10.0	0	110	1.0
(*Little Bear* Original							
Reduced Fat)	140	2.0	18.0	7.0	0	140	1.0
(*Snyder's*), 1.5 oz. . .	240	2.0	24.0	14.0	0	240	n.a.
(*Utz*)	240	3.0	25.0	15.0	0	240	1.0
(*Wahoos* Original) . . .	140	1.0	18.0	8.0	0	350	0
barbecue:							
(*Bachman*), 1.1 oz.	150	4.0	19.0	7.0	0	200	1.0
(*Bugles* Smokin),							
1.1 oz.	150	1.0	19.0	8.0	0	330	0
(*Fritos*)	150	2.0	15.0	10.0	0	170	1.0
(*Snyder's*), 1.5 oz.	240	2.0	28.0	14.0	0	270	n.a.
(*Utz*)	160	2.0	16.0	10.0	0	180	1.0
(*Wahoos*)	140	1.0	19.0	7.0	0	300	1.0
honey (*Fritos* Texas							
Grill)	150	2.0	17.0	9.0	0	250	1.0
cheese:							
(*Barbara's* Puffs) . .	150	2.0	16.0	10.0	0	130	0
(*Barbara's* Puffs							
Bakes)	160	2.0	13.0	11.0	0	190	0
(*Boston's Cheez*							
Bopps Puffs) . . .	130	2.0	17.0	6.0	0	250	0
(*Chee•tos* Crunchy)	160	2.0	15.0	10.0	0	290	<1.0
(*Chee•tos* Curls) . .	150	2.0	15.0	10.0	0	290	<1.0
(*Chee•tos* Puffed							
Balls)	150	2.0	15.0	10.0	0	300	<1.0
(*Chee•tos* Puffs) . .	160	2.0	15.0	10.0	0	370	<1.0
(*Chee•tos* Puffs							
Jumbo)	160	2.0	13.0	10.0	0	350	0
(*Chee•tos* X's & O's)	160	2.0	15.0	11.0	<5	290	<1.0
(*Chee•tos* Zig Zags)	170	2.0	17.0	11.0	<5	370	<1.0
(*Herr's* Curls)	110	1.0	13.0	6.0	0	240	2.0
(*Jax* Baked)	140	2.0	18.0	7.0	<5	360	<1.0
(*Planters Cheez*							
Balls)	160	2.0	15.0	10.0	0	300	<1.0
(*Planters Cheez*							
Curls)	150	1.0	15.0	10.0	<5	310	<1.0

Food and Measure	cal.	prot. (gms)	carbo. (gms)	fat (gms)	chol. (mgs)	sod. (mgs)	fiber (gms)
(*Planters Cheez Mania*)	160	1.0	14.0	11.0	5	280	<1.0
(*Snyder's* Twist) . . .	170	2.0	15.0	12.0	<5	230	n.a.
(*Utz* Balls)	170	2.0	18.0	10.0	0	230	1.0
(*Utz* Curls)	160	2.0	16.0	9.0	0	210	1.0
(*Utz* Curls Reduced Fat)	140	3.0	18.0	6.0	0	300	2.0
crunchy (*Utz* Curls)	150	2.0	16.0	10.0	0	180	1.0
hot (*Chee•tos* Flamin')	160	2.0	15.0	10.0	0	280	<1.0
hot (*Chee•tos* Puff Rods)	150	2.0	16.0	9.0	0	160	<1.0
jalapeño (*Barbara's* Puffs)	150	2.0	16.0	10.0	0	130	0
nacho (*Bugles*), 1.1 oz.	160	1.0	18.0	9.0	0	300	0
nacho (*Corn Nuts*), ⅓ cup	130	2.0	19.0	5.0	0	200	2.0
nacho (*Wahoos* Fiesta)	140	1.0	18.0	8.0	0	380	0
nacho, cheesy (*Little Bear* Reduced Fat)	140	2.0	17.0	7.0	0	230	1.0
twists (*Jax* Crunchy)	160	2.0	14.0	11.0	<5	200	0
cheese, cheddar:							
(*Bearitos* Puffs), 2 cups, 1.1 oz.	170	2.0	16.0	11.0	3.5	300	1.0
(*Bearitos* Puffs Lite), 2 cups, 1.1 oz.	150	3.0	22.0	5.0	5	280	1.0
(*Little Bear* Puffs Lite), .75-oz. bag	110	2.0	16.0	3.5	<5	200	1.0
extra (*Bearitos* Crunchitos)	130	2.0	17.0	6.0	0	230	<1.0
white (*Barbara's* Puffs)	160	2.0	13.0	11.0	0	190	0
chili cheese:							
(*Bugles* Chili Con Queso), 1.1 oz.	160	2.0	18.0	9.0	0	310	0
(*Fritos*)	160	2.0	15.0	10.0	0	260	1.0
(*Little Bear*)	150	2.0	15.0	10.0	0	230	1.0
hot (*Fritos/Fritos Sabrositas* Flamin')	160	2.0	15.0	10.0	0	160	1.0
lime 'n chili (*Fritos Sabrositas*)	150	2.0	17.0	9.0	0	240	1.0

Food and Measure	cal.	prot. (gms)	carbo. (gms)	fat (gms)	chol. (mgs)	sod. (mgs)	fiber (gms)
Corn chips/crisps *(cont.)*							
pepperoni, toasted							
(*Corn Nuts*), ⅓ cup	130	3.0	20.0	4.0	0	190	2.0
sour cream/onion							
(*Corn Nuts*), ⅓ cup	120	2.0	19.0	4.5	0	300	2.0
tortilla:							
(*Air Crisps*)	130	2.0	20.0	5.0	0	240	1.0
(*Bachman* Restaurant)	130	2.0	18.0	6.0	0	100	1.0
(*Boston's* Baked), 1.1 oz.	110	2.0	23.0	1.5	0	200	2.0
(*Doritos* Toasted) . .	140	2.0	18.0	7.0	0	120	1.0
(*Garden of Eatin'*)	140	2.0	19.0	5.0	0	50	0
(*Garden of Eatin' California Bakes*)	110	2.0	23.0	1.0	0	65	1.0
(*Guiltless Gourmet*)	110	3.0	22.0	2.0	0	140	2.0
(*Herr's* Bite Size) . .	140	3.0	18.0	6.0	0	90	2.0
(*Kettle Little Dippers*)	140	2.0	19.0	6.0	0	80	2.0
(*Santitas* Restaurant)	130	2.0	19.0	6.0	0	110	1.0
(*Santitas* White) . . .	130	2.0	19.0	6.0	0	100	1.0
(*Snyder's* White) . .	140	2.0	23.0	4.5	0	110	n.a.
(*Tostitos* Baked/ Baked Bite Size)	110	3.0	24.0	1.0	0	200	2.0
(*Tostitos* Bite Size)	140	2.0	17.0	8.0	0	110	1.0
(*Tostitos* Crispy Rounds)	140	2.0	18.0	7.0	0	120	1.0
(*Tostitos* Restaurant)	140	2.0	19.0	6.0	0	80	1.0
(*Tostitos* Santa Fe Gold)	140	2.0	19.0	6.0	0	80	1.0
(*Tostitos* WOW) . .	90	2.0	20.0	1.0	0	105	1.0
(*Utz* Baked)	120	2.0	23.0	1.5	0	170	1.0
(*Utz* Restaurant/ Round)	140	2.0	18.0	7.0	0	120	1.0
bite size (*Garden of Eatin'* Mini Corns)	150	2.0	19.0	7.0	0	45	<1.0
black bean (*Garden of Eatin'*)	150	3.0	18.0	7.0	0	55	1.0
black bean, spicy (*Guiltless Gourmet*)	110	3.0	22.0	2.0	0	200	2.0
black bean chili (*Garden of Eatin'*)	140	2.0	18.0	7.0	0	90	2.0

Food and Measure	cal.	prot. (gms)	carbo. (gms)	fat (gms)	chol. (mgs)	sod. (mgs)	fiber (gms)
black bean and salsa (*Bachman*)	140	3.0	18.0	7.0	0	160	3.0
brown rice and black bean (*Kettle*) . . .	120	3.0	16.0	6.0	0	85	2.0
cheddar quesadilla (*Tostitos* Baked Bite Size)	120	2.0	22.0	3.0	0	220	1.0
chili and lime (*Garden of Eatin'*)	140	2.0	20.0	5.0	0	75	<1.0
chili and lime (*Guiltless Gourmet*) . . .	110	2.0	22.0	2.0	0	200	2.0
hot and smoky chipotle (*Garden of Eatin' California Bakes*)	120	2.0	23.0	2.0	0	80	1.0
jalapeño cheddar (*Doritos 3D's*) . .	130	2.0	20.0	4.0	0	240	1.0
lime or roasted red pepper (*Tostitos* Restaurant Hint of)	140	2.0	19.0	6.0	0	160	1.0
picante (*Doritos* Baja)	140	2.0	18.0	7.0	0	220	1.0
quesadilla, spicy (*Tostitos* Bite Size)	150	2.0	16.0	9.0	0	200	1.0
ranch (*Doritos Cooler Ranch*) . .	140	2.0	18.0	7.0	0	170	1.0
ranch (*Doritos 3D's Cooler Ranch*) . .	140	2.0	18.0	6.0	<5	350	1.0
ranch, picante (*Guiltless Gourmet*)	110	3.0	22.0	2.0	0	200	2.0
salsa (*Barbara's Pinta*) 1.1 oz. . .	130	2.0	19.0	6.0	0	210	2.0
salsa/black bean (*Utz*)	140	2.0	19.0	6.0	0	230	1.0
salsa/cream cheese (*Tostitos* Baked Bite Size)	120	2.0	21.0	3.0	0	190	1.0
salsa verde (*Doritos*)	140	1.0	19.0	7.0	0	210	1.0
sesame rye w/caraway (*Kettle*)	140	3.0	17.0	6.0	0	80	2.0
sour cream (*Doritos* Sonic)	140	2.0	17.0	7.0	0	170	1.0
taco (*Doritos*)	140	2.0	18.0	7.0	0	170	1.0

Food and Measure	cal.	prot. (gms)	carbo. (gms)	fat (gms)	chol. (mgs)	sod. (mgs)	fiber (gms)
Corn chips/crisps, tortilla *(cont.)*							
yogurt green onion *(Garden of Eatin' California Bakes)*	120	2.0	23.0	2.0	0	70	1.0
tortilla, blue corn:							
(Barbara's), 1.1 oz.	140	3.0	16.0	7.0	0	40	1.0
(Barbara's No Salt), 1.1 oz.	140	3.0	16.0	7.0	0	0	1.0
(Garden of Eatin') . .	150	2.0	18.0	7.0	0	55	1.0
(Garden of Eatin' No Salt)	150	2.0	18.0	7.0	0	10	1.0
(Garden of Eatin' California Bakes Sunny Salsa) . . .	120	3.0	21.0	2.0	0	80	<1.0
(Garden of Eatin' Little Soy Blues)	140	3.0	18.0	6.0	0	55	2.0
(Garden of Eatin' Red Hot Blues) .	140	3.0	18.0	7.0	0	80	2.0
(Garden of Eatin' Sesame Blues) . .	150	3.0	16.0	8.0	0	65	1.0
(Guiltless Gourmet)	110	3.0	22.0	2.0	0	140	2.0
(Kettle)	140	3.0	18.0	6.0	0	80	2.0
(Kettle Sesame Blue Moons)	150	3.0	19.0	8.0	0	80	2.0
sesame, roasted *(Garden of Eatin' California Bakes)*	120	4.0	20.0	2.0	0	35	1.0
sunflower *(Garden of Eatin' Sunny Blues)*	160	3.0	16.0	8.0	0	70	1.0
tortilla, nacho:							
(Air Crisps), 1.1 oz.	130	1.0	21.0	5.0	0	340	1.0
(Bachman)	140	2.0	19.0	6.0	0	150	2.0
(Doritos Nacho Cheesier)	140	2.0	18.0	7.0	0	200	1.0
(Doritos Spicier) . .	140	2.0	18.0	7.0	0	210	1.0
(Doritos 3D's Nacho Cheesier)	140	2.0	17.0	7.0	<5	360	1.0
(Doritos WOW) . . .	90	2.0	18.0	1.0	0	240	1.0
(Guiltless Gourmet)	110	2.0	22.0	2.0	0	200	2.0
(Snyder's)	150	2.0	24.0	5.0	0	240	n.a.
(Utz Cheesier)	140	2.0	19.0	6.0	0	200	1.0

Food and Measure	cal.	prot. (gms)	carbo. (gms)	fat (gms)	chol. (mgs)	sod. (mgs	fiber (gms)
tortilla, red corn:							
(*Garden of Eatin'* Red Chips)	150	3.0	18.0	7.0	0	65	1.0
(*Garden of Eatin'* Salsa Reds)	150	3.0	17.0	7.0	0	80	1.0
(*Guiltless Gourmet*)	110	3.0	22.0	2.0	0	140	2.0
tortilla, yellow corn:							
(*Bearitos*)	140	2.0	18.0	7.0	0	120	2.0
(*Garden of Eatin'* Yellow Chips) ...	140	2.0	19.0	6.0	0	40	<1.0
(*Guiltless Gourmet*)	110	3.0	22.0	2.0	0	160	2.0
(*Guiltless Gourmet* No Salt)	110	3.0	22.0	1.0	0	26	2.0
(*Kettle*)	140	2.0	19.0	6.0	0	80	2.0
(*Snyder's*)	140	2.0	23.0	4.5	0	135	n.a.
five grain (*Kettle*) ...	140	2.0	18.0	6.0	0	80	2.0
Corn chips/dip kit:							
cheese dip:							
(*Fritos Scoops* Fiesta), ½ kit ...	430	8.0	42.0	28.0	15	860	3.0
(*Tostitos*), 1 kit ...	480	10.0	43.0	31.0	15	1090	3.0
chili dip (*Fritos Scoops*), ½ kit	380	10.0	36.0	22.0	15	700	4.0
salsa dip (*Tostitos*), 1 kit	320	5.0	43.0	15.0	0	990	5.0
Corn dog, see "Frankfurter, wrapped"							
Cornflake crumbs (*Kellogg's*), 2 tbsp.	40	1.0	9.0	0	0	80	0
Corn flour:							
(*Mascoa*), 1.1 oz. ...	110	2.0	23.0	1.5	0	0	2.0
whole-grain, 1 oz. ...	102	2.0	21.8	1.1	0	1	3.8
whole-grain, 1 cup ...	422	8.1	89.9	4.5	0	6	15.7
masa, 1 oz.	103	2.6	21.6	1.1	0	1	2.7
masa, 1 cup	416	10.7	87.0	4.3	0	6	10.9
Corn fritter, frozen (*Mrs. Paul's*), 1 pc.	130	4.0	15.0	6.0	<5	310	1.0
Corn fritter mix, dry (*Casbah*), mix for 2 fritters	130	3.0	25.0	2.0	0	265	2.0
Corn grits, 1 pkt., except as noted:							
(*Quaker* Instant)	95	2.0	22.0	0	0	305	1.0

Food and Measure	cal.	prot. (gms)	carbo. (gms)	fat (gms)	chol. (mgs)	sod. (mgs)	fiber (gms)
Corn grits *(cont.)*							
butter flavor (*Quaker* Instant)	100	2.0	20.0	1.0	0	370	1.0
w/cheddar, zesty (*Quaker* Instant) ..	100	3.0	20.0	1.5	<1	460	1.5
w/cheddar flavor, real (*Quaker* Instant) ..	105	2.5	20.0	2.0	<1	515	1.0
w/redeye gravy, ham bits (*Quaker* Instant)	95	3.0	21.0	.5	0	490	1.0
white, ¼ cup: (*Arrowhead Mills*)	140	3.0	30.0	0	0	0	1.0
(*Quaker* Quick Hominy)	130	3.0	29.0	.5	0	0	2.0
yellow, ¼ cup: (*Arrowhead Mills*)	130	3.0	29.0	0	0	0	1.0
hominy (*Quaker* Quick)	125	3.0	29.0	.5	0	0	2.0
Corn relish:							
(*Aunt Nellie's*), 1 tbsp.	20	0	5.0	0	0	40	0
(*Mrs. Renfro's*), 1 tbsp.	15	0	4.0	0	0	45	0
(*Nance's*), 2 tbsp. ...	25	2.0	6.0	0	0	75	0
Corn soufflé, frozen (*Stouffer's*), ½ cup	170	5.0	21.0	7.0	65	490	1.0
Corn syrup, 2 tbsp.:							
dark (*Karo*)	120	0	31.0	0	0	45	0
light (*Karo*)	120	0	31.0	0	0	35	0
Cornish hen, fresh or frozen:							
raw (*Tyson* Rock Cornish), 4 oz. ...	180	18.0	0	12.0	130	65	0
whole, cooked: dark (*Perdue*), 3 oz.	200	17.0	0	14.0	125	55	0
white (*Perdue*), 3 oz.	160	21.0	0	8.0	100	40	0
Cornmeal (see also "Corn flour" and "Polenta"):							
(*Goya* Fine), 3 tbsp. .	100	2.0	23.0	0	0	0	1.0
blue (*Arrowhead Mills*), ¼ cup	130	3.0	25.0	1.5	0	0	3.0
masa harina: (*Quaker*), ¼ cup ..	110	3.0	24.0	1.5	0	0	2.5

Food and Measure	cal.	prot. (gms)	carbo. (gms)	fat (gms)	chol. (mgs)	sod. (mgs)	fiber (gms)
(*Quaker* Preparada para Tortillas), ⅓ cup	160	4.0	27.0	4.5	0	400	1.0
white:							
(*Hodgson Mill*), ¼ cup	100	3.0	22.0	1.0	0	0	3.0
(*Quaker* Enriched), 3 tbsp.	90	2.0	21.0	.5	0	0	1.0
yellow:							
(*Arrowhead Mills*), ¼ cup	120	3.0	27.0	1.0	0	0	3.0
(*Hodgson Mill*), ¼ cup	100	3.0	28.0	1.0	0	0	3.0
(*Hodgson Mill* Self-rising), ¼ cup . .	90	3.0	21.0	10.0	0	260	3.0
(*Quaker* Enriched), 3 tbsp.	90	2.0	21.0	.5	0	0	1.5
Cornstarch:							
(*Argo*), 1 tbsp.	30	0	7.0	0	0	0	0
(*Hodgson Mill*), 2 tsp.	35	0	9.0	0	0	0	0
Cottonseed flour, partially defatted, 1 cup	337	38.5	38.1	5.8	8	33	2.8
Cottonseed kernels, roasted, 1 tbsp. . .	51	3.3	2.2	3.6	0	3	.6
Cottonseed meal, partially defatted, 1 oz.	104	13.9	10.9	1.4	0	10	<1.0
Country gravy mix, ¼ cup*:							
(*Loma Linda Gravy Quik/Natural Touch*)	20	<1.0	4.0	.5	0	290	0
(*McCormick* Low Fat)	40	0	5.0	0	0	280	0
(*McCormick* Original)	50	0	4.0	3.5	0	260	0
sausage flavor (*McCormick*)	45	0	4.0	3.0	0	200	0
Couscous:							
dry:							
(*Arrowhead Mills*), ¼ cup	170	6.0	35.0	0	0	0	2.0
(*Frieda's*), ¼ cup . .	210	7.0	43.0	0	0	5	3.0
(*Near East*), ⅓ cup	220	8.0	46.0	1.0	0	5	2.0

Food and Measure	cal.	prot. (gms)	carbo. (gms)	fat (gms)	chol. (mgs)	sod (mgs)	fiber (gms)
Couscous *(cont.)*							
cooked:							
(*Near East*), 1 cup .	230	8.0	46.0	2.0	0	5	2.0
½ cup	101	3.4	20.9	.1	0	4	1.3
Couscous, dried, 1 oz.:							
(*AlpineAire*)	100	3.0	20.0	.5	0	0	1.0
whole wheat (*Alpine-Aire*)	100	4.0	20.0	.5	0	0	1.0
Couscous dish, mix, 1 cup*, except as noted:							
almondine (*Nile Spice*), 1 pkg.	200	7.0	37.0	2.5	0	490	2.0
broccoli and cheese:							
(*Near East*)	240	8.0	42.0	5.0	10	710	3.0
chicken, herbed (*Near East*)	220	7.0	42.0	3.5	0	440	3.0
cranberry (*Marrakesh Express Calypso*) . .	200	7.0	42.0	0	0	220	1.0
curry (*Near East* Mediterranean*)	220	7.0	42.0	3.5	0	530	3.0
garlic, roasted (*Marrakesh Express Grande*)	250	8.0	51.0	1.0	0	450	2.0
garlic, roasted, and olive oil:							
(*Casbah*), ¼ cup . .	230	9.0	38.0	0	0	410	3.0
(*Near East*)	230	7.0	41.0	4.5	0	480	2.0
(*Near East* Meal Cup), 1 pkg. . . .	280	11.0	59.0	2.0	0	600	4.0
(*Nile Spice* Cup), 2.8 oz.	310	11.0	59.0	2.5	0	720	4.0
lemon spinach (*Casbah*), ¼ cup . .	220	8.0	40.0	0	0	420	3.0
lentil curry:							
(*Marrakesh Express*)	170	7.0	35.0	0	0	290	1.0
(*Nile Spice*), 1 pkg.	200	10.0	36.0	1.5	0	730	4.0
mango salsa (*Marrakesh Express*)	190	6.0	40.0	0	0	270	1.0
minestrone (*Nile Spice*), 1 pkg.	180	8.0	34.0	1.5	0	590	2.0
mushroom, wild:							
(*Casbah*), ¼ cup . .	220	9.0	35.0	0	0	420	3.0
(*Marrakesh Express*)	190	8.0	38.0	0	0	310	1.0

Food and Measure	cal.	prot. (gms)	carbo. (gms)	fat (gms)	chol. (mgs)	sod. (mgs)	fiber (gms)
and herb (*Near East*)	230	8.0	42.0	4.0	10	610	3.0
nutted, w/currants and spice (*Casbah*), ¼ cup	240	8.0	42.0	1.5	0	420	3.0
olive garlic (*Marrakesh Express*)	170	6.0	34.0	1.0	0	400	1.0
onion, toasted (*Marrakesh Express Grand*)	250	8.0	52.0	1.0	0	620	2.0
Parmesan:							
(*Near East*)	220	8.0	41.0	4.0	10	550	2.0
(*Nile Spice*), 1 pkg.	200	8.0	34.0	3.0	10	570	2.0
pilaf (*Casbah*), ¾ cup	220	8.0	40.0	.5	0	480	.5
pine nut, toasted (*Near East*)	230	7.0	40.0	6.0	0	450	2.0
red pepper, roasted (*Marrakesh Express Grand*)	250	8.0	52.0	.5	0	690	2.0
sesame ginger (*Marrakesh Express*)	180	7.0	36.0	1.0	0	350	0
sun-dried tomato:							
(*Marrakesh Express*)	190	8.0	36.0	1.0	0	230	1.0
(*Marrakesh Express Grande*)	250	8.0	51.0	1.0	0	630	2.0
tomato lentil (*Near East*)	220	8.0	42.0	3.5	0	650	3.0
vegetable (*Marrakesh Express Lucky 7*)	190	7.0	38.0	.5	0	300	1.0
***Cousins Subs*:**							
cold subs, 7½":							
BLT	613	17.0	45.0	42.0	35	917	1.0
chicken salad	569	25.0	61.0	26.0	51	1081	3.0
club sub	744	43.0	48.0	43.0	107	2004	2.0
ham/cheese	644	28.0	47.0	39.0	67	1333	2.0
provolone	685	25.0	46.0	45.0	63	957	2.0
roast beef	618	33.0	46.0	34.0	75	883	1.0
seafood w/crab	554	15.0	53.0	32.0	20	957	1.0
tuna	832	28.0	46.0	60.0	67	939	1.0
turkey breast	559	25.0	48.0	32.0	50	1493	1.0
veggie	365	20.0	49.0	11.0	30	661	2.0
hot subs, 7½":							
cheese steak	540	36.0	46.0	24.0	80	1126	1.0
cheese steak, double	851	61.0	46.0	46.0	160	1593	1.0
cheese steak, Philly	680	42.0	50.0	36.0	100	1250	1.0

Food and Measure	cal.	prot. (gms)	carbo. (gms)	fat (gms)	chol. (mgs)	sod. (mgs)	fiber (gms)
Cousins Subs, hot subs *(cont.)*							
chicken breast	618	35.0	46.0	34.0	73	1172	1.0
gyro	680	31.0	55.0	40.0	58	1539	2.0
Italian sausage	478	22.0	50.0	22.0	50	1227	3.0
meatball/cheese ...	586	36.0	50.0	27.0	80	1386	2.0
pepperoni melt ...	784	33.0	47.0	52.0	102	1803	2.0
veggie	491	25.0	49.0	23.0	50	1100	2.0
Italian subs, 7½":							
cappacolla/Genoa ..	630	23.0	48.0	40.0	64	1680	1.0
cappacolla/cheese .	637	28.0	48.0	39.0	60	1420	1.0
Genoa/cheese	730	29.0	48.0	49.0	83	1678	1.0
Italian regular	683	28.0	48.0	44.0	75	1722	1.0
Italian special	797	36.0	48.0	53.0	107	2168	1.0
mini subs, 4":							
chicken salad	319	14.0	37.0	13.0	26	601	2.0
ham/cheese	382	15.0	30.0	23.0	35	738	1.0
Italian special	431	18.0	31.0	27.0	49	1089	1.0
meatball/cheese ...	329	22.0	32.0	14.0	40	756	1.0
provolone	422	15.0	30.0	27.0	38	597	1.0
seafood w/crab ...	311	9.0	33.0	16.0	10	538	1.0
tuna	476	15.0	30.0	33.0	35	541	1.0
turkey breast	347	15.0	31.0	19.0	30	890	1.0
hot dog	300	12.0	29.0	16.0	15	830	0
french fries:							
large	525	7.0	72.0	24.0	21	460	1.0
medium	400	5.0	55.0	19.0	16	350	1.0
small	275	4.0	38.0	14.0	11	240	1.0
soup, regular:							
cheese	240	7.0	18.0	16.0	20	1350	2.0
cheese broccoli ...	192	6.0	15.0	12.0	15	940	3.0
clam chowder	190	8.0	19.0	5.0	10	1060	3.0
chicken dumpling .	170	11.0	19.0	5.0	50	970	3.0
chicken wild rice ..	230	10.0	21.0	12.0	30	1210	2.0
chili	250	18.0	26.0	9.0	35	1220	14.0
potato, cream of ..	190	5.0	24.0	9.0	5	860	3.0
soup, large:							
cheese	360	11.0	27.0	24.0	30	2025	3.0
cheese broccoli ...	285	9.0	23.0	18.0	23	1410	5.0
clam chowder	225	12.0	29.0	8.0	15	1590	5.0
chicken dumpling .	255	17.0	29.0	8.0	75	1455	5.0
chicken wild rice ..	345	15.0	32.0	18.0	45	1815	3.0
chili	375	27.0	39.0	14.0	53	1830	21.0
potato, cream of ..	285	8.0	36.0	14.0	8	1290	5.0
chocolate chip cookie	210	2.0	25.0	11.0	10	115	1.0

Food and Measure	cal.	prot. (gms)	carbo. (gms)	fat (gms)	chol. (mgs)	sod. (mgs)	fiber (gms)
Cowpeas, fresh, ½ cup:							
raw:							
immature seeds ...	65	2.1	13.7	.3	0	3	3.6
leafy tips, chopped	5	.7	.9	<.1	0	1	n.a.
pods, w/seeds	21	1.6	4.5	.1	0	2	n.a.
boiled, drained:							
immature seeds ...	80	2.6	16.8	.3	0	3	4.1
leafy tips, chopped	6	1.2	.7	0	0	2	n.a.
pods, w/seeds	16	1.2	3.3	.1	0	1	n.a.
Cowpeas, canned or frozen, see "Black-eyed peas"							
Cowpeas, catjang, see "Catjang"							
Crab, meat only, 4 oz.:							
Alaska king:							
raw	95	20.8	0	.7	47	948	0
boiled, poached, or steamed	110	21.9	0	1.7	60	1216	0
blue:							
raw	99	20.5	.1	1.2	89	332	0
boiled, poached, or steamed	116	22.9	0	2.0	113	316	0
Dungeness:							
raw	98	19.8	.8	1.1	67	335	0
boiled, poached, or steamed	125	25.3	1.1	1.4	86	429	0
queen:							
raw	102	21.0	0	1.4	62	611	0
boiled, poached, or steamed	130	26.9	0	1.7	81	784	0
Crab, canned, 2 oz., except as noted:							
(*Bumble Bee* Fancy Lump)	40	8.0	0	1.0	50	300	0
(*Chicken of the Sea* Fancy)	40	7.0	1.0	0	50	400	0
(*Orleans* Fancy White)	28	6.0	1.0	0	43	403	0
(*Reese*), ½ cup	45	10.0	0	.5	55	370	0
blue, 4 oz.	112	23.3	0	1.4	101	378	0
lump (*Chicken of the Sea*)	35	7.0	1.0	.5	50	400	0

Food and Measure	cal.	prot. (gms)	carbo. (gms)	fat (gms)	chol. (mgs)	sod. (mgs)	fiber (gms)
Crab, canned *(cont.)*							
white *(Chicken of the Sea)*	30	7.0	1.0	0	50	400	0
white lump *(Crown Prince Natural)*	45	10.0	1.0	0	50	210	1.0
"Crab," imitation, frozen:							
chunk or flakes *(Louis Kemp Crab Delights)*, ½ cup, 3 oz.	80	8.0	11.0	0	10	470	0
leg style *(Louis Kemp Crab Delights)*, ½ cup, 3 oz.	80	8.0	11.0	0	10	470	0
shreds *(Louis Kemp)*, ½ cup, 3 oz.	80	7.0	10.0	0	5	620	0
from surimi, 1 oz.	29	3.4	3.0	.4	6	238	0
Crab apple, fresh:							
(Frieda's), 5 oz.	110	1.0	28.0	0	0	0	0
1 oz.	22	.1	5.7	.1	0	<1	n.a.
sliced, ½ cup	42	.2	11.0	.2	0	1	n.a.
Crab cake, see "Crab dish"							
Crab cake seasoning *(Old Bay Classic)*, ⅙ pkg.	30	0	2.0	1.0	0	290	0
Crab dip mix, dry *(Watkins)*, 1 tsp.	10	0	2.0	0	0	140	0
Crab dish, frozen:							
cakes, 1 pc.:							
(Chesapeake Bay)	60	7.0	7.0	.5	15	360	<1.0
(Fisher Boy)	110	8.0	11.0	4.0	25	330	0
(Van de Kamp's)	190	6.0	20.0	9.0	20	560	0
deviled *(Mrs. Paul's)*	180	6.0	20.0	10.0	20	440	0
lightly breaded *(Chincoteague Maryland Style)*, 4 oz.	280	14.0	28.0	12.0	80	910	3.0
unbreaded *(Chincoteague Maryland Style)*	170	12.0	8.0	9.0	85	310	0
cakes, mini:							
(Van de Kamp's), 4 pcs.	260	9.0	31.0	12.0	35	890	1.0

Food and Measure	cal.	prot. (gms)	carbo. (gms)	fat (gms)	chol. (mgs)	sod. (mgs	fiber (gms)
deviled (*Mrs. Paul's*), 6 pcs.	220	7.0	22.0	12.0	15	480	0
nuggets:							
lightly breaded (*Chincoteague* Cocktail), 3 oz.	210	11.0	21.0	9.0	60	680	2.0
unbreaded (*Chincoteague* Cocktail), 6 pcs., 3 oz. . . .	180	13.0	8.0	10.0	90	340	0
poppers, cheese and (*Mrs. Paul's/Van de Kamp's* Bites), 4 pcs., 4 oz.	320	17.0	27.0	16.0	35	800	<1.0
Cracker:							
bacon (*Nabisco* Flavor Crisps), 15 pcs. . .	160	3.0	19.0	8.0	0	460	0
(*Barbara's* Rite Lite Rounds), 5 pcs., .5 oz.	55	1.0	12.0	<1.0	0	150	0
butter/butter flavor:							
(*Goya*), .25-oz. pc.	30	1.0	5.0	0	0	50	0
(*Harvest Bakery* Country), 2 pcs., .6 oz.	70	1.0	9.0	3.5	0	110	0
(*Hi Ho*), 4 pcs., .5 oz.	70	1.0	8.0	4.0	0	130	<1.0
(*Hi Ho* Reduced Fat), 5 pcs., .5 oz. . . .	70	1.0	10.0	2.5	0	140	<1.0
(*Keebler Club*), 4 pcs., .5 oz. . . .	70	1.0	9.0	3.0	0	160	0
(*Keebler Club* Reduced Fat), 5 pcs., .6 oz. . . .	70	1.0	12.0	2.0	0	200	0
(*Keebler Club* Reduced Sodium), 4 pcs., .5 oz. . . .	70	1.0	9.0	3.0	0	80	0
(*Pepperidge Farm*), 4 pcs., .5 oz. . . .	70	1.0	10.0	3.0	10	95	0
(*Ritz*), 5 pcs., .6 oz.	80	1.0	10.0	4.0	0	135	0
(*Ritz* Low Sodium), 5 pcs., .6 oz.	80	1.0	10.0	4.0	0	35	0
(*Ritz* Mini), 34 pcs., 1.1 oz.	150	1.0	19.0	8.0	0	260	<1.0

Food and Measure	cal.	prot. (gms)	carbo. (gms)	fat (gms)	chol. (mgs)	sod. (mgs)	fiber (gms)
Cracker, butter/butter flavor *(cont.)*							
(*Ritz* Reduced Fat), 5 pcs., .6 oz. . . .	70	1.0	11.0	2.0	0	140	0
(*Ritz Air Crisps*), 24 pcs., 1 oz. . .	140	2.0	22.0	5.0	0	240	<1.0
(*Town House*), 5 pcs., .6 oz. . . .	80	1.0	9.0	4.5	0	150	<1.0
(*Town House* Low Salt), 5 pcs., .6 oz.	80	1.0	10.0	4.5	0	75	<1.0
(*Town House* Reduced Fat), 6 pcs., .5 oz.	70	1.0	11.0	2.0	0	180	<1.0
w/cheese (*Ritz*), 1.4-oz. pkg. . . .	200	2.0	22.0	11.0	<56	400	<1.0
crisp (*Toasteds*), 5 pcs., .6 oz. . . .	80	<1.0	10.0	3.5	0	150	0
w/peanut butter (*Ritz*), 1.4-oz. pkg.	190	3.0	24.0	9.0	0	370	1.0
cheddar:							
(*Better Cheddars*), 22 pcs., 1.1 oz.	150	3.0	17.0	8.0	5	290	<1.0
(*Better Cheddars* Low Sodium), 22 pcs., 1.1 oz.	150	3.0	18.0	7.0	5	75	<1.0
(*Better Cheddars* Reduced Fat), 24 pcs., 1.1 oz.	140	4.0	19.0	6.0	5	350	<1.0
(*Cheese Nips* Reduced Fat), 31 pcs., 1.1 oz.	130	3.0	21.0	3.5	0	310	<1.0
(*Combos*), 1 oz. . .	140	2.0	18.0	6.0	0	290	0
(*Combos*), 1.7-oz. bag	240	3.0	31.0	11.0	0	490	1.0
(*Goldfish*), 55 pcs., 1.1 oz.	140	4.0	19.0	6.0	10	250	<1.0
(*Munch'ems*), 39 pcs., 1.1 oz.	140	3.0	19.0	6.0	<5	370	1.0
(*Ritz* Mini), 33 pcs., 1.1 oz.	150	2.0	19.0	7.0	0	340	<1.0
(*Snax Stix*), 20 pcs., 1 oz.	130	2.0	20.0	4.5	0	280	<1.0
(*Sportz*), 40 pcs., 1.1 oz.	150	3.0	19.0	7.0	0	260	<1.0

Food and Measure	cal.	prot. (gms)	carbo. (gms)	fat (gms)	chol. (mgs)	sod. (mgs)	fiber (gms)
extra (*Cheese Nips*), 27 pcs., 1.1 oz.	140	3.0	19.0	6.0	<1	350	<1.0
extra (*Goldfish Flavor Blaster*), 51 pcs., 1.1 oz.	150	3.0	19.0	6.0	<5	250	<1.0
golden (*Hain* Bites), 22 pcs., 1.1 oz.	120	3.0	23.0	1.5	0	460	1.0
mild (*Krispy*), 5 pcs., .5 oz.	60	2.0	10.0	2.0	0	180	<1.0
white (*Cheez-It*), 26 pcs., 1.1 oz.	150	3.0	18.0	7.0	<5	280	<1.0
white (*Goldfish*), 58 pcs., 1.1 oz.	150	3.0	18.0	7.0	<5	270	<1.0
white (*Hain* Bites), 22 pcs., 1.1 oz.	120	3.0	23.0	1.5	0	440	1.0
cheese:							
(*Barbara's* Bites), 26 pcs., 1.1 oz.	120	3.0	24.0	1.5	0	290	1.0
(*BIG Cheez-It*), 13 pcs., 1 oz. . .	150	4.0	16.0	8.0	0	230	<1.0
(*Cheez-It*), 27 pcs., 1.1 oz.	160	4.0	16.0	8.0	0	240	<1.0
(*Cheez-It* Mini), 44 pcs., 1 oz. . .	140	5.0	13.0	7.0	0	230	<1.0
(*Cheez-It* Reduced Fat), 29 pcs., 1.1 oz.	140	4.0	20.0	4.5	0	280	<1.0
(*Cheese Nips*), 29 pcs., 1.1 oz.	150	3.0	18.0	6.0	0	310	<1.0
(*Cheese Nips* Reduced Fat), 31 pcs., 1.1 oz.	130	3.0	21.0	3.5	0	310	<1.0
(*Cheese Nips* Air Crisps), 32 pcs., 1.1 oz.	130	3.0	21.0	4.0	<5	300	<1.0
(*Pepperidge Farm*), 2 pcs., .6 oz. . . .	80	2.0	8.0	4.0	<5	180	0
(*SnackWell's* Zesty), 38 pcs., 1.1 oz.	130	2.0	23.0	3.0	0	320	<1.0
(*Tid-Bit*), 32 pcs., 1.1 oz.	160	2.0	16.0	9.0	0	360	<1.0
hot, spicy (*Cheez-It*), 26 pcs., 1.1 oz.	150	4.0	17.0	8.0	0	300	<1.0

Food and Measure	cal.	prot. (gms)	carbo. (gms)	fat (gms)	chol. (mgs)	sod. (mgs)	fiber (gms)
Cracker, cheese *(cont.)*							
Parmesan *(Goldfish)*, 60 pcs., 1.1 oz.	140	4.0	19.0	5.0	0	300	1.0
pizza *(Cheese Nips)*, 29 pcs., 1.1 oz.	140	3.0	19.0	6.0	0	330	<1.0
and sesame *(Twigs)*, 15 pcs., 1.1 oz.	150	4.0	17.0	7.0	0	300	1.0
Swiss *(Nabisco* Flavor Crisps), 15 pcs., 1.1 oz.	140	2.0	18.0	7.0	0	350	1.0
cheese sandwich, 1 pkg., except as noted:							
(Chee•tos Golden Toast)	240	4.0	25.0	14.0	5	440	1.0
(Keebler Club Bite Size), 14 pcs., 1.1 oz.	160	2.0	17.0	9.0	<5	300	<1.0
(Ritz Bits), 14 pcs., 1.1 oz.	170	2.0	17.0	10.0	5	300	0
bacon *(Chee•tos)* ..	190	3.0	25.0	9.0	<5	410	1.0
cheddar *(Chee•tos)*	210	3.0	23.0	11.0	<5	390	1.0
cheddar *(Keebler Club)*	190	3.0	20.0	11.0	10	320	<1.0
cheddar, toast *(Nabisco)*	200	4.0	23.0	10.0	5	300	<1.0
cheddar, wheat *(Keebler)*	160	3.0	17.0	9.0	5	310	<1.0
jalapeño *(Doritos)*	230	3.0	26.0	13.0	<5	450	1.0
nacho *(Doritos Cheesier)*	240	4.0	25.0	14.0	<5	390	1.0
peanut butter *(Keebler)*	190	4.0	23.0	10.0	0	290	1.0
peanut butter *(Planters)*	190	4.0	22.0	10.0	0	370	1.0
peanut butter *(Peter Pan)*	210	6.0	23.0	10.0	0	350	1.0
chicken flavor *(Chicken in a Biskit)*, 12 pcs., 1.1 oz. ...	160	2.0	17.0	9.0	0	270	<1.0
corn bread *(Harvest Bakery)*, 2 pcs., .6 oz.	70	1.0	11.0	2.5	5	100	0

Food and Measure	cal.	prot. (gms)	carbo. (gms)	fat (gms)	chol. (mgs)	sod. (mgs)	fiber (gms)
croissant (*Carr's*), 3 pcs., .5 oz.	70	1.0	10.0	3.0	<5	115	0
garlic, roasted (*Health Valley*), 6 pcs., .5 oz.	60	2.0	10.0	1.5	0	140	1.0
(*Goldfish* Original), 55 pcs., 1.1 oz. ...	140	3.0	19.0	6.0	0	230	<1.0
(*Goya*), .3-oz. pc. ...	40	1.0	6.0	1.0	0	80	0
graham cracker, see "Cookie"							
herb:							
(*Hain*), 11 pcs., 1.1 oz.	110	3.0	23.0	0	0	190	1.0
garden (*Health Valley*), 6 pcs. .5 oz.	60	2.0	10.0	1.5	0	140	1.0
garden, whole wheat (*Triscuit*), 6 pcs., 1 oz.	130	3.0	20.0	4.5	0	130	3.0
Italian (*Harvest Crisp*), 13 pcs., 1 oz.	130	3.0	22.0	3.5	0	320	1.0
lavasch:							
(*Cedar's* Giant), 1 oz.	40	3.0	5.0	0	0	200	0
soy, all varieties (*Tofutti*), .5 oz.	60	3.0	10.0	1.0	0	57	1.0
matzo:							
(*Manischewitz* Everything!), 1-oz. pc.	110	3.0	22.0	.5	0	150	1.0
(*Manischewitz* No Salt), 1-oz. pc. ..	110	3.0	24.0	0	0	0	0
(*Manischewitz* Tam Tam), 10 pcs., 1.1 oz.	140	3.0	22.0	4.0	10	100	<1.0
garlic, savory (*Manischewitz*), 1-oz. pc.	100	3.0	23.0	0	0	200	1.0
tea thins (*Manischewitz*), .9-oz. pc.	100	3.0	22.0	0	0	0	0
whole wheat (*Manischewitz*), 1-oz. pc.	110	4.0	22.0	.5	0	0	4.0

Food and Measure	cal.	prot. (gms)	carbo. (gms)	fat (gms)	chol. (mgs)	sod. (mgs)	fiber (gms)
Cracker *(cont.)*							
multigrain:							
(*Harvest Bakery*),							
2 pcs., .6 oz.	70	1.0	10.0	2.5	0	80	<1.0
(*Harvest Crisps*),							
13 pcs., 1.1 oz.	130	3.0	23.0	3.5	0	270	1.0
7 (*Wheatables*),							
12 pcs., 1.1 oz.	140	2.0	20.0	6.0	0	250	1.0
(*Munch'ems* Original),							
41 pcs., 1.1 oz. ...	140	2.0	21.0	5.0	0	220	1.0
nori maki (*Eden*),							
15 pcs., 1.1 oz. ...	110	3.0	24.0	0	0	160	2.0
onion (*Toasteds*),							
5 pcs., .6 oz.	80	1.0	10.0	3.0	0	150	0
onion, French:							
(*Health Valley*),							
10 pcs., .5 oz. ..	60	2.0	10.0	1.5	0	140	1.0
(*SnackWell's*),							
38 pcs., 1.1 oz.	130	2.0	23.0	3.0	0	270	<1.0
whole wheat (*Triscuit Thin Crisps*),							
14 pcs., 1.1 oz.	130	3.0	20.0	4.5	0	160	3.0
peanut butter sandwich:							
(*Keebler Club* Bite Size), 14 pcs., 1.1 oz.	150	3.0	18.0	8.0	0	270	<1.0
(*Ritz Bits*), 14 pcs., 1.1 oz.	150	3.0	18.0	8.0	0	200	1.0
cheese, see "cheese sandwich," above							
toast (*Keebler*), 1 pkg.	190	4.0	23.0	10.0	0	290	1.0
toast (*Peter Pan*), 1 pkg.	210	5.0	23.0	11.0	0	280	<1.0
toast (*Planters*), 1.4-oz. pkg. ...	190	4.0	23.0	10.0	0	330	1.0
pepper, cracked:							
(*Health Valley*), 5 pcs., .5 oz. ...	60	2.0	10.0	1.5	0	140	1.0
(*SnackWell's*), 5 pcs., .5 oz. ...	60	1.0	10.0	1.5	0	115	0
pizza flavor:							
(*Goldfish*), 55 pcs., 1.1 oz.	140	3.0	19.0	6.0	0	160	1.0

Food and Measure	cal.	prot. (gms)	carbo. (gms)	fat (gms)	chol. (mgs)	sod. (mgs)	fiber (gms)
(*Sportz*) 39 pcs. . . .	150	3.0	19.0	7.0	0	230	0
poppy, savory (*Barbara's* Rite Lite), 5 pcs., .5 oz.	70	<1.0	11.0	2.0	0	135	0
potato:							
barbecue (*Air Crisps*), 22 pcs., 1 oz. . .	120	2.0	21.0	3.5	0	220	2.0
sour cream/onion (*Air Crisps*), 1 oz.	120	1.0	21.0	3.5	0	300	1.0
ranch, 1.1 oz.:							
(*Munch'ems*), 40 pcs.	140	3.0	20.0	5.0	0	260	1.0
(*Wheat Thins*), 14 pcs.	150	2.0	19.0	7.0	0	390	1.0
(*Wheat Thins Air Crisps*), 23 pcs.	130	2.0	21.0	4.5	0	300	<1.0
rice, brown:							
(*Eden*), 5 pcs., 1.1 oz.	120	3.0	22.0	2.0	0	230	2.0
seaweed (*Eden* Nori Maki), 15 pcs., 1.1 oz.	110	3.0	24.0	0	0	160	2.0
sesame (*San-J*), 5 pcs., 1 oz. . . .	130	3.0	19.0	5.0	0	170	1.0
sesame, black (*San-J*), 5 pcs., 1 oz.	140	4.0	17.0	6.0	0	180	1.0
tamari (*San-J*), 6 pcs., 1.1 oz. . .	120	3.0	26.0	1.0	0	170	1.0
rice bran (*Health Valley*), 6 pcs., 1 oz.	110	3.0	19.0	3.0	0	70	3.0
rice wafer, 7 pcs., .5 oz.: brown (*Westbrae Natural* No Salt)	50	1.0	11.0	.5	0	0	0
brown, onion garlic (*Westbrae Natural*)	50	1.0	11.0	0	0	55	0
5-spice or tamari (*Westbrae Natural*)	50	1.0	11.0	0	0	65	0
sesame (*Westbrae Natural*)	50	1.0	11.0	0	0	70	0
rye, whole wheat (*Triscuit*), 7 pcs., 1.1 oz.	140	3.0	22.0	5.0	0	170	4.0

Food and Measure	cal.	prot. (gms)	carbo. (gms)	fat (gms)	chol. (mgs)	sod. (mgs)	fiber (gms)
Cracker *(cont.)*							
saltine, 5 pcs., .5 oz.:							
(*Hain*)	60	2.0	13.0	0	0	130	0
(*Krispy*)	60	2.0	10.0	1.5	0	180	<1.0
(*Krispy* Fat Free)	50	1.0	11.0	0	0	150	0
(*Krispy* Unsalted Top)	60	2.0	10.0	1.5	0	120	<1.0
(*Premium*)	60	1.0	10.0	1.5	0	180	0
(*Premium* Fat Free)	60	2.0	12.0	0	0	200	0
(*Premium* Low Sodium)	60	1.0	10.0	1.5	0	35	0
(*Premium* Unsalted Top)	60	1.0	10.0	1.5	0	105	0
(*Zesta*)	60	1.0	10.0	2.0	0	190	<1.0
(*Zesta* Fat Free)	50	1.0	11.0	0	0	150	0
(*Zesta* Low Salt)	70	1.0	11.0	2.0	0	95	<1.0
(*Zesta* Unsalted Top)	70	1.0	10.0	2.0	0	90	<1.0
sesame:							
(*Hain*), 11 pcs., 1.1 oz.	140	3.0	19.0	6.0	0	170	1.0
(*Health Valley*), 5 pcs., .5 oz.	60	2.0	10.0	1.5	0	140	1.0
(*Toasteds*), 5 pcs., .6 oz.	80	<1.0	10.0	4.0	0	135	<1.0
tamari (*Barbara's* Rite Lite Rounds), 5 pcs., .5 oz.	70	1.0	12.0	2.0	0	160	0
sesame sticks, spelt:							
Cajun (*VitaSpelt*), 21 pcs., 1.1 oz.	160	5.0	14.0	10.0	0	160	2.0
garlic (*VitaSpelt*), 28 pcs., 1.1 oz.	170	5.0	13.0	11.0	0	230	3.0
salted (*VitaSpelt*), 28 pcs., 1.1 oz.	150	5.0	13.0	9.0	0	210	2.0
sour cream/onion (*VitaSpelt*), 22 pcs., 1.1 oz.	150	5.0	14.0	8.0	0	170	5.0
(*Snax Stix* Original), 21 pcs., 1 oz.	130	2.0	17.0	5.0	0	320	<1.0
(*Sociables*), 7 pcs., .5 oz.	80	1.0	9.0	4.0	0	150	0
soda/water:							
(*Crown Pilot*), .6-oz. pc.	70	2.0	13.0	1.5	0	85	0

Food and Measure	cal.	prot. (gms)	carbo. (gms)	fat (gms)	chol. (mgs)	sod. (mgs)	fiber (gms)
(*Royal Lunch*), .4-oz. pc.	60	<1.0	8.0	2.0	0	70	0
cracked pepper (*Carr's*), 5 pcs., .6 oz.	70	2.0	13.0	1.5	0	100	<1.0
poppy-sesame seeds (*Carr's*), 4 pcs., .6 oz. . . .	80	2.0	9.0	5.0	<5	135	<1.0
roasted garlic/herbs (*Carr's*), 5 pcs., .6 oz.	70	2.0	13.0	1.5	0	140	<1.0
soup/oyster, .5 oz.:							
(*Hain*), 36 pcs. . . .	60	2.0	13.0	0	0	130	0
(*Krispy*), 17 pcs.	60	2.0	11.0	1.5	0	200	<1.0
(*Premium*), 23 pcs.	60	1.0	11.0	1.5	0	230	0
(*Zesta*), 45 pcs. . .	70	1.0	9.0	3.0	0	220	0
sour cream/onion:							
(*Munch'ems*), 28 pcs., 1.1 oz.	140	3.0	20.0	5.0	0	280	1.0
(*Ritz* Mini), 33 pcs., 1.1 oz.	150	1.0	19.0	8.0	0	280	<1.0
(*Uneeda* Biscuit), 2 pcs., .5 oz. . . .	60	1.0	11.0	1.5	0	110	0
vegetable:							
(*Hain*), 11 pcs., 1.1 oz.	140	3.0	19.0	6.0	0	230	1.0
(*Health Valley* Bruschetta), 6 pcs. .5 oz. . . .	60	2.0	10.0	1.5	0	140	1.0
(*Health Valley* Bruschetta No Salt), 6 pcs. .5 oz. . . .	60	2.0	10.0	1.5	0	40	1.0
(*Vegetable Thins*), 14 pcs., 1.1 oz.	160	2.0	19.0	9.0	0	310	1.0
garden (*Harvest Crisps*), 15 pcs., 1.1 oz.	130	2.0	22.0	3.5	0	230	1.0
wheat:							
(*Pepperidge Farm*), 3 pcs., .6 oz. . . .	80	2.0	10.0	3.5	0	100	1.0
(*SnackWell's*), 5 pcs., .5 oz.	70	1.0	11.0	1.5	0	150	<1.0
(*Snax Stix*), 20 pcs., 1.1 oz.	130	2.0	18.0	5.0	0	260	<1.0

Food and Measure	cal.	prot. (gms)	carbo. (gms)	fat (gms)	chol. (mgs)	sod. (mgs)	fiber (gms)
Cracker, wheat *(cont.)*							
(*Toasteds*), 5 pcs., .6 oz.	80	1.0	10.0	3.0	0	150	<1.0
(*Toasteds* Reduced Fat), 5 pcs., .5 oz.	60	1.0	10.0	2.0	0	160	<1.0
(*Waverly*), 5 pcs., .5 oz.	70	1.0	10.0	3.0	0	135	0
(*Wheat Thins* Big), 11 pcs., 1.1 oz.	140	3.0	20.0	6.0	0	260	1.0
(*Wheat Thins* Low Sodium), 16 pcs., 1.1 oz.	140	2.0	20.0	6.0	0	75	2.0
(*Wheat Thins* Multigrain), 17 pcs., 1.1 oz.	130	2.0	21.0	4.5	0	290	2.0
(*Wheat Thins* Original 10 oz.), 16 pcs., .8 oz.	140	2.0	19.0	6.0	0	260	1.0
(*Wheat Thins* Original 1 lb.), 16 pcs., .8 oz.	150	2.0	21.0	6.0	0	270	1.0
(*Wheat Thins* Reduced Fat), 16 pcs., 1 oz.	130	2.0	21.0	4.0	0	260	1.0
(*Wheat Thins Air Crisps*), 24 pcs., 1.1 oz.	130	2.0	21.0	4.5	0	290	1.0
(*Wheatables*), 12 pcs., 1.1 oz.	140	2.0	19.0	6.0	0	210	1.0
(*Wheatables* Reduced Fat), 13 pcs., 1.1 oz.	130	2.0	21.0	4.0	0	230	2.0
(*Wheatsworth*), 5 pcs., .6 oz.	80	2.0	10.0	3.5	0	170	1.0
all varieties (*Barbara's Wheatines*), .5-oz. sq.	50	1.0	10.0	1.5	0	110	1.0
honey (*Wheatables*), 12 pcs., 1.1 oz.	140	2.0	20.0	6.0	0	200	1.0
savory (*Monterey*), 3 pcs., .5 oz.	70	1.0	9.0	2.5	0	95	<1.0
sesame (*Breton*), 3 pcs., .5 oz.	60	2.0	7.0	3.0	0	100	0

Food and Measure	cal.	prot. (gms)	carbo. (gms)	fat (gms)	chol. (mgs)	sod. (mgs)	fiber (gms)
stoned (*Health Valley*), 5 pcs., .5 oz.	60	2.0	10.0	1.0	0	140	1.0
stoned (*Red Oval Farms* Thins), 2 pcs.	60	2.0	10.0	1.5	0	140	<1.0
stoned, cracked wheat (*Red Oval Farms*), 4 pcs., .6 oz.	70	1.0	10.0	2.5	0	190	<1.0
wheat, whole:							
(*Hain*), 11 pcs., 1.1 oz.	110	3.0	24.0	0	0	190	1.0
(*Hain* Rich), 11 pcs., 1.1 oz.	130	3.0	18.0	6.0	0	135	1.0
(*Health Valley*), 5 pcs., .5 oz.	60	2.0	10.0	1.5	0	140	2.0
(*Krispy*), 5 pcs., .5 oz.	60	2.0	10.0	1.5	0	130	<1.0
(*Ritz*), 5 pcs., .6 oz.	70	1.0	11.0	2.5	0	120	<1.0
(*Triscuit* Original), 7 pcs., 1.1 oz.	140	3.0	22.0	5.0	0	170	4.0
(*Triscuit* Reduced Fat), 8 pcs., 1.2 oz.	130	3.0	24.0	3.0	0	170	4.0
(*Triscuit* Thin Crisps), 15 pcs., 1.1 oz.	130	3.0	21.0	5.0	0	170	3.0
zwieback (*Nabisco*), 1 pc., .3 oz.	35	1.0	6.0	1.0	0	10	0
Cracker crumbs/meal:							
crumbs:							
(*Ritz*), ⅓ cup	140	2.0	17.0	7.0	0	270	1.0
saltine (*Premium* Fat Free), ¼ cup	100	3.0	23.0	0	0	0	1.0
meal, ¼ cup:							
(*Golden Dipt*)	130	2.0	23.0	1.0	0	10	0
(*Nabisco*)	110	3.0	22.0	0	0	15	<1.0
matzo (*Manischewitz*)	130	3.0	28.0	.5	0	0	1.0
matzo (*Streit's*)	110	3.0	24.0	.5	0	0	1.0
Cranberry, fresh, ½ cup:							
(*Dole*)	23	0	6.0	0	0	1	6.0

Food and Measure	cal.	prot. (gms)	carbo. (gms)	fat (gms)	chol. (mgs)	sod. (mgs)	fiber (gms)
Cranberry, fresh *(cont.)*							
(*Ocean Spray*)	30	0	7.0	0	0	0	0
whole	23	.2	6.0	.1	0	1	2.0
chopped	27	.2	7.0	.1	0	1	2.3
Cranberry, can or jar, see "Cranberry fruit blend" and "Cranberry sauce"							
Cranberry, dried, ⅓ cup, 1.4 oz.:							
(*Craisins*)	130	0	33.0	0	0	0	2.0
(*Frieda's*)	120	0	28.0	0	0	0	3.0
(*Setton Farm*)	130	0	33.0	0	0	0	2.0
(*Sonoma*)	120	0	29.0	0	0	0	2.0
(*Sunsweet Fruitlings*) .	140	0	34.0	0	0	0	2.0
cherry flavor (*Craisins*)	130	0	34.0	0	0	0	2.0
orange flavor:							
(*Craisins*)	130	0	33.0	0	0	0	2.0
(*Setton Farm*)	130	0	33.0	0	0	6	2.0
(*Sunsweet Fruitlings*)	120	1.0	31.0	0	0	0	3.0
Cranberry bean:							
boiled, ½ cup	120	8.2	21.5	.4	0	1	3.0
canned, ½ cup	108	7.2	19.7	.4	0	431	n.a.
Cranberry drink, 8 fl. oz., except as noted:							
(*Langers* Diet)	30	0	9.0	0	0	10	0
(*Snapple* Twist)	100	0	26.0	0	0	10	0
cocktail:							
(*Dole*)	140	0	34.0	0	0	35	0
(*Dole*), 10 fl. oz. . . .	160	1.0	40.0	0	0	15	0
(*Dole*), 11.5 fl. oz.	200	0	49.0	0	0	50	0
(*Langers*)	140	0	35.0	0	0	10	0
(*Ocean Spray*)	140	0	34.0	0	0	35	0
(*Ocean Spray* Plus)	160	0	41.0	0	0	35	0
(*Ocean Spray* Light-style)	40	0	10.0	0	0	75	0
(*Season's Best*) . . .	140	0	34.0	0	0	35	0
cocktail, frozen*:							
(*Welch's*)	140	0	36.0	0	0	0	0
(*Welch's* Light) . . .	50	0	13.0	0	0	5	0
white (*Ocean Spray*) .	120	0	29.0	0	0	35	0

Food and Measure	cal.	prot. (gms)	carbo. (gms)	fat (gms)	chol. (mgs)	sod. (mgs)	fiber (gms)
Cranberry drink blends, 8 fl. oz.:							
(*Cran•Cherry*)	160	0	39.0	0	0	35	0
(*Cran•Currant*)	140	0	33.0	0	0	35	0
(*Cran•Mango*)	130	0	33.0	0	0	35	0
(*Cran•Mango Lightstyle*)	40	0	10.0	0	0	75	0
(*Cran•Strawberry*) ...	140	0	36.0	0	0	35	1.0
(*Cran•Tangerine*)	130	0	33.0	0	0	35	0
(*Langers* Caribbean)	135	0	34.0	0	0	10	0
(*Santa Cruz Organic* Nectar)	110	<1.0	27.0	0	0	25	0
apple:							
(*Cranapple*)	160	0	41.0	0	0	35	1.0
(*Langers* Fuji)	160	0	39.0	0	0	10	0
berry (*Langers*)	135	0	34.0	0	0	10	0
concentrate* (*R. W. Knudsen*)	65	0	13.0	0	0	10	0
grape:							
(*Cran•Grape*)	170	0	41.0	0	0	35	0
(*Cran•Grape Lightstyle*)	40	0	10.0	0	0	75	0
(*Dole*)	170	0	41.0	0	0	10	0
(*Langers*)	165	0	41.0	0	0	10	0
(*Season's Best*) ...	170	0	41.0	0	0	10	0
hibiscus (*R. W. Knudsen*)	120	<1.0	30.0	0	0	35	0
orange (*Langers*)	130	0	33.0	0	0	10	0
raspberry:							
(*Cran•Raspberry*) .	140	0	36.0	0	0	35	0
(*Cran•Raspberry Lightstyle*)	40	0	10.0	0	0	75	0
(*Langers*)	150	0	36.0	0	0	10	0
(*Langers* Diet)	30	0	9.0	0	0	10	0
(*R. W. Knudsen*) ..	140	0	36.0	0	0	35	0
(*Snapple*)	120	0	29.0	0	0	10	0
Cranberry fruit blend, orange or raspberry (*Cran•Fruit* for Chicken), ¼ cup ..	120	0	29.0	0	0	35	1.0
Cranberry juice, 8 fl. oz., except as noted:							
(*Langers*)	140	0	35.0	0	0	15	0

Food and Measure	cal.	prot. (gms)	carbo. (gms)	fat (gms)	chol. (mgs)	sod. (mgs)	fiber (gms)
Cranberry juice *(cont.)*							
(*R. W. Knudsen* Just Cranberry)	60	<1.0	14.0	0	0	25	0
Cranberry juice blends, 8 fl. oz., except as noted:							
(*After the Fall* Cape Cod)	100	0	24.0	0	0	20	0
(*Apple & Eve Naturally Cranberry*)	120	1.0	30.0	0	0	20	.5
(*Cranberry Echinacea*), 16 fl. oz.	230	1.0	57.0	0	0	25	0
(*Season's Best* Medley)	120	<1.0	29.0	0	0	20	0
apple (*Ocean Spray* Granny Smith)	130	0	32.0	0	0	35	0
berry (*Langers*)	135	0	34.0	0	0	10	0
grape:							
(*Langers*)	150	0	38.0	0	0	15	0
(*Ocean Spray* Concord)	150	0	39.0	0	0	35	0
grapefruit (*After the Fall Ruby of the Cape*)	110	1.0	29.0	0	0	10	0
kiwi (*After the Fall Ruby of the Cape*)	100	1.0	26.0	0	0	18	0
lime, Key (*Ocean Spray*)	140	0	35.0	0	0	35	0
nectar (*R. W. Knudsen*)	150	<1.0	38.0	0	0	45	0
orange (*After the Fall Ruby of the Cape*)	110	1.0	28.0	0	0	15	0
peach, Georgia:							
(*After the Fall*)	100	1.0	27.0	0	0	20	0
(*Ocean Spray*)	140	0	35.0	0	0	35	0
raspberry:							
(*After the Fall*)	90	1.0	23.0	0	0	20	0
(*Langers*)	145	0	35.0	0	0	15	0
(*Ocean Spray* Pacific)	140	0	34.0	0	0	35	0
raspberry grape (*Nantucket Nectars*)	150	0	38.0	0	0	45	0
strawberry (*After the Fall Ruby of the Cape*)	100	1.0	26.0	0	0	15	0

Food and Measure	cal.	prot. (gms)	carbo. (gms)	fat (gms)	chol. (mgs)	sod. (mgs)	fiber (gms)
Cranberry juice cocktail, see "Cranberry drink"							
Cranberry relish, ¼ cup:							
(*Country Sides*)	200	1.0	43.0	4.0	0	0	1.0
orange (*New England*)	120	0	31.0	0	0	0	0
Cranberry sauce, ¼ cup, except as noted:							
(*Kraft*), .5 oz. pkt. . . .	25	0	6.0	0	0	0	0
(*Marzetti* Homestyle Refrigerated)	100	0	25.0	0	0	0	1.0
(*R. W. Knudsen*), 1 tbsp.	25	0	6.0	0	0	0	0
whole (*Ocean Spray*)	110	0	28.0	0	0	35	1.0
whole or jellied (*S&W*)	100	0	26.0	0	0	15	1.0
jellied (*Ocean Spray*)	110	0	27.0	0	0	35	1.0
Crawfish, frozen, tail meat, cooked (*Ecrevisse Acadienne USA*), 3 oz.	90	13.0	<1.0	4.0	100	580	<1.0
Crayfish, mixed species:							
farmed, meat only:							
raw, 4 oz.	82	16.8	0	1.1	122	70	0
raw, 8 pcs., .95 oz.	19	4.0	0	.3	29	17	0
boiled or steamed, 4 oz.	99	19.9	0	1.5	155	110	0
wild, meat only:							
raw, 4 oz.	87	18.1	0	1.1	129	66	0
raw, 8 pcs., .95 oz.	21	4.3	0	.3	31	16	0
boiled or steamed, 4 oz.	93	19.0	0	1.4	151	107	0
Cream:							
all purpose (*Hood*), 1 tbsp.	45	0	<1.0	4.5	20	5	0
clotted (*The Devon Cream Company*), 2 tbsp.	150	0	<1.0	17.0	50	5	0
half-and-half:							
(*Darigold*), 2 tbsp.	40	1.0	1.0	3.0	15	15	0
(*Hood*), 2 tbsp. . .	40	1.0	1.0	3.5	15	20	0

Food and Measure	cal.	prot. (gms)	carbo. (gms)	fat (gms)	chol. (mgs)	sod. (mgs)	fiber (gms)
Cream, half-and-half *(cont.)*							
1 cup	315	7.2	10.4	27.8	89	98	0
1 tbsp.	20	.4	.6	1.7	6	6	0
light, coffee or table:							
(*Hood*), 1 tbsp. . .	30	0	<1.0	3.0	10	10	0
1 cup	469	6.5	8.8	46.3	159	95	0
1 tbsp.	29	.4	.6	2.9	10	6	0
medium (25% fat):							
1 cup	583	5.9	8.3	59.8	209	88	0
1 tbsp.	37	.4	.5	3.8	13	6	0
sour, see "Cream, sour"							
whipped topping, see							
"Cream topping"							
whipping[1], light:							
1 cup	699	5.2	7.1	73.9	265	82	0
1 tbsp.	44	.3	.4	4.6	17	5	0
whipping[1], heavy:							
(*Darigold*), 1 tbsp. . .	50	0	1.0	6.0	20	0	0
(*Darigold* Ultra-pasteurized),							
1 tbsp.	50	0	1.0	5.0	20	0	0
(*Hood*), 1 tbsp. . . .	50	0	0	5.0	20	0	0
1 cup	821	4.9	6.6	88.1	326	89	0
1 tbsp.	52	.3	.4	5.6	21	6	0
Cream, sour, 2 tbsp., except as noted:							
(*Breakstone's*)	60	<1.0	1.0	5.0	20	10	0
(*Crowley*)	70	1.0	1.0	7.0	30	15	0
(*Friendship*)	60	1.0	1.0	5.0	20	15	0
(*Hood*)	60	1.0	2.0	5.0	20	20	0
(*Knudsen Hampshire*)	60	<1.0	1.0	6.0	25	15	0
(*Land O Lakes*)	60	1.0	2.0	6.0	15	15	0
1 cup	493	7.3	9.8	48.2	102	123	0
light:							
(*Breakstone's* Reduced Fat)	45	1.0	2.0	3.5	15	20	0
(*Crowley*)	60	1.0	2.0	5.0	20	15	0
(*Friendship*)	40	1.0	3.0	2.5	10	25	0
(*Hood*)	40	1.0	2.0	2.5	5	20	0
(*Knudsen Light*) . .	40	2.0	2.0	2.5	10	20	0
(*Land O Lakes*) . . .	35	1.0	4.0	2.0	10	30	0

1. Unwhipped, volume approximately doubled when whipped.

Food and Measure	cal.	prot. (gms)	carbo. (gms)	fat (gms)	chol. (mgs)	sod. (mgs)	fiber (gms)
nonfat:							
(Breakstone's Free)	35	1.0	6.0	0	<5	25	0
(Crowley)	25	1.0	4.0	0	0	50	0
(Friendship)	25	2.0	4.0	0	0	20	0
(Hood)	25	1.0	4.0	0	0	25	0
(Knudsen Free) ...	30	2.0	5.0	0	<5	25	0
(Land O Lakes) ...	30	1.0	5.0	0	<5	40	0
Cream, sour, flavored, 2 tbsp.:							
roasted garlic (Friendship)	60	1.0	2.0	5.0	20	130	0
onion (Crowley)	60	1.0	2.0	5.0	20	140	0
salsa (Friendship) ...	50	1.0	2.0	4.0	15	120	0
"Cream," sour, non-dairy (Tofutti Sour Supreme), 2 tbsp.	50	1.0	1.0	5.0	0	120	0
Cream, sour, powder (AlpineAire), 2 oz.	310	13.0	20.0	20.0	80	200	0
Cream cheese dip, see "Fruit dip"							
Cream of tartar, 1 tsp.	7	0	1.9	0	0	2	0
Cream topping, 2 tbsp.:							
(Cool Whip)	25	0	2.0	1.5	0	0	0
(Cool Whip Extra Creamy)	25	0	2.0	2.0	0	5	0
(Cool Whip Free)	15	0	3.0	0	0	5	0
(Cool Whip Lite)	20	0	3.0	1.0	0	0	0
(Crowley Real)	25	0	2.0	2.0	5	0	0
(Kraft Dairy Whip) ...	10	0	<1.0	1.0	<5	0	0
(Reddi-wip Original)	20	0	<1.0	2.0	5	0	0
(Reddi-wip Extra Creamy)	30	0	<1.0	3.0	10	0	0
(Reddi-wip Fat Free)	10	0	2.0	0	0	0	0
(Reddi-wip Light) ...	15	<1.0	2.0	1.0	<5	0	0
(Reddi-wip Nondairy)	20	0	2.0	1.5	0	5	0
chocolate (Reddi-wip)	20	0	2.0	1.5	<5	0	0
Cream topping mix (Dream Whip), 1/16 pkt.	10	0	2.0	0	0	0	0
Creamer, nondairy:							
fluid, 1 tbsp.:							
(Coffee-Mate)	20	0	2.0	1.0	0	0	0
(Coffee-Mate Fat Free)	10	0	2.0	0	0	0	0

Food and Measure	cal.	prot. (gms)	carbo. (gms)	fat (gms)	chol. (mgs)	sod. (mgs)	fiber (gms)
Creamer, fluid *(cont.)*							
(*Coffee-Mate* Low Fat)	10	0	1.0	.5	0	5	0
(*Silk*)	15	0	1.0	1.0	0	5	0
(*WestSoy* Lite)	10	0	2.0	0	0	10	0
(*WestSoy* Crème de la Soy)	20	0	2.0	1.5	0	0	0
powder, 1 tsp.							
(*Coffee-Mate*)	10	0	1.0	.5	0	0	0
(*Coffee-Mate* Fat Free/Lite)	10	0	2.0	0	0	0	0
(*Cremora*)	15	0	2.0	.5	0	10	0
(*Cremora* Fat Free)	10	0	2.0	0	0	5	0
(*Cremora* Lite)	10	0	2.0	0	0	0	0
(*Cremora* Royale)	15	0	1.0	1.0	0	10	0
Creamer, flavored, nondairy:							
fluid, 1 tbsp.:							
all flavors (*Coffee-Mate* Fat Free) ..	25	0	5.0	0	0	0	0
all flavors, except chocolate raspberry (*Coffee-Mate*)	40	0	5.0	2.0	0	5	0
amaretto (*WestSoy* Crème de la Soy)	25	0	4.0	1.0	0	0	0
chocolate raspberry (*Coffee-Mate*) ..	40	0	5.0	2.0	0	10	0
vanilla (*Silk*)	20	0	3.0	1.0	0	5	0
vanilla, French (*WestSoy* Crème de la Soy)	25	0	3.0	1.0	0	0	0
powder, 4 tsp.:							
all flavors, except Swiss chocolate (*Coffee-Mate*) ..	60	0	9.0	3.0	0	15	0
chocolate, Swiss (*Coffee-Mate*) ..	50	0	10.0	1.0	0	25	0
chocolate, Swiss (*Coffee-Mate* Fat Free)	50	0	10.0	0	0	25	0
hazelnut or French vanilla (*Coffee-Mate* Fat Free) ..	50	0	11.0	0	0	15	0

Food and Measure	cal.	prot. (gms)	carbo. (gms)	fat (gms)	chol. (mgs)	sod. (mgs)	fiber (gms)
Crème fraîche (Santè), 2 tbsp.	100	<1.0	<1.0	11.0	40	10	0
Creole seasoning (McCormick), ¼ tsp.	0	0	0	0	0	150	0
Crepes (Frieda's), 2 pcs., .8 oz.	50	1.0	9.0	1.0	5	90	0
Cress, garden, ½ cup:							
raw	8	.7	1.4	.2	0	4	.3
boiled, drained	16	1.3	2.6	.4	0	5	.5
Cress, water, see "Watercress"							
Croaker, meat only, raw, Atlantic, 4 oz.	119	20.2	0	3.6	69	63	0
Croissant, 1 pc.:							
(Viola), 2.75 oz.	290	4.0	30.0	17.0	0	340	0
butter:							
(Awrey's), 1 oz. ...	80	2.0	10.0	4.0	10	140	0
(Awrey's), 1.5 oz. .	120	3.0	15.0	5.0	10	210	<1.0
(Awrey's), 2 oz. ...	170	4.0	19.0	8.0	25	250	<1.0
(Awrey's), 3 oz. ...	250	6.0	29.0	13.0	35	370	<1.0
1-oz. pc.	115	2.3	13.0	6.0	19	211	.7
apple, 2-oz. pc.	144	4.2	21.0	4.9	18	155	1.4
cheese, 1.5-oz. pc. ..	174	3.9	19.7	8.8	24	233	1.1
margarine, sandwich:							
(Awrey's), 1.5 oz.	130	3.0	15.0	6.0	0	115	<1.0
(Awrey's), 2 oz. ...	170	4.0	19.0	8.0	0	150	<1.0
(Awrey's), 2.5 oz.	210	5.0	24.0	11.0	0	190	<1.0
Croissant, frozen:							
French style (Sara Lee), 1 pc.	170	4.0	20.0	8.0	<5	200	1.0
French style, petite (Sara Lee), 2 pcs.	230	6.0	26.0	11.0	<5	260	1.0
Crookneck squash:							
baby (Frieda's), ⅔ cup, 3 oz.	15	1.0	3.0	0	0	0	1.0
sliced, ½ cup:							
raw, ends trimmed .	12	.6	2.6	.2	0	1	.7
boiled, drained	18	.8	3.9	.3	0	1	1.3
Crookneck squash, canned, cut, drained, no salt, ½ cup	14	.7	3.2	.1	0	5	1.1

Food and Measure	cal.	prot. (gms)	carbo. (gms)	fat (gms)	chol. (mgs)	sod. (mgs)	fiber (gms)
Crookneck squash, frozen, boiled, sliced, ½ cup	24	1.2	5.3	.2	0	6	1.2
Croutons (see also "Salad toppers"), 2 tbsp. or ¼ cup, except as noted:							
buttermilk ranch (*Pepperidge Farm*), 6 pcs., .3 oz.	30	<1.0	5.0	1.0	0	80	0
Caesar:							
(*Brownberry* Homestyle)	30	1.0	5.0	1.5	0	85	1.0
(*Chatham Village*)	35	1.0	4.0	1.5	0	60	0
(*Pepperidge Farm*), 6 pcs., .3 oz. . . .	35	1.0	4.0	1.5	0	90	0
(*Pepperidge Farm* Fat Free), 6 pcs., .3 oz.	30	1.0	5.0	0	0	80	0
(*Reese* Salad)	30	1.0	5.0	1.0	0	90	0
cheddar (*Reese*)	30	1.0	5.0	1.0	0	85	0
cheese, sourdough (*Brownberry* Homestyle)	30	<1.0	5.0	1.0	0	100	0
cheese and garlic:							
(*Chatham Village*)	40	1.0	3.0	2.5	0	55	0
(*Pepperidge Farm*), 9 pcs., .3 oz. . . .	30	1.0	4.0	1.5	0	80	0
garden herb (*Chatham Village*)	35	1.0	4.0	1.5	0	60	0
garlic, roasted (*Pepperidge Farm*), 6 pcs., .3 oz.	30	<1.0	5.0	1.0	0	90	0
garlic and butter (*Chatham Village*)	35	1.0	4.0	1.5	0	55	0
garlic herb (*Brownberry* Homestyle) . .	30	1.0	5.0	1.0	0	80	<1.0
garlic and onion (*Chatham Village* Fat Free)	25	1.0	6.0	0	0	50	0
Italian:							
(*Arnold* Classic) . . .	30	1.0	5.0	1.5	0	85	1.0

Food and Measure	cal.	prot. (gms)	carbo. (gms)	fat (gms)	chol. (mgs)	sod. (mgs	fiber (gms)
spicy (*Pepperidge Farm* Fat Free), 6 pcs., .3 oz.	30	1.0	5.0	0	0	90	0
zesty (*Arnold/ Brownberry* Homestyle)	30	<1.0	5.0	1.0	0	70	0
onion and garlic:							
(*Brownberry* Homestyle)	30	1.0	5.0	1.0	0	75	<1.0
(*Pepperidge Farm*), 9 pcs., .3 oz. ...	30	<1.0	5.0	1.5	0	80	0
(*Reese*)	30	1.0	5.0	1.0	0	115	0
seasoned:							
(*Arnold* Classic) ..	30	1.0	5.0	1.0	0	75	<1.0
(*Brownberry* Homestyle)	30	1.0	5.0	1.0	0	75	<1.0
(*Pepperidge Farm*), 9 pcs., .3 oz. ...	35	1.0	4.0	1.5	0	85	0
(*Reese*)	30	<1.0	5.0	1.0	0	105	0
sun-dried tomato (*Chatham Village* Fat Free)	30	1.0	5.0	0	0	80	0
Cucumber, w/peel:							
1 medium, 8¼" long .	38	2.1	8.3	.4	0	6	2.4
sliced, ½ cup	7	.4	1.4	.1	0	1	.4
Cucumber, Japanese (*Frieda's* Hothouse), ⅔ cup, 3 oz.	10	1.0	2.0	0	0	0	1.0
Cucumber, pickled, see "Pickles"							
Cucumber-dill dip mix (*Watkins*), 1 tsp. ..	10	0	2.0	0	0	230	0
Cucuzza squash (*Frieda's*), ¾ cup, 3 oz.	10	1.0	3.0	0	0	0	0
Cumin seed, ground:							
1 tsp.	8	.4	.9	.5	0	4	.2
Cupcake, see "Cake, snack"							
Currants:							
fresh, ½ cup:							
black, Europe	36	.8	8.6	.2	0	1	3.0
red or white	31	.8	7.7	.1	0	1	2.4

Food and Measure	cal.	prot. (gms)	carbo. (gms)	fat (gms)	chol. (mgs)	sod. (mgs)	fiber (gms)
Currants, dried *(cont.)*							
dried, Zante:							
(*Sun•Maid*), ¼ cup,							
1.4 oz.	130	1.0	31.0	0	0	10	2.0
½ cup	204	2.9	53.3	.2	0	6	4.9
Curry, vegetable, see "Vegetable dish, can or jar"							
Curry paste (see also "Curry sauce base"):							
hot:							
(*Patak's*), 2 tbsp.	160	1.0	4.0	16.0	0	1130	0
(*Patak's* Garam Masala), 2 tsp.	130	1.0	4.0	12.0	0	1080	0
(*Patak's* Kashmiri Masala), 1 tsp.	15	<1.0	<1.0	1.0	0	270	0
(*Patak's* Madras), 2 tbsp.	160	1.0	4.0	16.0	0	1010	0
(*Patak's* Vindaloo), 2 tbsp.	160	1.0	4.0	16.0	0	1020	0
medium, 2 tbsp.:							
(*Patak's* Balti)	115	2.0	6.0	10.0	0	640	<1.0
(*Patak's* Biryani Paste)	170	1.0	3.0	17.0	0	920	0
(*Patak's* Tikka Masala)	110	1.0	5.0	9.0	0	700	<1.0
mild (*Patak's*), 2 tbsp.	170	1.0	5.0	16.0	0	900	0
red (*Thai Kitchen*), 1 tbsp.	10	0	2.0	0	0	140	0
Curry powder:							
1 tbsp.	20	.8	3.7	.9	0	3	1.0
1 tsp.	6	.3	1.2	.3	0	1	.3
Curry oil, see "Oil"							
Curry sauce, cooking (see also "Thai sauce"), ½ cup:							
chili, hot:							
w/coriander (*Patak's* Vindaloo)	320	3.0	15.0	28.0	0	790	1.0
w/cumin (*Patak's* Madras 10 oz.)	280	3.0	15.0	23.0	0	770	1.0
w/cumin (*Patak's* Madras 15 oz.)	140	2.0	13.0	9.0	0	550	1.0

Food and Measure	cal.	prot. (gms)	carbo. (gms)	fat (gms)	chol. (mgs)	sod. (mgs)	fiber (gms)
coconut, rich creamy:							
mild (*Patak's* Korma 10 oz.)	210	4.0	11.0	17.0	0	670	2.0
mild (*Patak's* Korma 15 oz.)	110	2.0	11.0	6.0	0	520	1.0
coriander and lemon, tangy, medium:							
(*Patak's* Tikka Masala 10 oz.) . .	210	3.0	13.0	16.0	0	1030	2.0
(*Patak's* Tikka Masala 15 oz.) . .	110	2.0	13.0	6.0	0	760	1.0
sweet peppers and coconut, hot (*Patak's* Jalfrezi) . .	140	2.0	12.0	9.0	0	340	2.0
tomato:							
rich, mild (*Patak's* Dopiaza)	110	2.0	13.0	5.0	0	800	1.0
spicy, and cardamom (*Patak's* Rogan Josh 10 oz.) . . .	180	2.0	12.0	13.0	0	840	1.0
spicy, and cardamon (*Patrak's* Rogan Josh 15 oz.) . . .	110	2.0	12.0	6.0	0	600	1.0
Curry sauce base (see also "Curry paste"), 1 tsp.:							
green (*A Taste of Thai*)	15	0	1.0	1.5	0	200	1.0
Mussaman (*A Taste of Thai*)	20	0	1.0	1.5	0	170	0
Panang (*A Taste of Thai*)	25	0	2.0	2.0	0	170	0
red (*A Taste of Thai*) .	20	0	1.0	1.5	0	260	0
yellow (*A Taste of Thai*)	30	0	1.0	3.0	0	135	1.0
Curry seasoning mix, dinner (see also "Thai sauce"), 3.5 fl. oz.:							
green (*A Taste of Thai* Kit Lite)	90	1.0	6.0	7.0	0	930	0
Panang (*A Taste of Thai* Kit Lite)	110	1.0	7.0	8.0	0	700	0
red (*A Taste of Thai* Kit Lite)	90	1.0	6.0	7.0	0	980	0

Food and Measure	cal.	prot. (gms)	carbo. (gms)	fat (gms)	chol. (mgs)	sod. (mgs)	fiber (gms)
Curry seasoning mix *(cont.)*							
Mussaman (*A Taste of Thai* Kit Lite)	100	1.0	7.0	6.0	0	900	2.0
yellow (*A Taste of Thai* Kit Lite)	110	1.0	6.0	9.0	0	840	1.0
Cusk, meat only:							
raw, 4 oz.	99	21.6	0	.8	47	36	0
baked, broiled, or microwaved, 4 oz.	127	27.6	0	1.0	60	45	0
Custard, see "Pudding"							
Custard apple, trimmed, 1 oz.	29	.5	7.1	.2	0	1	1.0
Custard marrow, see "Chayote"							
Cuttlefish, meat only, 4 oz.:							
raw	90	18.4	.9	.8	127	422	0
boiled or steamed	179	36.8	1.9	1.6	254	844	0
Cuttlefish, canned, in ink (*Goya*), ¼ cup	120	8.0	2.0	9.0	15	350	0

D

Food and Measure	cal.	prot. (gms)	carbo. (gms)	fat (gms)	chol. (mgs)	sod. (mgs)	fiber (gms)
Daikon, see "Radish, Oriental"							
Dahl, see "Lentil dish mix"							
Daiquiri mixer:							
(*Trader Vic's* Hawaiian), 4 fl. oz.	170	0	42.0	0	0	20	0
strawberry (*Mr & Mrs T*), 3.5 fl. oz.	150	0	34.0	0	0	20	0
Daiquiri mixer, frozen (*Bacardi*), 2 fl. oz.	120	0	33.0	0	0	0	0
Dairy Queen/Brazier, 1 serving:							
burger/sandwiches:							
chicken, grilled . . .	310	24.0	30.0	10.0	50	1040	3.0
chicken breast fillet	430	24.0	37.0	20.0	55	760	2.0
chili 'n' cheese dog	330	14.0	22.0	21.0	45	1090	2.0
DQ Homestyle:							
cheeseburger . . .	340	20.0	29.0	17.0	55	850	2.0
cheeseburger, double	540	35.0	30.0	31.0	115	1130	2.0
cheeseburger, double, bacon	610	41.0	31.0	36.0	130	1380	2.0
hamburger	290	17.0	29.0	12.0	45	630	2.0
DQ Ultimate	670	40.0	29.0	43.0	135	1210	2.0
hot dog	240	9.0	19.0	14.0	25	730	1.0
Chicken Strip Basket	1000	35.0	102.0	50.0	55	2260	5.0
The Great Steakmelt basket	770	32.0	72.0	38.0	75	2290	5.0
side dishes:							
fries, medium	440	5.0	53.0	23.0	0	1110	4.0
fries, small	350	4.0	42.0	18.0	0	880	3.0
onion rings	320	5.0	39.0	16.0	0	180	3.0

Food and Measure	cal.	prot. (gms)	carbo. (gms)	fat (gms)	chol. (mgs)	sod. (mgs)	fiber (gms)
Dairy Queen/Brazier, side dishes *(cont.)*							
desserts and shakes:							
banana split	510	8.0	96.0	12.0	30	180	3.0
Blizzard, medium:							
chocolate chip							
cookie dough	950	17.0	143.0	36.0	75	660	1.0
chocolate sand-							
wich cookie . .	640	12.0	97.0	23.0	45	500	1.0
Blizzard, small:							
chocolate chip							
cookie dough	660	12.0	99.0	24.0	55	440	1.0
chocolate sand-							
wich cookie . .	520	10.0	79.0	18.0	40	380	1.0
Breeze yogurt:							
Heath, medium	710	15.0	123.0	18.0	20	580	1.0
Heath, small . . .	470	11.0	85.0	10.0	10	380	1.0
strawberry,							
medium	460	13.0	99.0	1.0	10	270	1.0
strawberry, small	320	10.0	68.0	.5	5	190	1.0
Buster Bar	450	10.0	41.0	28.0	15	280	2.0
Chocolate Dilly	210	3.0	21.0	13.0	10	75	0
cone, chocolate:							
DQ soft, ½ cup	150	4.0	22.0	5.0	15	75	0
medium	340	8.0	53.0	11.0	30	160	0
small	240	6.0	37.0	8.0	20	115	0
cone, dipped:							
medium	490	8.0	59.0	24.0	30	190	1.0
small	340	6.0	42.0	17.0	20	130	1.0
cone, vanilla:							
DQ soft, ½ cup	140	3.0	22.0	4.5	15	70	0
large	410	10.0	65.0	12.0	40	200	0
medium	330	8.0	53.0	9.0	30	160	0
small	230	6.0	38.0	7.0	20	115	0
DQ cake, ⅛ cake:							
frozen	370	7.0	56.0	13.0	25	280	<1.0
layered	330	6.0	49.0	12.0	15	350	0
DQ fudge bar	50	4.0	13.0	0	0	70	0
DQ sandwich	200	4.0	31.0	6.0	10	140	1.0
DQ Treatzza Pizza:							
Heath, ⅛ pizza . .	180	3.0	28.0	7.0	5	160	1.0
M&M's, ⅛ pizza	190	3.0	29.0	7.0	5	160	1.0
DQ vanilla orange							
bar	60	2.0	.17.0	0	0	40	0

Food and Measure	cal.	prot. (gms)	carbo. (gms)	fat (gms)	chol. (mgs)	sod. (mgs)	fiber (gms)
hot chocolate, frozen	860	14.0	127.0	35.0	50	350	3.0
Lemon DQ Freez'r, ½ cup	80	0	20.0	0	0	10	0
malt, chocolate:							
medium	880	19.0	153.0	22.0	70	500	0
small	650	15.0	111.0	16.0	55	370	0
Misty slush:							
medium	290	0	74.0	0	0	30	0
small	220	0	56.0	0	0	20	0
Peanut Buster parfait	730	16.0	99.0	31.0	35	400	2.0
Pecan Mudslide	650	11.0	85.0	30.0	35	420	2.0
shake, chocolate:							
medium	770	17.0	130.0	20.0	70	420	0
small	560	13.0	94.0	15.0	50	310	0
S'Mores Galore	730	11.0	111.0	30.0	30	340	3.0
Starkiss	80	0	21.0	0	0	10	0
strawberry short-cake	430	7.0	70.0	14.0	60	360	1.0
sundae, chocolate:							
medium	400	8.0	71.0	10.0	30	210	0
small	280	5.0	49.0	7.0	20	140	0
yogurt, frozen:							
cone, medium	260	9.0	56.0	1.0	5	160	0
cup, medium	230	8.0	48.0	.5	5	150	0
DQ nonfat, ½ cup	100	3.0	21.0	0	<5	70	0
yogurt sundae, strawberry, medium	280	8.0	61.0	.5	5	160	1.0
Dandelion greens:							
raw:							
(Frieda's), 2 cups, 3 oz.	40	2.0	8.0	0	0	65	3.0
½ cup chopped, 1 oz.	13	.8	2.6	.2	0	22	1.0
boiled, drained, chopped, ½ cup	17	1.0	3.3	.3	0	23	1.5
Danish, 1 pc.:							
all varieties (Awrey's Petite), 1.5 oz.	160	3.0	21.0	7.0	5	150	<1.0
apple:							
(Awrey's), 2.75 oz.	290	5.0	38.0	13.0	10	270	<1.0

Food and Measure	cal.	prot. (gms)	carbo. (gms)	fat (gms)	chol. (mgs)	sod. (mgs)	fiber (gms)
Danish, apple *(cont.)*							
(*Awrey's* Grande),							
4.5 oz.	470	4.0	51.0	28.0	20	370	1.0
(*Gourmet*), 2.5 oz.	240	3.0	46.0	12.0	10	210	<1.0
cheese:							
(*Awrey's*), 2.75 oz.	290	5.0	38.0	13	10	270	<1.0
(*Awrey's* Grande),							
4.5 oz.	470	4.0	51.0	28.0	20	370	1.0
(*Entenmann's*)	170	5.0	34.0	19.0	55	300	<1.0
(*Gourmet*), 2.5 oz.	250	4.0	46.0	12.0	10	210	<1.0
(*Sara Lee*), 4.75 oz.	520	8.0	54.0	30.0	35	650	3.0
cinnamon:							
(*Awrey's* Grande),							
4.5 oz.	480	8.0	68.0	19.0	20	620	n.a.
roll (*Awrey's* Home-							
style), 3 oz.	270	4.0	45.0	9.0	10	240	1.0
swirl (*Awrey's*),							
2.75 oz.	300	5.0	42.0	12.0	10	380	<1.0
swirl (*Awrey's*							
Grande), 3.75 oz.	400	7.0	57.0	16.0	14	520	2.0
raspberry cheese swirl							
(*Awrey's* Grande),							
3.75 oz.	360	5.0	44.0	18.0	20	260	1.0
strawberry:							
(*Awrey's*), 2.75 oz.	290	5.0	38.0	13.0	10	270	<1.0
(*Awrey's* Grande),							
4.5 oz.	470	4.0	51.0	28.0	20	370	1.0
Danish, frozen, crumb							
(*Sara Lee*), 1 pc. . .	370	5.0	41.0	15.0	40	300	1.0
Danish cake, see							
"Cake"							
Dasheen, see "Taro"							
Date, dried:							
(*Dole*), 5–6 pcs.	120	1.0	31.0	0	0	0	3.0
(*Frieda's* Medjool),							
2–3 pcs., 1.4 oz. . .	120	1.0	31.0	0	0	0	3.0
(*Setton Farm*), 1.4 oz.	120	1.0	31.0	0	0	0	3.0
(*Sonoma* Organic),							
5 pcs., 1.4 oz.	110	1.0	30.0	0	0	15	5.0
(*Sunsweet*), ¼ cup . .	120	1.0	32.0	0	0	0	3.0
10 pcs. , 2.9 oz.	228	1.6	61.0	.4	0	2	6.2
chopped:							
(*Dole*), 1 oz.	120	1.0	33.0	0	0	10	3.0

Food and Measure	cal.	prot. (gms)	carbo. (gms)	fat (gms)	chol. (mgs)	sod. (mgs)	fiber (gms)
(*Sunsweet*), ¼ cup	120	1.0	32.0	0	0	0	3.0
pitted, ½ cup	245	1.8	65.4	.5	0	3	6.7
Delicata squash							
(*Frieda's*), ¾ cup,							
3 oz.	30	1.0	7.0	0	0	0	1.0
Denny's, general menu,							
1 serving:							
breakfast dishes, no							
bread or syrup:							
All American Slam	712	38.0	9.0	62.0	686	1281	1.0
Big Texas Chicken							
Fajita Skillet	1217	49.0	25.0	70.0	518	1817	8.0
Breakfast Dagwood	1251	75.0	35.0	90.0	802	3597	1.0
Cinnamon Swirl							
Slam	1105	38.0	68.0	78.0	635	1374	2.0
country fried steak							
and eggs	430	22.0	9.0	36.0	440	861	4.0
eggs Benedict	695	34.0	34.0	46.0	515	1718	1.0
Farmer's Slam	1200	51.0	82.0	80.0	704	3204	3.0
French Slam	1029	44.0	58.0	71.0	777	1428	2.0
French toast, 2 . . .	507	16.0	54.0	24.0	219	594	3.0
French toast, cin-							
namon swirl	1030	23.0	124.0	49.0	280	675	4.0
Grand Slam							
Slugger	789	32.0	58.0	46.0	487	1438	2.0
grits, 4 oz.	80	2.0	18.0	0	0	520	0
ham 'n cheddar							
omelette	581	37.0	4.0	45.0	672	1180	0
hash browns	218	2.0	20.0	14.0	0	424	2.0
covered	318	9.0	21.0	23.0	30	604	2.0
covered,							
smothered . . .	359	9.0	26.0	26.0	30	790	2.0
covered,							
smothered,							
double	460	12.0	48.0	26.0	30	1213	5.0
hotcakes, plain, 3 . .	491	12.0	95.0	7.0	0	1818	3.0
Lumberjack Slam . .	1259	54.0	118.0	70.0	481	4028	5.0
Meat Lover's Skillet	1147	41.0	24.0	93.0	460	2507	7.0
Moons Over My							
Hammy	922	54.0	42.0	59.0	581	2810	2.0
oatmeal 'n' fixins . .	460	13.0	95.0	6.0	11	87	7.0
Original Grand Slam	795	34.0	65.0	50.0	460	2237	2.0
sirloin steak and							
eggs	622	43.0	1.0	49.0	572	632	1.0

Food and Measure	cal.	prot. (gms)	carbo. (gms)	fat (gms)	chol. (mgs)	sod. (mgs)	fiber (gms)
Denny's, breakfast dishes *(cont.)*							
Slim Slam	495	34.0	98.0	12.0	34	1746	1.0
T-bone steak and							
eggs	991	73.0	1.0	77.0	657	1003	1.0
tortillas and salsa ..	281	6.0	50.5	8.0	0	1031	4.0
Ultimate Omelette	564	30.0	9.0	47.0	639	939	2.0
veggie-cheese							
omelette	480	26.0	9.0	39.0	644	535	2.0
waffle, plain, 1	304	7.0	23.0	21.0	146	200	0
breakfast items:							
bacon, 4 strips ...	162	12.0	1.0	18.0	36	640	0
bagel, dry	235	9.0	46.0	1.0	0	495	0
biscuit, buttered ...	272	5.0	39.0	11.0	0	790	0
biscuit and sausage							
gravy	398	8.0	45.0	21.0	12	1267	0
cream cheese, 1 oz.	100	2.0	1.0	10.0	31	90	0
egg, 1	120	6.0	1.0	10.0	210	120	0
egg breakfast, 2 ...	825	31.0	24.0	67.0	538	1765	2.0
Egg Beaters	71	5.0	1.0	5.0	1.0	138	0
English muffin, dry	125	5.0	24.0	1.0	0	198	1.0
ham, grilled sliced	94	15.0	2.0	3.0	23	761	0
margarine, whipped	87	0	0	10.0	0	117	0
oatmeal, *Quaker* ...	100	5.0	18.0	2.0	0	175	3.0
potatoes, country							
fried	515	3.0	23.0	35.0	8	805	9.0
sausage, 4 links ...	354	16.0	0	32.0	64	944	0
sausage gravy	126	3.0	6.0	10.0	12	477	0
syrup, 1.5 oz.:							
blueberry	102	0	26.0	0	0	15	0
maple flavor	143	0	36.0	0	0	26	0
maple flavor, no							
sugar	23	0	9.0	0	0	71	0
strawberry	91	0	23.0	0	0	36	0
toast, dry, 1 slice ..	90	3.0	17.0	1.0	0	166	1.0
topping, 3 oz.:							
blueberry	106	0	26.0	0	0	15	0
cherry	86	0	21.0	0	0	5	0
strawberry	115	1.0	26.0	1.0	0	12	1.0
whipped cream ...	23	0	2.0	2.0	7	3	0
sandwiches:							
bacon/lettuce/							
tomato	634	18.0	37.0	46.0	54	1116	2.0
burger:							
bacon cheddar ..	875	53.0	58.0	52.0	163	1672	5.0

Food and Measure	cal.	prot. (gms)	carbo. (gms)	fat (gms)	chol. (mgs)	sod. (mgs	fiber (gms)
big Texas BBQ ..	929	53.0	53.0	58.0	163	2271	3.0
Boca Burger	616	29.0	66.0	28.0	14	861	10.0
chicken	632	35.0	53.0	32.0	81	1967	4.0
chicken, Buffalo	803	37.0	67.0	45.0	77	2143	5.0
classic	673	37.0	42.0	40.0	106	1142	3.0
classic w/cheese	836	47.0	43.0	53.0	137	1595	3.0
classic double decker	1377	62.0	81.0	92.0	210	2209	7.0
garlic mushroom Swiss	872	48.0	58.0	51.0	116	1529	5.0
chicken, grilled ...	520	35.0	64.0	14.0	77	1613	3.0
club	718	32.0	62.0	38.0	75	1666	3.0
ham/Swiss, rye ...	533	23.0	40.0	31.0	36	1638	5.0
Reuben	580	27.0	37.0	35.0	69	2726	5.0
The Super Bird ...	620	35.0	48.0	32.0	60	1880	2.0
turkey, multigrain ..	476	23.0	39.0	26.0	57	1107	5.0
soup, 8 oz.:							
broccoli, cream of	193	4.0	15.0	12.0	0	818	2.0
chicken noodle ...	60	2.0	8.0	2.0	10	640	0
clam chowder	214	5.0	22.0	11.0	5	903	1.0
potato, cream of ..	222	4.0	23.0	12.0	0	761	2.0
vegetable beef	79	6.0	11.0	1.0	5	820	2.0
chili w/cheese, 11 oz.	401	26.0	21.0	19.0	57	1039	7.0
appetizers, w/out condiments:							
cheese fries, chili ..	816	29.0	77.0	44.0	74	917	3.0
cheese fries, smothered	767	27.0	69.0	48.0	78	875	0
chicken strips, 5 ..	720	47.0	56.0	33.0	95	1666	0
chicken strips, Buffalo, 5	734	48.0	43.0	42.0	96	1673	0
Buffalo wings, 12 ..	856	92.0	1.0	54.0	500	5552	1.0
Sampler	1405	47.0	124.0	80.0	75	5305	4.0
entree, w/out sides:							
Charleston Chicken Dinner	327	25.0	16.0	18.0	65	993	1.0
chicken, grilled ...	130	24.0	0	4.0	67	560	0
chicken strips	635	47.0	55.0	25.0	95	1510	0
chicken stir-fry ...	864	43.0	149.0	10.0	67	3653	10.0
pot roast w/gravy ..	292	42.0	5.0	11.0	87	927	5.0
salmon, Alaskan, grilled	210	43.0	1.0	4.0	101	103	0
shrimp, fried	219	17.0	18.0	10.0	135	1114	3.0

Food and Measure	cal.	prot. (gms)	carbo. (gms)	fat (gms)	chol. (mgs)	sod. (mgs)	fiber (gms)
Denny's, entree, w/out sides (cont.)							
shrimp scampi							
skillet	289	25.0	3.0	19.0	192	766	3.0
sirloin steak	337	18.0	1.0	28.0	687	344	1.0
steak, chicken fried	265	15.0	14.0	17.0	27	668	1.0
steak and shrimp ..	645	36.0	31.0	42.0	150	1143	2.0
T-bone steak	860	65.0	0	65.0	196	867	0
turkey, roast,							
w/stuffing, gravy	388	46.0	38.0	3.0	116	2467	2.0
Western wing							
round-up	1517	89.0	89.0	88.0	465	3328	3.0
sides:							
applesauce	60	0	15.0	0	0	13	1.0
bread stuffing, plain	100	3.0	19.0	1.0	0	405	1.0
carrots, honey glaze	80	1.0	12.0	3.0	0	220	3.0
corn, butter sauce .	120	3.0	19.0	4.0	5	260	5.0
cottage cheese	72	9.0	2.0	3.0	10	281	0
fries, no salt	323	5.0	44.0	14.0	0	130	0
fries, seasoned ...	261	5.0	35.0	12.0	0	556	0
gravy, 1 oz.:							
brown	13	0	2.0	0	0	184	0
chicken	14	0	2.0	.5	2	139	0
country	17	0	2.0	1.0	0	93	0
green beans							
w/bacon	60	1.0	6.0	4.0	5	390	3.0
green peas, butter							
sauce	100	5.0	14.0	2.0	5	360	4.0
herb toast	170	2.0	15.0	11.0	<1	325	1.0
mushrooms, grilled	14	2.0	2.0	0	0	0	1.0
onion rings	381	5.0	38.0	23.0	6	1003	1.0
potato, baked, plain	220	5.0	51.0	0	0	16	5.0
potato, mashed,							
plain	105	3.0	21.0	1.0	0	378	2.0
potato, mashed,							
w/cheddar	117	3.0	22.0	2.0	2	405	2.0
rice pilaf, vegetable	85	2.0	16.0	1.0	0	325	1.0
tomato, 3 slices ...	13	1.0	3.0	0	0	6	1.0
salad, no dressing,							
except as noted:							
Caesar, grilled							
chicken,							
w/dressing	600	37.0	19.0	41.0	101	1792	4.0
garden deluxe:							
chicken breast ..	264	32.0	10.0	11.0	89	714	4.0

Food and Measure	cal.	prot. (gms)	carbo. (gms)	fat (gms)	chol. (mgs)	sod. (mgs)	fiber (gms)
Buffalo chicken strips	516	33.0	26.0	35.0	79	1197	4.0
fried chicken strips	438	33.0	26.0	26.0	78	1030	4.0
salmon fillet	389	67.0	10.0	9.0	124	349	4.0
turkey and ham	322	43.0	12.0	11.0	100	1706	4.0
side, Caesar, w/dressing	338	8.0	20.0	25.0	7	725	3.0
side, garden	113	3.0	16.0	4.0	0	147	3.0
dressings, 1 oz.:							
blue cheese	163	1.0	1.0	18.0	20	205	0
Caesar	133	1.0	1.0	14.0	2	380	0
French	106	0	3.0	10.0	7	274	0
honey mustard ...	38	0	9.0	0	0	121	0
Italian, low cal	15	0	3.0	.5	0	390	0
ranch	129	0	1.0	14.0	8	189	0
Thousand Island ..	118	0	5.0	11.0	15	170	0
condiments/sauces:							
BBQ sauce, 1.5 oz.	47	0	11.0	1.0	0	595	0
marinara, 1.5 oz. ..	48	1.0	7.0	2.0	0	206	1.0
salsa, 2 oz.	10	0	2.5	0	0	221	1.0
sour cream, 1.5 oz.	91	1.0	2.0	9.0	19	23	0
tartar, 1.5 oz.	230	0	5.0	24.0	17	185	0
dessert/shakes:							
chocolate layer cake	275	4.0	42.0	12.0	26	62	0
float, root beer/cola	280	3.0	47.0	10.0	39	109	0
grasshopper blender blaster	735	13.0	92.0	37.0	140	299	0
malted milkshake ..	583	12.0	82.0	26.0	100	278	<1.0
milkshake.	560	11.0	76.0	26.0	100	272	<1.0
peaches and cream parfait	568	5.0	91.0	22.0	81	227	1.0
pie, no topping:							
apple	470	3.0	64.0	24.0	0	470	1.0
apple, Dutch ...	440	3.0	65.0	19.0	0	290	1.0
cherry	630	3.0	101.0	25.0	0	550	2.0
chocolate peanut butter	653	15.0	64.0	39.0	27	319	3.0
cheesecake	470	6.0	48.0	27.0	90	280	0
cheesecake, peachy	590	8.0	74.0	30.0	105	306	.6
Hershey's chocolate chunks n' chips	600	6.0	58.0	36.0	10	270	3.0

Food and Measure	cal.	prot. (gms)	carbo. (gms)	fat (gms)	chol. (mgs)	sod. (mgs)	fiber (gms)
Denny's, dessert/shakes, pie, no topping *(cont.)*							
Oreo cookies and creme	651	6.0	67.0	40.0	20	401	2.0
sherbet, rainbow . .	120	1.0	25.0	1.5	5	30	0
sundae:							
banana split	894	15.0	121.0	43.0	78	177	6.0
double scoop . . .	375	6.0	29.0	27.0	74	86	0
grasshopper . . .	734	13.0	97.0	34.0	118	290	1.0
hot fudge cake . .	620	7.0	73.0	35.0	60	170	1.0
single scoop . . .	188	3.0	14.0	14.0	37	43	0
toppings, 2 oz.:							
blueberry	71	0	17.0	0	0	10	0
cherry	57	0	14.0	0	0	3	0
chocolate	317	2.0	27.0	25.0	0	83	0
fudge	201	1.0	30.0	10.0	3	96	1.0
strawberry	77	1.0	17.0	1.0	0	8	1.0
whipped cream, 2 tbsp.	23	0	2.0	2.0	7	3	0
yogurt, chocolate/ chocolate chip . .	110	4.0	19.0	2.0	5	60	1.0
Dessert, dried, 1 serving:							
apple almond crisp (*AlpineAire*)	260	6.0	55.0	2.0	0	80	7.0
apple blueberry cobbler (*AlpineAire*) . .	210	6.0	38.0	4.0	0	550	4.0
bananas Foster (*AlpineAire*)	250	2.0	47.0	5.0	0	75	2.0
cheesecake:							
blackberry (*Alpine-Aire Mountain*) . .	670	6.0	134.0	13.0	n.a.	490	1.0
blueberry (*Mountain House*)	220	4.0	37.0	6.0	10	330	1.0
chocolate hazelnut Bavarian cream (*AlpineAire*)	300	7.0	36.0	14.0	n.a.	60	4.0
raspberry crumble (*Mountain House*) . .	150	1.0	31.0	3.0	0	75	2.0
rice pudding (*Alpine-Aire*)	360	7.0	76.0	3.0	n.a.	190	0
Dill dip, 2 tbsp.: (*Marzetti Veggie Dip*)	140	1.0	2.0	14.0	25	190	0
(*Marzetti Veggie Dip Fat Free*)	30	1.0	6.0	0	0	410	0

Food and Measure	cal.	prot. (gms)	carbo. (gms)	fat (gms)	chol. (mgs)	sod. (mgs)	fiber (gms)
Dill dip mix, garden							
(*Knorr*), ½ tsp. ...	5	0	0	0	0	110	0
Dill seed, 1 tsp.	6	.3	1.2	.3	0	<1	.4
Dill weed, fresh:							
5 sprigs	<1	<1.0	.1	<.1	0	1	<.1
1 cup	4	.3	.6	.1	0	5	.2
Dill weed, dried,							
1 tsp.	3	.2	.6	<.1	0	2	.1
Dip (see also specific							
listings), 4-layer							
(*Ortega*), 2 tbsp. ...	50	3.0	5.0	2.0	5	170	1.0
Dock:							
raw, chopped, 1 cup	29	2.6	4.3	.9	9	5	3.9
boiled, drained, 4 oz.	23	2.1	3.3	.7	0	3	<1.0
Dolphin fish, meat							
only, 4 oz.:							
raw	97	21.0	0	.8	83	99	0
baked, broiled, or							
microwaved	124	26.9	0	1.0	107	128	0
Domino's:							
deep dish, ¼ of							
12" pie, cheese ...	482	18.7	56.2	21.7	30	1123	3.3
w/anchovy	516	24.9	56.2	23.2	43	1716	3.3
w/bacon	584	24.1	56.2	30.4	45	1406	3.3
w/banana pepper ..	487	18.9	57.0	21.8	30	1260	3.3
w/beef	560	22.4	56.2	28.6	44	1339	3.3
w/cheddar	539	22.2	56.3	26.4	44	1211	3.3
w/extra cheese	531	22.0	56.9	25.5	41	1286	3.5
w/green pepper ...	486	18.9	57.0	21.8	30	1124	3.5
w/ham	505	21.9	56.6	22.7	39	1338	3.3
w/mushrooms	488	19.2	57.3	21.8	30	1124	3.6
w/olives, green ...	501	18.9	56.4	23.7	30	1506	3.7
w/olives, ripe	503	18.9	57.1	23.5	30	1230	4.1
w/onion	488	18.9	57.3	21.7	30	1123	3.4
w/pepperoni	556	22.0	56.4	28.2	45	1397	3.3
w/pineapple	494	18.8	59.4	21.7	30	1124	3.5
w/sausage	559	22.1	58.4	27.8	45	1362	3.8
deep dish, ¼ of							
14" pie, cheese ...	677	26.4	80.3	29.7	41	1575	4.7
w/anchovy	722	34.6	80.3	31.6	59	2366	4.7
w/bacon	830	34.5	80.5	42.8	63	2000	4.7
w/banana pepper ..	684	26.6	81.5	29.8	41	1758	4.7
w/beef	788	31.7	80.3	39.6	62	1884	4.7
w/cheddar	748	30.8	80.6	35.6	59	1686	4.7

Food and Measure	cal.	prot. (gms)	carbo. (gms)	fat (gms)	chol. (mgs)	sod. (mgs)	fiber (gms)
***Domino's*, deep dish ¼ of 14" pie** *(cont.)*							
w/extra cheese	745	31.0	81.4	35.0	57	1804	5.0
w/green pepper . . .	682	26.6	81.5	29.8	41	1576	5.0
w/ham	708	30.7	80.9	31.0	53	1868	4.7
w/mushrooms . . .	686	27.1	82.0	29.8	41	1577	5.1
w/olives, green . . .	701	26.7	80.6	32.4	41	2085	4.9
w/olives, ripe	705	26.6	81.6	32.1	41	1718	5.7
w/onion	684	26.6	81.9	29.8	41	1576	4.8
w/pepperoni	775	30.8	80.7	38.4	61	1940	4.7
w/pineapple	696	26.5	85.3	29.7	41	1577	5.0
w/sausage	787	31.2	83.5	38.4	64	1917	5.4
deep dish, 1 whole							
6" pie, cheese . . .	598	22.9	68.4	27.6	36	1341	3.9
w/anchovy	643	31.1	68.4	29.6	55	2132	3.9
w/bacon	680	27.2	68.5	34.6	48	1568	3.9
w/banana pepper . .	601	23.0	68.9	27.7	36	1415	3.9
w/beef	642	25.0	68.4	31.6	45	1465	3.9
w/cheddar	684	28.2	68.6	34.7	59	1473	3.9
w/extra cheese	656	26.9	69.3	32.2	50	1537	4.1
w/green pepper . . .	600	23.0	68.8	27.7	36	1342	4.0
w/ham	615	25.2	68.7	28.3	43	1497	3.9
w/mushrooms	600	23.1	68.8	27.7	30	1342	4.0
w/olives, green . . .	608	23.0	68.5	28.7	36	1546	4.0
w/olives, ripe	609	23.0	68.9	28.6	36	1399	4.3
w/onion	601	23.0	67.6	27.6	36	1342	4.0
w/pepperoni	647	25.1	68.5	32.0	47	1524	3.9
w/pineapple	602	22.9	69.6	27.6	36	1342	4.0
w/sausage	642	24.8	69.6	31.1	45	1478	4.2
hand tossed, ¼ of							
12" pie, cheese . . .	375	15.4	54.7	11.1	23	776	3.0
w/anchovy	408	21.6	54.7	12.6	36	1369	3.0
w/bacon	477	20.8	54.8	19.8	38	1058	3.0
w/banana pepper . .	380	15.6	55.6	11.2	23	913	3.0
w/beef	452	19.1	54.8	18.0	37	992	3.0
w/cheddar	432	18.9	54.9	15.8	37	864	3.0
w/extra cheese	423	18.7	55.5	14.9	34	939	3.2
w/green pepper . . .	378	15.6	55.6	11.2	23	776	3.2
w/ham	398	18.6	55.1	12.1	32	990	3.0
w/mushrooms	381	15.9	55.9	11.2	23	777	3.3
w/olives, green . . .	393	15.6	54.9	23.7	30	1506	3.7
w/olives, ripe	395	15.6	55.6	13.1	23	1159	3.1
w/onion	380	15.6	55.9	11.1	23	776	3.1
w/pepperoni	448	18.7	55.0	17.6	38	1049	3.0
w/pineapple	387	15.5	57.9	11.1	23	1124	3.2

Food and Measure	cal.	prot. (gms)	carbo. (gms)	fat (gms)	chol. (mgs)	sod. (mgs)	fiber (gms)
w/sausage	451	18.8	56.9	17.2	39	777	3.4
hand tossed, ¼ of							
14" pie, cheese . . .	515	21.3	75.0	15.4	32	1080	4.1
w/anchovy	561	29.5	75.0	17.4	50	1870	4.1
w/bacon	669	29.4	75.1	28.5	54	1504	4.1
w/banana pepper . .	523	21.6	76.2	15.5	32	1263	4.1
w/beef	627	26.6	75.0	25.3	53	1389	4.1
w/cheddar	587	25.7	75.2	21.3	50	1190	4.1
w/extra cheese	584	26.0	76.0	20.8	47	1308	4.4
w/green pepper . . .	521	21.5	76.1	15.5	32	1081	4.4
w/ham	547	25.6	75.5	16.7	44	1372	4.1
w/mushrooms	525	22.1	76.6	15.8	32	1082	4.5
w/olives, green . . .	541	21.6	75.2	18.1	32	1591	4.3
w/olives, ripe	544	21.6	76.2	17.9	32	1223	5.1
w/onion	523	21.6	76.5	15.5	32	1081	4.2
w/pepperoni	614	25.8	75.3	24.1	52	1444	4.2
w/pineapple	535	21.5	79.9	15.4	32	1082	4.4
w/sausage	626	26.1	78.1	24.1	54	1422	4.8
thin crust, ¼ of							
12" pie, cheese . . .	273	12.0	31.0	11.9	23	835	1.8
w/anchovy	307	18.1	31.0	13.3	36	1428	1.8
w/bacon	375	17.4	31.1	20.6	38	1118	1.8
w/banana pepper . .	278	12.2	31.9	11.9	23	973	1.8
w/beef	350	15.7	31.1	18.8	37	1051	1.8
w/cheddar	330	15.5	31.2	16.5	37	923	1.8
w/extra cheese	321	15.3	31.8	15.7	34	998	1.9
w/green pepper . . .	277	12.1	31.9	11.9	23	836	1.9
w/ham	296	15.1	31.5	12.8	32	1050	1.8
w/mushrooms	279	12.5	32.2	12.0	23	836	2.1
w/olives, green . . .	291	12.2	31.3	13.9	23	1218	1.9
w/olives, ripe	294	12.2	31.9	13.7	23	942	2.5
w/onion	276	12.2	32.2	11.9	23	836	1.8
w/pepperoni	347	15.3	31.3	18.4	38	1109	1.8
w/pineapple	285	12.1	34.3	11.9	23	837	1.9
w/sausage	350	15.4	33.3	17.9	39	1074	2.2
thin crust, ¼ of							
14" pie, cheese . . .	382	16.8	43.5	16.6	32	1172	2.5
w/anchovy	427	25.0	43.5	18.5	50	1962	2.5
w/bacon	535	24.9	43.7	29.7	54	1596	2.5
w/banana pepper . .	389	17.0	44.7	16.7	32	1355	2.5
w/beef	493	22.1	43.6	26.5	52	1480	2.5
w/cheddar	453	21.2	43.7	22.5	50	1282	2.5
w/extra cheese	450	21.4	44.6	21.9	47	1400	2.7
w/green pepper . . .	387	17.0	44.6	16.7	32	1172	2.7

Food and Measure	cal.	prot. (gms)	carbo. (gms)	fat (gms)	chol. (mgs)	sod. (mgs)	fiber (gms)
***Domino's*, thin crust ¼ of 14" pie** *(cont.)*							
w/ham	414	21.1	44.0	17.9	44	1464	2.5
w/mushrooms	391	17.5	45.1	16.7	32	1173	2.9
w/olives, green	407	17.1	43.8	19.3	32	1682	2.7
w/olives, ripe	410	17.0	44.7	19.0	32	1314	3.5
w/onion	389	17.0	45.1	16.7	32	1172	2.5
w/pepperoni	481	21.2	43.8	25.3	52	1536	2.5
w/pineapple	401	16.9	48.5	16.6	32	1173	2.7
w/sausage	492	21.6	46.6	25.3	54	1513	3.1
Donut, 1 pc., except as noted:							
(*Entenmann's* Donut Dippers)	160	1.0	19.0	9.0	10	130	<1.0
plain:							
(*Awrey's*), 1.5 oz.	150	2.0	18.0	8.0	5	180	0
(*Awrey's*), 2 oz.	210	3.0	31.0	8.0	3	290	<1.0
chocolate iced/frosted:							
(*Awrey's* Ring), 3 oz.	300	4.0	33.0	17.0	0	270	1.0
(*Entenmann's* Rich)	280	2.0	27.0	19.0	10	200	1.0
(*Hostess Donettes*), 3 pcs., 1.75 oz.	230	2.0	24.0	14.0	0	210	0
(*Popems*), 4 pcs.	280	2.0	24.0	20.0	10	180	2.0
chocolate (*Awrey's*)	190	2.0	25.0	10.0	5	150	<1.0
custard (*Awrey's* Bismark)	330	3.0	44.0	16.0	0	300	1.0
milk chocolate (*Entenmann's*)	320	3.0	35.0	19.0	15	190	1.0
mini (*Entenmann's*)	150	1.0	12.0	11.0	<5	90	<1.0
sour cream (*Awrey's*), 3 oz.	310	3.0	47.0	12.0	20	270	1.0
sour cream (*Awrey's*), 3.75 oz.	430	3.0	54.0	22.0	0	350	<1.0
cinnamon sugar sour cream (*Awrey's*)	260	3.0	39.0	11.0	20	260	0
coconut topped (*Awrey's*)	210	2.0	25.0	12.0	10	190	0
cruller (*Entenmann's*)	220	2.0	26.0	13.0	15	190	<1.0
crumb (*Entenmann's*)	260	3.0	34.0	13.0	15	230	1.0
crunch:							
(*Awrey's*), 2.5 oz.	280	3.0	35.0	10.0	15	320	<1.0
topped (*Awrey's*), 1.75 oz.	160	2.0	19.0	8.0	10	190	0

Food and Measure	cal.	prot. (gms)	carbo. (gms)	fat (gms)	chol. (mgs)	sod. (mgs	fiber (gms)
devil's food:							
frosted (*Entenmann's*)	310	3.0	34.0	19.0	15	170	2.0
glazed (*Awrey's*) . .	300	4.0	41.0	14.0	5	400	1.0
glazed:							
(*Awrey's* Ring)	270	3.0	30.0	16.0	0	250	1.0
(*Awrey's* Twin Pack Sticks), 2.75 oz.	300	3.0	41.0	15.0	15	260	0
(*Entenmann's Little Bites*), 4 pcs. . .	220	2.0	28.0	11.0	15	210	<1.0
(*Entenmann's Popems*), 4 pcs.	210	2.0	28.0	10.0	15	190	1.0
raised (*Hostess*) . .	150	0	19.0	8.0	0	130	0
raised (*Rolling Pin Donuts*), 2.4 oz.	250	4.0	37.0	10.0	<5	340	<1.0
sour cream (*Awrey's*), 3 oz.	240	3.0	34.0	10.0	3	290	0
sour cream (*Awrey's*), 3.75 oz.	420	3.0	55.0	21.0	0	310	0
jelly:							
powdered sugar (*Awrey's* Bismark)	250	3.0	30.0	13.0	0	210	1.0
vanilla iced (*Awrey's* Bismark)	320	3.0	43.0	15.0	0	250	1.0
powdered sugar:							
(*Awrey's*), 1.5 oz.	160	2.0	21.0	8.0	5	180	0
(*Awrey's*), 2 oz. . . .	210	3.0	31.0	8.0	3	290	0
(*Drake's Donut Delites*), 3 pcs., 1.5 oz.	180	2.0	23.0	8.0	5	200	0
(*Entenmann's*)	220	2.0	27.0	12.0	20	240	<1.0
(*Hostess*)	150	2.0	19.0	8.0	10	180	0
(*Hostess Donettes*), 3 pcs., 2.2 oz. . .	250	3.0	34.0	11.0	0	280	1.0
mini (*Entenmann's Popettes*), 4 pcs.	280	3.0	30.0	17.0	20	250	<1.0
sour cream (*Awrey's*) .	370	4.0	41.0	22.0	0	340	0
sprinkle topped (*Awrey's*)	160	2.0	19.0	8.0	10	190	0
vanilla iced (*Awrey's* Long John)	370	4.0	44.0	20.0	0	320	1.0
white iced (*Awrey's*) .	200	2.0	24.0	10.0	15	240	0

Food and Measure	cal.	prot. (gms)	carbo. (gms)	fat (gms)	chol. (mgs)	sod. (mgs)	fiber (gms)
Dow gok, see "Yard-long bean"							
Drum, freshwater, meat only:							
raw, 4 oz.	135	19.9	0	5.6	73	85	0
baked, broiled, or microwaved, 4 oz.	173	25.5	0	7.2	93	109	0
Duck, domesticated, roasted, 4 oz.:							
meat w/skin	382	21.5	0	32.1	95	67	0
meat only	228	26.6	0	12.7	101	74	0
young, Peking:							
breast, meat w/skin	229	27.8	0	12.3	154	95	0
leg, meat w/skin . .	246	30.3	0	12.9	129	125	0
Duck, wild, raw:							
meat w/skin, 4 oz. . .	239	19.8	0	17.2	91	64	0
breast meat, 4 oz. . . .	139	22.5	0	4.8	87	65	0
Dulce de leche topping (*Smucker's*), 2 tbsp.	110	2.0	23.0	1.5	10	45	0
Dumpling, see "Pasta"							
Dumpling entree, Oriental style, frozen (*Lean Cuisine Everyday Favorites*), 9 oz.	290	9.0	49.0	6.0	15	560	2.0
Dumpling squash, see "Sweet dumpling squash"							
***Dunkin' Donuts*:**							
Omwich, 1 pc:							
bagel/bacon cheddar	600	26.0	79.0	21.0	295	1630	<1.0
bagel/pizza	560	25.0	74.0	19.0	255	1305	2.0
bagel, Spanish	570	24.0	79.0	18.0	280	1370	<1.0
biscuit/bacon cheddar	500	21.0	33.0	32.0	300	1660	1.0
biscuit/pizza	500	19.0	39.0	30.0	255	1475	<1.0
biscuit/Spanish . . .	470	19.0	34.0	29.0	285	1400	1.0
croissant, bacon/ cheddar	560	21.0	33.0	38.0	295	1190	1.0
croissant/pizza	510	18.0	33.0	34.0	260	895	<1.0
croissant/Spanish	530	19.0	33.0	36.0	285	930	1.0
English muffin/ bacon/cheddar . .	400	21.0	33.0	21.0	295	1440	2.0

Food and Measure	cal.	prot. (gms)	carbo. (gms)	fat (gms)	chol. (mgs)	sod. (mgs	fiber (gms)
English muffin/ham/ egg/cheese	320	22.0	31.0	12.0	195	1340	2.0
English muffin/pizza	350	17.0	33.0	17.0	255	1145	1.0
English muffin/ Spanish	370	18.0	34.0	18.0	280	1180	2.0
biscuit sandwich, 1 pc.:							
egg/cheese	380	17.0	30.0	22.0	180	1250	<1.0
sausage/egg/cheese	590	25.0	31.0	42.0	220	1620	<1.0
bagels, 1 pc.:							
plain	340	12.0	67.0	2.5	0	680	2.0
berry berry	340	11.0	69.0	3.0	0	540	4.0
blueberry	340	11.0	69.0	3.0	0	630	2.0
cinnamon raisin ...	340	11.0	69.0	3.5	0	600	3.0
everything	360	11.0	74.0	2.0	0	710	0
garlic	360	11.0	76.0	1.0	0	720	0
onion	350	12.0	66.0	4.0	0	660	3.0
poppy seed	360	11.0	74.0	2.5	0	710	<1.0
salt	340	10.0	73.0	1.0	0	3030	0
sesame	380	12.0	74.0	4.5	0	720	0
sun-dried tomato ..	330	13.0	66.0	2.5	0	700	3.0
wheat	330	13.0	67.0	4.5	0	640	4.0
cream cheese, 1 pkt.:							
plain	200	4.0	3.0	13.0	60	230	0
chive	190	3.0	3.0	19.0	55	220	<1.0
lite	130	5.0	3.0	7.0	30	250	0
garden vegetable	180	3.0	3.0	17.0	45	310	<1.0
salmon	180	5.0	2.0	11.0	50	150	0
strawberry	180	2.0	9.0	16.0	0	170	0
biscuit, 1 pc.	280	6.0	32.0	14.0	0	850	<1.0
cinnamon bun, 1 pc. .	510	8.0	85.0	15.0	10	420	0
croissant, 1 pc.	290	5.0	26.0	18.0	5	270	<1.0
cookies, 1 pc.:							
chocolate chocolate chunk	210	3.0	26.0	11.0	35	110	2.0
chocolate chunk ..	220	3.0	28.0	11.0	35	105	1.0
chocolate chunk w/nuts	230	3.0	27.0	12.0	35	110	1.0
oatmeal raisin pecan	220	3.0	29.0	10.0	30	110	1.0
peanut butter choco- late chunk w/nuts	240	4.0	24.0	14.0	25	125	2.0
peanut butter w/nuts	240	5.0	24.0	14.0	30	150	1.0
white chocolate chunk	230	3.0	28.0	12.0	35	120	1.0

Food and Measure	cal.	prot. (gms)	carbo. (gms)	fat (gms)	chol. (mgs)	sod. (mgs)	fiber (gms)
Dunkin' Donuts, **donuts** (cont.)							
donuts, 1 pc.:							
apple crumb	230	3.0	34.0	10.0	0	270	<1.0
apple fritter	300	4.0	41.0	14.0	0	360	1.0
apple n' spice	200	3.0	29.0	8.0	0	270	<1.0
Bavarian kreme ...	210	3.0	30.0	9.0	0	270	<1.0
black raspberry ...	210	3.0	32.0	8.0	0	280	<1.0
blueberry cake	290	3.0	35.0	16.0	10	400	<1.0
blueberry crumb ..	240	3.0	36.0	10.0	0	260	<1.0
Boston kreme	240	3.0	36.0	9.0	0	280	<1.0
bow tie	300	4.0	34.0	17.0	0	340	<1.0
butternut cake	300	3.0	36.0	16.0	0	360	<1.0
caramel apple krunch	300	4.0	41.0	14.0	0	310	<1.0
chocolate:							
cake, double ...	310	3.0	37.0	17.0	0	370	2.0
cake, glazed	290	3.0	33.0	16.0	0	370	1.0
coconut cake ...	300	4.0	31.0	19.0	0	370	1.0
frosted	200	3.0	29.0	9.0	0	260	<1.0
frosted cake	300	3.0	38.0	16.0	0	370	<1.0
frosted coffee roll	290	4.0	36.0	15.0	0	340	1.0
iced, Bismark ...	340	3.0	50.0	15.0	0	290	<1.0
kreme filled	270	3.0	35.0	13.0	0	260	<1.0
cinnamon cake ...	270	3.0	31.0	15.0	0	360	<1.0
coconut cake	290	3.0	33.0	17.0	0	360	<1.0
coconut cake, toasted	300	3.0	35.0	17.0	0	370	<1.0
coffee roll	270	4.0	33.0	14.0	0	340	1.0
cruller, chocolate, glazed	280	3.0	35.0	15.0	0	360	1.0
cruller, glazed	290	3.0	37.0	15.0	0	350	<1.0
cruller, plain	240	3.0	25.0	15.0	0	340	<1.0
cruller, powdered ..	270	3.0	30.0	15.0	0	340	<1.0
cruller, sugar	250	3.0	27.0	15.0	0	340	<1.0
Dunkin' Donut	240	3.0	25.0	15.0	0	340	<1.0
éclair	270	3.0	39.0	11.0	0	290	<1.0
glazed	180	3.0	25.0	8.0	0	250	<1.0
glazed cake	270	3.0	33.0	15.0	0	360	1.0
glazed fritter	260	4.0	31.0	14.0	0	330	1.0
jelly filled	210	3.0	32.0	8.0	0	280	<1.0
jelly stick	290	3.0	44.0	12.0	0	390	<1.0
lemon	200	3.0	28.0	9.0	0	270	<1.0
maple frosted	210	3.0	30.0	9.0	0	260	<1.0

Food and Measure	cal.	prot. (gms)	carbo. (gms)	fat (gms)	chol. (mgs)	sod. (mgs)	fiber (gms)
maple frosted coffee roll	290	4.0	36.0	14.0	0	340	1.0
marble frosted	200	3.0	29.0	9.0	0	260	<1.0
old-fashioned cake	250	3.0	26.0	15.0	0	360	<1.0
powdered cake . . .	270	3.0	32.0	15.0	0	350	<1.0
powdered cruller . .	270	3.0	30.0	15.0	0	340	<1.0
strawberry	210	3.0	32.0	8.0	0	260	<1.0
strawberry frosted	210	3.0	30.0	9.0	0	340	<1.0
sugar raised	170	3.0	22.0	8.0	0	250	<1.0
sugared cake	250	3.0	27.0	15.0	0	350	<1.0
vanilla frosted	210	3.0	30.0	9.0	0	260	<1.0
vanilla frosted coffee roll	290	4.0	36.0	14.0	0	340	1.0
vanilla kreme	270	3.0	36.0	13.0	0	250	<1.0
whole wheat glazed	310	4.0	32.0	19.0	0	380	2.0
Munchkins, cake:							
plain, 4 pcs.	220	2.0	22.0	14.0	0	310	<1.0
butternut, 3 pcs. . .	200	2.0	25.0	11.0	0	240	<1.0
chocolate, glazed, 3 pcs.	200	2.0	26.0	10.0	0	250	<1.0
cinnamon, 4 pcs.	250	3.0	30.0	14.0	0	330	<1.0
coconut, 3 pcs. . .	200	2.0	23.0	12.0	0	240	<1.0
coconut, toasted, 3 pcs.	200	2.0	24.0	11.0	0	250	<1.0
glazed, 3 pcs.	200	2.0	27.0	10.0	0	250	0
powdered, 4 pcs.	250	2.0	29.0	14.0	0	310	<1.0
sugared, 4 pcs. . .	240	2.0	28.0	14.0	0	310	<1.0
Munchkins, yeast:							
glazed, 5 pcs.	200	3.0	27.0	9.0	0	220	<1.0
jelly, 5 pcs.	210	3.0	30.0	9.0	0	240	<1.0
lemon, 4 pcs.	170	2.0	23.0	8.0	0	190	0
sugar raised, 7 pcs.	220	4.0	26.0	12.0	0	290	<1.0
muffins, 1 pc.:							
apple cinnamon pecan	510	8.0	74.0	21.0	70	590	1.0
blueberry	490	8.0	76.0	17.0	75	610	2.0
banana nut	530	10.0	72.0	23.0	75	540	2.0
blueberry, reduced fat	450	8.0	77.0	12.0	65	590	2.0
chocolate chip . .	590	9.0	88.0	24.0	75	560	3.0
corn	500	10.0	78.0	16.0	80	920	1.0
cranberry orange . .	470	8.0	76.0	15.0	75	600	2.0

Food and Measure	cal.	prot. (gms)	carbo. (gms)	fat (gms)	chol. (mgs)	sod. (mgs)	fiber (gms)
Dunkin' Donuts, muffins (cont.)							
honey bran raisin	490	7.0	84.0	16.0	30	880	5.0
lemon poppy							
seed	580	10.0	94.0	19.0	85	620	2.0
Coolatta, coffee,							
16 oz.:							
w/cream	410	3.0	51.0	22.0	75	65	0
w/cream, choco-							
late mint							
Whirl-Ins	460	4.0	58.0	24.0	75	120	0
w/cream, *Oreo*							
Whirl-Ins	460	4.0	58.0	24.0	75	150	0
w/milk	260	4.0	52.0	4.0	15	75	0
w/milk, *Oreo*							
Whirl-Ins	300	4.0	60.0	5.0	15	160	0
w/milk, chocolate							
mint *Whirl-Ins* ..	310	4.0	59.0	6.0	15	130	0
w/2% milk	240	4.0	52.0	2.0	10	80	0
w/skim milk	230	4.0	52.0	0	<5	80	0
Coolatta, orange							
mango,16 oz	290	<1.0	71.0	0	0	30	<1.0
Coolatta, piña,							
16 oz.	270	1.0	57.0	3.5	0	65	0
Coolatta, strawberry,							
16 oz.	280	0	70.0	0	0	30	1.0
Coolatta, vanilla bean:							
16 oz.	450	1.0	94.0	7.0	0	170	0
w/chocolate mint							
Whirl-Ins,							
16 oz.	500	2.0	82.0	19.0	0	150	0
w/*Oreo Whirl-Ins*,							
16 oz.	500	2.0	83.0	18.0	0	170	<1.0
Dunkaccino, 10 oz. ..	250	2.0	34.0	11.0	10	240	<1.0
hot cocoa, 10 oz. ...	230	2.0	38.0	8.0	0	310	2.0
Durian, fresh:							
½ of 1.3-lb. fruit	442	4.4	81.5	16.0	0	3	11.4
chopped, ½ cup	179	1.8	32.9	6.5	0	2	4.6

E

Food and Measure	cal.	prot. (gms)	carbo. (gms)	fat (gms)	chol. (mgs)	sod. (mgs)	fiber (gms)
Éclair, chocolate (*Entenmann's*), 1 pc.	260	3.0	45.0	9.0	80	210	<1.0
Edamame (see also "Soybean"), fresh:							
(*Yoshinoya*), ½ cup ..	120	9.0	12.0	4.0	0	330	3.0
boiled, salted (*Hanjo*), 1.8 oz., 3.5 oz. in pod	120	9.0	12.0	4.0	0	330	3.0
shelled (*Frieda's*), ½ cup, 2.6 oz. ...	100	10.0	9.0	2.5	0	70	1.0
Edamame, frozen, in pod (*Cascadian Farm*), ⅔ cup, 3 oz.	120	10.0	9.0	5.0	0	10	4.0
Eel, meat only:							
raw, 4 oz.	209	20.9	0	3.2	143	58	0
baked, broiled, or microwaved, 4 oz.	268	26.8	0	17.0	183	74	0
Egg, chicken:							
raw, 1 extra large (*Land O Lakes*) ...	80	7.0	1.0	5.0	240	70	0
raw, 1 large:							
(*Land O Lakes*) ...	70	6.0	1.0	4.5	215	65	0
whole	75	6.3	.6	5.0	213	63	0
white only	17	3.5	.3	0	0	55	0
yolk only[1]	59	2.8	.3	5.1	213	7	0
cooked:							
hard-boiled, chopped, 1 cup	210	17.1	1.5	14.4	578	169	0
poached, 1 large ..	74	6.2	.6	5.0	212	140	0
Egg, chicken, dried:							
whole:							
1 oz.	168	13.0	1.4	11.9	544	148	0

1. Includes a small portion of white.

Food and Measure	cal.	prot. (gms)	carbo. (gms)	fat (gms)	chol. (mgs)	sod. (mgs)	fiber (gms)
Egg, chicken, dried, whole *(cont.)*							
stabilized, 1 oz. . . .	174	13.7	.7	12.5	572	155	0
white:							
(*Just Whites*), 2 tsp.	12	3.0	0	0	0	51	0
flakes, 1 oz.	100	21.8	1.2	<.1	0	328	0
yolk, 1 oz.	195	8.7	.1	17.4	830	26	0
Egg, duck, 1 egg	130	9.0	1.0	9.6	619	102	0
Egg, goose, 1 egg . . .	267	20.0	1.9	19.1	1227	199	0
Egg, quail, 1 egg . . .	14	1.2	<.1	1.0	76	13	0
Egg, substitute, ¼ cup:							
(*Egg Beaters*)	30	6.0	1.0	0	0	125	0
(*Healthy Choice*)	30	5.0	1.0	<1.0	0	90	0
(*Morningstar Farms Better'n Eggs*)	20	5.0	0	0	0	90	0
(*Morningstar Farm Scramblers*)	35	6.0	2.0	0	0	95	0
(*Tofutti Egg Watchers*)	30	6.0	1.0	0	0	80	0
Egg, turkey, 1 egg . . .	135	10.8	.9	9.4	737	119	0
Egg breakfast, dried, 1 serving:							
w/bacon:							
(*Mountain House*)	150	11.0	4.0	10.0	395	420	0
precooked (*Mountain House*)	160	12.0	5.0	10.0	295	590	0
omelette:							
cheese (*Mountain House*)	180	13.0	6.0	12.0	390	500	1.0
ranch, w/beef (*Alpine-Aire*)	390	28.0	17.0	24.0	n.a.	580	1.0
scrambled:							
(*AlpineAire*)	170	11.0	2.0	13.0	345	180	0
(*AlpineAire* Bandito)	220	11.0	19.0	11.0	n.a.	620	2.0
scrambling/omelette mix (*AlpineAire*) . . .	330	27.0	3.0	23.0	n.a.	300	0
Egg breakfast, frozen (see also "Breakfast sandwich" and specific listings), 1 pkg.:							
bacon, egg, and potato (*Uncle Ben's* Bowl), 8.25 oz.	290	17.0	26.0	13.0	20	790	2.0

Food and Measure	cal.	prot. (gms)	carbo. (gms)	fat (gms)	chol. (mgs)	sod. (mgs)	fiber (gms)
ham, egg, and peppers (*Uncle Ben's* Bowl), 8.25 oz.	230	17.0	22.0	9.0	220	900	3.0
omelette, ham and cheese (*Great Starts*), 5.2 oz.	250	12.0	24.0	12.0	245	530	2.0
sausage, egg, and biscuit (*Uncle Ben's* Bowl), 7.5 oz.	350	13.0	31.0	20.0	175	840	5.0
scrambled, w/sausage (*Great Starts*), 6.25 oz.	360	12.0	21.0	26.0	280	800	3.0
Egg roll, frozen or refrigerated:							
chicken:							
(*Chun King/La Choy* Restaurant Style), 3-oz. pc.	210	6.0	25.0	9.0	20	550	2.0
(*Yu Sing*), 6 pcs., 3 oz.	180	6.0	23.0	7.0	20	340	1.0
mini (*Chun King/La Choy*), 6 pcs.	210	6.0	25.0	9.0	15	650	2.0
sweet/sour (*Yu Sing*), 6 pcs., 3 oz. ...	190	6.0	26.0	7.0	20	290	1.0
pork, sweet/sour (*Yu Sing*), 6 pcs., 3 oz.	210	6.0	25.0	9.0	25	280	1.0
pork and shrimp:							
(*Yu Sing*), 6 pcs., 3 oz.	200	6.0	23.0	9.0	25	330	1.0
bite size (*La Choy*), 12 pcs.	210	6.0	25.0	10.0	10	540	2.0
mini (*Chun King/La Choy*), 6 pcs.	210	6.0	27.0	9.0	15	540	2.0
shrimp:							
(*Chun King/La Choy* Restaurant Style), 3-oz. pc.	180	5.0	25.0	7.0	15	490	2.0
(*Chung's*), 1 pc. w/sauce pkt. ...	140	6.0	23.0	3.0	15	470	4.0
(*Yu Sing*), 6 pcs., 3 oz.	180	5.0	24.0	7.0	20	280	2.0
mini (*Chun King/La Choy*), 6 pcs. ...	190	5.0	28.0	6.0	10	730	2.0

Food and Measure	cal.	prot. (gms)	carbo. (gms)	fat (gms)	chol. (mgs)	sod. (mgs)	fiber (gms)
Egg roll *(cont.)*							
vegetable:							
(*Chung's*), 1 pc., w/sauce pkt. . . .	130	4.0	24.0	3.0	0	500	4.0
w/lobster, mini (*La Choy*), 6 pcs.	190	5.0	27.0	7.0	5	440	3.0
Egg roll entree, frozen, vegetable (*Lean Cuisine Everyday Favorites*), 9 oz. . .	300	7.0	57.0	5.0	0	610	4.0
Egg roll wrapper (see also "Wrappers"):							
(*Frieda's*), 2 pcs.	130	5.0	28.0	.5	0	250	1.0
(*Nasoya*), 3 pcs.	170	7.0	35.0	.5	10	410	1.0
Eggnog, dairy (*Turkey Hill*), ½ cup	190	5.0	23.0	9.0	65	105	0
Eggnog, canned (*Borden*), ½ cup . .	160	4.0	17.0	9.0	75	80	0
Eggplant, fresh:							
raw:							
(*Frieda's* Chinese/ Japanese), ⅔ cup, 3 oz.	20	1.0	5.0	0	0	0	2.0
1" pcs., ½ cup	11	.4	2.5	.1	0	1	1.0
boiled, drained, 1" cubes, ½ cup . .	13	.4	3.2	.1	0	2	1.2
Eggplant appetizer:							
(*Alessi* Caponata), ⅓ cup	140	2.0	7.0	7.0	0	310	4.0
(*Cedar's* Baba Ghannouj), 2 tbsp.	50	2.0	5.0	2.0	0	80	3.0
(*Cento* Caponata), 2 tbsp.	30	0	2.0	2.0	0	130	2.0
(*Progresso* Caponata), 2 tbsp.	25	0	2.0	2.0	0	130	2.0
(*Sabra Salads* Babaganoush/Hungarian), 1 oz.	77	.3	1.5	7.7	8	110	.9
(*Yorgo* Baba Ghannouj), 2 tbsp.	50	1.0	3.0	2.0	0	60	1.0
marinated (*Casa Visco*), 1 oz.	15	0	1.0	1.0	0	170	0
Eggplant dip (*Victoria*), 2 tbsp.	30	0	2.0	2.0	0	310	1.0

Food and Measure	cal.	prot. (gms)	carbo. (gms)	fat (gms)	chol. (mgs)	sod. (mgs)	fiber (gms)
Eggplant dish, frozen, Parmesan (*Mrs. Paul's*), ½ cup	190	6.0	18.0	11.0	10	490	2.0
Eggplant entree, frozen, 1 pkg., except as noted:							
cutlets, breaded (*Dominex*), 3 oz. ...	100	2.0	14.0	9.0	0	160	2.0
Parmesan:							
(*Cedarlane*), ½ of 10-oz. pkg.	160	7.0	16.0	8.0	15	390	3.0
(*Wolfgang Puck's*), 9 oz.	300	23.0	17.0	17.0	35	630	6.0
parmigiana:							
(*Celentano*), 10 oz.	350	9.0	17.0	28.0	70	600	4.0
(*DeLuca* Refrigerated), 1 cup	220	10.0	19.0	13.0	30	1070	2.0
w/linguine (*Michelina's*), 8 oz.	270	8.0	42.0	7.0	5	780	3.0
rollettes:							
(*Celentano*), 10 oz.	290	7.0	17.0	20.0	50	690	4.0
(*Celentano*), ⅒ of 72-oz. pkg.	230	7.0	11.0	18.0	65	530	2.0
Eggplant relish, Indian (*Patak's* Brinjal), 1 tbsp.	50	<1.0	5.0	4.0	0	240	0
El Pollo Loco, 1 serving:							
chicken:							
breast	160	26.0	0	6.0	110	390	0
leg.............	90	11.0	0	5.0	75	150	0
thigh	180	16.0	0	12.0	130	230	0
wing	110	12.0	0	6.0	80	220	0
tortilla:							
corn, 4½"	32	1.0	6.0	.5	0	21	0
corn, 6"	70	1.0	14.0	1.0	0	35	1.0
flour, 6½"	90	3.0	13.0	3.0	0	224	0
flour, 11"	260	7.0	42.0	7.0	0	583	6.0
spicy tomato	254	7.0	42.0	6.0	0	577	2.0
burritos:							
BRC	503	17.0	73.0	16.0	17	1263	10.0
chicken lover's	476	29.0	47.0	19.0	143	1373	8.0
classic	580	31.0	66.0	22.0	108	1595	9.0

Food and Measure	cal.	prot. (gms)	carbo. (gms)	fat (gms)	chol. (mgs)	sod. (mgs)	fiber (gms)
***El Pollo Loco*, burritos** *(cont.)*							
Mexican chicken							
Caesar	734	36.0	65.0	35.0	79	1214	2.0
ranch	616	40.0	45.0	30.0	127	1356	7.0
spicy	633	31.0	80.0	21.0	69	1495	10.0
ultimate	633	39.0	66.0	23.0	89	1237	5.0
tacos:							
chicken soft	237	9.0	15.0	12.0	74	629	0
taco al carbon	180	7.0	20.0	8.0	19	152	2.0
bowls:							
pollo bowl	469	30.0	66.0	11.0	42	1868	8.0
flame-broiled							
chicken salad ...	357	25.0	39.0	13.0	42	1079	4.0
Mexican chicken							
Caesar salad ...	494	26.0	32.0	30.0	55	1175	3.0
nacho pollo	766	37.0	64.0	33.0	87	1358	11.0
smoky black bean							
pollo	604	29.0	75.0	23.0	54	1955	6.0
specialties:							
barbecue chicken							
tostada salad ...	543	27.0	55.0	24.0	55	1650	5.0
chicken taquito ...	370	15.0	43.0	17.0	25	690	3.0
chicken tostada							
salad w/out shell/							
sour cream	304	29.0	28.0	11.0	57	1175	4.0
french fries	444	6.0	61.0	19.0	0	605	0
tortilla chips, no salt	426	5.0	48.0	24.0	0	12	4.0
tostada shell only ..	440	7.0	42.0	27.0	0	610	0
kid's chicken sticks ..	226	17.3	14.6	12.9	53	787	0
side dishes:							
black beans	306	7.0	35.0	16.0	13	731	5.0
coleslaw	206	2.0	2.0	16.0	11	358	2.0
corn cobette	80	3.0	18.0	1.0	0	10	1.0
french fries	444	6.0	61.0	19.0	0	605	0
garden salad	105	5.0	7.0	7.0	15	99	1.0
gravy	13	.4	2.0	.5	1	16	0
macaroni and							
cheese	244	10.0	24.0	12.0	22	950	3.0
mashed potatoes ..	97	3.0	21.0	1.0	0	369	2.0
pinto beans	185	11.0	29.0	4.0	0	744	8.0
potato salad	256	3.0	30.0	14.0	15	527	3.0
Spanish rice	130	2.0	24.0	3.0	0	397	1.0
vegetables, fresh ..	57	2.0	8.0	2.0	0	79	3.0

Food and Measure	cal.	prot. (gms)	carbo. (gms)	fat (gms)	chol. (mgs)	sod. (mgs)	fiber (gms)
dressings, 1.5 oz., except as noted:							
blue cheese	230	2.0	2.0	24.0	30	450	0
creamy cilantro, 1.75 oz.	266	1.0	1.0	29.0	13	306	0
Italian, light	20	0	2.0	1.0	0	780	0
ranch	220	1.0	2.0	24.0	10	420	0
ranch, *Hidden Valley*	110	1.0	1.0	11.0	10	250	0
Thousand Island . .	220	0	7.0	21.0	30	360	0
condiments, 1 oz., except as noted:							
guacamole	30	0	3.0	2.0	0	160	0
hot sauce, .5 oz. . .	5	0	1.0	0	0	110	0
salsa, avocado	12	0	1.0	1.0	0	204	0
salsa, house	6	0	1.0	0	0	96	0
salsa, pico de gallo	11	0	1.5	.5	0	131	0
salsa, spicy chipotle	7	0	1.0	0	0	180	0
sour cream	60	1.0	1.0	5.0	20	15	0
desserts:							
banana split	717	12.0	107.0	28.0	56	310	3.0
churros	179	3.0	18.0	11.0	5	221	1.0
Foster's Freeze, w/out cone	180	4.0	30.0	5.0	20	100	0
smoothie:							
berry banana . . .	367	3.0	68.0	7.0	23	136	2.0
kiwi strawberry	357	5.0	66.0	7.0	23	141	2.0
Elderberries, ½ cup	53	.5	13.3	.4	0	4	5.1
Elderberry nectar (*R. W. Knudsen*), 8 fl. oz.	120	<1.0	28.0	0	0	20	0
Elk, meat only, roasted, 4 oz.	166	34.2	0	2.2	83	69	0
Empanada, frozen, 2 pcs.:							
beef (*Goya* Empanadas de Carne de Res) . .	380	11.0	58.0	12.0	15	800	2.0
cheese (*Goya* Empanadilla)	350	10.0	44.0	15.0	20	660	2.0
pizza (*Goya* Empanadilla)	370	11.0	56.0	12.0	15	930	4.0
Enchilada, frozen, w/sauce, 4.5-oz. pc.:							
beef (*El Monterey Family Classics*) . . .	180	8.0	17.0	9.0	25	610	2.0

Food and Measure	cal.	prot. (gms)	carbo. (gms)	fat (gms)	chol. (mgs)	sod. (mgs)	fiber (gms)
Enchilada *(cont.)*							
cheese (*El Monterey Family Classics*) . . .	210	10.0	15.0	13.0	35	530	1.0
chicken (*El Monterey Family Classics*) . . .	190	11.0	18.0	10.0	30	440	1.0
vegetable (*Cedarlane Low Fat*)	140	9.0	20.0	3.0	10	310	3.0
Enchilada dinner, frozen, 1 pkg.:							
beef (*Patio*), 11 oz. . .	370	10.0	54.0	12.0	25	1330	8.0
beef, and tamales (*Patio*), 12.25 oz.	480	12.0	54.0	24.0	35	2040	9.0
black bean (*Amy's*), 10 oz.	250	7.0	41.0	8.0	0	680	5.0
cheese:							
(*Amy's*), 9 oz.	330	15.0	38.0	14.0	30	680	6.0
(*Patio*), 11 oz.	350	15.0	54.0	10.0	20	1500	8.0
chicken:							
(*Healthy Choice*), 11.3 oz.	270	13.0	42.0	6.0	25	600	6.0
con queso (*Patio*), 11 oz.	350	12.0	49.0	12.0	25	1500	10.0
combination (*Patio*), 11 oz.	370	10.0	55.0	12.0	20	1390	8.0
Enchilada entree, frozen, 1 pkg., except as noted:							
beef:							
(*Banquet*), 11 oz.	370	10.0	54.0	12.0	25	1330	8.0
(*Ortega*), 9⅜ oz. . .	360	12.0	49.0	13.0	25	1460	5.0
(*Patio* Platter), 2 pcs.	190	5.0	27.0	7.0	15	1100	3.0
beef, and tamale:							
(*Banquet*), 11 oz.	450	10.0	56.0	20.0	35	1530	8.0
chili gravy w/ (*Morton*), 10 oz.	350	9.0	44.0	15.0	15	1400	8.0
black bean vegetable:							
(*Amy's*), ½ of 9.5-oz. pkg. . . .	130	4.0	20.0	4.0	0	390	2.0
(*Amy's* Family), ⅛ of 35-oz. pkg.	240	120	3.0	17.0	4.0	350	3.0
cheese:							
(*Amy's*), ½ of 9.5-oz. pkg. . . .	210	10.0	13.0	12.0	35	440	2.0

Food and Measure	cal.	prot. (gms)	carbo. (gms)	fat (gms)	chol. (mgs)	sod. (mgs	fiber (gms)
(*Amy's* Family), ⅟₇ of 35-oz. pkg. . .	240	11.0	13.0	13.0	35	490	2.0
(*Banquet*), 11 oz.	350	12.0	54.0	10.0	20	1500	8.0
(*Ortega*), 9.75 oz.	410	12.0	56.0	15.0	20	1780	4.0
chicken:							
(*Banquet*), 11 oz.	350	12.0	54.0	10.0	25	1580	9.0
(*Healthy Choice* Solos), 9 oz. . . .	310	16.0	46.0	7.0	40	600	6.0
(*Lean Cuisine Everyday Favorites*), 9 oz.	280	11.0	48.0	5.0	25	520	3.0
(*Ortega*), 9.5 oz. . .	400	13.0	51.0	16.0	35	1450	4.0
(*Stouffer's Family Style Favorites*), ⅟₁₂ of 57-oz. pkg.	220	8.0	22.0	11.0	30	570	2.0
chicken and cheese (*Michelina's*), 8 oz.	420	16.0	48.0	19.0	50	1170	2.0
combo:							
(*Patio Platter*), 2 pcs.	190	5.0	26.0	7.0	15.0	1120	3.0
Mexican style (*Banquet*), 11 oz.	370	10.0	55.0	12.0	20	1390	8.0
pie, 3-layer (*Cedarlane*), ½ of 10-oz. pkg. . .	216	13.0	27.0	7.0	16	595	3.0
vegetarian (*Cascadian Farm*), 10 oz.	370	14.0	54.0	12.0	20	610	9.0
Enchilada sauce, ¼ cup:							
(*La Victoria*)	25	0	2.0	1.5	0	330	0
green chili:							
(*La Victoria*)	15	0	3.0	0	0	270	0
(*Las Palmas*)	25	0	3.0	1.5	0	260	0
fire-roasted (*El Torito*)	15	0	4.0	0	0	350	0
medium, mild, or hot (*Hatch*)	20	<1.0	3.0	1.0	0	320	0
mild (*Old El Paso*)	30	<1.0	3.0	1.5	0	330	0
hot or mild (*Old El Paso*)	20	0	3.0	1.0	0	220	0
medium (*Hatch*)	35	1.0	5.0	1.0	0	300	1.0
mild or hot (*Hatch*) . .	25	0	3.0	1.5	0	260	<1.0
tomatillo (*El Torito*) . .	20	0	4.0	0	0	130	0

Food and Measure	cal.	prot. (gms)	carbo. (gms)	fat (gms)	chol. (mgs)	sod. (mgs)	fiber (gms)
Enchilada sauce *(cont.)*							
tomato, fire-roasted							
(*El Torito*)	·45	1.0	7.0	1.5	0	190	1.0
Enchilada sauce							
seasoning (*Lawry's*),							
2 tsp.	20	0	4.0	0	0	250	0
Endive, chopped,							
½ cup	4	.3	.8	.1	0	6	.8
Endive, Belgian,							
see "Chicory, witloof"							
Epazote, raw, 2 sprigs	1	0	.3	0	0	172	.2
Eppaw, raw, ½ cup ..	75	2.3	15.8	.9	0	6	n.a.
Escarole, see "Endive"							

F

Food and Measure	cal.	prot. (gms)	carbo. (gms)	fat (gms)	chol. (mgs)	sod. (mgs)	fiber (gms)
Fajita entree kit, frozen:							
beef (*Tyson* Meal Kit), ½ pkg.	480	31.0	60.0	13.0	55	1100	5.0
chicken:							
(*El Torito* Skillet), 3 oz.	50	5.0	5.0	1.5	15	230	1.0
(*Tyson* Meal Kit), ½ pkg.	460	28.0	61.0	11.0	45	1220	6.0
filling, ½ cup:							
chicken (*Ortega* Skillet)	35	4.0	3.0	1.0	10	130	1.0
steak (*Ortega* Skillet)	35	4.0	3.0	1.0	5	190	1.0
Fajita entree kit, pkg.:							
(*Chi-Chi's*), 2 shells and seasoning	300	6.0	54.0	7.0	0	1280	2.0
(*Old El Paso* No Fuss), 2 shells w/beef* ..	300	17.0	19.0	17.0	55	840	2.0
Fajita sauce, 2 tbsp.:							
chicken (*Lawry's* Weekday Gourmet)	20	1.0	3.0	1.0	0	600	0
marinade, Mexican (*World Harbors*) ..	45	0	10	0	0	290	0
Fajita seasoning (*McCormick*), ¼ tsp.	0	0	0	0	0	130	0
Fajita seasoning mix:							
(*Chi-Chi's*), ¼ pkg. ..	35	0	7.0	1.0	0	510	0
(*El Torito*), ¼ pkg. ..	35	0	7.0	0	0	560	0
(*Lawry's*), 2 tsp.	15	0	3.0	0	0	400	0
(*McCormick*), ⅛ pkg. .	15	0	2.0	0	0	290	0
chicken (*Lawry's*), 1 tsp.	10	0	2.0	0	0	320	0

Food and Measure	cal.	prot. (gms)	carbo. (gms)	fat (gms)	chol. (mgs)	sod. (mgs)	fiber (gms)
Falafel mix:							
(*Casbah*), 1.5 oz. . . .	160	6.0	20.0	3.0	0	530	2.0
(*Near East*), fried, about 5 patties* . . .	230	10.0	18.0	15.0	0	560	5.0
Farina, whole-grain (see also "Cereal"):							
dry, 1 oz.	105	3.0	22.1	.1	0	1	.8
cooked, 1 cup	116	3.4	24.6	.2	0	1	3.3
Farro, see "Spelt"							
Fava bean, see "Broad bean" and "Habas"							
Feijoa, raw:							
(*Frieda's*), 5 oz.	70	2.0	15.0	1.0	0	0	0
w/skin, 1 medium, 2.3 oz.	25	.6	5.3	.4	0	2	0
pureed, ½ cup	60	1.5	12.9	1.0	0	4	0
Fennel, bulb:							
(*Andy Boy D'Arrigo*), ⅛ bulb, 3.2 oz. . . .	30	1.0	7.0	0	0	50	3.0
(*Frieda's*), ¾ cup, 3 oz.	25	1.0	6.0	0	0	45	0
8.3-oz. bulb	72	2.9	17.1	.5	0	122	7.3
sliced, 1 cup	27	1.1	6.3	.2	0	45	2.7
Fennel seed, 1 tsp. . .	7	.3	1.1	.3	0	2	<1.0
Fenugreek seed, 1 tsp.	12	.9	2.2	.2	0	2	<1.0
Fettuccine:							
dry, see "Pasta"							
refrigerated:							
(*Buitoni*), 1¼ cups	240	10.0	45.0	2.5	90	20	2.0
(*Di Giorno*), 2.5 oz., ¼ pkg.	200	8.0	38.0	1.5	0	140	2.0
spinach (*Buitoni*), 1¼ cups	250	12.0	46.0	2.5	70	90	4.0
Fettuccine dish, dried (*AlpineAire* Leonardo da Fettuccine), 2.75 oz.	320	16.0	44.0	9.0	30	740	1.0
Fettuccine dish, mix:							
Alfredo:							
(*Knorr* Side Dish), ¾ cup	280	11.0	43.0	7.0	70	960	2.0
(*Knorr TasteBreaks* Cup), 1 cont. . .	230	7.0	41.0	4.0	10	980	1.0

Food and Measure	cal.	prot. (gms)	carbo. (gms)	fat (gms)	chol. (mgs)	sod. (mgs	fiber (gms)
(*Pasta Roni*), 1 cup*	460	12.0	48.0	25.0	5	1150	2.0
(*Pasta Roni* Reduced Fat), 1 cup*	310	12.0	49.0	8.0	10	1080	2.0
w/creamy basil sauce (*Knorr TasteBreaks* Cup), 1 cont.	220	6.0	40.0	4.0	10	850	2.0

Fettuccine entree,
frozen, 1 pkg.,
except as noted:
Alfredo:

Food and Measure	cal.	prot. (gms)	carbo. (gms)	fat (gms)	chol. (mgs)	sod. (mgs	fiber (gms)
(*Freezer Queen* Homestyle), 9 oz.	360	13.0	42.0	15.0	45	840	3.0
(*Healthy Choice* Solos), 8 oz. ...	240	11.0	37.0	5.0	20	560	2.0
(*Lean Cuisine Everyday Favorites*), 9.25 oz.	280	13.0	40.0	7.0	20	690	2.0
(*Master Choice*), 1 cup	330	13.0	53.0	7.0	20	200	3.0
(*Michelina's*), 9 oz.	380	15.0	45.0	15.0	40	670	2.0
(*Stouffer's*), 11.5 oz.	540	19.0	64.0	23.0	125	1190	4.0
w/broccoli and chicken (*Michelina's*), 8.5 oz. ..	310	16.0	37.0	10.0	45	660	2.0
w/broccoli and chicken (*Michelina's* Family), 1 cup	260	14.0	32.0	9.0	40	500	2.0
w/four cheeses (*Budget Gourmet*), 8 oz.	290	11.0	33.0	12.0	75	1010	2.0
w/garlic bread (*Marie Callender's*), 14 oz.	920	23.0	82.0	55.0	90	1270	3.0
w/mushrooms (*Cascadian Farm*), 10 oz.	360	14.0	42.0	16.0	40	630	1.0
vegetarian, w/"chicken" (*Quorn*), 10.6 oz.	360	17.0	40.0	16.0	45	920	4.0
w/broccoli and chicken (*Marie Callender's*), 13 oz.	710	26.0	53.0	43.0	85	910	6.0

Food and Measure	cal.	prot. (gms)	carbo. (gms)	fat (gms)	chol. (mgs)	sod. (mgs)	fiber (gms)
Fettuccine entree *(cont.)*							
carbonara *(Michelina's)*, 8 oz.	330	12.0	41.0	12.0	35	480	2.0
chicken, see "Chicken entree, frozen"							
w/chicken *(Michelina's)*, 8 oz.	280	13.0	37.0	9.0	25	570	3.0
w/creamy pesto and vegetables *(Michelina's)*, 8.5 oz.	250	10.0	37.0	6.0	20	580	3.0
primavera:							
(Lean Cuisine Everyday Favorites), 10 oz.	260	13.0	34.0	8.0	15	590	3.0
(Michelina's), 8 oz.	270	9.0	36.0	9.0	20	620	2.0
w/tortellini *(Marie Callender's)*, 14 oz.	750	19.0	57.0	49.0	65	1130	6.0
herb sauce w/chicken *(Budget Gourmet)*, 8.5 oz.	230	11.0	30.0	7.0	15.0	540	2.0
Fiddlehead fern, fresh, 4 oz.	39	5.2	6.3	.5	0	1	n.a.
Fig, fresh:							
1 large, 2.3 oz.	47	.5	12.3	.2	0	1	2.1
1 medium, 1.8 oz.	37	.4	9.6	.2	0	1	1.7
Fig, can or jar, ½ cup:							
in light syrup	87	.5	22.6	.1	0	1	2.3
in heavy syrup	114	.5	29.7	.1	0	2	2.8
Kadota, in heavy syrup *(Oregon)*	130	<1.0	30.0	1.0	0	5	3.0
Fig, dried:							
10 figs, 6.6 oz.	477	5.7	122.2	2.2	0	20	17.4
Calimyrna:							
(Blue Ribbon/Orchard Choice/Sun•Maid), 1.5 oz., about 2 pcs.	120	1.0	28.0	0	0	0	5.0
or Mission *(Sonoma)*, 3 pcs., 1.4 oz.	110	1.0	26.0	0	0	0	5.0
crown *(Frieda's)*, 3 pcs., 1.4 oz.	100	1.0	26.0	0	0	0	4.0
Kalamata *(Krinos)*, 3 pcs., 1.4 oz.	100	1.0	26.0	0	0	0	4.0

Food and Measure	cal.	prot. (gms)	carbo. (gms)	fat (gms)	chol. (mgs)	sod. (mgs)	fiber (gms)
Mission:							
(*Frieda's*), ¼ cup, 1.4 oz.	110	1.0	26.0	0	0	0	5.0
(*Orchard Choice*), 4–5 pcs., 1.5 oz.	120	1.0	28.0	0	0	0	5.0
(*Sun•Maid Fast Fruit*), 3–4 pcs., 1.5 oz.	120	1.0	28.0	0	0	0	5.0
Filberts:							
(*Setton Farm* Natural), .8 oz.	200	4.0	6.0	18.0	0	0	4.0
raw, diced (*Blue Diamond* Hazelnuts), ¼ cup	200	5.0	5.0	19.0	0	0	3.0
dried:							
1 oz.	179	3.7	4.4	17.8	0	1	1.7
chopped, 1 cup ...	727	15.0	17.6	72.0	0	3	7.0
dry-roasted salted, 1 oz.	188	2.8	5.1	18.8	0	221	<2.0
oil-roasted salted, 1 oz.	187	4.1	5.4	18.1	0	223	1.8
Fillo dough, frozen:							
(*Apollo/Athens*), 2 oz., ⅛ pkg.	180	5.0	35.0	1.0	0	300	1.0
(*Apollo/Athens* Twin Pack), 5 sheets, 2 oz.	180	5.0	35.0	1.0	0	300	1.0
shredded (*Apollo/ Athens*), 2 oz.	180	5.0	35.0	2.0	0	140	4.0
extra thick (*Apollo/ Athens*), 2-oz. sheet	170	4.0	26.0	5.0	0	440	0
Fireweed, leaves, fresh, 1 cup	24	1.1	4.4	.7	0	8	2.4
Fish, see specific listings							
"Fish," vegetarian:							
frozen (*Worthington* Fillets), 2 pcs.	180	16.0	8.0	9.0	0	750	4.0
mix (*Loma Linda Ocean Platter*), ⅓ cup	90	14.0	8.0	1.0	0	450	4.0
Fish cake, see "Fish entree" and specific listings							

Food and Measure	cal.	prot. (gms)	carbo. (gms)	fat (gms)	chol. (mgs)	sod. (mgs)	fiber (gms)
Fish dinner, frozen, 1 pkg.:							
w/chips (*Swanson Traditional Favorites* Fish-n-Chips), 10 oz.	490	19.0	59.0	20.0	45	1030	5.0
herb baked (*Healthy Choice*), 10.9 oz.	360	16.0	55.0	8.0	40	590	5.0
lemon pepper (*Healthy Choice*), 10.7 oz.	320	14.0	15.0	7.0	30	480	5.0
sticks (*Swanson Fun Feast*), 7 oz.	340	10.0	48.0	12.0	0	590	3.0
Fish entree, frozen (see also specific fish listings):							
baked:							
(*Lean Cuisine Cafe Classics*), 9-oz. pkg.	290	20.0	40.0	6.0	40	690	2.0
au gratin (*Gorton's*), 1 pc.	130	14.0	7.0	5.0	50	400	0
breaded (*Marie Callender's*), 12-oz. pkg.	550	22.0	53.0	28.0	60	1400	3.0
cakes (*Mrs. Paul's*), 2 pcs.	210	8.0	24.0	10.0	15	730	<1.0
w/cheese, salsa (*Oven Poppers*), ½ of 9-oz. pkg.	130	16.0	3.0	6.0	70	150	1.0
croquette (*Dr. Praeger's*), 2.2-oz. pc.	120	10.0	12.0	5.0	· 25	170	1.0
fillet, w/macaroni and cheese (*Stouffer's* HomeStyle), 9-oz. pkg.	410	23.0	44.0	16.0	60	1000	2.0
fillet, battered:							
(*Gorton's*), 2 pcs.	240	10.0	17.0	15.0	30	770	0
(*Mrs. Paul's*), 1 pc.	150	6.0	14.0	8.0	20	370	0
(*Mrs. Paul's* Hearty Size), 1 pc.	200	9.0	19.0	10.0	25	510	0
(*Van de Kamp's*), 1 pc.	170	8.0	13.0	10.0	20	390	0
lemon pepper (*Gorton's*), 2 pcs.	270	9.0	18.0	18.0	35	610	0

Food and Measure	cal.	prot. (gms)	carbo. (gms)	fat (gms)	chol. (mgs)	sod. (mgs	fiber (gms)
fillet, breaded:							
(*Dr. Praeger's*), 2.1-oz. pc.	113	6.5	11.0	4.0	24	211	1.0
(*Dr. Praeger's* Sandwich), 4-oz. pc.	210	12.0	19.0	9.0	60	230	1.0
(*Gorton's*), 2 pcs.	250	9.0	20.0	15.0	25	600	0
(*Mrs. Paul's*), 2 pcs.	280	10.0	19.0	18.0	25	430	0
(*Mrs. Paul's* Crisp & Healthy), 1 pc.	130	8.0	19.0	2.0	20	320	0
(*Van de Kamp's*), 2 pcs.	260	10.0	17.0	17.0	25	380	0
(*Van de Kamp's* Hearty Size), 1 pc.	150	6.0	10.0	10.0	15	220	0
(*Van de Kamp's* Crisp & Healthy), 2 pcs.	170	11.0	25.0	3.0	25	400	0
garlic and herb (*Gorton's*), 2 pcs.	270	9.0	22.0	16.0	25	630	0
lemon pepper (*Gorton's* Skillet), 1 pc...........	220	1.0	13.0	13.0	40	670	0
Parmesan (*Gorton's*), 2 pcs.	250	10.0	19.0	15.0	30	650	0
ranch (*Gorton's*), 2 pcs.	240	9.0	22.0	13.0	30	650	0
seasoned (*Gorton's* Skillet Traditional), 1 pc.	220	1.0	13.0	13.0	40	700	0
fillet, breaded, baked:							
garlic herb or lemon pepper (*Mrs. Paul's* Crisp & Healthy), 1 pc.	130	8.0	19.0	2.0	20	340	0
garlic herb (*Van de Kamp's* Crisp & Healthy), 2 pcs.	170	11.0	25.0	3.0	25	450	0
lemon pepper (*Van de Kamp's* Crisp & Healthy), 2 pcs.	170	11.0	24.0	3.0	25	450	0
fillet, grilled, 1 pc.:							
Cajun (*Mrs. Paul's*)	130	19.0	0	6.0	60	280	0
char-grilled (*Gorton's* Grilled Fillets*) ..	110	17.0	1.0	4.5	60	240	0

Food and Measure	cal.	prot. (gms)	carbo (gms)	fat (gms)	chol. (mgs)	sod. (mgs)	fiber (gms)
Fish entree, fillet, grilled (cont.)							
garlic butter (Mrs. Paul's)	130	19.0	0	6.0	60	220	0
garlic butter (Van de Kamp's)	120	17.0	0	6.0	60	210	0
Italian herb (Gorton's Grilled Fillets) ..	100	17.0	<1.0	3.0	60	380	0
lemon butter or lemon pepper (Van de Kamp's)	120	17.0	0	6.0	60	190	0
lemon pepper (Gorton's Grilled Fillets)	100	12.0	0	4.5	60	170	0
lemon pepper (Mrs. Paul's)	130	19.0	0	6.0	60	210	0
portions:							
battered (Van de Kamp's), 1 pc.	160	6.0	13.0	9.0	20	360	0
breaded (Fisher Boy), 2 pcs. ...	200	0	19.0	10.0	15	460	2.0
breaded (Van de Kamp's), 3 pcs. .	300	14.0	23.0	24.0	30	480	0
w/shrimp, crab, vegetables (Oven Poppers), ½ of 9-oz. pkg.	200	13.0	13.0	11.0	85	380	0
w/spinach, cheese (Oven Poppers), ½ of 9-oz. pkg.	160	15.0	8.0	8.0	70	310	0
sticks:							
(Banquet), 6.6 oz.	270	13.0	31.0	10.0	30	690	3.0
(Freezer Queen Meal), 6.5-oz. pkg. ...	290	5.0	47.0	9.0	75	540	3.0
(Kid Cuisine), 8.25-oz. pkg. ..	330	10.0	45.0	12.0	25	820	4.0
sticks, battered (Gorton), 5 pcs. ..	290	10.0	20.0	19.0	25	530	0
sticks, breaded, 6 pcs., except as noted:							
(Dr. Praeger's Fillet), 2.9 oz.	138	7.0	14.0	6.0	24	185	1.0
(Dr. Praeger's Minced), 1.7 oz.	90	7.5	9.0	3.5	18	127	1.0
(Fisher Boy)	190	9.0	15.0	11.0	10	370	1.0
(Gorton's)	260	9.0	21.0	14.0	20	390	0

Food and Measure	cal.	prot. (gms)	carbo. (gms)	fat (gms)	chol. (mgs)	sod. (mgs)	fiber (gms)
(Mrs. Paul's)	250	10.0	21.0	14.0	20	430	1.0
(Mrs. Paul's Hearty Size), 5 pcs. ...	300	11.0	25.0	17.0	25	510	1.0
(Mrs. Paul's Crisp & Healthy)	190	11.0	26.0	3.0	30	450	0
(Van de Kamp's) ..	290	12.0	22.0	17.0	30	420	0
(Van de Kamp's Club Pack)	240	10.0	19.0	14.0	25	330	0
(Van de Kamp's Snack/Value Pack)	260	11.0	20.0	15.0	25	360	0
mini (Gorton's), 13 pcs.	250	9.0	24.0	13.0	15	380	0
mini (Van de Kamp's), 13 pcs. ..	250	11.0	19.0	14.0	30	330	0
strips, breaded, 4 pcs.:							
(Mrs. Paul's)	310	12.0	25.0	18.0	25	530	0
(Van de Kamp's) ..	270	12.0	25.0	14.0	25	400	0
tenders, 4 oz.:							
(Gorton's Original Batter)	260	10.0	22.0	15.0	25	620	0
breaded (Gorton's Extra Crunchy) ..	270	9.0	30.0	12.0	30	720	0
lemon herb, breaded (Gorton's)	260	11.0	26.0	12.0	30	660	0
tenders, battered, 4 pcs.:							
(Mrs. Paul's)	280	8.0	26.0	17.0	25	560	0
(Van de Kamp's) ..	290	11.0	24.0	17.0	25	570	0
Fish sandwich, fillet, frozen (Hormel Quick Meal), 1 pc.	420	15.0	49.0	18.0	40	960	1.0
Fish seasoning, see specific listings							
Fish seasoning and coating mix:							
(Old Bay Better Batter), ¼ cup	110	2.0	13.0	.5	0	690	<1.0
(Shake 'n Bake), ¼ pkt.	80	2.0	13.0	1.5	0	350	<1.0
fish and chips (Don's Chuck Wagon), ¼ cup	95	4.0	21.0	0	0	940	1.0
fish fry (Sylvia's), 3 tbsp.	100	3.0	10.0	1.0	0	710	0

Food and Measure	cal.	prot. (gms)	carbo. (gms)	fat (gms)	chol. (mgs)	sod. (mgs)	fiber (gms)
Fish seasoning and coating mix *(cont.)*							
garlic herb (*Golden Dipt Bag'n Season*), ¼ pkg.	25	0	3.0	0	0	370	0
lemon dill (*Golden Dipt Bag'n Season*), ¼ pkg.	35	0	6.0	0	0	190	0
seafood (*Don's Chuck Wagon* Bake & Fry), ¼ cup	95	2.0	21.0	0	0	690	1.0
Flatfish, meat only:							
raw, 4 oz.	104	21.4	0	1.4	54	92	0
baked, broiled, or microwaved, 4 oz.	133	27.4	0	1.7	77	119	0
Flax powder (*Arrowhead Mills* Nutri), 2 tbsp.	70	6.0	6.0	2.0	0	10	6.0
Flax seeds (*Arrowhead Mills*), 3 tbsp.	140	5.0	11.0	10.0	0	0	6.0
Flounder, fresh, see "Flatfish"							
Flounder entree, frozen:							
au gratin (*Oven Poppers*), 5-oz. pc.	220	24.0	5.0	11.0	75	450	1.0
fillet, breaded, 1 pc.:							
(*Mrs. Paul's* Premium), 2.8 oz.	170	11.0	11.0	9.0	30	220	0
(*Van de Kamp's* Premium), 4 oz.	230	14.0	18.0	11.0	40	390	0
stuffed, 5-oz. pc.:							
w/broccoli and cheese (*Oven Poppers*)	150	20.0	4.0	6.0	55	330	1.0
w/crab (*Oven Poppers*)	250	17.0	15.0	13.0	70	400	1.0
w/garlic, shrimp, almonds (*Oven Poppers*)	250	19.0	15.0	13.0	80	430	2.0
Flour, see "Wheat flour" and specific listings							
Focaccia, see "Bread"							
Focaccia, stuffed, frozen, 5.5 oz.:							
Italian (*Cedarlane*) . .	410	18.0	52.0	14.0	30	750	2.0

Food and Measure	cal.	prot. (gms)	carbo. (gms)	fat (gms)	chol. (mgs)	sod. (mgs)	fiber (gms)
Mediterranean (*Cedarlane*)	410	18.0	51.0	14.0	30	670	2.0
Roma tomato (*Cedarlane*)	380	19.0	46.0	13.0	2	730	2.5
Fondue:							
cheese, ¼ cup:							
(*Swiss Knight*)	120	9.0	2.0	9.0	25	390	0
(*Swissrose*)	140	10.0	0	10.0	20	440	0
chocolate (*Swiss Knight*), 1 oz.	160	2.0	15.0	10.0	0	30	2.0
Fradiavolo sauce, see "Pasta sauce"							
Frankfurter, 1 link, except as noted:							
(*Ball Park* Fat Free)	50	6.0	6.0	0	10	520	0
(*Ball Park* Lite)	100	6.0	3.0	7.0	25	540	0
(*Ball Park* Singles)	150	5.0	3.0	13.0	30	490	0
(*Boar's Head* Natural Casing/Skinless)	150	7.0	0	14.0	25	460	0
(*Healthy Choice* 10 Pack), 1.4 oz.	70	6.0	6.0	2.5	20	440	0
(*Healthy Choice* 8 Pack), 1.75 oz.	60	5.0	5.0	2.0	15	350	0
(*Hormel* Fat Free Hot Dogs)	45	5.0	5.0	0	15	580	0
(*Johnsonville* Wieners), 1.7 oz.	150	6.0	1.0	14.0	40	410	0
(*Light & Lean*)	45	5.0	4.0	1.0	15	490	0
(*Louis Rich* Original 50% less Fat), 1.6 oz.	90	5.0	2.0	6.0	40	510	0
(*Nathan's Famous*)	160	7.0	1.0	15.0	30	490	0
(*Oscar Mayer* Wieners)	140	5.0	1.0	13.0	35	440	0
beef:							
(*Ball Park*)	180	6.0	3.0	16.0	35	620	0
(*Ball Park* Fat Free)	55	6.0	7.0	0	10	490	0
(*Ball Park* Kosher)	140	6.0	2.0	12.0	30	440	0
(*Ball Park* Lite)	100	6.0	3.0	3.0	20	510	0
(*Ball Park* Singles)	150	5.0	2.0	13.0	30	500	0
(*Boar's Head* Lite)	90	7.0	0	6.0	25	270	0
(*Boar's Head* Natural Casing)	160	7.0	1.0	14.0	30	440	0
(*Boar's Head* Skinless)	120	6.0	0	11.0	20	350	0

Food and Measure	cal.	prot. (gms)	carbo. (gms)	fat (gms)	chol. (mgs)	sod. (mgs)	fiber (gms)
Frankfurter, beef *(cont.)*							
(*Healthy Choice*) . .	70	6.0	7.0	2.5	15	440	0
(*Hebrew National*)	150	6.0	1.0	14.0	30	370	0
(*Hebrew National* Family/Party Pack)	180	7.0	1.0	16.0	40	450	0
(*Hebrew National* 99% Fat Free) . .	45	6.0	3.0	1.5	15	400	0
(*Hebrew National* Reduced Fat) . . .	120	6.0	0	10.0	25	360	0
(*Hormel* Fat Free Hot Dogs)	45	6.0	5.0	0	10	590	0
(*Hormel* Natural Casing)	210	8.0	0	19.0	40	550	0
(*Nathan's Famous*)	170	7.0	1.0	15.0	35	470	0
(*Oscar Mayer*)	140	5.0	1.0	13.0	30	460	0
(*Oscar Mayer* Bun-Length)	180	6.0	2.0	17.0	30	580	0
(*Wranglers*)	170	7.0	1.0	15.0	40	560	0
dinner (*Hebrew National* ¼ Pound)	350	13.0	1.0	32.0	70	990	0
beef, cocktail.							
(*Boar's Head*), 5 pcs.	170	8.0	0	15.0	30	430	0
(*Hebrew National*), 5 pcs., 2 oz. . . .	180	7.0	1.0	16.0	40	450	0
cheese:							
(*Oscar Mayer*)	140	6.0	1.0	13.0	35	460	0
(*Wranglers*)	170	7.0	1.0	15.0	40	630	0
chicken, 2 oz.:							
(*Empire* Kosher) . .	100	8.0	1.0	7.0	70	465	0
(*Wampler*)	120	7.0	0	11.0	60	480	1.0
smoked:							
(*Oscar Mayer* Big & Juicy Smokie), 2.7 oz.	210	9.0	1.0	19.0	50	800	0
(*Wranglers*)	170	7.0	1.0	15.0	40	560	0
turkey:							
(*Jennie-O*)	80	4.0	0	7.0	25	360	0
(*Jennie-O* Jumbo)	130	7.0	0	11.0	40	600	0
(*Wampler*), 1.6 oz.	90	6.0	0	8.0	35	430	2.0
Frankfurter, canned (*Vienna* Big Foot Hot Dog), 2 oz. . . .	150	7.0	2.0	13.0	30	570	0

Food and Measure	cal.	prot. (gms)	carbo. (gms)	fat (gms)	chol. (mgs)	sod. (mgs)	fiber (gms)
"Frankfurter," vegetarian, 1 link or pc., except as noted:							
canned:							
(*Loma Linda* Big) ..	110	10.0	2.0	7.0	0	240	2.0
(*Loma Linda* Big Lowfat)	80	11.0	3.0	3.0	0	220	2.0
(*Loma Linda* Linketts)	70	7.0	1.0	4.5	0	160	1.0
(*Worthington* Super Links)	110	7.0	2.0	8.0	0	350	1.0
(*Worthington* Veja-Links)	50	5.0	1.0	3.0	0	180	0
(*Worthington* Veja-Links Lowfat) ...	40	5.0	1.0	1.5	0	190	0
frozen or refrigerated:							
(*Loma Linda* Corn Dog)	150	7.0	22.0	4.0	0	500	3.0
(*Morningstar Farms* Corn Dog)	150	7.0	22.0	4.0	0	500	3.0
(*Morningstar Farms* Veggie Dog)	80	11.0	6.0	.5	0	580	1.0
(*Natural Touch* Veggie Corn Dog)	170	8.0	22.0	6.0	0	530	3.0
(*Natural Touch* Veggie Dog)	90	11.0	6.0	2.0	0	680	1.0
(*Veggie Master* Vege Hot Dog), ¼ pkg.	134	7.0	6.2	7.5	0	135	6.2
(*Worthington* Leanies)	100	7.0	2.0	7.0	0	430	1.0
(*Yves* Chili Dogs) ..	50	10.0	3.0	0	0	360	2.0
(*Yves* The Good Dog)	70	13.0	2.0	1.5	0	460	1.0
(*Yves* Tofu Dogs) ..	45	9.0	2.0	.5	0	240	0
(*Yves* Veggie Dogs)	60	11.0	1.0	0	0	400	1.0
jumbo (*Yves* Veggie Dogs)	100	16.0	7.0	1.5	0	480	2.0
mini (*Morningstar Farms* Corn Dog), 4 pcs.	170	11.0	21.0	4.5	0	580	1.0
Frankfurter, wrapped, 1 pc., except as noted:							

Food and Measure	cal.	prot. (gms)	carbo. (gms)	fat (gms)	chol. (mgs)	sod. (mgs)	fiber (gms)
Franfurter, wrapped (cont.)							
beef (*Hebrew National Franks-in-a-Blanket*), 5 pcs.	290	9.0	8.0	24.0	40	690	1.0
corn dog:							
(*Hormel Quick Meal*)	272	7.0	32.9	12.5	35	590	1.0
(*State Fair*)	170	5.0	16.0	10.0	25	540	1.0
(*State Fair* Individually Wrapped)	180	4.0	15.0	12.0	15	560	0
beef (*State Fair*) . .	180	4.0	15.0	12.0	15	560	0
cheese (*State Fair*)	180	5.0	16.0	11.0	25	530	0
corn dog, mini:							
(*Hormel Quick Meal*), 10 pcs.	490	6.0	47.0	29.0	90	1130	1.0
(*State Fair*), 4 pcs.	230	7.0	22.0	13.0	30	460	3.0
beef (*State Fair*), 4 pcs.	250	6.0	21.0	16.0	25	510	2.0
cheese (*State Fair*), 4 pcs.	250	7.0	22.0	15.0	30	450	2.0
Franks and beans, see "Beans and franks"							
French toast, frozen:							
(*Aunt Jemima* Homestyle), 2 pcs.	240	10.0	35.0	7.0	95	310	2.0
(*Pepperidge Farm* Homestyle), 1 pc.	160	5.0	23.0	5.0	35	200	1.0
cinnamon:							
(*Aunt Jemima*), 2 pcs.	240	10.0	35.0	7.0	90	330	2.0
(*Pepperidge Farm*), 1 pc.	170	5.0	24.0	6.0	35	190	2.0
sticks (*Aunt Jemima*), 4 pcs.	350	5.0	52.0	13.0	<5	520	1.0
cinnamon raisin (*Pepperidge Farm*), 1 pc.	190	5.0	26.0	8.0	30	160	2.0
French toast breakfast, frozen, 1 pkg.:							
w/sausage:							
(*Great Starts*), 5.5 oz.	410	12.0	36.0	24.0	95	490	3.0
(*Uncle Ben's* Breakfast Bowl), 6 oz.	420	11.0	45.0	22.0	90	620	3.0
cinnamon swirl (*Great Starts*), 5.5 oz.	440	14.0	35.0	28.0	150	580	2.0

Food and Measure	cal.	prot. (gms)	carbo. (gms)	fat (gms)	chol. (mgs)	sod. (mgs)	fiber (gms)
sticks, w/syrup (*Great Starts*), 4.25 oz. ..	420	5.0	67.0	15.0	60	410	0
Frosting, ready-to-spread, 2 tbsp.:							
banana creme (*Pillsbury* Creamy Supreme)	150	0	23.0	6.0	0	70	0
butter cream:							
(*Creamy Deluxe*) ..	140	0	23.0	5.0	0	75	0
(*Duncan Hines*) ...	140	0	22.0	5.0	0	60	0
chocolate (*Duncan Hines*)	130	0	20.0	5.0	0	95	0
whipped (*Betty Crocker*)	100	0	16.0	4.5	0	25	0
caramel (*Duncan Hines*)	140	0	22.0	5.0	0	60	0
cherry (*Creamy Deluxe*)	140	0	23.0	5.0	0	75	0
cherry, wild, vanilla (*Duncan Hines*) ...	140	0	22.0	5.0	0	60	0
chocolate:							
(*Creamy Deluxe*) ..	130	0	21.0	5.0	0	90	0
(*Duncan Hines*) ...	130	0	20.0	5.0	0	95	0
(*Pillsbury* Creamy Supreme)	140	0	21.0	6.0	0	80	0
(*Sweet Rewards*) ..	120	1.0	24.0	2.0	0	50	1.0
dark (*Creamy Deluxe*)	130	1.0	20.0	5.0	0	95	1.0
fudge (*Duncan Hines*)	130	0	20.0	5.0	0	95	0
fudge (*Pillsbury* Creamy Supreme)	140	0	21.0	6.0	0	80	0
milk (*Creamy Deluxe*)	130	0	21.0	5.0	0	90	0
milk (*Duncan Hines*)	130	0	20.0	5.0	0	95	0
milk (*Pillsbury* Creamy Supreme)	140	0	21.0	6.0	0	60	<1.0
milk (*Sweet Rewards*)	120	0	25.0	2.0	0	45	0
milk, w/sprinkles (*Creamy Deluxe*)	130	0	22.0	5.0	0	85	0
milk, whipped (*Betty Crocker*)	100	0	14.0	4.5	0	50	0
mocha (*Duncan Hines*)	130	0	20.0	5.0	0	95	0

Food and Measure	cal.	prot. (gms)	carbo. (gms)	fat (gms)	chol. (mgs)	sod. (mgs)	fiber (gms)
Frosting, chocolate *(cont.)*							
whipped (*Betty Crocker*)	90	<1.0	14.0	4.5	0	55	0
coconut (*Duncan Hines*)	150	0	20.0	6.0	0	70	0
coconut pecan:							
(*Creamy Deluxe*) ..	140	<1.0	17.0	8.0	0	50	0
(*Duncan Hines*) ...	150	0	18.0	9.0	0	70	0
(*Pillsbury* Creamy Supreme)	160	0	17.0	10.0	0	60	<1.0
cookies and cream (*Pillsbury* Creamy Supreme)	150	0	23.0	6.0	0	70	0
cream cheese:							
(*Creamy Deluxe*) ..	140	0	23.0	5.0	0	80	0
(*Duncan Hines*) ...	140	0	22.0	5.0	0	60	0
(*Pillsbury* Creamy Supreme)	150	0	24.0	6.0	0	70	0
whipped (*Betty Crocker*)	100	0	15.0	4.5	0	45	0
fudge, hot (*Pillsbury* Creamy Supreme) .	140	0	21.0	6.0	0	55	0
Funfetti:							
chocolate (*Pillsbury* Creamy Supreme)	140	0	22.0	6.0	0	80	0
pink vanilla (*Pillsbury* Creamy Supreme)	150	0	24.0	6.0	0	70	0
vanilla (*Pillsbury* Creamy Supreme)	150	0	25.0	6.0	0	75	0
lemon:							
(*Creamy Deluxe*) ..	140	0	23.0	5.0	0	85	0
(*Duncan Hines*) ...	140	0	22.0	5.0	0	60	0
whipped (*Betty Crocker*)	100	0	15.0	5.0	0	25	0
rainbow chip (*Creamy Deluxe*) ..	140	0	23.0	5.0	0	65	0
sour cream:							
chocolate (*Creamy Deluxe*)	130	0	21.0	5.0	0	90	0
white (*Creamy Deluxe*)	140	0	23.0	5.0	0	70	0
strawberries 'n cream (*Duncan Hines*) ...	140	0	22.0	5.0	0	60	0

Food and Measure	cal.	prot. (gms)	carbo. (gms)	fat (gms)	chol. (mgs)	sod. (mgs	fiber (gms)
strawberry:							
cream cheese							
(*Creamy Deluxe*)	140	0	23.0	5.0	0	80	0
creme (*Pillsbury*							
Creamy Supreme)	150	0	24.0	6.0	0	75	0
whipped (*Betty*							
Crocker)	100	0	15.0	5.0	0	25	0
vanilla:							
(*Creamy Deluxe*) ..	140	0	23.0	5.0	0	70	0
(*Duncan Hines*) ...	140	0	22.0	5.0	0	60	0
(*Pillsbury* Creamy							
Supreme)	150	0	23.0	6.0	0	70	0
(*Sweet Rewards*) ..	130	0	27.0	2.0	0	60	0
French (*Creamy*							
Deluxe)	140	0	23.0	5.0	0	70	0
French (*Duncan*							
Hines)	140	0	22.0	5.0	0	60	0
French (*Pillsbury*							
Creamy Supreme)	160	0	26.0	6.0	0	75	0
French, whipped							
(*Betty Crocker*)	100	0	16.0	4.5	0	25	0
w/sprinkles							
(*Creamy Deluxe*)	140	0	24.0	5.0	0	70	0
whipped (*Betty*							
Crocker)	100	0	15.0	4.5	0	25	0
white, fluffy, whipped							
(*Betty Crocker*) ...	100	0	15.0	4.5	0	25	0
Frosting mix:							
fudge (*"Jiffy"*), ¼ cup	150	<1.0	28.0	4.0	0	150	<1.0
white:							
(*"Jiffy"*), ¼ cup ...	150	0	27.0	4.5	0	150	0
fluffy (*Betty*							
Crocker),							
6 tbsp.*	100	<1.0	24.0	0	0	60	0
Frozen desserts, see							
"Ice cream" and							
specific listings							
Fructose:							
(*Estee*), 1 tsp.	15	0	4.0	0	0	0	0
(*Estee*), 1 pkt.	10	0	3.0	0	0	0	0
(*Featherweight*), 1 tsp.	15	0	4.0	0	0	0	0
Fruit, see specific							
listings							

Food and Measure	cal.	prot. (gms)	carbo. (gms)	fat (gms)	chol. (mgs)	sod. (mgs)	fiber (gms)
Fruit, mixed, can or jar (see also "Fruit cocktail"), ½ cup, except as noted:							
in juice:							
(*Del Monte* Fruit Naturals Chunky)	60	0	15.0	0	0	10	1.0
(*Del Monte* Fruit Naturals Snack Cup), 4 oz.	50	0	13.0	0	0	10	<1.0
(*Libby's Natural Lite* Chunky)	60	0	14.0	0	0	5	1.0
(*S&W* Chunky) . . .	80	<1.0	19.0	0	0	20	3.0
tropical salad, in pineapple and passion fruit juices (*Del Monte*)	60	0	16.0	0	0	15	1.0
in extra light syrup:							
(*Del Monte* Lite Chunky)	60	0	15.0	0	0	10	1.0
(*Del Monte* Lite Snack Cup), 4 oz.	50	0	13.0	0	0	10	<1.0
(*Sunfresh* Fruit Salad Chilled) . .	70	1.0	22.0	0	0	5	2.0
Ambrosia (*Sunfresh* Chilled)	70	0	16.0	0	0	25	1.0
citrus (*Sunfresh* Chilled)	80	0	20.0	0	0	20	0
tropical (*Sunfresh* Chilled)	80	1.0	20.0	0	0	10	0
in light syrup:							
(*Del Monte* Fruit-to-Go Fruity Combo), 4 oz.	70	<1.0	18.0	0	0	10	<1.0
(*Sunfresh* Chilled Mixed Fruit)	90	1.0	20.0	0	0	25	2.0
California (*Del Monte Orchard Select*)	80	<1.0	19.0	0	0	10	<1.0
cherry flavored (*Del Monte Fruit Pleasures*)	90	<1.0	22.0	0	0	10	<1.0

Food and Measure	cal.	prot. (gms)	carbo. (gms)	fat (gms)	chol. (mgs)	sod. (mgs)	fiber (gms)
cherry flavored (*Del Monte Fruitageous Crazy Cherry*), 4 oz.	90	<1.0	22.0	0	0	10	<1.0
citrus (*Sunfresh Can*)	50	0	12.0	0	0	0	1.0
tropical salad, w/passion fruit juice (*Del Monte*)	80	0	21.0	0	0	10	1.0
tropical (*Dole*)	80	0	20.0	0	0	10	1.0
in heavy syrup:							
(*Del Monte* Chunky)	100	0	24.0	0	0	10	1.0
(*Del Monte* Snack Cup), 4 oz.	80	0	20.0	0	0	10	<1.0
tropical salad	110	.5	28.6	.1	0	3	1.7
Fruit, mixed, candied:							
(*Paradise/Queen Anne* Fruit Cake Mix), 2 tbsp.	100	0	25.0	0	0	20	1.0
(*Paradise* Old English/ White Swan*), 1 tbsp.	70	0	18.0	0	0	15	1.0
(*Seneca* Glacé Deluxe), 2 tbsp.	70	0	18.0	0	0	15	1.0
(*S&W* Glacé Cake Mix), 2 tbsp.	90	0	25.0	0	0	30	2.0
(*White Swan* Deluxe), 2 tbsp.	100	0	25.0	0	0	20	1.0
Fruit, mixed, dried:							
(*Setton Farm* Ambrosia), 1.1 oz. . . .	100	1.0	21.0	1.5	0	0	2.0
(*Sonoma*), 7 pcs., 1.4 oz.	120	1.0	30.0	0	0	0	3.0
(*Sun•Maid*), ¼ cup . .	110	1.0	26.0	0	0	55	3.0
(*Sunsweet* Fruit Morsels), 1.4 oz., ¼ cup	120	1.0	28.0	0	0	55	2.0
diced (*Sonoma*), ⅓ cup, 1.4 oz. . . .	120	1.0	31.0	0	0	0	3.0
Island mix (*Sunsweet Fruitlings*), ⅓ cup, 1.4 oz.	120	1.0	31.0	0	0	0	3.0
and nuts, see "Trail mix"							
tropical (*Sunsweet Fruitlings*), ¼ cup, 1.4 oz.	140	0	32.0	1.0	0	50	2.0

Food and Measure	cal.	prot. (gms)	carbo. (gms)	fat (gms)	chol. (mgs)	sod. (mgs)	fiber (gms)
Fruit, mixed, frozen:							
(*Big Valley*), ⅔ cup ..	60	1.0	14.0	0	0	0	2.0
(*Birds Eye*), ½ cup ..	90	.5	23.0	0	0	5	n.a.
(*McKenzie's*), ⅓ of							
16-oz. pkg.	60	1.0	13.0	0	0	20	2.0
Fruit bar, frozen (see							
also "Ice bar," and							
"Sorbet bar"), 1 pc.:							
all flavors:							
(*Ocean Spray*)	45	0	12.0	0	0	25	0
(*Ocean Spray* No							
Sugar)	25	0	6.0	0	0	0	0
(*Popsicle* Fruit							
Juicee)	60	0	15.0	0	0	0	0
banana cream:							
(*FrozFruit*)	150	1.0	20.0	8.0	30	20	<1.0
chocolate dipped							
(*Dreyer's/Edy's*							
Whole Fruit) ...	190	3.0	23.0	10.0	5	30	0
chocolate dipped							
(*FrozFruit*)	210	1.0	22.0	14.0	20	15	1.0
cantaloupe (*FrozFruit*)	60	0	15.0	0	0	5	0
cherry (*FrozFruit*) ...	70	1.0	16.0	0	0	55	<1.0
coconut cream:							
(*FrozFruit*)	200	2.0	18.0	14.0	35	25	2.0
chocolate dipped							
(*FrozFruit*)	240	2.0	24.0	17.0	20	35	8.0
lemon (*FrozFruit*) ...	80	0	19.0	0	0	75	0
lemonade (*Dreyer's/*							
Edy's Whole Fruit)	80	0	20.0	0	0	0	0
lime:							
(*Dreyer's/Edy's*							
Whole Fruit) ...	80	0	20.0	0	0	0	0
(*FrozFruit*)	90	0	22.0	0	0	85	0
lime, strawberry, and							
wildberry (*Dreyer's/*							
Edy's Whole Fruit)	60	0	14.0	0	0	0	0
mango (*FrozFruit*) ...	110	0	26.0	0	0	5	<1.0
peach (*FrozFruit*							
Smoothie.Yum Give							
Peach a Chance) ..	80	0	21.0	0	0	15	0
piña colada cream							
(*FrozFruit*)	180	2.0	22.0	10.0	30	20	1.0
pineapple (*FrozFruit*) .	80	0	20.0	0	0	0	0

Food and Measure	cal.	prot. (gms)	carbo. (gms)	fat (gms)	chol. (mgs)	sod. (mgs)	fiber (gms)
strawberry:							
(*Dreyer's/Edy's* Whole Fruit) ...	80	0	21.0	0	0	0	0
(*FrozFruit*)	90	0	23.0	0	0	5	<1.0
strawberry banana (*FrozFruit Smoothie. Yum Yumtonic*) ...	130	1.0	34.0	0	0	15	1.0
strawberry cream:							
(*FrozFruit*)	150	1.0	22.0	7.0	25	20	<1.0
chocolate dipped (*Dreyer's/Edy's* Whole Fruit) ...	190	2.0	22.0	10.0	0	25	0
chocolate dipped (*FrozFruit*)	200	2.0	18.0	17.0	20	15	1.0
tropical (*FrozFruit*) ...	90	0	21.0	.5	0	55	<1.0
watermelon (*Froz-Fruit*)	70	0	17.0	0	0	0	0
Fruit cocktail, can or jar, ½ cup:							
(*Del Monte Very Cherry*)	90	<1.0	22.0	0	0	10	<1.0
in juice:							
(*Del Monte* Fruit Naturals)	60	0	15.0	0	0	10	1.0
(*Libby's Lite*)	60	0	15.0	0	0	10	1.0
(*S&W*)	80	0	20.0	0	0	20	2.0
w/liquid	55	.6	14.1	0	0	5	1.2
in light syrup	72	.5	18.8	.1	0	7	1.4
in extra light syrup (*Del Monte* Lite) ..	60	0	15.0	0	0	10	1.0
in heavy syrup:							
(*Del Monte*)	100	0	24.0	0	0	10	1.0
(*S&W*)	90	0	23.0	0	0	15	1.0
w/liquid	91	.5	23.4	.1	0	7	1.2
Fruit dip (see also "Apple dip"), 2 tbsp.:							
chocolate:							
(*Marzetti* Fat Free)	100	1.0	25.0	0	0	150	0
(*Marzetti* Natural)	120	1.0	21.0	4.0	0	50	0
cream cheese:							
(*Marzetti*)	70	1.0	10.0	3.0	10	85	0
strawberry flavor (*Marzetti*)	70	1.0	9.0	3.0	15	95	0

Food and Measure	cal.	prot. (gms)	carbo. (gms)	fat (gms)	chol. (mgs)	sod. (mgs)	fiber (gms)
Fruit drink blends							
(see also specific listings), 8 fl. oz., except as noted:							
(*Capri Sun All Natural Mountain Cooler*), 6.75 fl. oz.	90	0	23.0	0	0	25	0
(*Capri Sun All Natural Pacific Cooler*), 6.75 fl. oz.	100	0	26.0	0	0	20	0
(*Dole* Paradise Blend)	120	<1.0	29.0	0	0	10	0
(*Dole* Paradise Blend), 11.5 fl. oz.	170	0	41.0	0	0	14	0
(*Hawaiian Punch* Juicy Red)	120	0	29.0	0	0	95	0
(*Simply Nutritious* Mega Green)	120	1.0	30.0	0	0	35	0
(*Snapple* Vitamin Supreme)	150	0	44.0	0	0	30	0
citrus, see "Citrus drink blends"							
punch:							
(*AriZona*)	110	0	28.0	0	0	25	0
(*Capri Sun All Natural*), 6.75 fl. oz.	100	0	26.0	0	0	20	0
(*Capri Sun All Natural Splash/ Surfer Cooler*), 6.75 fl. oz.	100	0	27.0	0	0	20	0
(*Minute Maid*)	120	0	31.0	0	0	25	0
(*Snapple*)	110	0	29.0	0	0	10	0
(*Tropicana*)	130	0	32.0	0	0	15	0
(*Tropicana*), 11.5 fl. oz.	200	0	50.0	0	0	45	0
canned	117	0	29.5	0	0	55	.3
frozen*	114	0	28.9	0	0	10	.4
tropical (*R. W. Knudsen*)	120	1.0	29.0	0	0	20	0
tropical:							
(*Capri Sun All Natural Tropical Punch Cooler*), 6.75 fl. oz.	90	0	25.0	0	0	20	0

Food and Measure	cal.	prot. (gms)	carbo. (gms)	fat (gms)	chol. (mgs)	sod. (mgs	fiber (gms)
(*Dole*)	160	0	30.0	0	0	30	0
(*Kool-Aid Bursts*), 6.75 fl. oz.	100	0	24.0	0	0	35	0
(*R. W. Knudsen*) . .	120	<1.0	29.0	0	0	20	0
(*Tang Tropical Tremor*)	100	0	25.0	0	0	30	0
(*Tropicana Twister*)	140	0	35.0	0	0	30	0
tropical, frozen* (*Minute Maid*)	100	0	28.0	0	0	5	0
Fruit drink mix*, 8 fl. oz.:							
all flavors (*Kool-Aid Magic Twists*).	60	0	16.0	0	0	0	0
tropical punch (*Kool-Aid* Sugar Sweetened)	60	0	16.0	0	0	0	0
Fruit juice blends (see also specific listings), 8 fl. oz., except as noted:							
(*Ceres*), 5.25 fl. oz. . .	87	0	21.0	0	0	n.a.	0
(*R. W. Knudsen* Natural Breakfast)	110	<1.0	27.0	0	0	35	0
(*Simply Nutritious* Morning Blend) . . .	120	1.0	31.0	0	0	15	0
(*Simply Nutritious* Mega C)	140	<1.0	31.0	0	0	15	0
(*Simply Nutritious* VitaJuice)	120	2.0	29.0	0	0	35	0
punch: (*Juicy Juice*)	120	1.0	29.0	0	0	10	0
(*Juicy Juice*), 12 fl. oz.	170	0	42.0	0	0	15	0
tropical: (*After the Fall* Kiwi Bear)	100	1.0	24.0	0	0	15	0
(*After the Fall* Maui Grove)	90	1.0	23.0	0	0	15	0
(*Juicy Juice*)	130	1.0	31.0	0	0	10	0
Fruit pectin, ⅛ tsp.: (*Sure•Jell/Slim Set*)	0	0	0	0	0	0	0
(*Sure•Jell* for Lower Sugar Recipes) . . .	0	0	0	0	0	5	0

Food and Measure	cal.	prot. (gms)	carbo. (gms)	fat (gms)	chol. (mgs)	sod. (mgs)	fiber (gms)
Fruit protector (*Sure•Jell Ever Fresh*), ⅛ tsp.	5	0	<1.0	0	0	0	0
Fruit sauce, Asian, four (*Heaven and Earth*), 1 tbsp. . . .	20	<1.0	9.0	<1.0	0	10	0
Fruit snack (see also specific listings), all varieties:							
(*Fruit by the Foot*), ¾-oz. roll	80	0	17.0	1.5	0	50	0
(*Fruit Gushers*), .9-oz. pouch	90	0	20.0	1.0	0	55	0
(*Fruit Roll-Ups*), ½-oz. roll	50	0	12.0	1.0	0	55	0
(*Fruit Shapes*), .9-oz. pouch	80	0	21.0	0	0	50	0
(*Sunkist* Fruit Roll), .75-oz. roll	70	0	18.0	0	0	20	1.0
Fruit spread (see also "Jam and pre- serves"), 1 tbsp., except as noted: all fruits:							
(*Cascadian Farm*) . .	40	0	10.0	0	0	0	0
(*Dickenson's*), 2 tbsp.	50	0	13.0	0	0	0	0
(*Kraft*), .5 oz. pkt. . .	30	0	8.0	0	0	0	0
(*Polaner*)	40	0	10.0	0	0	0	0
(*Smucker's Simply Fruit*)	40	0	10.0	0	0	0	0
grape (*Featherweight*)	15	0	4.0	0	0	15	0
Fruit-nut mix, see "Trail mix"							
Fudge, see "Candy"							
Fudge topping, see "Chocolate topping"							
Fuki, see "Butterbur"							
Fusilli pasta dish mix: w/creamy pesto sauce (*Knorr*), ⅔ cup . . .	250	9.0	46.0	3.5	<5	860	3.0

Food and Measure	cal.	prot. (gms)	carbo. (gms)	fat (gms)	chol. (mgs)	sod. (mgs)	fiber (gms)
w/red beans (*Marrakesh Express*), 1 cup*	210	9.0	41.0	1.0	<5	450	2.0
Fuzzy navel drink mixer, frozen (Bacardi), 2 fl. oz.	110	0	29.0	0	0	0	0

G

Food and Measure	cal.	prot. (gms)	carbo. (gms)	fat (gms)	chol. (mgs)	sod. (mgs)	fiber (gms)
Gai choy, see "Cabbage, mustard"							
Gai lan, see "Kale, Chinese"							
Galanga (*Frieda's*), ⅔ cup, 3 oz.	60	1.0	13.0	.5	0	10	2.0
Garbanzo beans:							
dry:							
(*Arrowhead Mills*), ¼ cup	170	10.0	29.0	2.0	0	10	6.0
(*Frieda's*), ⅓ cup	150	7.0	23.0	3.0	0	230	n.a.
boiled, ½ cup	134	7.3	22.5	2.1	0	6	2.9
Garbanzo beans, canned, ½ cup:							
(*Allens/East Texas Fair*)	120	5.0	19.0	2.5	0	330	8.0
(*Bush's Best* Chick Peas)	130	6.0	22.0	2.0	0	500	9.0
(*Eden*)	120	7.0	19.0	1.5	0	10	5.0
(*Goya* Chick Peas) . . .	100	6.0	20.0	2.0	0	360	7.0
(*Hain* Chick Peas) . . .	120	5.0	20.0	2.5	0	140	7.0
(*Progresso* Chickpeas)	120	5.0	20.0	2.5	0	280	5.0
(*S&W* Chick Peas) . . .	80	6.0	18.0	1.5	0	460	7.0
(*S&W* Garbanzo)	80	7.0	18.0	1.5	0	490	7.0
(*S&W* Garbanzo 50% Salt)	110	7.0	9.0	1.0	0	220	4.0
(*Westbrae Natural*) . .	110	6.0	18.0	2.0	0	10	5.0
Garbanzo flour (*Arrowhead Mills*), ¼ cup	90	5.0	15.0	1.0	0	0	3.0
Garlic, fresh:							
(*Frieda's* Elephant), 1 tbsp.	5	0	1.0	0	0	0	0
trimmed, 1 oz.	42	1.8	9.4	.1	0	5	.6
1 clove, .1 oz.	4	.2	1.0	<.1	0	1	.1

Food and Measure	cal.	prot. (gms)	carbo. (gms)	fat (gms)	chol. (mgs)	sod. (mgs)	fiber (gms)
granulated/minced:							
1 tsp.	13	.7	2.9	0	0	1	0
Garlic, in jars:							
chopped (*Italian Rose*),							
1 tbsp.	15	1.0	0	3.0	0	0	0
marinated (*Frieda's*),							
1 oz.	30	1.0	7.0	0	0	140	0
roasted (*Christopher*							
Ranch), 2–3 cloves	10	0	2.0	0	0	5	0
Garlic, crushed (*Mc-*							
Cormick), 1 tsp. ...	10	0	4.0	0	0	0	0
Garlic bread, see							
"Bread, frozen"							
Garlic juice (*Mc-*							
Cormick), ¼ tsp. .	0	0	0	0	0	0	0
Garlic oil (*Watkins*							
Liquid Spice), 1 tsp.	40	0	0	4.5	0	0	0
Garlic paste (*Italia In*							
Tavola), 1 tbsp. ...	60	0	3.0	6.0	0	520	0
Garlic pepper:							
(*Lawry's*), ¼ tsp. ...	0	0	0	0	0	70	0
(*McCormick*), ¼ tsp.	0	0	0	0	0	105	0
1 tsp.	8	.3	1.8	0	0	360	.3
Garlic powder:							
1 tsp.	10	.5	2.3	0	0	1	0
w/parsley (*Lawry's*),							
¼ tsp.	0	0	1.0	0	0	0	0
Garlic relish, medium,							
Indian (*Patak's*),							
1 tbsp.	40	1.0	3.0	3.0	0	55	0
Garlic salt, ¼ tsp.:							
(*Lawry's*)	0	0	0	0	0	240	0
(*McCormick*)	0	0	0	0	0	242	0
(*McCormick SeasonAll*)	0	0	0	0	0	260	0
(*Watkins*)	0	0	0	0	0	320	0
and parsley (*Mc-*							
Cormick)	0	0	0	0	0	225	0
w/parsley (*McCormick*							
California)	0	0	0	0	0	220	0
Garlic sauce (*Maille*							
Dipping), 2 tbsp. ..	130	0	4.0	14.0	0	350	0
Garlic spread:							
(*Lawry's* Concentrate),							
2 tsp.	50	0	1.0	6.0	0	80	0

Food and Measure	cal.	prot. (gms)	carbo. (gms)	fat (gms)	chol. (mgs)	sod. (mgs)	fiber (gms)
Garlic spread *(cont.)*							
(*Lawry's* Ready-to-Spread), 1 tbsp. ...	100	0	2.0	10.0	0	190	0
(*McCormick*), ½ tbsp.	45	0	1.0	4.0	0	140	0
and parsley (*Badia*), 1 tsp.	35	0	<1.0	5.0	0	25	0
Garlic sprouts, fresh (*Jonathan's*), 1 cup	70	5.0	14.0	.5	0	10	3.0
Garlic-chive seasoning (*Watkins*), 1 tbsp.	25	1.0	2.0	2.0	5	280	0
Garlic-dill dip mix (*Watkins*), 1 tsp. ..	10	0	2.0	0	0	100	0
Garlic-sesame seasoning (*Eden Shake*), ½ tsp.	10	0	0	.5	0	35	0
Gefilte fish, in jars, 1.5-oz. pc., except as noted:							
(*Rokeach*)	45	4.0	1.0	2.0	25	220	0
(*Rokeach* Old Vienna)	40	4.0	2.0	2.5	20	180	0
(*Rokeach* Old Vienna Can), 1.7-oz. pc. ..	45	5.0	3.0	1.5	25	200	1.0
in jellied broth (*Manischewitz*), 2.5-oz. pc.	70	7.0	3.0	3.0	15	540	<1.0
sweet (*Manischewitz*), 2.4-oz. pc.	50	5.0	4.0	2.0	15	340	<1.0
whitefish and pike: (*Manischewitz*), 2.2-oz. pc.	50	7.0	3.0	1.5	35	300	<1.0
(*Mother's*)	40	5.0	2.0	2.0	15	170	1.0
(*Mother's* Old World)	45	4.0	3.0	2.0	15	170	1.0
(*Rokeach*)	35	4.0	1.0	1.5	25	190	1.0
Gefilte fish, frozen (*BenZ's*), 3 oz.	140	10.0	19.0	2.0	0	160	0
Gelatin, unflavored (*Knox*), 1 pkt.	25	6.0	0	0	0	15	0
Gelatin dessert, all flavors, 3.5-oz. cont.:							
(*Jell-O*)	70	1.0	17.0	0	0	40	0
(*Jell-O* Sugar Free) ..	10	1.0	0	0	0	45	0
(*Jell-O* X-Treme)	100	0	24.0	0	0	45	0

Food and Measure	cal.	prot. (gms)	carbo. (gms)	fat (gms)	chol. (mgs)	sod. (mgs)	fiber (gms)
Gelatin dessert mix*, all flavors, ½ cup:							
(*Jell-O*)	80	2.0	19.0	0	0	—[1]	0
(*Jell-O* Gelatina) ...	140	6.0	20.0	4.0	15	60	0
(*Jell-O* Sugar Free)	10	1.0	0	0	0	—[2]	0
strawberry (*Jell-O 1-2-3*), ⅔ cup	130	2.0	26.0	1.5	0	50	0
Gelatin drink mix, orange (*Knox Nutra Joint*+), .4-oz. scoop	40	9.0	<1.0	0	0	30	0
Gemelli pasta dish mix, and white beans (*Marrakesh Express*), 1 cup* ..	220	10.0	43.0	1.0	<5	590	3.0
Gil choy (*Frieda's*), 1 tbsp.	0	0	0	0	0	0	0
Ginger, trimmed root:							
(*Frieda's*), 1 tbsp.	0	0	1.0	0	0	0	0
1 oz.	20	.5	4.3	.2	0	4	.6
sliced:							
¼ cup	17	.4	3.6	.2	0	3	.5
(*Ka•Me*), 20 pcs., ½ oz.	0	0	0	0	0	70	0
Ginger, candied or crystallized:							
(*Frieda's*), 9 pcs., 1.1 oz.	100	0	26.0	0	0	10	0
(*The Ginger People* Baker's Cut), .5 oz.	48	0	12.0	0	0	3	.2
(*The Ginger People* Premium Cut), 1 oz.	85	0	22.0	0	0	5	.4
(*McCormick*), 1 tsp.	15	0	3.0	0	0	0	0
(*Sonoma*), 1.5-oz. pkt.	140	0	34.0	0	0	5	1.0
Ginger, ground, 1 tsp.	6	.2	1.3	.1	0	1	.2
Ginger, pickled:							
(*Eden*), 1 tbsp.	15	0	3.0	0	0	340	1.0
(*Shirakiku*), 1 tbsp. ..	5	0	1.0	0	0	55	0
(*Sushi Chef*), 1 tbsp.	30	0	7.0	0	0	65	0
Japanese, 1 oz.	10	.1	2.1	<.1	0	105	0
Ginger, Thai, see "Galanga"							

[1]*Sodium values vary between 75 and 140 mgs. according to flavor.*
[2]*Sodium values vary between 50 and 80 mgs. according to flavor.*

Food and Measure	cal.	prot. (gms)	carbo. (gms)	fat (gms)	chol. (mgs)	sod. (mgs)	fiber (gms)
Ginger drink (*Santa Cruz Organic* Hawaiian Nectar) 8 fl. oz.	110	<1.0	27.0	0	0	35	0
Ginger mint sauce (*Heaven and Earth*), 1 tbsp.	35	0	9.0	0	0	10	0
Ginger preserves, see "Jam and preserves"							
Ginger-garlic oil (*Watkins* Liquid Spice), 1 tsp.	40	0	0	4.5	0	0	0
Ginkgo nut, shelled:							
raw, 1 oz.	52	1.2	10.7	.5	0	2	<1.0
canned, drained, 1 oz.	32	.6	6.3	.5	0	87	2.6
dried, 1 oz.	99	2.9	20.6	.8	0	4	n.a.
Glacé, cake, see "Fruit, mixed, candied"							
Glaze, see "Ham glaze" and "Strawberry pie glaze"							
Glaze sauce, see "Grilling sauce" and "Marinade"							
Gluten, see "Wheat gluten"							
Gnocchi, frozen or refrigerated:							
(*Celentano*), 1 cup ...	210	8.0	38.0	.5	0	236	0
(*Italian Village*), 1 cup	260	8.0	54.0	1.0	15	920	4.0
(*Mount Rose*), 1 cup	214	8.0	38.0	1.0	0	236	0
(*Rienzi*), 1½ cups ...	280	5.0	30.0	.5	0	590	2.0
tomato (*Rienzi*), 1½ cups	320	5.0	30.0	1.0	0	590	0
Goat, meat only, roasted, 4 oz.	162	30.7	0	3.4	85	98	
Gobo root, see "Burdock root"							
***Godfather's Pizza*,** 1 slice:							
original, cheese:							
medium, ⅛ pie ...	230	11.0	34.0	6.0	20	440	0
large, ⅒ pie	260	13.0	35.0	7.0	25	500	0

Food and Measure	cal.	prot. (gms)	carbo. (gms)	fat (gms)	chol. (mgs)	sod. (mgs)	fiber (gms)
original, combo:							
medium, ⅛ pie ...	320	16.0	36.0	12.0	30	800	<1.0
large, ⅒ pie	350	18.0	38.0	14.0	35	890	<1.0
original, veggie:							
medium, ⅛ pie ...	250	12.0	36.0	6.0	20	520	1.0
large, ⅒ pie	270	13.0	38.0	8.0	25	590	1.0
golden, cheese:							
medium, ⅛ pie ...	200	9.0	25.0	7.0	15	380	0
large, ⅒ pie	210	10.0	27.0	6.0	20	390	0
golden, combo:							
medium, ⅛ pie ...	250	12.0	27.0	11.0	25	600	<1.0
large, ⅒ pie	280	14.0	29.0	11.0	30	700	<1.0
golden, veggie:							
medium, ⅛ pie ...	210	9.0	27.0	7.0	15	410	<1.0
large, ⅒ pie	210	11.0	29.0	6.0	20	450	<1.0
Golden nugget squash (*Frieda's*), ¾ cup, 3 oz.	30	1.0	7.0	0	0	0	1.0
Goose, roasted:							
meat w/skin, 4 oz. ...	346	28.5	0	24.9	103	79	0
meat only, 4 oz.	270	32.9	0	14.4	109	86	0
Goose fat, 1 oz.	255	0	0	28.3	28	0	0
Goose liver, see "Liver" and "Pâté"							
Gooseberries, fresh, ½ cup	34	.7	7.6	.4	0	1	3.2
Gooseberries, canned, in light syrup (*Oregon*), ½ cup ..	90	<1.0	22.0	0	0	5	3.0
Gordita dinner kit, (*Old El Paso*), 1 tsp. seasoning, 1 shell:							
w/ranch sauce	300	4.0	34.0	3.0	0	1010	1.0
w/chicken breast*	390	20.0	34.0	19.0	45	1070	1.0
w/red sauce	210	4.0	36.0	5.0	0	950	1.0
w/chicken breast*	310	21.0	36.0	19.0	45	1010	1.0
Gourd, boiled, ½ cup:							
dishcloth, 1" slices ..	50	.6	12.8	.3	0	18	<1.0
white-flower, 1" cubes	11	.4	2.7	<.1	0	1	<1.0
Gourd, dried, see "Kanpyo"							

Food and Measure	cal.	prot. (gms)	carbo. (gms)	fat (gms)	chol. (mgs)	sod. (mgs)	fiber (gms)
Grains, mixed, dish, mix (see also specific listings), 1 cup*:							
chicken and herbs w/rice, barley, and wheat (*Near East Creative Grains*) . . .	270	8.0	51.0	6.0	0	760	6.0
garlic, roasted, w/rice, wheat, and bulgur (*Near East Creative Grains*) . . .	220	6.0	41.0	5.0	0	560	5.0
Parmesan, creamy, w/rice and wheat (*Near East Creative Grains*) . . .	280	8.0	48.0	7.0	20	820	3.0
pecan, roasted, and garlic, w/rice and wheat (*Near East Creative Grains*) . . .	240	6.0	37.0	9.0	0	540	4.0
Granadilla, see "Passion fruit"							
Granola, see "Cereal"							
Granola/cereal bar, 1 bar, except as noted:							
(*Chex*)	160	6.0	26.0	4.0	0	150	0
(*Kudos M&M's*)	100	1.0	17.0	1.5	0	115	0
(*Kudos Snickers*)	100	1.0	16.0	4.0	0	105	0
(*Rice Krispies Treats* Squares Original) . .	90	1.0	18.0	2.0	0	100	0
(*Rice Krispies Treats* Squares Singles) . .	160	1.0	30.0	3.5	0	170	0
all fruits:							
(*Barbara's Nature's Choice* Cereal) . .	120	2.0	27.0	1.5	0	75	2.0
(*Hain* Breakfast) . . .	140	2.0	29.0	2.5	0	110	1.0
(*Health Valley* Cobbler Cereal)	130	2.0	27.0	2.0	0	50	1.0
(*Health Valley* Fat Free Bakes)	70	2.0	19.0	0	0	30	3.0

Food and Measure	cal.	prot. (gms)	carbo. (gms)	fat (gms)	chol. (mgs)	sod. (mgs)	fiber (gms)
(*Health Valley* Fat Free Breakfast Bakes)	110	2.0	26.0	0	0	25	3.0
(*Health Valley* Fat Free Fruit/Granola)	140	2.0	35.0	0	0	10	3.0
(*Health Valley* Low Fat Cereal)	130	2.0	27.0	2.0	0	50	1.0
(*Health Valley* Low Fat Tarts)	130	2.0	28.0	2.0	0	80	1.0
(*Nutri-Grain* Cereal Bars/Yogurt) ...	140	2.0	27.0	3.0	0	110	1.0
apple:							
(*Health Valley* Moist & Chewy Granola)	100	2.0	22.0	1.0	0	15	2.0
cobbler (*Nutri-Grain* Twists)	140	1.0	27.0	3.0	0	105	1.0
apple cinnamon:							
(*Entenmann's* Multi-Grain)	140	9.0	24.0	3.0	0	80	1.0
(*Nabisco* Fruit 'n Grain)	130	2.0	25.0	2.5	0	60	<1.0
(*Quaker* Fruit & Oatmeal)	135	1.5	26.0	3.0	0	95	1.0
apple raisin (*Entenmann's* Multi-Grain)	140	2.0	27.0	3.0	0	130	1.0
Bavarian creme (*Health Valley* Low Fat Sandwich Bar)	130	2.0	28.0	2.0	0	80	1.0
berry:							
(*Health Valley* Moist & Chewy Granola)	100	2.0	22.0	1.0	0	5	2.0
(*Quaker* Fruit & Oatmeal)	135	2.0	27.0	3.0	0	125	1.0
mixed (*Nabisco* Fruit 'n Grain)	130	2.0	25.0	2.5	0	85	<1.0
blueberry:							
(*Entenmann's* Multi-Grain)	140	1.0	25.0	3.0	0	90	1.0
cheesecake (*Quaker* Fruit & Oatmeal)	135	1.5	26.0	3.0	0	130	1.0
w/*Butterfinger* pieces (*Quaker* Chewy Granola)	120	1.5	22.0	3.0	0	75	1.0

Food and Measure	cal.	prot. (gms)	carbo. (gms)	fat (gms)	chol. (mgs)	sod. (mgs)	fiber (gms)
Granola/cereal bar *(cont.)*							
caramel:							
chewy (*Hain* Mini							
Munchie)	90	1.0	20.0	1.5	0	100	1.0
chocolate (*Kellogg's*							
Rice Krispies							
Treats Squares)	10	1.0	19.0	3.0	0	100	<1.0
carob chip (*Barbara's*							
Nature's Choice							
Granola)	80	2.0	16.0	2.0	0	5	2.0
cherry:							
(*SnackWell's* Hearty							
Fruit 'n Grain) . .	130	1.0	26.0	2.5	0	90	1.0
cobbler (*Quaker*							
Fruit & Oatmeal)	135	1.5	26.0	3.0	0	120	1.0
chocolate:							
(*Health Valley* Low							
Fat Tarts)	130	2.0	28.0	2.0	0	80	1.0
double (*Hain* Mini							
Munchie)	90	1.0	20.0	1.5	0	100	1.0
chocolate chip:							
(*Health Valley* Fat							
Free Granola) . . .	140	2.0	35.0	0	0	10	3.0
(*Kudos*)	120	1.0	20.0	4.5	0	75	1.0
(*Quaker* Chewy							
Granola)	120	1.5	20.0	4.0	0	70	1.0
raisin (*Entenmann's*							
Multi-Grain)	140	2.0	28.0	3.0	0	110	1.0
chocolate chunk:							
(*Kellogg's Rice*							
Krispies Treats							
Squares Choco-							
lately)	100	1.0	15.0	4.0	0	75	<1.0
s'mores (*Golden*							
Grahams Treats)	90	1.0	17.0	2.5	0	100	0
s'mores (*Golden*							
Grahams Treats							
King Size)	190	1.0	34.0	5.0	0	210	1.0
chocolate fudge							
(*Kudos*)	120	1.0	20.0	4.5	0	75	1.0
chocolate peanut							
butter:							
(*Kashi GoLean*) . . .	290	13.0	50.0	6.0	0	150	6.0

Food and Measure	cal.	prot. (gms)	carbo. (gms)	fat (gms)	chol. (mgs)	sod. (mgs)	fiber (gms)
(*Kellogg's Rice Krispies Treats* Squares Chocolately)	100	2.0	16.0	3.5	0	100	<1.0
cinnamon:							
(*Cinnamon Toast Crunch*)	180	6.0	26.0	4.0	0	160	1.0
(*Nature Valley*), 2 bars	180	4.0	29.0	6.0	0	160	2.0
cinnamon raisin (*Barbara's Nature's Choice* Granola) ...	80	2.0	16.0	2.0	0	5	3.0
cocoa (*Rice Krispies Treats* Squares) ...	100	1.0	16.0	3.5	0	105	0
cookies and cream (*Kashi GoLean*) ...	290	13.0	54.0	6.0	0	100	7.0
w/Crunch (*Quaker Chewy Granola*) ...	120	1.5	22.0	3.5	0	70	1.0
fruit and nut (*Nature Valley* Trail Mix) ...	140	3.0	24.0	4.0	0	95	2.0
honey nut (*Cheerios*)	160	6.0	26.0	4.0	0	150	1.0
honey vanilla yogurt (*Kashi GoLean*) ...	290	11.0	53.0	5.0	0	70	6.0
malted chocolate crisp (*Kashi GoLean*) ...	280	13.0	51.0	5.0	20	85	6.0
maple brown sugar (*Nature Valley*), 2 bars	180	4.0	29.0	6.0	0	160	2.0
marshmallow:							
all varieties (*Health Valley* Fat Free)	100	1.0	24.0	0	0	20	1.0
graham (*Golden Graham Treats*)	90	1.0	17.0	2.0	0	110	0
oats 'n honey:							
(*Barbara's Nature's Choice* Granola)	80	2.0	15.0	2.0	0	5	2.0
(*Nature Valley*), 2 bars	180	4.0	29.0	6.0	0	160	2.0
peanut (*Health Valley* Moist & Chewy Granola)	110	3.0	19.0	3.0	0	80	2.0
peanut butter:							
(*Barbara's Nature's Choice* Granola)	80	2.0	14.0	3.0	0	5	2.0

Food and Measure	cal.	prot. (gms)	carbo. (gms)	fat (gms)	chol. (mgs)	sod. (mgs)	fiber (gms)
Granola/cereal bar, peanut butter *(cont.)*							
(*Kudos*)	130	2.0	19.0	5.0	0	85	1.0
(*Nature Valley*), 2 bars	180	5.0	29.0	6.0	0	170	2.0
(*Quaker* Chewy Granola)	110	2.5	18.0	3.5	0	105	1.0
chocolate (*Golden Graham Treats*)	90	1.0	15.0	3.5	0	105	0
chocolate (*Rice Krispies Treats Squares*)	110	2.0	16.0	4.0	0	100	0
crunch (*Hain* Mini Munchie)	90	1.0	20.0	1.5	0	100	1.0
raspberry:							
(*Entenmann's* Multi-Grain)	140	1.0	25.0	3.0	0	100	1.0
(*Nabisco* Fruit 'n Grain)	130	2.0	25.0	2.5	0	120	<1.0
s'mores (*Quaker* Chewy Granola Low Fat)	110	1.5	22.0	2.0	0	80	1.0
strawberry:							
(*Nabisco* Fruit 'n Grain)	130	2.0	25.0	2.5	0	105	<1.0
cheesecake (*Nutri-Grain Twists*) . . .	140	2.0	26.0	3.0	0	125	1.0
and creme (*Nutri-Grain Twists Cereal*)	140	2.0	26.0	3.0	0	125	1.0
banana or cheese-cake (*Quaker* Fruit & Oatmeal)	135	1.5	26.0	3.0	0	120	1.0
vanilla yogurt (*Kashi* GoLean)	290	11.0	53.0	5.0	0	75	6.0
vanilla creme (*Health Valley* Low Fat Sandwich Bar)	130	2.0	28.0	2.0	0	80	1.0
vanilla spice cake (*Kashi* GoLean) . . .	280	14.0	47.0	5.0	0	100	7.0
Grape, fresh:							
(*Dole*), 1½ cups	90	1.0	24.0	1.0	0	0	1.0
American type (slipskin):							
10 medium	15	.2	4.1	.1	0	tr.	.3

Food and Measure	cal.	prot. (gms)	carbo. (gms)	fat (gms)	chol. (mgs)	sod. (mgs）	fiber (gms)
peeled and seeded, ½ cup	29	.3	7.9	.2	0	1	.6
champagne (*Frieda's*), ½ cup, 3 oz.	50	1.0	15.0	0	0	0	1.0
European type (adherent skin): seeded, 1 lb.	287	2.7	72.0	2.3	0	7	2.7
seedless, 10 medium	36	.3	8.9	.3	0	1	.3
seedless or seeded, ½ cup	57	.5	14.2	.5	0	2	.5
Grape, can or jar, seedless, ½ cup:							
in light syrup (*Oregon* Thompson)	100	<1.0	23.0	0	0	0	1.0
in heavy syrup w/liquid	94	.6	25.1	.1	0	6	.5
Grape drink, 8 fl. oz., except as noted:							
(*Capri Sun All Natural*), 6.75 fl. oz.	100	0	25.0	0	0	20	0
(*Hawaiian Punch* Geyser)	120	0	30.0	0	0	100	0
(*Kool-Aid Bursts*), 6.75 fl. oz.	100	0	24.0	0	0	35	0
(*R. W. Knudsen* Aseptic)	140	1.0	35.0	0	0	30	0
(*Snapple* Grapeade) .	120	0	29.0	0	0	10	0
(*Tropicana*), 11.5 fl. oz.	200	0	49.0	0	0	35	0
canned	113	0	28.8	0	0	15	0
cocktail, frozen*: (*Welch's*)	150	0	37.0	0	0	0	0
white (*Welch's*) ...	150	0	36.0	0	0	40	0
Grape drink blends, 8 fl. oz.:							
(*After the Fall Hearty* Grape)	150	<1.0	37.0	0	0	30	0
punch (*Minute Maid*)	120	0	32.0	0	0	25	0
raspberry (*Dole*)	130	<1.0	32.0	0	0	25	0
Grape drink mix, 8 fl. oz.*:							
(*Kool-Aid* Sugar Sweetened)	60	0	16.0	0	0	0	0
(*Kool-Aid* Slushies) ..	140	0	35.0	0	0	60	2.0

Food and Measure	cal.	prot. (gms)	carbo. (gms)	fat (gms)	chol. (mgs)	sod. (mgs)	fiber (gms)
Grape juice, 8 fl. oz.:							
(*Juicy Juice*)	130	1.0	32.0	0	0	10	0
(*Langer's*)	160	0	40.0	0	0	15	0
(*Nantucket Nectars*) . .	160	0	39.0	0	0	20	0
(*R. W. Knudsen*)	150	<1.0	37.0	0	0	30	0
(*R. W. Knudsen*							
Concord)	160	<1.0	40.0	0	0	15	0
(*Season's Best*)	160	1.0	39.0	0	0	25	0
(*Welch's*)	170	0	42.0	0	0	20	0
canned or bottled . . .	154	1.4	37.9	.2	0	8	.3
frozen*, sweetened . . .	128	.5	31.9	.2	0	5	.3
sparkling, red or white							
(*R. W. Knudsen*) . .	130	<1.0	31.0	0	0	10	0
white:							
(*Santa Cruz Organic*)	160	<1.0	39.0	0	0	10	0
(*Welch's*)	160	0	39.0	0	0	20	0
Grape leaves, fresh:							
1 cup	13	.8	2.4	.3	0	1	1.5
1 leaf	3	.2	.5	<.1	0	<1	.3
Grape leaves, in jar							
(*Krinos*), 1 leaf . . .	5	0	0	0	0	200	1.0
Grape leaves, stuffed:							
(*Aegean*), 5 pcs.	205	5.0	23.0	11.0	0	571	3.0
(*Cedar's*), 6 pcs.	180	4.0	22.0	8.0	0	870	8.0
Grapefruit, fresh:							
(*Dole*), ½ medium . . .	60	1.0	16.0	0	0	0	6.0
all areas/varieties:							
½ large, 4.7 oz. . . .	53	1.1	13.4	.2	0	0	1.8
sections, 1 cup . . .	74	1.5	18.6	.2	0	0	2.5
all areas, pink/red:							
½ medium, 3¾" . . .	37	.7	9.5	.1	0	0	n.a.
sections, 1 cup . . .	69	1.3	17.7	.2	0	0	n.a.
all areas, white:							
½ medium, 3¾" . . .	39	.8	9.9	.1	0	0	1.3
sections, 1 cup . . .	76	1.3	17.7	.2	0	0	2.5
California/Arizona:							
pink/red, ½							
medium, 3¾" . .	46	.6	11.9	.1	0	1	1.4
pink/red, sections							
w/juice, 1 cup . .	85	1.2	22.3	.2	0	2	2.6
white, ½ medium,							
3¾"	43	1.0	10.7	.1	0	0	1.3
white, sections,							
w/juice, 1 cup . .	85	2.0	20.9	.2	0	0	2.6

Food and Measure	cal.	prot. (gms)	carbo. (gms)	fat (gms)	chol. (mgs)	sod. (mgs)	fiber (gms)
Florida:							
pink/red, ½							
medium, 3¾" ..	37	.7	9.2	.1	0	0	1.4
pink/red, sections							
w/juice, 1 cup ..	69	1.3	17.3	.2	0	0	2.5
white, ½ medium,							
3¾"	38	.7	9.7	.1	0	0	.2
white, sections							
w/juice, 1 cup ..	74	1.5	18.8	.2	0	0	.4
Grapefruit, can or jar,							
½ cup:							
in juice	46	.9	11.4	.1	0	9	.5
in juice, red or white							
(*Sunfresh* Chilled)	45	1.0	9.0	0	0	15	2.0
in extra light syrup, red							
(*Sunfresh* Chilled)	70	1.0	19.0	0	0	10	2.0
in light syrup:							
w/liquid	76	.7	19.6	.1	0	3	.5
red or white (*Sun-*							
fresh Can)	70	1.0	17.0	0	0	0	1.0
Grapefruit, Chinese,							
see "Pummelo"							
Grapefruit drink, ruby							
red:							
(*Dole*), 8 fl. oz.	130	1.0	31.0	0	0	10	0
(*Dole*), 10 fl. oz.	160	1.0	40.0	0	0	15	0
(*Dole*), 11.5 fl. oz. ..	185	1.0	44.0	0	0	15	0
(*Ocean Spray*), 8 fl. oz.	130	0	33.0	0	0	35	0
(*Season's Best* Cock-							
tail), 8 fl. oz.	130	1.0	31.0	0	0	10	0
(*Season's Best* Cock-							
tail), 10 fl. oz.	160	<1.0	41.0	0	0	40	0
(*Season's Best* Cock-							
tail), 11.5 fl. oz. ..	185	<1.0	47.0	0	0	45	0
(*Snapple*), 8 fl. oz. ..	120	0	30.0	0	0	10	0
(*Tropicana Twister*),							
10 fl. oz.	160	<1.0	42.0	0	0	40	0
Grapefruit drink blend,							
ruby red, 8 fl. oz.:							
mango (*Ocean Spray*)	130	0	33.0	0	0	35	0
strawberry (*Ocean*							
Spray)	130	0	34.0	0	0	35	0
tangerine (*Ocean*							
Spray)	130	0	32.0	0	0	35	0

Food and Measure	cal.	prot. (gms)	carbo. (gms)	fat (gms)	chol. (mgs)	sod. (mgs)	fiber (gms)
Grapefruit juice, 8 fl. oz.:							
(*Nantucket Nectars*) ..	100	1.0	23.0	0	0	0	0
(*Natalie's Orchard Island*)	100	1.0	24.0	0	0	0	0
(*R. W. Knudsen*)	100	2.0	23.0	0	0	35	0
(*Season's Best*)	90	<1.0	22.0	0	0	15	0
canned, unsweetened	94	1.3	22.1	.3	0	3	.3
fresh, pink or white ..	96	1.2	22.7	.3	0	3	.3
frozen*:							
(*Cascadian Farm*)	100	1.0	23.0	0	0	0	0
unsweetened	101	1.4	24.0	.3	0	3	.3
golden or ruby red (*Tropicana Pure Premium*)	90	1.0	22.0	0	0	0	0
pink (*Ocean Spray*) ..	110	0	28.0	0	0	35	0
red (*R. W. Knudsen*) .	140	1.0	35.0	0	0	0	0
ruby red:							
(*Florida's Natural* w/or w/out Calcium)	100	1.0	24.0	0	0	0	0
(*Horizon*)	90	1.0	22.0	0	0	0	0
(*Minute Maid*)	110	0	27.0	0	0	25	0
(*Nantucket Nectars*)	100	0	25.0	0	0	5	0
white (*Ocean Spray*)	100	0	24.0	0	0	35	0
Gravlax, see "Salmon, marinated"							
Gravy, see specific listings							
Gravy seasoning, see "Browning sauce"							
Great northern bean:							
dry (*Jack Rabbit*), ¼ cup	70	8.0	22.0	0	0	20	13.0
boiled, ½ cup	104	7.3	18.6	.4	0	2	6.2
Great northern bean, canned, ½ cup:							
(*Allens*)	100	6.0	19.0	.5	0	310	7.0
(*Bush's Best*)	110	7.0	18.0	.5	0	400	7.0
(*Westbrae Natural* Fat Free)	90	6.0	16.0	0	0	140	4.0
w/pork (*Bush's Best*)	110	6.0	17.0	1.5	5	460	6.0
w/sausage (*Trappey's*)	100	6.0	18.0	1.0	0	460	7.0

Food and Measure	cal.	prot. (gms)	carbo. (gms)	fat (gms)	chol. (mgs)	sod. (mgs)	fiber (gms)
seasoned (*Glory Foods*)	90	6.0	15.0	.5	0	850	3.0
Green bean, fresh:							
raw, ½ cup	17	1.0	3.9	.1	0	3	1.9
boiled, drained,							
½ cup	22	1.2	4.9	.2	0	2	2.0
Green bean, can or jar, ½ cup:							
(*Allens* Shell Outs) . . .	30	2.0	6.0	0	0	460	2.0
(*Green Giant* Kitchen Sliced)	20	<1.0	4.0	0	0	400	1.0
all styles:							
(*Del Monte* No Salt)	20	1.0	4.0	0	0	10	2.0
(*Libby's*)	25	1.0	5.0	0	0	380	2.0
(*Libby's* No Salt) . .	25	1.0	5.0	0	0	10	2.0
except seasoned French style (*Del Monte*)	20	1.0	4.0	0	0	390	2.0
whole, small (*S&W*)	20	1.0	4.0	0	0	390	2.0
cut:							
(*Allens* No Salt) . . .	15	0	3.0	0	0	10	2.0
(*Allens/Alma/Crest Top/GaBelle/Stone Mountain/Sunshine*)	30	0	6.0	0	0	320	3.0
(*Bonduelle*)	15	1.0	3.0	0	0	430	3.0
(*Bush's Best*)	25	1.0	5.0	0	0	430	2.0
(*Green Giant*)	20	<1.0	4.0	0	0	400	1.0
(*Green Giant* 50% Less Sodium) . .	20	<1.0	4.0	0	0	200	1.0
(*Greene's Farm*) . . .	20	<1.0	4.0	0	0	370	2.0
(*Greenleaf*)	15	1.0	3.0	0	0	430	3.0
(*Hain* Blue Lake) . .	20	1.0	4.0	0	0	370	1.0
(*Veg-All*)	20	<1.0	4.0	0	0	400	2.0
cut or French style:							
(*Blue Boy*)	25	1.0	5.0	0	0	380	2.0
(*S&W*)	20	1.0	4.0	0	0	340	2.0
drained	14	.8	3.0	<.1	0	177	1.3
French style:							
(*Allens*)	25	1.0	4.0	0	0	300	2.0
(*Bush's Best*)	25	1.0	5.0	0	0	430	2.0
(*Green Giant*)	20	<1.0	4.0	0	0	390	1.0
(*Greene's Farm*) . . .	26	<1.0	4.0	0	0	330	2.0
(*Hain*)	20	1.0	4.0	0	0	370	1.0

Food and Measure	cal.	prot. (gms)	carbo (gms)	fat (gms)	chol. (mgs)	sod. (mgs)	fiber (gms)
Green bean, can or jar, French style *(cont.)*							
(*Veg-All*)	20	<1.0	4.0	0	0	400	2.0
seasoned (*Del Monte*)	20	1.0	4.0	0	0	360	2.0
Italian cut:							
(*Allens/Sunshine*)	35	1.0	7.0	0	0	320	3.0
(*Del Monte*)	30	1.0	6.0	0	0	390	3.0
w/liquid	18	1.0	4.2	.1	0	311	1.8
seasoned (*Glory Foods*)	30	1.0	6.0	.5	0	410	2.0
Green bean, dried:							
(*Mountain House*), ½ cup	30	1.0	6.0	0	0	0	2.0
amandine, french cut (*AlpineAire*), .9 oz.	100	4.0	13.0	3.0	0	560	5.0
Green bean, frozen:							
whole:							
(*Green Giant Select*), 1 cup	20	1.0	4.0	0	0	10	2.0
(*Seabrook Farms*), ¾ cup	25	1.0	4.0	0	0	10	2.0
extra fine (*Bonduelle* Haricot Vert), 3 oz.	30	2.0	6.0	0	0	0	2.0
boiled, drained, ½ cup	19	1.0	4.4	.1	0	6	2.0
cut:							
(*Birds Eye*), ½ cup	25	1.0	6.0	0	0	0	2.0
(*Cascadian Farm*), ⅔ cup	40	1.0	6.0	0	0	0	3.0
(*Green Giant*), ¾ cup	20	1.0	4.0	0	0	10	2.0
(*John Cope's* 1"), ⅔ cup	25	1.0	4.0	0	0	10	2.0
(*Tree of Life* Organic), ⅔ cup	25	1.0	4.0	0	0	10	2.0
Italian (*Birds Eye* Deluxe), ½ cup . . .	35	2.0	8.0	0	0	0	3.0
Szechuan (*Cascadian Farm*), 1 cup	60	2.0	5.0	2.5	0	290	2.0
Green bean combinations, canned, ½ cup:							
w/potatoes:							
(*Allens/Sunshine*)	35	1.0	7.0	0	0	220	2.0

Food and Measure	cal.	prot. (gms)	carbo. (gms)	fat (gms)	chol. (mgs)	sod. (mgs	fiber (gms)
(*Glory Foods*)	50	2.0	10.0	.5	0	580	2.0
and shelly beans							
(*Bush's Best*) ...	45	3.0	7.0	0	0	400	3.0
Green bean combi-							
nations, frozen:							
(*Green Giant* Cas-							
serole), ⅔ cup	90	2.0	9.0	5.0	0	460	2.0
w/almonds:							
(*Cascadian Farm*),							
⅔ cup	70	3.0	10.0	3.0	0	115	3.0
(*Green Giant*),							
⅔ cup	50	2.0	4.0	3.0	0	100	2.0
mushroom casserole:							
(*Stouffer's Family*							
Style Favorites),							
½ cup	130	3.0	12.0	8.0	2	450	2.0
w/mushroom garlic							
sauce (*Casca-*							
dian Farm),							
¾ cup	90	3.0	10.0	5.0	10	360	2.0
stir-fry (*Birds Eye*							
Whole), ⅓ of							
16-oz. pkg.	100	4.0	19.0	.5	0	25	2.0
Green peas, see							
"Peas, green"							
Greens, mixed, fresh,							
see "Salad blend"							
Greens, mixed,							
canned (see also							
specific listings),							
½ cup:							
(*Allens/Sunshine*) ...	30	1.0	8.0	.5	0	10	4.0
(*Bush's Best*)	25	2.0	3.0	0	0	300	2.0
seasoned (*Glory*							
Foods)	50	4.0	7.0	.5	0	470	3.0
Grenadine syrup,							
2 tbsp.:							
(*Rose's*)	90	0	22.0	0	0	10	0
(*Trader Vic's*)	90	0	23.0	0	0	15	0
unsweetened							
(*Rose's*)	10	0	2.0	0	0	0	0
Grill seasoning							
(*Watkins*), ¼ tsp.	0	0	0	0	0	210	0

Food and Measure	cal.	prot. (gms)	carbo. (gms)	fat (gms)	chol. (mgs)	sod. (mgs)	fiber (gms)
Grilling sauce (see also "Barbecue sauce," "Marinade," and specific listings), 2 tbsp., except as noted:							
(*French's* Grill & Glaze)	60	<1.0	13.0	0	0	380	0
(*Jack Daniel's* Original No. 7 Barbecue Recipe)	50	0	12.0	0	0	270	1.0
(*Jack Daniel's* Sizzling Smokehouse Recipe)	45	0	11.0	0	0	320	1.0
(*San-J*)	40	2.0	8.0	0	0	860	0
Cajun, hot (*Bull's Eye*)	60	<1.0	12.0	0	0	320	<1.0
chipotle:							
(*Chi-Chi's*)	60	0	15.0	0	0	530	0
(*Texas Best* Sedona)	50	0	13.0	0	0	350	0
garlic, roasted, and herb (*Bull's Eye*) ..	60	<1.0	13.0	0	0	420	0
garlic herb (*McCormick* Flavor Medleys) ...	60	0	5.0	4.0	0	390	0
ginger sesame, sweet (*House of Tsang* Hibachi), 1 tbsp. ...	40	0	9.0	0	0	400	0
habanero mustard (*Texas Best* Mesa)	60	0	14.0	0	0	280	1.0
hickory mesquite (*Jack Daniel's* Tennessee)	45	0	10.0	0	0	310	1.0
Italian, Mediterranean style (*World Harbors* Amalfi Coast)	25	0	4.0	0	0	300	0
Italian herb (*Mc-Cormick* Flavor Medleys)	50	0	4.0	4.0	0	370	0
lemon pepper (*Mc-Cormick* Flavor Medleys)	50	0	4.0	3.5	0	450	0
pepper:							
cracked (*San-J*) ...	35	1.0	8.0	0	0	720	<1.0
lemon (*San-J*)	45	1.0	9.0	.5	0	410	0
peanut (*San-J*) ...	80	3.0	9.0	.5	0	540	4.0
tomato (*San-J*) ...	45	2.0	9.0	0	0	900	<1.0
rib sauce (*Texas Best*)	50	0	11.0	0	0	390	0

Food and Measure	cal.	prot. (gms)	carbo. (gms)	fat (gms)	chol. (mgs)	sod. (mgs)	fiber (gms)
roasted pepper (*Texas Best* Pueblo)	50	0	12.0	0	0	350	0
salsa (*Chi-Chi's*)	50	0	12.0	0	0	360	0
serrano (*Texas Best* Santa Fe)	35	1.0	8.0	0	0	250	0
sun-dried tomato and basil (*McCormick* Flavor Medleys) . . .	50	0	4.0	3.0	0	400	0
teriyaki: (*House of Tsang*), 1 tbsp.	40	0	10.0	0	0	520	0
tangy (Bull's Eye) . .	60	<1.0	13.0	0	0	420	0
Tex-Mex (*Chi-Chi's*) . .	35	5	8.0	0	0	280	0
Grits, see "Corn grits"							
Grog mixer, see "Navy grog drink mixer"							
Ground cherry, ½ cup	37	1.3	7.8	.5	0	n.a.	2.0
Grouper, meat only:							
raw, 4 oz.	104	22.0	0	1.2	42	60	0
baked, broiled, or microwaved, 4 oz.	134	28.2	0	1.5	53	60	0
Guacamole, 2 tbsp.:							
(*Calavo* Fiesta)	60	<1.0	4.0	5.0	0	140	2.0
(*Calavo* Mild)	50	<1.0	4.0	4.0	0	120	2.0
(*Dean's*)	80	1.0	1.0	8.0	5	170	0
(*Herr's*)	50	1.0	4.0	3.0	0	210	0
(*Kraft Dips*)	60	1.0	3.0	4.5	0	250	0
(*Marie's*)	90	1.0	1.0	9.0	4	190	<1.0
(*Marzetti*)	120	1.0	2.0	12.0	20	230	0
Southwestern (*El Monterey*)	57	1.0	3.0	5.0	0	147	2.0
Guacamole, frozen, 2 tbsp.:							
(*Simplot* Grande Zesty)	40	0	3.0	3.5	0	110	1.0
(*Simplot* Ranchero Grande)	40	0	3.0	3.0	0	170	1.0
(*Simplot* Ranchero Grande Low Fat) . .	35	0	5.0	1.5	0	190	1.0
(*Simplot* Western) . . .	50	1.0	2.0	5.0	0	170	2.0
Guacamole seasoning mix:							
(*Bearitos*), ½ tsp. . . .	5	0	1.0	0	0	220	0
(*El Torito*), 1/12 pkg. . .	5	0	1.0	0	0	50	0
(*Lawry's*), ½ tsp.	5	0	1.0	0	0	130	0

Food and Measure	cal.	prot. (gms)	carbo. (gms)	fat (gms)	chol. (mgs)	sod. (mgs)	fiber (gms)
Guanabana nectar, canned (*Goya*), 6 fl. oz.	110	0	27.0	0	0	20	<1.0
Guava (see also "Feijoas"):							
(*Frieda's*), 3-oz. fruit	45	1.0	10.0	.5	0	0	5.0
1 medium, 4 oz.	45	.7	10.7	.5	0	2	4.9
½ cup	42	.7	9.8	.5	0	2	4.5
strawberry, ½ cup ...	85	.7	21.2	.7	0	45	7.8
Guava drink:							
(*Goya* Nectar), 6 fl. oz.	110	0	27.0	0	0	10	1.0
(*Libby's* Nectar), 11.5-fl.oz. can	210	0	52.0	0	0	10	0
Guava juice blends:							
(*After the Fall Guava Maya*), 8 fl. oz. ...	110	1.0	26.0	0	0	20	0
blend (*Ceres*), 5.25 fl. oz.	87	0	21.0	0	0	n.a.	0
Guava nectar, see "Guava drink"							
Guava sauce, ½ cup	43	.4	11.3	.2	0	4	4.3
Guava-strawberry drink (*R. W. Knudsen*), 8 fl. oz.	110	<1.0	27.0	0	0	25	0
Guavadilla, see "Passion fruit"							
Guinea hen, raw:							
meat w/skin, 4 oz. ..	179	26.5	0	7.3	84	86	0
meat only, 4 oz.	125	23.4	0	2.8	71	78	0
Gyros mix, dry (*Casbah*), .65 oz. .	64	2.0	12.0	0	0	470	0

H

Food and Measure	cal.	prot. (gms)	carbo. (gms)	fat (gms)	chol. (mgs)	sod. (mgs)	fiber (gms)
Habas (*Frieda's*), ½ cup, 3 oz.	100	6.0	17.0	0	0	5	4.0
Haddock, meat only:							
raw, 4 oz.	99	21.5	0	.8	65	78	0
baked, broiled, or microwaved, 4 oz.	127	27.5	0	1.1	84	99	0
smoked, 4 oz.	132	28.6	0	1.1	87	865	0
Haddock entree, fillet, frozen:							
battered (*Van de Kamp's*), 2 pcs. . .	220	11.0	17.0	11.0	25	480	0
breaded, 1 pc.:							
(*Mrs. Paul's* Premium)	240	16.0	17.0	12.0	35	330	0
(*Van de Kamp's* Premium)	230	14.0	18.0	1.0	35	410	0
w/shrimp, crab, vege-tables (*Oven Pop-pers*), 4.5 oz.	210	19.0	12.0	9.0	85	310	1.0
Hake, see "Whiting"							
Halibut, meat only:							
Atlantic/Pacific, 4 oz.:							
raw	124	23.6	0	2.6	37	61	0
baked, broiled, or microwaved . . .	159	30.3	0	3.3	46	78	0
Greenland, 4 oz.							
raw	211	16.3	0	15.7	52	91	0
baked, broiled, or microwaved . . .	271	20.9	0	20.1	67	117	0
Halibut entree, frozen, battered:							
(*Van de Kamp's*), 3 pcs.	220	13.0	19.0	10.0	25	530	0
bites (*Mrs. Friday's*), 4 oz., about 8 pcs. .	180	17.0	11.0	7.0	30	370	2.0

Food and Measure	cal.	prot. (gms)	carbo. (gms)	fat (gms)	chol. (mgs)	sod. (mgs)	fiber (gms)
Halibut entree *(cont.)*							
fillets (*Mrs. Friday's*),							
2 pcs., 4 oz.	180	17.0	11.0	7.0	30	370	2.0
Halvah, 2 oz.:							
chocolate, vanilla, or							
marble (*Joyva*) ...	390	6.0	18.0	25.0	0	120	2.0
chocolate covered							
(*Joyva*)	380	5.0	20.0	25.0	0	95	3.0
Ham, fresh, meat only,							
4 oz., except as							
noted:							
whole leg, roasted:							
lean w/fat	310	30.4	0	20.0	107	68	0
lean w/fat, diced,							
1 cup	369	36.2	0	23.8	127	81	0
lean only	239	33.4	0	10.7	107	73	0
lean only, diced,							
1 cup	285	39.7	0	12.7	127	86	0
rump half, roasted:							
lean w/fat	286	32.7	0	16.2	109	70	0
lean only	235	35.1	0	9.2	109	74	0
shank half, roasted:							
lean w/fat	328	28.7	0	22.7	104	67	0
lean only	244	32.0	0	11.9	104	73	0
Ham, cured:							
whole leg, lean w/fat:							
unheated, 4 oz.	279	21.0	.1	21.0	64	1456	0
unheated, chopped							
or diced, 1 cup	344	25.9	.1	25.9	78	1798	0
roasted, 4 oz.	276	24.5	0	19.0	70	1346	0
roasted, chopped							
or diced, 1 cup	341	30.2	0	23.5	86	1661	0
whole leg, lean only:							
unheated, 4 oz.	167	25.3	.1	6.5	59	1719	0
unheated, chopped							
or diced, 1 cup	206	31.3	0	8.0	73	2122	0
roasted, 4 oz.	178	28.4	0	6.2	62	1505	0
roasted, chopped or							
diced, 1 cup	219	35.1	0	7.7	77	1858	0
boneless (11% fat):							
unheated, 4 oz. ...	206	19.9	3.5	12.0	65	1493	0
roasted, 4 oz.	202	25.7	0	10.2	67	1701	0
roasted, chopped or							
diced, 1 cup	249	31.7	0	12.6	83	2100	0

Food and Measure	cal.	prot. (gms)	carbo. (gms)	fat (gms)	chol. (mgs)	sod. (mgs)	fiber (gms)
boneless, extra lean (5% fat):							
unheated, 4 oz. ...	149	21.9	1.1	5.6	53	1620	0
roasted, 4 oz.	164	23.7	1.7	6.3	60	1364	0
roasted, chopped or diced, 1 cup	203	29.3	2.1	7.7	74	1684	0
Ham, deviled, see "Ham spread"							
Ham, refrigerated or canned, 3 oz., except as noted:							
(*Always Tender*), 4 oz.	270	18.0	0	22.0	75	400	0
(*Black Label* Refrigerator Can)	100	16.4	.7	4.5	47	1231	0
(*Black Label* Shelf Can)	100	17.3	0	4.7	50	1177	0
(*Boar's Head* 10") ...	90	14.0	2.0	2.0	30	840	0
(*Cure 81*)	100	15.0	0	4.5	45	870	0
(*Curemaster*)	80	14.0	0	3.0	40	940	0
(*Jones Dairy Farm* Country Carved/ Dainty/Country Club)	100	17.0	0	4.0	50	930	0
(*Jones Dairy Farm* Fully Cooked)	240	13.0	0	21.0	65	740	0
(*Jones Dairy Farm* Homestead)	140	16.0	0	8.0	55	750	0
(*Jones Dairy Farm* Old Fashioned)	220	15.0	0	18.0	65	1200	0
(*Jones Dairy Farm* Semi-Boneless) ...	180	16.0	0	13.0	60	800	0
(*Jones Dairy Farm* Skinless/Spiral Sliced)	160	16.0	0	11.0	60	680	0
(*Krakus* Polish), 2 oz.	50	10.0	0	1.5	25	730	0
(*Light & Lean* 97 Half)	90	14.0	2.0	2.5	35	950	0
(*Plumrose* Danish), 2 oz.	60	10.0	0	2.0	30	760	0
(*Spiral Cure 81*)	150	15.0	1.0	9.0	50	1090	0
butt or shank portion (*Cook's*), 4 oz. ...	220	14.0	3.0	17.0	50	1150	0
chunk (*Hormel*), 2 oz.	90	9.0	0	6.0	30	620	0
extra lean (4% fat):							
unheated, 4 oz. ...	136	21.0	0	5.2	43	1423	0
unheated, 1 cup ...	202	25.2	0	10.4	53	1786	0

Food and Measure	cal.	prot. (gms)	carbo. (gms)	fat (gms)	chol. (mgs)	sod. (mgs)	fiber (gms)
Ham, refrigerated or canned, extra lean *(cont.)*							
roasted, 4 oz.	154	24.0	.6	5.5	34	1287	0
roasted , 1 cup . . .	234	29.3	.7	11.8	57	1495	0
honey (*Jones Dairy Farm* Country Carved Family)	100	16.0	0	4.0	45	950	0
maple (*Jones Dairy Farm*)	100	15.0	1.0	4.0	45	810	0
maple glaze (*Boar's Head Honey Coat*)	90	7.0	1.0	1.5	35	870	0
roast, eye of pork (*Armour*), 4 oz. . .	140	20.0	0	6.0	45	460	0
slice:							
(*Boar's Head Sweet Slice*)	100	15.0	1.0	3.5	30	780	0
(*Jones Dairy Farm* Lean Choice), 2 slices, 1.6 oz. . .	50	9.0	0	1.5	30	420	0
(*Oscar Mayer* Dinner)	80	14.0	0	3.0	40	1020	0
maple glazed honey coat (*Boar's Head Sweet Slice*)	110	15.0	4.0	3.5	45	780	0
smoked (*Boar's Head*)	130	15.0	1.0	7.0	50	820	0
steak:							
(*Cook's*), 4 oz. . . .	150	14.0	3.0	9.0	50	1150	0
(*Jones Dairy Farm* Lean Choice) . . .	100	15.0	1.0	4.0	50	960	0
(*Oscar Mayer*), 2 oz.	60	10.0	0	2.0	30	750	0
"Ham," vegetarian, frozen:							
roll (*Worthington Wham*), 3/8" slice . .	110	10.0	3.0	6.0	0	390	0
sliced:							
(*Worthington Wham*), 2 slices	90	8.0	2.0	5.0	0	320	0
(*Yves* Deli Slices), 2.2 oz.	80	14.0	6.0	0	0	480	1.0
steak (*Veggie Master Vege*), 1/4 pkg.	88	2.0	5.0	4.0	0	238	3.0
Ham bologna (*Boar's Head*), 2 oz.	80	9.0	2.0	4.0	30	660	0

Food and Measure	cal.	prot. (gms)	carbo. (gms)	fat (gms)	chol. (mgs)	sod. (mgs	fiber (gms)
Ham entree, frozen, 1 pkg.:							
and cheese (*Healthy Choice* Bread Stuffs), 6.1 oz.	320	21.0	48.0	5.0	20	590	1.0
steak, w/honey-brown sugar glaze (*Marie Callender's*), 14 oz.	490	29.0	63.0	13.0	80	2310	5.0
Ham glaze:							
(*Boar's Head*), 2 tbsp.	120	0	30.0	0	0	95	0
(*Crosse & Blackwell*), 1 tbsp.	30	0	8.0	0	0	25	0
(*Reese's*), 1 tbsp. ...	20	0	5.0	0	0	55	0
Ham lunch meat, 2 oz., except as noted:							
(*Boar's Head* Deluxe) .	60	9.0	2.0	1.0	25	590	0
(*Boar's Head* Deluxe Lower Sodium) ...	60	10.0	2.0	1.0	25	460	0
(*Boar's Head* Tavern) .	60	10.0	2.0	1.0	30	580	0
(*Carl Buddig* 6 oz.) ..	85	10.0	1.0	5.0	35	760	0
(*Citterio Fresca* Rosmarino)	90	11.0	1.0	3.0	25	400	0
(*Healthy Deli* Deluxe) .	60	9.0	1.0	1.5	20	480	0
(*Healthy Deli* Olde Tyme Tavern)	60	10.0	1.0	1.5	20	470	0
(*Healthy Deli* Shattuck)	60	9.0	2.0	1.5	20	480	0
(*Light & Lean* 97), 1-oz. slice	25	4.0	0	1.0	15	340	0
(*Louis Rich*)	50	9.0	0	1.5	25	700	0
(*Louis Rich*), 2 slices, 1.6 oz.	40	8.0	0	1.0	20	570	0
(*Louis Rich*), 5 slices, 2.1 oz.	50	10.0	0	1.5	30	740	0
(*Oscar Mayer*)	50	9.0	<1.0	1.5	25	770	0
(*Oscar Mayer* Lower Sodium), 3 slices, 2.3 oz.	70	10.0	2.0	2.0	30	530	0
baked:							
(*Healthy Choice*), 1-oz. slice	30	5.0	1.0	1.0	10	240	0
(*Healthy Choice* Deli-Traditions*), 6 slices, 1.9 oz.	60	9.0	1.0	1.5	25	470	0

Food and Measure	cal.	prot. (gms)	carbo. (gms)	fat (gms)	chol. (mgs)	sod. (mgs)	fiber (gms)
Ham lunch meat, baked *(cont.)*							
(*Louis Rich*), 2 slices, 1.6 oz.	45	8.0	<1.0	1.0	25	550	0
(*Sara Lee* Home-style)	60	10.0	2.0	2.0	25	500	0
Black Forest:							
(*Boar's Head*)	60	10.0	2.0	1.0	30	580	0
(*Healthy Deli*)	60	10.0	1.0	1.5	20	480	0
boiled:							
(*Oscar Mayer*)	60	9.0	<1.0	2.0	25	730	0
(*Oscar Mayer*), 3 slices, 2.2 oz.	60	10.0	<1.0	2.0	30	820	0
(*Sara Lee*), 2 slices, 1.6 oz.	40	9.0	1.0	.5	20	610	0
brown sugar:							
(*Louis Rich*)	70	10.0	4.0	1.5	25	820	0
(*Louis Rich*), 5 slices, 2.1 oz.	70	10.0	4.0	1.5	30	860	0
(*Sara Lee*)	70	10.0	5.0	1.5	15	500	0
(*Sara Lee*), 2 slices, 1.6 oz.	60	8.0	4.0	1.0	10	490	0
cappicola:							
(*Boar's Head* Capocollo), 1 oz.	80	7.0	0	5.0	15	590	0
(*Daniele* Capocollo), 3 slices, 1 oz. . .	80	8.0	<1.0	5.0	17	540	0
(*Healthy Deli* Cappi)	60	9.0	2.0	1.5	20	480	0
chopped:							
(*Black Label*)	140	7.0	2.0	12.0	35	720	0
(*Oscar Mayer*), 1-oz. slice	50	4.0	2.0	3.5	15	320	0
(*Oscar Mayer*), 2 slices, 1.6 oz.	80	7.0	3.0	5.0	25	520	0
cinnamon apple (*Healthy Deli* Grove)	70	9.0	4.0	1.5	20	480	0
cooked:							
(*Alpine Lace*)	60	9.0	2.0	1.5	25	400	0
(*Healthy Choice*) . .	60	9.0	1.0	1.5	25	460	0
(*Healthy Choice*), 1-oz. slice	30	5.0	1.0	1.0	15	240	0
(*Healthy Choice Deli Traditions*), 6 slices, 1.9 oz.	60	9.0	1.0	1.5	25	470	0

Food and Measure	cal.	prot. (gms)	carbo. (gms)	fat (gms)	chol. (mgs)	sod. (mgs)	fiber (gms)
(*Healthy Choice* Virginia), 1-oz. slice	30	5.0	1.0	1.0	15	240	0
(*Healthy Deli* Fat Free)	50	10.0	1.0	0	5	480	0
(*Hormel* Deli)	60	8.0	2.0	2.5	20	680	0
(*Oscar Mayer*), 3 slices, 2.2 oz. .	60	10.0	<1.0	2.0	35	770	0
(*Sara Lee* Old Fashioned)	50	10.0	1.0	1.0	25	750	0
honey:							
(*Alpine Lace*)	60	9.0	2.0	1.0	25	530	0
(*Carl Buddig* 6 oz.) .	90	10.0	2.0	5.0	35	590	0
(*Healthy Choice*) ..	60	9.0	2.0	1.5	25	480	0
(*Healthy Choice*), 1-oz. slice	30	5.0	1.0	1.0	10	240	0
(*Healthy Choice* Savory Selections*), 6 slices, 1.9 oz.	60	9.0	2.0	1.5	25	470	0
(*Healthy Deli* Honey Valley)	60	9.0	2.0	1.5	20	480	0
(*Louis Rich*), 2 slices, 1.6 oz.	45	8.0	2.0	1.0	25	570	0
(*Louis Rich*), 6 slices, 2.1 oz.	60	10.0	2.0	1.5	30	760	0
(*Oscar Mayer*), 3 slices, 1.7 oz. .	35	7.0	2.0	0	20	580	0
(*Oscar Mayer*), 3 slices, 2.2 oz. .	70	10.0	2.0	2.0	30	770	0
(*Sara Lee* Bavarian)	70	9.0	2.0	3.5	40	560	0
baked (*Carl Buddig*), 2.5-oz. pkg. ...	90	13.0	3.0	2.0	25	830	0
cured (*Healthy Choice*), 1-oz. slice	30	5.0	1.0	1.0	15	240	0
cured (*Sara Lee*) ..	60	10.0	2.0	1.5	25	520	0
cured (*Sara Lee*), 2 slices, 1.6 oz.	45	8.0	1.0	1.0	20	420	0
maple (*Healthy Choice Savory Selections*), 1-oz. slice	30	5.0	2.0	1.0	15	170	0

Food and Measure	cal.	prot. (gms)	carbo. (gms)	fat (gms)	chol. (mgs)	sod. (mgs)	fiber (gms)
Ham lunch meat, honey *(cont.)*							
maple (*Healthy Choice Savory Selections*), 6 slices, 1.9 oz.	60	10.0	3.0	1.5	25	400	0
maple (*Sara Lee*)	70	9.0	4.0	2.0	20	550	0
mustard (*Healthy Choice Savory Selections*), 6 slices, 1.9 oz.	60	9.0	3.0	1.5	25	470	0
jalapeño (*Healthy Deli*)	60	8.0	3.0	1.5	15	480	0
hot (*Healthy Deli Rodeo*)	60	9.0	1.0	1.5	20	480	0
maple:							
(*Healthy Deli*)	60	9.0	3.0	1.5	20	460	0
flame seared (*Heathy Deli*)	70	11.0	3.0	2.0	25	480	0
glazed (*Boar's Head Honey Coat*)	60	10.0	3.0	1.0	20	570	0
minced, 1 oz.	75	4.6	.5	5.9	20	353	0
pepper:							
(*Boar's Head*)	70	9.0	3.0	2.0	30	590	0
(*Boar's Head Gourmet*)	60	10.0	2.0	1.0	20	610	0
(*Healthy Deli* Tutta Bella)	70	9.0	3.0	2.0	20	420	0
pesto Parmesan oven roasted (*Boar's Head*)	90	14.0	0	4.0	30	320	0
prosciutto, see "Prosciutto"							
rosemary:							
(*Black Bear*)	70	11.0	1.0	2.5	30	520	0
sun-dried tomato (*Boar's Head*)	70	10.0	2.0	2.5	10	590	0
smoked:							
(*Boar's Head Honey Coat*)	60	10.0	2.0	2.0	25	650	0
(*Carl Buddig*), 2.5-oz. pkg.	80	13.0	1.0	2.0	25	830	0
(*Healthy Choice*)	60	9.0	2.0	1.5	30	430	0
(*Healthy Choice*), 1-oz. slice	30	5.0	1.0	1.0	10	240	0

Food and Measure	cal.	prot. (gms)	carbo. (gms)	fat (gms)	chol. (mgs)	sod. (mgs	fiber (gms)
(*Healthy Choice Deli Traditions*), 2 slices, 1.9 oz. .	60	9.0	2.0	1.5	25	470	0
(*Louis Rich* Fat Free), 2 slices, 1.8 oz. .	35	7.0	<1.0	0	20	560	0
(*Oscar Mayer*)	50	9.0	0	2.0	25	680	0
(*Oscar Mayer*), 3 slices, 2.2 oz. .	60	10.0	0	2.5	30	760	0
(*Oscar Mayer* Fat Free), 3 slices, 1.7 oz.	35	7.0	<1.0	0	15	530	0
(*Sara Lee* Smoke-house)	50	10.0	1.0	1.5	20	620	0
double (*Healthy Deli*)	60	10.0	1.0	1.5	20	470	0
mesquite (*Healthy Choice*)	60	10.0	1.0	1.5	25	480	0
Virginia (*Boar's Head*)	60	9.0	2.0	1.0	25	590	0
spiced (*Boar's Head*)	120	7.0	1.0	10.0	30	570	0
sweet (*Healthy Deli* Dona Flor*)	60	8.0	5.0	1.0	10	480	0
tomato basil (*Black Bear*)	70	11.0	1.0	2.5	30	520	0
Virginia:							
(*Black Bear*)	50	9.0	2.0	1.0	25	580	0
(*Boar's Head*)	60	9.0	3.0	1.0	25	590	0
(*Healthy Choice*) . .	60	9.0	2.0	1.5	25	480	0
(*Healthy Choice Deli Traditions*), 5 slices, 1.9 oz. .	60	9.0	2.0	1.5	25	450	0
(*Healthy Choice Savory Selections*), 1-oz. slice	30	5.0	1.0	1.0	15	170	0
(*Healthy Deli* Less Sodium)	70	9.0	3.0	1.5	20	330	0
(*Sara Lee*), 3 slices, 1.8 oz.	60	8.0	2.0	2.0	20	560	0
baked (*Healthy Deli*)	70	10.0	3.0	1.5	20	480	0
fruited or smoked (*Healthy Deli*) . .	60	9.0	2.0	1.5	20	480	0
smoked (*Alpine Lace*)	60	9.0	2.0	1.0	25	400	0
Ham and cheese loaf (*Oscar Mayer*), 1-oz. slice	60	4.0	<1.0	4.5	20	350	0

Food and Measure	cal.	prot. (gms)	carbo. (gms)	fat (gms)	chol. (mgs)	sod. (mgs)	fiber (gms)
Ham and cheese pocket/sandwich, frozen, 4.5-oz. pc., except as noted:							
(*Deli Stuffs*)	320	12.0	44.0	11.0	40	630	2.0
(*Hot Pockets*)	310	12.0	40.0	12.0	35	550	2.0
(*Hot Pockets Toaster Melts*), 2.2 oz. ...	160	4.0	21.0	6.0	10	290	2.0
(*Lean Pockets*)	280	13.0	42.0	7.0	30	600	2.0
cheddar (*Croissant Pockets*)	330	13.0	40.0	14.0	40	610	2.0
croissant (*Sara Lee*), 3.7 oz.	300	12.0	27.0	16.0	45	570	2.0
"Ham" and cheese sandwich, vegetarian, frozen, stuffed (*Morningstar Farms* Meat-Free), 4.5-oz. pc.	300	15.0	45.0	7.0	10	520	1.0
Ham patty, 2-oz. patty:							
(*Hormel*)	180	7.0	1.0	16.0	40	620	0
and cheese (*Hormel*) .	180	7.0	0	17.0	40	520	0
Ham spread, deviled, ¼ cup:							
(*Cure 81*)	150	9.0	2.0	12.0	40	430	0
(*Underwood*)	160	8.0	1.0	14.0	30	410	0
Hamburger, see "Beef sandwich"							
"Hamburger," vegetarian, see "Burger, vegetarian"							
Hamburger entree mix (*Hamburger Helper*), 1 cup*:							
bacon cheeseburger .	380	23.0	34.0	17.0	65	1100	<1.0
beef pasta	270	20.0	26.0	10.0	50	910	1.0
beef Romanoff	300	21.0	29.0	11.0	55	950	0
beef stew	260	18.0	26.0	10.0	50	760	2.0
beef taco	300	19.0	31.0	12.0	50	880	1.0
beef teriyaki	290	18.0	34.0	10.0	50	990	2.0
cheddar/broccoli	350	22.0	32.0	15.0	55	840	0
cheddar melt	300	19.0	31.0	12.0	55	850	<1.0
cheese, three	340	21.0	32.0	15.0	55	830	<1.0
cheeseburger macaroni	360	23.0	32.0	16.0	65	940	1.0

Food and Measure	cal.	prot. (gms)	carbo. (gms)	fat (gms)	chol. (mgs)	sod. (mgs)	fiber (gms)
cheesy hash browns .	400	21.0	39.0	19.0	60	520	2.0
cheesy shells	340	21.0	30.0	15.0	55	850	<1.0
chili macaroni	300	20.0	30.0	12.0	55	820	1.0
fettuccine Alfredo . . .	300	20.0	26.0	13.0	55	860	0
Italian, zesty	300	20.0	32.0	10.0	50	850	2.0
Italian Parmesan	300	20.0	31.0	11.0	50	870	1.0
lasagna	270	19.0	29.0	10.0	50	1000	2.0
lasagna, 4-cheese . . .	350	23.0	31.0	15.0	60	800	0
pizza, double cheese .	320	21.0	35.0	12.0	55	1000	1.0
pizza, pepperoni	310	20.0	31.0	12.0	55	850	1.0
pizza pasta, w/cheese topping	280	19.0	31.0	10.0	50	750	2.0
Philly cheesesteak . . .	330	21.0	25.0	17.0	60	910	0
potatoes Stroganoff . .	260	18.0	24.0	11.0	50	880	2.0
ravioli w/cheese topping	310	20.0	34.0	10.0	50	960	1.0
rice Oriental	280	18.0	32.0	10.0	50	990	0
Salisbury	270	19.0	26.0	10.0	50	790	1.0
spaghetti	270	19.0	27.0	10.0	50	940	1.0
Stroganoff	320	21.0	30.0	13.0	55	830	0
Hard sauce (*Crosse & Blackwell*), 2 tbsp.	180	0	24.0	9.0	25	20	0
Hardee's, 1 serving:							
breakfast:							
biscuit:							
apple cinnamon 'n' raisin	250	2.0	42.0	8.0	0	350	n.a.
bacon, egg, cheese	520	17.0	45.0	30.0	210	1420	n.a.
Biscuit 'n Gravy .	530	10.0	56.0	30.0	15	1550	n.a.
chicken	590	24.0	62.0	27.0	45	1820	n.a.
ham	410	13.0	45.0	20.0	25	1200	n.a.
ham, country . . .	440	14.0	44.0	22.0	30	1710	n.a.
jelly	440	6.0	57.0	21.0	0	1000	n.a.
Made from Scratch	390	6.0	44.0	21.0	0	1000	n.a.
Omelet Biscuit . .	550	20.0	45.0	32.0	225	1350	n.a.
sausage	550	12.0	44.0	36.0	25	1310	n.a.
sausage and egg	620	19.0	45.0	41.0	225	1370	n.a.
steak	580	15.0	56.0	32.0	30	1580	n.a.
Frisco sandwich, ham	450	22.0	42.0	22.0	225	1290	n.a.
Hash Rounds, regular	230	3.0	24.0	14.0	0	560	n.a.

Food and Measure	cal.	prot. (gms)	carbo. (gms)	fat (gms)	chol. (mgs)	sod. (mgs)	fiber (gms)
Hardee's, *(cont.)*							
sandwiches:							
bacon Swiss crispy							
chicken	670	24.0	45.0	44.0	55	1600	n.a.
Big Roast Beef	410	24.0	26.0	24.0	40	1140	n.a.
burger:							
All Star	660	29.0	41.0	43.0	100	1260	n.a.
hamburger	270	13.0	29.0	11.0	35	550	n.a.
Famous Star . . .	570	24.0	41.0	35.0	80	860	n.a.
Frisco	720	31.0	37.0	49.0	95	1180	n.a.
Monster Burger .	1060	49.0	37.0	79.0	185	1860	n.a.
Super Star	790	40.0	41.0	53.0	145	970	n.a.
chicken, grilled . . .	350	23.0	28.0	16.0	65	860	n.a.
chicken fillet	480	24.0	44.0	23.0	55	1190	n.a.
Fisherman's Fillet . .	530	25.0	45.0	28.0	75	1280	n.a.
hot dog,							
w/condiments . .	450	15.0	25.0	32.0	55	1240	n.a.
Hot Ham 'N Cheese	300	16.0	34.0	12.0	50	1390	n.a.
roast beef, monster	610	35.0	26.0	39.0	105	1940	n.a.
roast beef, regular .	310	17.0	26.0	16.0	40	800	n.a.
chicken:							
breast	370	29.0	29.0	15.0	75	1190	n.a.
leg	170	13.0	15.0	7.0	45	570	n.a.
thigh	330	19.0	30.0	15.0	60	1000	n.a.
wing	200	10.0	23.0	8.0	30	740	n.a.
sides:							
coleslaw, 4 oz. . . .	240	2.0	13.0	20.0	10	340	n.a.
Crispy Curls:							
large	520	7.0	62.0	28.0	0	1450	n.a.
medium	340	5.0	41.0	18.0	0	950	n.a.
monster	590	8.0	70.0	31.0	0	1640	n.a.
fries, large	440	5.0	59.0	21.0	0	520	n.a.
fries, monster	510	6.0	67.0	24.0	0	590	n.a.
fries, regular	340	4.0	45.0	16.0	0	390	n.a.
gravy, 1.5 oz.	20	<1.0	3.0	<1.0	0	260	n.a.
mashed potatoes,							
small	70	2.0	14.0	<1.0	0	330	n.a.
desserts/shakes:							
apple turnover	270	4.0	38.0	12.0	0	250	n.a.
peach cobbler	310	2.0	60.0	7.0	0	360	n.a.
shake, chocolate . .	370	13.0	67.0	5.0	30	270	0
shake, vanilla	350	12.0	65.0	5.0	20	300	0
twist cone	180	4.0	34.0	2.0	10	120	0

Food and Measure	cal.	prot. (gms)	carbo. (gms)	fat (gms)	chol. (mgs)	sod. (mgs	fiber (gms)
Hash, see "Beef hash" and "Sausage hash"							
Hazelnut, see "Filberts"							
Hazelnut spread							
(*Nutella*), 2 tbsp. . .	160	2.0	19.0	9.0	0	30	0
Hazelnut syrup							
(*Ferrara*), 2 oz. . . .	130	0	32.0	0	0	12	0
Head cheese (*Boar's Head*), 2 oz.	90	10.0	<1.0	5.0	65	420	0
Heart, braised or simmered, 4 oz.:							
beef	199	32.6	.5	6.4	219	71	0
chicken, broiler-fryer .	210	30.0	.1	9.0	274	54	0
lamb	210	28.3	2.2	9.0	282	71	0
pork	168	26.8	.5	5.7	251	40	0
turkey	201	30.3	2.3	6.9	256	62	0
veal	211	33.0	.1	7.7	200	66	0
Herbs, see specific listings							
Herbs, mixed (*Lawry's* Pinch of Herbs), ¼ tsp.	0	0	0	0	0	80	0
Herring, fresh:							
Atlantic, meat only:							
raw, 4 oz.	180	20.4	0	10.3	68	102	0
baked, broiled, or microwaved, 4 oz.	230	26.1	0	13.1	87	130	0
kippered, 4 oz. . . .	246	27.9	0	14.0	93	1041	0
pickled, 4 oz.	297	16.1	10.9	20.4	15	987	0
lake, see "Cisco"							
Pacific, meat only:							
raw, 4 oz.	224	18.6	0	15.8	87	84	0
baked, broiled, or microwaved, 4 oz.	284	23.8	0	20.2	112	108	0
Herring, canned, see "Sardine"							
Herring, kippered, canned, ¼ cup, except as noted:							
(*Crown Prince* Snacks), 3.25-oz. can	190	19.0	0	13.0	60	390	0

Food and Measure	cal.	prot. (gms)	carbo. (gms)	fat (gms)	chol. (mgs)	sod. (mgs)	fiber (gms)
Herring, kippered *(cont.)*							
in mustard (*Crown Prince Natural*) ...	100	9.0	0	8.0	40	290	0
in salsa picante (*Crown Prince*)	90	6.0	3.0	6.0	15	200	0
smoked (*Crown Prince Natural*)	110	11.0	0	8.0	35	40	0
Herring, pickled, in jars, ¼ cup, except as noted:							
slices (*Vita* Lunch), 2 oz.	130	9.0	5.0	8.0	40	600	0
in sour cream:							
(*Elf*), ¼ cup	110	8.0	5.0	6.0	25	520	0
(*Vita*), ¼ cup	120	7.0	8.0	7.0	35	600	0
in wine sauce, 2 oz.:							
(*Nathan's*)	90	5.0	7.0	4.0	25	420	0
(*Skansen* Tidbits) ..	85	8.0	7.0	3.0	18	550	<1.0
(*Vita* Party Snacks Tastee Bits)	120	9.0	10.0	5.0	30	480	0
rollmops (*Elf*)	100	7.0	8.0	4.0	20	520	0
Herring oil, see "Oil"							
Herring salad, pickled (*Blue Ridge Farms*), ⅓ cup, 3 oz.	150	9.0	17.0	6.0	50	250	1.0
Hickory nut, dried, shelled, 1 oz.	187	3.6	5.2	18.3	0	tr.	1.8
Hickory smoked salt (*McCormick*), ¼ tsp.	0	0	0	0	0	455	0
Hiziki, see "Seaweed"							
Hoisin sauce:							
(*House of Tsang*), 1 tsp.	15	0	4.0	0	0	120	0
(*Ka•Me*), 2 tbsp.	70	1.0	15.0	0	0	370	0
Hollandaise sauce, in jars, 2 tbsp.:							
(*Melba*)	90	1.0	1.0	9.0	80	410	0
(*Reese's*)	90	1.0	1.0	9.0	75	380	0
Hollandaise sauce mix:							
(*Knorr* Classic), 1 tsp.	10	0	2.0	0	0	85	0
(*McCormick Produce Partners*), ⅒ pkt. .	20	0	2.0	.5	0	160	0

Food and Measure	cal.	prot. (gms)	carbo. (gms)	fat (gms)	chol. (mgs)	sod. (mgs)	fiber (gms)
Home-style gravy mix (*McCormick*), ¼ cup*	25	0	4.0	1.0	0	280	0
Hominy, dry, white (*Goya*), ¼ cup	180	4.0	39.0	0	0	0	0
Hominy, canned, ½ cup:							
golden:							
(*Allens/Uncle William*)	120	2.0	27.0	.5	0	340	4.0
(*Bush's Best*)	60	1.0	13.0	.5	0	550	3.0
w/red and green pepper (*Bush's Best*)	70	2.0	14.0	1.0	0	570	3.0
Mexican (*Allens/Uncle William* Pepi)	120	2.0	25.0	1.0	0	340	3.0
white:							
(*Allens/Uncle William*)	100	2.0	22.0	.5	0	340	4.0
(*Bush's Best* Pozole Blanco)	70	1.0	14.0	1.0	0	530	4.0
(*Juanitas* Mexican)	60	2.0	10.0	.5	0	190	6.0
w/red and green pepper (*Bush's Best*)	80	2.0	16.0	1.0	0	500	4.0
Hominy grits, see "Corn grits"							
Honey, 1 tbsp.:							
(*Aunt Sue's/Grandma's/ Sue Bee*)	60	0	17.0	0	0	0	0
(*Miel H*)	70	0	17.0	0	0	0	0
Honey bun, see "Bun, sweet"							
Honey butter, see "Butter, flavored"							
Honey Dijon sauce (*Kraft*), 1 oz.	180	0	10.0	4.5	<5	230	0
Honey loaf, see "Lunch meat"							
Honey mustard, see "Mustard blend" and "Pretzel dip"							

Food and Measure	cal.	prot. (gms)	carbo. (gms)	fat (gms)	chol. (mgs)	sod. (mgs)	fiber (gms)
Honey mustard sauce Dijon (*World Harbors* Mont St. Michel), 2 tbsp.	30	0	7.0	0	0	230	0
Honey roll sausage, beef, 1 oz.	52	5.3	.6	3.0	14	375	0
Honey spread, flavored, all varieties (*Bigelow*), 1 tbsp.	70	0	17.0	0	0	0	0
Honeycomb (*Frieda's*), ½ cup, 3 oz.	260	0	70.0	0	0	0	0
Honeydew:							
(*Dole*), ⅒ melon	50	1.0	13.0	0	0	35	1.0
⅒ melon, 7" x 2"	46	.6	11.8	.1	0	13	.8
cubed, 1 cup	60	.8	15.6	.2	0	17	1.0
Horned melon (*Frieda's*), 3.5 oz.	25	0	0	0	0	0	1.0
Horseradish, fresh: leafy tips, ½ cup:							
raw, chopped	6	.9	.8	.1	0	1	.2
boiled, drained, chopped	13	1.1	2.3	.2	0	2	.4
pods, ½ cup:							
raw, sliced	19	1.1	4.3	.1	0	21	1.6
boiled, drained, sliced	21	1.2	4.8	.1	0	25	2.5
Horseradish, prepared, 1 tsp.:							
(*Boar's Head*)	0	0	0	0	0	30	0
(*Kraft/Kraft* Cream Style)	0	0	0	0	0	50	0
w/beets (*Gold's*)	0	0	0	0	0	30	0
Horseradish mustard, see "Mustard blend"							
Horseradish root (*Frieda's*), 1 tbsp. . .	0	0	1.0	0	0	0	0
Horseradish sauce:							
(*Bennetts*), 1 tbsp. . .	50	0	3.0	5.0	<5	130	0
(*Boar's Head* Pub Style), 1 tsp.	15	0	1.0	1.5	5	15	0
(*Heinz*), 1 tsp.	20	0	1.0	2.0	0	35	0
(*Kraft*), 1 tsp.	20	0	<1.0	1.5	<5	35	0
(*Marzetti*), 1 tbsp. . .	90	0	1.0	10.0	5	80	0

Food and Measure	cal.	prot. (gms)	carbo. (gms)	fat (gms)	chol. (mgs)	sod. (mgs)	fiber (gms)
Hot dog, see "Frankfurter"							
Hot dog sauce, see "Chili sauce"							
Hot fudge sauce, see "Chocolate topping"							
Hot sauce, 1 tsp., except as noted:							
(*Cholula* Mexican) . . .	0	0	0	0	0	20	0
(*Frank's RedHot*)	0	0	0	0	0	230	0
(*Glory Foods*)	0	0	0	0	0	45	0
(*Goya* Salsa Picante) .	0	0	0	0	0	125	0
(*Grace* Jamaican) . . .	0	0	0	0	0	125	0
(*Helen's Tropical Exotics* Pepper Sauce)	0	0	1.0	0	0	40	0
(*Lottie's* Barbados) . .	5	0	1.0	0	0	70	0
(*Louisiana*)	0	0	0	0	0	240	0
(*Tabasco*)	0	0	0	0	0	30	0
(*Texas Best*)	0	0	0	0	0	125	0
(*Trappey's* Indi-Pep West Indian)	0	0	<1.0	0	0	140	0
(*Trappey's* Mexi-Pep/ Bull Louisiana)	0	0	<.10	0	0	115	0
(*Trappey's* Red Devil) .	0	0	0	0	0	150	0
(*Watkins* Calypso) . . .	10	0	3.0	0	0	25	0
(*Watkins* Inferno), 2 tbsp.	35	0	8.0	0	0	790	0
chili:							
(*Heaven and Earth* Dragon Fire), 1 tbsp.	25	0	6.0	0	0	50	0
(*Sun Luck*)	0	0	<1.0	0	0	125	0
green pepper (*Tabasco*)	0	0	0	0	0	140	0
habanero:							
(*D. L. Jardine's* Blazin' Saddle XXX Hot)	0	0	0	0	0	100	0
(*Shotgun Willie's* XXXX Hot), 2 tbsp.	10	0	2.0	0	0	220	0
jalapeño:							
(*Búfalo*)	0	0	0	0	0	115	0
(*D. L. Jardine's* Texa-peppa)	0	0	0	0	0	70	0

Food and Measure	cal.	prot. (gms)	carbo. (gms)	fat (gms)	chol. (mgs)	sod. (mgs)	fiber (gms)
Hot sauce, jalapeño *(cont.)*							
(*Trappey's* Chef Magic)	0	0	0	0	0	140	0
(*Watkins*)	0	0	0	0	0	70	0
picante, medium							
(*Búfalo*)	0	0	0	0	0	140	0
Hubbard squash:							
raw:							
(*Frieda's*), ¾ cup, 3 oz.	35	2.0	7.0	0	0	0	2.0
1 cup	46	2.3	10.1	.6	0	8	2.7
baked, cubed, ½ cup .	51	2.5	11.0	.6	0	8	2.9
boiled, drained, mashed, ½ cup . . .	35	1.8	7.6	.4	0	6	3.4
Hummus, 2 tbsp., except as noted:							
(*Athenos* Original) . . .	60	2.0	5.0	3.5	0	180	1.0
(*Sabra Salads* Chumus), 1 oz. . . .	69	4.0	1.5	4.8	0	32	2.0
(*Telma*), ½ cup	160	7.0	13.0	9.0	0	450	3.0
(*Tribe of Two Sheiks*) .	50	2.0	4.0	3.0	– 0	105	1.0
all varieties:							
(*Cedar's*)	50	3.0	5.0	2.0	0	120	3.0
(*Yorgo*)	50	2.0	5.0	2.0	0	60	3.0
cucumber dill (*Athenos*)	60	2.0	5.0	4.0	0	240	1.0
eggplant, roasted (*Athenos*)	45	2.0	4.0	2.5	0	280	1.0
garlic, roasted (*Athenos*)	50	2.0	5.0	3.5	0	200	1.0
olive, black (*Athenos*)	50	2.0	5.0	3.0	0	200	1.0
pesto (*Athenos*)	50	2.0	6.0	3.5	0	170	2.0
red pepper, roasted (*Athenos*)	60	2.0	6.0	3.5	0	210	1.0
scallion (*Athenos*) . . .	50	2.0	6.0	3.5	0	230	2.0
spicy, three pepper (*Athenos*)	60	2.0	5.0	3.5	0	270	1.0
Hummus mix							
(*Casbah*), 1 oz. . . .	160	5.0	14.0	8.0	0	180	1.0
Hummus and pita, 2 tbsp. hummus and 2 pcs. pita.:							
(*Athenos* Travelers Original)	130	3.0	17.0	6.0	0	360	1.0

Food and Measure	cal.	prot. (gms)	carbo. (gms)	fat (gms)	chol. (mgs)	sod. (mgs)	fiber (gms)
eggplant, roasted							
(*Athenos* Travelers)	120	3.0	16.0	5.0	0	440	2.0
garlic, roasted							
(*Athenos* Travelers)	130	3.0	17.0	6.0	0	370	2.0
red pepper, roasted							
(*Athenos* Travelers)	140	3.0	19.0	6.0	0	410	2.0
spicy three pepper							
(*Athenos* Travelers)	130	3.0	7.0	6.0	0	460	2.0
Hunter gravy mix, see "Mushroom gravy mix"							
Hush puppies, frozen							
(*McKenzie's*), 2 oz.	190	2.0	23.0	10.0	0	470	2.0
Hush puppies, mix							
(*Sylvia's*), ⅓ cup . .	130	3.0	24.0	2.0	0	500	0
Hyacinth bean, immature, boiled, drained, ½ cup . . .	22	1.3	4.1	.1	0	1	n.a.
Hyacinth bean, dried, boiled, ½ cup	114	7.9	20.1	.6	0	7	n.a.

I

Food and Measure	cal.	prot. (gms)	carbo. (gms)	fat (gms)	chol. (mgs)	sod. (mgs)	fiber (gms)
Ice:							
cherry (*Popsicle* Zone),							
12 fl. oz.	240	0	62.0	0	0 .	10	0
chocolate:							
(*Marinos*), 1 cup . .	120	1.0	29.0	0	0	70	0
(*Rosati*), 6 fl. oz.	180	0	37.0	0	0	15	0
lemon:							
(*Chill* Double), ¾ of							
6-oz. cup	100	0	26.0	0	0	20	0
(*Luigi's*), 6 fl. oz.	120	0	30.0	0	0	10	<1.0
(*Popsicle* Zone),							
12 fl. oz.	230	0	60.0	0	0	10	0
orange (*Chill Orange Overload*), ¾ of							
6-oz. cup	100	0	24.0	0	0	20	0
strawberry (*Chill Verry Strawberry*), ¾ of							
6-oz. cup	90	0	23.0	0	0	20	0
Ice bar (see also "Fruit bar" and "Iced confection bar"), 1 pc., except as noted:							
all flavors:							
(*Blue Bell* Mini Rainbows)	40	0	10.0	0	0	5	0
(*Blue Bell Bullets*)	60	0	14.0	0	0	5	0
(*Blue Bell Bullets* Sugar Free)	15	2.0	4.0	0	0	0	0
(*Kool-Aid Kool-Pops*), 2 pcs.	50	0	13.0	0	0	20	0
(*Popsicle Micro Pops* Multipack)	40	0	10.0	0	0	5	0
(*Popsicle Micro Pops* Single) . . .	60	0	13.0	0	0	10	0

Food and Measure	cal.	prot. (gms)	carbo. (gms)	fat (gms)	chol. (mgs)	sod. (mgs)	fiber (gms)
(*Blue Bell Megabite*)	140	0	35.0	0	0	10	0
(*Blue Bell Rainbow Freeze*)	120	0	30.0	0	0	10	0
cherry:							
(*Blue Bell Frostbite*)	120	0	29.0	0	0	10	0
(*Popsicle Torpedo*)	35	0	8.0	0	0	10	0
banana (*Blue Bell Frostbite*)	80	0	20.0	0	0	5	0
orange (*Popsicle Pop*)	45	0	11.0	0	0	0	0
pineapple (*Popsicle Big Stick*)	50	0	12.0	0	0	5	0
(*Firecracker* Red, White & Blue)	80	0	20.0	0	0	0	0
(*Good Humor Bubble Play* Sports Bar) . .	110	0	27.0	0	0	0	0
(*Good Humor The Great White*)	70	0	18.0	0	0	0	0
(*Good Humor Hyper Stripe* Pop)	80	0	21.0	0	0	0	0
(*Good Humor Towering Tornedo*)	90	0	21.0	0	0	0	0
grape and cherry (*Blue Bell* Twin)	80	0	20.0	0	0	5	0
lemonade (*Blue Bell* Mini)	40	0	10.0	0	0	5	0
orange cherry (*Blue Bell* Pop 'n Fudge)	60	0	14.0	0	0	5	0
orange cherry grape (*Popsicle* Multipack)	45	0	11.0	0	0	0	0
(*Popsicle Big Stick Pop/Lick-a-Color* Single)	90	0	22.0	0	0	0	0
(*Popsicle* Great White/ Tingle Twister Pop)	45	0	11.0	0	0	0	0
(*Popsicle La Fruta Loca*)	90	0	22.0	0	0	5	0
(*Popsicle Scribblers*)	60	0	15.0	0	0	0	0
(*Popsicle Super Twin*)	70	0	16.0	0	0	5	0
rainbow:							
(*Popsicle* Multipack)	45	0	11.0	0	0	0	0
(*Popsicle* Single) . .	90	0	22.0	0	0	0	0
tamarind (*Los Kitos*) .	90	0	22.0	0	0	n.a.	0

Food and Measure	cal.	prot. (gms)	carbo. (gms)	fat (gms)	chol. (mgs)	sod. (mgs)	fiber (gms)
Ice bar (cont.)							
tutti-fruitti (*Blue Bell Big Shot*)	140	0	35.0	0	0	15	0
Ice cream, ½ cup:							
almond:							
(*Darigold* Avalanche)	170	3.0	17.0	10.0	25	50	1.0
praline (*Dreyer's* Grand)	170	3.0	21.0	8.0	25	85	0
toasted (*Dreyer's* Grand)	150	3.0	15.0	9.0	25	30	0
apple pie:							
(*Dreyer's* Grand) . .	140	2.0	18.0	7.0	25	40	0
(*Dreyer's/Edy's* Homemade a la Mode)	140	2.0	19.0	6.0	25	55	0
deep dish (*Dreamery*)	280	3.0	34.0	15.0	75	95	0
banana:							
(*Dreamery Banana Boogie*)	290	6.0	27.0	17.0	55	110	1.0
nut (*Blue Bell* Pint)	170	3.0	17.0	9.0	30	55	0
banana fudge chunk (*Breyers* Special Edition)	170	2.0	22.0	9.0	20	40	<1.0
banana pudding:							
(*Blue Bell* Half Gallon)	190	3.0	24.0	9.0	35	60	0
(*Blue Bell* Pint) . . .	180	3.0	24.0	8.0	30	65	0
banana split:							
(*Blue Bell*)	170	3.0	22.0	8.0	30	50	0
(*Blue Bell* Light) . . .	110	3.0	20.0	2.0	10	65	0
(*Blue Bell* No Sugar Lowfat)	100	4.0	15.0	3.0	10	70	0
(*Breyers Ice Cream Parlor*)	180	3.0	22.0	9.0	15	55	0
(*Healthy Choice*) . .	130	3.0	24.0	2.0	2	60	<1.0
(*Ben & Jerry's* Peanut Turtles)	320	6.0	33.0	19.0	45	115	2.0
(*Ben & Jerry's* Aloha Macadamia)	330	5.0	30.0	21.0	45	75	2.0
(*Ben & Jerry's* Apple Crumble)	280	3.0	35.0	14.0	65	125	0
(*Ben & Jerry's* Bovinity Divinity*)	290	4.0	30.0	18.0	40	65	1.0

Food and Measure	cal.	prot. (gms)	carbo. (gms)	fat (gms)	chol. (mgs)	sod. (mgs)	fiber (gms)
(*Ben & Jerry's Chubby Hubby*)	350	6.0	33.0	21.0	55	250	1.0
(*Ben & Jerry's Chunky Monkey*)	310	5.0	32.0	19.0	55	55	3.0
(*Ben & Jerry's Concession Obsession*)	300	4.0	31.0	18.0	75	95	0
(*Ben & Jerry's Festivus*)	300	4.0	37.0	15.0	60	160	0
(*Ben & Jerry's KaBerry KaBoom!*)	240	3.0	27.0	13.0	55	45	0
(*Ben & Jerry's Nutty Waffle Cone*)	310	5.0	32.0	19.0	75	65	0
(*Ben & Jerry's Phish Food*)	300	4.0	41.0	14.0	35	80	3.0
(*Ben & Jerry's 2-Twisted Everything But the . . .*)	320	5.0	30.0	19.0	60	80	1.0
(*Ben & Jerry's 2-Twisted Half Baked*)	290	4.0	36.0	15.0	60	115	1.0
(*Ben & Jerry's 2-Twisted Monkey Wrench*)	310	5.0	28.0	20.0	65	80	1.0
(*Ben & Jerry's 2-Twisted S.N.A.F.U.*)	250	4.0	28.0	14.0	65	55	1.0
(*Ben & Jerry's 2-Twisted This Is Nuts*)	300	6.0	26.0	20.0	55	90	2.0
(*Ben & Jerry's 2-Twisted Urban Jumble*)	310	5.0	28.0	21.0	55	60	2.0
(*Ben & Jerry's Wavy Gravy*)	340	7.0	32.0	20.0	60	120	9.0
birthday cake (*Blue Bell*)	190	4.0	23.0	9.0	30	70	0
Black Forest (*Breyers Ice Cream Parlor*)	150	3.0	22.0	6.0	20	55	0
black raspberry, see "raspberry," below							
black walnut:							
(*Baldwin*)	170	2.0	37.0	11.0	35	55	0
(*Blue Bell* Half Gallon)	160	3.0	16.0	9.0	40	50	0
(*Blue Bell* Pint) ...	150	4.0	16.0	8.0	30	55	0

Ice cream *(cont.)*
blackberry:

Food and Measure	cal.	prot. (gms)	carbo. (gms)	fat (gms)	chol. (mgs)	sod (mgs)	fiber (gms)
pie (*Dreyer's/Edy's Grand Light*) ...	110	2.0	17.0	4.0	15	45	0
swirl (*Edy's* Grand)	140	2.0	17.0	7.0	25	35	0
(*Blue Bell Moo-llennium Crunch*) ..	190	4.0	20.0	11.0	25	70	0
blueberry cobbler (*Dreyer's/Edy's* Fat/Sugar Free)	100	3.0	22.0	0	<5	60	0
brownies (*Dreyer's Edy's Homemade* a la Mode)	150	3.0	18.0	7.0	30	65	0
butter almond:							
(*Breyers*)	160	3.0	14.0	11.0	25	110	0
(*Turkey Hill*)	180	4.0	15.0	12.0	35	105	0
butter pecan:							
(*Baldwin*)	180	3.0	36.0	12.0	35	120	1.0
(*Blue Bell*)	180	4.0	17.0	11.0	30	90	0
(*Blue Bell* Light) ...	150	5.0	22.0	5.0	10	120	0
(*Blue Bell* No Sugar Lowfat)	110	4.0	16.0	3.0	<5	100	0
(*Breyers*)	170	3.0	14.0	12.0	25	110	0
(*Breyers* No Sugar Reduced Fat) ...	110	3.0	11.0	7.0	20	100	0
(*Breyers Home-made*)	170	3.0	16.0	11.0	50	70	0
(*Dreyer's/Edy's* Grand)	170	3.0	16.0	10.0	25	70	0
(*Dreyer's/Edy's* No Sugar)	110	3.0	14.0	5.0	10	45	0
(*Dreyer's/Edy's* Grand Light) ...	120	3.0	16.0	5.0	20	100	0
(*Dreyer's/Edy's* Homemade)	160	3.0	15.0	10.0	30	90	0
(*Häagen-Dazs*)	310	5.0	21.0	23.0	110	110	<1.0
(*Turkey Hill*)	170	2.0	16.0	11.0	30	50	0
(*Turkey Hill* Light)	130	3.0	17.0	6.0	15	80	0
crunch (*Healthy Choice*)	120	3.0	22.0	2.0	5	60	<1.0
candy bar:							
(*Blue Bell*)	200	4.0	22.0	10.0	30	95	0
(*Darigold* Classic) .	160	3.0	21.0	8.0	20	105	1.0

Food and Measure	cal.	prot. (gms)	carbo. (gms)	fat (gms)	chol. (mgs)	sod. (mgs	fiber (gms)
sundae (*Breyers Ice Cream Parlor*) ..	170	3.0	21.0	8.0	15	120	0
cappuccino:							
(*Cascadian Farm*) ..	175	4.0	21.0	11.0	33	55	0
(*Häagen-Dazs* Gelato)	240	4.0	39.0	7.0	75	75	0
(*Häagen-Dazs Cappuccino Commotion*)	310	5.0	25.0	21.0	100	90	1.0
cappuccino chocolate crunch (*Healthy Choice*)	120	3.0	22.0	2.0	10	60	1.0
cappuccino mocha crunch (*Healthy Choice*)	140	3.0	25.0	2.0	5	60	<1.0
caramel:							
(*Darigold* Colossal)	140	2.0	19.0	7.0	25	70	0
(*Darigold* Killer) ...	140	2.0	21.0	6.0	25	65	0
(*Darigold* To the Max)	160	2.0	21.0	7.0	25	90	0
(*Dreyer's/Edy's Crazy for Caramel Grand Light*) ...	120	3.0	19.0	4.0	15	55	0
chunk (*Ben & Jerry's Triple Caramel Chunk*)	290	4.0	32.0	17.0	40	105	0
creme, pecan (*Häagen-Dazs*) ..	320	5.0	29.0	20.0	95	120	0
creme (*Stonyfield Farm*)	250	3.0	26.0	15.0	65	75	0
s'mores (*Darigold*)	160	2.0	21.0	7.0	20	95	0
triple (*Blue Bell*) ..	200	4.0	26.0	10.0	30	110	0
caramel crunch:							
praline (*Breyers*) ..	170	2.0	22.0	9.0	20	75	0
sundae (*Blue Bell*)	190	3.0	24.0	10.0	30	125	0
caramel fudge:							
(*Turkey Hill* Fat/ Sugar Free)	100	3.0	23.0	0	0	75	0
pecan (*Blue Bell*) ..	200	3.0	21.0	11.0	30	85	0
caramel toffee (*Dreamery* Heaven)	270	5.0	32.0	14.0	65	95	0
cashew praline (*Dreamery Parfait*)	260	5.0	30.0	13.0	65	90	0

Food and Measure	cal.	prot (gms)	carbo. (gms)	fat (gms)	chol. (mgs)	sod. (mgs)	fiber (gms)
Ice cream *(cont.)*							
cherry:							
(*Baldwin* New York)	160	3.0	38.0	9.0	35	50	0
black, chunk							
(*Darigold*)	140	2.0	18.0	7.0	25	50	0
black sweet							
(*Baldwin*)	150	2.0	17.0	8.0	30	45	0
cherry chocolate:							
chip (*Breyers*							
Special Edition)	160	3.0	16.0	8.0	20	35	0
chip (*Edy's* Grand)	160	2.0	19.0	8.0	25	40	0
chunk (*Healthy*							
Choice)	120	3.0	21.0	2.0	5	70	<1.0
covered (*Blue Bell*)	190	4.0	24.0	9.0	30	65	0
cherry, fudge flakes:							
(*Ben & Jerry's*							
Cherry Garcia) . .	260	5.0	26.0	16.0	70	60	0
brownie (*Ben &*							
Jerry's 2-Twisted							
Jerry's Jubilee)	260	4.0	29.0	14.0	55	70	<1.0
cherry vanilla:							
(*Blue Bell*)	160	3.0	19.0	8.0	35	55	0
(*Breyers*)	140	2.0	17.0	8.0	20	30	0
(*Häagen-Dazs*)	240	4.0	23.0	15.0	100	60	0
(*Healthy Choice*) . .	120	2.0	22.0	2.0	5	50	<1.0
(*Stonyfield Farm*) . .	250	2.0	24.0	16.0	60	35	0
black (*Edy's* Grand)	140	2.0	17.0	7.0	25	35	0
black (*Turkey Hill*)	140	2.0	18.0	7.0	25	30	0
fudge (*Turkey Hill*							
Fat/Sugar Free)	90	3.0	20.0	0	0	80	0
sweet (*Turkey Hill*)	160	3.0	18.0	8.0	30	50	0
chocolate:							
(*Ben & Jerry's*							
World's Best) . . .	280	5.0	27.0	17.0	45	55	2.0
(*Blue Bell* Deca-							
dence)	190	3.0	20.0	10.0	20	55	<1.0
(*Breyers*)	160	2.0	18.0	9.0	30	20	<1.0
(*Breyers* Rainbow)	140	3.0	16.0	7.0	20	40	0
(*Darigold* Death By)	150	3.0	19.0	8.0	25	70	1.0
(*Darigold* Totally) . .	140	2.0	17.0	7.0	25	70	<1.0
(*Dreyer's/Edy's*							
Grand)	150	3.0	16.0	8.0	25	35	0
(*Häagen-Dazs*)	270	5.0	22.0	18.0	115	60	1.0

Food and Measure	cal.	prot. (gms)	carbo. (gms)	fat (gms)	chol. (mgs)	sod. (mgs)	fiber (gms)
(*Häagen-Dazs* Gelato)	240	5.0	37.0	8.0	80	70	2.0
(*Turkey Hill*)	170	3.0	18.0	10.0	35	40	0
(*Turkey Hill* Death By Chocolate) ..	160	2.0	21.0	8.0	30	35	0
dark (*Godiva* Belgian)	280	5.0	26.0	17.0	65	40	3.0
double (*Cascadian Farm*)	195	4.0	29.0	11.0	29	60	1.0
Dutch (*Blue Bell* Half Gallon)	160	3.0	18.0	8.0	35	70	0
Dutch (*Blue Bell* Light)	140	3.0	23.0	4.5	15	100	0
Dutch (*Blue Bell* Pint)	160	3.0	18.0	8.0	30	65	0
Dutch (*Turkey Hill*)	150	2.0	19.0	8.0	30	30	0
Dutch (*Turkey Hill* Fat/Sugar Free)	90	3.0	20.0	0	0	70	0
French (*Breyers* Light)	140	3.0	21.0	5.0	30	55	<1.0
triple (*Blue Bell*) ..	180	3.0	21.0	9.0	35	60	0
triple (*Edy's Triple Chocolate Thunder* Grand)	160	2.0	18.0	9.0	25	40	0
triple (*Dreyer's/ Edy's* No Sugar)	100	3.0	15.0	3.0	10	60	0
chocolate almond: (*Breyers Hershey's Ice Cream Parlor*)	170	3.0	21.0	8.0	25	15	<1.0
bar (*Dreamery*) ...	300	5.0	32.0	17.0	50	70	1.0
marshmallow (*Blue Bell*)	200	3.0	23.0	10.0	30	85	<1.0
Swiss (*Häagen-Dazs*)	300	5.0	24.0	20.0	100	55	2.0
white (*Blue Bell*) ..	190	4.0	17.0	12.0	35	65	0
chocolate brownie walnut (*Häagen-Dazs*)	290	5.0	25.0	19.0	100	75	1.0
chocolate cake, German (*Häagen-Dazs*)	290	5.0	28.0	18.0	100	120	<1.0
chocolate w/candy (*Dreyer's/Edy's* M&M's)	170	3.0	22.0	8.0	20	50	0

Food and Measure	cal.	prot. (gms)	carbo (gms)	fat (gms)	chol. (mgs)	sod. (mgs)	fiber (gms)
Ice cream *(cont.)*							
chocolate caramel:							
(*Breyers* No Sugar Light)	100	3.0	14.0	4.0	25	65	0
brownie (*Starbucks Brownies au Caramel*)	270	4.0	31.0	14.0	60	70	1.0
nut (*Breyers* Special Edition)	190	3.0	24.0	9.0	20	35	1.0
swirl (*Dreyer's/Edy's* Grand)	170	2.0	19.0	9.0	25	40	0
chocolate cheesecake (*Häagen-Dazs*)	300	5.0	29.0	18.0	110	160	1.0
chocolate chip:							
(*Blue Bell*)	170	3.0	18.0	10.0	35	65	0
(*Breyers*)	170	2.0	17.0	10.0	25	35	0
(*Dreyer's/Edy's* Grand Chips!) . .	170	3.0	18.0	9.0	25	45	0
(*Dreyer's/Edy's* Homemade Cookie Jar) .	170	3.0	18.0	9.0	30	85	0
chocolate (*Häagen-Dazs*)	300	5.0	26.0	20.0	105	55	2.0
chocolate (*Sharon's Custard*)	260	4.0	26.0	14.0	180	35	2.0
cookie (*Breyers Chips Ahoy! Ice Cream Parlor*) . .	160	3.0	19.0	8.0	25	55	0
cookie dough (*Ben & Jerry's*)	300	5.0	34.0	16.0	65	95	0
cookie dough (*Blue Bell* Half Gallon)	190	3.0	23.0	10.0	25	90	0
cookie dough (*Blue Bell* Pint)	190	3.0	23.0	10.0	30	85	0
cookie dough (*Breyers*)	180	3.0	20.0	10.0	25	45	0
cookie dough (*Turkey Hill*) . . .	190	2.0	23.0	10.0	30	80	0
cookie dough, double (*Blue Bell*)	210	3.0	25.0	10.0	25	110	0
chocolate chunk:							
chocolate (*Healthy Choice*)	120	3.0	21.0	2.0	5	45	2.0

Food and Measure	cal.	prot. (gms)	carbo. (gms)	fat (gms)	chol. (mgs)	sod. (mgs	fiber (gms)
double (*Dreyer's/ Edy's Homemade*)	170	3.0	19.0	9.0	30	55	0
w/nuts (*Ben & Jerry's* New York Super Fudge Chunk)	320	5.0	28.0	21.0	50	65	4.0
chocolate cream pie (*Dreyer's/Edy's Homemade*)	170	3.0	19.0	9.0	30	60	0
chocolate fudge: (*Dreyer's/Edy's* Fat/ Sugar Free)	100	4.0	22.0	0	0	60	0
brownie (*Ben & Jerry's*)	280	5.0	32.0	15.0	45	90	2.0
brownie (*Healthy Choice*)	110	4.0	20.0	2.0	5	60	0
mousse (*Dreyer's/ Edy's Grand Light*)	120	3.0	17.0	4.0	20	45	0
mousse (*Edy's Grand*)	160	2.0	19.0	8.0	25	45	0
sundae (*Edy's Grand*)	170	3.0	20.0	9.0	20	50	0
chocolate hazelnut truffle (*Godiva*) ...	340	5.0	31.0	22.0	55	210	2.0
chocolate malt, double (*Breyers Ice Cream Parlor*)	160	3.0	21.0	7.0	15	60	0
chocolate marsh- mallow (*Turkey Hill*)	160	2.0	24.0	7.0	30	30	0
chocolate mint chip: (*Turkey Hill* Half Gallon)	180	2.0	18.0	11.0	30	40	0
(*Turkey Hill* Light)	140	3.0	19.0	5.0	15	75	0
(*Turkey Hill* Pint) ..	160	2.0	18.0	9.0	30	35	0
chocolate mint cookie (*Dreyer's/ Edy's Girl Scouts* Thin Mint)	170	2.0	18.0	10.0	30	45	0
chocolate peanut butter (*Häagen-Dazs*)	360	8.0	27.0	24.0	100	100	2.0

Food and Measure	cal.	prot. (gms)	carbo. (gms)	fat (gms)	chol. (mgs)	sod. (mgs)	fiber (gms)
Ice cream *(cont.)*							
chocolate raspberry:							
(*Dreyer's/Edy's Escape Grand Light*)	120	3.0	19.0	4.0	15	45	0
(*Stonyfield Farm*) ..	250	3.0	25.0	15.0	55	30	1.0
truffle (*Godiva*) ...	280	4.0	31.0	16.0	60	55	2.0
chocolate swirl:							
(*Dreamery Galactic*)	280	5.0	37.0	12.0	45	150	1.0
double (*Stonyfield Farm*)	260	3.0	26.0	16.0	60	35	2.0
chocolate truffle (*Dreamery* Explo-sion)	280	5.0	30.0	15.0	55	75	1.0
cinnamon:							
(*Häagen-Dazs*)	250	4.0	20.0	17.0	110	65	0
swirl (*Edy's* Grand)	150	2.0	19.0	7.0	25	35	0
coconut:							
(*Häagen-Dazs* Gelato)	240	4.0	38.0	8.0	75	75	0
nutty (*Blue Bell*) .	190	3.0	16.0	13.0	25	50	0
coffee:							
(*Blue Bell*)	160	3.0	18.0	8.0	35	55	0
(*Breyers*)	140	2.0	14.0	9.0	25	35	0
(*Dreyer's/Edy's* Grand)	140	2.0	15.0	8.0	25	40	0
(*Häagen-Dazs*)	270	5.0	21.0	18.0	120	70	0
(*Starbucks* Classic)	230	5.0	26.0	12.0	65	50	0
(*Stonyfield Farm* Decaf)	250	3.0	21.0	18.0	65	40	0
(*Turkey Hill* Colom-bian)	140	2.0	16.0	8.0	30	35	0
almond fudge (*Healthy Choice*)	110	3.0	21.0	2.0	5	55	0
almond fudge (*Starbucks*)	250	5.0	28.0	13.0	60	65	1.0
chocolate chunk (*Starbucks* Java Chip)	250	4.0	29.0	13.0	60	55	0
chocolate toffee (*Starbucks* Java Toffee)	260	4.0	30.0	14.0	60	95	0
crunch (*Ben & Jerry's* Heath) ..	310	4.0	32.0	18.0	65	125	0

Food and Measure	cal.	prot. (gms)	carbo. (gms)	fat (gms)	chol. (mgs)	sod. (mgs)	fiber (gms)
espresso fudge chips (*Ben & Jerry's 2-Twisted From Russia with Buzz*)	280	4.0	26.0	18.0	70	65	<1.0
fudge (*Häagen-Dazs Low Fat*)	170	5.0	32.0	2.5	25	95	0
mocha chip (*Häagen-Dazs*) ..	290	5.0	25.0	19.0	110	75	<1.0
mousse crunch (*Edy's Grand Light*)	120	3.0	17.0	4.0	20	45	0
cookie creme de menthe (*Healthy Choice*)	130	3.0	24.0	2.0	5	60	<1.0
cookie dough: (*Dreyer's/Edy's Grand*)	180	3.0	21.0	9.0	25	65	0
(*Dreyer's/Edy's Grand Light*) ...	120	3.0	19.0	4.0	20	65	0
chip (*Häagen-Dazs*)	310	4.0	29.0	20.0	95	125	0
cookies and cream: (*Blue Bell* Half Gallon)	170	4.0	21.0	8.0	30	100	0
(*Blue Bell* Light) ...	150	5.0	26.0	3.5	10	110	0
(*Blue Bell* No Sugar Lowfat)	110	4.0	18.0	3.0	10	95	0
(*Blue Bell* Pint) ...	170	4.0	21.0	8.0	30	95	0
(*Breyers*)	170	3.0	18.0	9.0	20	45	0
(*Breyers Oreo Ice Cream Parlor*) ..	160	3.0	19.0	8.0	25	80	0
(*Darigold*)	140	2.0	18.0	7.0	25	65	0
(*Dreyer's/Edy's Grand*)	160	3.0	19.0	8.0	25	55	0
(*Dreyer's/Edy's Grand Light*) ...	120	3.0	17.0	4.0	20	50	0
(*Häagen-Dazs*)	270	5.0	23.0	17.0	105	95	0
(*Healthy Choice*) ..	120	3.0	21.0	2.0	5	90	<1.0
(*Turkey Hill*)	160	2.0	19.0	9.0	30	60	0
(*Dreamery Coney Island Waffle Cone*)	300	4.0	31.0	18.0	65	60	1.0
(*Dreamery Grandma's Cookie Jar*) ..	270	5.0	32.0	14.0	65	100	0

Food and Measure	cal.	prot. (gms)	carbo. (gms)	fat (gms)	chol. (mgs)	sod. (mgs)	fiber (gms)
Ice cream *(cont.)*							
(*Dreamery Nuts About Malt*)	280	6.0	29.0	15.0	60	75	1.0
(*Dreamery White Out*)	320	6.0	29.0	20.0	65	140	1.0
(*Dreyer's/Edy's Chips 'N Swirls No Sugar*)	100	3.0	16.0	3.0	10	60	0
(*Dreyer's/Edy's Dexter's Amazing Creation*)	160	3.0	21.0	7.0	20	60	0
(*Dreyer's/Edy's French Silk Grand Light*)	120	3.0	19.0	4.0	15	50	0
(*Dreyer's/Edy's Fudge 'N Cups Grand*)	180	3.0	18.0	11.0	25	60	0
(*Dreyer's/Edy's Girl Scouts Samoas Cookie*)	170	3.0	21.0	8.0	20	50	0
(*Dreyer's/Edy's Girl Scouts Tagalongs Cookie Light*)	130	3.0	17.0	5.0	20	60	0
(*Dreyer's/Edy's M&M's Chills 'n Thrills!*)	180	3.0	22.0	9.0	25	50	0
(*Dreyer's/Edy's Milky Way*)	160	3.0	21.0	7.0	25	70	0
(*Dreyer's/Edy's Scooby Doo Dough Grand Light*)	130	3.0	19.0	4.5	20	55	0
(*Dreyer's/Edy's Scooby Snack Grand*)	170	3.0	19.0	9.0	25	60	0
(*Dreyer's/Edy's S'mores & more Grand Light*)	130	3.0	20.0	3.5	15	60	0
(*Dreyer's/Edy's Snickers*)	180	3.0	21.0	9.0	25	70	0
(*Dreyer's/Edy's 3 Musketeers*)	160	3.0	22.0	7.0	20	50	0
(*Dreyer's/Edy's Twix*) .	190	3.0	23.0	9.0	25	70	0

Food and Measure	cal.	prot. (gms)	carbo. (gms)	fat (gms)	chol. (mgs)	sod. (mgs)	fiber (gms)
dulce de leche:							
(*Blue Bell*)	170	3.0	22.0	8.0	35	65	0
(*Breyers*)	160	2.0	21.0	7.0	20	80	0
(*Dreamery*)	270	4.0	32.0	14.0	70	70	0
(*Edy's* Grand)	150	2.0	20.0	8.0	25	50	0
(*Häagen-Dazs*)	290	5.0	28.0	17.0	100	95	0
(*Healthy Choice*) ..	110	2.0	21.0	2.0	10	70	1.0
eggnog (*Dreyer's/Edy's* Homemade)	140	3.0	17.0	7.0	30	55	0
espresso chip:							
(*Edy's* Grand)	150	2.0	17.0	8.0	25	50	0
fudge (*Dreyer's/ Edy's Grand Light*)	120	3.0	18.0	4.0	15	55	0
fudge brownie:							
(*Baldwin*)	180	2.0	21.0	10.0	30	60	0
(*Breyers Ice Cream Parlor Sundae*) ..	200	3.0	27.0	10.0	30	85	1.0
(*Healthy Choice*) ..	120	3.0	22.0	2.0	5	55	<1.0
double (*Dreyer's/ Edy's* Grand) ...	170	2.0	19.0	9.0	30	45	0
double (*Edy's* No Sugar)	100	3.0	16.0	3.0	10	60	0
nut (*Blue Bell*)	170	3.0	21.0	9.0	25	105	0
fudge ripple (*Turkey Hill*)	140	2.0	20.0	7.0	30	70	0
fudge sundae, hot (*Blue Bell*)	180	3.0	20.0	9.0	30	60	0
gingerbread man (*Dreyer's/Edy's Grand Light*)	120	3.0	19.0	4.0	20	65	0
hazelnut (*Häagen-Dazs* Gelato)	260	5.0	33.0	12.0	75	55	<1.0
honey almond (*Häagen-Dazs* Gelato)	250	6.0	34.0	10.0	75	60	<1.0
ice cream sandwich:							
(*Breyers Ice Cream Parlor*)	160	3.0	21.0	7.0	20	65	0
(*Edy's* Grand)	150	3.0	19.0	7.0	25	75	0
Irish cream (*Häagen-Dazs Baileys*)	270	5.0	23.0	17.0	115	70	0
latte (*Starbucks* Low Fat)	170	5.0	30.0	3.0	10	60	0
macadamia brittle (*Häagen-Dazs*)	300	4.0	25.0	20.0	110	110	0
mango (*Häagen-Dazs*)	250	4.0	28.0	14.0	85	50	<1.0

Ice cream (cont.)

Food and Measure	cal.	prot. (gms)	carbo. (gms)	fat (gms)	chol. (mgs)	sod. (mgs)	fiber (gms)
marionberry (*Darigold Northwest*)	140	2.0	21.0	6.0	20	50	0
mint:							
(*Dreamery* Cool Mint)	280	5.0	34.0	14.0	55	95	1.0
chip (*Darigold* Cool)	140	2.0	17.0	7.0	25	55	0
chip (*Häagen-Dazs*)	300	5.0	26.0	19.0	105	85	<1.0
chocolate (*Blue Bell*)	180	5.0	22.0	9.0	35	85	0
mint chocolate chip:							
(*Baldwin*)	170	3.0	18.0	10.0	30	45	0
(*Ben & Jerry's*) ...	280	4.0	28.0	17.0	70	130	1.0
(*Blue Bell* Pint) ...	170	3.0	17.0	10.0	40	60	0
(*Breyers*)	170	2.0	17.0	10.0	25	35	0
(*Breyers* Light) ...	130	3.0	20.0	5.0	15	50	0
(*Dreyer's/Edy's* Grand Chips!) ..	170	3.0	18.0	9.0	25	45	0
(*Dreyer's/Edy's* Grand Light Chips!)	120	3.0	17.0	4.0	20	50	0
(*Healthy Choice*) ..	120	3.0	21.0	2.0	5	50	<1.0
(*Turkey Hill*)	180	3.0	18.0	11.0	35	50	0
chunk (*Dreyer's/ Edy's Homemade*)	170	3.0	18.0	9.0	25	65	0
mint chocolate cookie (*Breyers Oreo Ice Cream Parlor*)	160	3.0	22.0	7.0	25	75	0
Mississippi mud:							
(*Breyers Ice Cream Parlor*)	180	2.0	23.0	9.0	20	80	<1.0
pie (*Blue Bell*)	180	3.0	22.0	9.0	25	70	0
mocha almond fudge:							
(*Blue Bell* Half Gallon)	180	4.0	21.0	9.0	30	70	<1.0
(*Blue Bell* Pint) ...	180	4.0	21.0	9.0	30	65	<1.0
(*Breyers* Special Edition)	180	3.0	20.0	10.0	15	75	1.0
(*Darigold*)	140	2.0	18.0	7.0	25	55	1.0
(*Dreyer's* Grand) ..	160	3.0	17.0	9.0	25	45	0
(*Dreyer's Grand Light*)	120	3.0	16.0	4.5	20	45	0
mocha biscotti (*Stonyfield Farm*)	260	3.0	28.0	15.0	55	45	<1.0

Food and Measure	cal.	prot. (gms)	carbo. (gms)	fat (gms)	chol. (mgs)	sod. (mgs)	fiber (gms)
mud pie:							
(*Darigold*)	140	2.0	21.0	6.0	20	65	1.0
(*Starbucks*)	240	4.0	32.0	11.0	55	85	1.0
Neapolitan:							
(*Baldwin*)	160	3.0	40.0	9.0	35	50	0
(*Blue Bell*)	160	3.0	17.0	9.0	40	55	0
(*Darigold*)	130	2.0	16.0	7.0	25	55	0
(*Dreyer's/Edy's* Grand)	140	2.0	16.0	7.0	25	35	0
(*Dreyer's/Edy's* No Sugar)	80	3.0	13.0	3.0	10	45	0
(*Turkey Hill*)	150	2.0	18.0	8.0	30	30	0
peach:							
(*Baldwin* Georgia)	150	2.0	17.0	6.0	25	40	0
(*Breyers*)	130	2.0	17.0	6.0	15	25	0
(*Dreamery* Harvest)	220	4.0	26.0	11.0	60	45	0
(*Dreyer's/Edy's* Homemade)	110	2.0	15.0	5.0	25	40	0
cobbler (*Darigold* Plantation)	140	2.0	19.0	6.0	20	50	0
and homemade vanilla (*Blue Bell*)	160	3.0	23.0	7.0	30	50	0
peanut butter:							
(*Dreyer's/Edy's* Grand Blitz) ...	170	3.0	16.0	10.0	25	45	0
(*Dreyer's/Edy's* All About PB No Sugar)	130	4.0	15.0	6.0	10	85	0
(*Dreyer's/Edy's* Twix)	210	4.0	21.0	12.0	25	85	0
chunk, chocolate (*Dreamery*)	310	7.0	29.0	18.0	50	110	2.0
fudge chunk (*Häagen-Dazs*) ..	340	7.0	25.0	23.0	95	95	1.0
ripple (*Turkey Hill*)	170	3.0	16.0	11.0	30	60	0
peanut butter cup:							
(*Ben & Jerry's*) ...	380	7.0	32.0	25.0	65	130	2.0
(*Breyers Reese's Ice Cream Parlor*)	180	4.0	22.0	9.0	25	75	0
(*Healthy Choice*) ..	110	3.0	19.0	2.0	5	65	<1.0
(*Dreyer's/Edy's* Grand Light Cups!*)	130	3.0	17.0	5.0	20	50	0

Food and Measure	cal.	prot. (gms)	carbo. (gms)	fat (gms)	chol. (mgs)	sod. (mgs)	fiber (gms)
Ice cream, peanut butter cup *(cont.)*							
chocolate (*Turkey Hill*)	180	3.0	18.0	11.0	30	60	0
peanut and toffee crunch (*Dreyer's/ Edy's Cracker Jack*)	170	3.0	20.0	9.0	25	60	0
pecan caramel (*Ben & Jerry's Southern Pecan Pie*)	290	4.0	26.0	19.0	45	90	0
pecan praline: and cream (*Blue Bell*)	190	3.0	22.0	10.0	35	75	0
sundae (*Dreyer's/ Edy's* Grand) ...	160	3.0	18.0	9.0	25	50	0
peppermint: (*Blue Bell*)	160	3.0	20.0	8.0	35	60	0
(*Dreyer's/Edy's* Grand)	150	2.0	17.0	8.0	25	40	0
candy (*Darigold*) ..	140	2.0	17.0	7.0	25	50	0
pineapple coconut (*Häagen-Dazs*)	230	4.0	25.0	13.0	90	55	0
pineapple passion fruit (*Ben & Jerry's Island Paradise*) ...	240	3.0	31.0	12.0	55	50	0
pineapple upside-down cake (*Blue Bell*) ...	180	3.0	21.0	7.0	25	75	0
pistachio: (*Ben & Jerry's Pista- chio Pistachio*) ..	240	4.0	20.0	15.0	40	50	0
(*Häagen-Dazs*)	290	5.0	22.0	20.0	110	80	<1.0
almond (*Blue Bell*)	170	4.0	17.0	10.0	30	80	0
praline caramel: (*Breyers* Light) ...	140	3.0	24.0	3.5	15	75	0
(*Healthy Choice*) ..	130	3.0	25.0	2.0	5	70	<1.0
cluster (*Healthy Choice*)	140	2.0	27.0	2.0	5	80	<1.0
pralines and cream (*Baldwin*)	180	3.0	21.0	9.0	25	65	0
pumpkin (*Dreyer's/ Edy's* Grand) ...	140	2.0	17.0	7.0	25	50	0
raspberry: (*Häagen-Dazs* Gelato)	240	4.0	40.0	7.0	80	75	<1.0

Food and Measure	cal.	prot. (gms)	carbo. (gms)	fat (gms)	chol. (mgs)	sod. (mgs	fiber (gms)
black (*Dreamery* Avalanche)	250	5.0	27.0	14.0	70	60	1.0
black (*Turkey Hill*)	140	2.0	18.0	7.0	30	35	0
wild, truffle (*Healthy Choice*)	130	2.0	25.0	2.0	5	50	<1.0
raspberry brownie (*Dreamery* a la Mode)	270	4.0	33.0	14.0	70	60	1.0
raspberry cheesecake (*Dreyer's/Edy's* Grand)	150	2.0	20.0	7.0	20	50	0
raspberry vanilla swirl (*Dreyer's/Edy's* No Sugar Fat Free) ...	90	3.0	19.0	0	0	50	0
rocky road:							
(*Blue Bell* Half Gallon)	180	3.0	18.0	10.0	35	70	0
(*Blue Bell* Light) ...	110	3.0	18.0	3.0	5	75	<1.0
(*Blue Bell* No Sugar Lowfat)	100	4.0	15.0	3.0	5	80	<1.0
(*Blue Bell* Pint) ...	180	3.0	18.0	10.0	30	70	<1.0
(*Breyers*)	180	3.0	24.0	9.0	25	25	<1.0
(*Breyers* Light) ...	140	3.0	21.0	4.5	10	50	<1.0
(*Darigold*)	160	3.0	19.0	8.0	25	65	<1.0
(*Dreyer's/Edy's* Grand)	170	3.0	17.0	10.0	25	30	0
(*Dreyer's/Edy's* Grand Light) ...	120	3.0	17.0	4.0	20	40	0
(*Healthy Choice*) ..	140	3.0	28.0	2.0	5	60	<1.0
(*Turkey Hill*)	170	3.0	23.0	8.0	30	40	0
rum raisin (*Häagen-Dazs*)	270	4.0	22.0	17.0	110	60	0
spumoni (*Edy's* Grand)	150	3.0	16.0	8.0	25	40	0
strawberries and cream:							
(*Dreyer's/Edy's* Home-made)	120	2.0	15.0	6.0	25	45	0
(*Turkey Hill*)	140	2.0	19.0	6.0	25	30	0
strawberries and home-made vanilla:							
(*Blue Bell* Half Gallon)	160	3.0	23.0	7.0	30	50	0
(*Blue Bell* Light) ...	140	3.0	24.0	3.0	15	55	0
(*Blue Bell* Pint) ...	150	3.0	22.0	6.0	25	45	0

Food and Measure	cal.	prot. (gms)	carbo. (gms)	fat (gms)	chol. (mgs)	sod. (mgs)	fiber (gms)
Ice cream *(cont.)*							
strawberry:							
(*Blue Bell* Half Gallon)	150	3.0	20.0	6.0	25	45	0
(*Blue Bell* Pint) ...	140	3.0	19.0	6.0	25	45	0
(*Breyers*)	130	2.0	15.0	7.0	20	25	0
(*Breyers* Light) ...	100	3.0	17.0	3.0	15	45	0
(*Breyers Ice Cream Parlor Sundae*) ..	140	2.0	20.0	6.0	20	40	0
(*Darigold* Summer)	120	2.0	16.0	6.0	25	45	0
(*Dreamery Strawberry Fields*) ...	220	4.0	25.0	12.0	65	40	1.0
(*Dreyer's/Edy's* Grand Real)	130	2.0	16.0	6.0	20	30	0
(*Dreyer's/Edy's* No Sugar)	90	3.0	13.0	3.0	10	45	0
(*Häagen-Dazs*)	250	4.0	23.0	16.0	95	65	<1.0
(*Healthy Choice*) ..	110	2.0	20.0	2.0	0	35	1.0
cheesecake (*Blue Bell*)	170	3.0	22.0	8.0	35	115	0
shortcake (*Breyers Ice Cream Parlor*)	160	2.0	24.0	6.0	15	40	0
shortcake (*Dreamery New York*)	250	5.0	27.0	13.0	70	80	0
shortcake (*Dreyer's/ Edy's Grand Light*)	110	2.0	18.0	3.5	20	40	0
tin Lizzie sundae (*Turkey Hill* Light)	140	3.0	21.0	5.0	10	120	0
tin roof:							
(*Blue Bell* Half Gallon)	200	4.0	22.0	10.0	30	65	0
(*Blue Bell* Pint) ...	200	4.0	21.0	11.0	35	65	0
(*Darigold* Classic) .	150	2.0	19.0	7.0	25	70	0
sundae (*Healthy Choice*)	120	3.0	21.0	2.0	10	55	<1.0
sundae (*Turkey Hill*)	160	2.0	19.0	9.0	30	70	0
tiramisu:							
(*Dreamery*)	270	4.0	33.0	14.0	80	170	0
(*Häagen-Dazs* Gelato)	250	5.0	35.0	10.0	95	140	0
toffee:							
brownie (*Dreyer's/ Edy's Grand* a la Mode)	160	2.0	21.0	8.0	25	70	0

Food and Measure	cal.	prot. (gms)	carbo. (gms)	fat (gms)	chol. (mgs)	sod. (mgs)	fiber (gms)
English (*Breyers Heath Ice Cream Parlor*)	180	3.0	22.0	9.0	30	115	0
turtle fudge cake (*Healthy Choice*) ..	130	3.0	25.0	2.0	<5	60	2.0
turtle sundae (*Breyers Ice Cream Parlor*)	170	3.0	20.0	8.0	20	80	0
vanilla:							
(*Baldwin*)	160	3.0	38.0	9.0	35	55	0
(*Ben & Jerry's World's Best*) ..	250	4.0	22.0	16.0	75	60	0
(*Blue Bell* Homemade Half Gallon)	180	5.0	21.0	8.0	35	75	0
(*Blue Bell* Homemade Light Half Gallon)	140	5.0	22.0	4.0	20	75	0
(*Blue Bell* Homemade Pint)	160	4.0	19.0	8.0	35	65	0
(*Blue Bell* Homemade Light Pint)	130	4.0	20.0	4.0	15	70	0
(*Blue Bell* Gallon) ..	180	4.0	20.0	9.0	40	70	0
(*Blue Bell* Country)	160	3.0	16.0	9.0	40	50	0
(*Blue Bell* Country No Sugar Lowfat)	100	4.0	15.0	3.0	15	75	0
(*Breyers*)	150	3.0	15.0	9.0	25	35	0
(*Breyers* Calcium Rich Natural) ...	130	3.0	14.0	7.0	20	35	0
(*Breyers* Fat Free)	90	3.0	19.0	0	0	65	<1.0
(*Breyers* Light) ...	130	3.0	18.0	4.5	35	45	0
(*Breyers* Light Natural)	110	3.0	17.0	3.0	15	50	0
(*Breyers* No Sugar Light)	90	3.0	11.0	4.5	25	50	0
(*Breyers* Homemade)	140	2.0	16.0	8.0	40	60	0
(*Cascadian Farm*) ..	180	4.0	22.0	12.0	35	55	0
(*Darigold* Very) ...	130	2.0	16.0	7.0	25	50	0
(*Dreamery*)	260	5.0	25.0	15.0	70	55	0
(*Dreyer's* Grand) ..	150	2.0	14.0	10.0	35	35	0
(*Dreyer's/Edy's* No Sugar)	90	3.0	13.0	3.0	10	50	0
(*Dreyer's/Edy's* Fat/ Sugar Free)	90	3.0	19.0	0	0	50	0
(*Dreyer's/Edy's* Grand Light) ...	100	3.0	15.0	3.0	20	45	0

Food and Measure	cal.	prot. (gms)	carbo. (gms)	fat (gms)	chol. (mgs)	sod. (mgs)	fiber (gms)
Ice cream, vanilla *(cont.)*							
(*Dreyer's/Edy's Homemade* All Natural)	130	3.0	14.0	7.0	30	55	0
(*Edy's Grand*)	140	2.0	15.0	8.0	25	30	0
(*Häagen-Dazs*)	270	5.0	21.0	18.0	120	70	0
(*Healthy Choice*) ..	100	3.0	18.0	2.0	5	50	<1.0
(*Stonyfield Farm*) ..	250	3.0	20.0	18.0	65	40	0
(*Turkey Hill*)	170	3.0	16.0	10.0	35	50	0
(*Turkey Hill* Original)	140	2.0	16.0	8.0	30	35	0
bean (*Blue Bell*) ...	190	4.0	20.0	10.0	40	55	0
bean (*Blue Bell* Fat/ Sugar Free)	80	4.0	17.0	0	<5	75	0
bean (*Dreyer's/Edy's* Grand)	140	2.0	15.0	8.0	25	35	0
bean (*Healthy Choice*)	110	2.0	21.0	2.0	5	50	<1.0
bean (*Turkey Hill*) .	140	2.0	16.0	8.0	30	35	0
bean (*Turkey Hill* Fat/ Sugar Free)	90	3.0	20.0	0	0	60	0
bean, (*Turkey Hill* Light)	110	3.0	18.0	3.0	15	65	0
custard (*Dreyer's/ Edy's Homemade*)	140	4.0	15.0	8.0	55	65	0
French (*Blue Bell* Half Gallon)	170	3.0	18.0	9.0	80	50	0
French (*Breyers*) ..	160	3.0	15.0	10.0	75	35	0
French (*Breyers* Light)	120	3.0	18.0	4.0	35	50	0
French (*Darigold*)	140	2.0	17.0	7.0	45	55	0
French (*Dreyer's/ Edy's* Grand) ...	160	2.0	17.0	9.0	50	40	0
French (*Turkey Hill*)	140	2.0	16.0	8.0	55	40	0
vanilla w/candy:							
(*Ben & Jerry's* Heath Bar)	310	4.0	30.0	19.0	70	135	0
(*Dreyer's/Edy's* M&M's)	180	3.0	22.0	9.0	25	50	0
vanilla caramel:							
almond (*Cascadian Farm*)	210	4.0	27.0	12.0	30	70	<1.0
fudge (*Ben & Jerry's*)	300	4.0	33.0	17.0	70	115	1.0
fudge (*Dreyer's/ Edy's* Grand) ...	150	2.0	18.0	8.0	25	45	0

Food and Measure	cal.	prot. (gms)	carbo. (gms)	fat (gms)	chol. (mgs)	sod. (mgs	fiber (gms)
vanilla chocolate:							
(*Breyers* Take Two)	150	2.0	16.0	9.0	25	30	0
(*Dreyer's/Edy's* Grand)	150	3.0	16.0	8.0	25	30	0
(*Turkey Hill*)	150	2.0	17.0	8.0	30	35	0
(*Turkey Hill* Light)	110	3.0	18.0	3.0	15	60	0
vanilla chocolate strawberry:							
(*Breyers*)	140	2.0	16.0	8.0	25	30	0
(*Breyers* Light) ...	110	3.0	18.0	3.0	15	50	0
(*Breyers* No Sugar Light)	90	3.0	11.0	4.5	25	45	0
(*Edy's* Grand)	140	2.0	16.0	7.0	25	35	0
vanilla crème brûlée or w/raspberry (*Sharon's* Custard)	230	3.0	24.0	14.0	190	35	0
vanilla fudge:							
(*Breyers* Ice Cream Parlor* Sundae) ..	160	3.0	19.0	7.0	20	60	0
brownie (*Stonyfield Farm*)	260	3.0	28.0	15.0	55	60	0
twirl (*Breyers*)	150	3.0	18.0	8.0	20	35	<1.0
twirl (*Breyers* No Sugar Light) ...	100	3.0	14.0	4.5	25	55	0
vanilla Swiss almond (*Häagen-Dazs*)	300	5.0	24.0	20.0	105	75	<1.0
"Ice cream," nondairy, ½ cup:							
all flavors, soft-serve (*Tofutti*)	190	2.0	20.0	4.0	0	95	0
(*Tofutti* Lite)	90	2.0	20.0	1.0	0	80	0
almond pecan (*Soy Delicious*)	160	2.0	24.0	6.0	0	75	1.0
Better Pecan (*Tofutti* Premium)	220	1.0	22.0	13.0	0	200	0
cappuccino:							
(*Rice Dream*)	150	0	23.0	6.0	0	100	1.0
almond fudge (*Rice Dream* Supreme)	170	1.0	24.0	8.0	0	95	2.0
carob:							
(*Rice Dream*)	150	1.0	24.0	6.0	0	100	2.0
almond (*Rice Dream*)	170	1.0	24.0	8.0	0	95	2.0

Food and Measure	cal.	prot. (gms)	carbo. (gms)	fat (gms)	chol. (mgs)	sod. (mgs)	fiber (gms)
"Ice cream," nondairy, carob *(cont.)*							
peppermint (*Soy Delicious*)	130	2.0	24.0	3.0	0	30	1.0
cherry:							
(*Soy Delicious Purely Decadent*)	190	1.0	32.0	9.0	0	15	5.0
chocolate chunk (*Rice Dream Supreme*)	170	1.0	27.0	7.0	0	85	1.0
vanilla (*Rice Dream*)	150	0	24.0	6.0	0	90	1.0
chocolate:							
(*Rice Dream*)	150	1.0	24.0	7.0	0	100	2.0
(*Soy Delicious Awesome*)	130	2.0	24.0	3.0	0	25	1.0
(*Soy Delicious Purely Decadent*)	210	2.0	36.0	9.0	0	15	5.0
(*Soy Delicious Velvet*)	130	2.0	23.0	4.0	0	35	2.0
(*Soy Dream*)	140	1.0	18.0	7.0	0	70	1.0
(*Tofutti* Premium Supreme)	180	3.0	18.0	11.0	0	180	0
chocolate almond:							
(*Soy Delicious*) . . .	160	3.0	24.0	6.0	0	65	2.0
brownie (*Soy Delicious* Purely Decadent)	210	3.0	34.0	10.0	0	75	6.0
chunk (*Rice Dream* Supreme)	170	2.0	25.0	8.0	0	95	2.0
chocolate chip (*Rice Dream*)	170	1.0	26.0	8.0	0	95	1.0
chocolate cookie crunch (*Tofutti* Premium)	210	3.0	21.0	11.0	0	100	0
chocolate fudge:							
(*Tofutti* Low Fat Supreme)	120	2.0	25.0	2.0	0	98	0
brownie (*Rice Dream* Supreme)	170	1.0	28.0	7.0	0	95	2.0
sundae (*Tofutti* Fat/ Sugar Free)	80	<1.0	20.0	0	0	105	0
chocolate peanut butter (*Soy Delicious*) . . .	150	2.0	23.0	5.0	0	65	1.0
cocoa marble fudge (*Rice Dream*)	150	1.0	25.0	6.0	0	100	2.0

Food and Measure	cal.	prot. (gms)	carbo. (gms)	fat (gms)	chol. (mgs)	sod. (mgs)	fiber (gms)
coffee marshmallow swirl (*Tofutti* Low Fat Supreme)	100	1.0	24.0	1.0	0	77	0
cookie:							
(*Rice Dream* Cookie N' Dream)	170	1.0	26.0	7.0	0	100	1.0
(*Soy Delicious* Purely Decadent)	200	2.0	34.0	9.0	0	70	5.0
espresso:							
(*Soy Delicious*) ...	130	2.0	25.0	3.0	0	30	1.0
double (*Rice Dream* Supreme)	160	1.0	24.0	7.0	0	95	1.0
honey vanilla chamomile (*Tofutti*)	190	2.0	20.0	11.0	0	210	0
mint carob chip (*Rice Dream*)	170	1.0	26.0	8.0	0	95	1.0
mint chocolate:							
chip (*Rice Dream*)	170	1.0	26.0	8.0	0	95	1.0
chunky (*Soy Delicious* Purely Decadent)	200	2.0	35.0	8.0	0	30	6.0
cookie (*Rice Dream* Supreme)	170	1.0	26.0	8.0	0	100	1.0
marble fudge (*Soy Delicious*)	140	2.0	25.0	3.0	0	35	1.0
Neapolitan:							
(*Rice Dream*)	150	1.0	24.0	6.0	0	100	2.0
(*Soy Delicious*) ...	130	2.0	23.0	4.0	0	40	1.0
orange vanilla swirl (*Rice Dream*)	150	0	24.0	6.0	0	90	1.0
peach mango (*Tofutti* Low Fat Supreme) .	100	1.0	23.0	1.0	0	102	0
peanut butter:							
(*Soy Delicious* Purely Decadent)	230	3.0	32.0	13.0	0	50	5.0
cup (*Rice Dream* Supreme)	180	2.0	25.0	8.0	0	105	2.0
praline:							
(*Rice Dream* Supreme)	180	1.0	24.0	9.0	0	95	1.0
pecan (*Soy Delicious* Purely Decadent)	210	2.0	33.0	10.0	0	50	5.0

Food and Measure	cal.	prot. (gms)	carbo. (gms)	fat (gms)	chol. (mgs)	sod. (mgs)	fiber (gms)
"Ice cream," nondairy *(cont.)*							
raspberry (*Soy Delicious*)	130	1.0	25.0	3.0	0	25	1.0
strawberry:							
(*Rice Dream*)	140	0	24.0	5.0	0	85	1.0
(*Soy Delicious*) ...	130	2.0	23.0	4.0	0	55	1.0
strawberry banana (*Tofutti* Low Fat Supreme)	100	1.0	23.0	1.0	0	92	0
vanilla:							
(*Rice Dream*)	150	0	23.0	6.0	0	100	1.0
(*Soy Delicious*) ...	130	2.0	23.0	4.0	0	55	1.0
(*Soy Delicious* Fruit Sweetened)	130	2.0	25.0	3.0	0	30	1.0
(*Soy Delicious* Purely Decadent)	170	1.0	29.0	8.0	0	20	6.0
(*Tofutti*)	190	<2.0	20.0	11.0	0	90	0
(*Tofutti* Premium)	190	2.0	20.0	11.0	0	210	0
vanilla almond:							
(*Tofutti* Vanilla Almond Bark*)	210	3.0	21.0	13.0	0	130	0
Swiss (*Rice Dream*)	180	1.0	25.0	8.0	0	95	1.0
vanilla fudge:							
(*Tofutti* Low Fat Supreme)	120	2.0	24.0	2.0	0	90	0
sundae (*Tofutti* Fat/ Sugar Free)	80	<1.0	20.0	0	0	105	0
vanilla strawberry sundae (*Tofutti* Fat/ Sugar Free)	80	<1.0	19.0	0	0	95	0
wild berry supreme (*Tofutti* Premium)	190	2.0	24.0	9.0	0	190	0
Ice cream bar (see also "Iced confection bar"), 1 pc.:							
all flavors (*Blue Bell* Créme Pops Reduced Fat)	60	<0	12.0	1.0	<5	20	0
almond:							
(*Blue Bell*)	240	4.0	19.0	17.0	20	65	<1.0
(*Klondike Big Bear*)	310	5.0	26.0	21.0	30	70	0
toasted (*Good Humor* Multipack)	180	2.0	22.0	10.0	5	25	<1.0

Food and Measure	cal.	prot. (gms)	carbo. (gms)	fat (gms)	chol. (mgs)	sod. (mgs	fiber (gms)
toasted (*Good Humor* Single) ..	230	2.0	30.0	12.0	10	35	1.0
(*Ben & Jerry's Phish Stick*)	260	3.0	29.0	16.0	20	60	2.0
(*Ben & Jerry's Phish Stick* Single)	290	3.0	32.0	18.0	25	70	2.0
candy bar swirl (*Klondike*)	320	5.0	29.0	21.0	25	150	<1.0
candy center (*Good Humor* Crunch) ...	300	3.0	22.0	23.0	15	80	<1.0
cappuccino (*Klondike*)	290	4.0	26.0	20.0	30	65	<1.0
caramel:							
crunch (*Klondike*)	290	4.0	30.0	17.0	30	95	0
soft (*Breyers Magnum*)	360	4.0	35.0	22.0	30	125	<1.0
cherry, dark chocolate (*Cascadian Farm*) ..	220	3.0	22.0	13.0	10	50	<1.0
cherry fudge flakes (*Ben & Jerry's Cherry Garcia*)	250	3.0	25.0	16.0	30	55	1.0
chocolate:							
(*Klondike* Variety Pack)	240	3.0	21.0	16.0	20	40	<1.0
and almonds (*Häagen-Dazs* Single)	380	6.0	27.0	27.0	90	65	2.0
chocolate (*Klondike*)	280	3.0	25.0	19.0	25	50	1.0
dark chocolate (*Cascadian Farm*)	230	4.0	25.0	14.0	10	45	1.0
dark chocolate (*Häagen-Dazs* Single)	350	5.0	28.0	24.0	85	45	2.0
chocolate éclair:							
(*Col. Crunch*)	150	1.0	21.0	7.0	5	70	1.0
(*Good Humor* Multi-pack)	160	2.0	20.0	8.0	5	60	<1.0
(*Good Humor* Single)	220	2.0	30.0	10.0	10	90	<1.0
coffee:							
(*Frappuccino*)	110	4.0	20.0	2.0	10	50	0
almond, milk chocolate (*Cascadian Farm*)	230	4.0	22.0	15.0	15	35	1.0

Food and Measure	cal.	prot. (gms)	carbo. (gms)	fat (gms)	chol. (mgs)	sod. (mgs)	fiber (gms)
Ice cream bar, coffee *(cont.)*							
almond crunch (*Häagen-Dazs* Single)	370	5.0	27.0	27.0	90	80	<1.0
coconut, tropical (*Häagen-Dazs*)	340	5.0	25.0	24.0	90	70	0
cookie dough (*Ben & Jerry's*)	410	5.0	45.0	24.0	45	140	<1.0
cookies and cream: (*Good Humor*) . . .	190	2.0	21.0	12.0	10	120	<1.0
crunch (*Häagen-Dazs* Single)	370	5.0	30.0	26.0	85	100	<1.0
dulce de leche (*Häagen-Dazs* Single)	370	4.0	34.0	24.0	75	90	0
fudge (*Blue Bell* Lowfat)	45	2.0	6.0	1.0	<5	40	0
(*Good Humor* Number 1)	190	2.0	22.0	11.0	10	45	<1.0
(*Klondike Krunch*) . . .	270	4.0	26.0	17.0	25	75	<1.0
mocha (*Frappuccino*) .	120	4.0	21.0	2.0	10	50	0
Neapolitan (*Klondike*)	280	4.0	25.0	19.0	25	60	<1.0
peanut butter cup: (*Good Humor* Multipack)	250	3.0	24.0	16.0	15	70	1.0
(*Good Humor Reese's* Single)	310	4.0	31.0	19.0	20	80	1.0
(*Popsicle* No Sugar)	190	4.0	19.0	10.0	5	65	4.0
(*Popsicle* Sprinklers Multipack)	130	1.0	18.0	6.0	10	25	0
(*Popsicle* Sprinklers Single)	180	1.0	26.0	8.0	10	35	0
(*Popsicle* Wildlife Single)	100	2.0	14.0	4.0	15	40	0
(*Popsicle* Wildlife Multipack)	110	2.0	14.0	6.0	20	40	0
(*Popsicle* Scribblers Multipack)	120	4.0	12.0	7.0	25	35	0
(*Popsicle* Snoopy) . . .	150	2.0	18.0	8.0	20	50	0
(*Popsicle* WWF)	200	2.0	25.0	10.0	15	90	0
raspberry, dark chocolate (*Cascadian Farm*)	220	3.0	21.0	13.0	10	50	<1.0

Food and Measure	cal.	prot. (gms)	carbo. (gms)	fat (gms)	chol. (mgs)	sod. (mgs	fiber (gms)
s'mores:							
(*Ben & Jerry's S'Mores Pop*) ..	280	4.0	30.0	16.0	25	60	1.0
(*Ben & Jerry's S'Mores Pop Single*)	330	5.0	34.0	19.0	30	85	1.0
strawberry:							
shortcake (*Col. Crunch*)	70	1.0	21.0	8.0	5	50	<1.0
shortcake (*Good Humor* Multipack)	170	1.0	21.0	9.0	5	60	0
shortcake (*Good Humor* Single) ..	220	2.0	31.0	10.0	10	80	<1.0
soft (*Breyers Magnum*)	360	3.0	35.0	22.0	30	80	<1.0
swirl (*Klondike*) ...	290	4.0	28.0	19.0	25	80	0
vanilla w/chocolate:							
(*Blue Bell* Belle) ...	180	2.0	15.0	12.0	20	45	0
(*Dove Bar* Single)	320	4.0	32.0	21.0	35	40	2.0
(*Good Humor* Premium)	240	3.0	24.0	15.0	20	45	<1.0
(*Klondike* Original) .	290	4.0	26.0	20.0	30	65	<1.0
(*Klondike* Reduced Fat/No Sugar) ..	190	4.0	19.0	10.0	5	65	<1.0
(*Klondike* Variety Pack)	240	3.0	21.0	16.0	20	65	0
(*Popsicle*)	160	2.0	15.0	11.0	15	35	1.0
w/crisps (*Klondike* Krispy Krunch) ..	300	4.0	28.0	19.0	30	65	1.0
dark (*Cascadian Farm*)	220	4.0	23.0	14.0	10	55	<1.0
dark (*Good Humor*)	180	2.0	16.0	13.0	15	25	1.0
dark (*Häagen-Dazs* Single)	350	5.0	27.0	24.0	85	50	1.0
dark (*Klondike*) ...	290	4.0	25.0	20.0	30	55	<1.0
milk (*Ben & Jerry's*)	330	5.0	29.0	14.0	60	65	<1.0
milk (*Good Humor*)	180	2.0	16.0	12.0	15	35	<1.0
milk (*Häagen-Dazs* Single)	340	5.0	25.0	24.0	90	65	<1.0
milk, w/almond (*Cascadian Farm*)	230	4.0	23.0	15.0	15	40	1.0
milk, w/crisps (*Blue Bell* Krunch)	220	2.0	20.0	15.0	20	70	0

Food and Measure	cal.	prot. (gms)	carbo. (gms)	fat (gms)	chol. (mgs)	sod. (mgs)	fiber (gms)
Ice cream bar, vanilla w/chocolate *(cont.)*							
w/toffee (*Ben & Jerry's Heath*) ..	320	4.0	32.0	21.0	50	105	<1.0
w/toffee (*Klondike Heath*)	300	4.0	27.0	20.0	30	110	0
(*York* Peppermint Pattie Bar)	290	4.0	24.0	20.0	30	65	<1.0
"Ice cream" bar, non-dairy, 1 bar:							
chocolate:							
(*Rice Dream*)	270	2.0	32.0	15.0	0	95	2.0
w/nuts (*Rice Dream Nutty*)	270	4.0	23.0	18.0	0	55	2.0
chocolate fudge (*Tofutti* Treats)	30	1.0	6.0	0	0	86	0
fruit, mixed, chocolate coated (*Tofutti Frutti*)	120	1.0	15.0	5.0	0	20	0
fudge:							
(*Soy Delicious*) ...	140	3.0	25.0	4.0	0	25	2.0
(*Tofutti Teddy Fudge*)	90	1.0	19.0	1.0	0	50	0
peanut butter (*Tofutti* Monkey Bars)	220	3.0	22.0	13.0	0	105	<1.0
strawberry:							
(*Rice Dream*)	250	1.0	31.0	13.0	0	80	1.0
crumb (*Tofutti* Crumb Cakes) ..	220	<1.0	20.0	15.0	0	90	0
vanilla:							
(*Rice Dream*)	270	1.0	33.0	14.0	0	95	1.0
(*Soy Delicious*) ...	250	3.0	31.0	13.0	0	25	1.0
and almonds (*Soy Delicious*)	300	4.0	32.0	17.0	0	30	2.0
w/nuts (*Rice Dream Nutty*)	260	4.0	23.0	18.0	0	55	2.0
vanilla fudge, crumb coated (*Tofutti Crumb Cake*)	230	2.0	20.0	16.0	0	125	0
Ice cream cake, ⅙ of 15-oz. cake:							
cappuccino (*Viennetta*)	190	3.0	19.0	11.0	35	35	0
chocolate, triple (*Viennetta*)	180	3.0	16.0	12.0	25	14	0
vanilla (*Viennetta*) ...	190	3.0	19.0	11.0	40	40	0

Food and Measure	cal.	prot. (gms)	carbo. (gms)	fat (gms)	chol. (mgs)	sod. (mgs)	fiber (gms)
Ice cream cone, filled (see also "Iced confection cone"), 1 pc.:							
caramel (*Klondike Big Bear*)	370	7.0	40.0	21.0	20	135	<1.0
cookies and cream (*Blue Bell Country*)	280	4.0	37.0	13.0	20	100	<1.0
fudge (*Klondike Big Bear*)	370	7.0	40.0	21.0	15	105	<1.0
(*Good Humor Giant King Cone*)	390	7.0	45.0	21.0	40	140	1.0
(*Klondike Kone*)	330	6.0	35.0	19.0	25	115	<1.0
praline (*Blue Bell Country*)	310	6.0	33.0	17.0	25	60	0
rocky road sundae (*Turkey Hill*)	310	5.0	35.0	17.0	25	105	2.0
sundae:							
(*Good Humor*) . . .	140	4.0	32.0	16.0	15	90	1.0
(*Turkey Hill* Super)	290	6.0	31.0	17.0	25	160	1.0
caramel center (*Klondike Big Bear*)	340	5.0	39.0	18.0	20	130	<1.0
fudge center (*Klondike Big Bear*) . .	340	5.0	39.0	18.0	15	130	<1.0
vanilla (*Klondike Big Bear*)	330	6.0	35.0	19.0	25	115	<1.0
tin roof sundae (*Turkey Hill*)	290	5.0	30.0	17.0	25	135	1.0
vanilla:							
(*Blue Bell Country*)	290	6.0	29.0	16.0	20	50	0
(*Good Humor King Cone*)	270	4.0	33.0	14.0	20	100	1.0
(*Klondike Big Bear*)	350	7.0	35.0	21.0	20	110	<1.0
vanilla fudge (*Blue Bell Country*)	310	6.0	33.0	17.0	20	55	<1.0
Ice cream cone/cup, unfilled, 1 pc.:							
bowl, waffle (*Keebler*)	50	<1.0	10.0	1.0	0	25	0
cone:							
chocolate (*Oreo*) . .	50	0	10.0	1.0	0	90	<1.0
fudge dipped (*Keebler*)	35	0	6.0	1.5	0	20	0
sugar (*Comet*)	60	0	12.0	0	0	5	0

Food and Measure	cal.	prot. (gms)	carbo. (gms)	fat (gms)	chol. (mgs)	sod. (mgs)	fiber (gms)
Ice cream cone *(cont.)*							
sugar (*Keebler*) ...	50	<1.0	10.0	.5	0	15	0
waffle (*Keebler*) ...	50	<1.0	10.0	1.0	0	25	0
cup:							
(*Comet*)	20	0	4.0	0	0	10	0
(*Keebler*)	15	0	4.0	0	0	20	0
rainbow (*Comet*) ..	20	0	4.0	0	0	5	0
Ice cream cup, filled, 1 pc.:							
chocolate, Dutch (*Blue Bell*), 3 fl. oz.	180	4.0	20.0	9.0	35	75	0
cookies and cream (*Popsicle* Zone) ...	360	5.0	50.0	16.0	45	180	2.0
fudge (*Fudgsicle Frostee*)	280	7.0	41.0	11.0	35	95	2.0
(*Good Humor Sundae Twist*)	160	2.0	33.0	2.5	10	100	0
sundae (*Klondike*) ...	280	6.0	26.0	17.0	35	125	<1.0
vanilla (*Blue Bell* Homemade)	170	4.0	19.0	8.0	35	70	0
"Ice cream" dessert roll, nondairy (*Tofutti* Rock), 2.4-oz. slice	180	1.0	22.0	10.0	0	160	0
Ice cream mix, ½ cup:							
chocolate (*Junket*) ..	110	1.0	26.0	0	0	20	0
vanilla and strawberry (*Junket*)	110	5.0	27.0	0	0	10	0
Ice cream pie, see "Ice cream sandwich"							
Ice cream sandwich, 1 pc:							
cookie:							
(*Good Humor Premium*)	290	4.0	44.0	11.0	20	210	1.0
(*Klondike Oreo*) ...	240	4.0	35.0	10.0	15	310	2.0
chocolate chip (*Klondike Big Bear Multipack*)	290	3.0	41.0	13.0	15	200	1.0

Food and Measure	cal.	prot. (gms)	carbo. (gms)	fat (gms)	chol. (mgs)	sod. (mgs)	fiber (gms)
chocolate chip (*Klondike Big Bear Single*)	460	6.0	70.0	18.0	30	390	1.0
oatmeal (*Blue Bell Country*)	310	5.0	45.0	13.0	25	350	2.0
cookies and cream							
(*Blue Bell* Single) ..	190	3.0	30.0	7.0	15	160	<1.0
(*Blue Bell* 12 Pack)	180	3.0	27.0	6.0	15	150	<1.0
(*Klondike* Choco Taco)	300	4.0	38.0	15.0	15	150	1.0
mint chocolate chip							
(*Turkey Hill*)	200	3.0	27.0	8.0	25	180	0
Mississippi mud							
(*Good Humor* Giant)	310	7.0	39.0	15.0	35	220	<1.0
Neapolitan:							
(*Blue Bell*)	210	4.0	32.0	8.0	25	150	1.0
(*Good Humor* Giant)	250	4.0	38.0	10.0	25	200	1.0
(*Klondike*)	200	4.0	30.0	7.0	20	160	<1.0
(*Klondike Big Bear* Multipack)	200	4.0	30.0	7.0	20	160	<1.0
(*Klondike Big Bear* Single)	300	5.0	45.0	11.0	30	220	1.0
vanilla:							
(*Blue Bell* Single) ..	180	3.0	28.0	7.0	20	140	0
(*Blue Bell* 12 Pack)	170	3.0	25.0	6.0	15	130	0
(*Good Humor* Family Pack) ...	160	2.0	25.0	6.0	10	140	<1.0
(*Good Humor* Single)	180	3.0	29.0	6.0	15	160	0
(*Good Humor* Giant)	250	4.0	38.0	9.0	25	190	1.0
(*Klondike Big Bear* Multipack)	200	3.0	31.0	7.0	20	170	<1.0
(*Klondike Big Bear* Single)	290	5.0	45.0	10.0	30	230	1.0
(*Turkey Hill*)	190	3.0	26.0	8.0	25	180	0
mini (*Blue Bell* 24 Pack)	100	2.0	15.0	4.0	0	80	0
vanilla chocolate (*Turkey Hill* Double Decker)	200	3.0	29.0	8.0	20	170	1.0
"Ice cream" sandwich nondairy, 1 pc.:							
chocolate:							
(*Rice Dream*)	320	3.0	39.0	18.0	0	80	0
wafer (*Tofutti Cuties*)	130	2.0	16.0	5.0	0	110	0

Food and Measure	cal.	prot. (gms)	carbo. (gms)	fat (gms)	chol. (mgs)	sod. (mgs)	fiber (gms)
"Ice cream," sandwich, nondairy *(cont.)*							
chocolate chip cookie:							
(*Soy Delicious*) . . .	260	3.0	41.0	10.0	0	60	2.0
mint (*Soy Delicious*)	260	3.0	41.0	10.0	0	70	2.0
mint (*Rice Dream*) . . .	320	3.0	39.0	18.0	0	80	2.0
mocha (*Rice Dream*) .	320	3.0	40.0	17.0	0	80	1.0
peanut butter, wafer							
(*Tofutti Cuties*)	165	3.0	20.0	8.0	0	135	0
vanilla:							
(*Rice Dream*)	320	3.0	40.0	17.0	0	80	1.0
cookie (*Tofutti Too-Too's*)	215	3.0	28.0	10.0	0	141	0
dark chocolate							
(*Tofutti* Cutie Pies)	250	2.0	18.0	19.0	0	130	0
wafer (*Tofutti Cuties*)	120	2.0	17.0	5.0	0	121	0
vanilla chocolate chip							
(*Tofutti* Too-Too's) .	230	3.0	30.0	11.0	0	155	0
wafer (*Soy Delicious* Big Buddy)	240	4.0	47.0	8.0	0	190	2.0
wild berry, wafer							
(*Tofutti Cuties*)	120	2.0	17.0	5.0	0	121	0
Ice cream and sherbet or sorbet, see "Sherbet" and "Sorbet"							
Iced confection bar (see also "Ice bar"), 1 pc.:							
banana fudge:							
(*Blue Bell* Single) . .	120	3.0	19.0	4.0	0	80	0
(*Blue Bell* 12 Pack)	100	3.0	16.0	2.5	0	40	0
(*Blue Bell* Pop 'n Fudge)	100	3.0	16.0	3.5	0	70	0
(*Fudgsicle* Banana Bananza!)	60	0	14.0	0	0	10	0
chocolate (*Blue Bell* Fudge Blast) . . .	190	4.0	28.0	7.0	0	105	<1.0
chocolate (*Blue Bell* Fudge Bombstick*)	210	5.0	31.0	7.0	0	120	<1.0
mini (*Blue Bell*) . . .	60	2.0	10.0	1.5	0	25	0
chocolate fudge:							
(*Blue Bell* Multipack)	120	2.0	17.0	4.5	0	65	<1.0
(*Blue Bell* Pop 'n Fudge)	120	2.0	17.0	4.5	0	65	<1.0

Food and Measure	cal.	prot. (gms)	carbo. (gms)	fat (gms)	chol. (mgs)	sod. (mgs)	fiber (gms)
(*Blue Bell* Texas Double Fudge) . .	260	6.0	34.0	11.0	0	130	0
(*Fudgsicle* 8 Pack)	90	3.0	17.0	1.5	5	55	<1.0
(*Fudgsicle* Fat Free)	60	3.0	13.0	0	0	50	<1.0
(*Fudgsicle* No Sugar)	45	1.0	9.0	.5	0	45	<1.0
(*Fudgsicle* Original Pop)	60	2.0	12.0	1.0	<5	40	0
(*Fudgsicle* Single)	90	3.0	18.0	1.5	<5	60	<1.0
(*Fudgsicle* Variety 18 Pack)	120	4.0	24.0	1.5	5	75	<1.0
(*Popsicle* Fudge Pop)	60	2.0	12.0	1.0	<5	40	0
double (*Firecracker*) <1.0		150	5.0	29.0	2.0	10	95
mini (*Blue Bell*) . . .	70	2.0	9.0	2.5	0	30	0
chocolate vanilla: (*Popsicle* Pop)	100	1.0	10.0	6.0	10	20	0
swirl (*Fudgsicle* Variety Pack) . . .	120	4.0	23.0	1.5	5	70	<1.0
vanilla (*Fudgsicle* Variety 18 Pack) . .	120	3.0	22.0	2.0	5	65	<1.0
vanilla, w/chocolate: (*Blue Bell Mooo*) . .	190	1.0	14.0	14.0	0	45	0
(*Blue Bell Mini Mooos*)	90	<1.0	7.0	6.0	0	25	0
w/crisps (*Blue Bell Krunch* Pack) . . .	190	1.0	16.0	13.0	0	60	0
w/crisps, mini (*Blue Bell Krunch*)	110	<1.0	9.0	7.0	0	35	0
Iced confection cone (see also "Ice cream cone"), 1 pc.:							
mini (*Blue Bell Country Variety 12 Pack*) . .	90	1.0	12.0	4.5	0	40	0
vanilla, w/chocolate, mini (*Blue Bell Country* 12 Pack) . .	90	1.0	11.0	4.5	0	40	0
Icing, cake, see "Frosting"							
Irish cream syrup (*Ferrara*), 2 oz. . . .	130	0	32.0	0	0	12	0
Italian seasoning (*Wyler's Shakers*), 1 tsp.	10	0	2.0	0	0	630	0

J

Food and Measure	cal.	prot. (gms)	carbo. (gms)	fat (gms)	chol. (mgs)	sod. (mgs)	fiber (gms)
***Jack-in-the-Box*,**							
1 serving:							
breakfast items:							
bacon	20	2.0	0	1.5	5	95	0
biscuit, sausage . . .	380	11.0	25.0	27.0	35	730	2.0
biscuit, sausage,							
egg, cheese	760	25.0	33.0	60.0	280	1390	2.0
Breakfast Jack	310	14.0	34.0	14.0	210	770	1.0
croissant, sausage	680	18.0	41.0	50.0	250	760	2.0
croissant, supreme	540	18.0	37.0	35.0	240	860	1.0
French toast sticks	430	8.0	57.0	18.0	10	460	2.0
hash browns	150	1.0	13.0	10.0	0	230	2.0
sausage sandwich,							
extreme	720	26.0	35.0	53.0	280	1180	2.0
sourdough sand-							
wich	450	18.0	36.0	26.0	220	830	2.0
ultimate sandwich .	650	28.0	52.0	37.0	440	1390	1.0
syrup	130	0	32.0	0	0	30	0
burgers:							
cheeseburger:							
big	630	24.0	46.0	39.0	70	1100	1.0
big Texas	540	24.0	41.0	31.0	65	1040	1.0
bacon bacon . . .	820	34.0	44.0	56.0	95	1410	2.0
double	410	20.0	32.0	22.0	70	920	1.0
Jack's Western . .	600	22.0	46.0	36.0	60	860	2.0
ultimate	980	39.0	42.0	73.0	140	1270	1.0
ultimate, bacon .	1050	45.0	42.0	78.0	160	1640	1.0
hamburger	250	12.0	30.0	9.0	30	610	2.0
hamburger							
w/cheese	300	14.0	31.0	13.0	40	840	2.0
Jumbo Jack	560	20.0	45.0	33.0	45	800	2.0
Jumbo Jack							
w/cheese	650	25.0	47.0	40.0	75	1180	2.0
Sourdough Jack . .	660	27.0	33.0	47.0	75	950	3.0

Food and Measure	cal.	prot. (gms)	carbo. (gms)	fat (gms)	chol. (mgs)	sod. (mgs)	fiber (gms)
chicken and fish:							
chicken breast, 5 pcs.	360	27.0	24.0	17.0	80	970	1.0
chicken fajita pita	330	24.0	35.0	11.0	55	910	3.0
chicken fillet, grilled	430	23.0	34.0	22.0	60	910	2.0
chicken sandwich	410	15.0	39.0	21.0	35	740	2.0
chicken supreme	710	30.0	62.0	39.0	70	1440	4.0
chicken teriyaki bowl	550	26.0	103.0	3.0	35	1720	3.0
fish & chips	610	18.0	66.0	31.0	40	1240	5.0
Jack's Spicy Chicken	580	24.0	53.0	31.0	60	950	3.0
sourdough grilled chicken club	490	31.0	33.0	26.0	80	1190	3.0
taco	180	7.0	16.0	10.0	20	310	2.0
taco, monster	280	10.0	22.0	17.0	35	560	3.0
snacks/sides:							
bacon cheddar potato wedges	770	21.0	52.0	53.0	45	1330	3.0
cheddar wedges, spicy	730	16.0	51.0	52.0	45	1340	<1.0
cheese sticks, 3	240	11.0	21.0	12.0	25	420	1.0
cheese sticks, 5	400	18.0	35.0	21.0	40	700	2.0
egg rolls, 1	130	5.0	15.0	6.0	5	310	2.0
egg rolls, 3	400	14.0	44.0	19.0	15	920	6.0
fries	330	3.0	44.0	16.0	0	550	3.0
fries, jumbo	410	4.0	55.0	20.0	0	690	4.0
fries, super scoop	580	6.0	77.0	28.0	0	960	6.0
fries, curly: chili cheese	630	13.0	54.0	40.0	30	1640	6.0
seasoned	400	6.0	45.0	23.0	0	890	5.0
jalapeño, stuffed, 3	230	7.0	22.0	13.0	20	690	2.0
jalapeño, stuffed, 7	530	15.0	51.0	30.0	45	1600	4.0
onion rings	500	6.0	51.0	30.0	0	420	3.0
side salad	50	3.0	5.0	3.0	10	65	2.0
condiments:							
cheese, 1 slice: American	45	2.0	1.0	3.5	10	180	0
Swiss style	40	2.0	1.0	3.0	10	150	0
Country Crock Spread	25	0	0	2.5	0	45	0
croutons	50	1.0	8.0	2.0	0	105	0

Food and Measure	cal.	prot. (gms)	carbo. (gms)	fat (gms)	chol. (mgs)	sod. (mgs)	fiber (gms)
***Jack-in-the-Box*, condiments** *(cont.)*							
dipping sauces, 1 oz.:							
barbecue	45	1.0	11.0	0	0	330	0
buttermilk house	130	<1.0	3.0	13.0	10	210	0
Frank's Red Hot							
Buffalo	10	0	2.0	0	0	840	0
sweet and sour	45	0	11.0	0	0	160	0
dressing, 2 oz.:							
blue cheese	260	1.0	5.0	26.0	30	670	0
buttermilk house	310	1.0	3.0	33.0	20	470	0
Italian, low-cal . .	15	0	4.0	0	0	510	0
Thousand Island	160	1.0	12.0	12.0	15	490	0
grape jelly	35	0	9.0	0	0	10	0
ketchup	10	0	2.0	0	0	105	0
marinara sauce . . .	15	0	3.0	0	0	210	0
mustard	0	0	1.0	0	0	50	0
salsa	10	0	2.0	0	0	220	0
sour cream	60	1.0	2.0	5.0	15	20	0
soy sauce	5	0	1.0	0	0	480	0
tartar sauce	210	1.0	2.0	22.0	20	370	0
taco sauce , ...	0	0	0	0	0	80	0
desserts/shakes:							
apple turnover	320	3.0	41.0	16.0	0	370	2.0
cheesecake	310	7.0	34.0	16.0	55	220	0
double fudge cake	310	3.0	49.0	11.0	25	270	4.0
shakes, 16 oz.:							
cappuccino	640	10.0	85.0	28.0	110	220	0
chocolate	660	11.0	89.0	29.0	115	270	1.0
Oreo cookie	670	11.0	81.0	33.0	110	350	1.0
strawberry	640	10.0	84.0	28.0	110	220	0
vanilla	570	12.0	65.0	29.0	115	220	0
Jackfruit, fresh,							
trimmed, 1 oz. . . .	27	.4	6.8	.1	0	1	.5
Jackfruit, canned, in							
syrup, ½ cup	82	.3	21.3	.1	0	10	.8
Jackfruit, dried							
(*Frieda's*), ½ cup,							
3 oz.	80	1.0	20.0	0	0	0	1.0
Jalapeño, see "Pepper,							
jalapeño"							
Jalapeño dip mix							
(*Watkins*), 1 tsp. . . .	10	0	1.0	0	0	80	0
Jalapeño sauce, see							
"Hot sauce"							

Food and Measure	cal.	prot. (gms)	carbo. (gms)	fat (gms)	chol. (mgs)	sod. (mgs)	fiber (gms)
Jam and preserves (see also "Fruit spreads"), 1 tbsp or .5 oz.:							
all fruits:							
(*Hero*)	60	0	15.0	0	0	0	0
(*Kraft*)	35	0	9.0	0	0	0	0
(*Smucker's*)	50	0	13.0	0	0	0	0
(*Smucker's* Low Sugar)	25	0	6.0	0	0	0	0
(*Smucker's* Sugar Free)	10	0	5.0	0	0	0	0
amaretto, peach, or pecan (*D. L. Jardine's*)	80	0	19.0	0	0	0	0
berry, twin (*Watkins* Preserves)	50	0	12.0	0	0	0	0
ginger (*Chivers*)	50	0	13.0	0	0	0	0
kiwi (*Frieda's*)	35	0	9.0	0	0	0	1.0
lingonberry, wild (*D'arbo*)	45	0	11.0	0	0	0	0
mango (*Goya*)	40	0	10.0	0	0	0	0
orange marmalade (*Crosse & Blackwell*)	60	0	16.0	0	0	0	0
papaya (*Goya*)	45	0	9.5	0	0	0	0
raspberry cherry (*Watkins*)	40	0	11.0	0	0	0	0
raspberry or strawberry (*Cascadian Farm* Conserve) . . .	40	0	10.0	0	0	0	0
Java plum:							
3 medium, .4 oz. . . .	5	.1	1.4	<.1	0	1	<1.0
seeded, ½ cup	41	.5	10.5	.2	0	9	<1.0
Jelly, fruit, 1 tbsp., except as noted:							
all fruits:							
(*Kraft*), 5-oz. pkt. . .	35	0	9.0	0	0	0	0
(*Smucker's*)	50	0	13.0	0	0	0	0
apple:							
(*Musselman's*)	50	0	13.0	0	0	0	0
mint (*Crosse & Blackwell*)	60	0	14.0	0	0	0	0
guava (*Goya*)	50	0	12.0	0	0	0	0

Food and Measure	cal.	prot. (gms)	carbo. (gms)	fat (gms)	chol. (mgs)	sod. (mgs)	fiber (gms)
Jelly *(cont.)*							
guava or red currant:							
(*Crosse & Blackwell*)	60	0	14.0	0	0	0	0
Jelly, pepper, 2 tbsp., except as noted:							
habanero (*D. L. Jardine's* Hotter) ..	70	0	19.0	0	0	0	0
hot (*Reese*), 1 tbsp.	50	0	13.0	0	0	35	0
jalapeño (*D. L. Jardine's* Hotter) ..	80	0	20.0	0	0	0	0
jalapeño cherry (*D. L. Jardine's*)	70	0	21.0	0	0	0	0
Jerk sauce (see also "Marinade"), 2 tbsp.:							
dipping (*Helen's Tropical Exotics* Jamaican)	45	1.0	10.0	0	0	640	1.0
Jamaican style (*World Harbors*)	70	0	18.0	0	0	200	0
Jerk seasoning:							
(*Helen's Tropical Exotics*), 1 tbsp. ..	30	1.0	7.0	0	0	210	1.0
(*McCormick* Caribbean), ¼ tsp.	0	0	0	0	0	70	0
Jerusalem artichoke:							
(*Frieda's Sunchoke*), ½ cup, 3 oz.	70	2.0	14.0	0	0	0	1.0
sliced, ½ cup	57	1.5	13.1	<.1	0	3	1.2
Jew's ear, see "Pepeao"							
Jicama, see "Yam bean"							
Jujube:							
raw, seeded, 1 oz.	22	.3	5.7	.1	0	1	n.a.
dried, 1 oz.	81	1.0	20.1	.3	0	3	n.a.
Jute, potherb, ½ cup:							
raw	5	.7	.8	<.1	0	1	n.a.
boiled, drained	16	1.6	3.1	.1	0	5	.9

K

Food and Measure	cal.	prot. (gms)	carbo. (gms)	fat (gms)	chol. (mgs)	sod. (mgs)	fiber (gms)
Kabocha squash (*Frieda's*), ¾ cup, 3 oz.	30	1.0	7.0	0	0	0	1.0
Kale, fresh, ½ cup:							
raw, chopped	17	1.1	3.4	.2	0	15	.7
boiled, drained, chopped	18	1.2	3.7	.3	0	5	3.6
Kale, canned, ½ cup:							
(*Allens/Sunshine*) . . .	30	1.0	3.0	.5	0	20	2.0
chopped (*Bush's Best*)	30	2.0	4.0	0	0	330	2.0
seasoned (*Glory Foods*)	50	4.0	6.0	.5	0	440	3.0
Kale, frozen, boiled, drained, chopped, ½ cup	20	1.9	3.4	.3	0	10	1.3
Kale, Chinese, fresh:							
raw (*Frieda's* Gai Lan), 1 cup, 3 oz.	15	2.0	3.0	0	0	15	n.a.
cooked, 1 cup	19	1.0	3.3	.6	0	6	2.2
Kale, Scotch, ½ cup:							
raw, chopped	14	1.0	2.8	.2	0	24	.6
boiled, drained, chopped	18	1.2	3.7	.3	0	29	.8
Kamranga, see "Carambola"							
Kamut flakes, see "Cereal"							
Kamut flour (*Arrowhead Mills*), ¼ cup	110	4.0	25.0	.5	0	0	4.0
Kanpo, dried:							
.2-oz. strip	16	.5	4.1	<.1	0	1	n.a.
½ cup	70	2.3	15.6	.1	0	4	n.a.
Kasha, see "Buckwheat groats"							

Food and Measure	cal.	prot. (gms)	carbo. (gms)	fat (gms)	chol. (mgs)	sod. (mgs)	fiber (gms)
Kefir, 8 fl. oz.:							
plain (*Lifeway* Lowfat)	110	14.0	8.0	2.5	10	125	0
all fruit flavors (*Lifeway* Lowfat)	160	14.0	21.0	2.0	10	125	0
Ketchup, 1 tbsp., except as noted:							
(*Del Monte*)	15	0	4.0	0	0	190	0
(*Estee* Smart Treats) .	15	0	5.0	– 0	0	190	0
(*Heinz*)	15	0	4.0	0	0	190	0
(*Heinz* Hot)	20	0	4.0	0	0	220	0
(*Hunt's*)	15	0	3.5	0	0	200	0
(*Muir Glen*)	15	0	3.0	0	0	190	0
(*New Organics*)	20	0	5.0	0	0	220	0
(*Red Gold*)	20	0	5.0	0	0	180	0
(*Smucker's*)	25	0	7.0	0	0	110	0
(*Westbrae Natural* Fruit Sweetened)	20	0	4.0	0	0	210	0
(*Westbrae Natural* Unsweetened)	5	0	1.0	0	0	60	0
KFC, 1 serving:							
chicken, 1 pc.:							
Original Recipe:							
breast	400	29.0	16.0	24.0	135	1110	1.0
drumstick	140	13.0	4.0	9.0	75	422	0
thigh	250	16.0	6.0	18.0	95	747	1.0
whole wing	140	9.0	5.0	10.0	55	414	0
Extra Crispy:							
breast	470	39.0	17.0	28.0	160	874	<1.0
drumstick	195	15.0	7.0	12.0	77	375	<1.0
thigh	380	21.0	14.0	27.0	118	625	<1.0
whole wing	250	16.0	6.0	18.0	95	747	1.0
Hot & Spicy:							
breast	505	38.0	23.0	29.0	162	1170	1.0
drumstick	175	13.0	9.0	10.0	77	360	<1.0
thigh	355	19.0	13.0	26.0	126	630	1.0
whole wing	210	10.0	9.0	15.0	55	350	<1.0
chicken pot pie	770	29.0	69.0	42.0	70	2160	5.0
chicken *Twister*	600	22.0	52.0	34.0	50	1430	4.0
Crispy Strips, 3 pcs.:							
Colonel's	300	26.0	18.0	16.0	56	1165	1.0
spicy	335	25.0	23.0	15.0	70	1140	<1.0
honey barbecue, 6 pcs.	607	33.0	33.0	38.0	193	1145	1.0
Hot Wings, 6 pcs.	471	27.0	18.0	33.0	150	1230	2.0

Food and Measure	cal.	prot. (gms)	carbo. (gms)	fat (gms)	chol. (mgs)	sod. (mgs)	fiber (gms)
popcorn chicken:							
large	620	30.0	36.0	40.0	73	1046	0
small	362	17.0	21.0	23.0	43	610	0
sandwiches:							
Original Recipe ...	450	29.0	33.0	22.0	70	940	2.0
Original Recipe,							
w/out sauce	360	29.0	21.0	13.0	60	890	<1.0
honey barbecue ...	310	28.0	37.0	6.0	125	560	2.0
honey barbecue							
crunch melt	556	33.0	48.0	26.0	60	1010	2.0
Tender Roast	350	32.0	26.0	15.0	75	880	1.0
Tender Roast,							
w/out sauce	270	31.0	23.0	5.0	65	690	1.0
Triple Crunch	490	28.0	39.0	29.0	70	710	2.0
Triple Crunch,							
w/out sauce	390	25.0	29.0	15.0	50	650	2.0
Triple Crunch							
Zinger	550	28.0	39.0	32.0	85	830	2.0
Triple Crunch							
Zinger, w/out							
sauce	390	25.0	36.0	15.0	50	650	2.0
sides and vegetables:							
baked beans, BBQ .	190	6.0	33.0	3.0	5	760	6.0
biscuit, 1 pc.	180	4.0	20.0	10.0	0	560	<1.0
coleslaw, 5 oz. ...	232	2.0	26.0	13.5	8	284	3.0
corn on the cob ...	150	5.0	35.0	1.5	0	20	2.0
macaroni & cheese	180	7.0	21.0	8.0	10	860	2.0
potato salad	230	4.0	23.0	14.0	15	540	3.0
potato wedges	280	5.0	28.0	13.0	5	750	5.0
potatoes, mashed,							
w/gravy	120	1.0	17.0	6.0	<1	440	2.0
desserts:							
Colonel's pie:							
apple	310	2.0	23.0	14.0	0	280	0
pecan	490	5.0	66.0	23.0	65	510	2.0
strawberry creme	280	4.0	32.0	15.0	15	130	2.0
double chocolate							
chip cake	320	4.0	41.0	16.0	55	230	1.0
Little Bucket parfait:							
chocolate cream	290	3.0	37.0	15.0	15	330	2.0
fudge brownie ..	280	3.0	44.0	10.0	145	190	1.0
lemon creme ...	410	7.0	62.0	14.0	20	290	4.0
strawberry							
shortcake	200	1.0	33.0	7.0	10	220	1.0

Food and Measure	cal.	prot. (gms)	carbo. (gms)	fat (gms)	chol. (mgs)	sod. (mgs)	fiber (gms)
Kidney beans:							
dry (*Arrowhead Mills*),							
¼ cup	160	11.0	29.0	.5	0	0	10.0
boiled, ½ cup	112	7.6	20.1	.4	0	2	6.5
Kidney beans, canned,							
½ cup:							
red:							
(*Blue Boy*)	120	7.0	21.0	0	0	360	6.0
(*Eden* Organic) . . .	100	8.0	18.0	0	0	15	10.0
(*Progresso*)	110	7.0	20.0	.5	0	280	8.0
(*S&W*)	100	7.0	23.0	.5	0	460	6.0
(*S&W* 50% Salt) . .	120	7.0	21.0	.5	0	220	6.0
(*Trappey's* Creole							
Style)	100	6.0	19.0	0	0	370	6.0
(*Westbrae Natural*)	80	6.0	15.0	0	0	140	4.0
dark (*Allens/*							
Trappey's)	130	8.0	22.0	.5	0	310	8.0
dark (*Bush's Best*) .	130	8.0	21.0	1.0	0	260	7.0
dark (*Hain* Organic)	120	8.0	18.0	0	0	140	8.0
dark (*Progresso*) . .	110	8.0	20.0	0	0	340	6.0
dark (*S&W*)	100	7.0	23.0	.5	0	460	6.0
light (*Allens/*							
Trappey's)	120	6.0	22.0	.5	0	340	8.0
light (*Bush's Best*) .	110	7.0	20.0	0	0	260	7.0
light (*Joan of Arc*) .	110	8.0	20.0	0	0	340	6.0
w/bacon (*Trappey's*							
New Orleans) . . .	110	6.0	20.0	1.0	0	410	6.0
w/chili gravy							
(*Trappey's*)	110	6.0	20.0	1.0	0	510	7.0
w/jalapeño, light							
(*Trappey's*)	110	6.0	19.0	1.0	0	420	6.0
Spanish style (*Goya*)	110	6.0	18.0	1.0	0	620	5.0
white:							
(*Eden* Organic) . . .	100	6.0	17.0	1.0	0	40	5.0
(*Progresso*							
Cannellini)	100	5.0	18.0	.5	0	270	5.0
Kidney beans, dried							
(*AlpineAire*), 1 oz. .	110	7.0	19.0	0	0	0	5.0
Kidney beans,							
sprouted, raw,							
½ cup	27	3.9	3.8	.5	0	6	<1.0
Kidneys, braised:							
beef, 4 oz.	163	28.9	1.1	3.9	439	152	0
lamb, 4 oz.	155	26.8	1.1	4.1	641	171	0

Food and Measure	cal.	prot. (gms)	carbo. (gms)	fat (gms)	chol. (mgs)	sod. (mgs	fiber (gms)
pork, 4 oz.	171	28.8	0	5.3	544	91	0
pork, chopped, 1 cup .	211	35.6	0	6.6	673	111	0
veal, 4 oz.	185	29.8	0	6.4	897	125	0
Kielbasa (see also "Polish sausage"):							
(*Boar's Head*), 2 oz. .	120	9.0	0	10.0	50	440	0
(*Healthy Choice* Polska), 2 oz.	80	7.0	6.0	2.5	25	480	0
(*Thorn Apple Valley*), 3.2-oz. link	280	11.0	4.0	25.0	55	700	0
grilled (*Johnsonville*), 3-oz. link	290	14.0	1.0	25.0	65	800	0
turkey, 2 oz.:							
(*Jennie-O*)	70	9.0	0	3.0	55	500	0
(*Louis Rich* Polska)	90	8.0	2.0	6.0	35	850	0
Kimchee (*Frieda's*), ¼ cup, 2 oz.	15	1.0	2.0	0	0	340	1.0
Kippers, see "Herring, kippered"							
Kiwi:							
(*Dole*), 2 medium, 5.2 oz.	100	2.0	24.0	1.0	0	0	4.0
(*Frieda's*), 5 oz.	90	1.0	21.0	.5	0	5	5.0
1 large, 3.7 oz.	55	.9	13.5	.4	0	4	3.1
1 medium, 3.1 oz. . .	46	.8	11.3	.3	0	4	2.6
Kiwi, dried (*Sonoma*), 7–8 pcs., 1 oz. . . .	90	1.0	19.0	1.0	0	0	2.0
Kiwi lime topping (*Smucker's Plate Scrapers*), 2 tbsp. .	100	0	25.0	0	0	10	0
Kiwi-strawberry drink, 8 fl. oz.:							
(*R. W. Knudsen*)	120	<1.0	30.0	0	0	25	0
(*Snapple*)	110	0	28.0	0	0	10.	0
Knockwurst, 1 link:							
(*Ball Park*), 4 oz. . . .	360	12.0	4.0	33.0	80	1320	0
beef:							
(*Ball Park*), 4 oz. .	340	13.0	1.0	32.0	75	1120	0
(*Boar's Head*), 4 oz.	310	15.0	1.0	27.0	50	950	0
(*Hebrew National*), 3 oz.	260	10.0	1.0	24.0	55	670	0
(*Karl Ehmer*), 4 oz.	250	15.0	1.0	20.0	65	850	0
(*Shofar*), 3 oz. . . .	210	10.0	1.0	17.0	40	530	0

Food and Measure	cal.	prot. (gms)	carbo. (gms)	fat (gms)	chol. (mgs)	sod. (mgs)	fiber (gms)
Knockwurst, beef *(cont.)*							
jalapeño (*Hebrew National*), 3 oz. . . .	260	10.0	1.0	24.0	55	670	0
Kohlrabi:							
raw:							
(*Frieda's*), ⅔ cup, 3 oz.	25	1.0	5.0	0	0	15	3.0
sliced, ½ cup	19	1.2	4.3	.1	0	14	2.5
boiled, drained, sliced, ½ cup	24	1.5	5.5	.1	0	17	.9
Kreplach, frozen, meat (*Cohen's*), 3 pcs.	130	8.0	18.0	3.0	20	580	1.0
Krispy Kreme dough-nuts, 1 pc.:							
blueberry, glazed	300	2.0	37.0	15.0	5	200	1.0
blueberry filled, powdered	270	5.0	33.0	13.0	<5	170	1.0
cake, traditional	200	3.0	22.0	11.0	<5	280	<1.0
cinnamon apple filled .	280	5.0	35.0	13.0	<5	180	3.0
cinnamon bun	220	5.0	26.0	11.0	0	160	4.0
cinnamon twist	220	4.0	27.0	11.0	5	150	<1.0
creme filled, glazed . .	350	4.0	39.0	20.0	<5	135	1.0
cruller, glazed	250	2.0	24.0	16.0	5	190	0
devil's food, glazed . .	390	2.0	41.0	24.0	<5	250	5.0
fudge iced:							
cake	230	3.0	28.0	12.0	15	280	<1.0
creme filled	340	5.0	39.0	18.0	<5	160	4.0
custard filled	310	4.0	39.0	16.0	<5	170	5.0
glazed	280	3.0	36.0	14.0	<5	75	1.0
glazed cruller	240	2.0	31.0	12.0	10	160	<1.0
sprinkles	220	2.0	31.0	10.0	<5	95	<1.0
lemon filled, glazed . .	280	5.0	33.0	14.0	<5	160	1.0
maple iced glazed . . .	200	3.0	28.0	9.0	0	100	2.0
original glazed	210	2.0	22.0	12.0	<5	65	0
raspberry filled, glazed	270	4.0	37.0	12.0	<5	170	2.0
Kumquat:							
(*Frieda's*), 5 oz.	90	1.0	23.0	0	0	10	9.0
1 medium, .7 oz. . . .	12	.2	3.1	<.1	0	1	1.3
seeded, 1 oz.	18	.3	4.7	<.1	0	2	1.9
Kun choy, see "Celery, Chinese"							
Kuri squash, see "Red kuri squash"							

L

Food and Measure	cal.	prot. (gms)	carbo. (gms)	fat (gms)	chol. (mgs)	sod. (mgs)	fiber (gms)
Lamb, choice grade, meat only[1], 4 oz., except as noted:							
cubed, leg/shoulder:							
braised or stewed	253	38.2	0	10.0	122	79	0
broiled	211	31.8	0	8.3	102	86	0
foreshank, braised:							
lean w/fat	276	32.2	0	15.3	120	82	0
lean only	212	35.2	0	6.8	118	84	0
ground:							
raw	320	18.8	0	26.5	83	67	0
broiled	321	28.1	0	22.3	110	92	0
broiled, 1 cup	328	28.7	0	23.1	113	94	0
leg, whole, roasted:							
lean w/fat	293	29.0	0	18.7	105	75	0
lean w/fat, 1 slice, 3" diam. x ¼"	73	7.2	0	4.7	26	19	0
lean only	217	32.1	0	8.8	101	77	0
lean only, 3" slice	54	8.0	0	2.2	25	19	0
leg, shank, roasted:							
lean w/fat	255	29.9	0	14.1	102	74	0
lean w/fat, 1 slice, 3" diam. x ¼"	64	7.5	0	3.5	26	18	0
lean only	204	31.9	0	7.6	99	75	0
lean only, 3" slice	51	8.0	0	1.9	25	19	0
leg, sirloin, roasted:							
lean w/fat	331	27.9	0	23.4	110	77	0
lean w/fat, 1 slice, 3" diam. x ¼"	83	7.0	0	5.9	27	19	0
lean only	231	32.1	0	10.4	104	81	0
lean only, 3" slice	58	8.0	0	2.6	26	20	0

1. Retail cuts trimmed to ¼" fat.

Food and Measure	cal.	prot. (gms)	carbo. (gms)	fat (gms)	chol. (mgs)	sod. (mgs)	fiber (gms)
Lamb *(cont.)*							
loin chop, broiled:							
lean w/fat, 2¼ oz.							
(4.2 oz. raw							
w/bone)	201	16.1	0	14.7	64	49	0
lean w/fat	358	28.5	0	26.2	113	87	0
lean only, 1.6 oz.							
(4.2 oz. raw							
w/bone and fat)	100	13.9	0	4.5	44	39	0
lean only	245	34.0	0	11.0	108	95	0
loin, roasted:							
lean w/fat	350	25.6	0	26.8	108	73	0
lean only	229	30.2	0	11.1	99	75	0
rib:							
broiled, lean w/fat	409	25.1	0	33.6	112	86	0
broiled, lean only ..	266	31.5	0	14.7	103	96	0
roasted, lean w/fat	407	24.0	0	33.8	110	83	0
roasted, lean only	263	29.7	0	15.1	100	92	0
shoulder, whole:							
braised, lean w/fat	390	32.5	0	27.8	132	85	0
braised, lean only	321	37.2	0	10.0	133	90	0
roasted, lean w/fat	313	25.5	0	22.6	104	75	0
roasted, lean only	231	28.3	0	12.2	99	77	0
Lamb, New Zealand,							
meat only, 4 oz.:							
foreshank:							
braised, lean w/fat	293	30.6	0	18.0	116	53	0
braised, lean only	211	34.9	0	6.8	115	56	0
leg, whole:							
roasted, lean w/fat	279	28.1	0	17.6	115	49	0
roasted, lean only	205	31.4	0	7.9	113	51	0
loin chop:							
broiled, lean w/fat	357	26.6	0	27.1	127	56	0
broiled, lean only ..	226	33.2	0	9.3	129	62	0
rib:							
roasted, lean w/fat	386	21.5	0	32.6	113	49	0
roasted, lean only	222	27.7	0	11.5	107	54	0
shoulder:							
braised, lean w/fat	405	32.0	0	29.8	139	58	0
braised, lean only	323	38.6	0	17.6	144	64	0
Lamb's quarters,							
boiled, drained,							
chopped, ½ cup ..	29	2.9	4.5	.6	0	26	1.9
Lard, pork, 1 tbsp. ...	115	0	0	12.8	12	<1	0

Food and Measure	cal.	prot. (gms)	carbo. (gms)	fat (gms)	chol. (mgs)	sod. (mgs	fiber (gms)
Lasagna:							
dried, see "Pasta"							
frozen:							
(*Aunt Vi's*), 4 oz. . . .	210	8.0	43.0	.5	0	10	0
roll-ups (*Aunt Vi's*),							
3 oz.	180	9.0	24.0	5.0	20	410	1.0
Lasagna entree, can							
or pkg.:							
(*Dinty Moore American*							
Classics), 1 bowl . .	340	22.0	28.0	16.0	60	990	3.0
meat sauce, 1 cup:							
(*Chef Boyardee*) . . .	270	9.0	41.0	8.0	30	830	2.0
(*Hormel* Microcup)	210	9.0	31.0	6.0	20	840	2.0
Lasagna entree, dried,							
1 serving:							
(*Mountain House*							
Double/Four)	310	17.0	31.0	13.0	35	800	4.0
(*Mountain House*							
Single)	380	21.0	39.0	16.0	45	990	5.0
vegetable (*Mountain*							
House)	210	10.0	33.0	4.0	5	700	6.0
Lasagna entree,							
frozen, 1 pkg.,							
except as noted:							
Alfredo (*Michelina's*),							
9 oz.	360	14.0	38.0	16.0	45	630	2.0
bake:							
(*Healthy Choice*							
Solos), 13.5 oz.	280	15.0	43.0	6.0	40	600	5.0
(*Stouffer's*),							
11.5 oz.	450	25.0	51.0	16.0	45	1110	4.0
cheese:							
(*Amy's*), 10.25 oz.	310	19.0	37.0	11.0	35	680	6.0
(*Celentano* Low Fat),							
10 oz.	290	13.0	40.0	6.0	50	630	3.0
(*Lean Cuisine Every-*							
day Favorites),							
10 oz.	240	13.0	37.0	4.5	10	570	5.0
(*Lean Cuisine Every-*							
day Favorites							
Classic), 11.5 oz.	290	18.0	39.0	7.0	25	630	4.0
extra (*Marie Cal-*							
lender's), 15 oz.	590	27.0	61.0	27.0	50	1230	7.0

Food and Measure	cal.	prot. (gms)	carbo. (gms)	fat (gms)	chol. (mgs)	sod. (mgs)	fiber (gms)
Lasagna entree, frozen, cheese *(cont.)*							
five (*Lean Cuisine Everyday Favorites*), 1/12 of 96-oz. pkg.	210	14.0	27.0	5.0	20	690	3.0
five (*Stouffer's*), 10¾ oz.	340	20.0	39.0	11.0	30	1100	6.0
four (*Marie Callender's*), 10.75 oz.	330	15.0	37.0	13.0	40	1290	5.0
four (*Michelina's*), 8 oz.	290	14.0	43.0	7.0	25	550	3.0
four (*Wolfgang Puck's*), 12 oz.	480	28.0	43.0	22.0	85	680	10.0
chicken:							
(*Lean Cuisine Cafe Classics*), 10 oz.	270	16.0	34.0	8.0	35	690	3.0
(*Lean Cuisine Everyday Favorites*), 10 oz.	280	20.0	34.0	7.0	40	590	2.0
(*Lean Cuisine Everyday Favorites*), 1/12 of 96-oz. pkg.	200	15.0	26.0	4.5	20	690	3.0
(*Michelina's*), 8 oz.	280	17.0	33.0	10.0	45	480	2.0
(*Stouffer's Family Style Favorites*), 1 cup or 1/5 of 39-oz. pkg.	310	15.0	29.0	15.0	30	760	3.0
spicy (*Wolfgang Puck's*), 12 oz.	470	26.0	45.0	21.0	85	680	13.0
ground beef, marinara (*Mamma Rita's*), 1/2 of 18-oz. pkg.	370	27.0	24.0	19.0	70	410	2.0
meat:							
(*Healthy Choice Medley*), 10.6 oz.	360	23.0	46.0	9.0	30	600	7.0
(*Marie Callender's*), 10.5 oz.	350	20.0	33.0	16.0	55	1190	6.0
(*Marie Callender's* 21 oz.), 1 cup ..	280	15.0	26.0	12.0	45	830	4.0
(*Marie Callender's* Family 40/96 oz.), 1 cup	310	13.0	27.0	16.0	45	600	2.0
(*Wolfgang Puck's*), 12 oz.	490	24.0	51.0	22.0	55	800	4.0

Food and Measure	cal.	prot. (gms)	carbo. (gms)	fat (gms)	chol. (mgs)	sod. (mgs)	fiber (gms)
meat sauce:							
(*Banquet*), 11 oz. . .	320	15.0	46.0	9.0	20	1170	7.0
(*Banquet* Family), 1 cup	270	14.0	33.0	10.0	45	600	2.0
(*Budget Gourmet*), 8.5 oz.	250	12.0	34.0	7.0	20	580	3.0
(*Freezer Queen* Homestyle), 10 oz.	290	13.0	42.0	8.0	15	1530	5.0
(*Freezer Queen* Deluxe Family), 1 cup	270	12.0	39.0	8.0	15	930	4.0
(*Lean Cuisine Everyday Favorites*), 10.5 oz.	300	19.0	38.0	8.0	30	590	4.0
(*Marie Callender's*), 15 oz.	630	29.0	59.0	31.0	75	1230	3.0
(*Michelina's*), 8 oz.	240	15.0	29.0	7.0	25	930	3.0
(*Michelina's*), 9 oz.	290	16.0	39.0	8.0	35	810	3.0
(*Michelina's*), 10 oz.	410	23.0	47.0	13.0	55	1250	4.0
(*Stouffer's*), 10.5 oz.	370	27.0	35.0	14.0	45	1050	4.0
(*Stouffer's*), 21 oz., 1 cup or ⅓ pkg.	270	18.0	28.0	9.0	35	720	3.0
w/meat and sauce:							
(*Stouffer's Family Style Favorites*), ⅕ of 40-oz. pkg.	270	16.0	28.0	10.0	30	620	3.0
(*Stouffer's Family Style Favorites*), 1/12 of 96-oz. pkg.	270	16.0	28.0	10.0	30	620	3.0
mozzarella (*Budget Gourmet*), 8 oz. . .	300	11.0	45.0	8.0	10	590	3.0
mushroom (*Wolfgang Puck's*), 12 oz. . . .	410	18.0	49.0	16.0	25	320	9.0
pomodoro (*Michelina's*), 8 oz.	270	13.0	29.0	11.0	30	720	1.0
primavera:							
(*Celentano*), 10 oz.	260	11.0	39.0	4.5	40	410	4.0
(*Michelina's*), 8 oz.	270	10.0	35.0	10.0	25	670	2.0
spinach (*Cascadian Farm*), 11 oz.	330	18.0	42.0	10.0	30	670	4.0
tomato sauce, sausage (*Stouffer's*), 10⅞ oz.	420	20.0	43.0	19.0	50	1190	4.0
vegetable:							
(*Amy's*), 9.5 oz. . .	300	15.0	39.0	10.0	15	680	5.0

Food and Measure	cal.	prot. (gms)	carbo. (gms)	fat (gms)	chol. (mgs)	sod. (mgs)	fiber (gms)
Lasagna entree, frozen, vegetable *(cont.)*							
(*Amy's* Family), ⅙ of 42-oz. pkg. ...	200	10.0	26.0	8.0	10	480	3.0
(*Lean Cuisine Everyday Favorites*), 10.5 oz.	260	17.0	33.0	7.0	20	580	4.0
(*Michelina's*), 8 oz.	210	12.0	30.0	5.0	15	670	3.0
(*Michelina's*), 8.5 oz.	240	13.0	35.0	6.0	25	690	3.0
(*Stouffer's*), 10.5 oz.	410	19.0	42.0	18.0	30	870	4.0
(*Stouffer's Family Style Favorites*), ¹⁄₁₂ of 96-oz. pkg.	320	7.0	30.0	16.0	20	820	4.0
garden (*Cedarlane*), 10 oz.	280	21.0	48.0	2.0	5	680	5.0
Italian (*Wolfgang Puck's*), 12 oz.	440	20.0	53.0	16.0	30	430	9.0
tofu (*Amy's*), 9.5 oz.	300	13.0	41.0	10.0	0	630	6.0
vegetarian:							
(*Quorn*), 10.6 oz. .	360	23.0	43.0	12.0	15	910	4.0
(*Yves* Veggie), 10.5 oz.	300	17.0	51.0	3.0	0	650	4.0
Lasagna entree, refrigerated, 1 cup:							
cheese (*DeLuca*)	200	11.0	16.0	10.0	40	740	1.0
meat (*DeLuca*)	260	14.0	18.0	18.0	65	840	2.0
Lasagna mix (*Lipton Sizzle & Stir*), 3 oz. mix	190	7.0	32.0	4.0	<5	890	2.0
Lavash, see "Cracker"							
Leek, w/lower leaf portion, fresh:							
raw:							
(*Frieda's*), 1 cup, 3 oz.	50	1.0	12.0	0	0	15	2.0
9.9-oz. leek	76	1.9	17.6	.4	0	25	2.2
chopped, ½ cup ..	32	.8	7.4	.2	0	10	.9
boiled, drained:							
4.4-oz. leek	38	.2	9.5	.3	0	12	1.2
chopped, ½ cup ..	16	.4	4.0	.1	0	5	.5
Leek, freeze-dried, 1 tbsp.	1	<.1	.2	tr.	0	<1	<1.0
Lemon, fresh:							
(*Dole*), 1 medium ...	15	0	5.0	0	0	5	1.0
2⅛" lemon, 3.8 oz. ..	22	1.3	11.6	.3	0	3	n.a.

Food and Measure	cal.	prot. (gms)	carbo. (gms)	fat (gms)	chol. (mgs)	sod. (mgs)	fiber (gms)
1 wedge, ¼ medium .	5	.3	2.9	.1	0	1	n.a.
peeled, 2⅛" lemon . . .	17	.6	5.4	.2	0	1	1.6
Lemon butter dill sauce, 2 tbsp.:							
(*Golden Dipt*)	120	0	4.0	10.0	0	210	0
(*Golden Dipt* Fat Free)	35	0	7.0	0	0	210	0
Lemon curd:							
(*Crosse & Blackwell*), 1 tbsp.	50	0	13.0	0	0	0	0
(*Dickenson's*), 2 tbsp.	65	0	15.0	0	15	15	2.0
(*Grant's*), 1 tbsp. . . .	40	0	10.0	0	0	15	0
(*Laird's Larder*), 1 tbsp.	60	0	25.0	1.0	0	25	0
Lemongrass, fresh:							
1 tbsp.	5	.1	1.2	<.1	0	<1	n.a.
1 cup	66	.5	16.9	.3	0	4	n.a.
Lemongrass, in jar, hearts (*A Taste of Thai*), .3-oz. pc. . .	0	0	1.0	0	0	0	1.0
Lemon herb sauce mix (*Knorr* Classic), 1 tbsp.	30	<1.0	4.0	1.0	0	260	0
Lemon juice, fresh:							
½ cup	31	.5	10.5	0	0	1	.5
1 tbsp.	4	.1	1.3	0	0	<1	.1
Lemon juice, can or jar:							
(*Santa Cruz Organic*), 1 tsp.	0	0	0	0	0	0	0
½ cup	26	.5	7.9	.4	0	1	.5
Lemon peel, fresh, 1 tbsp.	—¹	.1	1.0	<.1	0	0	.6
Lemon peel, candied diced:							
(*Seneca* Glacé), 2 tbsp.	70	0	18.0	0	0	20	1.0
(*S&W* Glacé), 58 pcs., 1.1 oz.	80	0	23.0	0	0	25	2.0
Lemon pepper:							
(*Lawry's*), ¼ tsp. . . .	0	0	0	0	0	80	0
(*McCormick*), ¼ tsp.	0	0	0	0	0	30	0
1 tsp.	7	.2	1.5	0	0	425	.3

1. *Cannot be calculated; no digestibility value for fresh peel.*

Food and Measure	cal.	prot. (gms)	carbo. (gms)	fat (gms)	chol. (mgs)	sod. (mgs)	fiber (gms)
Lemon pepper salt (*McCormick*), ¼ tsp.	0	0	0	0	0	130	0
Lemon sauce, Oriental (*Ka•Me*), 1 tbsp. . .	45	0	11.0	0	0	125	0
Lemonade, 8 fl. oz., except as noted:							
(*After the Fall*)	90	0	23.0	0	0	10	0
(*Crystal Light*)	5	0	0	0	0	5	0
(*Horizon*)	110	0	27.0	0	0	0	0
(*R. W. Knudsen* Natural)	120	<1.0	29.0	0	0	35	0
(*R. W. Knudsen* Aseptic)	110	1.0	27.0	0	0	35	0
(*Newman's Own*)	110	0	27.0	0	0	40	0
(*Santa Cruz Organic*) .	100	<1.0	24.0	0	0	0	0
(*Snapple*)	120	0	30.0	0	0	10	0
(*Tropicana*)	110	<1.0	28.0	0	0	20	0
(*Turkey Hill*)	120	0	29.0	0	0	10	0
pink:							
(*AriZona*)	110	0	28.0	0	0	25	0
(*Snapple*)	110	0	26.0	0	0	10	0
frozen*:							
(*Cascadian Farm*) .	110	0	28.0	0	0	9	0
(*Minute Maid*)	110	0	30.0	0	0	0	0
pink	99	.3	25.9	0	0	7	0
white	99	.3	26.0	0	0	7	.3
Lemonade fruit blends, 8 fl. oz.:							
cherry or cranberry (*R. W. Knudsen*) . .	120	<1.0	29.0	0	0	35	0
raspberry:							
(*Santa Cruz Organic*)	100	0	24.0	0	0	0	0
(*Turkey Hill*)	120	0	29.0	0	0	10	0
strawberry:							
(*Santa Cruz Organic*)	100	<1.0	24.0	0	0	0	0
kiwi (*Turkey Hill*) . .	120	0	29.0	0	0	10	0
Lemonade, mix*, 8 fl. oz.:							
(*Country Time*)	70	0	17.0	0	0	25	0
(*Country Time* Sugar Free)	5	0	0	0	0	0	0
(*Crystal Light*)	5	0	0	0	0	0	0
(*Kool-Aid* Sugar Sweetened)	70	0	17.0	0	0	0	0

Food and Measure	cal.	prot. (gms)	carbo. (gms)	fat (gms)	chol. (mgs)	sod. (mgs)	fiber (gms)
(*Kool-Aid Slushies* Lemon Ice)	140	0	35.0	0	0	70	1.0
blue raspberry:							
(*Kool-Aid* Sugar Sweetened)	70	0	17.0	0	0	5	0
(*Kool-Aid Slushies*)	140	0	35.0	0	0	70	1.0
raspberry (*Country Time Lem'n Berry Sippers*)	80	0	19.0	0	0	0	0
strawberry:							
(*Country Time Lem'n Berry Sippers*) . .	80	0	20.0	0	0	0	0
(*Kool-Aid Soarin' Strawberry*)	70	0	17.0	0	0	15	0
Lemon-lime drink mix* (*Kool-Aid* Unsweetened), 8 fl. oz.	0	0	0	0	0	5	0
Lentil:							
dry, ¼ cup:							
(*Goya*)	70	8.0	19.0	0	0	5	9.0
green	162	13.5	27.4	.5	0	5	14.6
green or red (*Arrowhead Mills*)	150	11.0	27.0	0	0	15	9.0
pink	166	11.9	28.4	1.0	0	3	5.2
cooked, ½ cup	115	8.9	19.9	.4	0	2	7.8
Lentil, canned, ½ cup:							
(*Eden* Organic)	90	8.0	13.0	0	0	210	4.0
(*Westbrae Natural*) . .	80	6.0	13.0	0	0	140	5.0
Lentil, dehydrated (*AlpineAire*), 1 oz. . .	80	7.0	0	6.0	0	0	6.0
Lentil, sprouted, raw, ½ cup	40	3.4	8.4	.2	0	4	n.a.
Lentil dish, mix:							
chili (*Taste Adventure*), ¾ cup	230	19.0	40.0	1.0	0	500	18.0
dahl, 1 cup*:							
(*Neera's* Chaunk) . .	140	11.0	23.0	1.0	0	4	12.0
(*Neera's* Urad and Channa)	105	8.0	18.0	1.0	0	4	9.0
pilaf:							
(*Casbah*), ¾ cup . .	240	9.0	38.0	.5	0	400	2.0
(*Near East*), 1 cup*	200	11.0	36.0	3.5	10	660	8.0

Food and Measure	cal.	prot. (gms)	carbo. (gms)	fat (gms)	chol. (mgs)	sod. (mgs)	fiber (gms)
Lentil entree, packaged, w/rice, 1 pkg.:							
chili (*Tamarind Tree Dal Makhani*)	330	14.0	55.0	6.0	5	670	14.0
w/vegetables (*Tamarind Tree Channa Dal Masala*)	340	13.0	62.0	5.0	0	700	10.0
Lentil rice dish mix, curry (*Taste Adventure Quick Cuisine Bombay*), ⅓ cup . .	150	5.0	32.0	.5	0	250	3.0
Lentil rice loaf, frozen (*Natural Touch*), 1" slice, 3.2 oz . . .	160	8.0	16.0	7.0	0	370	4.0
Lettuce (see also "Salad blend" and "Salad kit"):							
(*Dole* Greener Selection), 3 oz.	15	1.0	3.0	0	0	10	1.0
(*Dolo* Just I ettuce), 3 oz.	15	1.0	3.0	0	0	10	1.0
bibb or Boston:							
1 head, 5" diam. . .	21	2.1	3.8	.4	0	8	1.6
2 inner leaves	2	.2	.4	<.1	0	1	.5
butterhead (*Frieda's* Limestone), ⅔ cup, 3 oz.	10	1.0	2.0	0	0	10	1.0
iceberg:							
(*Dole*), ⅙ medium head	15	1.0	3.0	0	0	10	1.0
(*Dole* Classic Salad), 3 oz.	15	1.0	4.0	0	0	15	1.0
1 head, 6" diam. . .	70	5.4	11.3	1.0	0	48	7.5
1 leaf, .7 oz.	3	.2	.4	<.1	0	2	.3
iceberg, shredded:							
(*Dole*), 3 oz.	15	1.0	3.0	0	0	10	1.0
(*Fresh Express Shreds!*), 1½ cups	15	1.0	3.0	0	0	10	1.0
1 cup	7	.6	1.2	.1	0	3	.8
leaf, shredded (*Dole*), 1½ cups	15	1.0	4.0	0	0	30	2.0
loose-leaf, shredded, ½ cup	5	.4	1.0	.1	0	3	.5

Food and Measure	cal.	prot. (gms)	carbo. (gms)	fat (gms)	chol. (mgs)	sod. (mgs)	fiber (gms)
romaine or cos:							
(*Dole*), 6 leaves,							
3 oz.	20	1.0	3.0	0	0	0	1.0
(*Dole* Classic Salad),							
3 oz.	15	1.0	4.0	0	0	10	1.0
(*Fresh Express*),							
3 oz.	15	1.0	2.0	0	0	5	1.0
(*Ready Pac* Bella),							
1½ cups, 3 oz. . .	15	1.0	2.0	0	0	5	1.0
(*Ready Pac* Organic							
Caesar), 2¾ cups,							
3 oz.	15	<1.0	2.0	0	0	10	<1.0
1 inner leaf	1	.2	.2	0	0	1	.2
shredded, ½ cup . .	4	.5	.7	.1	0	2	.5
romaine hearts:							
(*Dole*), 3 oz.	15	1.0	3.0	0	0	5	1.0
(*Dole* Organic Blend							
Mix), 3 oz.	15	1.0	3.0	0	0	10	1.0
(*Fresh Express*) . . .	15	1.0	2.0	0	0	5	1.0
jumbo (*Andy Boy*),							
6 leaves, 3 oz. . .	20	1.0	3.0	.5	0	0	1.0
Lima beans:							
immature, ½ cup:							
raw, trimmed	88	5.3	15.7	.7	0	6	3.8
boiled, drained	104	5.8	20.1	.3	0	14	4.5
mature:							
dry (*Frieda's*),							
⅓ cup, 3 oz. . . .	120	8.0	20.0	0	0	530	8.0
baby, dry (*Goya*),							
¼ cup	70	8.0	23.0	0	0	15	15.0
baby, dry (*Jack							
Rabbit*), ¼ cup	70	8.0	23.0	0	0	15	15.0
baby, boiled, ½ cup	115	7.3	21.2	.3	0	2	7.0
large, dry (*Jack							
Rabbit*), ¼ cup	70	7.0	22.0	0	0	20	12.0
large, boiled, ½ cup	108	7.3	19.6	.4	0	2	6.6
Lima beans, can or jar,							
½ cup:							
(*Aunt Nellie's* Reber							
Butter Beans)	140	7.0	25.0	1.0	0	530	6.0
(*Libby's* Lima)	80	3.0	18.0	0	0	280	5.0
(*S&W* Butterbeans) . .	80	6.0	19.0	0	0	500	5.0
baby:							
(*Allens* Butterbeans)	120	7.0	22.0	.5	0	460	6.0

Lima beans, can or jar, baby *(cont.)*

Food and Measure	cal.	prot. (gms)	carho. (gms)	fat (gms)	chol. (mgs)	sod. (mgs)	fiber (gms)
(*Bush's Best* Butterbeans)	120	7.0	19.0	.5	0	510	5.0
(*Eden* Organic) ...	100	6.0	17.0	1.0	0	35	4.0
green:							
(*Allens/East Texas Fair* Limas)	120	7.0	23.0	0	0	370	8.0
(*Bush's Best* Butterbeans)	110	6.0	19.0	1.0	0	340	6.0
(*Del Monte*)	80	4.0	15.0	0	0	390	4.0
(*Sunshine* Butterbeans)	120	7.0	23.0	0	0	370	8.0
baby (*Veg-All* Limas)	90	4.0	15.0	1.0	0	330	3.0
medium (*Bush's Best* Green Limas)	110	6.0	17.0	1.0	0	310	5.0
small (*Bush's Best* Green Limas) ...	100	5.0	16.0	1.0	0	320	5.0
small (*S&W* Limas)	80	4.0	15.0	0	0	390	4.0
green and white (*Allens* Limas)	110	6.0	20.0	1.0	0	280	9.0
large:							
(*Allens* Butterbeans)	120	7.0	20.0	1.0	0	290	7.0
(*Bush's Best* Butterbeans)	100	6.0	18.0	.5	0	450	5.0
speckled (*Bush's Best* Butterbeans)	110	6.0	19.0	.5	0	420	5.0
w/bacon, baby:							
green (*Trappey's* Limas)	120	6.0	22.0	1.0	0	330	6.0
white (*Trappey's* Limas)	130	8.0	21.0	1.5	0	350	6.0
w/sausage, large white (*Trappey's* Butterbeans)	110	6.0	21.0	1.0	0	300	6.0
seasoned:							
(*Glory Foods* Butter Beans)	120	7.0	20.0	1.0	0	530	5.0
(*Glory Foods* Limas) 140		8.0	24.0	1.0	0	620	7.0

Lima beans, frozen,
½ cup, except as
noted:

Food and Measure	cal.	prot. (gms)	carbo. (gms)	fat (gms)	chol. (mgs)	sod. (mgs)	fiber (gms)
(*Birds Eye* Southern Butter Beans/ Speckled Butter Beans)	100	6.0	22.0	0	0	140	5.0
(*McKenzie's* Baby) ...	110	6.0	22.0	.5	0	140	5.0
(*McKenzie's* Butter Beans/Speckled Butter Beans)	100	6.0	20.0	0	0	130	4.0
baby:							
(*Birds Eye*)	130	7.0	24.0	0	0	115	6.0
(*Green Giant*)	80	5.0	16.0	0	0	140	3.0
(*John Cope's*)	110	6.0	22.0	0	0	140	5.0
(*Seabrook Farms* Petite)	110	6.0	22.0	0	0	140	5.0
boiled, drained	95	6.0	17.5	.3	0	26	5.4
Fordhook (*Birds Eye*) .	100	6.0	19.0	0	0	10	5.0
Lime, fresh:							
(*Frieda's* Key), 3-oz. lime	25	1.0	9.0	0	0	0	2.0
2"-diam. lime	20	.5	7.1	.1	0	1	1.9
peeled, seeded, 1 oz.	9	.2	3.0	.1	0	1	.8
Lime curd (*Crosse & Blackwell*), 1 tbsp.	50	0	13.0	0	0	0	0
Lime drink (*Kool-Aid Bursts*), 6.75 fl. oz.	100	0	24.0	0	0	35	0
Lime drink blends, 8 fl. oz.:							
(*After the Fall* Key West)	100	1.0	25.0	0	0	10	0
(*R. W. Knudsen* Cactus Quencher)	120	<1.0	29.0	0	0	35	0
frozen* (*Minute Maid* Limeade)	100	0	26.0	0	0	0	0
Lime juice, fresh:							
½ cup	33	.5	11.1	.1	0	1	.5
1 tbsp.	4	.1	1.4	<.1	0	tr.	.1
Lime juice, in jars:							
sweetened (*Rose's*), 1 tbsp.	90	0	22.0	0	0	10	0
unsweetened:							
(*Key Largo*), 1 tsp.	0	0	0	0	0	0	0
(*Rose's*), 2 tbsp. ..	10	0	2.0	0	0	0	0
(*Santa Cruz Organic*), 1 tsp.	0	0	0	0	0	0	0
2 tbsp.	6	<.1	2.0	<.1	0	5	.1

Food and Measure	cal.	prot. (gms)	carbo. (gms)	fat (gms)	chol. (mgs)	sod. (mgs)	fiber (gms)
Lime relish, Indian, 1 tbsp.:							
hot (*Patak's*)	30	<1.0	.5	3.0	0	520	<1.0
mild (*Patak's*)	30	0	0	3.0	0	530	0
Limeade, see "Lime drink"							
Ling, meat only:							
raw, 4 oz.	99	21.5	0	.7	45	153	0
baked, broiled, micro- waved, 4 oz.	126	27.6	0	.9	58	196	0
Ling cod, meat only:							
raw, 4 oz.	96	20.0	0	1.2	59	67	0
baked, broiled, or microwaved, 4 oz.	124	25.7	0	1.5	76	86	0
Linguica sausage (*Caspar's*), 2 oz. . .	120	10.0	1.0	9.0	30	360	0
Linguine:							
dry, see "Pasta"							
refrigerated:							
(*Buitoni*), 1¼ cups	240	10.0	45.0	2.5	90	20	2.0
(*Di Giorno*), 2.5 oz., ¼ pkg.	200	8.0	38.0	1.5	0	140	2.0
Linguine dish, mix, 1 cup*:							
chicken and broccoli (*Pasta Roni*)	380	11.0	49.0	15.0	5	990	2.0
chicken Parmesan, creamy (*Pasta Roni*)	410	13.0	51.0	18.0	10	1250	3.0
Linguine entree, frozen, 1 pkg.:							
w/clams and sauce (*Michelina's*), 8.5 oz.	290	11.0	51.0	3.0	10	550	2.0
w/clams and shrimp (*Budget Gourmet*), 8 oz.	300	13.0	48.0	6.0	45	240	2.0
Liquor[1], 1 fl. oz.:							
80 proof	64	0	0	0	0	tr.	0
90 proof	73	0	0	0	0	tr.	0
100 proof	82	0	0	0	0	tr.	0
Litchi, see "Lychee"							

---

1. *Includes all pure distilled liquors: bourbon, brandy, gin, rum, Scotch, tequila, vodka, etc.*

Food and Measure	cal.	prot. (gms)	carbo. (gms)	fat (gms)	chol. (mgs)	sod. (mgs)	fiber (gms)
Liver:							
beef, panfried, 4 oz. . .	246	30.3	8.9	9.1	547	120	0
chicken, simmered:							
4 oz.	178	27.6	1.0	6.2	716	58	0
chopped, 1 cup . . .	219	34.1	1.2	7.6	883	71	0
duck, raw, 1 oz.	39	5.3	1.0	1.3	146	n.a.	0
goose, raw, 1 oz. . . .	38	4.6	1.8	1.2	146	40	0
lamb, panfried, 4 oz. .	270	29.0	4.3	14.3	559	141	0
pork, braised, 4 oz. . .	187	29.5	4.3	5.0	403	56	0
turkey, simmered:							
4 oz.	192	27.2	3.9	6.7	710	73	0
chopped, 1 cup . . .	237	33.6	4.8	8.3	876	89	0
veal (calves),							
braised, 4 oz.	187	24.5	3.1	7.8	636	60	0
panfried, 4 oz. . . .	278	33.8	4.5	12.9	374	150	0
Liver cheese (*Oscar Mayer*), 1.3-oz. slice	120	6.0	<1.0	10.0	80	420	0
Liver pâté, see "Pâté"							
Liver spread, frozen, chopped (*Weinberg's*), 2 oz.	100	6.0	4.0	7.0	110	230	0
"Liver" spread, vegetarian (*Sabra Salads*), 1 oz.	70	.9	1.4	6.7	14	87	.9
Liverwurst (see also "Braunschweiger" and "Pâté"), 2 oz.:							
(*Boar's Head* Strassburger)	170	8.0	1.0	15.0	85	560	0
(*Hansel 'n Gretel*) . . .	170	9.0	4.0	13.0	95	730	0
smoked (*Boar's Head*)	170	8.0	1.0	15.0	45	620	0
Lo bok, see "Radish, Oriental"							
Lobster, northern, meat only:							
raw, 4 oz.	102	21.3	.6	1.0	108	n.a.	0
boiled or steamed:							
4 oz.	111	23.2	1.5	.7	82	431	0
1 cup, 5.1 oz.	142	29.7	1.9	.9	104	551	0
"Lobster," imitation, frozen:							
chunk style (*Louis Kemp Lobster Delights*), ½ cup, 3 oz.	80	8.0	12.0	0	10	420	0

Food and Measure	cal.	prot. (gms)	carbo. (gms)	fat (gms)	chol. (mgs)	sod. (mqs)	fiber (gms)
"Lobster," imitation *(cont.)*							
salad (*Louis Kemp Lobster Delights*), ½ cup, 3 oz.	80	8.0	12.0	0	10	420	0
Lobster, spiny, see "Spiny lobster"							
Lobster sauce (*Progresso*), ½ cup . . .	100	3.0	6.0	7.0	5	430	2.0
Loganberries, fresh, 1 cup	89	1.4	21.5	.9	0	1	n.a.
Loganberries, canned in light syrup (*Oregon*), ½ cup	105	<1.0	25.0	.5	0	0	5.0
Longanberries, frozen, ½ cup	40	1.1	9.6	.2	0	1	3.6
Long bean, see "Yardlong bean"							
Long John Silver's:							
entrees:							
clams, breaded, 2.5 oz.	250	9.0	26.0	14.0	35	580	n.a.
chicken plank, battered, 1.85-oz. pc. . . .	140	8.0	9.0	8.0	20	400	n.a.
crab cake, 2-oz. pc.	150	4.0	12.0	9.0	15	180	n.a.
fish:							
battered, 3.25-oz. pc.	230	12.0	16.0	13.0	30	700	n.a.
battered, Jr. . . . 1.6-oz. pc. . . .	120	12.0	8.0	8.0	15	410	n.a.
breaded, chunky 2.8-oz. pc. . .	200	10.0	17.0	10.0	10	300	n.a.
lemon crumb, 2 pcs., 5.3 oz.	210	23.0	10.0	12.0	55	790	n.a.
lemon crumb, a la carte, 2 pcs. w/rice, 10.3 oz.	480	27.0	52.0	17.0	55	1490	n.a.
lemon crumb, Add-a-Piece, 1 pc. w/rice, 3.15 oz.	150	12.0	9.0	7.0	30	460	n.a.
lemon crumb meal, 16.6 oz.	730	31.0	89.0	29.0	60	1720	n.a.

Food and Measure	cal.	prot. (gms)	carbo. (gms)	fat (gms)	chol. (mgs)	sod. (mgs)	fiber (gms)
shrimp:							
battered, 1 pc.	45	2.0	3.0	2.5	15	125	n.a.
popcorn, 4 oz.	320	15.0	33.0	15.0	85	1440	n.a.
sandwiches, 1 pc.:							
chicken	340	13.0	40.0	14.0	25	840	n.a.
chicken, w/cheese	390	16.0	40.0	19.0	40	1090	n.a.
fish	340	11.0	40.0	15.0	20	800	n.a.
fish, w/cheese	480	19.0	46.0	25.0	50	1390	n.a.
Ultimate Fish	480	19.0	46.0	25.0	50	1400	n.a.
wrap, 12.5 oz.	840	20.0	99.0	41.0	10	2180	n.a.
soup, 8-oz.cup:							
broccoli-cheese ...	180	5.0	13.0	12.0	15	1240	n.a.
clam chowder	260	12.0	26.0	12.0	35	1020	n.a.
salads, no dressing:							
chicken, grilled ...	140	20.0	10.0	2.5	45	260	n.a.
garden	45	3.0	9.0	0	0	25	n.a.
ocean chef	130	14.0	15.0	2.0	60	540	4.0
side salad	20	1.0	3.0	0	0	10	<1.0
salad dressing, 1 pkt.:							
French, fat free ...	40	0	10.0	0	0	240	0
ranch	170	0	1.0	18.0	10	260	0
ranch, fat free	40	0	9.0	0	0	290	0
Thousand Island ..	120	0	5.0	10.0	15	290	0
sides and soup:							
cheese sticks, 3 ...	160	6.0	12.0	9.0	10	360	<1.0
coleslaw, 4 oz. ...	170	2.0	23.0	7.0	0	310	n.a.
corn cobbette:							
plain	80	3.0	19.0	.5	0	0	0
w/butter	140	3.0	19.0	8.0	0	0	0
fries, large, 5 oz. ..	420	5.0	46.0	24.0	0	830	n.a.
fries, regular, 3 oz.	250	3.0	28.0	15.0	0	500	3.0
hush puppy, 1 pc.	60	1.0	9.0	2.5	0	25	0
rice, 4 oz.	180	3.0	34.0	4.0	0	560	n.a.
sauces/condiments, 1 pkt.:							
honey mustard ...	20	0	5.0	0	0	65	0
ketchup	10	0	2.0	0	0	110	0
malt vinegar	0	0	0	0	0	15	0
shrimp sauce	15	0	3.0	0	0	180	0
sweet and sour ...	20	0	5.0	0	0	45	0
tartar sauce	40	0	2.0	3.5	5	105	0
dessert pie:							
apple, Dutch	290	2.0	44.0	13.0	0	250	n.a.
banana split sundae	300	4.0	34.0	17.0	15	130	n.a.

Food and Measure	cal.	prot. (gms)	carbo. (gms)	fat (gms)	chol. (mgs)	sod. (mgs)	fiber (gms)
Long John Silver's, dessert pie *(cont.)*							
chocolate creme ..	280	4.0	29.0	17.0	15	125	n.a.
lemon, double	350	6.0	41.0	18.0	40	180	n.a.
pecan	390	3.0	53.0	19.0	40	250	n.a.
pineapple creme							
cheesecake	310	4.0	36.0	17.0	5	105	n.a.
strawberry creme	280	4.0	32.0	15.0	15	130	n.a.
Longan, fresh:							
1 medium	2	<.1	.5	0	0	0	tr.
seeded, 1 oz.	17	.4	4.3	<.1	0	<1	.3
Longan, dried, 1 oz.	81	1.4	21.0	.1	0	14	<1.0
Loquat:							
(*Frieda's*), 5 oz.	70	1.0	17.0	0	0	0	2.0
1 large, .7 oz.	9	<.1	2.4	0	0	tr.	.3
cubed, 1 cup	70	.6	18.1	.3	0	1	2.5
peeled, seeded, 1 oz.	13	.1	3.4	.1	0	<1	.5
Lotus root:							
raw:							
(*Frieda's*), 3 oz.	50	2.0	15.0	0	0	35	4.0
10 slices	60	2.1	14.0	.1	0	32	4.0
trimmed, 1 oz. ...	16	.7	4.9	<.1	0	11	1.4
boiled, drained, ½ cup	40	1.0	9.6	< 1	0	27	1.9
Lotus seed:							
raw, 1 oz.	25	1.2	4.9	.2	0	<1	n.a.
dried, 1 oz.	94	4.4	18.3	.6	0	1	n.a.
fried, 1 cup	106	4.9	20.6	.6	0	1	n.a.
Lox, see "Salmon, smoked"							
Lunch meat, loaf (see also specific listings), 1 oz., except as noted:							
Dutch brand (*Oscar Mayer*), 2 oz.	150	7.0	2.0	12.0	25	610	0
honey (*Oscar Mayer*)	35	5.0	1.0	1.0	15	380	0
mother's loaf, pork ..	80	3.4	2.1	6.3	13	320	0
olive:							
(*Boar's Head*), 2 oz.	130	6.0	<1.0	12.0	20	630	0
(*Oscar Mayer*)	70	3.0	2.0	6.0	20	350	0
pickle and pepper (*Boar's Head*), 2 oz.	150	6.0	2.0	13.0	30	500	0
pickle and pimiento (*Oscar Mayer*)	70	3.0	2.0	6.0	20	350	0
spiced (*Oscar Mayer*)	60	4.0	2.0	4.5	20	340	0

Food and Measure	cal.	prot. (gms)	carbo. (gms)	fat (gms)	chol. (mgs)	sod. (mgs)	fiber (gms)
Lunch meat, canned, 2 oz.:							
(*Spam/Spam* Smoked)	170	7.0	0	16.0	40	750	0
(*Spam* Less Salt)	170	7.0	0	16.0	40	560	0
(*Spam* Lite)	110	9.0	0	8.0	45	560	0
turkey (*Spam*)	70	10.0	1.0	3.0	30	420	0
pork (*Goya*)	180	8.0	1.0	16.0	45	590	0
Lupin, boiled, ½ cup .	98	12.9	8.2	2.4	0	3	2.3
Lupin, in jars (*Pastene* Lupini), 2 oz.	30	1.0	8.0	0	0	460	1.0
Lychee, fresh:							
1 fruit	6	.1	1.6	0	0	0	.1
shelled:							
1 cup	125	1.6	31.4	.8	0	2	2.5
1 oz.	19	.2	4.7	.1	0	<1	.4
Lychee, dried, 1 oz. .	78	1.1	20.0	.3	0	1	1.3
Lychee juice blend (*Ceres*), 5.25 fl. oz.	87	0	21.0	0	0	n.a.	0
Lyonnaise gravy mix (*Knorr*), 2 tsp. ...	20	<1.0	4.0	.5	0	370	0

M

Food and Measure	cal.	prot. (gms)	carbo. (gms)	fat (gms)	chol. (mgs)	sod. (mgs)	fiber (gms)
Macadamia nuts:							
(*Frieda's*), 1.1 oz. . . .	210	2.0	4.0	22.0	0	0	3.0
(*Mauna Loa*), 1 oz. . .	210	2.0	5.0	20.0	0	70	2.0
raw, whole or halves:							
1 oz.	204	2.2	3.9	21.5	0	1	2.4
¼ cup	241	2.7	4.6	25.4	0	2	2.9
dried, shelled:							
1 oz.	199	2.4	3.9	20.9	0	1	2.6
¼ cup	235	2.8	4.6	24.7	0	2	3.1
dry-roasted:							
1 oz.	204	2.2	3.8	21.8	0	1	2.3
whole or halves,							
¼ cup	241	2.6	4.5	25.5	0	1	2.7
diced (*Blue Dia-*							
mond), ¼ cup . .	240	3.0	5.0	24.0	0	0	3.0
oil-roasted, 1 oz. . . .	204	2.1	3.7	21.7	0	2	n.a.
honey-roasted (*Mauna*							
Loa), 1 oz.	210	2.0	6.0	21.0	0	35	2.0
onion-garlic (*Mauna*							
Loa), 1.4-oz. pkg. .	320	3.0	5.0	31.0	0	190	3.0
Macaroni (see also							
"Pasta"):							
uncooked:							
(*Mueller's*), 2 oz. . .	210	7.0	42.0	1.0	0	0	1.0
2 oz.	210	7.3	42.4	.9	0	4	1.4
elbow, 1 cup	389	13.4	78.4	1.7	0	8	2.5
enriched, 2 oz. . . .	213	11.3	38.3	1.3	0	5	1.4
whole wheat, 2 oz. .	198	.3	42.8	.8	0	5	4.7
cooked, 1 cup:							
enriched, elbows . .	197	6.7	39.7	.9	0	1	1.8
enriched, spirals . .	189	6.4	38.0	.9	0	1	1.7
small shells, 1 cup .	162	5.5	32.6	.8	0	1	1.8
vegetable, enriched,							
spirals	172	6.1	35.7	.2	0	8	5.8

Food and Measure	cal.	prot. (gms)	carbo. (gms)	fat (gms)	chol. (mgs)	sod. (mgs)	fiber (gms)
whole-wheat, elbows	174	7.5	37.2	.8	0	4	3.9
Macaroni entree, can or pkg., 1 cup, except as noted:							
and beef:							
(*Chef Boyardee Beefaroni*)	260	10.0	37.0	7.0	25	870	5.0
(*Chef Boyardee Beefaroni*), 7-oz. can	190	8.0	30.0	5.0	20	720	3.0
(*Kid's Kitchen* Beefy)	190	11.0	23.0	6.0	25	800	2.0
w/cheese (*Kid's Kitchen* Cheezy) .	260	15.0	33.0	7.0	30	910	1.0
and cheese:							
(*Bowl Appétit!*), 1 bowl	370	11.0	56.0	12.0	10	930	1.0
(*Chef Boyardee*), ½ of 15-oz. can	180	8.0	35.0	1.5	20	1090	2.0
(*Hormel*), 7.5-oz. can	270	12.0	30.0	11.0	35	670	1.0
(*Hormel* Microcup)	270	12.0	30.0	11.0	35	670	1.0
(*Kid's Kitchen*)	260	12.0	30.0	11.0	35	660	1.0
(*Kraft* Easy Mac Microwavable), 1 pouch	250	7.0	38.0	8.0	10	570	<1.0
w/ham (*Dinty Moore American Classics/ Cure 81*), 1 bowl	330	16.0	30.0	16.0	35	1090	1.0
and franks, w/cheese (*Kid's Kitchen*)	310	13.0	30.0	15.0	40	930	1.0
Macaroni entree, freeze-dried, and cheese, 1 serving:							
(*AlpineAire* Forever Young)	370	17.0	54.0	9.0	n.a.	1420	1.0
w/beef (*Mountain House*)	240	10.0	38.0	5.0	15	710	3.0
Macaroni entree, frozen, 1 pkg., except as noted:							
and beef:							
(*Healthy Choice* Solos), 8.5 oz.	220	12.0	34.0	4.0	20	450	5.0

Food and Measure	cal.	prot. (gms)	carbo. (gms)	fat (gms)	chol. (mgs)	sod. (mgs)	fiber (gms)
Macaroni entree, frozen, and beef *(cont.)*							
(*Lean Cuisine Every-day Favorites*),							
10 oz.	250	16.0	36.0	5.0	20	630	4.0
(*Michelina's*), 8 oz.	250	12.0	36.0	5.0	20	700	2.0
(*Michelina's* Family),							
1 cup	200	9.0	28.0	5.0	15	550	2.0
(*Stouffer's*), 11.5 oz.	380	23.0	37.0	15.0	45	1210	4.0
and cheese:							
(*Amy's*), 9 oz.	410	16.0	47.0	16.0	50	590	3.0
(*Banquet*), 12 oz.	420	15.0	57.0	14.0	20	1330	5.0
(*Banquet* Family),							
1 cup	230	8.0	33.0	7.0	10	1290	3.0
(*Boston Market* Home Style),							
10 oz.	430	12.0	58.0	15.0	20	1210	2.0
(*Budget Gourmet* Homestyle), 8 oz.	340	14.0	41.0	13.0	25	610	2.0
(*Freezer Queen* Family Side Dish),							
1 cup	250	10.0	43.0	4.0	5	780	2.0
(*Freezer Queen* Homestyle), 8 oz.	350	15.0	46.0	11.0	25	720	4.0
(*Healthy Choice* Solos), 9 oz. . . .	250	12.0	36.0	6.0	25	600	3.0
(*Lean Cuisine Every-day Favorites*),							
10 oz.	290	15.0	42.0	7.0	20	630	2.0
(*Marie Callender's*),							
12 oz.	540	25.0	55.0	24.0	50	1930	5.0
(*Marie Callender's* Family), 1 cup . .	350	16.0	36.0	16.0	45	1500	2.0
(*Michelina's*), 8 oz.	270	12.0	41.0	6.0	15	590	2.0
(*Morton*), 1 cup . . .	240	9.0	34.0	8.0	20	1190	3.0
(*Stouffer's*), 12 oz.,							
1 cup	320	13.0	31.0	16.0	30	990	3.0
(*Stouffer's*), 20 oz.,							
1 cup	340	13.0	32.0	18.0	30	980	2.0
(*Stouffer's Family Style Favorites*),							
⅕ of 40-oz. pkg.	270	16.0	40.0	17.0	35	1020	2.0
(*Stouffer's Family Style Favorites*),							
⅑ of 76-oz. pkg.	360	15.0	37.0	17.0	30	940	2.0

Food and Measure	cal.	prot. (gms)	carbo. (gms)	fat (gms)	chol. (mgs)	sod. (mgs)	fiber (gms)
(*Swanson*), 6 oz.	200	9.0	25.0	7.0	10	700	1.0
w/broccoli (*Stouffer's*), 10.5 oz.	350	16.0	38.0	15.0	25	980	4.0
cheddar, sharp (*Michelina's*), 10 oz.	430	19.0	50.0	16.0	35	810	2.0
cheddar/Romano (*Budget Gourmet*), 8 oz.	270	12.0	40.0	7.0	20	640	2.0
four (*Wolfgang Puck's*), 12 oz.	650	27.0	50.0	38.0	115	870	2.0
w/ham (*Michelina's*), 8 oz.	340	19.0	33.0	14.0	45	860	1.0
and "cheese," nondairy: (*Amy's* Soy Cheeze), 9 oz.	360	16.0	42.0	14.0	0	500	4.0
(*Tofutti*), 6 oz. ...	194	7.0	31.0	5.0	0	552	1.0
and cheese pie: (*Banquet*), 6.5 oz.	210	7.0	34.0	5.0	10	750	1.0
(*Morton*), 6.5 oz.	210	7.0	34.0	5.0	10	750	1.0
vegetarian (*Yves Veggie*), 10.5 oz. ...	230	14.0	38.0	2.0	0	580	3.0
Macaroni entree, refrigerated, and cheese (*DeLuca*), 1 cup	340	16.0	35.0	13.0	35	940	1.0
Macaroni entree mix (see also "Shells, pasta, mix"), and cheese: (*Annie's* Microwavable Single), ¾ cup* ...	230	9.0	38.0	5.0	15	690	<1.0
(*Annie's* Original Shells), 1 cup* ...	270	10.0	49.0	3.5	10	360	2.0
(*Kraft* Deluxe Dinner Original), 3.5 oz. ..	320	13.0	44.0	10.0	20	900	2.0
(*Kraft* Deluxe Dinner w/2% Milk Cheese), 3.5 oz.	290	13.0	49.0	4.5	15	870	2.0
(*Kraft* Dinner Original/ Shapes), 2.5 oz. ..	260	11.0	48.0	2.5	10	560	1.0

Food and Measure	cal.	prot. (gms)	carbo. (gms)	fat (gms)	chol. (mgs)	sod. (mgs)	fiber (gms)
Macaroni entree mix *(cont.)*							
(*Kraft* Premium Dinner Thick 'n Creamy), 2.5 oz.	260	10.0	48.0	2.5	10	580	2.0
(*Land O Lakes*), 2.5 oz.	260	9.0	49.0	2.0	5	550	2.0
(*Land O Lakes* Deluxe Plus), 3.5 oz.	360	13.0	46.0	12.0	20	700	3.0
Alfredo:							
(*Annie's*), ⅔ cup . .	270	11.0	46.0	5.0	15	380	2.0
(*Annie's* Organic), 1 cup*	280	11.0	46.0	5.0	15	630	2.0
cheesy (*Kraft* Premium Dinner), 2.5 oz.	260	10.0	48.0	2.5	10	620	2.0
bunny shape (*Annie's*), 1 cup*	270	10.0	47.0	3.5	10	370	2.0
cheddar:							
(*Annie's* Cheddar Mac), 1 cup* . . .	270	10.0	47.0	5.0	10	550	2.0
mild (*Annie's*), 1 cup*	270	10.0	49.0	4.5	5	170	2.0
white (*Annie's* Organic Shells), 1 cup*	280	11.0	45.0	6.0	15	530	2.0
white (*Kraft* Premium Dinner), 2.5 oz.	260	11.0	48.0	2.5	10	570	2.0
whole wheat shells (*Annie's* Organic), 1 cup*	270	12.0	46.0	5.0	15	530	8.0
four cheese (*Kraft* Deluxe Dinner), 3.5 oz.	320	13.0	44.0	10.0	20	910	2.0
three cheese:							
(*Knorr TasteBreaks* Cup), 1 cont. . .	230	8.0	41.0	3.5	10	940	1.0
(*Kraft* Premium Dinner), 2.5 oz.	260	11.0	48.0	2.5	10	610	2.0
Mexican (*Annie's*), ⅔ cup	270	11.0	47.0	4.5	10	370	2.0
whole wheat (*Hodgson Mill*), ⅓ pkg.	250	11.0	45.0	1.5	<5	570	6.0

Food and Measure	cal.	prot. (gms)	carbo. (gms)	fat (gms)	chol. (mgs)	sod. (mgs)	fiber (gms)
Macaroni and cheese, see "Macaroni entree"							
Macaroni salad:							
(*Blue Ridge Farms*), ½ cup	230	4.0	28.0	11.0	10	640	1.0
(*Chef's Express*), 4 oz.	210	4.0	21.0	12.0	10	360	1.0
Mace, ground, 1 tsp.	8	.1	.9	.6	0	1	.1
Mackerel, meat only:							
Atlantic, 4 oz.:							
raw	230	21.1	0	15.8	80	102	0
baked, broiled, or microwaved ...	297	27.0	0	20.2	85	94	0
king, 4 oz.:							
raw	119	23.0	0	2.3	61	179	0
baked, broiled, or microwaved	152	29.5	0	2.9	77	230	0
Pacific/jack, 4 oz.:							
raw	179	22.8	0	9.0	53	98	0
baked, broiled, or microwaved	228	29.2	0	11.5	68	125	0
Spanish, 4 oz.:							
raw	158	21.9	0	7.2	86	67	0
baked, broiled, or microwaved	179	26.8	0	7.2	83	75	0
Mackerel, canned:							
jack (*Chicken of the Sea*), 2 oz.	90	13.0	0	4.0	55	280	0
fillets (*Crown Prince*), 1 can, 3.1 oz.	130	23.0	0	4.0	45	450	0
in oil:							
(*Reese*), 4.375-oz. can drained	240	20.0	0	18.0	40	470	0
(*Royal Crown*), ¼ cup	80	13.0	0	3.0	64	200	0
smoked (*3 Diamonds*), 2 oz. ..	160	11.0	0	12.0	30	250	0
in water (*Crown Prince*), ⅓ cup	80	13.0	0	3.0	64	200	0
Mackerel, smoked, fillets, 2 oz.:							
(*Belweder*)	150	11.0	0	14.0	20	400	0
(*Spence & Co.*)	180	13.0	0	15.0	30	840	0
herb (*Ducktrap River*)	110	12.0	0	6.0	10	560	0

Food and Measure	cal.	prot. (gms)	carbo. (gms)	fat (gms)	chol. (mgs)	sod. (mgs)	fiber (gms)
Mackerel, smoked *(cont.)*							
peppered *(Ducktrap River)*	120	12.0	0	8.0	10	520	0
Mahimahi, see "Dolphin fish"							
Mai Tai mixer:							
(Mr & Mrs T), 4.5 fl. oz.	140	0	33.0	0	0	65	0
(Trader Vic's), 4 fl. oz.	130	0	32.0	0	0	20	0
Malanga, fresh:							
(Frieda's), ⅔ cup, 3 oz.	90	1.0	23.0	0	0	10	2.0
sliced, 1 cup	132	2.0	32.0	.5	0	28	2.0
Malt cooler *(Bartles & Jaymes)*, 12 fl. oz.:							
original	190	0	29.0	0	0	0	0
berry	210	0	33.0	0	0	5	0
cherry, black	200	0	32.0	0	0	5	0
Fuzzy Navel	230	0	39.0	0	0	5	0
kiwi strawberry	214	0	39.0	0	0	4	0
lemonade, hard	230	0	39.0	0	0	0	0
Margarita	260	0	46.0	0	0	40	0
peach	210	0	33.0	0	0	5	0
piña colada	270	0	48.0	0	0	5	0
strawberry daiquiri . .	220	0	36.0	0	0	5	0
tropical	230	0	37.0	0	0	5	0
Malt syrup, 1 tbsp.:							
barley *(Eden Organic)*	60	1.0	14.0	0	0	0	0
rye *(Eden Organic)* . .	50	1.0	13.0	0	0	30	0
wheat *(Eden Organic)*	60	1.0	14.0	0	0	5	0
Malted milk powder, 3 tbsp.:							
natural *(Carnation)* . .	90	3.0	15.0	2.0	5	85	<1.0
chocolate *(Carnation)*	90	1.0	18.0	1.0	0	40	<1.0
Mammy apple:							
½ of 25-oz. fruit	216	2.1	52.9	2.1	0	63	12.7
peeled, seeded, 1 oz.	14	.1	3.5	.1	0	4	.9
Mandarin orange, see "Tangerine"							
Mango, fresh:							
(Dole), ½ medium, 3.7 oz.	70	0	17.0	.5	0	0	1.0
(Frieda's), 5 oz.	90	1.0	24.0	0	0	0	3.0
10.6-oz. fruit, 7.3 oz. trimmed	135	1.1	35.2	.6	0	4	3.7
sliced, 1 cup	107	8.4	28.1	.5	0	2	3.0

Food and Measure	cal.	prot. (gms)	carbo. (gms)	fat (gms)	chol. (mgs)	sod. (mgs)	fiber (gms)
Mango, can or jar:							
in extra light syrup (*Sunfresh* Chilled), ½ cup	100	0	25.0	.5	0	5	0
in light syrup (*Sunfresh* Can), ½ cup .	90	0	22.0	0	0	0	0
in syrup (*Herdez*), 2 pcs.	170	0	30.0	0	0	10	1.0
Mango, dried:							
(*Frieda's*), 4 pcs., 1.4 oz.	130	0	32.0	1.0	0	35	0
(*Setton Farm*), 6 pcs., 1.4 oz.	160	0	40.0	0	0	25	2.0
(*Sonoma*), 6 pcs., 1.1 oz.	100	0	23.0	0	0	25	0
Mango orange topping (*Smucker's Plate Scrapers*), 2 tbsp. .	100	0	24.0	0	0	0	0
Mango relish, Indian, 1 tbsp.:							
hot (*Patak's*)	40	<1.0	1.5	4.0	0	640	<1.0
mild (*Patak's*)	40	0	1.0	4.0	0	660	0
Mango drink, 8 fl. oz., except as noted:							
(*AriZona* Mucho) ...	100	0	27.0	0	0	20	0
(*Goya* Nectar), 6 fl. oz.	110	<1.0	27.0	0	0	15	1.0
(*Libby's*) ....,	140	0	36.0	0	0	5	0
(*Libby's*), 11.5 fl. oz. .	210	0	51.0	0	0	10	0
(*Snapple* Mango Madness)	110	0	29.0	0	0	10	0
Mango juice blend (*After the Fall Mango Montage*), 8 fl. oz.	110	1.0	27.0	0	0	10	0
Mango juice blend:							
(*Ceres*), 5.25 fl. oz. ..	87	0	21.0	0	0	n.a.	0
orange guanabana (*Nantucket Nectars*), 8 fl. oz.	130	1.0	31.0	0	0	25	0
Mango-peach drink (*R. W. Knudsen*), 8 fl. oz.	120	<1.0	30.0	0	0	50	0
Mangosteen, canned in syrup, ½ cup ...	70	.4	6.7	5.7	0	7	1.8

Food and Measure	cal.	prot. (gms)	carbo. (gms)	fat (gms)	chol. (mgs)	sod. (mgs)	fiber (gms)
Manicotti entree, frozen, 1 pkg.: cheese:							
(*Celentano*), 10 oz.	340	13.0	34.0	16.0	60	810	3.0
(*Stouffer's*), 9 oz.	360	19.0	34.0	16.0	40	850	4.0
three (*Healthy Choice* Solos), 11 oz.	300	15.0	40.0	9.0	35	600	5.0
three, marinara (*Budget Gourmet*), 8.5 oz.	290	.0	33.0	14.0	40	760	3.0
cheese/spinach (*Lean Cuisine Hearty Portions*), 15.5 oz.	350	19.0	50.0	8.0	40	910	6.0
Manioc, see "Yuca"							
Maple syrup (*Cary's/ Maple Orchard's/ MacDonald's*), ¼ cup	210	0	52.0	0	0	15	0
Maple syrup granules (*AlpineAire*), 1.2 oz.	90	0	23.0	0	0	0	0
Margarine, 1 tbsp., except as noted:							
(*I Can't Believe It's Not Butter*)	90	0	0	10.0	0	95	0
(*I Can't Believe It's Not Butter* Squeeze)	80	0	0	8.0	0	95	0
(*Hain* Safflower)	100	0	0	11.0	0	140	0
(*Land O Lakes* Stick)	100	0	0	11.0	0	115	0
(*Land O Lakes* Tub)	100	0	0	11.0	0	110	0
(*Land O Lakes* Country Morning Blend Stick)	100	0	0	11.0	0	90	0
(*Land O Lakes* Country Morning Blend Tub)	100	0	0	11.0	<5	80	0
(*Mazola* Premium)	100	0	0	11.0	0	100	0
light:							
(*I Can't Believe It's Not Butter* Light/ Sweet Cream/ Calcium)	50	0	0	6.0	0	85	0
(*Land O Lakes* Country Morning Blend Stick)	50	0	0	6.0	10	110	0

Food and Measure	cal.	prot. (gms)	carbo. (gms)	fat (gms)	chol. (mgs)	sod. (mgs)	fiber (gms)
(*Land O Lakes* Country Morning Blend Tub)	50	0	0	6.0	5	90	0
(*Mazola* 40% Corn Oil Diet Reduced Calorie)	50	0	0	6.0	0	130	0
(*Mazola* Unsalted) .	100	0	0	11.0	0	0	0
(*Smart Balance*) ...	45	0	0	5.0	0	100	0
(*Smart Beat* Trans-Fat Free)	20	0	0	2.0	0	105	0
(*Smart Beat* Unsalted)	25	0	0	2.5	0	0	0
(*Weight Watchers* Lite)	45	0	2.0	4.0	0	70	0
(*Weight Watchers* Lite Sodium Free)	45	0	2.0	4.0	0	0	0
soft:							
(*Hain* Safflower) ..	100	0	0	11.0	0	170	0
(*Land O Lakes*) ...	100	0	0	11.0	0	105	0
spread:							
(*Country Morning* Soft)	100	0	0	11.0	<5	80	0
(*Country Morning* Soft Light)	50	0	0	6.0	5	90	0
(*Country Morning* Stick)	100	0	0	11.0	0	90	0
(*Country Morning* Stick Light)	50	0	0	6.0	10	110	0
(*Land O Lakes* w/Sweet Cream Soft)	80	0	0	8.0	0	70	0
(*Land O Lakes* w/Sweet Cream Stick)	90	0	0	10.0	0	95	0
(*Mazola* 40% Corn Oil Light)	50	0	0	6.0	0	100	0
(*Smart Balance* 37% Light)	45	0	0	5.0	0	100	0
(*Smart Balance* 67% Buttery)	80	0	0	9.0	0	90	0
unsalted (*Country Morning* Stick)	100	0	0	11.0	0	0	0

Food and Measure	cal.	prot. (gms)	carbo. (gms)	fat (gms)	chol. (mgs)	sod. (mgs)	fiber (gms)
Margarine, spread *(cont.)*							
unsalted (*Land O Lakes* w/Sweet Cream Stick) . . .	90	0	0	10.0	0	0	0
squeeze (*Smart Beat* Fat Free)	5	0	1.0	0	0	100	0
Margarita mix, dry (*Bar-Tender's*), 2 pouches	90	0	21.0	0	0	70	0
Margarita mixer, 4 fl. oz., except as noted:							
bottled:							
(*D. L. Jardine's*), .5 oz.	90	0	22.0	0	0	10	0
(*Mr & Mrs T*)	130	0	29.0	0	0	40	0
peach (*Daily's*)	190	0	48.0	0	0	75	2.0
raspberry (*Daily's*) .	180	0	46.0	0	0	75	2.0
strawberry (*Mr & Mrs T*), 3.5 fl. oz.	150	0	34.0	0	0	20	0
strawberry (*Trader Vic's*)	160	0	40.0	0	0	20	0
frozen (*Bacardi*), 2 fl. oz.	90	0	25.0	0	0	0	0
Marinade (see also "Grilling sauce" and specific listings), 1 tbsp., except as noted:							
(*House of Tsang Mandarin*)	25	0	6.0	0	0	680	0
Cajun:							
(*Golden Dipt*), 2 tbsp.	60	0	2.0	4.5	0	230	0
spicy (*Cardini's*) . . .	10	0	2.0	0	0	350	0
citrus grill w/orange juice (*Lawry's*)	15	0	3.0	0	0	210	0
chipotle pepper (*Cardini's*)	10	0	2.0	0	0	330	0
coriander and ginger, mild (*Patak's* Tikka Marinade/Grill), 2 tbsp.	40	1.0	4.0	2.0	0	800	0

Food and Measure	cal.	prot. (gms)	carbo. (gms)	fat (gms)	chol. (mgs)	sod. (mgs	fiber (gms)
Dijon, white wine (*Golden Dipt*)	10	0	1.0	0	0	125	0
Dijon and honey w/lemon juice (*Lawry's*)	20	0	3.0	0	0	0	0
fajitas, meat (*D. L. Jardine's*)	5	0	1.0	0	0	270	0
garlic, roasted, and herb (*Cardini's*) ...	10	0	2.0	0	0	430	0
garlic herb (*Golden Dipt*)	60	0	1.0	6.0	0	140	0
ginger, 2 tbsp.:							
hickory (*The Ginger People*)	30	0	8.0	0	0	240	0
lemon (*The Ginger People*)	90	0	3.0	9.0	0	90	0
lime (*The Ginger People*)	35	0	9.0	0	0	440	0
peanut (*The Ginger People*)	50	2.0	5.0	3.0	0	120	0
teriyaki (*Golden Dipt*)	60	0	5.0	3.0	0	560	0
ginger and garlic, spicy (*Patak's* Tandoori Marinade/ Grill), 2 tbsp.	35	<1.0	7.0	.5	0	1060	0
Hawaiian w/tropical fruit juice (*Lawry's*)	20	0	4.0	0	0	250	0
herb and garlic w/lemon juice (*Lawry's*)	10	0	2.0	0	0	400	0
hickory w/apple cider (*Lawry's*)	20	0	5.0	0	0	420	0
honey:							
hickory (*World Harbors* Ember Wisp), 2 tbsp. ...	45	0	10	0	0	230	0
Dijon (*Cardini's*) ...	20	0	4.0	0	0	430	0
mustard (*Golden Dipt* Fat Free) ...	25	0	4.0	0	0	60	0
soy (*Golden Dipt*), 2 tbsp.	30	0	7.0	0	0	390	0

Food and Measure	cal.	prot. (gms)	carbo. (gms)	fat (gms)	chol. (mgs)	sod. (mgs)	fiber (gms)
Marinade (cont.)							
Indian style, Bombay mango (*World Harbors Bengali*), 2 tbsp.	45	0	10.0	0	0	220	0
jerk:							
(*Helen's Tropical Exotics*)	10	0	1.0	.5	0	30	0
Caribbean, w/papaya juice (*Lawry's*) ..	25	0	6.0	0	0	430	0
lemon herb (*Golden Dipt*), 2 tbsp.	80	0	0	8.0	0	125	0
lemon pepper:							
w/lemon juice (*Lawry's*)	10	0	2.0	0	0	380	0
and garlic (*World Harbors* Maine's Own), 2 tbsp. ...	35	0	8.0	0	0	140	0
zesty (*Cardini's*) ...	15	0	4.0	0	0	340	0
lemongrass herb (*Annie Chun's*), 2 tbsp.	60	0	6.0	3.0	0	75	0
London broil (*Lawry's Weekday Gourmet*)	10	0	2.0	0	0	510	0
Mediterranean w/lemon juice (*Lawry's*)	10	0	2.0	0	0	320	0
mesquite:							
(*Golden Dipt*)	10	0	1.0	.5	0	250	0
(*S&W* Cooking Sauce)	10	0	3.0	0	0	400	0
w/lime juice (*Lawry's*)	5	0	1.0	0	0	350	0
fajita (*Cardini's*) ...	10	0	2.0	0	0	270	0
Oriental style (*World Harbors Cheriyaki Glaze/Marinade*), 2 tbsp.	50	0	14.0	0	0	390	0
Southwestern/fajita (*S&W* Cooking Sauce)	10	0	2.0	0	0	230	<1.0
steak:							
(*A1 Classic Steakhouse*)	15	0	3.0	0	0	270	0
hickory (*A1*)	10	0	3.0	0	0	640	0

Food and Measure	cal.	prot. (gms)	carbo. (gms)	fat (gms)	chol. (mgs)	sod. (mgs)	fiber (gms)
Italian herb (*A1*) ..	15	0	4.0	0	0	480	0
tequila lime w/lime juice (*Lawry's*)	15	0	4.0	0	0	410	0
teriyaki:							
(*Annie Chun's*)	25	1.0	5.0	0	0	350	0
(*S&W* Cooking Sauce)	25	<1.0	5.0	0	0	480	0
w/pineapple juice (*Lawry's*)	25	0	6.0	0	0	570	0
and sauce (*Kikkoman*)	15	1.0	2.0	0	0	610	0
and sauce (*Kikkoman* Lite)	15	<1.0	3.0	0	0	320	0
and sauce, roasted garlic (*Kikkoman*)	25	1.0	5.0	0	0	730	0
steak (*Lawry's* Weekday Gourmet) ..	25	0	5.0	1.0	0	600	0
tangy (*Cardini's*) ..	20	1.0	4.0	0	0	550	0
Thai ginger w/lime juice (*Lawry's*)	10	0	2.0	0	0	400	0
Marinade seasoning mix (see also specific listings):							
beef (*Lawry's*), ¾ tsp.	0	0	1.0	0	0	540	0
Cajun, spicy (*Adolph's For the Grill*), 1 tsp.	5	0	1.0	0	0	230	0
chicken (*Adolph's Marinade in Minutes*), ¾ tsp.	5	0	1.0	0	0	290	0
garlic (*Adolph's Marinade in Minutes*), ¾ tsp.	5	0	1.0	0	0	430	0
lemon herb w/black pepper (*Adolph's For the Grill*), ½ tsp.	5	0	1.0	0	0	150	0
meat:							
(*Adolph's Marinade in Minutes*), ¾ tsp.	5	0	1.0	0	0	380	0
(*Adolph's Marinade in Minutes* Sodium Free), ¾ tsp.	5	0	2.0	0	0	0	0
(*McCormick*), ½ cup*	15	0	2.0	0	0	240	0

Food and Measure	cal.	prot. (gms)	carbo. (gms)	fat (gms)	chol. (mgs)	sod. (mgs)	fiber (gms)
Marinade seasoning mix *(cont.)*							
mesquite (*Adolph's For the Grill*), ¾ tsp. . . .	5	0	1.0	0	0	230	0
roasted garlic (*Adolph's For the Grill*), 1 tsp.	5	0	1.0	0	0	230	0
steak sauce (*Adolph's Marinade in Minutes*), ¾ tsp.	5	0	1.0	0	0	460	0
Marjoram, dried, 1 tsp.	2	.1	.4	<.1	0	<1	.1
Marmalade, see "Jam and preserves"							
Marrow beans, dried (*Frieda's*), ½ cup . .	120	7.0	22.0	0	0	0	9.0
Marrow squash, raw, trimmed, 1 oz. . . .	4	.2	1.0	<.1	0	n.a.	<1.0
Marshmallow topping, 2 tbsp.:							
(*Marshmallow Fluff*) .	60	0	15.0	0	0	10	0
(*Smucker's*)	120	0	29.0	0	0	0	0
raspberry or strawberry (*Marshmallow Fluff*)	60	0	15.0	0	0	10	0
Masa, see "Cornmeal"							
Matai, see "Water chestnut"							
Matzo, see "Cracker"							
Matzo ball, in jars:							
(*Manischewitz*), 1 cup	220	7.0	27.0	9.0	80	880	3.0
(*Mrs. Adler's*), 1 cup, 3 pcs. w/liquid	190	5.0	24.0	8.0	0	710	1.0
Matzo ball mix, dry (*Manischewitz*), 1½ tbsp.	45	1.0	9.0	0	0	660	<1.0
Matzo meal, see "Cracker crumbs/ meal"							
Mayonnaise, 1 tbsp.:							
in jars:							
(*Hain*)	100	0	0	11.0	5	100	0
(*Hain* Lite)	45	0	2.0	4.0	5	130	0
(*Hellmann's/Best Foods* Real)	100	0	0	11.0	5	90	0
(*Hellman's/Best Foods* Extra Heavy)	100	0	0	11.0	10	85	0

Food and Measure	cal.	prot. (gms)	carbo. (gms)	fat (gms)	chol. (mgs)	sod. (mgs)	fiber (gms)
(Hellmann's/Best Foods Light) ...	50	0	1.0	5.0	5	120	0
(Henri's)	100	0	0	11.0	5	85	0
(Hollywood Canola)	100	0	0	11.0	5	100	0
(Kraft Extra Heavy)	100	2.0	0	11.0	5	45	0
(Kraft Light)	45	0	2.0	4.0	<5	90	0
(Kraft Signature) ..	100	0	0	10.0	5	80	0
(Smart Balance Light)	50	0	2.0	5.0	5	125	0
(Smart Beat Fat Free)	10	0	3.0	0	0	135	0
w/lime juice (Kraft)	100	0	0	11.0	10	85	0
refrigerated:							
(Delouis Fils)	110	0	0	12.0	30	70	0
garlic (Delouis Fils Aioli)	102	0	0	11.2	27	97	0
Mayonnaise dressing, 1 tbsp.:							
(Hain Eggless)	100	0	1.0	11.0	0	0	0
(Hellmann's/Best Foods Deli Blend Whipped)	60	0	2.0	6.0	10	100	0
(Hellmann's/Best Foods Deli Blend Whipped Fat Free)	20	0	5.0	0	0	140	0
(Hellmann's/Best Foods Low Fat) ...	15	0	2.0	1.0	0	120	0
(Hellmann's/BestFoods/ Just 2 Good Reduced Fat)	25	0	2.0	2.0	0	130	0
(Kraft Salad)	50	0	2.0	4.5	5	110	0
(Kraft Fat Free)	10	0	2.0	0	0	120	0
(Miracle Whip)	60	0	2.0	6.0	5	100	0
(Miracle Whip Light) .	35	0	2.0	3.0	<5	130	0
(Miracle Whip Free Nonfat)	15	0	3.0	0	0	125	0
tofu (Nayonaise)	35	0	1.0	3.5	0	115	0
McDonald's, 1 serving: breakfast bagel:							
ham, egg, cheese ..	550	26.0	58.0	23.0	255	1490	2.0
Spanish omelette ..	690	27.0	60.0	38.0	275	1570	3.0
steak, egg, and cheese	700	38.0	57.0	35.0	290	1290	2.0
breakfast biscuit:							
plain	240	4.0	30.0	11.0	0	640	1.0

Food and Measure	cal.	prot. (gms)	carbo. (gms)	fat (gms)	chol. (mgs)	sod. (mgs)	fiber (gms)
McDonald's, breakfast biscuit *(cont.)*							
bacon, egg, cheese	480	20.0	31.0	31.0	250	1410	1.0
sausage	410	10.0	30.0	28.0	35	930	1.0
sausage and egg . .	490	16.0	31.0	33.0	245	1010	1.0
breakfast burrito	290	13.0	24.0	16.0	170	680	2.0
breakfast dishes:							
eggs, scrambled, 2	160	13.0	1.0	11.0	425	170	0
hash browns	130	1.0	14.0	8.0	0	330	1.0
hotcakes:							
plain	340	9.0	58.0	8.0	20	630	2.0
w/syrup, margarine	600	9.0	104.0	17.0	20	770	2.0
sausage	170	6.0	0	16.0	35	290	0
breakfast muffin:							
English, plain	150	5.0	27.0	2.0	0	260	2.0
Egg McMuffin	300	18.0	29.0	12.0	235	830	2.0
Sausage McMuffin	370	14.0	28.0	23.0	45	790	2.0
Sausage McMuffin, w/egg	450	20.0	29.0	28.0	255	930	2.0
Danish and muffin:							
apple bran muffin, low fat	300	6.0	61.0	3.0	0	380	3.0
apple Danish	340	5.0	47.0	15.0	20	340	2.0
cheese Danish	400	7.0	45.0	21.0	40	400	2.0
cinnamon roll	390	6.0	50.0	18.0	65	310	2.0
sandwiches:							
Big Mac	590	24.0	47.0	34.0	85	1090	3.0
Big N' Tasty	540	24.0	39.0	32.0	80	970	2.0
Big N' Tasty w/cheese	590	27.0	40.0	37.0	95	1210	4.0
cheeseburger	330	15.0	36.0	14.0	45	830	2.0
Chicken flatbread . .	540	28.0	56.0	24.0	70	1620	n.a.
no cheese	410	21.0	54.0	13.0	35	960	n.a.
no cheese/sauce	340	21.0	52.0	7.0	30	800	n.a.
no sauce	460	28.0	53.0	16.0	65	1450	n.a.
Chicken McGrill . . .	400	25.0	37.0	17.0	60	890	2.0
Chicken McGrill w/out mayo	300	24.0	37.0	6.0	50	800	2.0
crispy chicken	500	22.0	46.0	26.0	50	1100	2.0
Filet-O-Fish	470	15.0	45.0	26.0	50	890	2.0
hamburger	280	12.0	35.0	10.0	30	590	2.0
Quarter Pounder . .	430	23.0	37.0	21.0	70	840	2.0
Quarter Pounder, w/cheese	530	28.0	38.0	30.0	95	1310	2.0

Food and Measure	cal.	prot. (gms)	carbo. (gms)	fat (gms)	chol. (mgs)	sod. (mgs)	fiber (gms)
Chicken McNuggets:							
4 pcs.	210	10.0	12.0	13.0	35	460	1.0
6 pcs.	310	15.0	18.0	20.0	50	680	2.0
9 pcs.	460	22.0	27.0	29.0	75	1020	2.0
McNuggets sauce pkt.:							
barbeque	45	0	10.0	0	0	250	0
honey	45	0	12.0	0	0	0	0
honey mustard ...	50	0	3.0	4.5	10	85	0
hot mustard	60	1.0	7.0	3.5	5	240	<1.0
mayonnaise, light .	45	0	1.0	4.5	10	100	0
sweet and sour ...	50	0	11.0	0	0	140	0
french fries:							
large	540	8.0	68.0	26.0	0	350	6.0
medium	450	6.0	57.0	22.0	0	290	5.0
small	210	3.0	26.0	10.0	0	135	2.0
Super Size	610	9.0	77.0	29.0	0	390	7.0
McSalad Shaker salads:							
chef	150	17.0	5.0	8.0	95	740	2.0
garden	100	7.0	4.0	6.0	75	120	2.0
grilled chicken							
Caesar	100	17.0	3.0	2.5	40	240	2.0
croutons, 1 pkt. ..	50	1.0	9.0	1.0	0	105	0
dressing, 1 pkt.:							
Caesar	150	1.0	5.0	13.0	10	400	0
herb vinaigrette, fat							
free	35	0	8.0	0	0	260	0
honey mustard ...	160	1.0	13.0	11.0	15	260	0
ranch	170	0	3.0	18.0	15	460	0
red French, reduced							
calorie	130	0	18.0	6.0	0	360	0
Thousand Island ..	130	1.0	11.0	9.0	15	350	0
desserts/shakes:							
baked apple pie ...	260	3.0	34.0	13.0	0	200	<1.0
cookies, 1 pkg.:							
chocolate chip ..	280	3.0	37.0	14.0	40	170	1.0
McDonaldland ..	230	3.0	38.0	8.0	0	250	1.0
Fruit 'n Yogurt							
Parfait	380	10.0	76.0	5.0	15	240	2.0
Fruit 'n Yogurt							
Parfait, w/out							
granola	280	8.0	53.0	4.0	15	115	<1.0
McFlurry:							
Butterfinger	620	16.0	90.0	22.0	70	260	1.0
M&M's	630	16.0	90.0	23.0	75	210	<1.0

Food and Measure	cal.	prot. (gms)	carbo. (gms)	fat (gms)	chol. (mgs)	sod. (mgs)	fiber (gms)
McDonald's, desserts/shakes, McFlurry *(cont.)*							
Nestlé Crunch . .	630	16.0	89.0	24.0	75	230	<1.0
Oreo	570	15.0	82.0	20.0	70	280	<1.0
shake, *Triple Thick*, 16 fl. oz.:							
chocolate	580	15.0	94.0	17.0	65	280	1.0
strawberry	560	14.0	89.0	16.0	65	190	<1.0
vanilla	570	14.0	89.0	16.0	65	400	0
sundae, hot caramel	360	7.0	61.0	10.0	35	180	0
sundae, hot fudge .	340	8.0	52.0	12.0	30	170	1.0
sundae, strawberry	290	7.0	50.0	7.0	30	95	<1.0
sundae nuts	40	2.0	2.0	3.5	0	55	<1.0
vanilla cone, reduced fat	150	4.0	23.0	4.5	20	75	0
Meat, potted, see "Meat spread"							
Meat loaf, refrigerated (*Always Tender*), 5 oz.	240	19.0	14.0	12.0	55	790	0
Meat loaf dinner, frozen, 1 pkg.:							
(*Healthy Choice*), 12 oz.	330	15.0	52.0	7.0	35	460	6.0
(*Stouffer's* HomeStyle), 17 oz.	560	29.0	38.0	32.0	95	1420	5.0
(*Swanson Traditional Favorites*), 10.75 oz.	380	19.0	37.0	14.0	35	730	5.0
Meat loaf entree, frozen, 1 pkg.:							
(*Banquet*), 9.5 oz. . . .	240	14.0	20.0	11.0	30	1040	4.0
(*Freezer Queen Meal*), 9.5 oz.	310	18.0	26.0	15.0	30	930	7.0
(*Stouffer's* HomeStyle), 9⅞ oz.	390	22.0	28.0	21.0	90	840	3.0
in gravy (*Stouffer's Family Style Favorites*), ⅙ of 33-oz. pkg.	220	16.0	10.0	13.0	50	710	1.0
and gravy:							
(*Marie Callender's*), 14 oz.	540	23.0	42.0	30.0	95	1570	5.0
w/mashed potato (*Michelina's*), 8 oz.	340	13.0	20.0	23.0	85	1230	2.0

Food and Measure	cal.	prot. (gms)	carbo. (gms)	fat (gms)	chol. (mgs)	sod. (mgs)	fiber (gms)
w/mashed potato (*Michelina's*), 10.5 oz.	390	17.0	25.0	24.0	70	1730	3.0
savory (*Banquet Family*), 1 patty w/gravy	190	10.0	7.0	13.0	35	750	1.0
w/mashed potato, gravy (*Marie Callender's* Family), 1 patty, gravy, ½ cup potato	280	11.0	19.0	17.0	60	960	1.0
in port wine sauce (*Wolfgang Puck's*), 12 oz.	540	25.0	38.0	30.0	130	840	5.0
tomato sauce and: (*Freezer Queen* Family), 1 patty w/gravy, ⅙ pkg.	200	8.0	10.0	14.0	25	650	4.0
(*Morton*), 9 oz. ...	250	9.0	24.0	13.0	20	1200	3.0
w/whipped potato (*Lean Cuisine Cafe Classics*), 9⅜ oz.	260	20.0	28.0	7.0	45	690	4.0
Meat loaf seasoning: (*Adolph's Meal Makers*), 1 tbsp.	25	<1.0	5.0	0	0	380	0
(*Lawry's*), 1 tbsp. ...	35	<1.0	7.0	0	0	430	0
(*McCormick*), ⅒ pkg.	15	0	2.0	0	0	350	0
(*McCormick Bag'n Season*), ⅛ pkg. ..	15	1.0	2.0	0	0	390	0
(*Tempo*), 3 tbsp.	70	2.0	13.0	1.0	0	700	1.0
Meat spread (see also specific listings): (*Spam* Spread), 4 tbsp.	140	8.0	1.0	12.0	40	570	0
potted meat: (*Armour*), ¼ cup ..	80	8.0	0	5.0	55	550	0
(*Goya*), ¼ cup	80	8.0	0	5.0	55	550	0
(*Hormel*), 4 tbsp., 2 oz.	100	7.0	0	8.0	50	610	0
Meat tenderizer (*Adolph's* Original No MSG), ¼ tsp.	0	0	0	0	0	420	0
(*Adolph's* Original No Sodium), ½ tsp. ..	0	0	<1.0	0	0	0	0

Food and Measure	cal.	prot. (gms)	carbo. (gms)	fat (gms)	chol. (mgs)	sod. (mgs)	fiber (gms)
Meat tenderizer *(cont.)*							
(*Tone's*), 1 tsp.	7	0	1.2	.2	0	1760	tr.
seasoned, ¼ tsp.:							
(*Adolph's*)	0	0	0	0	0	450	0
(*Adolph's* No Sodium)	0	0	<1.0	0	0	0	0
Meatball, frozen or refrigerated:							
baked (*DeLuca*), 2 pcs., ¼ cup sauce	180	10.0	12.0	11.0	55	420	2.0
chicken, Italian style (*Tyson* Family Pack), 6 pcs., 3 oz.	150	13.0	6.0	8.0	45	540	2.0
Italian, 3 oz.:							
(*Home Market*), 3 pcs.	230	14.0	5.0	17.0	50	440	1.0
(*Master Choice*), about 4 pcs. . . .	230	13.0	3.0	18.0	45	670	0
(*Rosina*), 6 small or 1 large	250	14.0	5.0	19.0	55	620	3.0
Swedish (*Rosina*), 6 pcs., 3 oz.	260	12.0	5.0	19.0	45	630	3.0
turkey, 3 oz.:							
(*Rosina*), 3 pcs. . . .	170	15.0	7.0	9.0	65	670	3.0
Italian (*Shady Brook Farms*), 3 pcs. .	130	12.0	5.0	7.0	45	350	1.0
sweet/sour, appetizer (*Shady Brook Farms*), 5 pcs. w/sauce	130	10.0	10.0	6.0	40	370	0
"Meatball," vege-tarian, canned, w/gravy (*Loma Linda Tender Rounds*), 6 pcs. . . .	120	14.0	5.0	5.0	0	330	3.0
Meatball entree, canned, stew (*Dinty Moore*), 1 cup	250	13.0	17.0	15.0	40	1120	2.0
Meatball entree, frozen, 1 pkg.:							
Italian style (*Healthy Choice* Bread Stuffs), 6.1 oz.	330	18.0	52.0	5.0	20	600	4.0

Food and Measure	cal.	prot. (gms)	carbo. (gms)	fat (gms)	chol. (mgs)	sod. (mgs)	fiber (gms)
mashed potatoes and (*Michelina's*), 8.5 oz.	280	10.0	26.0	14.0	35	1130	3.0
Stroganoff (*Country Skillet*), ¼ of 32-oz. pkg.	340	14.0	29.0	19.0	45	1130	1.0
Swedish:							
(*Banquet*), 10.25 oz.	400	22.0	33.0	19.0	80	1040	5.0
(*Budget Gourmet*), 10 oz.	530	18.0	44.0	30.0	140	1030	4.0
(*Lean Cuisine Every-day Favorites*), 9⅛ oz.	290	22.0	35.0	7.0	45	590	4.0
(*Marie Callender's*), 10.25 oz.	450	22.0	43.0	21.0	53	740	5.0
(*Stouffer's*), 10.5 oz.	520	25.0	49.0	25.0	75	1280	4.0
w/gravy (*Michelina's*), 10 oz. ..	400	17.0	37.0	18.0	50	1000	2.0
w/gravy (*Michelina's Family*), 1 cup ..	290	12.0	30.0	12.0	30	620	2.0
Meatball pocket, frozen 4.5-oz. pc.:							
(*Lean Pockets*)	300	13.0	44.0	7.0	30	600	2.0
and mozzarella (*Hot Pockets*)	320	13.0	41.0	11.0	35	660	2.0
Meatball seasoning:							
Italian (*Tempo*), 2½ tbsp.	70	2.0	13.0	1.0	0	670	1.0
Swedish (*Tempo*), 3 tbsp.	70	2.0	13.0	1.0	0	620	1.0
Melon, see specific listings							
Melon, mixed, dried (*Sunsweet Fruitlings*), 1.4 oz., ⅓ cup	130	1.0	33.0	0	0	50	3.0
Melon balls, frozen, cantaloupe/honey-dew, ½ cup	28	.7	6.9	.2	0	27	.6
Melon salad, chilled, in extra light syrup (*Sunfresh*), ½ cup .	45	0	10.0	0	0	15	2.0
Melogold, fresh (*Frieda's*), ½ fruit, 5.9 oz.	50	0	13.0	0	0	0	2.0

Food and Measure	cal.	prot. (gms)	carbo. (gms)	fat (gms)	chol. (mgs)	sod. (mgs)	fiber (gms)
Menudo, see "Soup"							
Mesclun, see "Salad blend"							
Mexican beans (see also "Chili beans"), canned, ½ cup:							
(*Allens/Brown Beauty* Chili)	120	6.0	22.0	1.0	0	300	8.0
(*Old El Paso* Mexe) . .	110	7.0	19.0	0	0	630	7.0
Mexican dinner (see also specific listings), frozen, 1 pkg.:							
(*Swanson Hungry-Man*), 20 oz.	710	26.0	87.0	29.0	40	2160	13.0
combo (*Swanson Traditional Favorites*), 13.25 oz.	470	18.0	59.0	18.0	25	1610	5.0
Mexican dinner kit (see also specific listings), white or yellow (*Chi-Chi's*), 2 shells/seasoning	200	4.0	30.0	7.0	0	860	2.0
Mexican sauce (see also specific listings), 2 tbsp.:							
hot (*Mrs. Renfro's*) . .	10	0	2.0	0	0	210	0
mild (*Mrs. Renfro's*)	10	0	3.0	0	0	240	0
Mexican seasoning (*McCormick*), ¼ tsp.	0	0	0	0	0	50	0
Mexican squash (*Frieda's*), ½ cup, 3 oz.	35	1.0	9.0	0	0	0	2.0
Milk, 8 fl. oz.:							
buttermilk:							
(*Darigold* Lowfat) . .	110	9.0	13.0	2.5	15	270	0
(*Friendship* Lowfat)	120	9.0	12.0	4.0	15	125	0
cultured	99	8.1	11.7	2.2	9	257	0
whole:							
(*Darigold*)	150	8.0	12.0	8.0	35	125	0
(*Parmalat*)	160	9.0	13.0	8.0	35	130	0
(*Turkey Hill*)	160	8.0	12.0	8.0	35	120	0
3.3% fat	150	8.0	11.4	8.2	33	120	0
reduced/low fat:							
2% (*Darigold*)	130	8.0	13.0	5.0	20	125	0

Food and Measure	cal.	prot. (gms)	carbo. (gms)	fat (gms)	chol. (mgs)	sod. (mgs)	fiber (gms)
2% (*Parmalat*) ...	130	9.0	13.0	5.0	20	130	0
2% (*Turkey Hill*) ..	130	8.0	12.0	5.0	20	120	0
2% fat	121	8.1	11.7	4.7	18	122	0
2%, protein fortified	137	9.7	13.5	4.9	19	145	0
1% (*Darigold*)	110	9.0	13.0	2.5	15	130	0
1% (*Parmalat*) ...	110	9.0	13.0	2.5	15	135	0
1% (*Turkey Hill*) ..	100	8.0	12.0	2.5	10	125	0
1% fat	102	8.0	11.7	2.6	10	123	0
1%, protein fortified	119	9.7	13.6	2.9	10	143	0
skim/fat free:							
(*Darigold*)	90	9.0	13.0	0	<5	130	0
(*Darigold* Acidophi-lus/Trim Deluxe)	100	10.0	14.0	0	<5	140	0
(*Parmalat*)	90	8.0	13.0	.3	5	130	0
(*Turkey Hill*)	90	8.0	12.0	0	5	125	0
8 fl. oz.	86	8.4	11.9	.4	4	126	0
Milk, canned, 2 tbsp.:							
condensed, sweetened							
(*Carnation*)	130	3.0	22.0	3.0	10	45	0
evaporated:							
(*Carnation*)	40	2.0	3.0	2.0	10	30	0
(*Carnation* Fat Free)	25	2.0	4.0	0	0	40	0
(*Carnation* Lowfat)	25	2.0	3.0	.5	5	35	0
(*Pet*)	40	2.0	3.0	2.0	10	30	0
skim (*Pet*)	25	2.0	4.0	0	0	40	0
Milk, chocolate, see "Milk, flavored"							
Milk, dry:							
buttermilk:							
sweet cream, 1 cup	464	41.2	58.8	6.9	83	620	0
sweet cream, 1 tbsp.	25	2.2	3.2	.4	4	34	0
whole, 1 oz.	141	7.5	10.9	7.6	27	105	0
whole, 1 cup	635	33.7	49.2	34.2	124	475	0
nonfat:							
(*AlpineAire*), 1 oz.	100	10.0	0	0	n.a.	140	0
(*Carnation*), ⅓ cup	80	8.0	12.0	0	<5	125	0
regular, 1 cup	435	43.4	62.4	.9	24	642	0
instant, 3.2-oz. pkt.	244	23.9	35.5	.5	12	373	0
Milk, flavored, 8 fl. oz.:							
banana (*Nesquik* Re-duced Fat)	200	7.0	31.0	5.0	20	95	0
berry (*DariGo* Blast Re-duced Fat)	220	9.0	33.0	6.0	25	140	0

Food and Measure	cal.	prot. (gms)	carbo. (gms)	fat (gms)	chol. (mgs)	sod. (mgs)	fiber (gms)
Milk, flavored (cont.)							
chocolate:							
(*DariGo* Maximum)	240	8.0	33.0	9.0	40	260	0
(*Hershey's*)	230	8.0	28.0	9.0	30	140	<1.0
(*Hershey's* Fat Free)	150	9.0	29.0	0	<5	140	<1.0
(*Hershey's* Reduced Fat)	190	8.0	30.0	4.5	15	140	1.0
(*Nesquik*)	230	7.0	33.0	8.0	30	130	1.0
(*Nesquik* Fat Free)	160	8.0	31.0	0	0	140	1.0
(*Parmalat* 2%)	180	7.0	28.0	5.0	20	115	1.0
(*Turkey Hill* 1%) ...	180	8.0	32.0	2.5	10	180	0
orange cream (*Turkey Hill Cool Moos*) ...	190	8.0	33.0	2.5	10	135	0
strawberry:							
(*Hershey's* Reduced Fat)	200	8.0	31.0	4.5	15	130	0
(*Nesquik*)	230	7.0	33.0	8.0	30	100	0
(*Turkey Hill Cool Moos*)	160	8.0	27.0	2.5	10	125	0
vanilla (*Turkey Hill Cool Moos*)	160	8.0	26.0	2.5	10	125	0
Milk, goat, 1 cup:							
(*Meyenberg*)	140	8.0	11.0	7.0	25	115	0
fresh	168	8.7	10.9	10.1	28	122	0
"Milk," nondairy, see "Rice beverage" and "Soy beverage"							
Milk, human, 1 cup	171	2.9	16.9	10.8	32	42	0
Milk, sheep, 1 cup ..	264	14.7	13.1	17.2	66	108	0
Milkfish, meat only:							
raw, 4 oz.	168	23.3	0	7.6	59	82	0
baked, broiled, or microwaved, 4 oz.	215	29.8	0	9.8	76	104	0
Millet:							
raw, 1 oz.	107	3.1	20.7	1.2	0	1	2.4
cooked, 4 oz.	135	4.0	26.8	1.1	0	2	1.5
hulled (*Arrowhead Mills*), ¼ cup	150	5.0	34.0	1.5	0	0	3.0
Millet flour (*Arrowhead Mills*), ¼ cup	110	4.0	26.0	1.0	0	0	2.0
Mincemeat, see "Pie filling"							

Food and Measure	cal.	prot. (gms)	carbo. (gms)	fat (gms)	chol. (mgs)	sod. (mgs)	fiber (gms)
Mint sauce:							
(*Crosse & Blackwell*), 1 tsp.	5	0	1.0	0	0	0	0
honey (*Reese* Lamb), 1 tbsp.	20	0	5.0	0	0	15	0
Mirin (*Sushi Chef*), 1 tbsp.	50	0	11.0	0	0	0	0
Miso, soy, 1 tbsp., except as noted:							
(*Eden/Eden* Organic Hacho)	35	3.0	2.0	1.5	0	600	1.0
1 oz.	58	3.3	7.9	1.7	0	1034	1.5
½ cup	284	16.3	38.6	8.4	0	5032	7.6
w/barley (*Eden* Organic Mugi)	25	2.0	3.0	1.0	0	760	1.0
w/brown rice (*Eden* Organic Genmai)	25	2.0	3.0	1.0	0	810	<1.0
rice w/soy (*Eden* Organic Shiro)	35	2.0	5.0	1.0	0	410	1.0
Molasses, 1 tbsp.:							
(*Brer Rabbit* Full Flavored)	60	0	15.0	0	0	10	0
(*Grandma's*)	50	0	12.0	0	0	0	0
blackstrap:							
(*Brer Rabbit*)	60	1.0	13.0	0	0	65	0
(*New Morning*)	60	<1.0	13.0	0	0	20	0
mild:							
(*Brer Rabbit*)	60	0	15.0	0	0	10	0
(*Grandma's*)	50	0	14.0	0	0	0	0
robust (*Grandma's*)	50	0	12.0	0	0	0	0
Mole sauce, 2 tbsp.:							
(*Doña Maria*)	230	3.0	12.0	15.0	0	460	2.0
(*Doña Maria* Verde)	240	5.0	6.0	18.0	0	660	2.0
Monkfish, meat only:							
raw, 4 oz.	86	16.4	0	1.7	29	21	0
baked, broiled, or microwaved, 4 oz.	110	21.0	0	2.2	36	26	0
Monosodium glutamate (*Tone's*), 1 tsp.	0	0	0	0	0	638	0
Moose, meat only, roasted, 4 oz.	152	33.2	0	1.1	88	78	0
Mortadella, 2 oz.:							
(*Black Bear*)	240	8.0	0	23.0	45	610	0
(*Boar's Head*)	160	9.0	0	14.0	30	560	0

Food and Measure	cal.	prot. (gms)	carbo. (gms)	fat (gms)	chol. (mgs)	sod. (mgs)	fiber (gms)
Mortadella *(cont.)*							
(Daniele)	150	10.0	2.0	14.0	30	490	0
(Fiorucci)	240	8.0	0	23.0	45	610	0
w/pistachios *(Boar's Head)*	170	10.0	2.0	14.0	30	560	0
Mothbean, boiled, 4 oz.	133	8.9	23.8	.6	0	11	n.a.
Mudslide drink mixer *(Daily's)*, 4 fl. oz.	300	0	69.0	3.0	0	70	0
Muffin, 1 pc., except as noted:							
apple:							
(Awrey's), 1.5 oz.	130	2.0	18.0	6.0	20	220	0
(Awrey's), 2.5 oz.	230	3.0	30.0	10.0	40	310	0
banana:							
nut *(Awrey's)*, 1.5 oz.	130	2.0	22.0	5.0	10	125	<1.0
nut *(Awrey's Grande)*, 4 oz.	410	6.0	48.0	21.0	70	340	1.0
nut *(Awrey's Petite)*, 2 pcs.	160	3.0	22.0	7.0	10	170	<1.0
nut *(Old Spunk-meyer)*, ½ pc. ,	240	3.0	30.0	12.0	25	190	<1.0
walnut, mini *(Hostess)*, 3 pcs.	160	2.0	16.0	9.0	25	100	0
blueberry:							
(Awrey's), 1.5 oz.	130	2.0	19.0	5.0	10	180	<1.0
(Awrey's), 2.5 oz. .	210	3.0	30.0	9.0	25	250	1.0
(Awrey's Grande), 4 oz.	380	6.0	54.0	15.0	55	400	1.0
(Awrey's Petite), 2 pcs.	150	2.0	23.0	6.0	20	170	<1.0
(Entenmann's Light)	130	3.0	29.0	0	0	250	<1.0
mini *(Entenmann's Little Bites)*, 4 pcs.	190	2.0	26.0	8.0	30	180	1.0
mini *(Hostess)*, 3 pcs.	150	1.0	18.0	8.0	25	110	0
2-oz. pc.	127	3.1	27.2	3.7	17	253	1.5
cheese streusel *(Awrey's Grande)* ..	380	5.0	52.0	17.0	55	380	<1.0
chocolate chip: *(Old Spunkmeyer)*, ½ pc.	240	3.0	28.0	13.0	35	210	<1.0
chocolate *(Awrey's Grande)*	480	6.0	56.0	26.0	80	430	2.0

Food and Measure	cal.	prot. (gms)	carbo. (gms)	fat (gms)	chol. (mgs)	sod. (mgs)	fiber (gms)
mini (*Hostess*), 3 pcs.	160	2.0	17.0	9.0	20	100	0
cinnamon apple, mini (*Hostess*), 3 pcs.	160	1.0	16.0	9.0	25	110	0
corn:							
(*Awrey's*), 1.25 oz.	130	2.0	17.0	6.0	15	150	0
(*Awrey's*), 4 oz. ...	410	5.0	49.0	21.0	70	290	<1.0
(*Entenmann's*)	210	3.0	30.0	9.0	15	300	<1.0
2-oz.pc.	174	3.6	29.0	4.8	15	297	1.9
cranberry nut (*Awrey's*)	150	2.0	19.0	7.0	15	190	0
English:							
(*Awrey's*)	140	5.0	28.0	1.5	0	230	2.0
(*Bays*)	140	5.0	27.0	1.5	0	530	1.0
(*Thomas'*)	120	4.0	25.0	1.0	0	200	1.0
(*Thomas'* Super Size)	190	7.0	38.0	2.0	0	280	2.0
(*Vermont Bread*) ..	120	5.0	24.0	.5	0	190	<1.0
blueberry (*Thomas'*)	140	4.0	29.0	1.0	0	210	1.0
blueberry (*Vermont Bread*)	120	4.0	24.0	.5	0	180	<1.0
cinnamon (*Thomas'*)	150	4.0	31.0	1.0	0	200	1.0
cinnamon raisin (*Vermont Bread*)	130	4.0	28.0	.5	0	170	1.0
honey wheat (*Thomas'*)	130	4.0	27.0	.5	0	180	2.0
maple (*Vermont Bread*)	130	5.0	26.0	.5	0	200	<1.0
maple French toast (*Thomas'*)	150	5.0	30.0	1.5	20	220	<1.0
oat bran (*Thomas'*)	130	4.0	26.0	1.0	0	210	2.0
sourdough (*Bays*)	130	5.0	26.0	1.0	0	470	2.0
sourdough (*Thomas'*)	120	4.0	25.0	1.0	0	190	1.0
lemon poppy seed:							
(*Awrey's*), 4 oz. ...	420	6.0	45.0	24.0	70	310	1.0
(*Awrey's* Petite), 2 pcs.	160	2.0	24.0	6.0	20	160	<1.0
oat bran:							
(*Hostess*)	160	2.0	21.0	8.0	0	150	1.0
2-oz. pc.	154	4.0	27.5	4.2	0	224	2.6
raisin bran:							
(*Awrey's*), 1.5 oz.	110	2.0	18.0	4.0	15	170	1.0
(*Awrey's*), 2.5 oz.	200	3.0	31.0	7.0	25	220	2.0
(*Awrey's*), 4 oz. ...	350	5.0	45.0	17.0	75	340	4.0

Food and Measure	cal.	prot. (gms)	carbo. (gms)	fat (gms)	chol. (mgs)	sod. (mgs)	fiber (gms)
Muffin, frozen, 1 pc.:							
blueberry (*Sara Lee*)	220	3.0	27.0	11.0	15	170	<1.0
corn (*Sara Lee*)	260	3.0	30.0	14.0	25	220	1.0
Muffin mix (see also "Bread mix, sweet"), 1 pc.*, except as noted:							
apple cinnamon:							
(*Betty Crocker*) . . .	170	3.0	24.0	7.0	35	220	0
(*Duncan Hines* All Bran)	140	4.0	26.0	4.5	20	220	4.0
(*"Jiffy"*), ¼ cup . . .	170	2.0	28.0	5.0	0	300	1.0
(*Pillsbury*), ⅓ cup	170	2.0	30.0	5.0	<5	180	<1.0
(*Sweet Rewards*) . .	140	2.0	28.0	2.0	20	200	0
(*Sweet Rewards* Fat Free)	120	2.0	28.0	0	0	200	0
apple streusel (*Betty Crocker*)	210	3.0	33.0	8.0	20	220	0
banana nut:							
(*Betty Crocker* Box)	170	3.0	27.0	6.0	20	250	1.0
(*Betty Crocker* Pouch)	170	3.0	22.0	7.0	35	250	0
(*"Jiffy"*), ¼ cup . . .	160	2.0	25.0	5.0	0	300	2.0
(*Pillsbury*), ¼ cup	170	2.0	26.0	6.0	<5	210	<1.0
blueberry:							
(*Betty Crocker* Pouch)	160	3.0	25.0	6.0	35	220	0
(*Duncan Hines* All Bran)	140	4.0	25.0	4.5	20	230	5.0
(*Duncan Hines* Streusel)	190	2.0	32.0	6.0	15	260	0
(*"Jiffy"*), ¼ cup . . .	160	2.0	28.0	5.0	0	270	1.0
(*Pillsbury*), ⅓ cup .	170	2.0	30.0	5.0	<5	180	0
(*Pillsbury* Lowfat), ¼ cup	150	2.0	31.0	2.0	0	180	<1.0
twice (*Betty Crocker* Box)	140	2.0	25.0	4.0	20	180	1.0
wild (*Betty Crocker* Box)	170	2.0	28.0	5.0	20	210	<1.0
wild (*Sweet Rewards*)	130	2.0	26.0	2.0	20	190	0
wild (*Sweet Rewards* Fat Free)	110	2.0	26.0	0	0	190	0

Food and Measure	cal.	prot. (gms)	carbo. (gms)	fat (gms)	chol. (mgs)	sod. (mgs)	fiber (gms)
bran, ¼ cup:							
(*Hodgson Mill*) ...	130	4.0	27.0	.5	0	150	3.0
w/dates (*"Jiffy"*) ..	150	2.0	26.0	4.0	0	240	3.0
chocolate, double							
(*Betty Crocker*) ...	200	3.0	30.0	8.0	20	220	0
chocolate chip:							
(*Betty Crocker*) ...	170	3.0	23.0	8.0	35	220	0
(*Duncan Hines*) ...	190	3.0	30.0	7.0	20	250	1.0
(*Pillsbury*), ⅓ cup	180	2.0	30.0	6.0	<5	180	<1.0
cinnamon:							
(*Pillsbury*), ¼ cup	140	2.0	26.0	3.5	<5	160	<1.0
swirl (*Duncan Hines*)	200	3.0	33.0	6.0	20	250	0
corn:							
(*Glory Foods*),							
¼ cup	150	2.0	25.0	4.0	0	340	<1.0
(*"Jiffy"*), ¼ cup ...	160	2.0	28.0	4.0	0	320	1.0
golden (*Betty*							
Crocker)	160	3.0	25.0	5.0	35	260	0
cranberry orange:							
(*Betty Crocker*) ...	150	2.0	25.0	5.0	20	180	0
(*Duncan Hines*) ...	150	2.0	26.0	5.0	20	260	0
lemon poppy seed:							
(*Betty Crocker* Box)	190	2.0	30.0	7.0	20	230	0
(*Betty Crocker*							
Pouch)	180	3.0	25.0	8.0	35	190	0
oat bran (*Arrowhead*							
Mills) ⅓ cup	160	2.0	33.0	2.5	0	240	4.0
raspberry (*"Jiffy"*),							
¼ cup	170	2.0	26.0	6.0	0	310	<1.0
strawberry or wild-							
berry (*Pillsbury*),							
⅓ cup	170	2.0	30.0	5.0	<5	180	0
whole grain (*Arrow-*							
head Mills), ⅓ cup	150	7.0	26.0	2.0	0	160	7.0
whole wheat (*Hodgson*							
Mill), ¼ cup	130	4.0	27.0	.5	0	560	3.0
Muffin sandwich, see							
"Breakfast sandwich"							
Mulberries, fresh:							
10 berries, ½ oz. ...	7	.2	1.5	.1	0	2	.3
½ cup	31	1.0	6.9	.3	0	7	1.2
Mullet, striped, meat							
only, 4 oz.:							
raw	133	22.0	0	4.3	56	74	0

Food and Measure	cal.	prot (gms)	carbo. (gms)	fat (gms)	chol. (mgs)	sod. (mgs)	fiber (gms)
baked, broiled, or microwaved	170	28.1	0	5.5	71	81	0
Multigrain chips, see "Snack chips"							
Mung bean:							
dry (*Arrowhead Mills*), ¼ cup	160	11.0	28.0	.5	0	0	9.0
boiled, ½ cup	106	7.1	19.3	.4	0	2	7.7
Mung bean sprouts:							
raw:							
(*Jonathan's*), 1 cup	30	3.0	4.0	.5	0	5	.5
1 cup	31	3.2	6.2	.2	0	6	1.9
1 oz.	9	.9	1.7	.1	0	2	.5
boiled, drained, ½ cup	13	1.3	2.6	.1	0	6	.5
Mung bean sprouts, canned, drained, 1 cup	15	1.8	2.7	<.1	0	175	1.0
Mungo bean, boiled, ½ cup	95	6.8	16.5	.5	0	7	5.8
Mushroom (see also specific listings), common, ½ cup:							
raw, pcs. or slices ...	9	1.0	1.5	.2	0	1	.4
boiled, drained, pcs. .	21	1.7	4.0	.4	0	2	1.7
Mushroom, can or jar:							
whole or sliced drained, ½ cup ...	19	1.5	3.9	.5	0	332	1.9
w/liquid, ½ cup ...	20	2.0	3.0	0	0	400	<1.0
whole, sliced, or pcs. (*Green Giant*), ½ cup	30	3.0	4.0	0	0	440	2.0
whole, marinated (*Giorgio*), 1 oz., about 6 whole	10	1.0	2.0	0	0	90	<1.0
sliced (*BinB*), 1 can ..	30	3.0	4.0	0	<5	460	2.0
stems and pieces (*Libby's*), ½ cup ..	25	2.0	5.0	0	0	500	3.0
(*Libby's* Natural Pack), ½ cup ...	25	2.0	5.0	0	0	15	3.0
Mushroom, breaded, frozen (*Empire Kosher*), 7 pcs., 2.85 oz.	90	4.0	16.0	1.0	0	390	1.0

Food and Measure	cal.	prot. (gms)	carbo. (gms)	fat (gms)	chol. (mgs)	sod. (mgs)	fiber (gms)
Mushroom, chanterelle, dried (*Frieda's*), 2 pcs. . . .	15	1.0	2.0	0	0	0	1.0
Mushroom, cloud ear, dried:							
.2-oz. pc.	13	.4	3.3	<.1	0	2	3.2
½ cup	39	1.3	10.2	.1	0	5	9.8
Mushroom, crimini, brown, or Italian, raw, .5-oz. pc.	3	.4	.6	0	0	1	<.1
Mushroom, enoki, fresh:							
(*Frieda's*), ¼ pkg., .9 oz.	10	1.0	2.0	0	0	0	1.0
trimmed, 1 oz.	10	.2	2.0	.1	0	1	.7
1 large, 4⅛" long	2	.1	.4	<.1	0	<1	<1.0
Mushroom, morel, dried (*Frieda's*), 3 pcs.	15	1.0	2.0	0	0	0	0
Mushroom, oyster: fresh:							
(*Frieda's*), 3 oz. . . .	20	2.0	4.0	0	0	0	1.0
1 large, 5.2 oz. . . .	55	6.1	9.2	.8	0	46	3.6
1 small, .5 oz.	6	.6	.9	.1	0	5	.4
dried:							
(*Epicurean Specialty*), ⅓ oz.	12	1.0	2.0	0	0	6	0
(*Frieda's*), 3 pcs. . .	15	1.0	2.0	0	0	0	0
Mushroom, porcini, dried:							
(*Epicurean Specialty*), ⅓ oz.	12	1.0	2.0	0	0	6	0
(*Frieda's*), 5 pcs.	15	1.0	2.0	0	0	0	1.0
Mushroom, porto-bello:							
fresh, 1 oz.	7	.7	1.4	<.1	0	2	.4
dried (*Frieda's*), 7 pcs.	5	1.0	1.0	0	0	0	0
Mushroom, shiitake: fresh, cooked, 4 medium or ½ cup pcs.	40	1.1	10.4	.2	0	3	1.5
dried:							
(*Frieda's*), ¼ cup . .	10	0	3.0	0	0	0	0
4 medium, .5 oz. .	44	1.4	11.3	.2	0	2	1.7

Food and Measure	cal.	prot. (gms)	carbo. (gms)	fat (gms)	chol. (mgs)	sod. (mgs)	fiber (gms)
Mushroom, straw:							
canned, drained, ½ cup	29	3.5	4.2	.6	0	350	2.3
dried (*Frieda's* Padi Straw), 6 pcs.	15	1.0	2.0	0	0	0	0
Mushroom, wood ear:							
fresh (*Frieda's*), 3 oz.	20	2.0	4.0	0	0	0	1.0
dried (*Frieda's*), 3 pcs.	15	0	2.0	0	0	0	0
Mushroom batter mix (*Don's Chuck Wagon*), ¼ cup	95	3.0	21.0	0	0	990	1.0
Mushroom gravy, in jars, ¼ cup:							
(*Franco-American*)	20	1.0	3.0	1.0	<5	300	0
rich (*Heinz* Homestyle)	25	1.0	3.0	1.0	0	360	0
Mushroom gravy mix:							
(*Loma Linda Gravy Quik/Natural Touch*), ¼ cup*	15	<1.0	3.0	0	0	350	0
(*Knorr* Classic Hunter), 1 tbsp.	25	<1.0	4.0	.5	0	280	0
(*McCormick*), ¼ cup*	20	0	2.0	.5	0	260	0
Mushroom sauce:							
carciofi (*Italia In Tavola*), 2 tbsp.	110	0	2.0	12.0	0	360	<1.0
porcini (*Italia In Tavola*), 2 tbsp.	110	0	2.0	12.0	0	350	<1.0
shiitake (*Annie Chun's*), 1 tbsp.	15	1.0	3.0	0	0	190	0
Muskrat, meat only, roasted, 4 oz.	265	34.1	0	13.3	88	78	0
Mussels, blue, meat only:							
raw, 4 oz.	98	13.5	4.2	2.5	32	324	0
raw, 1 cup	129	17.9	3.4	5.5	42	429	0
boiled or steamed, 4 oz.	195	27.0	8.4	5.1	64	418	0
Mussels, canned, in red sauce (*Reese*), 4-oz. can drained	120	11.0	4.0	5.0	20	560	0
Mussels, smoked (*Ducktrap River*), ¼ cup	140	9.0	3.0	10.0	60	560	0

Food and Measure	cal.	prot. (gms)	carbo. (gms)	fat (gms)	chol. (mgs)	sod. (mgs)	fiber (gms)
Mussels dish, frozen:							
on half shell (*Southern Seafoods* New Zealand Greenshell), 3 oz. cooked	100	16.0	4.0	2.5	25	480	0
in tomato sauce (*Plumpy*), 3 oz. ..	100	12.0	6.0	2.5	30	410	<1.0
Mustard, prepared, 1 tsp.:							
(*Boar's Head* Deli) ...	0	0	0	0	0	40	0
(*French's* Classic Yellow)	0	0	0	0	0	55	0
(*French's* Deli)	5	0	0	0	0	80	0
(*Grey Poupon* Spicy Brown)	5	0	<1.0	0	0	50	0
(*Gulden's* Spicy Brown)	5	0	0	0	0	50	0
(*Hebrew National* Deli)	4	0	0	0	0	65	0
(*Hellmann's/Best Foods* Deli)	5	0	<1.0	0	0	50	0
(*Jack Daniel's* Old No. 7)	5	0	0	0	0	70	0
(*Plochman's* Premium Stoneground/Hearty Bavarian)	5	0	0	0	0	60	0
(*Kraft*)	0	0	0	0	0	60	0
(*Watkins* German) ...	10	0	1.0	0	0	110	0
Dijon:							
(*Bornier*)	5	0	0	.5	0	130	0
(*Jack Daniel's* Stoneground) ..	5	0	0	0	0	150	0
(*Plochman's* Premium)	5	0	0	0	0	80	0
extra strong (*Beaufor*), 1 tbsp.	9	.4	.3	.6	0	85	0
hickory smoke (*Jack Daniel's*)	5	0	0	0	0	125	0
w/white wine (*Grey Poupon*)	5	0	<1.0	0	0	120	0
hot:							
(*Eden* Organic) ...	0	0	<1.0	0	0	65	0
(*Nance's*)	15	0	2.0	1.0	0	90	0
(*Plochman's* Premium Spicy Peppa)	0	0	<1.0	0	0	50	0
sweet (*Napa Valley*)	5	0	2.0	0	0	15	0

Food and Measure	cal.	prot. (gms)	carbo. (gms)	fat (gms)	chol. (mgs)	sod. (mgs)	fiber (gms)
Mustard *(cont.)*							
jalapeño (*Watkins*) . . .	10	0	1.0	0	0	150	0
onion, sweet (*French's*)	10	0	2.0	0	0	70	0
sharp and creamy							
(*Nance's*)	15	0	2.0	1.0	0	100	0
spicy brown							
(*Kosciusko*)	0	0	0	0	0	60	0
yellow:							
mild (*Plochman's*)	0	0	0	0	0	55	0
Mustard blend (see also "Honey Dijon sauce"), 1 tsp.:							
chili (*Plochman's Premium Chili Dog*)	0	0	<1.0	0	0	50	0
honey:							
(*Boar's Head*)	10	0	2.0	0	0	25	0
(*French's*)	5	0	1.0	0	0	30	0
(*Grey Poupon*)	10	0	2.0	0	0	5	0
(*Hellmann's/Best Foods*)	10	0	1.0	0	0	20	0
(*Nance's*)	15	0	3.0	0	0	105	0
(*Watkins*)	15	0	2.0	.5	0	110	0
Dijon (*Jack Daniel's*)	10	0	2.0	0	0	70	0
Dijon (*Plochman's Premium*)	10	0	2.0	0	0	0	0
spicy (*Plochman's Premium*)	10	0	2.0	0	0	20	0
horseradish:							
(*Grey Poupon*)	5	0	0	0	0	50	0
(*Jack Daniel's*)	5	0	0	0	0	75	0
(*Kraft*)	0	0	0	0	0	55	0
(*Watkins*)	10	0	1.0	0	0	115	0
spicy (*Plochman's Premium*)	0	0	0	0	0	55	0
zesty (*Plochman's Premium*)	5	0	0	0	0	60	0
mayonnaise (*Dijon-naise*)	5	0	1.0	0	0	70	0
Mustard cabbage, see "Cabbage, mustard"							
Mustard greens, fresh:							
chopped, raw, 1 oz. or ½ cup	7	.8	1.4	.1	0	7	.6

Food and Measure	cal.	prot. (gms)	carbo. (gms)	fat (gms)	chol. (mgs)	sod. (mgs)	fiber (gms)
boiled, drained, ½ cup	11	1.6	1.5	.2	0	11	1.4
Mustard greens, canned, ½ cup:							
(*Allens/Sunshine*) ...	30	1.0	5.0	.5	0	10	3.0
chopped (*Bush's Best*)	25	2.0	3.0	0	0	400	2.0
seasoned (*Glory Foods*)	50	3.0	7.0	.5	0	460	3.0
Mustard greens, frozen, chopped:							
(*Birds Eye* Southern), 1 cup	30	2.0	2.0	0	0	20	2.0
boiled, drained, 1 cup	30	3.4	4.7	.4	0	38	4.2
Mustard powder, 1 tsp.	9	.5	.3	.6	0	<1	<1.0
Mustard seeds, 1 tsp.	15	.8	1.2	1.0	0	<1	<1.0
Mustard spinach:							
raw, chopped, 1 cup	33	3.3	5.9	.5	0	32	4.2
boiled, drained, chopped, 1 cup ...	29	3.1	5.0	.4	0	25	3.6
Mustard tallow, 1 tbsp.	115	0	0	12.8	13	0	0

N

Food and Measure	cal.	prot. (gms)	carbo. (gms)	fat (gms)	chol. (mgs)	sod. (mgs)	fiber (gms)
Nacho snack, frozen, stuffed, beef, 6 pcs.:							
(*Totino's* Grande)	210	6.0	27.0	9.0	10	560	2.0
and cheese (*Totino's*) .	210	6.0	27.0	9.0	10	540	1.0
nacho (*Totino's*)	220	7.0	27.0	9.0	10	660	1.0
taco flavor (*Totino's*) .	220	7.0	26.0	10.0	10	560	2.0
Nacho topping, ¼ cup:							
beef fiesta flavor (*Tostitos*)	120	4.0	6.0	8.0	10	500	<2.0
chicken quesadilla flavor (*Tostitos*) ...	90	4.0	6.0	6.0	10	600	<2.0
Name yam (*Frieda's*), ¾ cup, 3 oz.	100	1.0	24.0	0	0	10	3.0
Natto, ½ cup	187	15.6	12.6	9.7	0	6	4.8
Navy beans, boiled, ½ cup	129	7.9	24.0	.5	0	1	3.3
Navy beans, canned, ½ cup:							
(*Allens*)	110	6.0	19.0	1.0	0	380	6.0
(*Bush's Best*)	110	5.0	19.0	.5	0	450	6.0
(*Eden* Organic)	110	7.0	20.0	.5	0	15	7.0
(*Trappey's* Creole) ...	110	7.0	19.0	.5	0	380	5.0
w/bacon or bacon and jalapeño (*Trappey's*)	110	6.0	17.0	1.5	0	420	7.0
Navy beans, dehydrated (*AlpineAire*), 1 oz.	100	6.0	17.0	1.0	0	0	8.0
Navy beans, sprouted, ½ cup	35	3.2	6.8	.4	0	14	n.a.
Navy grog mixer (*Trader Vic's*), 2 fl. oz.	124	0	30.0	0	0	15	0
Nectarine:							
(*Dole*), 4.9-oz. fruit ..	70	1.0	16.0	.5	0	0	2.0

Food and Measure	cal.	prot. (gms)	carbo. (gms)	fat (gms)	chol. (mgs)	sod. (mgs)	fiber (gms)
1 medium, 2½" diam.	67	1.3	16.0	.6	0	<1	2.2
sliced, ½ cup	34	.7	8.1	.3	0	<1	1.1
Newburg sauce mix							
(*Knorr*), 1 tbsp.	35	1.0	5.0	1.0	0	350	0
Noodle, Asian, 2 oz.							
dry, except as noted:							
cellophane or long rice	200	.1	48.8	<.1	0	6	<1.0
Chinese style (*Nasoya*),							
1 cup............	210	8.0	43.0	.5	0	400	2.0
chow mein:							
(*Annie Chun's*							
Original)	200	8.0	39.0	1.0	0	350	3.0
(*La Choy*), ½ cup .	140	3.0	18.0	7.0	0	210	<1.0
(*Frieda's*), 4 oz. ...	270	10.0	40.0	1.0	0	550	4.0
½ cup	119	1.9	13.0	6.9	0	99	.9
crispy (*Frieda's*),							
½ cup, 1 oz.	160	1.0	17.0	6.0	0	160	1.0
Japanese style							
(*Nasoya*), 1 cup ...	210	8.0	43.0	.5	0	410	2.0
pad Thai, rice, basil, or							
original (*Annie*							
Chun's)	210	2.0	50.0	0	0	75	0
rice:							
(*Annie Chun's*							
Original/Hunan) .	210	2.0	50.0	0	0	75	0
(*A Taste of Thai*) ..	200	3.0	46.0	0	0	20	2.0
soba:							
(*Eden* Organic Tradi-							
tional)	200	8.0	38.0	1.5	0	70	2.0
(*Eden* Traditional) .	190	8.0	37.0	1.0	0	490	3.0
buckwheat (*Eden*) .	200	5.0	41.0	1.5	0	30	3.0
lotus root (*Eden*) ..	190	9.0	37.0	1.0	0	470	4.0
mugwort (*Eden*) ..	190	8.0	37.0	.5	0	550	2.0
wild yam (*Eden*							
Jinenjo)	190	9.0	37.0	.5	0	510	2.0
soba, cooked, 1 cup .	113	5.8	24.4	.1	0	40	n.a.
somen:							
(*Eden* Organic Tradi-							
tional)	200	8.0	38.0	1.5	0	80	3.0
uncooked	203	6.5	42.2	.5	0	1049	2.4
cooked, 1 cup	230	7.0	48.5	.3	0	284	n.a.
spinach (*Azumaya/*							
Nasoya), 1 cup ...	210	8.0	42.0	.5	0	370	2.0

Food and Measure	cal.	prot. (gms)	carbo. (gms)	fat (gms)	chol. (mgs)	sod. (mgs)	fiber (gms)
Noodle, Asian *(cont.)*							
thin cut *(Azumaya)*,							
1 cup	210	8.0	43.0	.5	0	400	2.0
udon:							
(Eden)	190	8.0	37.0	1.5	0	660	3.0
(Eden Organic Tradi-							
tional)	200	8.0	38.0	2.0	0	80	3.0
brown rice *(Eden)* .	190	8.0	38.0	1.0	0	510	2.0
udon, cooked, 4 oz. . .	115	2.8	23.0	.6	0	51	n.a.
wide cut *(Azumaya)*,							
1 cup	210	8.0	43.0	.5	0	410	2.0
Noodle, egg, dry:							
all styles *(Mueller's)*							
2 oz.	220	8.0	38.0	3.0	65	10	1.0
enriched, 2 oz.	216	7.9	40.3	2.4	54	12	1.5
four color *(Hodgson							
Mill)*, 2 oz.	200	9.0	37.0	2.0	35	25	2.0
whole wheat, 2 oz.:							
(Pastamania!)	190	10.0	34.0	2.0	30	20	4.0
spinach *(Pasta-							
mania!)*	190	10.0	32.0	2.0	30	45	5.0
Noodle, egg, cooked:							
1 cup	212	7.6	39.7	2.4	53	11	1.8
spinach, 1 cup	211	8.1	38.8	2.5	52	20	3.7
Noodle, egg, frozen,							
½ cup, except							
as noted:							
(Aunt Vi's), 2 oz.	150	8.0	26.0	2.0	20	60	2.0
(Reames)	170	4.0	32.0	2.0	85	10	1.0
(Reames Free)	160	5.0	32.0	0	0	10	1.0
(Reames Original) . . .	170	5.0	32.0	2.0	70	10	1.0
(Reames Quick Cook),							
1 cup	230	10.0	42.0	2.5	80	30	2.0
cooked *(Aunt Vi's*							
Heat-N-Serve), 4 oz.	150	8.0	26.0	2.0	20	60	2.0
flat dumpling *(Reames)*	190	6.0	35.0	2.0	75	15	2.0
yolk-free *(Aunt Vi's)*,							
4 oz.	80	7.0	29.0	0	0	15	0
Noodle, Chinese,							
Japanese, or Thai,							
see "Noodle, Asian"							
Noodle dish, mix,							
1 cup*, except as							
noted:							

Food and Measure	cal.	prot. (gms)	carbo. (gms)	fat (gms)	chol. (mgs)	sod. (mgs)	fiber (gms)
Alfredo							
(*Lipton* Noodles & Sauce), ½ pkg. .	250	10.0	39.0	7.0	75	940	2.0
broccoli (*Lipton* Noodles & Sauce)	340	12.0	43.0	14.0	80	970	2.0
butter:							
(*Lipton* Noodles & Sauce)	310	8.0	41.0	14.0	70	870	2.0
herb (*Lipton* Noodles & Sauce)	300	9.0	42.0	13.0	65	780	2.0
chicken:							
(*Lipton* Noodles & Sauce)	290	9.0	42.0	10.5	65	830	2.0
creamy (*Lipton* Noodles & Sauce), ½ pkg.	240	8.0	39.0	6.0	70	700	2.0
tetrazzini (*Lipton* Noodles & Sauce)	300	10.0	41.0	11.5	70	950	2.0
chow mein, garlic scallion (*Annie Chun's* Noodles & Sauce), ⅓ box	250	7.0	40.0	6.0	0	950	3.0
garlic black bean (*Annie Chun's* Noodles & Sauce), ⅓ box	260	8.0	43.0	6.0	0	950	3.0
Parmesan (*Lipton* Noodles & Sauce), ½ pkg.	250	10.0	37.0	8.0	70	750	2.0
soba, soy ginger (*Annie Chun's* Noodles & Sauce), ⅓ box	210	7.0	40.0	2.0	0	1020	3.0
sour cream and chive (*Lipton* Noodles & Sauce), ½ pkg. . . .	260	8.0	41.0	8.0	70	800	2.0
Stroganoff (*Lipton* Noodles & Sauce), ½ pkg.	210	8.0	38.0	4.0	65	800	2.0
Noodle entree, can or pkg., 1 cup:							
and beef, Stroganoff (*Dinty Moore* Microwave Cup)	240	11.0	16.0	14.0	65	920	0

Food and Measure	cal.	prot. (gms)	carbo. (gms)	fat (gms)	chol. (mgs)	sod. (mgs)	fiber (gms)
Noodle entree, can or pkg. *(cont.)*							
and chicken:							
(*Hormel* Microcup)	200	8.0	20.0	9.0	40	1140	1.0
rings (*Kid's Kitchen*)	150	10.0	17.0	4.0	30	1110	1.0
Noodle entree, frozen,							
1 pkg., except as							
noted:							
Alfredo (*Michelina's*),							
8 oz.	330	12.0	40.0	14.0	75	590	2.0
w/beef, 1 cup:							
(*Freezer Queen*							
Family)	200	8.0	33.0	4.0	30	1160	3.0
brown gravy							
(*Banquet* Family)	150	11.0	16.0	5.0	35	1120	2.0
w/chicken:							
(*Michelina's*), 8 oz.	300	16.0	38.0	11.0	85	690	2.0
(*Michelina's* Noodles							
'n Chicken), 8 oz.	290	13.0	38.0	9.0	70	700	2.0
creamy (*Kid Cuisine*							
Bowl), 8 oz. . . .	220	9.0	30.0	6.0	15	1040	2.0
escalloped (*Marie*							
Callender's),							
13 oz.	740	21.0	60.0	46.0	90	1600	5.0
escalloped (*Marie*							
Callender's Family),							
1 cup	280	8.0	22.0	17.0	40	680	1.0
home style (*Banquet*),							
12 oz.	390	12.0	44.0	19.0	50	1080	7.0
Japanese, and vege-							
tables (*Cascadian*							
Farm Veggie Bowl),							
9 oz.	180	3.0	28.0	2.5	0	630	4.0
Romanoff:							
(*Stouffer's*), 12 oz.	490	17.0	53.0	23.0	55	1260	5.0
w/meatballs (*Miche-*							
lina's), 10 oz. . .	310	14.0	45.0	7.0	65	1800	2.0
stir-fry, Asian (*Amy's*),							
10 oz.	240	12.0	41.0	4.5	0	680	6.0
Stroganoff (*Michelina's*),							
8 oz.	350	14.0	38.0	14.0	80	760	2.0
Nopales/Nopalitos,							
see "Cactus pads"							
Nori, see "Seaweed"							

Food and Measure	cal.	prot. (gms)	carbo. (gms)	fat (gms)	chol. (mgs)	sod. (mgs)	fiber (gms)
Nut topping, see specific nut listings							
Nutmeg, ground, 1 tsp.	12	.1	1.1	.8	0	tr.	.1
Nuts, see specific listings							
Nuts, mixed, 1 oz., except as noted:							
(*Bazzini Nut Club* Salted), 4 tbsp. . . .	210	5.0	8.0	8.0	0	40	3.0
(*Bazzini Nut Club* Unsalted), 4 tbsp.	210	5.0	8.0	8.0	0	5	3.0
(*Fisher*)	180	6.0	5.0	16.0	0	110	2.0
(*House of Bazzini* Raw), 4 tbsp.	210	5.0	8.0	16.0	0	0	3.0
(*Planters* Deluxe)	170	5.0	6.0	16.0	0	110	2.0
w/peanuts:							
(*Blue Diamond* Deluxe), ¼ cup	210	7.0	6.0	19.0	0	70	<1.0
(*Planters*)	170	5.0	6.0	15.0	0	115	3.0
(*Planters* Unsalted)	170	5.0	6.0	15.0	0	0	2.0
w/out peanuts:							
(*Blue Diamond* Extra Fancy), ¼ cup . .	210	5.0	7.0	20.0	0	70	<1.0
cinnamon flavor (*Planters* Sweet Roasts)	160	2.0	9.0	13.0	0	55	2.0
dry-roasted:							
w/peanuts	169	4.9	7.2	14.6	0	3	2.6
w/peanuts, salted . .	169	4.9	7.2	14.6	0	190	2.6
honey (*Planters* Sweet Roasts)	160	3.0	10.0	12.0	0	120	2.0
honey-roasted (*Planters*)	160	5.0	9.0	13.0	0	120	2.0
oil-roasted:							
w/peanuts	175	4.8	6.1	16.0	0	3	2.8
w/peanuts, salted . .	175	4.8	6.1	16.0	0	185	2.8
vanilla flavor (*Planters* Sweet Roasts)	160	3.0	10.0	12.0	0	55	2.0

O

Food and Measure	cal.	prot. (gms)	carbo. (gms)	fat (gms)	chol. (mgs)	sod. (mgs)	fiber (gms)
Oat (see also "Cereal"):							
whole-grain, 1 oz. . . .	110	4.8	18.8	2.0	0	1	n.a.
flakes, rolled (*Arrow-head Mills*), ⅓ cup	130	5.0	23.0	2.5	0	0	4.0
rolled or oatmeal:							
dry, 1 oz.	109	4.5	19.0	1.8	0	1	2.9
cooked, 1 cup	145	6.1	25.3	2.3	0	2	4.0
steel cut (*Arrowhead Mills*), ¼ cup	170	6.0	29.0	3.0	0	0	5.0
Oat beverage, original vanilla (*WestSoy* Oat Plus), 8 fl, oz.	150	6.0	26.0	3.0	0	80	4.0
Oat bran, dry:							
(*Arrowhead Mills*), ⅓ cup	150	8.0	23.0	2.5	0	0	7.0
1 oz.	70	4.9	18.8	2.0	0	1	4.5
Oat flour:							
(*Arrowhead Mills*), ⅓ cup	120	5.0	20.0	2.0	0	0	4.0
bran, ¼ cup:							
(*Hodgson Mill*) . . .	110	3.0	23.0	2.0	0	4	3.0
(*Hodgson Mill Organic*)	110	3.0	24.0	1.0	0	120	3.0
blend (*Hodgson Mill*)	110	3.0	24.0	1.0	0	3	3.0
Oat groats (*Arrowhead Mills*), ¼ cup	160	6.0	29.0	3.0	0	0	4.0
Oca (*Frieda's*), ½ cup, 3 oz.	70	2.0	15.0	0	0	5	1.0
Ocean perch, Atlantic, meat only:							
raw, 4 oz.	107	21.1	0	1.9	48	85	0
baked, broiled, or microwaved, 4 oz.	137	27.1	0	2.4	61	109	0

Food and Measure	cal.	prot. (gms)	carbo. (gms)	fat (gms)	chol. (mgs)	sod. (mgs)	fiber (gms)
Ocean perch entree, frozen, battered fillet (*Van de Kamp's*), 2 pcs., 3.7 oz.	220	10.0	18.0	12.0	25	460	0
Octopus, 4 oz.:							
raw	93	16.9	2.5	1.2	54	261	0
boiled or steamed . . .	186	33.8	5.0	2.4	109	522	0
Octopus, canned:							
(*Goya*), ¼ cup	140	11.0	3.0	9.0	25	410	0
spiced, in red sauce (*Reese*), 2 oz.	120	7.0	4.0	8.0	0	430	0
Oheloberry, ½ cup . .	20	.3	4.8	.2	0	1	n.a.
Oil, 1 tbsp., except as noted:							
(*Arrowhead Mills Essential Balance*)	130	0	0	14.0	0	0	0
(*House of Tsang Mongolian Fire*), 1 tsp.	45	0	0	5.0	0	0	0
all varieties (*Hain*) . . .	120	0	0	14.0	0	0	0
almond, canola, cocoa butter, corn, cottonseed, hazelnut, oat, palm, or poppy seed	120	0	0	13.6	0	0	0
avocado or mustard . .	124	0	0	14.0	0	0	0
butter oil	112	<.1	0	12.7	33	0	0
coconut	117	0	0	13.6	0	0	0
cod liver	123	0	0	13.6	78	0	0
flaxseed (*Arrowhead Mills*)	130	0	0	14.0	0	0	0
grape seed, plain or flavored (*Watkins*)	120	0	0	14.0	0	0	0
herring	123	0	0	13.6	104	0	0
olive, peanut, safflower, sesame, soybean, sunflower, vegetable, or walnut	120	0	0	14.0	0	0	0
salmon	123	0	0	13.6	66	0	0
sardine	123	0	0	13.6	97	0	0
wok (*House of Tsang*)	130	0	0	14.0	0	0	0
Oil, seasoned, see specific listings							
Okra, fresh:							
raw, sliced, ½ cup . . .	19	1.0	3.8	.1	0	4	1.3

Food and Measure	cal.	prot. (gms)	carbo. (gms)	fat (gms)	chol. (mgs)	sod. (mgs)	fiber (gms)
Okra *(cont.)*							
boiled, drained, 8 pods, 3" x ⅝"	27	1.6	6.1	.1	0	5	2.1
boiled, drained, sliced, ½ cup	25	1.5	5.8	.1	0	4	2.0
Okra, canned, ½ cup:							
cut (*Allens/Trappey's*)	25	1.0	6.0	0	0	400	3.0
gumbo (*Trappey's* Creole)	35	2.0	6.0	0	0	290	3.0
w/tomatoes (*Allens/ Trappey's*)	30	1.0	5.0	0	0	380	3.0
w/tomatoes and corn (*Allens/Trappey's*)	30	<1.0	6.0	0	0	280	4.0
Okra, cocktail, hot (*Trappey's*), 1.1 oz.	10	0	2.0	0	0	220	0
Okra, frozen:							
whole:							
(*Birds Eye*), 9 pods	25	1.0	5.0	0	0	35	3.0
(*McKenzie's*), 3 oz.	25	1.0	5.0	0	0	35	3.0
cut, ¾ cup:							
(*Birds Eye*)	25	1.0	5.0	0	0	35	3.0
(*McKenzie's*)	25	1.0	5.0	0	0	35	3.0
boiled, drained, sliced, ½ cup	34	1.9	7.5	.3	0	3	2.8
and tomato, ¾ cup:							
(*Birds Eye*)	25	1.0	4.0	0	0	15	3.0
(*McKenzie's*)	20	1.0	4.0	0	0	30	2.0
Olive, pickled:							
black, see "ripe," below							
Calamata (*Krinos*), 3 pcs., .5 oz.	45	0	2.0	4.0	0	230	0
Greek, black:							
10 medium	65	.4	1.7	6.9	0	631	0
10 extra large	89	.6	2.3	9.5	0	868	0
pitted, 1 oz.	96	.6	2.5	10.2	0	932	0
green, w/pits:							
10 small	33	.4	.4	3.6	0	686	.7
10 large	45	.5	.5	4.9	0	926	1.0
10 giant	76	.9	.9	8.3	0	1572	1.7
queen, Spanish (*Early California* 7 oz.), 2 pcs., .5 oz.	25	0	1.0	2.0	0	350	0

Food and Measure	cal.	prot. (gms)	carbo. (gms)	fat (gms)	chol. (mgs)	sod. (mgs)	fiber (gms)
Spanish (*Early California*), 14 pcs., .5 oz.	30	0	1.0	2.5	0	190	0
green, cracked (*Krinos*), 2 pcs., .5 oz.	20	0	2.0	1.0	0	220	0
green, pitted:							
1 oz.	33	.4	.4	3.6	0	680	.7
Spanish (*Early California*), 5 pcs., .5 oz.	25	0	1.0	2.0	0	350	0
ripe, pitted:							
(*Black Pearls*), 2 colossal	20	0	1.0	1.5	0	95	0
(*Black Pearls*), 3 jumbo or extra large, 4 large, 5 medium, or 6 small	25	0	1.0	2.0	0	95	0
(*Early California*), 2 colossal	20	0	1.0	2.0	0	110	0
(*Early California*), 3 jumbo	25	0	0	2.0	0	135	0
(*Early California*), 4 large, 3 extra large, 5 medium, or 6 small	25	0	1.0	2.5	0	115	0
(*Early California*), 1 supercolossal	15	0	1.0	1.0	0	75	0
(*Lindsay*), 6 small, 5 medium, 4 large, 1⅓ tbsp.							
chopped	25	0	1.0	2.5	0	115	0
chopped (*Black Pearls*), 1⅓ tbsp.	25	0	1.0	2.5	0	115	0
chopped or sliced (*Early California*), .5 oz.	25	0	1.0	2.5	0	115	0
sliced (*Black Pearls* 2.25 oz.), 2 tbsp.	25	0	1.0	2.5	0	125	0
sliced (*Black Pearls* 3.8 oz.), 2 tbsp.	25	0	1.0	2.0	0	95	0
sliced (*Lindsay*), 2 tbsp.	25	0	1.0	2.5	0	125	0

Food and Measure	cal.	prot. (gms)	carbo. (gms)	fat (gms)	chol. (mgs)	sod. (mgs)	fiber (gms)
Olive *(cont.)*							
stuffed, green:							
w/almonds (*Reese*),							
4 pcs., .5 oz. . . .	35	0	<1.0	3.5	0	310	0
w/anchovies (*Goya*),							
4 pcs., .5 oz. . . .	25	0	<1.0	2.5	<1	240	0
w/anchovies (*Reese*),							
4 pcs., .5 oz. . . .	20	0	<1.0	2.0	0	220	0
w/sun-dried tomato							
(*Byzantine*), 5 pcs.	17	.5	1.5	1.3	0	281	.7
stuffed, w/pimiento:							
(*Pompeian*), 6 pcs.,							
.5 oz.	25	0	1.0	2.5	0	240	0
queen (*Goya*), 1 pc.	20	0	1.0	1.5	0	160	0
queen, Spanish							
(*Early California*),							
2 pcs., .6 oz. . . .	20	0	1.0	1.5	0	380	0
Spanish (*Early Cali-*							
fornia), 3–4 pcs.,							
.5 oz.	25	0	1.0	2.0	0	330	0
Spanish (*Early Cali-*							
fornia), 5 pcs.,							
.5 oz.	25	0	1.0	2.0	0	350	0
Olive-jalapeño spread							
(*D. L. Jardine's*							
Texas Caviar), .5 oz.	15	0	0	1.5	0	510	0
Olive loaf, see "Lunch							
meat"							
Olive oil, see "Oil"							
Olive salad (*Progresso*),							
2 tbsp.	25	0	1.0	2.5	0	360	<1.0
Olive sauce, green							
(*Italia In Tavola*),							
2 tbsp.	90	0	0	10.0	0	970	0
Omelette, see "Egg							
breakfast"							
Onion, fresh/stored:							
raw:							
(*Frieda's* Boiler/Cipol-							
line), 3 pcs., 3 oz.	30	1.0	7.0	0	0	0	2.0
(*Frieda's* Hawaiian							
Maui), ⅓ cup,							
3 oz.	10	0	3.0	0	0	0	1.0

Food and Measure	cal.	prot. (gms)	carbo. (gms)	fat (gms)	chol. (mgs)	sod. (mgs	fiber (gms)
(*Frieda's* Pearl), ⅔ cup, 3 oz.	30	1.0	7.0	0	0	0	2.0
(*Lucinda's* Pearl Red/White), 1 oz., about 1 pc.	20	0	4.0	0	0	25	.4
1 oz.	11	.3	2.4	<.1	0	1	.5
chopped, ½ cup ..	30	.9	6.9	0.1	0	2	1.4
chopped, 1 tbsp. ...	4	.1	.9	<.1	0	tr.	.2
boiled, drained:							
chopped, ½ cup ..	46	1.4	10.7	.2	0	3	1.5
chopped, 1 tbsp. ...	7	.2	1.5	<.1	0	<1	.2
Onion, can or jar:							
whole, ½ cup:							
(*Aunt Nellie's/Lohmann*), ½ cup ..	35	<1.0	8.0	0	0	410	2.0
(*Hanover*), ½ cup .	25	1.0	6.0	0	0	420	1.0
2.2-oz. onion	12	.5	2.5	<.1	0	234	.8
cocktail (*Crosse & Blackwell*), 1 tbsp.	0	0	1.0	0	0	250	0
pickled, sour (*London Pub*), ¼ cup, 1.1 oz.	10	2.0	2.0	0	0	130	0
Onion, dehydrated, chopped (*Alpine-Aire*), 1.3 oz.	80	2.0	17.0	0	0	15	4.0
Onion, dried:							
flakes, 1 tbsp.	16	.5	4.2	<.1	0	1	.5
minced, 1 tsp.	7	.2	1.9	0	0	<1	.2
Onion, frozen:							
whole:							
boiled, drained, ½ cup	30	.7	7.0	0	0	8	1.5
small (*Birds Eye*), 17 pcs.	30	1.0	7.0	0	0	10	1.0
whole, pearl, in real cream sauce							
diced (*Birds Eye*), ⅔ cup	30	<1.0	6.0	0	0	30	1.0
chopped:							
(*Seabrook Farms*), ⅔ cup	30	<1.0	6.0	0	0	30	1.0
boiled, drained, 1 tbsp.	4	.1	1.0	<.1	0	2	.2

Food and Measure	cal.	prot. (gms)	carbo. (gms)	fat (gms)	chol. (mgs)	sod. (mgs)	fiber (gms)
Onion, frozen *(cont.)*							
in cream sauce, pearl							
(*Birds Eye*), ½ cup	60	2.0	8.0	2.0	10	280	1.0
rings, see "Onion rings"							
Onion, green, raw,							
trimmed, w/top:							
(*Dole*), ¼ cup	10	0	2.0	0	0	5	1.0
chopped, ½ cup	16	.9	3.7	.1	0	8	1.3
chopped, 1 tbsp.	2	.1	.4	<.1	0	1	.2
Onion, pickled, see							
"Onion, in jars"							
Onion, Welsh, 1 oz.	10	.5	1.8	.1	0	5	<1.0
Onion dip, 2 tbsp.:							
bold/spicy (*Heluva*							
Good Bodacious)	60	1.0	3.0	5.0	20	210	0
French:							
(*Frito-Lay*)	60	1.0	4.0	5.0	15	230	0
(*Heluva* Good)	60	1.0	2.0	5.0	20	170	0
(*Kraft Dips*)	60	1.0	3.0	4.5	0	210	0
(*Marzetti*)	130	1.0	2.0	13.0	25	220	0
(*Marzetti* Light)	70	1.0	3.0	6.0	10	250	0
green (*Kraft Dips*)	60	1.0	4.0	4.0	0	190	0
sour cream and:							
(*Marzetti* Fat Free)	35	1.0	6.0	0	0	300	0
(*Utz*)	60	1.0	2.0	5.0	15	220	0
Onion dip mix, 2 tbsp.*,							
except as noted:							
and chive (*Knorr*),							
½ tsp.	5	0	<1.0	0	0	110	0
French:							
(*McCormick*)	35	0	2.0	5.0	0	180	0
(*Ruffles*)	70	1.0	3.0	6.0	10	190	<1.0
spring (*McCormick*)	35	0	2.0	5.0	0	170	0
Onion gravy, zesty							
(*Heinz* Home Style),							
¼ cup	25	1.0	3.0	1.0	0	350	0
Onion gravy mix:							
(*Loma Linda* Gravy							
Quik/*Natural Touch*),							
¼ cup*	15	<1.0	3.0	0	0	240	<1.0
(*McCormick*), ¼ cup*	20	0	3.0	.5	0	340	0
Onion flavor chips,							
see "Snack chips"							

Food and Measure	cal.	prot. (gms)	carbo. (gms)	fat (gms)	chol. (mgs)	sod. (mgs)	fiber (gms)
Onion oil (*Watkins* Liquid Spice), 1 tsp.	40	0	0	4.5	0	0	0
Onion powder:							
(*Tone's*), ¼ tsp.	5	0	1.0	0	0	0	0
1 tsp.	7	.2	1.7	0	0	1	.1
Onion ring, canned (*French's Taste Toppers*), 2 tbsp.	45	0	3.0	3.5	0	60	0
Onion ring, frozen:							
(*McKenzie's*), 3.25 oz.	220	3.0	28.0	10.0	0	210	6.0
(*Mrs. Paul's*), 4 pcs., 2.9 oz.	190	3.0	22.0	10.0	<5	280	1.0
(*Ore-Ida Onion Ringers*), 6 pcs., 3.2 oz.	220	3.0	25.0	12.0	0	350	3.0
(*Ore-Ida Vidalia O's*), 5 pcs., 3.2 oz.	240	3.0	20.0	15.0	0	420	1.0
heated, 10 rings	289	3.8	27.1	19.0	0	17	2.9
Onion ring batter mix, ¼ cup:							
(*Don's Chuck Wagon/ Vidalia Sweet*)	100	3.0	21.0	0	0	690	1.0
(*Golden Dipt* Fry Easy)	100	1.0	20.0	0	0	660	0
(*McCormick Produce Partners*)	110	2.0	18.0	.5	0	610	0
Onion salt, ¼ tsp.:							
(*McCormick*)	0	0	0	0	0	450	0
(*Watkins*)	0	0	0	0	0	330	0
w/parsley (*McCormick California*)	0	0	0	0	0	170	0
Onion sauce (*Boar's Head* Vidalia), 1 tbsp.	10	0	2.0	0	0	15	0
Onion snack chips, see "Snack chips"							
Onion sprouts (*Jonathan's*), 1 cup	30	1.0	5.0	0	0	5	2.0
Opo squash (*Frieda's*), ⅔ cup, 3 oz.	10	1.0	3.0	0	0	0	0
Opossum, meat only, roasted, 4 oz.	251	34.3	0	11.6	146	66	0
Orange, fresh:							
(*Dole*), 5.4-oz. fruit . .	70	1.0	21.0	0	0	0	7.0
(*Frieda's* Blood/Cara Cara), 5 oz.	70	1.0	16.0	0	0	0	3.0
(*Frieda's* Seville), 3 oz.	40	1.0	10.0	0	0	0	2.0

Food and Measure	cal.	prot. (gms)	carbo. (gms)	fat (gms)	chol. (mgs)	sod. (mgs)	fiber (gms)
Orange *(cont.)*							
all varieties:							
3¹⁄₁₆" fruit, 6.5 oz.	87	1.7	21.6	.2	0	0	4.4
sections, 1 cup …	85	1.7	21.2	.2	0	0	4.3
California navel:							
2⅞" fruit, 5 oz. …	65	1.4	16.3	.1	0	1	3.4
sections, 1 cup …	76	1.7	19.2	.2	0	2	4.0
California Valencia:							
2⅞" fruit, 4.25 oz.	59	1.3	14.4	.4	0	0	3.0
sections, 1 cup …	88	1.9	21.4	.5	0	0	4.5
Florida:							
2¹¹⁄₁₆" fruit, 5 oz.	65	1.0	16.3	.3	0	1	3.4
sections, 1 cup …	85	1.3	21.4	.4	0	1	4.4
Orange, Mandarin, see "Tangerine"							
Orange dip mix (*Watkins* Mandarin), 1 tsp. …	20	0	5.0	0	0	35	0
Orange drink, 8 fl. oz., except as noted:							
(*Capri Sun All Natural*), 6.75 fl. oz. …	100	0	25.0	0	0	20	0
(*Hawaiian Punch* Orange Ocean) …	120	0	29.0	0	0	95	0
(*Snapple* Orangeade)	120	0	29.0	0	0	10	0
(*Sunny Delight* Calcium) …	140	0	34.0	0	0	75	0
(*Tang Orange Uproar*)	120	0	31.0	0	0	35	0
(*Turkey Hill* Orangeade)	120	0	30.0	0	0	10	0
(*WhipperSnapple* Dream), 10 fl. oz.	150	0	36.0	0	0	60	0
canned …	126	0	32.0	0	0	40	.3
Orange drink blends, 8 fl. oz., except as noted:							
apple, frozen* (*Cascadian Farm* Sunrise)	110	0	29.0	0	0	9	0
cranberry:							
(*Tropicana Twister*)	120	<1.0	30.0	0	0	45	0
(*Tropicana Twister*) 10 fl. oz. …	160	<1.0	40.0	0	0	60	0
(*Tropicana Twister*), 11.5 fl. oz. …	190	<1.0	46.0	0	0	65	0
mango (*R. W. Knudsen*)	120	<1.0	30.0	0	0	50	0

Food and Measure	cal.	prot. (gms)	carbo. (gms)	fat (gms)	chol. (mgs)	sod. (mgs)	fiber (gms)
pineapple (*Tropicana*), 11.5 fl. oz.	180	0	45.0	0	0	35	0
pineapple apple (*Welch's*)	140	0	35.0	0	0	20	0
strawberry banana:							
(*Dole*)	130	<1.0	32.0	0	0	45	0
(*Dole*), 11.5 fl. oz. .	180	<1.0	45.0	0	0	60	0
(*Tropicana Twister*)	130	<1.0	32.0	0	0	45	0
(*Tropicana Twister*), 10 fl. oz.	160	<1.0	40.0	0	0	60	0
(*Tropicana Twister*), 11.5 fl. oz.	190	<1.0	46.0	0	0	65	0
Orange drink mix, 8 fl. oz.*, except as noted:							
(*Kool-Aid* Sugar Sweetened)	60	0	16.0	0	0	5	0
(*Tang*)	90	0	23.0	0	0	25	0
creamy (*Watkins* Cooler), ½ tbsp. ...	25	0	4.0	1.0	0	10	0
pineapple (*Tang*)	100	0	24.0	0	0	45	0
Orange juice, 8 fl. oz.:							
(*Dole*)	110	1.0	27.0	0	0	15	0
(*Florida's Natural* Original/Home Squeezed w/Pulp) .	110	0	26.0	0	0	0	0
(*Florida's Natural* Calcium)	120	1.0	29.0	0	0	0	0
(*Hood*)	120	0	30.0	0	0	20	0
(*Horizon*)	110	2.0	26.0	0	0	0	0
(*Langers*)	120	0	29.0	0	0	15	0
(*Nantucket Nectars*) ..	120	0	27.0	0	0	0	0
(*R. W. Knudsen*)	100	2.0	23.0	0	0	25	0
(*R. W. Knudsen* Organic)	100	2.0	23.0	0	0	35	0
(*Season's Best* Calcium/ Vitamin C)	110	1.0	27.0	0	0	15	0
(*Season's Best* Glass)	110	1.0	26.0	0	0	15	0
(*Season's Best* Pulp/ Pulp Free)	110	<1.0	27.0	0	0	15	0
(*Simply Orange*)	110	2.0	26.0	0	0	0	0
(*Tropicana* Low Acid) .	110	2.0	26.0	0	0	0	0
(*Tropicana* Pure Premium)	110	1.0	26.0	0	0	0	0

Food and Measure	cal.	prot. (gms)	carbo. (gms)	fat (gms)	chol. (mgs)	sod. (mgs)	fiber (gms)
Orange juice *(cont.)*							
(*Turkey Hill*)	100	1.0	24.0	0	0	5	0
(*Uncle Matt's*)	110	2.0	26.0	0	0	0	0
canned	105	1.5	24.5	.4	0	5	.5
chilled	110	2.0	25.1	.7	0	3	.5
fresh	112	1.7	25.8	.5	0	2	.5
frozen*:							
(*Cascadian Farm*) .	120	1.0	29.0	0	0	5	0
(*Minute Maid*)	110	0	27.0	0	0	0	0
(*Minute Maid* Calcium)	120	0	27.0	0	0	0	0
Orange juice blends, 8 fl. oz.:							
(*After the Fall 24 Karrot Orange*)	120	1.0	29.0	0	0	45	0
(*Tropicana* Ruby Red)	110	2.0	26.0	0	0	0	0
apricot (*Snapple* Snapricot)	120	0	30.0	0	0	10	0
banana (*Tropicana*) ..	140	2.0	32.0	0	0	0	0
carrot (*Horizon*)	90	2.0	21.0	0	0	65	0
grapefruit, canned ...	106	1.5	25.4	.3	0	7	.3
guava (*Dole*)	120	0	30.0	0	0	35	0
kiwi passion (*Tropicana Pure Tropics*)	100	<1.0	26.0	0	0	15	0
peach mango:							
(*Dole*)	120	1.0	28.0	0	0	35	0
(*Tropicana Pure Tropics*)	110	<1.0	27.0	0	0	20	0
pineapple:							
(*Season's Best*) ...	110	<1.0	27.0	0	0	15	0
(*Tropicana* Calcium)	130	2.0	31.0	0	0	0	0
(*Tropicana Pure Tropics*)	120	2.0	27.0	0	0	20	0
strawberry (*Tropicana*)	130	2.0	30.0	0	0	0	0
strawberry banana:							
(*Dole*)	120	1.0	28.0	0	0	30	0
(*Tropicana Pure Tropics*)	110	<1.0	27.0	0	0	10	0
tangerine:							
(*Nantucket Nectars*)	120	0	29.0	0	0	35	0
(*Tropicana*)	110	2.0	25.0	0	0	0	0
Orange peel, fresh, 1 tbsp.	—[1]	.1	1.5	<.1	0	0	.2

1. Cannot be calculated; no digestibility value for peel.

Food and Measure	cal.	prot. (gms)	carbo. (gms)	fat (gms)	chol. (mgs)	sod. (mgs)	fiber (gms)
Orange peel, candied, diced, 2 tbsp.:							
(*Seneca* Glacé), 2 tbsp.	70	0	18.0	0	0	20	1.0
(*S&W* Glacé), 58 pcs., 1.1 oz.	80	0	23.0	0	0	35	2.0
Orange sauce, Oriental (*Ka•Me* Mandarin), 2 tbsp.	80	0	21.0	0	0	430	0
Oregano, dried, 1 tsp.	3	.1	.5	0	0	0	.1
Oriental 5-spice (*Tone's*), 1 tsp. . . .	9	.3	1.9	.3	0	2	.5
Oyster, meat only, 4 oz., except as noted:							
Eastern, wild:							
raw, 1 lb.	310	32.0	17.7	11.1	238	957	0
raw, 6 medium, 3 oz.	57	5.9	3.3	2.1	44	177	0
baked, broiled, or microwaved . . .	82	9.4	5.4	2.2	56	277	0
steamed or poached	155	16.0	8.9	5.6	119	478	0
Eastern, farmed:							
raw	67	5.9	6.3	1.8	29	202	0
baked, broiled, or microwaved	90	7.9	8.3	2.4	43	185	0
Pacific:							
raw	93	10.7	5.6	2.6	n.a.	120	0
raw, boiled, or steamed, 1 medium	41	4.7	2.5	1.2	n.a.	53	0
boiled or steamed	185	21.4	11.2	5.2	n.a.	240	0
Oyster, canned, 2 oz., except as noted:							
Eastern, wild:							
w/liquid, 4 oz.	78	8.0	4.4	2.8	62	127	0
w/liquid, 1 cup	170	17.5	9.7	6.1	136	277	0
whole:							
(*Bumble Bee* Fancy)	70	7.0	3.0	3.0	45	140	0
(*Chicken of the Sea*)	70	7.0	3.0	3.0	30	220	0
(*3 Diamonds*)	60	8.0	2.0	.5	45	210	0
boiled (*Crown Prince*), ⅓ cup . .	70	7.0	4.0	3.0	35	150	0
smoked:							
(*Bumble Bee*)	120	10.0	6.0	7.0	35	210	0
(*Chicken of the Sea*), 2.5 oz.	140	11.0	7.0	8.0	40	260	0

Food and Measure	cal.	prot. (gms)	carbo. (gms)	fat (gms)	chol. (mgs)	sod. (mgs)	fiber (gms)
Oyster, canned *(cont.)*							
(Chicken of the Sea),							
3 oz.	190	14.0	9.0	11.0	˙55	340	0
(Crown Prince							
Natural)	60	14.0	0	0	35	140	0
(3 Diamonds)	110	9.0	9.0	4.0	25	200	0
medium *(Reese)* . .	110	8.0	6.0	6.0	50	220	0
Oyster plant, see							
"Salsify"							
Oyster sauce, Asian							
(Ka•Me), 1 tbsp. . .	10	0	3.0	0	0	260	0
Oyster stew, see							
"Soup, condensed"							

P

Food and Measure	cal.	prot. (gms)	carbo. (gms)	fat (gms)	chol. (mgs)	sod. (mgs)	fiber (gms)
Pad Thai sauce, see "Thai sauce"							
Palm, hearts of, can or jar:							
1.2-oz. pc.	9	.8	1.5	.2	0	141	.8
1 cup	41	3.7	6.8	.9	0	622	3.5
Pancake, frozen, 3 pcs., except as noted:							
(*Aunt Jemima* Home-style)	210	6.0	40.0	3.5	20	560	2.0
(*Aunt Jemima* Low-fat)	170	4.0	33.0	2.5	<5	410	8.0
(*Aunt Jemima* Mini), 13 pcs.	240	6.0	46.0	4.0	25	640	2.0
(*Hungry Jack* Mini), 11 pcs.	270	5.0	45.0	8.0	10	570	<1.0
(*Hungry Jack* Original	270	6.0	51.0	4.5	10	600	1.0
blueberry:							
(*Aunt Jemima*)	210	6.0	40.0	3.5	20	590	2.0
(*Hungry Jack*)	250	5.0	49.0	4.0	10	590	1.0
buttermilk:							
(*Aunt Jemima*)	210	6.0	40.0	3.5	20	600	2.0
(*Eggo*)	270	7.0	44.0	8.0	15	610	1.0
(*Hungry Jack*)	270	6.0	51.0	4.5	10	630	1.0
Pancake batter, frozen, ½ cup:							
(*Aunt Jemima* Home-style)	260	7.0	50.0	3.5	40	820	3.0
blueberry (*Aunt Jemima*)	290	6.0	54.0	5.0	35	890	4.0
buttermilk (*Aunt Jemima*)	270	8.0	51.0	3.5	45	830	3.0

Food and Measure	cal.	prot. (gms)	carbo. (gms)	fat (gms)	chol. (mgs)	sod. (mgs)	fiber (gms)
Pancake breakfast, frozen, 1 pkg.:							
apple cinnamon (*Uncle Ben's*), 6 oz.	330	5.0	59.0	8.0	5	250	3.0
buttermilk, w/bacon, home fries (*Great Starts*), 6.8 oz. ...	450	12.0	70.0	13.0	40	910	3.0
w/sausage (*Great Starts*), 6 oz.	490	14.0	52.0	25.0	90	950	3.0
Pancake mix, ⅓ cup, except as noted:							
(*Aunt Jemima* Original)	150	4.0	34.0	.5	0	745	1.0
(*Aunt Jemima* Complete)	160	5.0	32.0	2.0	10	475	1.0
(*Betty Crocker* Original Complete), ⅓ cup or 3 cakes*	200	6.0	39.0	3.0	10	540	1.0
(*Betty Crocker* Original Pouch), 3 cakes* ..	250	9.0	39.0	7.0	70	660	1.0
(*Bisquick Shake 'N Pour* Original), 3 cakes*	210	5.0	39.0	4.0	0	710	<1.0
(*Hungry Jack* Original)	150	3.0	32.0	1.5	0	640	<1.0
(*Hungry Jack* Extra Light)	160	3.0	33.0	1.5	0	590	<1.0
(*Hungry Jack* Extra Light Complete) ...	150	4.0	30.0	2.0	0	600	<1.0
blue corn (*Arrowhead Mills*)	150	4.0	28.0	2.0	0	130	3.0
blueberry:							
(*AlpineAire*), 3¼ oz.	360	9.0	63.0	8.0	120	580	7.0
(*Bisquick Shake 'N Pour*), 3 cakes* .	210	6.0	40.0	3.5	0	640	1.0
buckwheat:							
(*Arrowhead Mills*) .	140	8.0	25.0	1.5	0	220	5.0
(*Aunt Jemima*), ¼ cup	100	4.0	23.0	1.0	0	580	4.0
(*Don's Chuck Wagon*)	160	5.0	33.0	1.0	0	550	1.0
(*Hodgson Mill*) ...	160	5.0	36.0	1.0	0	590	5.0
buttermilk:							
(*Arrowhead Mills*), ¼ cup	120	5.0	25.0	.5	<5	350	2.0

Food and Measure	cal.	prot. (gms)	carbo. (gms)	fat (gms)	chol. (mgs)	sod. (mgs)	fiber (gms)
(Aunt Jemima), ¼ cup	110	4.0	23.0	1.0	<5	480	1.0
(Aunt Jemima Complete)	160	5.0	30.0	2.5	10	460	1.0
(Aunt Jemima Complete Reduced Calorie)	130	7.0	28.0	1.5	15	630	5.0
(Betty Crocker Complete Box), ⅓ cup or 3 cakes* .	200	5.0	39.0	2.5	10	540	1.0
(Betty Crocker Pouch), 3 cakes*	210	6.0	37.0	4.0	25	780	1.0
(Bisquick Shake 'N Pour), 3 cakes* .	200	7.0	38.0	3.0	0	680	1.0
(Hungry Jack)	160	4.0	33.0	1.5	0	650	<1.0
(Hungry Jack Complete)	160	4.0	32.0	1.5	<5	570	<1.0
gluten free (Arrowhead Mills), ¼ cup	130	4.0	24.0	2.0	0	180	5.0
kamut (Arrowhead Mills), ¼ cup	130	7.0	26.0	1.0	0	330	4.0
multigrain:							
(Arrowhead Mills), ¼ cup	120	5.0	24.0	.5	0	260	3.0
5-grain (AlpineAire), 2 cakes*, 4"	120	5.0	18.0	3.0	n.a.	460	2.0
oat bran (Arrowhead Mills)	140	7.0	25.0	1.5	0	160	6.0
spelt (VitaSpelt Pancake/Muffin Mix) ..	140	5.0	22.0	2.5	0	220	5.0
wild rice (Arrowhead Mills)	140	3.0	30.0	1.0	0	65	0
whole grain (Arrowhead Mills), ¼ cup .	120	5.0	24.0	.5	0	260	4.0
whole wheat:							
(Aunt Jemima), ¼ cup	120	4.0	26.0	.5	0	625	3.0
(Hodgson Mill) ...	120	4.0	28.0	1.0	0	550	4.0
Pancake syrup, 4 tbsp. or ¼ cup:							
(Aunt Jemima)	210	0	53.0	0	0	120	0
(Aunt Jemima Lite) ..	100	0	26.0	0	0	180	0
(Golden Griddle Light)	90	0	24.0	0	0	135	0
(Hungry Jack)	210	0	52.0	0	0	90	0

Food and Measure	cal.	prot. (gms)	carbo. (gms)	fat (gms)	chol. (mgs)	sod. (mgs)	fiber (gms)
Pancake syrup *(cont.)*							
(*Hungry Jack* Lite) . . .	100	0	24.0	0	0	180	0
(*Karo*)	240	0	63.0	0	0	85	0
(*Kraft*)	180	0	45.0	0	0	50	0
(*Smucker's* Breakfast Sugar Free)	30	0	8.0	0	0	60	0
(*Vermont Maid*)	210	0	53.0	0	0	25	0
(*Vermont Maid* Lite) .	100	0	26.0	0	0	100	0
butter flavor:							
(*Aunt Jemima* Butter Rich)	210	0	52.0	0	0	170	0
(*Aunt Jemima* Butter-lite)	105	0	26.0	0	0	180	0
butter maple flavor:							
(*Hungry Jack*)	210	0	52.0	0	0	90	0
(*Hungry Jack* Lite) .	100	0	24.0	0	0	180	0
cinnamon flavor (*Golden Griddle*) . .	240	0	60.0	0	0	40	0
Pancetta, see "Bacon, Italian"							
Pancreas, braised:							
beef, 4 oz.	307	30.7	0	19.5	n.a.	68	0
lamb, 4 oz.	265	25.9	0	17.1	454	59	0
pork, 4 oz.	248	32.3	0	12.2	357	48	0
veal (calves), 4 oz. . .	290	33.0	0	16.6	n.a.	77	0
Papa John's:							
original crust, 1/8 of 14" pizza::							
All the Meats	390	18.0	37.0	19.0	41	1096	2.0
cheese	283	13.0	37.0	10.0	20	717	2.0
Garden Special . . .	280	12.0	38.0	10.0	16	713	2.0
pepperoni	303	13.0	37.0	12.0	23	793	2.0
sausage	322	14.0	37.0	14.0	28	877	2.0
The Works	342	16.0	38.0	15.0	32	943	2.0
thin crust, 1/8 of 14" pizza:							
All the Meats	393	19.0	22.0	26.0	50	1051	1.0
cheese	233	11.0	22.0	13.0	20	496	1.0
Garden Special . . .	226	10.0	24.0	12.0	16	496	2.0
pepperoni	266	11.0	22.0	16.0	26	621	1.0
sausage	283	12.0	22.0	17.0	30	697	1.0
The Works	322	15.0	24.0	20.0	37	871	2.0
bread stick, 1	140	4.0	26.0	2.0	0	260	1.0
cheese sticks, 2	180	8.0	20.0	8.0	13	380	1.0

Food and Measure	cal.	prot. (gms)	carbo. (gms)	fat (gms)	chol. (mgs)	sod. (mgs)	fiber (gms)
sauce, 1 tbsp.:							
cheese	30	1.5	0	2.0	8	115	0
garlic	75	0	0	8.5	0	115	0
pizza	10	0	1.0	.5	0	50	0
Papaya, fresh:							
(*Dole*), ½ medium, 4.9 oz.	70	0	19.0	0	0	10	2.0
(*Frieda's*), 1 cup, 5 oz.	50	1.0	14.0	0	0	0	3.0
1 lb., 3½" x 5⅛"	117	1.9	29.8	.4	0	8	5.5
cubed, 1 cup	55	.9	13.7	.2	0	4	2.5
mashed, 1 cup	90	1.4	22.6	.3	0	7	4.1
Papaya, in jars, in extra light syrup (*Sunfresh*), ½ cup	70	1.0	17.0	0	0	5	1.0
Papaya, dried:							
(*Frieda's*), ⅓ cup, 1.4 oz.	140	0	29.0	2.5	0	40	4.0
(*Sonoma*), 8 pcs., 1.4 oz.	110	2.0	26.0	0	0	10	5.0
Papaya, frozen (*Goya*), ⅓ pkg.	50	1.0	11.0	0	0	12	2.0
Papaya juice, concentrate* (*R. W. Knudsen*), 8 fl. oz.	40	<1.0	10.0	0	0	10	0
Papaya juice blends:							
(*After the Fall Pele's Papaya Nectar*), 8 fl. oz.	100	1.0	25.0	0	0	15	0
(*Ceres*), 5.25 fl. oz. . .	87	0	21.0	0	0	n.a.	0
nectar (*R. W. Knudsen*), 8 fl. oz.	130	<1.0	34.0	0	0	35	0
Papaya nectar:							
(*Libby's*), 11.5 fl. oz. .	210	<1.0	51.0	0	0	10	0
(*Santa Cruz Organic*), 8 fl. oz.	110	<1.0	28.0	0	0	35	0
canned, 8 fl. oz.	143	.4	36.3	.4	0	12	1.5
Paprika:							
(*McCormick*), ¼ tsp.	2	.1	.3	.1	0	<1	.2
1 tsp.	6	.3	1.2	.3	0	1	.6
Parsley, fresh:							
10 sprigs	4	.3	.6	.1	0	6	.3
chopped, ½ cup	11	.9	1.9	.2	0	17	1.0

Food and Measure	cal.	prot. (gms)	carbo. (gms)	fat (gms)	chol. (mgs)	sod. (mgs)	fiber (gms)
Parsley, dried:							
1 tsp.	1	.1	.2	.1	0	1	.2
freeze-dried, 1 tbsp.	1	.1	.2	<.1	0	2	.2
Parsley root:							
(*Frieda's*), ⅔ cup,							
3 oz.	10	2.0	2.0	.5	0	70	1.0
1 oz.	3	.8	.7	.2	0	28	.4
Parsnip:							
raw, sliced:							
(*Frieda's*), 1 cup ...	100	2.0	24.0	0	0	10	7.0
½ cup	50	.8	12.1	.2	0	7	3.3
boiled, drained:							
1 medium, 9"	130	2.1	31.3	.5	0	17	6.4
sliced, ½ cup	63	1.0	15.2	.2	0	8	3.1
Passion fruit, fresh:							
(*Frieda's*), 5 oz.	140	3.0	33.0	1.0	0	40	15.0
purple:							
1 medium	18	.4	4.2	.1	0	5	1.9
trimmed, ½ cup ...	115	.3	27.5	.8	0	33	12.2
Passion fruit, frozen							
(*Goya*), ⅓ pkg. ...	70	2.0	15.0	0	0	35	2.0
Passion fruit drink							
(*Tropicana Twister*							
Eruption) 8 fl. oz.	120	<1.0	29.0	0	0	15	0
Passion fruit juice,							
fresh, 8 fl. oz.:							
purple	126	1.0	33.6	.1	0	15	.5
yellow	148	1.7	35.7	.4	0	15	.5
Passion fruit juice							
blend (*After the Fall*							
Passion of the							
Island), 8 fl. oz. ..	100	1.0	26.0	0	0	10	0
Passion fruit syrup							
(*Trader Vic's*),							
2 tbsp.	80	0	21.0	0	0	15	0
Pasta (see also "Mac-							
aroni"), dry, 2 oz.,							
except as noted:							
plain	211	7.3	42.6	.9	0	4	1.4
all styles:							
(*Delverde*)	200	7.0	41.0	.5	0	0	1.0
(*Mueller's* Fiber/							
Calcium Fortified)	210	7.0	42.0	1.0	0	10	5.0

Food and Measure	cal.	prot. (gms)	carbo. (gms)	fat (gms)	chol. (mgs)	sod. (mgs)	fiber (gms)
(*Mueller's* Micro Quick)	210	7.0	42.0	1.0	0	0	1.0
four color (*Hodgson Mill*)	200	8.0	41.0	1.0	0	15	1.0
except noodle style (*Mueller's*)	210	7.0	42.0	1.0	0	0	1.0
alphabets, vegetable (*Eden*)	200	8.0	40.0	1.0	0	0	3.0
bow-ties, vegetable (*Westbrae Natural*), ½ cup	190	9.0	40.0	1.5	0	5	5.0
cavatappi, pesto (*Mueller's* Savory Collection)	210	7.0	41.0	1.5	0	350	2.0
elbow, plain or hot pepper (*Eden*)	210	8.0	41.0	1.0	0	0	4.0
fettuccine: (*Pastamania!*)	200	8.0	38.0	2.0	30	20	1.0
garlic-parsley or pesto (*Pastamania!*)	200	8.0	38.0	2.0	30	20	1.0
w/Jerusalem artichoke (*Pastamania!*)	210	8.0	41.0	1.5	0	10	2.0
lemon-pepper (*Pastamania!*) ..	220	8.0	40.0	2.5	35	15	2.0
w/mushroom (*Pastamania!*) ..	210	8.0	41.0	2.0	35	15	2.0
spinach (*Pastamania!*)	200	8.0	37.0	2.0	40	35	2.0
wheat and spinach (*Pastamania!*) ..	200	8.0	38.0	2.0	35	30	1.0
finbows, parsley garlic (*Eden* Organic) ...	210	8.0	41.0	1.0	0	0	4.0
kamut-quinoa, twisted (*Eden*)	210	8.0	40.0	2.0	0	0	5.0
kuzu and sweet potato or kiri (*Eden*)	190	0	47.0	0	0	0	0
lasagna, 20" pc.: spinach (*Westbrae Natural*), 1.8 oz. ..	180	9.0	35.0	2.0	0	20	5.0
whole wheat (*Westbrae Natural*), 1.8 oz.	200	8.0	36.0	1.5	0	10	7.0

Food and Measure	cal.	prot. (gms)	carbo. (gms)	fat. (gms)	chol. (mgs)	sod. (mgs)	fiber (gms)
Pasta *(cont.)*							
linguine:							
pesto (*Mueller's*							
Savory Collection)	210	7.0	41.0	1.5	0	350	2.0
thin (*Pastamania!*)	200	8.0	38.0	2.0	30	20	1.0
mung bean (*Eden*							
Harusame)	190	0	47.0	0	0	5	0
noodle style, yolk-free							
(*Mueller's*)	210	8.0	42.0	1.0	0	0	1.0
oat bran (*Pasta-*							
mania!)	209	8.0	41.0	1.4	0	7	2.0
penne, lemon pepper							
(*Mueller's* Savory							
Collection)	210	7.0	42.0	1.0	0	190	2.0
pennette, sun-dried							
tomato-basil							
(*Mueller's* Savory							
Collection)	210	7.0	41.0	1.0	0	35	2.0
ribbon:							
all varieties, except							
kluski and spinach							
(*Eden*)	210	9.0	40.0	1.5	0	0	3.0
kluski or spinach							
(*Eden*)	210	8.0	41.0	1.0	0	0	4.0
whole wheat (*West-*							
brae Natural),							
1 cup	200	9.0	38.0	1.5	0	10	7.0
whole wheat (*Pasta-*							
mania!)	190	10.0	34.0	1.0	0	15	5.0
rice pasta:							
(*Eden Bifun*)	200	5.0	44.0	.5	0	5	0
all styles (*Lund-*							
berg)	210	4.0	44.0	2.0	0	5	3.0
rotelle, roasted garlic							
herb (*Mueller's*							
Savory Collection)	210	7.0	41.0	1.0	0	300	2.0
shells:							
(*Mueller's*)	210	7.0	42.0	1.0	0	0	1.0
vegetable (*Eden*) ..	200	8.0	40.0	1.0	0	0	3.0
spaghetti:							
(*Eden*)	200	8.0	40.0	1.0	0	0	3.0
corn (*Westbrae*							
Natural)	210	4.0	46.0	1.5	0	15	0
kamut (*Eden*)	190	10.0	33.0	1.5	0	0	6.0

Food and Measure	cal.	prot. (gms)	carbo. (gms)	fat (gms)	chol. (mgs)	sod. (mgs)	fiber (gms)
lemon pepper (*Mueller's* Savory Collection)	210	7.0	42.0	1.0	0	190	2.0
parsley-garlic (*Eden*)	210	8.0	41.0	1.0	0	0	4.0
spinach (*Westbrae Natural*)	180	9.0	38.0	2.0	0	20	6.0
whole grain (*Eden*)	210	10.0	40.0	1.5	0	0	6.0
whole wheat, spinach (*Pastamania!*)	190	9.0	35.0	2.0	0	25	5.0
whole wheat, thin (*Pastamania!*) . .	190	9.0	34.0	1.0	0	25	6.0
spelt:							
white (*VitaSpelt*) . .	210	9.0	42.0	.5	0	0	2.0
whole grain (*VitaSpelt*)	190	8.0	40.0	1.5	0	0	5.0
spirals:							
kamut (*Eden*)	190	10.0	33.0	1.5	0	0	6.0
rye (*Eden*)	200	6.0	44.0	0	0	10	8.0
sesame rice (*Eden*)	200	9.0	37.0	2.0	0	0	6.0
sesame rice (*Westbrae Natural*), 1 cup	190	10.0	38.0	2.0	0	5	5.0
spinach (*Eden*) . . .	210	8.0	41.0	1.0	0	0	4.0
vegetable (*Eden*) . .	200	8.0	40.0	1.0	0	0	3.0
vegetable (*Westbrae Natural*), 1 cup .	210	10.0	43.0	2.0	0	10	5.0
tubes, endless (*Eden*)	210	8.0	41.0	1.0	0	0	4.0
twists, pesto (*Eden*) . .	200	8.0	40.0	1.0	0	0	3.0
whole wheat, all styles, except ribbons, spinach, and thin spaghetti (*Pastamania!*)	190	9.0	34.0	1.0	0	10	6.0
Pasta, cooked (see also "Macaroni"):							
corn, 1 cup	176	3.7	39.1	1.0	0	1	3.4
spaghetti, 1 cup:							
plain	197	6.7	39.7	.9	0	1	2.4
protein fortified . . .	230	11.3	44.3	.3	0	7	2.4
spinach	182	6.4	36.6	.9	0	20	n.a.
whole wheat	174	7.5	37.2	.6	0	4	6.3
Pasta, frozen, see specific listings							

Food and Measure	cal.	prot. (gms)	carbo. (gms)	fat (gms)	chol. (mgs)	sod. (mgs)	fiber (gms)
Pasta, refrigerated							
(see also specific listings) plain:							
uncooked, 2 oz.:							
w/egg	163	6.4	31.0	1.3	41	15	2.0
spinach, w/egg . . .	164	6.4	31.6	1.2	41	15	n.a.
cooked, 4 oz.:							
w/egg	149	5.8	28.3	1.2	37	7	n.a.
spinach, w/egg . . .	147	5.7	28.4	1.1	37	7	n.a.
Pasta dish, frozen							
(see also "Pasta entree, frozen" and specific listings):							
Alfredo:							
(*Green Giant*), 9 oz.	300	14.0	38.0	18.0	10	980	3.0
(*Green Giant Pasta Accents*), 2 cups	200	8.0	27.0	7.0	10	400	3.0
and vegetables (*Amy's* Skillet Meals), 1 cup . . .	220	11.0	27.0	8.0	20	460	4.0
cheddar:							
(*Amy's* Skillet Meals Country), 1 cup	250	9.0	27.0	11.0	5	480	3.0
creamy (*Green Giant Pasta Accents*), 2⅓ cups	250	9.0	36.0	8.0	15	640	3.0
white (*Birds Eye Pasta Secrets*), 2 cups	240	7.0	30.0	10.0	10	560	2.0
cheese, three:							
(*Birds Eye Pasta Secrets*), 2 cups .	230	9.0	31.0	8.0	5	590	2.0
(*Green Giant*), 9 oz.	270	10.0	40.0	8.0	25	1230	3.0
(*Green Giant Pasta Accents*), 2 cups	300	12.0	42.0	9.0	15	890	3.0
garden herb (*Green Giant Pasta Accents*), 2 cups	230	9.0	32.0	7.0	15	750	7.0
garlic:							
(*Green Giant Pasta Accents*), 2 cups	260	7.0	36.0	10.0	15	640	3.0
zesty (*Birds Eye Pasta Secrets*), 2 cups	240	7.0	31.0	10.0	5	310	2.0

Food and Measure	cal.	prot. (gms)	carbo. (gms)	fat (gms)	chol. (mgs)	sod. (mgs)	fiber (gms)
roasted (*Green Giant*), 9 oz. . . .	250	9.0	41.0	6.0	15	960	3.0
pesto, Italian (*Birds Eye Pasta Secrets*), 2⅓ cups, 6.4 oz. . .	240	9.0	32.0	9.0	5	700	2.0
primavera:							
(*Birds Eye Pasta Secrets*), 2⅓ cups, 6.7 oz.	230	9.0	26.0	10.0	10	430	3.0
(*Tree of Life Easy-Meal*), 1 pkg. . .	300	11.0	54.0	4.0	10	780	4.0
(*Tree of Life Easy-Meal*), 1 pkg.*							
w/tofu, oil	460	20.0	54.0	16.0	10	790	3.0
ranch (*Birds Eye Pasta Secrets*), 6.6 oz. . .	300	7.0	29.0	15.0	25	460	2.0
salad, w/vegetables (*Fitness Choice*), 4 oz.	130	5.0	26.0	0	0	50	1.0
Pasta dish, mix (see also specific pasta listings), 1 cup*, except as noted:							
Alfredo:							
(*Annie's*), ⅔ cup . .	270	12.0	46.0	4.5	10	500	2.0
garlic (*Pasta Roni*)	360	12.0	49.0	14.0	10	1110	2.0
broccoli:							
(*Pasta Roni*)	330	10.0	42.0	14.0	5	910	2.0
au gratin (*Pasta Roni*)	280	9.0	41.0	10.0	5	850	2.0
cheddar:							
broccoli (*Annie's*), ⅔ cup	260	10.0	48.0	3.0	5	450	2.0
broccoli (*Lipton* Pasta & Sauce), ½ pkg.	260	9.0	46.0	3.5	10	870	1.0
zesty (*Lipton* Pasta & Sauce)	290	9.0	42.0	10.0	10	930	2.0
cheese:							
four (*Annie's*), ⅔ cup	260	11.0	46.0	3.5	5	520	2.0
Italian (*Lipton* Pasta & Cheese), ½ pkg.	220	8.0	38.0	4.5	10	800	<1.0

Food and Measure	cal.	prot. (gms)	carbo. (gms)	fat (gms)	chol. (mgs)	sod. (mgs)	fiber (gms)
Pasta dish, mix, cheese *(cont.)*							
nacho (*Knorr Forkfulls*), 1 bowl ...	370	10.0	60.0	10.0	<5	1350	1.0
triple (*Knorr Forkfulls*), 1 bowl ...	360	11.0	59.0	8.0	10	1170	1.0
zesty (*Knorr Forkfulls*), 1 bowl ...	360	10.0	59.0	9.0	<5	1630	1.0
chicken:							
(*Pasta Roni*)	310	9.0	41.0	13.0	5	1030	2.0
(*Pasta Roni* Homestyle)	230	8.0	39.0	6.0	0	1020	3.0
flavor, creamy (*Knorr Forkfulls*), 1 bowl	300	10.0	54.0	5.0	0	1240	1.0
flavor, quesadilla (*Knorr Forkfulls*), 1 bowl	340	11.0	58.0	8.0	<5	1380	1.0
and garlic (*Pasta Roni* Low Fat) ..	300	8.0	40.0	11.0	5	950	2.0
primavera (*Lipton* Pasta & Sauce), ½ pkg.	220	7.0	40.0	3.0	5	720	1.0
garlic, creamy (*Lipton* Pasta & Sauce), ½ pkg.	270	8.0	47.0	6.0	10	880	1.0
garlic, roasted, and olive oil w/sundried tomato (*Lipton* Pasta & Sauce) ...	270	8.0	42.0	8.5	0	880	2.0
garlic and Parmesan (*Annie's*), ⅔ cup ..	180	8.0	34.0	3.0	5	430	1.0
mushroom, creamy (*Lipton* Pasta & Sauce)	320	10.0	46.0	10.5	15	870	0
Parmesano (*Pasta Roni*)	390	12.0	50.0	17.0	5	930	2.0
pesto (*Taste Adventure* Quick Cuisine), ⅓ cup	160	6.0	30.0	1.0	0	350	4.0
pizza flavor (*Knorr Forkfulls*), 1 bowl ..	330	9.0	60.0	5.0	<5	1230	2.0
Romanoff (*Pasta Roni*)	400	11.0	48.0	19.0	10	1060	2.0

Food and Measure	cal.	prot. (gms)	carbo. (gms)	fat (gms)	chol. (mgs)	sod. (mgs)	fiber (gms)
salad:							
Caesar (*Suddenly Salad*)	250	6.0	34.0	10.0	0	650	1.0
classic (*Suddenly Salad*)	240	6.0	37.0	7.0	0	880	2.0
Italian (*Kraft*), ¼ box	160	7.0	30.0	1.5	<5	320	2.0
garlic, roasted, Parmesan (*Suddenly Salad*), ¾ cup*	240	7.0	32.0	10.0	10	740	1.0
Parmesan, creamy (*Suddenly Salad*)	360	7.0	30.0	24.0	20	520	1.0
ranch w/bacon (*Kraft*), ⅕ box ..	130	6.0	26.0	.5	0	240	1.0
ranch and bacon (*Suddenly Salad*), ¾ cup*	330	7.0	31.0	20.0	15	480	1.0
sour cream and chives (*Pasta Roni*)	320	9.0	39.0	15.0	5	880	2.0
Stroganoff (*Pasta Roni*)	370	12.0	49.0	14.0	10	980	2.0
tomato:							
(*Ragú Express* Traditional), ½ pkg.*	190	6.0	36.0	2.5	0	490	2.0
and basil (*Annie's*), ⅔ cup	260	10.0	49.0	2.5	5	390	2.0
meat flavored (*Ragú Express*), ½ pkg.*	200	7.0	39.0	3.0	0	320	3.0
Parmesan, creamy (*Lipton* Pasta & Sauce), ½ pkg.	240	5.0	41.0	5.0	10	840	2.0
spicy (*Near East* Meal Cup), 1 pkg.	230	7.0	48.0	2.0	0	320	3.0
sweet, and garlic (*Ragú Express*), ½ pkg.*	200	7.0	39.0	2.5	0	320	3.0
Pasta entree, can or pkg. (see also specific listings), 1 cup, except as noted:							
(*Annie's BernieOs/ P'Sghetti Loops/*All Stars)	150	4.0	31.0	1.0	0	680	<1.0

Food and Measure	cal.	prot (gms)	carbo. (gms)	fat (gms)	chol. (mgs)	sod. (mgs)	fiber (gms)
Pasta entree, can or pkg. *(cont.)*							
Alfredo (*Bowl Appétit!*), 1 bowl	360	13.0	51.0	12.0	15	830	1.0
chicken flavor (*Bowl Appétit!*), 1 bowl . .	260	10.0	42.0	6.0	10	830	2.0
w/meatballs:							
(*Chef Boyardee Junior* Dinosaurs)	290	8.0	39.0	11.0	35	990	2.0
(*Chef Boyardee Junior* ABC's/ 123's)	200	5.0	43.0	.5	<5	900	2.0
w/soy meatballs (*Annie's P'Sghetti Loops*)	200	9.0	32.0	3.5	0	860	2.0
Pasta entree, dried, 1 serving:							
(*AlpineAire* Roma) . . .	370	18.0	53.0	10.0	25	730	2.0
primavera:							
(*Mountain House* Double/Four) . . .	320	12.0	47.0	9.0	25	900	4.0
(*Mountain House* Single)	370	14.0	56.0	11.0	30	1070	3.0
Pasta entree, frozen (see also "Pasta dish, frozen" and specific listings), 1 pkg., except as noted:							
(*Kid Cuisine* Fun), 10.6 oz.	340	10.0	57.0	8.0	25	1100	6.0
Alfredo:							
w/chicken (*Marie Callender's* Bowl), 10.5 oz.	410	26.0	38.0	17.0	70	1070	5.0
primavera (*Lean Cuisine Everyday Favorites*), 10 oz.	280	12.0	44.0	6.0	10	580	4.0
cheddar, w/beef, to- matoes (*Stouffer's*), 11 oz.	500	26.0	44.0	24.0	40	1200	2.0
cheese, three:							
w/broccoli (*Cedar- lane*), 9 oz.	430	21.0	43.0	19.0	55	410	3.0

Food and Measure	cal.	prot. (gms)	carbo. (gms)	fat (gms)	chol. (mgs)	sod. (mgs	fiber (gms)
w/sweet red pepper (*Cascadian Farm*), 10 oz.	340	15.0	42.0	13.0	30	680	1.0
marinara (*Cascadian Farm Veggie Bowl*), 9 oz.	180	11.0	30.0	3.0	0	600	3.0
and meatballs: (*Country Skillet*), ¼ of 32-oz. pkg.	320	12.0	32.0	16.0	30	850	2.0
(*Marie Callender's* Skillet Meals), ½ of 24-oz. pkg.	570	26.0	50.0	30.0	70	1360	4.0
(*Swanson Fun Feast*), 12 oz.	410	12.0	65.0	12.0	15	520	7.0
primavera: (*Amy's*), 9.5 oz. . .	320	15.0	39.0	12.0	29	680	3.0
(*Cascadian Farm Veggie Bowl*), 9 oz.	220	11.0	37.0	8.0	6	620	2.0
and Stroganoff sauce, w/meatballs (*Freezer Queen* Deluxe Family), 1 cup	240	11.0	30.0	9.0	30	570	3.0
stuffed, trio (*Marie Callender's*), 10.5 oz.	380	15.0	40.0	18.0	50	950	5.0
wheels and cheese (*Michelina's*), 8 oz.	300	13.0	43.0	8.0	20	590	2.0
wrap (*Wolfgang Puck's*), 12 oz. . . .	340	14.0	76.0	3.0	65	740	9.0
Pasta flour, see "Semolina flour"							
Pasta salad, see "Pasta dish, mix"							
Pasta salad dressing mix, vinaigrette (*Mc-Cormick*), ⅙ pkg.	15	0	2.0	0	0	590	0
Pasta salad seasoning Meditarranean (*Mc-Cormick*), ¼ pkg.	25	1.0	4.0	0	0	460	0
Pasta sauce, tomato (see also "Tomato sauce" and specific listings), ½ cup:							

Food and Measure	cal.	prot. (gms)	carbo. (gms)	fat (gms)	chol. (mgs)	sod. (mgs)	fiber (gms)
Pasta sauce *(cont.)*							
(*Aunt Millie's* Traditional)	90	2.0	17.0	1.5	0	400	3.0
(*Del Monte* Traditional)	60	2.0	15.0	.5	0	590	3.0
(*Eden*)	80	3.0	12.0	2.5	0	320	3.0
(*Eden* No Salt)	80	3.0	12.0	2.5	0	10	3.0
(*Emeril's Kicked Up Tomato*)	70	1.0	9.0	3.0	0	400	2.0
(*Healthy Choice* Traditional)	50	2.0	11.0	0	0	390	2.0
(*Patsy's* Pizzaiola)	100	3.0	9.0	6.0	0	423	3.0
(*Prego* Traditional)	120	2.0	22.0	3.0	0	660	2.0
(*Progresso* Spaghetti)	100	3.0	12.0	4.5	<5	620	2.0
(*Ragú Old World Style* Traditional)	70	2.0	8.0	3.0	0	820	2.0
Alfredo, tomato, ¼ cup:							
(*Classico* Di Liguria)	60	2.0	6.0	3.5	10	270	1.0
sun-dried (*Classico* Di Capri)	110	2.0	4.0	9.0	40	450	0
Amatriciana (*Patsy's*)	120	2.0	8.0	8.0	5	351	2.0
balsamic roasted onion (*Muir Glen*)	50	2.0	10.0	.5	0	320	2.0
basil:							
(*Amy's*)	80	2.0	11.0	3.0	0	580	3.0
(*Classico* Di Napoli)	50	2.0	9.0	1.0	0	390	2.0
(*Del Monte*)	70	2.0	16.0	1.0	0	600	3.0
(*Five Brothers*)	70	3.0	12.0	1.5	0	470	3.0
(*Muir Glen*)	50	2.0	12.0	1.0	0	370	0
(*Newman's Own* Bombolina)	100	1.0	15.0	4.0	0	590	5.0
(*Patsy's*)	90	2.0	7.0	6.0	0	430	2.0
(*Ragú* Light)	50	2.0	10.0	0	0	370	2.0
(*Ragú* Light No Sugar)	50	3.0	7.0	1.5	0	350	2.0
and Italian cheese (*Ragú* Gardenstyle)	110	3.0	17.0	3.0	5	620	2.0
beef, w/mushroom (*Ragú Robusto!*)	70	3.0	8.0	3.0	5	680	2.0
beef, sauteed, onion and garlic (*Ragú Robusto!*)	90	3.0	11.0	4.5	5	540	2.0

Food and Measure	cal.	prot. (gms)	carbo. (gms)	fat (gms)	chol. (mgs)	sod. (mgs)	fiber (gms)
cheese, see "Cheese sauce, cooking":							
w/cheese:							
four (*Classico* Di Parma)	80	2.0	8.0	4.0	<5	500	1.0
four (*Del Monte*) . .	70	2.0	15.0	1.5	0	680	3.0
four (*Master Choice*)	70	2.0	13.0	1.0	0	610	3.0
five (*Five Brothers*)	90	4.0	11.0	3.0	5	660	3.0
five (*Newman's Own*)	90	2.0	14.0	3.0	<5	510	3.0
six (*Ragú Robusto!*)	80	3.0	9.0	3.0	5	570	2.0
diced (*Hunt's*)	50	2.0	10.0	1.0	0	770	2.0
fra diavolo:							
(*Newman's Own* Hot & Spicy)	70	0	10.0	3.0	0	510	3.0
(*Patsy's*)	100	3.0	9.0	6.0	0	423	3.0
garden combination (*Ragú* Gardenstyle)	100	2.0	17.0	3.0	0	550	2.0
garden:							
(*Master Choice*) . . .	70	3.0	13.0	1.0	0	540	3.0
(*Ragú* Mama's Special)	110	3.0	18.0	3.0	0	530	2.0
combination (*Ragú* Gardenstyle) . . .	100	2.0	17.0	3.0	0	550	2.0
garlic, super (*Ragú* Gardenstyle)	100	2.0	17.0	3.0	0	580	2.0
garlic, roasted:							
(*Classico* Di Sorrento)	60	2.0	9.0	1.5	0	390	2.0
(*Emeril's Roasted Gaaahlic*)	70	2.0	10.0	3.0	0	430	2.0
(*Muir Glen*)	50	2.0	10.0	.5	0	320	0
(*Ragú Robusto!*) . .	90	2.0	12.0	3.0	0	540	2.0
and peppers (*Newman's Own*)	70	2.0	11.0	2.5	0	460	4.0
primavera (*Ragú* Light)	45	2.0	9.0	0	0	370	2.0
and Romano (*Healthy Choice*)	60	2.0	11.0	1.0	0	390	3.0
and Vidalia onion (*Five Brothers*) . .	80	3.0	12.0	1.5	0	480	3.0
garlic and basil (*Prego* Pasta Bake), ⅛ jar	80	1.0	11.0	3.5	0	530	2.0

Food and Measure	cal.	prot. (gms)	carbo. (gms)	fat (gms)	chol. (mgs)	sod. (mgs)	fiber (gms)
Pasta sauce *(cont.)*							
garlic and herb:							
(*Del Monte* Chunky)	60	2.0	11.0	1.5	0	490	<1.0
(*Healthy Choice*) ..	50	2.0	10.0	0	0	390	2.0
garlic mushroom							
(*Amy's*)	120	3.0	10.0	7.0	5	680	3.0
garlic and onion:							
(*Del Monte*)	80	2.0	16.0	1.0	0	490	2.0
(*Muir Glen*)	55	2.0	12.0	.5	0	320	0
(*Ragú* Gardenstyle)	110	2.0	18.0	3.0	0	520	2.0
green pepper mush-							
room (*Del Monte*) .	80	2.0	16.0	1.0	0	490	3.0
hamburger (*Prego*) ..	120	3.0	17.0	4.0	10	580	3.0
herb:							
(*Lydia's* Sugo al							
Pomodoro Fresco)	80	3.0	9.0	3.0	0	420	3.0
(*Muir Glen* Chunky)	50	2.0	10.0	.5	0	320	0
Italian (*Del Monte*							
Chunky)	60	2.0	12.0	1.0	0	520	<1.0
Italian (*Muir Glen*) .	55	2.0	12.0	.5	0	320	0
seven (*Ragú*							
Robusto!*)	80	2.0	11.0	3.5	0	540	2.0
marinara:							
(*Amy's*)	50	1.0	8.0	1.0	0	590	3.0
(*Muir Glen* Cabernet)	50	2.0	11.0	.5	0	330	0
(*Newman's Own*) ..	60	2.0	9.0	2.0	0	590	3.0
(*Patsy's*)	100	3.0	9.0	6.0	0	423	3.0
(*Progresso* Authen-							
tic)	100	4.0	12.0	4.0	<5	590	3.0
(*Ragú Old World*							
Style)	80	2.0	8.0	4.5	0	780	2.0
w/Burgundy (*Five*							
Brothers)	80	3.0	11.0	3.0	0	490	3.0
w/Burgundy							
(*Healthy Choice*							
Mediterranean) .	50	1.0	11.0	.5	0	390	2.0
mushroom (*Muir*							
Glen)	45	2.0	10.0	0	0	320	0
mushroom (*New-*							
man's Own)	60	2.0	9.0	2.0	0	590	3.0
w/pizza paste (*Aunt*							
Millie's)	70	2.0	10.0	2.5	0	330	3.0
sweet basil (*Classico*							
Di Campania) ...	70	2.0	11.0	2.0	0	500	2.0

Food and Measure	cal.	prot. (gms)	carbo. (gms)	fat (gms)	chol. (mgs)	sod. (mgs)	fiber (gms)
meat/meat flavor:							
(*Aunt Millie's*)	100	3.0	17.0	2.0	<5	400	3.0
(*Del Monte*)	60	3.0	14.0	1.0	<5	720	3.0
(*Master Choice* Bolognese)	80	3.0	14.0	1.0	0	620	3.0
(*Prego*)	140	2.0	21.0	5.0	5	540	3.0
(*Prego* Pasta Bake), ⅛ jar	120	4.0	12.0	6.0	10	790	2.0
(*Ragú Old World Style*)	80	2.0	8.0	3.5	<5	760	2.0
Italian (*Ragú Robusto!* Classic)	90	3.0	9.0	4.0	5	690	2.0
meatball, mini (*Prego*)	160	4.0	20.0	7.0	10	660	3.0
mushroom:							
(*Aunt Millie's*)	90	2.0	17.0	1.5	0	400	3.0
(*Del Monte*)	60	2.0	14.0	.5	0	630	2.0
(*Prego*)	150	2.0	23.0	5.0	0	670	3.0
(*Ragú Old World Style*)	70	2.0	8.0	3.0	0	750	2.0
garlic (*Five Brothers*)	80	3.0	12.0	3.0	0	490	3.0
and garlic (*Healthy Choice*)	45	2.0	10.0	0	0	390	2.0
garlic and onion (*Prego* Pasta Bake), ⅛ jar	90	2.0	13.0	3.0	0	650	2.0
green pepper (*Ragú* Gardenstyle) ...	100	3.0	17.0	3.0	0	580	2.0
and olives (*Classico Di Sicilia*)	70	2.0	11.0	1.5	0	430	2.0
and olives (*Master Choice* Siciliano)	70	3.0	12.0	1.0	0	620	4.0
portobello (*Classico Di Toscana*)	70	2.0	11.0	1.5	0	420	2.0
portobello (*Muir Glen*)	50	2.0	11.0	0	0	330	0
super chunky (*Ragú* Gardenstyle) ...	110	3.0	18.0	3.5	0	610	2.0
olive, green (*Muir Glen*)	60	2.0	11.0	1.5	0	350	0
onion, roasted (*Muir Glen*)	50	2.0	12.0	.5	0	320	0
onion and:							
garlic (*Prego*)	120	2.0	18.0	4.0	0	430	3.0
garlic, sauteed (*Aunt Millie's*)	90	2.0	17.0	1.5	0	410	3.0

Food and Measure	cal.	prot (gms)	carbo. (gms)	fat (gms)	chol. (mgs)	sod. (mgs)	fiber (gms)
Pasta sauce, onion *(cont.)*							
garlic, sauteed (*Ragú Robusto!*)	90	2.0	11.0	4.5	0	530	2.0
mushroom, sauteed (*Ragú Robusto!*)	90	3.0	11.0	4.0	0	610	3.0
pepper (*Lydia's Sugo Capricciosa*)	75	2.0	10.0	3.0	0	380	3.0
Parmesan/Romano (*Ragú Robusto!*)	90	3.0	12.0	4.0	5	600	2.0
pepper and tomato (*Sacla Pasta Gusto*), ⅓ cup	100	2.0	7.0	17.0	0	380	2.0
pepperoni (*Prego*)	120	3.0	20.0	4.5	10	570	3.0
peppers and spice (*Newman's Own*)	60	2.0	9.0	2.0	0	590	3.0
pizza (*Eden*)	80	3.0	12.0	2.5	0	320	3.0
puttanesca:							
(*Emeril's*)	80	2.0	9.0	5.0	0	760	2.0
(*Francesco Rinaldi*)	70	2.0	8.0	4.0	0	720	<1.0
red pepper, spicy (*Classico Di Roma Arrabbiata*)	60	2.0	7.0	2.5	0	270	2.0
red pepper, roasted:							
(*Emeril's*)	60	1.0	7.0	3.0	0	390	2.0
and onion (*Classico Di Salerno*)	60	2.0	9.0	2.0	0	410	2.0
and onion (*Ragú Gardenstyle*)	110	2.0	18.0	3.0	0	510	2.0
Romano, pecorino, and herb (*Classico Di Palermo*)	80	4.0	8.0	3.0	<5	410	2.0
sausage, Italian:							
and garlic (*Prego*)	120	3.0	16.0	5.0	10	500	3.0
w/peppers and onions (*Classico D'Abruzzi*)	70	3.0	8.0	3.0	10	500	2.0
sweet, and cheese (*Ragú Robusto!*)	90	4.0	11.0	4.5	5	670	3.0
sausage flavored (*Aunt Millie's*)	100	3.0	17.0	2.0	<5	400	3.0
spinach and cheese, Florentine (*Classico Di Firenze*)	80	3.0	8.0	4.5	<5	490	2.0

Food and Measure	cal.	prot. (gms)	carbo. (gms)	fat (gms)	chol. (mgs)	sod. (mgs)	fiber (gms)
tomato:							
chopped, olive oil and garlic (*Ragú Robusto!*)	100	2.0	9.0	5.0	0	710	3.0
fire-roasted, and garlic (*Classico Di Siena*)	60	2.0	10.0	1.0	0	390	2.0
spicy, and pesto (*Classico Di Genoa*)	90	3.0	9.0	5.0	0	530	2.0
sun-dried (*Classico Di Capri*)	80	2.0	8.0	4.0	0	430	2.0
sun-dried (*Muir Glen*)	55	2.0	10.0	1.0	0	370	0
sun-dried and herb (*Healthy Choice* Mediterranean) .	60	3.0	12.0	.5	0	390	3.0
sun-dried, and basil (*Ragú* Garden-style)	110	2.0	18.0	3.0	0	510	2.0
vegetable:							
garden (*Muir Glen*)	50	2.0	10.0	1.0	0	320	0
garden and herb (*Lydia's* Sugo all'Ortolana)	80	2.0	10.0	3.0	0	380	3.0
primavera (*Healthy Choice* Chunky) .	45	2.0	9.0	0	0	390	2.0
summer, grilled (*Five Brothers*) . .	80	3.0	11.0	3.0	0	530	3.0
super (*Ragú* Garden-style)	100	2.0	16.0	3.0	0	500	2.0
vodka sauce:							
(*Emeril's*)	130	2.0	13.0	8.0	10	490	2.0
(*Patsy's*)	110	2.0	7.0	7.0	5	390	2.0
Pasta sauce, refrigerated (see also specific listings), tomato:							
herb Parmesan (*Buitoni*), ½ cup . .	140	3.0	12.0	9.0	10	720	4.0
marinara, ½ cup:							
(*Buitoni*)	80	2.0	10.0	3.5	0	650	2.0
(*Di Giorno*)	70	2.0	15.0	0	0	220	2.0

Food and Measure	cal.	prot. (gms)	carbo. (gms)	fat (gms)	chol. (mgs)	sod. (mgs)	fiber (gms)
Pasta sauce, refrigerated, marinara *(cont.)*							
garlic, roasted (*Buitoni*)	60	2.0	10.0	2.0	0	550	1.0
mushroom (*Di Giorno*)	60	2.0	13.0	0	0	260	2.0
Pasta sauce mix (see also specific listings), ½ cup*, except as noted:							
(*Hain* Spaghetti), 1 tbsp.	20	0	4.0	0	0	440	0
(*Knorr* Parma Rosa), 2 tbsp.	60	2.0	8.0	2.5	<5	550	0
(*McCormick* Pasta Rosa)	40	1.0	4.0	2.0	0	540	0
(*Spatini* Spaghetti) ...	20	0	3.0	0	0	560	0
garlic herb (*Knorr* Pasta Sauces), 2 tbsp.	70	1.0	8.0	3.5	0	860	0
herb and garlic (*McCormick*)	20	1.0	2.0	0	0	500	0
Italian style (*McCormick* Spaghetti)	25	0	5.0	0	0	490	0
mild (*McCormick* Spaghetti)	25	1.0	5.0	.5	0	410	0
primavera (*McCormick*)	30	0	4.0	1.0	0	490	0
thick, zesty (*McCormick* Spaghetti)	25	0	6.0	0	0	620	0
Pastrami, 2 oz., except as noted:							
(*Boar's Head* Choice)	140	11.0	0	11.0	35	750	0
(*Boar's Head* First Cut)	90	12.0	2.0	4.0	30	620	0
(*Boar's Head* Navel) ..	180	10.0	0	15.0	30	570	0
(*Boar's Head* Red Round)	80	12.0	1.0	3.0	35	460	0
(*Boar's Head* Round)	70	12.0	<1.0	2.5	30	530	0
(*Carl Buddig*), 2.5-oz. pkg.	100	14.0	1.0	5.0	50	750	0
(*Healthy Choice*)	60	10.0	2.0	1.5	30	410	0
(*Healthy Choice* Savory Selections), 6 slices, 1.9 oz. ..	70	11.0	2.0	1.5	25	400	0
(*Healthy Deli*)	80	11.0	3.0	3.0	30	480	0

Food and Measure	cal.	prot. (gms)	carbo. (gms)	fat (gms)	chol. (mgs)	sod. (mgs)	fiber (gms)
(*Hebrew National* Thin Sliced)	90	13.0	1.0	4.0	35	500	0
(*Sara Lee*), 3 slices, 2.2 oz.	70	12.0	0	2.0	35	520	0
turkey, see "Turkey pastrami"							
Pastry shell, puff (see also "Pie crust"):							
patty shell (*Pepperridge Farm*), 1 pc.	190	4.0	16.0	13.0	0	230	<1.0
sheet (*Pepperidge Farm*), ⅛ sheet ...	170	3.0	14.0	11.0	0	200	<1.0
Pastry filling (see also "Pie filling"), canned, 2 tbsp.:							
almond (*Solo*)	120	1.0	23.0	2.5	0	45	2.0
almond paste (*Blue Diamond* Baker's)	150	4.0	11.0	10.0	0	0	2.0
apple, Dutch (*Solo*) ..	80	0	20.0	0	0	45	1.0
apricot (*Solo*)	80	0	17.0	0	0	20	1.0
blueberry (*Solo*)	80	0	17.0	0	0	25	1.0
cherry (*Solo*)	80	0	20.0	0	0	25	1.0
date (*Solo*)	100	0	22.0	0	0	40	3.0
nut, fancy (*Solo*)	140	1.0	25.0	5.0	0	55	5.0
pecan (*Solo*)	130	1.0	24.0	4.0	0	50	1.0
pineapple (*Solo*)	80	0	19.0	0	0	20	1.0
poppy seed (*Solo*) ...	140	2.0	30.0	4.0	0	30	3.0
prune plum (*Solo*) ...	70	0	18.0	0	0	25	1.0
raspberry (*Solo*)	80	0	19.0	0	0	25	1.0
strawberry (*Solo*) ...	70	0	18.0	0	0	20	1.0
Pâté, can or jar:							
1 oz.	90	4.0	.4	7.9	72	198	0
1 tbsp.	41	1.9	.2	3.6	33	91	0
chicken liver:							
1 oz.	57	3.8	1.9	3.7	111	109	0
1 tbsp.	26	1.8	.9	1.7	51	51	0
goose liver:							
smoked, 1 oz.	131	3.2	1.3	12.4	43	198	0
smoked, 1 tbsp. ..	60	1.5	.6	5.7	20	91	0
Pâté, refrigerated, 2 oz.:							
(*Boar's Head* Liverwurst)	150	9.0	0	12.0	70	470	0

Food and Measure	cal.	prot. (gms)	carbo. (gms)	fat (gms)	chol. (mgs)	sod. (mgs)	fiber (gms)
Pâté, refrigerated *(cont.)*							
(*Charcuterie de Bretagne* de Campagne)	200	6.0	2.0	18.0	60	300	0
duck and pork mousse w/truffles (*Marcel & Henri*)	240	6.0	<1.0	24.0	95	340	0
glazed, w/truffles (*Tour Eiffel Campagnard Française*)	210	8.0	2.0	19.0	75	390	0
Pea pods, see "Peas, edible-podded"							
Peach, fresh:							
(*Dole*), 1 medium, 3.5 oz.	40	1.0	10.0	0	0	0	2.0
(*Frieda's* Donut/Late Season), 5 oz. . . .	60	1.0	16.0	0	0	0	3.0
2½" peach, 4 per lb.	37	.6	9.7	.1	0	0	1.7
sliced, 1 cup.	73	1.2	18.9	.2	0	0	3.4
Peach, can or jar, halves or slices, ½ cup, except as noted:							
(*Del Monte Fruitrageous* Peachy Peach Pie), 4 oz.	80	<1.0	21.0	0	0	10	<1.0
in juice:							
(*Del Monte* Fruit Naturals)	60	0	15.0	0	0	10	1.0
(*Libby's*)	70	1.0	17.0	0	0	10	1.0
(*S&W*)	80	1.0	19.0	0	0	20	1.0
w/liquid	55	.8	14.5	<.1	0	5	1.6
in juice or extra light syrup (*Del Monte* Fruit Snack Cup), 4 oz.	50	0	13.0	0	0	10	<1.0
in extra light syrup:							
(*Del Monte* Lite Cling)	60	0	15.0	0	0	10	1.0
(*Del Monte* Lite Freestone)	60	0	14.0	0	0	10	1.0
in light syrup:							
(*Del Monte* Orchard Select)	80	<1.0	20.0	0	0	10	<1.0
w/liquid	68	.6	18.3	<.1	0	5	1.6

Food and Measure	cal.	prot. (gms)	carbo. (gms)	fat (gms)	chol. (mgs)	sod. (mgs)	fiber (gms)
(S&W White California Snow)	80	<1.0	20.0	0	0	15	1.0
diced (S&W California Sun)	80	<1.0	20.0	0	0	20	1.0
diced, w/passion fruit (S&W)	80	<1.0	19.0	0	0	15	0
banana berry (Del Monte Fruit-to-Go), 4 oz.	70	<1.0	17.0	0	0	10	<1.0
cinnamon (Del Monte Chunky Cut)	80	0	20.0	0	0	10	1.0
cinnamon (S&W Sweet Memory) .	80	<1.0	19.0	0	0	15	1.0
peach flavored (Del Monte Fruit-to-Go), 4 oz.	70	<1.0	17.0	0	0	10	<1.0
raspberry flavored (Del Monte/Del Monte Fruit Pleasures)	80	<1.0	20.0	0	0	10	<1.0
spiced (Del Monte)	80	<1.0	21.0	0	0	10	<1.0
wild raspberry flavored (Del Monte Fruit-rageous), 4 oz.	80	<1.0	22.0	0	0	10	<1.0
in heavy syrup: (Del Monte/Del Monte Melba) . .	100	0	24.0	0	0	10	1.0
(S&W)	100	1.0	24.0	0	0	10	1.0
w/liquid	97	.6	26.1	.1	0	8	1.7
diced (Del Monte Snack Cup), 4 oz.	80	0	20.0	0	0	10	<1.0
spiced, whole (Del Monte)	100	0	24.0	0	0	10	<1.0
Peach, dried:							
(Sonoma Organic), 4 pcs., 1.4 oz.	130	2.0	31.0	0	0	0	3.0
(Sun•Maid), ¼ cup . .	100	2.0	25.0	0	0	0	3.0
(Sunsweet), 1.4 oz., about 3 pcs.	110	2.0	25.0	0	0	0	3.0
freeze-dried, diced (AlpineAire), .4 oz.	40	1.0	9.0	0	0	0	0

Food and Measure	cal.	prot. (gms)	carbo. (gms)	fat (gms)	chol. (mgs)	sod. (mgs)	fiber (gms)
Peach, dried *(cont.)*							
sulfured:							
halves, ½ cup	191	2.9	49.1	.6	0	6	6.6
10 halves, 4.6 oz.	311	4.7	79.7	1.0	0	9	10.7
Peach, frozen:							
(*Big Valley*), ⅔ cup ..	50	1.0	13.0	0	0	0	2.0
sliced, sweetened,							
½ cup	118	.8	30.0	.2	0	8	1.8
Peach butter							
(*Smucker's*), 1 tbsp.	45	0	11.0	0	0	10	0
Peach drink blends:							
(*Snapple* Summer							
Peach), 8 fl. oz. ..	120	0	30.0	0	0	10	0
mango (*Whipper-*							
Snapple), 10 fl. oz.	150	0	39.0	0	0	60	0
Peach juice (*Nan-*							
tucket Nectars),							
8 fl. oz.	120	0	30.0	0	0	15	0
Peach juice blends							
(*Ceres*), 5.25 fl. oz. ...	87	0	21.0	0	0	n.a.	0
mango, frozen*							
(*Cascadian Farm*),							
8 fl. oz.	120	0	29.0	0	0	9	0
Peach nectar:							
(*Goya*), 6 fl. oz.	110	<1.0	27.0	0	0	30	1.0
(*Libby's*),							
5.5-fl.-oz. can	90	0	23.0	0	0	5	0
(*Libby's*), 8 fl. oz. ...	140	<1.0	34.0	0	0	5	0
(*Libby's*),							
11.5-fl.-oz. can ...	200	<1.0	49.0	0	0	10	0
(*R. W. Knudsen*),							
8 fl. oz.	120	<1.0	30.0	0	0	25	0
canned	135	.7	34.7	<.1	0	17	1.5
Peach orange juice							
(*Nantucket Nectars*),							
8 fl. oz.	130	1.0	31.0	0	0	25	0
Peach and pear,							
canned, in light							
syrup, wild berry							
(*Del Monte*							
Fruit-to-Go							
Jumble), 4 oz. ...	80	<1.0	20.0	0	0	10	<1.0
Peach salsa, see							
"Salsa"							

Food and Measure	cal.	prot. (gms)	carbo. (gms)	fat (gms)	chol. (mgs)	sod. (mgs	fiber (gms)
Peanut, shelled, 1 oz., except as noted:							
(*Frito-Lay* Salted), 1.1 oz.	200	7.0	5.0	16.0	0	180	2.0
(*House of Bazzini* Unsalted)	170	7.0	8.0	12.0	0	5	4.0
(*Planters* Cocktail) . . .	170	7.0	6.0	14.0	0	115	2.0
(*Planters* Cocktail Unsalted)	170	7.0	6.0	14.0	0	0	2.0
(*Planters* Salted)	170	6.0	5.0	15.0	0	135	2.0
boiled, salted	90	3.8	6.0	6.2	0	213	2.5
dry-roasted:							
(*Fisher*)	170	7.0	6.0	14.0	0	190	2.0
(*Planters*)	160	7.0	6.0	13.0	0	190	2.0
(*Planters*), 1.75-oz. pkg. . .	290	8.0	9.0	26.0	0	230	4.0
diced (*Blue Diamond*), ¼ cup . .	190	7.0	7.0	16.0	0	0	2.0
½ cup	428	17.3	15.7	36.3	0	4	5.8
honey-roasted:							
(*Fisher*)	170	7.0	7.0	13.0	0	70	2.0
(*Frito-Lay*), 1.1 oz.	180	7.0	9.0	13.0	0	170	2.0
(*Planters*)	160	6.0	8.0	13.0	0	95	2.0
(*Weight Watchers*), .7-oz. pouch . . .	100	7.0	7.0	5.0	0	100	2.0
hot:							
(*D. L. Jardine's* Texacali), ¼ cup, 1 oz.	160	8.0	5.0	13.0	0	290	2.0
(*Frito-Lay*), 1.1 oz.	190	7.0	6.0	16.0	0	250	2.0
(*Planters* Heat) . . .	160	6.0	6.0	13.0	0	210	2.0
(*Planters* Heat), 1-oz. pkg.	160	6.0	5.0	14.0	0	190	2.0
oil-roasted:							
(*Fisher*)	170	7.0	5.0	15.0	0	130	2.0
½ cup	419	19.0	13.6	35.5	0	4	6.6
roasted:							
(*Planters*)	150	6.0	5.0	13.0	0	240	2.0
blanched (*Blue Diamond*), ¼ cup . .	200	9.0	6.0	17.0	0	0	2.0
Peanut bake mix, spicy (*A Taste of Thai*), ¼ pkt.	45	1.0	7.0	1.5	0	190	1.0

Food and Measure	cal.	prot. (gms)	carbo. (gms)	fat (gms)	chol. (mgs)	sod. (mgs)	fiber (gms)
Peanut butter, 2 tbsp., except as noted:							
(*Estee* Low Sodium)	190	7.0	7.0	15.0	0	0	2.0
(*Kettle Roaster Fresh*), 1 oz.	165	4.0	9.0	14.0	0	4	0
(*Peanut Wonder*) . . .	100	4.0	13.0	2.5	0	95	0
(*Simply Jif*)	190	8.0	6.0	16.0	0	50	2.0
chunky or creamy:							
(*Arrowhead Mills* Easy Spread) . . .	200	8.0	7.0	15.0	0	100	2.0
(*Arrowhead Mills* Valencia)	200	9.0	6.0	15.0	0	0	1.0
(*Smucker's* Natural)	200	7.0	7.0	16.0	0	120	2.0
(*Smucker's* Natural No Salt)	200	7.0	7.0	16.0	0	0	2.0
chunky/crunchy:							
(*Jif* Reduced Fat) . .	190	8.0	15.0	12.0	0	270	2.0
(*Peter Pan*)	190	8.0	6.0	16.0	0	115	3.0
(*Reese's*)	200	8.0	7.0	15.0	0	110	2.0
extra (*Jif*)	190	8.0	7.0	16.0	0	130	2.0
super (*Skippy*) . . .	190	7.0	7.0	16.0	0	140	2.0
super (*Skippy* Reduced Fat Spread)	190	7.0	14.0	12.0	0	170	2.0
creamy/smooth:							
(*Jif*)	190	8.0	7.0	16.0	0	150	2.0
(*Jif* Reduced Fat) . .	190	8.0	15.0	12.0	0	250	2.0
(*Peter Pan*)	190	8.0	6.0	17.0	0	150	2.0
(*Reese's*)	200	7.0	8.0	15.0	0	140	2.0
(*Skippy*)	190	7.0	7.0	16.0	0	150	2.0
(*Skippy* Reduced Fat Spread)	190	7.0	15.0	12.0	0	190	2.0
(*Smucker's* Natural Reduced Fat) . . .	200	9.0	12.0	12.0	0	120	2.0
honey nut, roasted:							
chunky (*Skippy*) . .	190	7.0	7.0	16.0	0	125	2.0
creamy (*Skippy*) . .	190	7.0	7.0	17.0	0	125	2.0
Peanut butter, baking, 1 tbsp.:							
bits (*Reese's*)	70	<1.0	10.0	3.0	0	40	0
chips (*Reese's*)	80	3.0	7.0	4.0	0	35	0
Peanut butter blend (see also "Peanut butter-jelly"), 2 tbsp.:							
apple cinnamon (*Jif*) .	200	6.0	11.0	16.0	0	115	2.0

Food and Measure	cal.	prot. (gms)	carbo. (gms)	fat (gms)	chol. (mgs)	sod. (mgs)	fiber (gms)
berry (*Jif*)	200	6.0	10.0	17.0	0	115	1.0
chocolate:							
(*Jif* Silk)	190	5.0	14.0	15.0	0	115	1.0
(*Skippy Doubly Delicious*)	210	7.0	12.0	15.0	0	130	2.0
(*Skippy Doubly Delicious Buncha Crunch*)	210	7.0	12.0	15.0	0	135	2.0
Peanut butter sprinkles, 2 tbsp.:							
(*Hershey's Reese's Chocolate Shoppe*)	160	4.0	17.0	8.0	<5	45	1.0
candy coated (*Hershey's Reese's Chocolate Shoppe*)	150	2.0	19.0	7.0	<5	50	<1.0
Peanut butter topping, 2 tbsp.:							
(*Hershey's* Shell)	220	<1.0	17.0	17.0	0	70	1.0
(*Reese's* Pourable) ..	220	7.0	7.0	18.0	0	160	2.0
(*Smucker's Magic Shell*)	220	2.0	16.0	17.0	0	50	0
Peanut butter-jelly:							
(*Goober's*), 3 tbsp. ..	230	7.0	24.0	13.0	0	140	2.0
w/crackers (*Smucker's Snackers*), 1 pkg.	410	11.0	47.0	20.0	0	480	3.0
Peanut butter-jelly sandwich, grape or strawberry (*Smucker's Uncrustables*), 1 pc.	200	7.0	27.0	8.0	0	260	2.0
Peanut flour, 1 cup:							
defatted	196	31.3	20.8	.3	0	9	9.5
low fat	257	20.3	18.8	13.1	0	0	9.5
Peanut sauce, Thai:							
(*Annie Chun's*), 2 tbsp.	120	4.0	10.0	7.0	0	230	1.0
(*Heaven and Earth*), 1 tbsp.	100	10.0	5.0	16.0	0	90	0
(*San-J* Thai), 2 tbsp.	70	3.0	7.0	3.0	0	710	1.0
satay, 2 tbsp.:							
(*Ka•Me*)	80	2.0	9.0	4.0	0	340	1.0
(*A Taste of Thai*) ..	50	0	5.0	3.0	0	60	1.0
Peanut sauce mix (*A Taste of Thai*), ¼ pkt.	45	1.0	7.0	1.5	0	190	1.0

Food and Measure	cal.	prot. (gms)	carbo. (gms)	fat (gms)	chol. (mgs)	sod. (mgs)	fiber (gms)
Pear, fresh, w/peel:							
(*Dole*), 1 medium,							
5.9 oz.	100	1.0	25.0	1.0	0	0	4.0
1 large, 2 per lb.	123	.8	31.6	.8	0	0	5.0
Bartlett, 1 medium,							
2½ per lb.	98	.7	25.1	.7	0	1	4.0
sliced, ½ cup	49	.3	12.5	.3	0	1	2.0
Pear, Asian:							
(*Frieda's*), 5 oz.	60	1.0	15.0	0	0	0	5.0
1 medium, 2¼" x							
2½" diam.	51	.6	13.0	.3	0	0	4.4
Pear, can or jar, halves							
or slices, ½ cup,							
except as noted:							
in juice:							
(*Del Monte* Fruit							
Naturals)	60	0	15.0	0	0	10	1.0
(*Libby's Lite*)	60	0	13.0	0	0	10	1.0
(*S&W* Halves)	80	0	21.0	1.0	0	10	2.0
(*S&W* Slices)	80	0	20.0	1.0	0	25	2.0
w/liquid	62	.4	16.0	.1	0	5	2.0
in extra light syrup:							
(*Del Monte* Lite) ..	60	0	15.0	0	0	10	1.0
(*Del Monte* Lite							
Snack Cup), 4 oz.	50	0	13.0	0	0	10	<1.0
in light syrup:							
(*Del Monte Orchard*							
Select Bartlett) ..	80	<1.0	20.0	0	0	10	2.0
w/liquid	72	.2	19.0	<.1	0	6	2.0
diced (*S&W* Sun) ..	80	<1.0	20.0	0	0	10	<1.0
cinnamon flavor							
(*Del Monte*)	80	0	21.0	0	0	10	1.0
in heavy syrup:							
(*Del Monte*)	100	0	24.0	0	0	10	1.0
(*S&W*)	90	0	23.0	0	0	15	1.0
w/liquid	98	.3	25.5	.2	0	7	2.1
diced (*Del Monte*							
Snack Cup), 4 oz.	80	0	20.0	0	0	10	<1.0
ginger flavor, natural							
(*Del Monte*)	90	0	22.0	0	0	10	1.0
Pear, dried:							
(*Sonoma* Organic),							
4 pcs., 1.4 oz.	140	1.0	32.0	0	0	0	7.0
2 oz.	149	1.1	39.5	.4	0	4	4.3

Food and Measure	cal.	prot. (gms)	carbo. (gms)	fat (gms)	chol. (mgs)	sod. (mgs)	fiber (gms)
sulfured:							
halves, ½ cup	236	1.7	62.7	.6	0	5	6.8
stewed, ½ cup	162	1.2	43.1	.4	0	4	8.2
Pear butter (*Sonoma*),							
2 tbsp.	50	0	11.0	0	0	0	2.0
Pear juice, 8 fl. oz.:							
(*After the Fall* Alle-							
gany)	90	0	22.0	0	0	30	0
(*R. W. Knudsen*							
Organic)	120	<1.0	30.0	0	0	25	0
Pear juice blends:							
(*After the Fall* Rouge							
River), 8 fl. oz. ...	100	1.0	24.0	0	0	20	0
(*Ceres*), 5.25 fl. oz. ..	87	0	21.0	0	0	n.a.	0
Pear nectar:							
(*Goya*), 12 fl. oz. ...	240	1.0	59.0	0	0	20	2.0
(*Libby's*),							
5.5-fl.-oz. can	100	0	25.0	0	0	0	0
(*Libby's*), 8 fl. oz. ...	150	0	36.0	0	0	5	0
(*Libby's*),							
11.5-fl.-oz. can ...	210	0	51.0	0	0	5	3.0
(*Santa Cruz Organic*),							
8 fl. oz.	110	<1.0	28.0	0	0	35	0
canned, 8 fl. oz.	150	.3	39.4	<.1	0	10	1.5
Peas, see specific							
listings							
Peas, black-eyed, see							
"Black-eyed peas"							
Peas, butter, frozen							
(*Birds Eye* Southern),							
½ cup	110	7.0	20.0	.5	0	10	4.0
Peas, cream, canned,							
½ cup:							
(*Bush's Best*)	110	7.0	18.0	1.0	0	500	5.0
(*East Texas Fair*)	100	6.0	17.0	1.0	0	460	5.0
Peas, crowder, canned,							
½ cup:							
(*Allens/East Texas*							
Fair)	110	6.0	19.0	1.0	0	460	8.0
(*Bush's Best*)	110	7.0	18.0	1.0	0	500	5.0
Peas, crowder, frozen							
(*Birds Eye* Southern),							
½ cup	120	8.0	22.0	1.0	0	10	4.0

Food and Measure	cal.	prot. (gms)	carbo. (gms)	fat (gms)	chol. (mgs)	sod. (mgs)	fiber (gms)
Peas, edible-podded, fresh:							
raw:							
(*Dole* Sugar), ½ cup, 2.5 oz.	30	2.0	5.0	0	0	0	2.0
(*Frieda's* Snow), 1 cup, 3 oz. . . .	35	2.0	6.0	0	0	0	2.0
(*Frieda's* Sugar Snap), ⅔ cup, 3 oz.	35	2.0	6.0	0	0	0	2.0
(*Mann's* Stringless Sugar Snap), 4 oz.	50	3.0	9.0	0	0	0	3.0
1 cup	41	2.7	7.4	.2	0	4	2.6
raw, w/sauce, ½ cup:							
(*Frieda's* Snow) . . .	40	2.0	8.0	0	0	180	2.0
(*Frieda's* Sugar Snap)	35	2.0	8.0	0	0	180	2.0
boiled, drained, ½ cup	34	2.6	5.6	.2	0	3	2.2
Peas, edible podded, frozen:							
(*Cascadian Farm* Sugar Snap), ¾ cup	35	2.0	6.0	0	0	0	2.0
(*Green Giant Select* Sugar Snap), ¾ cup	35	2.0	7.0	0	0	0	3.0
(*John Cope's* Sugar Snap), ⅔ cup	45	2.0	6.0	0	0	10	2.0
(*La Choy* Snow Pea), 3 oz., about 42 pods	35	2.0	4.0	1.5	0	0	2.0
boiled, drained, ½ cup	42	2.8	7.2	.3	0	4	2.5
stir-fry blend (*Birds Eye* Sugar Snap), ¾ cup	35	1.0	5.0	0	0	20	1.0
Peas, field, canned, (see also "Peas, crowder" and "Peas, purple hull"), ½ cup:							
(*Bush's Best*)	110	7.0	18.0	1.0	0	500	5.0

Food and Measure	cal.	prot. (gms)	carbo. (gms)	fat (gms)	chol. (mgs)	sod. (mgs)	fiber (gms)
(Glory Foods)	80	6.0	14.0	0	0	830	4.0
(Sunshine)	120	7.0	21.0	1.0	0	300	6.0
w/snaps:							
(Allens/East Texas Fair/Homefolks)	120	6.0	21.0	1.0	0	300	6.0
(Bush's Best)	110	7.0	17.0	.5	0	550	5.0
(Glory Foods)	70	5.0	12.0	0	0	830	5.0
w/bacon (Trappey's)	90	6.0	15.0	1.0	0	380	5.0
w/bacon and snaps (Trappey's)	110	6.0	19.0	1.0	0	380	4.0
Peas, field, frozen, w/snaps:							
(Birds Eye), ⅔ cup ..	130	9.0	24.0	1.0	0	15	4.0
(McKenzie's), ½ cup	110	7.0	21.0	.5	0	10	4.0
Peas, green, fresh: raw:							
in pod, 1 lb.	140	9.3	24.9	.7	0	8	8.8
shelled, ½ cup	59	3.9	10.4	.3	0	3	3.7
boiled, drained, ½ cup	67	4.3	12.5	.2	0	2	4.4
Peas, green, can or jar, ½ cup: early or sweet:							
(Blue Boy)	70	4.0	12.0	0	0	370	4.0
(Bush's Best Early June)	80	5.0	12.0	1.0	0	340	4.0
(Bush's Best Small Early)	70	4.0	11.0	1.0	0	340	3.0
(Del Monte)	60	3.0	13.0	0	0	390	4.0
(Del Monte No Salt)	60	3.0	11.0	0	0	10	4.0
(Green Giant)	60	4.0	11.0	0	0	380	4.0
(Greenleaf Early June)	45	6.0	8.0	0	0	310	3.0
(Hain)	60	4.0	10.0	0	0	360	3.0
(Libby's)	70	4.0	12.0	0	0	370	4.0
(Libby's No Salt) ..	70	4.0	12.0	0	0	15	4.0
(LeSueur)	60	4.0	12.0	0	0	380	3.0
(Veg-All)	60	4.0	10.0	.5	0	370	3.0
drained	59	3.8	10.7	.3	0	214	3.5
medium/small or petite (S&W)	70	4.0	12.0	0	0	330	4.0
seasoned, w/liquid ...	57	3.5	10.5	.3	0	288	2.8
very young, small (Del Monte)	60	3.0	10.0	0	0	360	4.0

Food and Measure	cal.	prot. (gms)	carbo. (gms)	fat (gms)	chol. (mgs)	sod. (mgs)	fiber (gms)
Peas, green, dried:							
(*Frieda's*), ⅓ cup, 3 oz.	130	9.0	22.0	0	0	290	9.0
freeze-dried (*Alpine-Aire*), 1.3 oz.	80	5.0	14.0	0	0	115	5.0
Peas, green, frozen, ⅔ cup, except as noted:							
(*Birds Eye*)	70	5.0	12.0	.5	0	105	4.0
(*Greene's Farm* Garden)	60	4.0	10.0	0	0	250	3.0
(*John Cope's*)	70	5.0	12.0	.5	0	105	4.0
(*Richfood* Petite)	70	5.0	12.0	.5	0	105	4.0
(*Seabrook Farms*) . . .	70	5.0	12.0	.5	0	105	4.0
(*Tree of Life* Organic)	70	5.0	12.0	0	0	100	4.0
boiled, drained, ½ cup	62	4.1	11.4	.2	0	70	4.4
extra fine (*Bonduelle* Petite), 3 oz.	68	4.0	12.0	.5	0	n.a.	6.0
garden (*Cascadian Farm*)	70	4.0	12.0	0	0	55	5.0
sweet (*Green Giant*), ¾ cup	70	5.0	12.0	.5	0	135	4.0
sweet, baby:							
(*Birds Eye*)	70	5.0	12.0	.5	0	105	4.0
(*Green Giant LeSueur*)	70	4.0	12.0	.5	0	190	4.0
(*Green Giant Select LeSueur*)	60	4.0	11.0	.5	0	150	4.0
tiny:							
(*John Cope's*)	70	5.0	12.0	0	0	105	4.0
(*Seabrook Farms* Petite)	70	5.0	12.0	.5	0	105	4.0
Peas, green, combinations, fresh, and carrots (*Mann's*), 3 oz.	40	2.0	8.0	0	0	60	2.0
Peas, green, combinations, can or jar, ½ cup:							
and carrots:							
(*Del Monte*)	60	2.0	11.0	0	0	360	2.0
(*Green Giant*)	50	2.0	11.0	0	0	410	3.0
(*Libby's*)	60	3.0	10.0	0	0	330	4.0
(*S&W*)	60	2.0	11.0	0	0	360	2.0

Food and Measure	cal.	prot. (gms)	carbo. (gms)	fat (gms)	chol. (mgs)	sod. (mgs)	fiber (gms)
(*Veg-All*)	60	2.0	12.0	0	0	320	2.0
baby (*Bonduelle*) . .	45	6.0	6.0	0	0	310	3.0
w/liquid	48	2.8	10.8	.3	0	332	2.6
w/mushrooms and onions (*LeSueur*) .	60	3.0	11.0	0	0	380	2.0
and onions:							
(*S&W*)	40	3.0	11.0	0	0	530	3.0
w/liquid	31	2.0	5.1	.2	0	265	1.4
pearl onions (*Green Giant*)	60	4.0	11.0	0	0	440	3.0
Peas, green, combinations, frozen:							
baby, blend (*Birds Eye Tiny Tender*), ¾ cup	40	2.0	7.0	0	0	40	2.0
and carrots:							
(*Cascadian Farm*), ⅔ cup	50	5.0	9.0	0	0	160	0
(*John Cope's*), ½ cup	50	3.0	9.0	0	0	80	3.0
boiled, drained, ½ cup	38	2.7	8.1	.3	0	54	2.5
and onions, pearl:							
(*Birds Eye*), ⅔ cup	90	5.0	18.0	.5	0	520	5.0
(*Cascadian Farm*), ¾ cup	60	4.0	11.0	0	0	130	4.0
baby peas (*Birds Eye*), ⅔ cup	60	4.0	12.0	.5	0	85	4.0
boiled, drained, ½ cup	41	2.3	7.8	.2	0	33	2.0
and potatoes w/cream (*Birds Eye*), ½ cup	90	4.0	13.0	2.5	10	350	2.0
Peas, w/pork, see "Baked Beans" and specific listings							
Peas, pepper, canned (*East Texas Fair*), ½ cup	120	6.0	22.0	1.0	0	580	6.0
Peas, pigeon, see "Pigeon peas"							
Peas, purple hull, canned, ½ cup:							
(*Allens/East Texas Fair*)	120	7.0	21.0	1.0	0	350	6.0
(*Bush's Best*)	110	7.0	18.0	1.0	0	500	5.0

Food and Measure	cal.	prot. (gms)	carbo. (gms)	fat (gms)	chol. (mgs)	sod. (mgs)	fiber (gms)
Peas, purple hull, frozen, ½ cup:							
(*Birds Eye* Southern)	110	7.0	21.0	.5	0	10	4.0
(*McKenzie's*)	110	7.0	21.0	.5	0	10	4.0
Peas, split, see "Split peas"							
Peas, sprouted:							
raw, ½ cup	77	5.3	17.0	.4	0	12	n.a.
boiled, drained, 4 oz.	134	8.0	24.8	.6	0	3	3.7
Peas, sugar snap or snow, see "Peas, edible-podded"							
Peas, sweet, see "Peas, green"							
Peas, white acre, canned (*East Texas Fair*), ½ cup	100	6.0	17.0	1.0	0	460	5.0
Peas and carrots or onions, see "Peas, green, combinations"							
Pecan, shelled:							
(*Bazzini's Nut Club*), ¼ cup	210	3.0	2.0	22.0	0	?	3.0
(*Blue Diamond* Fancy Halves), ⅓ cup ...	220	3.0	5.0	22.0	0	0	3.0
(*Blue Diamond* Pieces), ¼ cup	210	3.0	5.0	22.0	0	0	5.0
(*Fisher*), 1 oz.	200	3.0	4.0	20.0	0	0	2.0
(*Planters*)	190	3.0	4.0	20.0	0	0	3.0
(*Planters* Halves), 2-oz. pkg.	390	3.0	7.0	40.0	0	5	7.0
dried:							
1 oz.	190	2.2	5.2	19.2	0	<1	2.2
halves, 1 cup	721	8.4	19.7	73.1	0	1	8.2
chopped, 1 cup ...	794	9.2	21.7	80.5	0	1	9.0
dry-roasted:							
unsalted, 1 oz. ...	201	2.7	3.8	21.1	0	<1	2.7
unsalted, 1 cup ...	781	10.5	14.9	81.7	0	11	10.5
oil-roasted:							
unsalted, 1 oz. ...	203	2.7	3.7	21.3	0	<1	2.7
unsalted, 1 cup ...	787	10.5	14.3	82.8	0	11	10.5
Pecan filling, see "Pastry filling"							
Pecan flour, 1 oz. ...	93	9.1	14.4	.4	0	tr.	n.a.

Food and Measure	cal.	prot. (gms)	carbo. (gms)	fat (gms)	chol. (mgs)	sod. (mgs)	fiber (gms)
Pecan topping, in syrup (*Smucker's*), 2 tbsp.	170	1.0	20.0	10.0	0	0	0
Pectin, see "Fruit pectin"							
Penne, plain, see "Pasta"							
Penne dish, mix:							
w/black beans (*Marrakesh Express*), 1 cup*	170	7.0	32.0	.5	0	520	1.0
Italian herb butter sauce (*Land O Lakes*), 2.5 oz. . . .	290	8.0	45.0	8.0	5	590	2.0
w/sausage flavor tomato sauce (*Classico It's Pasta Anytime*), 15.25-oz. cont.	540	17.0	100.0	8.0	<5	1100	12.0
tomato:							
and mushroom sauce (*Classico It's Pasta Anytime*), 15.25-oz. cont. .	510	15.0	98.0	6.0	0	970	12.0
sun-dried, Parmesan sauce (*Knorr* Side Dish), ½ cup . . .	270	9.0	50.0	3.5	<5	660	3.0
Penne entree, frozen, 1 pkg.:							
w/chunky tomatoes and Italian sausage (*Budget Gourmet*), 8 oz.	270	10.0	46.0	6.0	10	410	3.0
w/Italian sausage (*Michelina's*), 9 oz.	300	14.0	36.0	10.0	20	530	3.0
w/mushroom sauce (*Michelina's*), 8 oz.	280	10.0	42.0	8.0	15	380	3.0
w/mushrooms (*Michelina's*), 8 oz.	250	10.0	39.0	6.0	20	630	3.0
pollo (*Michelina's*), 8.5 oz.	290	16.0	39.0	8.0	40	580	2.0
primavera (*Michelina's*), 8.5 oz.	280	10.0	40.0	9.0	20	530	3.0
w/tomato (*Lean Cuisine Everyday Favorites*), 10 oz. .	260	9.0	47.0	3.5	0	390	5.0

Food and Measure	cal.	prot. (gms)	carbo. (gms)	fat (gms)	chol. (mgs)	sod. (mgs)	fiber (gms)
Penne dish, mix *(cont.)*							
vegetarian (*Yves Veggie Penne*), 10.5 oz.	220	12.0	36.0	1.5	0	730	4.0
Penne entree, pkg., tomato Parmesan (*Bowl Appétit!*), 1 bowl	350	12.0	59.0	8.0	5	870	2.0
Pepeao, raw, sliced, 1 cup	25	.5	6.7	0	0	9	n.a.
Pepeao, dried, 1 cup	72	1.2	19.5	.1	0	17	n.a.
Pepper, seasoning:							
black:							
ground, 1 tsp.	6	.3	1.7	.1	0	1	.7
whole, 1 tsp.	8	.3	1.9	0	0	1	.8
blend, Szechuan style (*McCormick*), ¼ tsp.	0	0	0	0	0	15	0
chili, 1 tsp.	9	.3	1.2	.3	0	<1	.7
red or cayenne, 1 tsp.	6	.2	1.0	.3	0	1	.7
seasoned (*Lawry's*), ¼ tsp.	0	0	1.0	0	0	0	0
white, 1 tsp.	7	.3	1.7	.1	0	0	.2
Pepper, nacho, dried, .6-oz. pepper	48	2.0	8.7	1.4	0	7	3.7
Pepper, banana, fresh, 1.2-oz. pc.	9	.6	1.8	.2	0	4	1.1
Pepper, banana, in jars, 1 oz.:							
hot or mild (*Vlasic*)	5	0	1.0	0	0	480	0
mild (*Trappey's*)	5	0	1.0	0	0	378	0
Pepper, bell, see "Pepper, sweet"							
Pepper, cherry:							
hot (*Progresso*), 1 oz.	10	0	2.0	0	0	150	<1.0
mild (*Trappey's*), 1.2 oz.	10	0	2.0	0	0	260	0
Pepper, cherry, stuffed, w/prosciutto and provolone:							
(*La Rosa D'Oro*), 2 oz.	60	2.0	1.0	5.0	10	490	0
(*Norpaco*), 1 pc. and 1 tsp. oil	70	2.0	1.0	6.0	5	240	0

Food and Measure	cal.	prot. (gms)	carbo. (gms)	fat (gms)	chol. (mgs)	sod. (mgs)	fiber (gms)
Pepper, chili, fresh, all varieties (*Frieda's Cucina*), 1-oz. pc.	10	1.0	3.0	0	0	0	0
green and red:							
1 medium, 1.6 oz.	18	.9	4.3	.1	0	3	.7
chopped, ½ cup	30	1.5	7.1	.2	0	5	1.1
Pepper, chili, can or jar:							
whole:							
chipotle (*Herdez*), 3 pcs., 1 oz.	30	0	3.0	1.0	0	360	0
chipotle in adobo sauce (*La Morena*), 2 pcs., 1 oz.	15	0	2.0	0	0	350	0
guerito (*Embasa*), 7 pcs., 1.1 oz.	10	0	1.0	.5	0	550	2.0
poblano (*Herdez*), ½ pc., 1.2 oz.	10	0	1.0	0	0	180	0
yellow quero (*Corona Real Chiles de Oro*), 1 pc.	6	0	1.0	0	0	27	2.0
whole, green:							
(*Chi-Chi's*), ¾ pc.	10	0	1.0	0	0	15	0
(*Embasa*), 1 pc.	15	<1.0	3.0	0	0	30	<1.0
(*Old El Paso*), 1 pc.	10	0	2.0	0	0	230	1.0
2.6-oz. pc.	15	.7	3.7	<.1	0	856	1.0
½ cup	15	.5	3.2	.1	0	276	1.2
peeled (*Hatch*), 2-oz. pc.	10	0	2.0	0	0	100	<1.0
chopped:							
chipotle in adobo sauce (*Embasa*), 2 tbsp. w/sauce	15	<1.0	2.0	.5	0	140	1.0
green (*Old El Paso*), 2 tbsp.	5	0	1.0	0	0	110	1.0
w/liquid, ½ cup	17	.6	4.2	.1	0	n.a.	1.3
diced, green, 2 tbsp.:							
(*Chi-Chi's*)	10	0	1.0	0	0	20	0
(*Hatch*)	10	0	2.0	0	0	40	<1.0
minced, red (*A Taste of Thai*), 2 tbsp.	40	1.0	1.0	0	0	15	0
Pepper, chili, sun-dried, hot, 2 pcs.	3	.1	.8	.1	0	1	.3

Food and Measure	cal.	prot. (gms)	carbo. (gms)	fat (gms)	chol. (mgs)	sod. (mgs)	fiber (gms)
Pepper, green or red, sweet, see "Pepper, sweet"							
Pepper, Hungarian, fresh, .94-oz. pc.	8	.2	1.8	.1	0	<1.	n.a.
pepper, jalapeño, fresh, .5-oz. pc. . .	4	.2	.8	.1	0	<1	.4
Pepper, jalapeño, can or jar:							
(*La Victoria* Marinated), 1.1 oz.	10	0	2.0	0	0	280	<1.0
(*La Victoria* Pickled), 1.1 oz.	10	0	2.0	0	0	115	<1.0
whole (*Chi-Chi's*), 2½ pcs.	10	0	2.0	0	0	120	0
chopped, w/liquid, ¼ cup	7	.2	1.2	.2	0	434	.8
diced (*La Victoria*), 1.1 oz.	10	0	2.0	0	0	100	<1.0
sliced:							
(*Hatch*), 2 tbsp. . .	5	0	1.0	0	0	320	0
(*Trappey's*), 1 oz.	5	0	<1.0	0	0	300	1.0
w/liquid, ¼ cup . . .	9	.3	1.6	.3	0	568	.9
nacho (*La Victoria*), 1.1 oz.	5	0	<1.0	0	0	350	<1.0
nacho, pickled (*La Costeña*), ¼ cup	20	0	1.0	1.5	0	480	1.0
wheels (*Chi-Chi's*), 19 pcs., 1 oz.	10	0	2.0	0	0	120	0
Pepper, jalapeno, stuffed, frozen, w/cream cheese, breaded (*Poppers*), .9-oz. pc.	70	1.0	6.0	4.0	10	150	<1.0
Pepper, pasilla, dried, .25-oz. pc.	24	.9	3.6	1.1	0	6	1.9
Pepper, poblano, see "Pepper, chili, can or jar"							
Pepper, roasted, see "Pepper, sweet, in jars"							
Pepper, seasoned, see "Pepper"							

Food and Measure	cal.	prot. (gms)	carbo. (gms)	fat (gms)	chol. (mgs)	sod. (mgs)	fiber (gms)
Pepper, serrano, fresh:							
whole, .2-oz. pc.	2	.1	.4	<.1	0	2	.2
chopped, ½ cup	17	.9	3.5	.5	0	5	1.9
Pepper, stuffed, entree, frozen:							
(*Stouffer's*), 10-oz. pkg.	210	10.0	25.0	8.0	20	840	3.0
(*Stouffer's*), ½ of 15.5-oz. pkg.	180	8.0	20.0	7.0	25	530	2.0
(*Stouffer's Family Style Favorites*), ¼ of 32-oz. pkg.	200	9.0	21.0	9.0	20	1130	2.0
Pepper, sweet, fresh: green and red:							
raw (*Dole*), 1 medium, 5.2 oz.	30	1.0	7.0	0	0	0	2.0
raw, 1 medium, 3¾" x 3" or ½ cup chopped ...	20	.7	4.8	.1	0	1	1.3
raw, sliced, 1 cup	25	.8	5.9	.2	0	2	1.7
boiled, drained, 1 medium	20	.7	4.9	.1	0	1	.9
boiled, drained, chopped, 1 tbsp.	3	.1	.8	<.1	0	<1	.1
boiled, drained, strips, ½ cup ...	19	.6	4.6	.1	0	1	.8
yellow, raw:							
1 large, 5" x 3" ...	50	1.9	11.8	.4	0	4	1.7
10 strips, 1.8 oz.	14	.5	3.3	.1	0	1	.5
Pepper, sweet, can or jar (see also "Pimiento"):							
drained, ½ cup	13	.6	2.7	.2	0	958	.8
fire-roasted:							
(*Frieda's*), 1-oz. pc.	35	1.0	5.0	0	0	280	0
(*Pompeian*), ½ cup	30	1.0	5.0	0	0	310	1.0
w/garlic, oil (*Paesana*), 2 tbsp.	20	0	2.0	1.0	0	125	0
roasted, in olive oil (*Haddon House*), 2 tbsp.	20	1.0	5.0	1.0	0	180	1.0
salad, w/oregano, garlic (*B&G*), 1 oz.	10	0	3.0	0	0	240	0
sun-dried, in oil (*Antica Italia*), 1 oz.	170	0	2.0	18.0	0	5	1.0

Food and Measure	cal.	prot. (gms)	carbo. (gms)	fat (gms)	chol. (mgs)	sod. (mgs)	fiber (gms)
Pepper, sweet, dried, red or green:							
dehydrated (*Alpine-Aire*), .5 oz.	15	2.0	1.0	.5	0	0	0
freeze-dried, ¼ cup . .	5	.3	1.1	<.1	0	3	.3
Pepper, sweet, frozen:							
chopped:							
(*Seabrook Farms*), 1 oz.	6	0	1.0	0	0	1	0
1 oz.	6	.3	1.2	.1	0	1	.5
green, diced (*Birds Eye Southern*), ¾ cup	20	1.0	4.0	0	0	10	2.0
stir-fry blend (*Birds Eye*), 3 oz.	25	1.0	5.0	0	0	15	2.0
Pepper, tabasco, in vinegar (*Trappey's*), 1 oz.	5	0	1.0	0	0	730	0
Pepper, tempero, see "Pepperoncini"							
Pepper, torrido (*Trappey's* Santa Fe Grande), 1.3 oz. . . .	10	0	3.0	0	0	630	0
Pepper dip, red (*Victoria*), ¼ cup	50	0	12.0	2.0	0	120	0
Pepper relish, 1 tbsp.:							
hot (*Cains*)	20	0	5.0	0	0	60	0
sweet (*Cains*)	20	0	5.0	0	0	45	0
Pepper salad:							
(*B&G*), 1 oz.	10	0	3.0	0	0	240	0
drained (*Progresso*), 2 tbsp.	15	0	1.0	1.0	0	160	<1.0
Pepper salt (see also specific listings), ¼ tsp.:							
(*McCormick Season-All*)	0	0	0	0	0	110	0
black (*Lawry's*)	0	0	0	0	0	160	0
red (*Lawry's*)	0	0	0	0	0	290	0
Pepper sauce, see "Hot sauce" and specific listings							
Pepper steak, see "Beef entree, frozen"							

Food and Measure	cal.	prot. (gms)	carbo. (gms)	fat (gms)	chol. (mgs)	sod. (mgs)	fiber (gms)
Peppercorn sauce mix (*Knorr* Classic), 2 tsp.	25	<1.0	3.0	1.0	0	380	0
Pepperoncini:							
(*Krinos*), ¼ cup	5	0	2.0	0	0	950	0
(*Progresso* Tuscan), 3 pcs., 1 oz.	10	0	1.0	0	0	450	0
(*Trappey's* Tempero), 1 oz.	5	0	1.0	0	0	470	0
(*Zorba*), 5 pcs., 1.1 oz.	15	1.0	2.0	0	0	450	0
Pepperoni:							
(*Boar's Head*), 1 oz.	140	6.0	1.0	13.0	25	490	0
(*Boar's Head* Sandwich Style), 1 oz.	130	5.0	1.0	12.0	25	460	0
(*Hormel* Chunk or Sliced), 1 oz.	140	5.0	0	13.0	35	470	0
(*Hormel* Twin), 1 oz.	140	5.0	0	13.0	35	500	0
(*Hormel* Pillow Pack), 14 slices, 1 oz. ...	140	5.0	0	13.0	35	470	0
(*Sara Lee*), 7 slices, 1.1 oz.	140	6.0	1.0	14.0	25	560	0
(*Sara Lee* Sandwich), 7 slices, .9 oz. ...	120	5.0	0	12.0	20	450	0
turkey, see "Turkey pepperoni"							
"Pepperoni," vegetar-ian, frozen (*Yves* Pizza Slices), 1.7 oz.	70	14.0	4.0	0	0	480	3.0
Pepperoni pocket, see "Pizza, stuffed/ pocket"							
Perch, meat only:							
raw, 4 oz.	103	22.0	0	1.1	102	70	0
baked, broiled, or microwaved, 4 oz.	133	28.2	0	1.3	130	90	0
ocean, see "Ocean perch"							
Persimmon, fresh:							
(*Frieda's* Fuyu/Hachiya/ Sharon), 5 oz.	100	1.0	26.0	0	0	0	5.0
Japanese, 1 medium .	118	1.0	31.2	.3	0	3	6.0
native, 1 medium, 1.1 oz.	32	.2	8.4	.1	0	<1	n.a.

Food and Measure	cal.	prot. (gms)	carbo. (gms)	fat (gms)	chol. (mgs)	sod. (mgs)	fiber (gms)
Persimmon, dried:							
(*Frieda's* Fuyu), ⅓ cup, 1.4 oz.	140	1.0	35.0	0	0	10	3.0
(*Sonoma*), 7 pcs., 1.4 oz.	140	1.0	35.0	0	0	10	3.0
Japanese, 1 oz.	78	.4	20.8	.2	0	1	4.1
Pesto paste (*Amore*), 2 tbsp.	110	<1.0	3.0	10.0	0	630	0
Pesto sauce, in jars, ¼ cup, except as noted:							
(*Cardini's* Pasta Dressing/Marinade), 2 tbsp.	140	0	1.0	14.0	0	270	0
(*Pastene*)	231	1.7	1.5	24.3	0	346	0
(*Sacla Pasta Gusto* Genovese)	240	2.0	5.0	24.0	<5	850	0
(*Watkins* Pasta Topper), 2 tbsp.	20	1.0	3.0	1.0	5	240	0
black (*Cora* Gourmet)	200	2.0	5.0	26.0	0	1050	1.0
Genovese (*Italia In Talvola*), 2 tbsp. . .	160	2.0	4.0	16.0	0	370	<1.0
green (*Cora* Gourmet)	140	3.0	2.0	13.0	0	460	2.0
red (*Cora* Gourmet), 2 tbsp.	190	2.0	3.0	20.0	0	240	1.0
tomato (*Sonoma*) . . .	110	3.0	6.0	9.0	2	125	1.0
white (*Cora* Gourmet)	120	1.0	1.0	12.0	0	260	0
Pesto sauce, refrigerated, ¼ cup:							
basil:							
(*Buitoni*)	290	6.0	12.0	24.0	20	580	3.0
(*Buitoni* Light)	230	6.0	11.0	18.0	15	580	2.0
(*Di Giorno*)	320	7.0	2.0	31.0	15	530	<1.0
sun-dried tomato (*Buitoni*)	190	3.0	10.0	15.0	5	380	3.0
Pesto sauce mix:							
(*Knorr* Pasta Sauces), 2 tsp.	15	<1.0	2.0	0	0	480	0
(*McCormick*), ¼ pkg.	10	1.0	1.0	0	0	480	0
creamy (*Knorr* Pasta Sauces), 1 tbsp. . .	25	<1.0	3.0	1.0	0	450	0
red pepper (*Knorr* Pasta Sauces), ⅔ tbsp.	25	<1.0	4.0	.5	0	510	<1.0

Food and Measure	cal.	prot. (gms)	carbo. (gms)	fat (gms)	chol. (mgs)	sod. (mgs)	fiber (gms)
sun-dried tomato (*Knorr* Pasta Sauces), 1 tbsp. . .	35	1.0	6.0	.5	0	530	1.0
Pheasant, raw:							
meat w/skin, 4 oz. . .	205	25.7	0	10.5	n.a.	45	0
meat only:							
4 oz.	151	26.7	0	4.1	n.a.	42	0
½ breast, 6.4 oz.	243	44.4	0	5.9	n.a.	60	0
1 leg, 3.8 oz.	143	23.8	0	4.6	n.a.	48	0
Phyllo, see "Fillo dough"							
Picante sauce (see also "Salsa"), 2 tbsp.:							
(*Pace*)	10	0	2.0	0	0	220	0
hot (*Chi-Chi's*)	10	0	2.0	0	0	200	0
hot or medium (*Shotgun Willie's* Texas)	10	0	2.0	0	0	260	0
w/jalapeño (*La Victoria*)	15	0	3.0	0	0	210	0
medium or mild *Chi-Chi's*)	10	0	2.0	0	0	230	0
Piccalilli, see "Tomato relish"							
Pickle, cucumber, 1 oz., except as noted:							
(*Hans Jurgen*)	5	0	1.0	0	0	240	0
bread and butter:							
(*B&G* Chips)	30	0	7.0	0	0	120	0
(*Cascadian Farm* Chips), 6 pcs., 1 oz.	25	0	6.0	0	0	180	0
(*Mrs. Fannings*), 3 pcs., 1 oz. . . .	25	0	6.0	0	0	190	0
cornichon (*Italica*), 7 pcs., 1.1 oz.	0	0	0	0	0	330	0
dill:							
whole (*Claussen*), ½ pc., 1 oz. . . .	5	0	1.0	0	0	330	0
whole (*Del Monte*) 1½ pcs., 1 oz.	5	0	1.0	0	0	370	<1.0
whole, baby (*Cascadian Farm*)	5	0	1.0	0	0	300	0

Food and Measure	cal.	prot (gms)	carbo. (gms)	fat (gms)	chol. (mgs)	sod. (mgs)	fiber (gms)
Pickle, dill *(cont.)*							
whole, garlic (*Ba-Tampte*)	0	0	<1.0	0	0	180	0
whole, gherkins (*B&G*), 1½ pcs., 1 oz.	0	0	0	0	0	270	0
halves (*Del Monte*), ¼ pc., 1 oz. ...	5	0	1.0	0	0	370	<1.0
hamburger chips (*B&G*), 6 pcs., 1 oz.	0	0	0	0	0	270	0
hamburger chips (*Del Monte*), 5½ pcs., 1 oz. ...	5	0	0	0	0	300	0
hamburger chips (*Vlassic*), 5 pcs., 1 oz.	10	0	3.0	0	0	390	0
slices (*Claussen Super Slices for Burgers*), .8-oz. slice	5	0	1.0	0	0	270	0
dill, kosher:							
(*B&G* Crunchy) ...	0	0	0	0	0	200	0
(*Cascadian Farm*) ..	5	0	1.0	0	0	300	0
(*Cascadian Farm Genuine*)	5	0	1.0	0	0	350	0
(*Cascadian Farm Low Sodium*) ...	5	0	1.0	0	0	135	0
(*Hebrew National*), 1 pc.	23	1.0	4.0	0	0	1570	0
chips (*B&G*), 4 pcs., 1 oz.	0	0	0	0	0	200	0
slices (*Cascadian Farm*), 2 pcs., 1 oz.	5	0	1.0	0	0	300	0
spears (*B&G*)	0	0	0	0	0	200	0
spears or spicy (*Cascadian Farm*)	5	0	1.0	0	0	300	0
spicy (*Cascadian Farm* Sodium Reduced)	5	0	1.0	0	0	135	0
tiny (*Del Monte*), 1½ pcs., 1 oz. ...	5	0	1.0	0	0	250	<1.0

Food and Measure	cal.	prot. (gms)	carbo. (gms)	fat (gms)	chol. (mgs)	sod. (mgs)	fiber (gms)
sweet:							
baby (*Cascadian Farm*), 1¾ pc., 1 oz.	30	0	8.0	0	0	180	0
chips (*Del Monte*), 5 pcs., 1 oz.	40	0	10.0	0	0	210	<1.0
gherkin (*Vlasic*), about 3 pcs., 1 oz.	35	0	8.0	0	0	170	0
gherkin (*Del Monte*), 2 pcs., 1 oz.	40	0	10.0	0	0	210	<1.0
midget (*Del Monte*), 3 pcs., 1 oz.	40	0	10.0	0	0	210	<1.0
Pickle relish (see also specific listings), cucumber, 1 tbsp.:							
(*Crosse & Blackwell* Branston)	25	0	6.0	0	0	125	0
dill (*Cascadian Farm*)	0	0	0	0	0	150	0
hamburger:							
(*B&G*)	20	0	5.0	0	0	75	0
(*Del Monte*)	20	0	6.0	0	0	220	<1.0
hot dog:							
(*B&G*)	15	0	4.0	0	0	95	0
(*Del Monte*)	15	0	4.0	0	0	140	<1.0
(*Heinz*)	15	0	4.0	0	0	150	0
India (*Heinz*)	20	0	5.0	0	0	100	0
sweet:							
(*Cascadian Farm*)	20	0	5.0	0	0	75	0
(*Del Monte*)	20	0	5.0	0	0	125	0
(*Heinz*)	20	0	5.0	0	0	95	0
Pickling spice (*Tone's*), 1 tsp.	10	.3	1.2	.6	0	1	.3
Pie:							
apple:							
(*Entenmann's* Homestyle), ⅙ pie	370	2.0	55.0	16.0	<5	250	3.0
(*Entenmann's* Ultimate), ⅛ pie	320	2.0	51.0	12.0	0	220	2.0
cherry (*Entenmann's*), ⅙ pie	360	3.0	55.0	16.0	0	260	1.0
coconut custard (*Entenmann's*), ⅕ pie	340	7.0	37.0	18.0	135	300	1.0
pumpkin (*Entenmann's*), ⅕ pie	270	4.0	38.0	12.0	40	290	2.0

Food and Measure	cal.	prot. (gms)	carbo. (gms)	fat (gms)	chol. (mgs)	sod. (mgs)	fiber (gms)
Pie *(cont.)*							
sweet potato (*Entenmann's*), ⅙ pie . . .	320	5.0	42.0	15.0	90	290	2.0
Pie, frozen (see also "Cobbler"), ⅛ pie, except as noted:							
apple:							
(*Amy's*), ½ pie	220	2.0	35.0	8.0	25	130	2.0
(*Mountain Top*), ⅙ pie	340	2.0	45.0	16.0	15	340	1.0
(*Mountain Top* Old Fashioned)	350	2.0	50.0	16.0	15	330	1.0
(*Mrs. Smith's* 9") . .	340	3.0	46.0	17.0	0	380	2.0
(*Mrs. Smith's* Special Recipe 10"), 1/12 pie	330	2.0	45.0	16.0	0	340	2.0
(*Mrs. Smith's* Unbaked 9")	350	3.0	42.0	20.0	0	440	3.0
(*Sara Lee* Homestyle)	340	3.0	46.0	16.0	0	310	1.0
(*Sara Lee* Reduced Fat), ⅙ pie	290	4.0	51.0	8.0	<5	400	2.0
crumb (*Mountain Top*), ⅙ pie	320	2.0	48.0	13.0	10	230	2.0
apple, Dutch:							
(*Mrs. Smith's* 9") . .	360	3.0	52.0	16.0	0	360	2.0
(*Mrs. Smith's* 10"), ⅒ pie	320	3.0	49.0	13.0	0	300	2.0
(*Sara Lee* Homestyle)	350	3.0	53.0	15.0	0	320	2.0
blueberry:							
(*Mountain Top*), ⅙ pie	330	2.0	43.0	16.0	15	380	2.0
(*Mrs. Smith's* 9") . .	330	3.0	43.0	17.0	0	500	3.0
(*Sara Lee* Homestyle)	360	3.0	54.0	15.0	0	340	2.0
blackberry (*Mountain Top*), ⅙ pie	330	3.0	44.0	16.0	15	450	3.0
Boston cream, see "Cake, frozen"							
cappuccino (*Mrs. Smith's* 10"), ⅑ pie	300	4.0	45.0	13.0	0	260	2.0
cherry:							
(*Mountain Top*), ⅙ pie	340	2.0	46.0	16.0	15	330	1.0

Food and Measure	cal.	prot. (gms)	carbo. (gms)	fat (gms)	chol. (mgs)	sod. (mgs	fiber (gms)
(*Mountain Top* Old Fashioned)	380	3.0	55.0	16.0	15	330	1.0
(*Mrs. Smith's* 9") . .	320	3.0	41.0	17.0	0	490	2.0
(*Mrs. Smith's* Special Recipe 10"), 1/12 pie	330	3.0	49.0	14.0	0	310	1.0
(*Sara Lee* Home-style)	320	3.0	42.0	16.0	0	290	2.0
cherry-berry (*Mrs. Smith's* Special Recipe 10"), 1/12 pie	340	3.0	48.0	16.0	0	340	2.0
chocolate cream: (*Mrs. Smith's* 8"), 1/3 pie	370	3.0	54.0	16.0	0	250	3.0
(*Pet-Ritz Chocolate Drizzle*), 1/4 pie . .	310	2.0	37.0	18.0	0	135	1.0
mint (*Mrs. Smith's* 9"), 1/6 pie	390	4.0	52.0	19.0	0	180	2.0
chocolate silk (*Sara Lee* Supreme), 1/5 pie	500	4.0	49.0	32.0	<5	440	<2.0
coconut: cream (*Sara Lee*), 1/5 pie	480	4.0	47.0	31.0	0	430	2.0
custard (*Mrs. Smith's* 9")	260	6.0	28.0	14.0	70	310	<1.0
cookies and cream (*Mrs. Smith's* 9"), 1/6 pie	360	4.0	52.0	16.0	0	290	2.0
French silk (*Mrs. Smith's* 10"), 1/9 pie	560	4.0	48.0	40.0	55	280	1.0
lime, Key (*Mrs. Smith's* 10"), 1/9 pie	430	5.0	62.0	18.0	15	290	1.0
lemon cream: (*Mrs. Smith's* 8"), 1/3 pie	440	3.0	49.0	26.0	0	180	<1.0
(*Pet-Ritz Razz*), 1/4 pie	320	2.0	39.0	18.0	0	270	<1.0
lemon meringue (*Sara Lee* Home-style), 1/6 pie . . .	350	2.0	59.0	11.0	0	460	5.0

Food and Measure	cal.	prot. (gms)	carbo. (gms)	fat (gms)	chol. (mgs)	sod. (mgs)	fiber (gms)
Pie, frozen, lemon meringue *(cont.)*							
lemonade (*Mrs. Smith's*), ⅙ pie	370	3.0	46.0	20.0	0	150	<1.0
mince/mincemeat:							
(*Mountain Top*), ⅙ pie	350	2.0	50.0	16.0	15	500	0
(*Mrs. Smith's* 9")	380	3.0	53.0	17.0	0	520	2.0
(*Sara Lee* Home-style)	390	3.0	56.0	17.0	0	450	3.0
peach:							
(*Mountain Top*), ⅙ pie	310	2.0	38.0	16.0	15	330	2.0
(*Mountain Top* Old Fashioned)	360	3.0	50.0	16.0	15	330	1.0
(*Mrs. Smith's* 9")	320	3.0	40.0	17.0	0	450	2.0
(*Mrs. Smith's* Special Recipe 10"), 1/12 pie	300	3.0	42.0	14.0	0	320	2.0
(*Sara Lee* Home-style)	320	3.0	46.0	14.0	0	250	2.0
pecan:							
(*Mrs. Smith's* 8"), ⅕ pie	560	6.0	75.0	27.0	65	450	2.0
(*Mrs. Smith's* 10")	550	7.0	75.0	26.0	85	510	2.0
(*Sara Lee* Home-style)	520	5.0	70.0	24.0	45	480	3.0
pumpkin:							
(*Mountain Top*), ⅙ pie	250	4.0	35.0	10.0	40	390	1.0
(*Mountain Top* Old Fashioned)	250	4.0	36.0	10.0	45	400	1.0
(*Sara Lee* Home-style)	260	4.0	37.0	11.0	30	460	2.0
custard (*Mrs. Smith's* 9")	280	5.0	37.0	12.0	45	320	3.0
custard (*Mrs. Smith's* 10"), 1/10 pie	290	4.0	42.0	12.0	40	370	2.0
raspberry:							
(*Mrs. Smith's* 9")	330	3.0	44.0	17.0	0	510	1.0
(*Sara Lee* Home-style)	380	3.0	48.0	19.0	<5	330	2.0
s'mores cream (*Mrs. Smith's* 9"), ⅙ pie	410	4.0	54.0	20.0	0	230	2.0

Food and Measure	cal.	prot. (gms)	carbo. (gms)	fat (gms)	chol. (mgs)	sod. (mgs)	fiber (gms)
strawberry-banana (*Mrs. Smith's 9"*), ⅛ pie	380	3.0	45.0	21.0	0	250	<1.0
sweet potato custard (*Mrs. Smith's 9"*) . .	340	4.0	44.0	17.0	40	240	2.0
Pie, mix* (*Jell-O* No Bake), ⅛ pie, except as noted:							
Chips Ahoy!	360	4.0	48.0	17.0	<5	480	1.0
chocolate lover's	310	4.0	44.0	14.0	<5	470	2.0
chocolate silk	280	4.0	37.0	15.0	5	520	2.0
lemon silk	270	4.0	36.0	13.0	<5	400	2.0
Oreos and creme	360	4.0	50.0	17.0	<5	570	2.0
peanut butter cup, ⅛ pie	360	5.0	36.0	22.0	<5	400	2.0
pumpkin, ⅛ pie	260	4.0	36.0	12.0	5	480	<1.0
Pie, snack, 1 pc.:							
apple:							
(*Drake's*), 4 oz. . . .	400	3.0	60.0	16.0	0	240	3.0
(*Entenmann's*), 5 oz.	370	4.0	45.0	21.0	0	360	3.0
(*Hostess*), 4.5 oz. .	480	3.0	67.0	22.0	15	390	2.0
(*Mr. Kipling*), 2.2 oz.	200	2.0	31.0	8.0	5	70	<1.0
blueberry:							
(*Entenmann's*), 5 oz.	440	3.0	61.0	20.0	0	340	3.0
(*Hostess*), 4.5 oz. .	480	3.0	70.0	20.0	20	460	2.0
cherry:							
(*Drake's*), 4 oz. . . .	420	3.0	60.0	18.0	0	260	3.0
(*Entenmann's*), 5 oz.	430	4.0	60.0	20.0	0	310	2.0
(*Hostess*), 4.5 oz. .	470	1.0	65.0	22.0	20	470	1.0
lemon:							
(*Entenmann's*), 5 oz.	430	4.0	60.0	20.0	20	400	<1.0
(*Hostess*), 4.5 oz. .	500	3.0	66.0	24.0	20	430	0
peach:							
(*Entenmann's*), 5 oz.	380	3.0	49.0	19.0	0	330	2.0
(*Hostess*), 4.5 oz. .	480	3.0	68.0	21.0	25	460	1.0
pineapple (*Entenmann's*), 5 oz.	400	3.0	55.0	19.0	0	350	1.0
Pie crust, ⅙ crust, except as noted:							
chocolate cookie:							
(*Oreo*), ⅙ crust . . .	140	1.0	18.0	7.0	0	170	1.0
graham:							
(*Honey Maid*), ⅙ crust	140	1.0	18.0	7.0	0	125	<1.0

Food and Measure	cal.	prot. (gms)	carbo. (gms)	fat (gms)	chol. (mgs)	sod. (mgs)	fiber (gms)
Pie crust, graham *(cont.)*							
(*Ready Crust*)	110	1.0	14.0	5.0	0	135	<1.0
(*Ready Crust* Reduced Fat)	90	1.0	14.0	3.5	0	85	0
(*Ready Crust* 2 Extra Servings), ⅒ crust	130	1.0	17.0	6.0	0	170	<1.0
chocolate (*Ready Crust*)	110	1.0	14.0	5.0	0	100	<1.0
shortbread (*Ready Crust*)	110	1.0	14.0	5.0	0	100	0
vanilla cookie (*Nilla*), ⅙ crust	140	1.0	18.0	8.0	<5	65	0
Pie crust, frozen or refrigerated (see also "Pastry shell"), ⅛ crust:							
(*Mrs. Smith's* 18 oz.)	100	1.0	9.0	6.0	0	90	0
(*Mrs. Smith's* 19.5 oz.)	110	1.0	10.0	7.0	0	95	0
(*Pet-Ritz* 9")	80	<1.0	9.0	4.0	<5	75	0
(*Pet-Ritz* Extra Large 9⅝")	110	1.0	13.0	6.0	5	110	0
(*Pillsbury* All Ready) .	120	<1.0	13.0	7.0	5	100	0
deep dish (*Pet-Ritz* 9")	90	1.0	11.0	5.0	0	60	0
all vegetable:							
(*Pet-Ritz* 9")	80	1.0	10.0	4.5	0	75	0
deep dish (*Pet-Ritz*)	90	1.0	11.0	5.0	0	80	0
Pie crust mix:							
(*Betty Crocker*), ⅛ of 9" crust*	110	1.0	9.0	8.0	0	135	0
(*Flako*), ¼ cup	130	2.0	13.0	8.0	5	170	1.0
("*Jiffy*"), ¼ cup	180	2.0	19.0	10.0	<5	250	<1.0
Pie filling (see also "Pastry filling"), 3 oz., except as noted:							
apple:							
(*Lucky Leaf*)	90	0	22.0	0	0	40	2.0
(*Lucky Leaf* Lite) ..	25	0	7.0	0	0	10	1.0
apricot (*Lucky Leaf*) .	90	0	22.0	0	0	55	0
berry, triple (*Crosse & Blackwell*), ⅓ cup	120	0	30.0	0	0	15	2.0
blueberry:							
(*Lucky Leaf*)	90	0	22.0	0	0	50	1.0

Food and Measure	cal.	prot. (gms)	carbo. (gms)	fat (gms)	chol. (mgs)	sod. (mgs)	fiber (gms)
(*Lucky Leaf* Premium)	100	0	24.0	0	0	45	1.0
cherry:							
(*Lucky Leaf*)	100	0	24.0	0	0	40	0
(*Lucky Leaf* Cherries Jubilee)	80	0	20.0	0	0	10	1.0
(*Lucky Leaf* Lite) ..	35	0	8.0	0	0	10	1.0
red tart, in water (*Oregon*), ⅔ cup	60	1.0	14.0	0	0	10	2.0
cherry blackberry (*Crosse & Blackwell*), ⅓ cup	100	0	26.0	0	0	15	0
lemon (*Lucky Leaf*) ..	120	0	30.0	1.0	0	200	0
mince/mincemeat:							
(*Crosse & Blackwell*), ¼ cup	180	<1.0	43.0	0	0	220	0
(*None Such*), ⅓ cup	190	0	45.0	.5	0	230	0
w/brandy, rum (*None Such*), ⅓ cup	200	0	47.0	1.0	0	250	0
w/brandy and rum (*Crosse & Blackwell*), ¼ cup ...	180	<1.0	43.0	0	0	230	0
condensed (*None Such*), 4 tsp.	150	0	36.0	.5	0	230	1.0
peach (*Lucky Leaf*) ..	80	0	21.0	0	0	30	0
pumpkin (*Libby's* Mix), ⅓ cup	90	<1.0	20.0	.5	0	115	2.0
raisin (*Lucky Leaf*) ..	90	0	22.0	0	0	75	1.0
strawberry (*Lucky Leaf*)	80	0	20.0	0	0	50	1.0
Pie filling mix, see "Pudding and pie filling mix"							
Pie glaze, see "Strawberry pie glaze"							
Pierogi, frozen, 3 pcs., except as noted:							
cheddar and potato (*Tofutti*), 4 pcs. ..	185	5.0	35.0	4.0	0	195	.5
cheese, American (*Mrs. T's*)	220	9.0	32.0	6.0	20	520	<1.0

Food and Measure	cal.	prot. (gms)	carbo. (gms)	fat (gms)	chol. (mgs)	sod. (mgs)	fiber (gms)
Pierogi *(cont.)*							
jalapeño cheddar:							
(*Mrs. T's*)	190	7.0	35.0	2.5	10	490	2.0
(*Mrs. T's 'Rogies*),							
7 pcs.	130	5.0	25.0	2.0	5	340	0
potato cheese:							
(*Empire* Kosher),							
½ pkg., 5.3 oz.	247	7.0	44.0	4.0	60	233	.7
cheddar (*Mrs. T's*)	180	7.0	34.0	2.5	10	430	2.0
cheddar (*Mrs. T's*							
'Rogies), 7 pcs.	130	5.0	24.0	1.5	10	310	0
potato onion:							
(*Empire* Kosher),							
½ pkg., 5.3 oz.	243	5.0	47.0	4.0	48	260	.7
(*Mrs. T's*)	180	6.0	34.0	2.0	<5	340	2.0
potato roasted garlic							
(*Mrs. T's*)	270	7.0	41.0	9.0	30	620	2.0
sauerkraut (*Mrs. T's*) .	170	6.0	32.0	1.5	5	770	3.0
Pig's feet:							
simmered, 4 oz.	220	21.8	0	14.1	113	34	0
pickled:							
(*Hormel*), 2 oz. . . .	80	7.0	0	6.0	45	530	0
cured, 1 oz.	58	3.8	<.1	4.6	26	262	0
Pigeon peas, fresh:							
raw, ½ cup	105	5.5	18.4	1.3	0	4	3.2
boiled, drained, ½ cup	86	4.6	15.0	1.1	0	3	2.5
Pigeon peas, dried:							
(*Jack Rabbit*), ¼ cup	70	8.0	24.0	0	0	20	14.0
boiled, ½ cup	102	5.7	19.5	.3	0	5	3.9
Pigeon peas, canned,							
green:							
(*El Jibarito*), ½ cup . .	80	5.0	18.0	0	0	490	5.0
(*Goya*), 8 oz.	110	10.0	26.0	0	0	560	8.0
(*Tupi*), ½ cup	70	4.0	14.0	0	0	390	4.0
Pignolia nuts, see							
"Pine nuts"							
Pike, meat only:							
northern, 4 oz.:							
raw	100	21.8	0	.8	44	44	0
baked, broiled, or							
microwaved	128	28.0	0	1.0	57	56	0
walleye, 4 oz.:							
raw	105	21.7	0	1.4	98	58	0

Food and Measure	cal.	prot. (gms)	carbo. (gms)	fat (gms)	chol. (mgs)	sod. (mgs	fiber (gms)
baked, broiled, or microwaved ...	135	27.8	0	1.8	125	74	0
Pili nuts, shelled:							
dried, 1 oz.	204	3.1	1.1	22.6	0	4	<1.0
dried, 1 cup	863	13.0	4.8	95.5	0	4	3.4
Pimiento, in jars, drained:							
(*Goya* Fancy), ¼ pc., .5 oz.	0	0	1.0	0	0	40	0
(*Roland*), ½ cup	30	1.0	5.0	0	0	310	1.0
Piña colada drink mixer, fluid:							
canned or bottled:							
(*Daily's*), 3 fl. oz.	160	0	37.0	2.0	0	115	1.0
(*Mr & Mrs T*), 4.5 fl. oz.	180	0	43.0	0	0	130	0
frozen (*Bacardi*), 2 fl. oz.	170	0	35.0	4.0	0	20	0
Pine nuts:							
raw (*Blue Diamond*), ¼ cup	190	8.0	5.0	17.0	0	0	2.0
pignolia, dried:							
(*Bazzini's Nut Club*), ¼ cup	190	4.0	9.0	15.0	0	0	4.0
(*Frieda's*), ¼ cup, 1.1 oz.	150	7.0	4.0	15.0	0	0	1.0
(*Krinos*), .5 oz. ...	90	5.0	0	7.5	0	5	1.0
(*Progresso*), 1 oz.	170	10.0	2.0	13.0	0	0	0
1 oz.	160	6.8	4.0	14.2	0	1	1.3
1 tbsp.	49	2.1	1.2	4.4	0	<1	.4
pinyon, dried:							
1 oz.	178	3.3	5.5	17.3	0	20	3.0
10 kernels	6	.1	.2	.6	0	1	.1
Pineapple, fresh:							
(*Frieda's* Baby), 3 oz.	70	1.0	17.0	0	0	15	0
(*Frieda's* South African Baby), 1 cup, 5 oz.	70	1.0	17.0	.5	0	0	2.0
whole, 1 lb.	231	1.8	58.5	2.0	0	5	5.7
diced, ½ cup	38	.3	9.6	.3	0	<1	.9
sliced (*Dole*), 2 slices, 3" diam., 4 oz. ...	60	1.0	16.0	0	0	10	1.0

Food and Measure	cal.	prot. (gms)	carbo. (gms)	fat (gms)	chol. (mgs)	sod. (mgs)	fiber (gms)
Pineapple, can or jar, ½ cup, except as noted:							
in juice:							
all styles, except sliced (*Del Monte*)	70	0	17.0	0	0	10	1.0
crushed (*Dole*)	70	1.0	17.0	0	0	10	1.0
crushed or chunks .	75	.5	19.6	.1	0	1	1.0
sliced (*Del Monte*), 4 oz., 2 slices ..	60	0	16.0	0	0	10	1.0
sliced (*Dole*), 4 oz., 2 slices	60	0	15.0	0	0	10	1.0
tidbits (*Del Monte* Snack Cup), 4 oz.	50	0	15.0	0	0	10	<1.0
tidbits or chunks (*Dole*)	60	0	15.0	0	0	10	1.0
in extra light syrup (*Sunfresh* Chilled) .	80	1.0	17.0	0	0	65	0
in light syrup, crushed or chunks	66	4.5	17.0	.2	0	1	1.0
in heavy syrup:							
all styles, except sliced (*Dole*) ...	90	1.0	24.0	0	0	10	1.0
crushed or chunks (*Del Monte*)	90	0	24.0	0	0	10	1.0
chunks, tidbits or crushed	100	.5	25.8	.1	0	2	.9
sliced (*Dole*), 2 slices	90	1.0	23.0	0	0	10	1.0
Pineapple, candied:							
all styles (*Seneca* Glacé), 1 oz.	90	0	21.0	0	0	20	0
sliced (*S&W* Glacé), 2.2-oz. pc.	180	0	46.0	0	0	40	0
wedged (*S&W* Glacé), 5 pcs., 1 oz.	80	0	21.0	0	0	20	0
w/cherries, see "Cherry, candied"							
Pineapple, dried:							
(*Setton Farm*), 1.4 oz.	140	0	35.0	0	0	90	1.0
(*Sonoma* Organic), ¼ cup, 1.4 oz. ...	110	1.0	25.0	0	0	0	2.0

Food and Measure	cal.	prot. (gms)	carbo. (gms)	fat (gms)	chol. (mgs)	sod. (mgs)	fiber (gms)
freeze-dried, chunks (*AlpineAire*), .4 oz.	45	0	10.0	0	0	0	1.0
Pineapple, frozen, sweetened, chunks, ½ cup ...	104	.5	27.1	.1	0	2	1.3
Pineapple drink blends, 8 fl. oz., except as noted:							
coconut:							
(*AriZona* Piña Colada)	140	0	34.0	1.0	0	30	0
(*R. W. Knudsen*) ..	130	<1.0	32.0	0	0	50	0
grapefruit, pink:							
(*Dole* Can)	130	1.0	32.0	0	0	20	0
(*Dole* Can), 6 fl. oz.	100	0	25.0	0	0	15	0
guava nectar (*Goya*) .	150	1.0	37.0	0	0	30	3.0
passion fruit nectar (*Goya*), 6 fl. oz.	120	1.0	28.0	0	0	20	0
Pineapple guava, see "Feijoas"							
Pineapple juice, 8 fl. oz., except as noted:							
(*Del Monte*)	130	1.0	32.0	0	0	10	1.0
(*Del Monte*), 6 fl. oz. .	80	<1.0	20.0	0	0	5	0
(*Del Monte* Not from Concentrate)	110	1.0	29.0	0	0	15	2.0
(*Dole*)	130	2.0	29.0	0	0	20	0
(*Dole* Can)	110	<1.0	29.0	0	0	10	2.0
(*Dole* Can Reconstituted)	120	<1.0	29.0	0	0	10	0
(*Goya*), 6 fl. oz.	90	1.0	21.0	0	0	25	<1.0
canned	140	.8	34.5	.2	0	3	.5
frozen*	130	1.0	31.9	<.1	0	3	.5
Pineapple juice blends, 8 fl. oz., except as noted:							
citrus (*Dole*)	120	1.0	29.0	0	0	40	0
(*Dole*), 11.5 fl. oz. .	170	1.0	41.0	0	0	55	0
grapefruit (*Dole* Can), 6 fl. oz.	100	1.0	24.0	0	0	15	0
nectar (*R. W. Knudsen*)	140	0	34.0	0	0	20	0
orange:							
(*Dole*)	120	2.0	27.0	0	0	20	0

Food and Measure	cal.	prot. (gms)	carbo. (gms)	fat (gms)	chol. (mgs)	sod. (mgs)	fiber (gms)
Pineapple juice blends, orange *(cont.)*							
(*Dole*), 10 fl. oz. . .	150	1.0	36.0	0	0	25	0
(*Dole* Can), 6 fl. oz.	100	1.0	24.0	0	0	15	0
orange banana							
(*Dole*)	120	2.0	29.0	0	0	20	0
(*Dole*), 10 fl. oz. . .	150	2.0	36.0	0	0	25	0
(*Dole* Can), 6 fl. oz.	100	1.0	25.0	0	0	15	0
(*Nantucket Nectars*)	140	<1.0	35.0	0	0	15	0
orange strawberry							
(*Dole*)	130	0	32.0	0	0	20	0
Pineapple topping, 2 tbsp.:							
(*Kraft*)	110	0	28.0	0	0	15	0
(*Smucker's*)	110	0	28.0	0	0	0	0
Pineapple-apricot sauce (*Sable & Rosenfeld*), 2 tbsp.	80	0	20.0	0	0	0	0
Pink beans, dried, boiled, ½ cup	125	7.6	23.5	.4	0	2	4.5
Pinquito beans (*S&W*), ½ cup	80	6.0	20.0	.5	0	480	6.0
Pinto beans:							
dry (*Arrowhead Mills*), ¼ cup	150	10.0	27.0	.5	0	0	8.0
boiled, ½ cup	117	7.0	21.8	.4	0	1	7.3
Pinto beans, canned (see also "Chili Beans" and "Refried beans"), ½ cup, except as noted:							
(*Allens/Brown Beauty*)	110	5.0	20.0	1.0	0	290	7.0
(*Bush's Best*)	110	6.0	18.0	.5	0	430	6.0
(*Eden* Organic)	100	6.0	18.0	0	0	15	6.0
(*Goya* Spanish), 7.5 oz.	140	11.0	31.0	1.0	0	860	10.0
(*Hain* Organic)	110	8.0	18.0	1.0	0	140	8.0
(*Westbrae Natural*) . .	90	5.0	16.0	0	0	140	6.0
w/bacon:							
(*Bush's Best*)	110	6.0	18.0	1.0	0	540	6.0
(*Trappey's*)	120	6.0	20.0	1.0	0	270	7.0
w/bacon, jalapeños:							
(*Bush's Best*)	110	7.0	17.0	1.5	5	550	6.0
(*Trappey's* Jalapinto)	120	6.0	22.0	1.0	0	540	8.0

Food and Measure	cal.	prot. (gms)	carbo. (gms)	fat (gms)	chol. (mgs)	sod. (mgs)	fiber (gms)
w/pork (*Bush's Best*)	120	6.0	17.0	2.5	5	530	6.0
seasoned (*Glory Foods*)	90	5.0	15.0	.5	0	850	5.0
Pinto beans, dehydrated (*AlpineAire*), 1 oz.	100	6.0	18.0	0	0	0	6.0
Pinto beans, frozen, boiled, drained, ⅓ of 10-oz. pkg.	152	8.8	29.0	.5	0	78	8.1
Pinto–great northern beans, canned (*Bush's Best* Mixed Beans), ½ cup	110	7.0	19.0	0	0	500	6.0
Pipian, in jars (*Doña Maria*), 2 tbsp. . . .	250	4.0	5.0	20.0	0	580	3.0
Pistachio nut, shelled, except as noted: (*AlpineAire* Raging Flame), 2.5 oz. . . .	440	10.0	22.0	35.0	0	270	7.0
(*AlpineAire* Wild West), 2.5 oz.	440	10.0	20.0	36.0	0	460	8.0
raw, ¼ cup: (*Bazzini's Nut Club*)	190	6.0	4.0	16.0	0	190	4.0
(*Blue Diamond*) . . .	200	7.0	10.0	15.0	0	15	3.0
dried: 1 oz.	164	5.8	7.1	13.7	0	2	3.1
salted (*Sonoma*), ¼ cup, 1.1 oz.	190	6.0	9.0	14.0	0	220	3.0
dried, in shell (*Sunkist*), ½ cup, ¼ cup shelled	180	6.0	9.0	14.0	0	220	3.0
dry-roasted: (*Planters*), ½ cup	160	5.0	7.0	14.0	0	180	3.0
unsalted, 1 oz. . . .	162	6.1	7.8	13.0	0	2	2.9
unsalted, ¼ cup . . .	183	6.8	8.9	14.7	0	3	3.3
roasted, in shell: (*Setton Farm*), 1 oz.	170	6.0	9.0	3.0	0	190	3.0
(*Setton Farm* Unsalted), 1 oz. . . .	170	6.0	9.0	3.0	0	0	3.0
Pita, see "Bread"							
Pitanga:							
1 medium, .3 oz. . . .	2	.1	.5	<.1	0	<1	<1.0
½ cup	29	.7	6.5	.3	0	3	<1.0

Food and Measure	cal.	prot. (gms)	carbo. (gms)	fat (gms)	chol. (mgs)	sod. (mgs)	fiber (gms)
Pizza, frozen, 1 pie, except as noted:							
artichoke heart (*Wolfgang Puck's*), ½ pie	340	15.0	34.0	17.0	25	450	3.0
bacon burger (*Totino's* Crispy Crust Party), ½ pie	390	14.0	35.0	21.0	15	810	2.0
bacon cheeseburger:							
(*Jack's Naturally Rising*), ⅙ pie ..	310	16.0	35.0	12.0	35	720	2.0
(*Jack's Original*), ¼ pie	300	16.0	29.0	14.0	40	770	2.0
Canadian bacon:							
(*Jack's Naturally Rising*), ⅙ pie ..	280	15.0	35.0	9.0	30	600	2.0
(*Jack's Original*), ¼ pie	260	14.0	29.0	10.0	30	610	2.0
(*Jeno's Crisp 'n Tasty*)	440	16.0	51.0	19.0	15	1120	2.0
(*Tombstone* Original 9"), ⅓ pie	250	13.0	28.0	10.0	25	570	3.0
(*Tombstone* Original 12"), ¼ pie	340	17.0	37.0	13.0	35	780	4.0
(*Totino's* Crisp Crust Party), ½ pie ...	330	13.0	35.0	15.0	10	860	1.0
cheese:							
(*Amy's*), ⅓ pie. ...	300	12.0	38.0	12.0	15	590	2.0
(*Celeste* Large), ¼ pie	300	14.0	33.0	13.0	20	620	3.0
(*Celeste* for One) ..	420	17.0	43.0	20.0	30	840	4.0
(*Jack's Naturally Rising*), ⅕ pie ..	340	16.0	41.0	12.0	30	600	3.0
(*Jack's Original*), ¼ pie	330	16.0	38.0	13.0	30	650	3.0
(*Michelina's* Single)	420	16.0	42.0	22.0	30	690	2.0
(*Michelina's That'za Pizza!*)	410	16.0	42.0	21.0	25	650	2.0
(*Tombstone* Cheese Stuffed), ⅕ pie	390	17.0	40.0	19.0	35	810	4.0
(*Tombstone* Deep Dish)	460	17.0	51.0	21.0	30	870	3.0
(*Totino's* Family Size), ⅓ pie	370	17.0	39.0	16.0	20	720	2.0

Food and Measure	cal.	prot. (gms)	carbo. (gms)	fat (gms)	chol. (mgs)	sod. (mgs)	fiber (gms)
(*Totino's* Crisp Crust Party), ½ pie ...	320	15.0	34.0	14.0	20	620	2.0
(*Wolfgang Puck's*), ¼ pie	300	18.0	33.0	10.0	25	620	1.0
mini deep dish (*Tombstone*), 2 pies	360	15.0	42.0	15.0	20	620	2.0
cheese, extra:							
(*Tombstone* Original 9"), ½ pie	370	17.0	42.0	15.0	30	720	4.0
(*Tombstone* Original 12"), ¼ pie	340	16.0	37.0	15.0	30	670	4.0
(*Tombstone For One*)	520	21.0	52.0	26.0	45	1040	3.0
cheese, five, tomato:							
(*California Pizza Kitchen 9"*), ⅓ pie	320	18.0	29.0	15.0	35	720	1.0
(*California Pizza Kitchen 12"*), ⅙ pie	350	18.0	35.0	15.0	35	770	2.0
cheese, four:							
(*Celeste* for One Original)	470	19.0	41.0	26.0	40	890	4.0
(*Celeste* for One Zesty)	470	19.0	43.0	25.0	40	920	4.0
(*Celeste* Rising Crust), ⅙ pie ...	320	14.0	42.0	11.0	20	690	4.0
(*Di Giorno Deep Dish*), ⅙ pie ...	360	17.0	32.0	18.0	40	810	3.0
(*Di Glorno Rising Crust 8"*), ⅓ pie .	270	13.0	34.0	9.0	20	700	2.0
(*Di Giorno Rising Crust 12"*), ⅙ pie	320	16.0	40.0	11.0	25	820	3.0
(*Freschetta* 11.15 oz.), ½ pie	390	19.0	47.0	14.0	30	820	2.0
(*Freschetta* 26.85 oz.), ⅕ pie	380	17.0	45.0	15.0	25	790	2.0
(*Freschetta* Sauce Stuffed Crust), ⅕ pie	370	15.0	43.0	16.0	20	780	2.0
(*Wolfgang Puck's*), ½ pie	360	17.0	40.0	15.0	25	530	5.0

Food and Measure	cal.	prot. (gms)	carbo. (gms)	fat (gms)	chol. (mgs)	sod. (mgs)	fiber (gms)
Pizza *(cont.)*							
cheese, super:							
(*Jack's Great Combinations* 9"), ½ pie	410	21.0	37.0	21.0	55	750	3.0
(*Jack's Great Combinations* 12"), ¼ pie	360	19.0	31.0	19.0	55	670	3.0
cheese, three:							
(*Tombstone* Thin Crust), ¼ pie	350	16.0	27.0	20.0	40	700	3.0
(*Tombstone* Oven Rising Crust), ⅙ pie	300	14.0	36.0	11.0	30	520	2.0
chicken:							
barbecue (*California Pizza Kitchen* 9"), ⅓ pie	280	17.0	33.0	9.0	30	700	1.0
barbecue (*California Pizza Kitchen* 12"), ⅙ pie	310	17.0	38.0	9.0	30	780	2.0
barbecue (*Wolfgang Puck's*), ¼ pie	370	20.0	41.0	13.0	50	640	2.0
garlic (*California Pizza Kitchen*), ⅓ pie	290	15.0	30.0	12.0	40	600	1.0
roasted garlic w/rosemary (*Freschetta*), ⅓ pie	260	14.0	32.0	9.0	25	550	1.0
rosemary potato (*California Pizza Kitchen*), ⅓ pie	290	13.0	35.0	11.0	35	540	1.0
Southwest (*Freschetta* Supreme), ½ pie	340	15.0	47.0	10.0	20	1140	2.0
supreme, spicy (*Di Giorno Rising Crust* 8"), ⅓ pie	280	15.0	35.0	9.0	30	790	2.0
supreme, spicy (*Di Giorno Rising Crust* 12"), ⅙ pie	320	17.0	40.0	10.0	30	890	3.0
Thai (*California Pizza Kitchen* 9"), ⅓ pie	290	16.0	33.0	10.0	20	740	3.0

Food and Measure	cal.	prot. (gms)	carbo. (gms)	fat (gms)	chol. (mgs)	sod. (mgs)	fiber (gms)
Thai (*California Pizza Kitchen* 12"), ⅙ pie	310	16.0	38.0	11.0	20	790	3.0
zesty (*Celeste* for One Supreme) ..	380	15.0	38.0	19.0	10	970	5.0
combination:							
(*Jeno's Crisp 'n Tasty*)	500	17.0	50.0	26.0	20	1100	2.0
(*Michelina's* Single)	430	15.0	41.0	24.0	30	830	2.0
(*Totino's* Crispy Crust Party), ½ pie	380	13.0	35.0	21.0	15	850	2.0
(*Totino's* Family Size), ¼ pie	310	11.0	29.0	17.0	15	700	1.0
deluxe:							
(*Celeste* Large), ¼ pie	340	13.0	34.0	17.0	10	850	5.0
(*Celeste* for One) ..	470	16.0	46.0	25.0	20	1100	5.0
(*Freschetta*), ⅙ pie	350	16.0	39.0	15.0	25	810	2.0
(*Freschetta* Special), ⅙ pie	350	15.0	40.0	15.0	25	810	2.0
(*Tombstone* Original 9"), ⅓ pie	280	13.0	29.0	13.0	25	600	3.0
(*Tombstone* Original 12"), ⅕ pie	300	14.0	31.0	14.0	30	650	3.0
ham/shrimp, Hawaiian style (*Contessa*), ⅓ pie	320	13.0	45.0	10.0	25	890	2.0
hamburger:							
(*Jack's Original*), ¼ pie	290	14.0	29.0	13.0	30	610	2.0
(*Jeno's Crisp 'n Tasty*)	500	18.0	51.0	25.0	25	1040	2.0
(*Tombstone* Original 9"), ⅓ pie	260	13.0	28.0	11.0	30	560	3.0
(*Tombstone* Original 12"), ⅕ pie	280	15.0	30.0	12.0	30	620	3.0
(*Totino's* Crisp Crust Party), ½ pie	380	14.0	35.0	20.0	15	790	2.0
Margherita (*Freschetta*), ½ pie	340	13.0	44.0	12.0	20	870	2.0
meat, four:							
(*Freschetta*), ⅙ pie	340	16.0	39.0	14.0	25	810	2.0

Food and Measure	cal.	prot. (gms)	carbo. (gms)	fat (gms)	chol. (mgs)	sod. (mgs)	fiber (gms)
Pizza, meat, four *(cont.)*							
combo (*Tombstone* Original), ⅕ pie	320	15.0	30.0	16.0	35	740	3.0
meat, three:							
(*Celeste* Rising Crust), ⅙ pie . . .	340	13.0	42.0	13.0	25	880	6.0
(*Di Giorno Rising Crust* 8"), ⅓ pie	320	15.0	35.0	14.0	30	860	2.0
(*Di Giorno Rising Crust* 12"), ⅙ pie	360	17.0	40.0	16.0	30	980	3.0
(*Jack's Naturally Rising*), ⅙ pie . .	320	14.0	35.0	14.0	30	630	2.0
(*Jeno's Crisp 'n Tasty*)	490	17.0	49.0	25.0	25	1150	2.0
(*Tombstone Cheese Stuffed*), ⅙ pie	360	15.0	33.0	19.0	40	830	3.0
(*Tombstone Oven Rising Crust*), ⅙ pie	310	14.0	35.0	13.0	30	660	2.0
(*Totino's* Crisp Crust Party), ½ pie . . .	360	13.0	34.0	19.0	15	860	2.0
Mexican style:							
(*Jack's Original*), ¼ pie	330	15.0	30.0	16.0	40	710	3.0
cheese quesadilla (*Tombstone*), ⅓ pie	360	16.0	37.0	17.0	40	730	3.0
chicken fajita (*Tombstone*), ¼ pie . . .	300	15.0	29.0	14.0	45	670	2.0
nacho grande (*Tombstone*), ¼ pie	380	15.0	37.0	19.0	45	890	3.0
taco supreme (*Tombstone* 9"), ½ pie	410	16.0	43.0	19.0	45	1080	3.0
taco supreme (*Tombstone* 12"), ¼ pie	360	14.0	37.0	17.0	40	950	3.0
mushroom, mixed, portobello (*California Pizza Kitchen*), ½ pie	350	17.0	45.0	12.0	20	720	2.0
mushroom/olive (*Amy's*), ⅓ pie	250	10.0	33.0	9.0	10	560	2.0

Food and Measure	cal.	prot. (gms)	carbo. (gms)	fat (gms)	chol. (mgs)	sod. (mgs)	fiber (gms)
mushroom/pepperoni/ sausage (*Jack's Naturally Rising*), ⅙ pie	330	14.0	35.0	15.0	35	630	2.0
mushroom/spinach (*Wolfgang Puck's*), ⅓ pie	230	11.0	29.0	8.0	20	350	2.0
nondairy (*Amy's* Soy Cheeze), ⅓ pie ...	280	12.0	37.0	11.0	0	490	2.0
pepperoni:							
(*Banquet Meal*), 6.75-oz. pkg. ..	480	11.0	56.0	23.0	35	870	5.0
(*Celeste* Large), ¼ pie	350	11.0	38.0	17.0	15	900	3.0
(*Celeste* for One) ..	470	14.0	43.0	27.0	20	1060	4.0
(*Celeste* Rising Crust), ⅙ pie ...	330	13.0	42.0	13.0	40	860	4.0
(*Di Giorno Deep Dish*), ⅙ pie ...	390	17.0	32.0	22.0	40	990	3.0
(*Di Giorno Rising Crust 8"*), ⅓ pie	310	14.0	35.0	14.0	30	850	2.0
(*Di Giorno Rising Crust 12"*), ⅙ pie	360	17.0	40.0	16.0	30	990	2.0
(*Freschetta* 11.58 oz.), ½ pie	430	21.0	48.0	17.0	35	1040	2.0
(*Freschetta* 28.15 oz.), ⅙ pie	350	16.0	39.0	15.0	25	840	2.0
(*Freschetta* Sauce Stuffed Crust), ⅕ pie	340	15.0	42.0	13.0	20	860	2.0
(*Jack's Naturally Rising*), ⅙ pie ..	330	14.0	34.0	15.0	35	650	2.0
(*Jack's Original 9"*), ½ pie	370	16.0	36.0	18.0	35	820	3.0
(*Jack's Original 12"*), ¼ pie	300	14.0	29.0	15.0	35	680	2.0
(*Jeno's Crisp 'n Tasty*)	510	16.0	50.0	27.0	25	1130	2.0
(*Michelina's* Single)	440	15.0	42.0	24.0	30	890	2.0
(*Tombstone* Cheese Stuffed), ⅙ pie	380	15.0	33.0	20.0	40	850	3.0
(*Tombstone* Deep Dish)	500	16.0	51.0	25.0	35	1030	3.0

Food and Measure	cal.	prot. (gms)	carbo. (gms)	fat (gms)	chol. (mgs)	sod. (mgs)	fiber (gms)
Pizza, pepperoni *(cont.)*							
(*Tombstone* Original 9"), ⅓ pie	290	13.0	28.0	15.0	30	650	3.0
(*Tombstone* Original 12"), ¼ pie	400	17.0	37.0	21.0	45	910	4.0
(*Tombstone* Thin Crust), ¼ pie . . .	400	16.0	27.0	25.0	50	920	2.0
(*Tombstone Double Top*), ⅕ pie	410	19.0	31.0	23.0	55	960	3.0
(*Tombstone For One*)	550	20.0	52.0	30.0	50	1230	3.0
(*Tombstone Oven Rising* Crust), ⅙ pie	330	14.0	35.0	15.0	35	720	2.0
(*Totino's* Crisp Crust Party), ½ pie . . .	380	13.0	35.0	21.0	20	860	1.0
(*Totino's* Family Size), ⅓ pie	420	14.0	38.0	23.0	20	940	2.0
(*Wolfgang Puck's*), ¼ pie	360	20.0	34.0	15.0	30	880	1.0
mini deep dish (*Tombstone*), 2 pies	450	18.0	42.0	23.0	35	880	2.0
supreme (*Jack's Naturally Rising*), ⅙ pie	330	14.0	35.0	15.0	35	660	2.0
pepperoni/cheese:							
(*Di Giorno Rising Crust Half & Half*), cheese, ⅙ pie . .	310	15.0	40.0	11.0	25	810	3.0
(*Di Giorno Rising Crust Half & Half*), pepperoni, ⅙ pie	390	18.0	40.0	18.0	40	1070	3.0
(*Jack's Original Half & Half*), cheese, ⅓ pie	330	16.0	38.0	13.0	30	640	3.0
(*Jack's Original Half & Half*), pepperoni, ⅓ pie	420	20.0	39.0	22.0	50	980	3.0
pepperoni/mushroom:							
(*Jack's Original*), ¼ pie	300	14.0	29.0	15.0	35	680	2.0
(*Wolfgang Puck's*), ⅓ pie	310	15.0	32.0	13.0	30	550	2.0

Food and Measure	cal.	prot. (gms)	carbo. (gms)	fat (gms)	chol. (mgs)	sod. (mgs)	fiber (gms)
pepperoni/sausage, see "sausage/ pepperoni," below							
pepperoni/supreme:							
(*Tombstone* Original Half & Half), pepperoni, ⅕ pie . . .	310	13.0	29.0	15.0	30	690	3.0
(*Tombstone* Original Half & Half), supreme, ⅕ pie .	350	15.0	31.0	19.0	40	810	3.0
pesto, w/tomato and broccoli (*Amy's*), ⅓ pie	300	12.0	40.0	11.0	10	480	2.0
sausage:							
(*Celeste* for One) . .	480	18.0	45.0	26.0	20	1140	4.0
(*Di Giorno Rising Crust 8"*), ⅓ pie .	310	14.0	35.0	13.0	25	810	2.0
(*Di Giorno Rising Crust 12"*), ⅙ pie	360	16.0	40.0	15.0	30	930	3.0
(*Freschetta*), ⅙ pie	350	15.0	39.0	14.0	25	780	2.0
(*Jack's Naturally Rising*), ⅙ pie . .	320	14.0	35.0	14.0	30	570	2.0
(*Jack's Original 9"*), ½ pie	340	15.0	37.0	15.0	35	690	3.0
(*Jack's Original 12"*), ¼ pie	290	13.0	29.0	14.0	30	590	2.0
(*Jeno's Crisp 'n Tasty*)	480	16.0	51.0	24.0	20	1050	2.0
(*Tombstone* Original 12"), ⅕ pie	300	13.0	30.0	15.0	30	650	3.0
(*Tombstone* Original Classic), ⅓ pie . .	270	12.0	28.0	13.0	25	570	3.0
(*Tombstone Double Top*), ⅙ pie	320	16.0	27.0	17.0	40	750	3.0
(*Totino's* Crispy Crust Party), ½ pie	380	13.0	36.0	20.0	15	820	2.0
(*Totino's* Family Size), ¼ pie	300	11.0	29.0	16.0	10	680	1.0
Italian (*Tombstone* Cheese Stuffed), ⅙ pie	360	14.0	34.0	19.0	35	790	3.0

Food and Measure	cal.	prot. (gms)	carbo. (gms)	fat (gms)	chol. (mgs)	sod. (mgs)	fiber (gms)
Pizza, sausage *(cont.)*							
Italian (*Tombstone* Thin Crust), ¼ pie	380	16.0	27.0	24.0	45	820	3.0
Italian, spicy (*Jack's Naturally Rising*), ⅙ pie	320	15.0	35.0	14.0	35	630	2.0
Italian, spicy (*Jack's Original*), ¼ pie .	290	13.0	29.0	13.0	30	610	2.0
mini deep dish (*Tombstone*), 2 pies	420	18.0	43.0	19.0	30	790	2.0
sausage/cheese:							
(*Jack's Original* Half & Half), cheese, ⅓ pie	330	16.0	38.0	13.0	30	640	3.0
(*Jack's Original* Half & Half), sausage, ⅓ pie	400	19.0	39.0	19.0	45	820	3.0
sausage/herb (*Wolfgang Puck's*), ⅓ pie	350	15.0	27.0	13.0	30	500	2.0
sausage/mushroom:							
(*Jack's Original*), ¼ pie	300	14.0	29.0	14.0	30	600	2.0
(*Tombstone* Original 12"), ⅕ pie	300	13.0	30.0	14.0	30	650	3.0
(*Totino's* Crispy Crust Party), ½ pie . . .	360	13.0	34.0	19.0	15	780	2.0
sausage/mushroom/ pepperoni (*California Pizza Kitchen*), ⅓ pie	290	14.0	30.0	13.0	25	730	2.0
sausage/pepperoni:							
(*Celeste* for One) . .	560	20.0	43.0	34.0	25	1370	4.0
(*Di Giorno Rising Crust* 8"), ⅓ pie .	320	14.0	35.0	14.0	30	850	2.0
(*Di Giorno Rising Crust* 12"), ⅙ pie	360	16.0	40.0	16.0	30	980	3.0
(*Freschetta*), ⅕ pie	350	15.0	38.0	15.0	30	820	2.0
(*Freschetta* Sauce Stuffed Crust), ⅕ pie	390	15.0	43.0	18.0	20	920	2.0
(*Jack's Naturally Rising*), ⅙ pie . .	330	14.0	35.0	15.0	35	620	2.0

Food and Measure	cal.	prot. (gms)	carbo. (gms)	fat (gms)	chol. (mgs)	sod. (mgs)	fiber (gms)
(*Jack's Original* 9"), ½ pie	380	16.0	36.0	18.0	40	820	3.0
(*Jack's Original* 12"), ¼ pie	310	14.0	29.0	16.0	35	680	2.0
(*Jack's Original* Half & Half), pepperoni, ¼ pie	310	14.0	29.0	16.0	35	710	2.0
(*Jack's Original* Half & Half), sausage, ¼ pie	290	14.0	29.0	14.0	30	600	2.0
(*Tombstone* Original Half & Half), pepperoni, ¼ pie . . .	400	17.0	37.0	20.0	40	900	4.0
(*Tombstone* Original Half & Half), sausage, ¼ pie .	380	17.0	38.0	18.0	35	830	4.0
(*Tombstone Double Top*), ⅙ pie	340	17.0	27.0	19.0	45	810	3.0
(*Tombstone* Original 9"), ⅓ pie	300	13.0	29.0	15.0	30	680	3.0
(*Tombstone* Original 12"), ⅕ pie	310	14.0	30.0	15.0	30	710	3.0
(*Totino's* Crisp Crust Party), ½ pie . . .	380	13.0	35.0	21.0	15	850	2.0
(*Totino's* Crisp Crust Party Zesty Italiano), ½ pie .	390	13.0	36.0	21.0	15	850	2.0
shrimp, ⅓ pie:							
basil pesto (*Contessa*)	300	12.0	37.0	11.0	20	700	2.0
roasted red pesto (*Contessa*)	300	11.0	38.0	12.0	15	690	2.0
roasted vegetables (*Contessa*)	280	10.0	38.0	9.0	15	650	2.0
spinach (*Amy's*), ⅓ pie	320	13.0	40.0	11.0	15	490	2.0
spinach/mushroom/ garlic:							
(*Di Giorno Rising Crust* 8"), ⅓ pie .	260	13.0	36.0	8.0	15	670	2.0
(*Di Giorno Rising Crust* 12"), ⅙ pie	300	14.0	40.0	9.0	20	760	3.0

Pizza *(cont.)*
supreme:

Food and Measure	cal.	prot. (gms)	carbo. (gms)	fat (gms)	chol. (mgs)	sod. (mgs)	fiber (gms)
(*Celeste* Rising Crust), ⅙ pie . . .	360	16.0	41.0	15.0	25	940	6.0
(*Celeste* Suprema for One)	530	20.0	48.0	29.0	25	1290	6.0
(*Di Giorno Deep Dish*), ⅛ pie	310	13.0	25.0	17.0	35	770	2.0
(*Di Giorno Rising Crust* 8"), ⅓ pie	330	15.0	35.0	14.0	30	880	2.0
(*Di Giorno Rising Crust* 12"), ⅙ pie	370	17.0	40.0	16.0	35	1000	3.0
(*Freschetta*), ⅓ pie	290	14.0	33.0	12.0	20	670	2.0
(*Freschetta* Sauce Stuffed Crust), ⅕ pie	400	15.0	44.0	19.0	20	930	2.0
(*Jack's Original*), ¼ pie	310	14.0	29.0	16.0	35	680	2.0
(*Jeno's Crisp 'n Tasty*)	500	17.0	50.0	26.0	20	1080	2.0
(*Michelina's Single*)	430	14.0	42.0	24.0	30	810	2.0
(*Tombstone* Cheese Stuffed), ⅙ pie	380	15.0	34.0	20.0	40	850	3.0
(*Tombstone* Deep Dish)	470	16.0	52.0	23.0	30	960	3.0
(*Tombstone* Original 12"), ⅕ pie	310	13.0	30.0	16.0	35	690	3.0
(*Tombstone* Oven Rising Crust), ⅙ pie	320	14.0	36.0	14.0	30	680	3.0
(*Totino's* Crisp Crust Party), ½ pie . . .	380	13.0	35.0	21.0	15	840	2.0
(*Wolfgang Puck's*), ½ of 12-oz. pie or ¼ of 24-oz. pie	400	22.0	37.0	17.0	40	920	2.0
vegetarian (*Morningstar Farms*), ½ pie	300	15.0	38.0	9.0	0	480	2.0
supreme/cheese: (*Di Giorno Rising Crust* Half & Half), cheese, ⅙ pie . .	340	17.0	41.0	13.0	30	890	3.0

Food and Measure	cal.	prot. (gms)	carbo. (gms)	fat (gms)	chol. (mgs)	sod. (mgs	fiber (gms)
(*Di Giorno Rising Crust* Half & Half), supreme, ⅙ pie	380	17.0	41.0	17.0	35	1030	3.0
(*Jack's Original* Half & Half), cheese, ¼ pie	250	12.0	29.0	10.0	25	480	2.0
(*Jack's Original* Half & Half), supreme, ¼ pie	330	15.0	30.0	18.0	40	750	3.0
(*Tombstone* Original Half & Half), cheese, ⅕ pie . .	300	15.0	30.0	14.0	35	620	3.0
(*Tombstone* Original Half & Half), supreme, ⅕ pie .	330	14.0	30.0	17.0	35	750	3.0
supreme/pepperoni:							
(*Di Giorno Rising Crust* Half & Half), pepperoni, ⅙ pie	400	19.0	40.0	19.0	40	1090	3.0
(*Di Giorno Rising Crust* Half & Half), supreme, ⅙ pie .	410	18.0	41.0	20.0	40	1140	3.0
vegetable:							
(*Celeste* for One) . .	430	16.0	45.0	22.0	5	1090	5.0
(*Di Giorno Rising Crust* 8"), ⅓ pie .	260	12.0	36.0	8.0	15	660	3.0
(*Di Giorno Rising Crust* 12"), ⅙ pie	300	14.0	40.0	9.0	15	750	3.0
(*Tombstone For One* ½ Less Fat)	370	18.0	53.0	10.0	20	930	4.0
(*Tombstone Light*), ⅕ pie	230	13.0	31.0	6.0	10	530	3.0
(*Wolfgang Puck's*), ¼ pie	360	18.0	37.0	14.0	25	620	2.0
combo (*Amy's*), . . ⅓ pie	250	9.0	34.0	9.0	10	530	2.0
grilled (*Freschetta* Medley Sauce Stuffed Crust), ⅕ pie	340	13.0	44.0	13.0	10	710	2.0
grilled, cheeseless (*Wolfgang Puck's*), ⅓ pie	150	6.0	31.0	2.0	0	340	2.0

Food and Measure	cal.	prot. (gms)	carbo. (gms)	fat (gms)	chol. (mgs)	sod. (mgs)	fiber (gms)
Pizza, vegetable *(cont.)*							
primavera *(Freschetta)*, ⅕ pie ..	350	15.0	45.0	13.0	20	660	2.0
roasted *(Amy's)*, ⅓ pie	270	6.0	43.0	8.0	0	470	3.0
the works *(Jack's Naturally Rising)*, ⅙ pie	320	14.0	35.0	14.0	30	580	3.0
Pizza, bagel, frozen:							
(Empire Kosher), 2.25-oz. pc.	100	5.0	14.0	3.0	10	170	1.0
mini, cheese, 4 pcs.:							
(Ore-Ida Bagel Bites Hot Bites)	200	9.0	27.0	6.0	15	570	1.0
pepperoni *(Ore-Ida Bagel Bites Hot Bites)*	200	9.0	26.0	7.0	20	630	1.0
sausage and pepperoni *(Ore-Ida Bagel Bites Hot Bites)*	200	9.0	27.0	6.0	15	600	1.0
nondairy *(Tofutti Cheese Pizzazz)*, 1 pc.	175	7.0	15.0	50	0	380	1.0
Pizza, French bread, frozen, 1 pc.:							
cheese:							
(Healthy Choice) ..	340	22.0	51.0	5.0	15	600	5.0
(Lean Cuisine)	310	16.0	48.0	6.0	15	520	4.0
(Stouffer's)	370	14.0	43.0	16.0	15	880	3.0
extra *(Stouffer's)* ..	400	16.0	49.0	16.0	25	950	4.0
four *(Marie Callender's)*	530	28.0	50.0	24.0	60	980	4.0
five *(Stouffer's)* ...	420	17.0	48.0	18.0	25	850	3.0
deluxe:							
(Lean Cuisine)	290	16.0	43.0	6.0	25	550	3.0
(Stouffer's)	420	15.0	48.0	19.0	30	880	3.0
meat, three *(Stouffer's)*	470	15.0	48.0	24.0	35	1110	6.0
pepperoni:							
(Healthy Choice) ..	340	24.0	49.0	5.0	20	600	6.0
(Lean Cuisine)	300	15.0	43.0	8.0	25	590	3.0
(Stouffer's)	390	12.0	47.0	17.0	25	990	3.0
hearty *(Marie Callender's)*	570	29.0	50.0	28.0	65	1160	4.0

Food and Measure	cal.	prot. (gms)	carbo. (gms)	fat (gms)	chol. (mgs)	sod. (mgs	fiber (gms)
pepperoni and mushroom (*Stouffer's*) ..	440	15.0	49.0	20.0	30	910	5.0
sausage:							
(*Healthy Choice*) ..	320	21.0	48.0	5.0	25	580	5.0
(*Stouffer's*)	420	17.0	48.0	18.0	20	1260	3.0
sausage and pepperoni (*Stouffer's*)	470	16.0	47.0	24.0	40	1050	4.0
sun-dried tomato (*Lean Cuisine*)	350	17.0	50.0	9.0	20	500	5.0
supreme:							
(*Healthy Choice*) ..	330	21.0	51.0	5.0	20	600	6.0
super (*Marie Callender's*)	510	26.0	50.0	23.0	50	1200	4.0
vegetable:							
(*Healthy Choice*) ..	280	17.0	44.0	4.0	10	600	5.0
grilled (*Stouffer's*) .	350	12.0	48.0	12.0	10	500	3.0
white (*Stouffer's*)	470	17.0	43.0	25.0	25	700	3.0
Pizza, stuffed/pocket, frozen, 4.5-oz. pc., except as noted:							
cheese:							
(*Amy's*)	300	14.0	42.0	9.0	15	450	4.0
double (*Hot Pockets Pizza Minis*), 7 pcs., 3.1 oz. ..	280	6.0	35.0	12.0	15	460	2.0
double (*Hot Pockets Toaster Pizza*), 2.2 oz.	170	4.0	21.0	8.0	10	300	2.0
four (*Hot Pockets*) .	360	13.0	45.0	15.0	45	680	3.0
deluxe (*Lean Pockets*)	290	13.0	45.0	7.0	30	600	2.0
pepperoni:							
(*Croissant Pockets*)	360	11.0	40.0	17.0	30	590	2.0
(*Deli Stuffs*)	350	11.0	45.0	14.0	40	630	2.0
(*Hot Pockets*)	340	11.0	43.0	14.0	40	650	2.0
(*Hot Pockets Pizza Minis*), 7 pcs., 3.1 oz.	280	6.0	33.0	14.0	20	540	2.0
(*Hot Pockets Toaster Pizza*), 2.2 oz. ..	180	4.0	22.0	9.0	10	370	2.0
pepperoni and sausage:							
(*Hot Pockets*)	340	11.0	39.0	16.0	35	480	2.0
(*Hot Pockets Pizza Minis*), 7 pcs., 3.1 oz.	280	6.0	34.0	13.0	15	510	2.0

Food and Measure	cal.	prot. (gms)	carbo. (gms)	fat (gms)	chol. (mgs)	sod. (mgs)	fiber (gms)
Pizza, stuffed/pocket *(cont.)*							
(*Hot Pockets Toaster* Pizza), 2.2 oz. . .	170	4.0	21.0	8.0	10	350	2.0
sausage (*Hot Pockets*)	370	11.0	40.0	18.0	40	540	2.0
supreme (*Croissant Pockets*)	350	10.0	41.0	17.0	35	560	2.0
vegetarian:							
(*Amy's*)	250	11.0	39.0	6.0	10	360	4.0
"cheese," soy (*Amy's* Cheeze)	270	9.0	39.0	8.0	0	590	2.0
"pepperoni" (*Morningstar Farms* Meat-Free Sandwich)	280	12.0	42.0	7.0	5	420	5.0
Pizza crust:							
(*Mama Mary's*), ½ of 7" crust	200	6.0	32.0	5.0	0	135	3.0
(*Pillsbury*), ⅕ crust . .	150	5.0	27.0	2.0	0	410	<1.0
Pizza crust mix, ⅛ pkg., except as noted:							
(*Betty Crockor*), ¼ crust*	160	4.0	33.0	2.0	0	340	1.0
(*Eagle Mills*)	160	5.0	29.0	2.0	0	170	1.0
white (*Watkins* Deep Dish)	180	6.0	36.0	1.0	0	60	2.0
whole wheat (*Watkins* Thin)	90	3.0	18.0	1.0	0	75	2.0
Pizza Hut, 1 slice of medium pie, except as noted:							
The Big New Yorker:							
beef	480	24.0	42.0	26.0	40	1380	8.0
cheese	380	19.0	41.0	17.0	20	1140	7.0
ham	340	18.0	41.0	13.0	25	1160	7.0
pepperoni	370	17.0	41.0	16.0	20	1150	7.0
pork topping	470	23.0	42.0	25.0	35	1470	8.0
sausage	570	27.0	42.0	33.0	55	1620	8.0
supreme	450	22.0	43.0	23.0	35	1350	8.0
Veggie Lover's	450	18.0	52.0	22.0	10	1340	9.0
hand-tossed:							
beef	330	16.0	29.0	17.0	25	880	3.0
cheese	240	12.0	28.0	10.0	10	650	2.0
chicken supreme . .	230	13.0	29.0	7.0	15	650	2.0

Food and Measure	cal.	prot. (gms)	carbo. (gms)	fat (gms)	chol. (mgs)	sod. (mgs)	fiber (gms)
ham	260	14.0	28.0	10.0	20	800	2.0
Meat Lover's	320	14.0	28.0	17.0	30	900	2.0
pepperoni	280	13.0	28.0	13.0	20	790	2.0
Pepperoni Lover's	250	11.0	27.0	11.0	15	730	2.0
pork topping	320	16.0	29.0	16.0	25	920	3.0
sausage, Italian	340	16.0	38.0	18.0	30	910	2.0
super supreme	290	13.0	29.0	14.0	25	850	2.0
supreme	270	13.0	29.0	12.0	20	730	3.0
Veggie Lover's	220	9.0	29.0	8.0	5	580	2.0
The Insider, cheese	370	17.0	41.0	16.0	30	890	3.0
The New Edge, 1 sq.:							
chicken supreme	90	7.0	9.0	3.5	15	290	<1.0
Meat Lover's	160	7.0	8.0	11.0	20	440	<1.0
Veggie Lover's	70	4.0	9.0	3.0	<5	180	<1.0
the works	110	5.0	9.0	6.0	10	270	<1.0
pan pizza:							
beef	330	14.0	29.0	18.0	20	690	3.0
cheese	290	12.0	28.0	14.0	10	590	2.0
chicken supreme	270	13.0	29.0	12.0	15	580	2.0
ham	260	11.0	28.0	12.0	15	610	2.0
Meat Lover's	360	14.0	29.0	21.0	30	840	3.0
pepperoni	280	11.0	28.0	14.0	15	610	2.0
Pepperoni Lover's	330	14.0	29.0	18.0	20	760	2.0
pork topping	320	13.0	29.0	17.0	20	730	3.0
sausage, Italian	340	13.0	29.0	20.0	25	720	2.0
super supreme	340	14.0	30.0	18.0	25	780	3.0
supreme	320	13.0	29.0	17.0	20	670	3.0
Veggie Lover's	270	10.0	30.0	12.0	5	510	3.0
Personal Pan Pizza, 1 pizza:							
beef	710	31.0	71.0	35.0	45	1580	6.0
cheese	630	28.0	71.0	28.0	25	1370	6.0
ham	580	27.0	70.0	23.0	35	1450	5.0
pepperoni	620	26.0	70.0	28.0	30	1430	5.0
pork topping	700	31.0	71.0	34.0	40	1670	6.0
sausage, Italian	740	31.0	71.0	39.0	55	1640	6.0
Sicilian:							
beef	260	11.0	31.0	11.0	15	640	2.0
cheese	290	12.0	31.0	13.0	10	630	2.0
chicken supreme	270	12.0	32.0	11.0	15	620	2.0
ham	257	11.0	30.0	10.0	14	745	2.6
Meat Lover's	350	14.0	31.0	19.0	25	830	2.0
pepperoni	280	10.0	31.0	13.0	15	630	2.0
Pepperoni Lover's	320	13.0	31.0	16.0	20	780	2.0

Food and Measure	cal.	prot. (gms)	carbo. (gms)	fat (gms)	chol. (mgs)	sod. (mgs)	fiber (gms)
Pizza Hut, Sicilian *(cont.)*							
pork topping	320	13.0	31.0	16.0	20	750	2.0
sausage, Italian ...	333	13.0	31.0	18.0	24	855	2.8
super supreme ...	340	13.0	32.0	18.0	20	780	2.0
supreme	310	12.0	32.0	15.0	15	690	2.0
Veggie Lover's	270	12.0	32.0	11.0	5	620	2.0
stuffed crust, 1 slice of large pizza:							
beef	390	19.0	40.0	18.0	30	1150	3.0
cheese	360	18.0	39.0	16.0	25	1090	3.0
chicken supreme ..	350	21.0	41.0	13.0	35	1130	3.0
ham	330	18.0	39.0	13.0	30	1130	3.0
Meat Lover's	470	22.0	40.0	25.0	50	1430	3.0
pepperoni	360	17.0	39.0	16.0	30	1120	3.0
Pepperoni Lover's .	420	21.0	40.0	21.0	40	1350	3.0
pork topping	380	19.0	40.0	18.0	30	1190	3.0
sausage, Italian ...	400	19.0	40.0	20.0	35	1180	3.0
super supreme ...	430	21.0	41.0	22.0	40	1360	3.0
supreme	410	20.0	41.0	20.0	35	1220	3.0
Veggie Lover's	340	16.0	42.0	14.0	20	1030	3.0
Thin 'n' Crispy:							
beef	270	13.0	22.0	15.0	25	750	2.0
cheese	200	10.0	22.0	9.0	25	590	2.0
chicken supreme ..	200	12.0	23.0	7.0	20	620	2.0
ham	170	9.0	21.0	7.0	15	610	2.0
Meat Lover's	310	14.0	22.0	19.0	35	910	2.0
pepperoni	190	9.0	21.0	9.0	20	610	2.0
Pepperoni Lover's .	250	12.0	22.0	13.0	20	760	2.0
pork topping	270	13.0	22.0	14.0	25	820	2.0
sausage, Italian ...	290	12.0	22.0	17.0	30	800	2.0
super supreme ...	280	13.0	23.0	15.0	25	840	2.0
supreme	250	12.0	23.0	13.0	20	710	2.0
Veggie Lover's	190	8.0	24.0	7.0	5	520	2.0
twisted crust, 1 slice of large pizza:							
cheese	450	20.0	58.0	16.0	15	1210	3.0
pepperoni	440	18.0	58.0	15.0	20	1230	3.0
supreme	470	20.0	59.0	18.0	25	1280	3.0
sauces, 1 cont.:							
marinara	60	2.0	12.0	1.0	0	491	2.0
ranch	440	2.0	4.0	48.0	20	840	0
appetizers:							
Buffalo wings:							
hot, 4 pcs.	210	22.0	4.0	12.0	130	900	<1.0

Food and Measure	cal.	prot. (gms)	carbo. (gms)	fat (gms)	chol. (mgs)	sod. (mgs)	fiber (gms)
mild, 5 pcs. . . .	200	23.0	<1.0	12.0	150	510	0
garlic bread, 1 slice	150	3.0	16.0	8.0	0	240	1.0
bread stick, 1 pc. .	130	3.0	20.0	4.0	0	170	1.0
bread stick dipping sauce	30	<1.0	5.0	.5	0	170	<1.0
pasta, 1 serving:							
Cavatini	480	22.0	66.0	14.0	8	1170	9.0
Cavatini Supreme . .	560	24.0	73.0	19.0	10	1400	10.0
spaghetti:							
w/marinara	490	18.0	91.0	6.0	0	730	8.0
w/meat sauce . .	600	23.0	98.0	13.0	8	910	9.0
w/meatballs	850	37.0	120.0	24.0	17	1120	10.0
sandwiches, 1 pc:							
ham & cheese	550	33.0	57.0	21.0	22	2150	4.0
supreme	640	34.0	62.0	28.0	28	2150	4.0
dessert pizza, 1 pc.:							
apple	250	3.0	48.0	4.5	0	230	2.0
cherry	250	3.0	47.0	4.5	0	220	3.0
Pizza pocket, see "Pizza, stuffed/ pocket"							
Pizza rolls, see "Pizza snack"							
Pizza sauce, ¼ cup:							
(*Contadina/Contadina Pizza Squeeze*)	30	1.0	6.0	0	0	340	1.0
(*Muir Glen*)	40	1.0	6.0	1.0	0	230	2.0
(*Prince* Traditional) . .	20	1.0	4.0	0	0	330	1.0
(*Progresso*)	20	<1.0	4.0	0	0	170	1.0
(*Ragú*)	25	1.0	3.0	1.0	0	250	<1.0
(*Ragú Pizza Quick* Traditional)	40	1.0	4.0	2.0	0	380	1.0
cheese, four (*Contadina*)	30	<1.0	6.0	.5	0	390	<1.0
garlic and basil (*Ragú Pizza Quick*)	40	1.0	5.0	2.0	0	380	1.0
pepperoni:							
(*Contadina*)	35	1.0	5.0	1.0	0	390	<1.0
(*Ragú Pizza Quick*)	50	2.0	5.0	2.0	5	470	1.0
Pizza snack (see also "Nacho snack"), frozen, 6 pcs.:							
cheese:							
(*Amy's*)	180	9.0	22.0	6.0	10	290	2.0

Food and Measure	cal.	prot. (gms)	carbo. (gms)	fat (gms)	chol. (mgs)	sod. (mgs)	fiber (gms)
Pizza snack, cheese *(cont.)*							
(*Michelina's* Rolls) .	230	8.0	23.0	12.0	30	380	1.0
(*Totino's Pizza Rolls*)	210	9.0	25.0	8.0	10	420	1.0
nacho (*Michelina's* Rolls)	220	8.0	25.0	10.0	25	300	1.0
combination:							
(*Michelina's* Rolls)	230	8.0	23.0	12.0	25	370	1.0
(*Totino's Pizza Rolls*)	230	8.0	22.0	12.0	15	470	1.0
hamburger:							
(*Michelina's* Rolls)	220	8.0	23.0	10.0	25	360	1.0
(*Totino's Pizza Rolls*)	210	8.0	23.0	9.0	10	490	1.0
meat, four (*Michelina's* Rolls)	230	8.0	22.0	12.0	30	400	1.0
meat, three (*Totino's Pizza Rolls*)	220	8.0	23.0	11.0	15	450	1.0
pepperoni:							
(*Jack's Pizza Bursts*)	260	8.0	25.0	15.0	15	550	1.0
(*Michelina's* Rolls) .	240	8.0	23.0	13.0	30	410	1.0
(*Totino's Pizza Rolls*)	230	8.0	23.0	12.0	15	540	1.0
supreme (*Totino's Pizza Rolls*)	220	8.0	23.0	11.0	10	450	1.0
sausage (*Totino's Pizza Rolls*)	220	8.0	23.0	11.0	10	380	1.0
supreme (*Totino's Pizza Rolls*)	220	7.0	25.0	10.0	10	350	1.0
Plantain:							
raw:							
(*Frieda's*), 3 oz. ...	100	1.0	27.0	0	0	0	2.0
1 medium, 6.3 oz. .	218	2.3	57.1	.6	0	7	4.1
sliced, ½ cup	91	1.0	23.6	.3	0	3	1.7
cooked, sliced, ½ cup	89	.6	24.0	.1	0	4	1.8
Plantain, frozen:							
baked, ripe (*Goya* Plátanos Maduros Horneados), 3 oz.	237	1.0	56.0	1.0	0	68	3.0
fried, 4 pcs.:							
(*Latin Fiesta*)	210	1.0	35.0	8.0	0	0	0
(*Goya* Plátanos Tostones)	210	1.0	35.0	8.0	0	0	0
Plum, fresh:							
(*Dole*), 2 medium ...	80	1.0	19.0	1.0	0	0	2.0
Japanese or hybrid, 2⅛" fruit	36	.5	8.6	.4	0	tr.	<1.0
sliced, ½ cup	46	.7	10.7	.5	0	1	1.2

Food and Measure	cal.	prot. (gms)	carbo. (gms)	fat (gms)	chol. (mgs)	sod. (mgs)	fiber (gms)
Plum, can or jar, purple:							
in juice:							
½ cup	73	.7	19.1	<.1	0	2	1.3
3 plums and 2 tbsp. liquid ...	55	.5	14.4	<.1	0	1	1.0
in light syrup:							
½ cup	79	.5	20.5	.1	0	25	1.3
3 plums and 2¾ tbsp. liquid	83	.5	21.7	.1	0	26	1.3
in heavy syrup:							
½ cup	115	.5	30.0	.1	0	25	1.3
purple (*Oregon*) ...	100	1.0	25.0	0	0	15	2.0
purple, whole (*S&W*), ½ cup	130	0	33.0	0	0	15	2.0
Plum, dried:							
(*Dole*), ¼ cup	110	1.0	26.0	0	0	5	2.0
w/pits:							
(*Sunsweet*), 3 large, 6 medium, 1.4 oz.	100	1.0	26.0	0	0	5	3.0
large (*Sonoma* Organic), ½ cup, 1.4 oz. edible ...	120	1.0	29.0	0	0	5	3.0
pitted:							
(*Sonoma* Organic), ¼ cup, 1.4 oz.	120	1.0	29.0	0	0	5	3.0
(*Sunsweet Lemon/ Orange Essence*), 1.4 oz., 5 pcs. ..	100	1.0	26.0	0	0	5	3.0
10 pcs.	201	2.2	52.7	.4	0	3	6.0
bite size (*Sunsweet*), 1.4 oz., 7 pcs. ..	100	1.0	25.0	0	0	5	3.0
stewed, w/pits, un- sweetened, ½ cup	113	1.2	29.8	.2	0	2	7.0
Plum, dried, canned, in heavy syrup:							
(*Sonoma* Organic), 3–4 pcs., 1.4 oz. ..	110	1.0	26.0	0	0	5	2.0
pitted, 4 oz.	119	1.0	31.5	.2	0	3	4.3
½ cup	123	1.0	32.5	.2	0	3	4.4
5 pcs., 2 tbsp. liquid	90	.8	23.9	.2	0	2	3.3
Plum butter:							
(*Lost Acres*), 1 tbsp.	45	0	11.0	0	0	0	0
(*Sonoma*), 2 tbsp. ..	50	<1.0	13.0	0	0	0	1.0

Food and Measure	cal.	prot. (gms)	carbo. (gms)	fat (gms)	chol. (mgs)	sod. (mgs)	fiber (gms)
Plum pudding (*Crosse & Blackwell*), 1/3 pkg.	460	6.0	87.0	10.0	0	240	5.0
Plum sauce:							
(*Ka•Me*), 2 tbsp.	70	0	16.0	0	0	360	0
dipping, 2 tbsp.:							
(*Sonoma*)	60	<1.0	15.0	0	0	75	1.0
(*Trader Vic's*)	70	0	16.0	0	0	220	0
Plum–passion fruit, dried (*Sunsweet Fruitlings*), 1.4 oz., 1/3 cup	110	1.0	28.0	0	0	5	3.0
Poi, 1/2 cup	134	.5	32.7	.2	0	14	.5
Pocket sandwich, see specific listings							
Poke greens, canned (*Allens*), 1/2 cup ...	35	2.0	5.0	1.0	0	7	3.0
Pokeberry shoots:							
raw, 1/2 cup	18	2.1	3.0	.3	0	18	1.4
boiled, drained, 1/2 cup	16	1.9	2.5	.3	0	15	1.2
Polenta (see also "Cornmeal"), instant (*Bellino*), 1/4 cup ...	140	3.0	32.0	0	0	0	4.0
Polenta, canned (*Greene's Farm*), 1/2 cup	80	2.0	17.0	0	0	400	0
Polenta, refrigerated:							
(*Frieda's*), 4 oz.	100	3.0	21.0	0	0	440	3.0
(*San Gennaro*), 2 slices, 1/2"	70	2.0	15.0	0	0	310	1.0
Polish sausage (see also "Kielbasa" and "Sausage, canned"):							
fresh, grilled (*Johnsonville*), 3-oz. link ...	290	14.0	1.0	25.0	65	800	0
precooked (*Johnsonville*), 2.7-oz. link ..	240	9.0	2.0	21.0	60	640	0
Pollock, meat only:							
Atlantic, 4 oz.:							
raw	104	22.1	0	1.1	80	98	0
baked, broiled, or microwaved ...	134	28.3	0	1.4	103	125	0
walleye, 4 oz.:							
raw	91	19.5	0	.9	81	112	0

Food and Measure	cal.	prot. (gms)	carbo. (gms)	fat (gms)	chol. (mgs)	sod. (mgs)	fiber (gms)
baked, broiled, or microwaved ...	128	26.7	0	1.3	109	132	0
Pomegranate:							
(*Dole*), 1 medium ...	104	2.0	26.0	0	0	0	1.0
(*Frieda's*), 5 oz.	100	1.0	24.0	0	0	0	1.0
w/peel, 9.7-oz. fruit ..	104	1.5	26.4	.5	0	5	.9
Pomegranate juice (*R. W. Knudsen*), 8 fl. oz.	150	<1.0	37.0	0	0	10	0
Pompano, Florida, meat only:							
raw, 4 oz.	186	21.0	0	10.7	57	74	0
baked, broiled, or microwaved, 4 oz.	239	26.4	0	13.8	73	86	0
Popcorn:							
(*Arrowhead Mills*), ¼ cup	180	6.0	36.0	2.5	0	0	6.0
(*Jolly Time* Sugar Corn), 3 cups*	120	6.0	20.0	7.0	0	0	9.0
(*Pop•Secret* Homestyle), 3 tbsp.	170	3.0	17.0	12.0	0	430	3.0
(*Pop Weaver* Premium Hybrid), 1 oz.	100	3.0	20.0	1.0	0	2	4.0
(*Pop Weaver Naks Paks* Coconut Oil), 3 tbsp.	140	3.0	19.0	8.0	0	260	3.0
(*Pop Weaver Naks Paks* Safflower Oil), 3 tbsp.	150	3.0	20.0	8.0	0	270	3.0
butter/butter flavor:							
(*America's Best*), 5 cups*	90	4.0	23.0	2.0	0	210	9.0
(*B. K. Heuermann's Exclusive*), 2 tbsp.	140	2.0	16.0	8.0	0	115	4.0
(*B. K. Heuermann's Exclusive* Intense Butter), 2 tbsp. .	160	2.0	16.0	9.0	0	270	4.0
(*B. K. Heuermann's Exclusive* Low Fat), 2 tbsp.	120	2.0	16.0	2.0	0	115	4.0
(*Healthy Choice*), 3 tbsp.	120	4.0	25.0	3.0	0	330	5.0
(*Jolly Time Blast O Butter*), 3½ cups*	150	3.0	19.0	11.0	0	340	9.0

Food and Measure	cal.	prot. (gms)	carbo. (gms)	fat (gms)	chol. (mgs)	sod. (mgs)	fiber (gms)
Popcorn, butter/butter flavor *(cont.)*							
(*Jolly Time Blast O Butter* Light), 4 cups*	130	3.0	21.0	6.0	0	340	6.0
(*Jolly Time Butter• Licious*), 4 cups*	140	3.0	18.0	9.0	0	320	6.0
(*Jolly Time Butter• Licious* Light), 5 cups*	120	3.0	21.0	6.0	0	290	7.0
(*Jolly Time Healthy Pop*), 5 cups*	90	4.0	23.0	2.0	0	210	9.0
(*Newman's Own*), 3½ cups*	170	2.0	16.0	11.0	0	180	2.0
(*Newman's Own* Butter Boom), 3½ cups*	170	2.0	15.0	11.0	0	630	3.0
(*Newman's Own* Light), 3½ cups*	110	2.0	20.0	3.0	0	90	3.0
(*Pop•Secret* Extra Butter), 3 tbsp.	180	2.0	17.0	13.0	0	360	3.0
(*Pop•Secret* Light), 3 tbsp.	140	3.0	23.0	6.0	0	390	4.0
(*Pop•Secret* Light), 6 cups*	120	3.0	20.0	5.0	0	290	4.0
(*Pop•Secret* Light Snack Size), ¼ cup	160	4.0	26.0	7.0	0	440	5.0
(*Pop•Secret* Light Snack Size) 1 cup*	20	<1.0	4.0	1.0	0	50	<1.0
(*Pop•Secret* Movie Theater), 3 tbsp.	180	2.0	17.0	13.0	0	300	3.0
(*Pop•Secret* 94% Fat Free), 3 tbsp.	120	4.0	26.0	2.0	0	380	4.0
(*Pop•Secret* 94% Fat Free), 6 cups*	110	4.0	23.0	2.0	0	230	4.0
(*Pop•Secret* Rev It Up), 3 tbsp.	180	2.0	17.0	13.0	0	300	3.0
(*Pop•Secret* Land O Lakes), 3 tbsp.	180	3.0	17.0	12.0	0	330	3.0
(*Pop•Secret* Land O Lakes), 1 cup*	35	<1.0	4.0	2.5	0	60	<1.0
(*Pop•Secret* Jumbo Pop), 3 tbsp.	170	2.0	18.0	11.0	0	280	3.0

Food and Measure	cal.	prot. (gms)	carbo. (gms)	fat (gms)	chol. (mgs)	sod. (mgs)	fiber (gms)
(*Pop•Secret Jumbo Pop* Movie Theater), 3 tbsp.	170	2.0	18.0	11.0	0	320	3.0
(*Pop Weaver* Microwave), ⅓ bag, 1.2 oz.	140	3.0	19.0	9.0	0	350	4.0
(*Pop Weaver* Microwave Extra Butter), ⅓ bag, 1.2 oz. .	160	2.0	17.0	10.0	0	375	3.0
(*Pop Weaver* Microwave Light), ⅓ bag, 1.2 oz. .	115	2.0	18.0	3.5	0	220	3.0
white, buttery (*Jolly Time*), 4 cups* ..	150	4.0	16.0	9.0	0	350	4.0
cheddar (*Jolly Time*), 3 cups*	160	3.0	17.0	10.0	0	350	4.0
crispy (*Jolly Time Light*), 5 cups* ...	120	3.0	20.0	5.0	0	320	7.0
natural flavor:							
(*B. K. Heuermann's Exclusive*)	120	2.0	16.0	8.0	0	115	4.0
(*Healthy Choice*), 3 tbsp.	120	4.0	26.0	2.5	0	330	5.0
(*Newman's Own*), 3½ cups*	170	2.0	16.0	11.0	0	180	3.0
(*Pop•Secret*), 3 tbsp.	170	3.0	17.0	12.0	0	340	3.0
(*Pop•Secret 94% Fat Free*), 3 tbsp. ..	120	4.0	26.0	2.0	0	380	4.0
(*Pop•Secret 94% Fat Free*), 6 cups* ..	110	4.0	23.0	2.0	0	230	4.0
(*Pop•Weaver* Microwave), ⅓ bag, 1.2 oz.	140	3.0	18.0	7.0	0	250	3.0
white, crispy (*Jolly Time*), 4 cups* ...	150	3.0	16.0	10.0	0	410	6.0
white/yellow (*Jolly Time*), 5 cups airpopped	100	4.0	24.0	.5	0	0	6.0
Popcorn, popped:							
(*Bachman*), 1 oz. ...	140	2.0	15.0	10.0	0	230	5.0
(*Bachman* Lite), 1 oz.	110	3.0	19.0	5.0	0	110	5.0
(*Bearitos* No Oil), 5 cups, 1.1 oz. ...	110	4.0	23.0	1.5	0	90	4.0

Food and Measure	cal.	prot. (gms)	carbo. (gms)	fat (gms)	chol. (mgs)	sod. (mgs)	fiber (gms)
Popcorn, popped *(cont.)*							
(*Bearitos* No Oil/Salt), 4¼ cups, 1.1 oz. ...	120	4.0	24.0	1.5	0	0	1.0
(*Boston's* Gourmet Super Premium), 2 cups	160	2.0	13.0	11.0	0	120	3.0
(*Boston's Lite*), 4 cups	140	3.0	19.0	6.0	0	90	4.0
(*Boston's Lite*), 1-oz. pkg.	130	3.0	18.0	6.0	0	80	3.0
(*Herr's*), 1 oz., 3 cups	140	2.0	11.0	11.0	0	250	3.0
butter/butter flavor:							
(*Bearitos* Buttery), 2½ cups, 1.1 oz.	170	2.0	14.0	12.0	0	210	1.0
(*Bearitos* Buttery Lite), 3½ cups, 1.1 oz.	140	3.0	19.0	6.0	0	140	1.0
(*Chester's*), 3 cups	170	2.0	16.0	12.0	0	330	3.0
(*Snyder's*), ⅝ oz.	110	1.0	6.0	10.0	0	150	n.a.
(*Utz*), 2 cups	170	2.0	13.0	12.0	0	210	3.0
caramel:							
(*Bearitos* Fat Free), 1 cup, 1.1 oz. ..	120	1.0	27.0	0	0	125	1.0
(*Boston's* Fat Free), ⅔ cup	100	<1.0	23.0	0	0	55	2.0
(*Cracker Jacks* Fat Free), ¾ cup ...	110	<1.0	26.0	0	0	70	1.0
(*Utz* Cluster), 1 oz.	142	.9	17.0	2.0	0	159	1.0
w/peanuts (*Cracker Jack*), ½ cup ...	120	2.0	23.0	2.0	0	70	1.0
cheese:							
(*Bachman*), 1 oz.	150	2.0	16.0	8.0	<5	210	4.0
(*Utz*), 2 cups	150	2.0	14.0	9.0	0	250	3.0
(*Utz* Hulless Puff'n Corn), 2 cups ...	160	2.0	13.0	12.0	0	210	0
cheddar, white:							
(*Bearitos*), 2⅓ cups, 1.1 oz.	170	3.0	14.0	11.0	5	230	1.0
(*Boston's* 40% Less Fat), 2¾ cups ..	140	3.0	17.0	6.0	<5	180	3.0
(*Chester's*), 3 cups	200	3.0	17.0	13.0	<5	340	2.0
(*Smartfood*), 1¾ cups	160	3.0	14.0	10.0	5	200	2.0
(*Smartfood* Reduced Fat), 3 cups	140	4.0	19.0	6.0	<5	280	3.0

Food and Measure	cal.	prot. (gms)	carbo. (gms)	fat (gms)	chol. (mgs)	sod. (mgs)	fiber (gms)
(*Utz*), 2 cups	150	3.0	15.0	8.0	0	250	3.0
toffee:							
butter (*Cracker Jack Fat Free*), ¾ cup	110	1.0	26.0	0	0	85	1.0
buttery, w/peanuts (*Crunch 'n Munch*), ⅔ cup, 1.1 oz.	150	2.0	22.0	6.0	5	170	<1.0
Popcorn cake:							
plain:							
(*Hain*), 1 pc.	35	1.0	8.0	0	0	55	<1.0
(*Hain* Mini), 8 pcs.	50	1.0	11.0	0	0	90	<1.0
barbecue (*Hain* Mini), 6 pcs.	50	1.0	11.0	1.0	0	150	<1.0
butter:							
(*Hain*), 1 pc.	50	1.0	10.0	0	0	85	<1.0
(*Hain* Mini), 7 pcs. .	50	1.0	10.0	1.0	0	85	<1.0
caramel:							
(*Hain*), 1 pc.	50	1.0	11.0	0	0	20	<1.0
(*Hain* Mini), 6 pcs.	50	1.0	12.0	0	0	15	<1.0
cheddar, 6 pcs.:							
mild (*Hain* Mini) ..	50	1.0	10.0	1.0	0	160	<1.0
white (*Hain* Mini)	50	1.0	10.0	1.0	0	170	<1.0
Popcorn seasoning (*Tone's*), ¼ tsp. ..	0	0	0	0	0	630	0
Poppy seeds, 1 tsp.	15	.5	.7	1.3	0	1	.8
Porgy, see "Scup"							
Pork (see also "Pork, refrigerated"), meat only, 4 oz.:							
back ribs, roasted, lean w/fat	420	27.5	0	33.5	134	115	0
ground, cooked	337	29.1	0	23.6	107	83	0
leg, see "Ham"							
loin, whole:							
braised, lean w/fat	271	30.9	0	15.4	90	54	0
braised, lean only	231	32.4	0	10.3	90	57	0
broiled, lean w/fat	274	30.9	0	15.8	90	70	0
broiled, lean only ..	238	32.4	0	11.1	90	73	0
roasted, lean w/fat	281	30.7	0	16.6	93	67	0
roasted, lean only	237	32.5	0	10.9	92	66	0
loin, blade:							
braised, lean w/fat	366	24.8	0	28.8	96	62	0
braised, lean only	255	28.4	0	14.8	94	70	0
broiled, lean w/fat	363	25.5	0	28.2	98	79	0

Food and Measure	cal.	prot. (gms)	carbo. (gms)	fat (gms)	chol. (mgs)	sod. (mgs)	fiber (gms)
Pork, loin, blade *(cont.)*							
broiled, lean only ..	265	28.8	0	15.8	95	91	0
roasted, lean w/fat	366	26.9	0	27.9	106	34	0
roasted, lean only	280	30.2	0	16.8	106	33	0
loin, center:							
braised, lean w/fat	•280	31.7	0	16.0	98	67	0
braised, lean only	229	33.8	0	9.4	96	70	0
broiled, lean w/fat	272	32.6	0	14.8	93	66	0
broiled, lean only ..	229	34.2	0	9.2	93	68	0
panfried, lean w/fat	314	33.9	0	18.8	104	91	0
panfried, lean only	263	36.5	0	11.9	104	97	0
roasted, lean w/fat	265	29.8	0	15.3	91	71	0
roasted, lean only	226	31.2	0	10.2	90	75	0
loin, center rib:							
braised, lean w/fat	284	30.2	0	17.1	83	45	0
braised, lean only	234	32.1	0	10.7	81	47	0
broiled, lean w/fat	298	32.6	0	17.6	93	70	0
broiled, lean only ..	248	34.9	.0	11.0	92	74	0
roasted, lean w/fat	289	31.1	0	17.3	83	52	0
roasted, lean only	253	32.6	0	12.6	81	53	0
loin, top, bone-in:							
braised, lean w/fat	264	31.5	0	14.4	85	48	0
braised, lean only	229	33.0	0	9.7	83	48	0
broiled, lean w/fat	260	34.0	0	12.7	92	71	0
broiled, lean only ..	230	35.3	0	8.8	91	74	0
roasted, lean w/fat	256	31.9	0	13.0	89	50	0
roasted, lean only.	220	34.3	0	8.2	89	51	0
loin, top, boneless:							
panfried, lean w/fat	291	32.9	0	16.8	89	62	0
panfried, lean only	255	34.6	0	11.9	87	65	0
ribs, country-style:							
braised, lean w/fat	336	27.1	0	24.4	99	67	0
braised, lean only	265	29.5	0	15.4	98	71	0
roasted, lean w/fat	372	26.5	0	28.7	104	59	0
roasted, lean only .	280	30.2	0	16.8	106	33	0
shoulder, whole:							
roasted, lean w/fat	331	26.4	0	24.3	102	77	0
roasted, lean only	261	28.7	0	15.4	102	85	0
shoulder, arm (picnic):							
braised, lean w/fat	374	31.7	0	26.3	124	100	0
braised, lean only	281	36.6	0	13.8	129	116	0
roasted, lean w/fat	360	26.6	0	27.2	107	79	0
roasted, lean only	259	30.3	0	14.3	108	91	0

Food and Measure	cal.	prot. (gms)	carbo. (gms)	fat (gms)	chol. (mgs)	sod. (mgs)	fiber (gms)
shoulder, Boston blade:							
braised, lean w/fat	362	32.5	0	24.7	128	79	0
braised, lean only	310	35.3	0	17.6	132	85	0
broiled, lean w/fat	294	29.0	0	18.8	108	78	0
broiled, lean only ..	257	30.3	0	14.2	107	84	0
roasted, lean w/fat	305	26.2	0	21.4	98	76	0
roasted, lean only	263	27.5	0	16.2	96	100	0
sirloin, bone-in:							
braised, lean w/fat	278	28.8	0	17.1	93	58	0
braised, lean only	223	30.6	0	10.2	92	60	0
broiled, lean w/fat	294	30.2	0	18.2	98	77	0
broiled, lean only ..	242	32.3	0	11.5	96	82	0
roasted, lean w/fat	296	30.9	0	28.2	99	68	0
roasted, lean only	245	32.7	0	11.7	98	71	0
sirloin, boneless:							
braised, lean w/fat	214	30.1	0	9.5	92	52	0
braised, lean only	198	30.6	0	7.5	92	52	0
broiled, lean w/fat	236	34.6	0	9.8	103	64	0
broiled, lean only ..	219	35.3	0	7.6	104	64	0
roasted, lean w/fat	235	32.3	0	10.7	98	64	0
roasted, lean only	225	32.7	0	9.4	98	64	0
spareribs, lean w/fat,							
braised	450	33.0	0	34.4	137	106	0
tenderloin:							
broiled, lean w/fat	228	33.9	0	9.2	107	73	0
roasted, lean w/fat	196	31.5	0	6.9	90	62	0
roasted, lean only	186	31.9	0	5.5	90	64	0
Pork, cured:							
arm (picnic), roasted:							
lean w/fat, 4 oz. ..	318	23.2	0	24.2	66	1216	0
lean w/fat, chopped							
or diced, 1 cup	392	28.6	0	29.9	81	1501	0
lean only, 4 oz. ...	193	28.3	0	8.0	54	1396	0
lean only, chopped							
or diced, 1 cup	238	34.9	0	9.9	67	1723	0
blade roll, lean w/fat,							
roasted, 4 oz.	325	19.6	.4	26.6	76	1103	0
leg, see "Ham"							
Pork, ground, raw							
(*Johnsonville*), 4 oz.	340	17.0	0	29.0	80	45	0
Pork, pickled (see also							
"Pig's feet"), 2 oz.:							
hocks (*Hormel*)	110	9.0	0	8.0	45	530	0
tidbits (*Hormel*)	100	8.0	0	8.0	45	530	0

Food and Measure	cal.	prot. (gms)	carbo. (gms)	fat (gms)	chol. (mgs)	sod. (mgs)	fiber (gms)
Pork, refrigerated, 4 oz., except as noted:							
blade steak:							
(*Always Tender*) ..	260	17.0	0	21.0	65	470	0
boneless (*Armour*)	200	17.0	0	15.0	40	660	0
loin (*Armour*)	210	20.0	0	15.0	45	390	0
boneless roast (*Always Tender* Chef's Prime)	160	21.0	0	9.0	60	470	0
bottom round (*Armour*)	120	23.0	0	4.0	45	470	0
chops, center cut (*Always Tender*) ..	190	20.0	0	12.0	65	460	0
chops, loin:							
(*Always Tender*) ..	190	20.0	0	12.0	65	470	0
(*Armour*)	210	20.0	0	15.0	45	390	0
boneless (*Armour*)	160	19.0	0	10.0	40	630	0
center cut (*Armour*)	190	20.0	0	12.0	45	470	0
center cut, boneless (*Always Tender*)	160	21.0	0	9.0	60	470	0
center cut, boneless (*Armour*)	160	19.0	0	10.0	40	630	0
chops, rib:							
center cut (*Armour*)	210	20.0	0	15.0	45	390	0
center cut, boneless, thin (*Armour*) ..	160	19.0	0	10.0	40	630	0
chops, sirloin, boneless (*Armour*)	150	22.0	1.0	6.0	55	480	0
cubed steak or kabob cubes (*Armour*) ..	160	19.0	0	10.0	40	630	0
loin, boneless (*Armour*)	150	22.0	0	8.0	35	460	0
loin back ribs (*Armour*)	250	18.0	0	20.0	55	560	0
loin half, onion and garlic (*Armour*) ...	170	21.0	2.0	9.0	55	600	0
loin ribs, country style (*Armour*)	210	20.0	0	15.0	45	390	0
loin roast, center cut (*Armour*)	190	20.0	0	12.0	45	470	0
loin fillet and roast:							
(*Always Tender* Original)	130	21.0	0	4.5	50	330	0
lemon garlic (*Always Tender*)	130	20.0	1.0	5.0	50	690	0

Food and Measure	cal.	prot. (gms)	carbo. (gms)	fat (gms)	chol. (mgs)	sod. (mgs)	fiber (gms)
honey mustard							
(*Always Tender*)	140	20.0	4.0	5.0	55	410	0
mesquite barbecue							
(*Always Tender*)	130	20.0	2.0	5.0	50	710	0
salsa (*Always Tender*)	140	20.0	2.0	5.0	55	610	0
roast:							
(*Armour*)	300	18.0	2.0	25.0	80	650	1.0
au jus (*Always Tender*), 5 oz. ..	180	29.0	0	7.0	85	570	0
Italian style (*Armour*)	150	19.0	3.0	7.0	70	390	1.0
onion and garlic (*Armour*)	190	19.0	1.0	12.0	75	580	0
porketta style (*Armour*)	190	19.0	1.0	12.0	75	580	0
teriyaki (*Armour*) .	160	20.0	2.0	8.0	70	560	0
shoulder butt:							
roast, smoked (*Boar's Head*), 3 oz.	170	13.0	<1.0	13.0	55	760	0
steak (*Armour*) ...	200	17.0	0	15.0	40	660	0
shoulder roast:							
(*Always Tender* Country Roast)	200	15.0	1.0	15.0	60	520	0
(*Armour*)	200	17.0	0	15.0	40	660	0
boneless (*Armour*)	160	23.0	0	8.0	50	60	0
onion garlic (*Always Tender*)	200	15.0	2.0	15.0	60	570	0
sirloin, boneless (*Armour*)	150	22.0	1.0	6.0	55	480	0
spareribs:							
(*Always Tender* Country style) ..	260	17.0	0	21.0	65	470	0
(*Always Tender* Ribs)	240	18.0	0	18.0	80	470	0
(*Always Tender* Spareribs/Special Trim Ribs)	280	17.0	0	23.0	80	470	0
(*Armour* for Barbecue)	220	17.0	0	17.0	45	710	0
(*Armour* St. Louis Style)	260	17.0	1.0	19.0	50	520	0
tenderloin:							
(*Armour*)	110	20.0	0	4.0	55	480	0

Food and Measure	cal.	prot. (gms)	carbo. (gms)	fat (gms)	chol. (mgs)	sod. (mgs)	fiber (gms)
Pork, refrigerated, tenderloin *(cont.)*							
lemon pepper (*Armour*)	120	22.0	1.0	3.0	60	340	0
garden herb (*Armour*)	120	21.0	2.0	3.0	60	640	1.0
mesquite and green chili (*Armour*) . .	100	18.0	3.0	2.0	40	550	0
peppercorn (*Always Tender*)	130	19.0	2.0	4.5	60	670	0
peppercorn (*Armour*)	120	22.0	1.0	3.0	60	340	0
teriyaki (*Always Tender*)	140	21.0	4.0	4.0	65	540	0
teriyaki (*Armour*) .	110	21.0	4.0	1.5	50	690	0
Pork back fat, 1 oz.	230	2.6	0	25.3	16	3	0
Pork belly, raw, 1 oz.	147	2.7	0	15.0	20	9	0
Pork dinner, frozen, 1 pkg.:							
boneless, rib-shape:							
(*Swanson Traditional Favorites*), 10.5 oz.	470	18.0	58.0	19.0	30	900	5.0
riblet (*Banquet Extra Helping*), 15.25 oz.	720	27.0	62.0	40.0	80	1590	7.0
and roast potato (*Stouffer's Home-Style*), 15⅝ oz. . . .	510	27.0	70.0	13.0	60	1650	8.0
Pork entree, dried, sweet/sour, w/rice, 1 serving:							
(*Mountain House Double*)	380	14.0	56.0	11.0	35	1060	3.0
(*Mountain House Single*)	480	18.0	70.0	14.0	40	1330	3.0
Pork entree, frozen (see also "Pork, refrigerated"), 1 pkg., except as noted:							
chop, country fried (*Marie Callender's*), 15 oz.	540	23.0	50.0	28.0	65	2240	8.0

Food and Measure	cal.	prot. (gms)	carbo. (gms)	fat (gms)	chol. (mgs)	sod. (mgs)	fiber (gms)
country breaded, w/cheddar bacon potato (*Healthy Choice* Duo), 8 oz.	280	18.0	38.0	6.0	30	600	4.0
country fried (*Banquet*), 10.25 oz.	430	15.0	38.0	25.0	50	1640	6.0
cutlet, breaded (*Stouffer's* Home-Style), 10 oz.	370	14.0	35.0	19.0	45	1250	4.0
fried rice:							
(*Yu Sing*), 8.5 oz. .	450	12.0	69.0	12.0	25	1050	2.0
and shrimp (*Yu Sing*), 8 oz.	400	12.0	65.0	10.0	40	860	2.0
honey roasted (*Lean Cuisine Cafe Classics*), 9.5 oz. .	240	17.0	31.0	5.0	45	590	3.0
rib patty, w/barbecue sauce (*Banquet Family*), 1 patty w/sauce	110	12.0	22.0	12.0	40	520	2.0
ribettes (*Kid Cuisine*), 7.55 oz.	390	16.0	39.0	19.0	50	760	3.0
riblet, boneless (*Banquet*), 10 oz. .	400	17.0	37.0	20.0	45	1070	4.0
Pork entree mix, chops, w/herb stuffing (*Campbell's* Supper Bakes), ⅙ pkg. . . .	160	5.0	31.0	1.0	<5	770	2.0
(*Campbell's* Supper Bakes), ⅙ pkg.* . .	380	24.0	31.0	18.0	70	850	2.0
Pork fat, roasted, 1 oz.	167	2.2	0	17.5	24	177	0
Pork gravy, in jars, ¼ cup:							
(*Franco-American* Gold/Roast Pork) . .	45	1.0	3.0	4.0	5	340	1.0
(*Heinz* Homestyle) . . .	25	1.0	3.0	1.0	0	350	0
Pork gravy mix, ¼ cup*:							
(*McCormick*)	20	0	4.0	0	0	370	0
roasted (*Knorr*)	25	1.0	4.0	.5	0	350	0
Pork lunch meat, 2 oz.:							
(*Boar's Head*)	80	14.0	0	3.0	35	310	0
(*Healthy Deli*)	70	13.0	1.0	1.0	25	340	0

Food and Measure	cal.	prot. (gms)	carbo. (gms)	fat (gms)	chol. (mgs)	sod. (mgs)	fiber (gms)
Pork lunch meat *(cont.)*							
roast, sirloin (*Black Bear*)	70	12.0	0	2.0	30	320	0
Pork rind snack, ½ oz.:							
(*Baken-ets*)	80	7.0	<1.0	5.0	20	330	<1.0
(*Baken-ets* Cracklins)	90	7.0	<1.0	6.0	15	550	<1.0
(*Herr's*)	80	9.0	0	5.0	20	270	0
(*Utz*)	80	9.0	0	5.0	15	230	0
barbecue:							
(*Baken-ets*)	70	7.0	<1.0	5.0	10	400	<1.0
(*Utz*)	80	6.0	0	7.0	15	300	0
hot/spicy (*Utz*)	80	6.0	0	6.0	15	390	0
hot and spicy:							
(*Baken-ets*)	80	7.0	<1.0	5.0	20	470	<1.0
(*Baken-ets* Cracklins)	80	7.0	<1.0	5.0	20	350	<1.0
Pork sandwich, frozen, barbecued, 1 pc.:							
(*Hormel Quick Meal*)	360	15.0	38.0	16.0	45	560	1.0
rib shaped (*Hormel Quick Meal*)	430	14.0	40.0	24.0	50	660	1.0
Pork seasoning and coating mix, ⅛ pkg., except as noted:							
(*Shake 'n Bake* Original)	45	1.0	8.0	.5	0	230	0
barbecue (*Shake 'n Bake* Glaze)	45	0	9.0	1.0	0	410	0
chops (*McCormick Bag'n Season*), ⅙ pkg.	15	0	4.0	0	0	590	0
extra crispy (*Oven Fry*)	60	2.0	11.0	1.5	0	340	0
honey, tangy, or honey mustard (*Shake 'n Bake* Glaze)	45	0	9.0	1.0	0	300	0
hot and spicy (*Shake 'n Bake*)	40	1.0	7.0	1.0	0	170	0
Italian (*Shake 'n Bake* Classic)	40	1.0	7.0	.5	0	270	0
tenderloin, herb roasted (*McCormick Bag'n Season*)	15	0	2.0	0	0	200	0

Food and Measure	cal.	prot. (gms)	carbo. (gms)	fat (gms)	chol. (mgs)	sod. (mgs)	fiber (gms)
Portugese sausage, see "Linguica sausage"							
Posole, see "Corn, dried"							
Pot pie, see specific entree listings							
Pot roast, see "Beef dinner, frozen" and "Beef entree, frozen"							
Potato:							
raw:							
(*Dole*), 1 medium, 5.2 oz.	100	4.0	26.0	0	0	0	3.0
(*Frieda's* Baby/Fingerling/Red/Purple/Yukon Gold/Yellow Finnish), ½ cup, 3 oz.	70	2.0	15.0	0	0	5	1.0
(*Frieda's* Fingerling Bag), 4 pcs., 5.2 oz.	100	4.0	25.0	0	0	0	3.0
unpeeled:							
1 large, 6.5 oz.	145	3.8	33.1	.2	0	11	2.9
1 long, 7.1 oz.	160	4.2	36.3	.2	0	12	3.2
peeled, 2½" potato	88	2.3	20.1	.1	0	7	1.8
peeled, diced, ½ cup	59	1.6	13.5	.1	0	5	1.2
baked:							
in skin, 4¾" x 2⅓"	220	4.7	51.0	.2	0	16	4.8
w/out skin, 2⅓" ..	145	3.1	33.6	.2	0	8	2.3
w/out skin, ½ cup	57	1.2	13.2	.1	0	3	.9
skin only, 1 oz.	56	1.2	13.1	0	0	6	2.2
boiled in skin, peeled:							
2½" potato, 4.8 oz.	118	2.5	27.4	.1	0	6	2.4
½ cup	68	1.5	15.7	.1	0	3	1.4
boiled w/out skin:							
2½" potato	116	2.3	27.0	.1	0	7	2.4
½ cup	67	1.3	15.6	.1	0	4	1.4
microwaved in skin:							
w/skin, 4¾" x 2⅓" potato	212	4.9	48.7	.2	0	16	4.7
peeled, ½ cup	78	1.6	18.2	.1	0	5	1.2
skin only, 2 oz. ...	75	2.5	16.8	.1	0	9	3.2

Food and Measure	cal.	prot. (gms)	carbo. (gms)	fat (gms)	chol. (mgs)	sod. (mgs)	fiber (gms)
Potato *(cont.)*							
mashed, w/whole milk:							
½ cup	81	2.0	18.4	.6	2	318	2.1
w/butter, ½ cup . . .	111	2.0	17.5	4.4	13	309	2.1
w/margarine,							
½ cup	111	2.0	17.5	4.4	2	309	2.1
Potato, can or jar:							
w/liquid, 1 cup	132	3.6	29.7	.3	0	651	4.2
drained:							
1 cup	108	2.5	24.5	.4	0	394	4.1
1.2-oz. potato	21	.5	4.8	.1	0	77	.8
whole:							
(*Butterfield/Sun-*							
shine), 5.6 oz.,							
2½ pcs.	90	2.0	20.0	0	0	330	2.0
new (*Del Monte*),							
2 medium							
w/liquid	60	1.0	13.0	0	0	360	2.0
small (*S&W*), 2 pcs.	60	1.0	13.0	0	0	360	2.0
white (*Libby's*),							
⅔ cup	80	2.0	17.0	0	0	300	2.0
sliced:							
(*Butterfield*), ½ cup	100	2.0	22.0	0	0	390	4.0
new (*Del Monte*),							
⅔ cup	60	1.0	13.0	0	0	360	2.0
diced (*Butterfield*),							
⅔ cup	100	2.0	22.0	0	0	350	3.0
Potato, dehydrated,							
(*AlpineAire*), 1.4 oz.	70	2.0	16.0	0	0	0	1.0
Potato, frozen (see							
also "Potato dish,							
frozen"), 3 oz.,							
except as noted:							
whole:							
(*Birds Eye Southern*),							
3 pcs.	50	1.0	13.0	0	0	25	1.0
(*Bonduelle* Parisian),							
3 oz., about 10 . .	80	2.0	15.0	1.0	0	0	1.0
whole, baby:							
(*Birds Eye* Gourmet),							
4 oz., about 7 pcs.	100	2.0	21.0	0	0	15	1.0
blend (*Birds Eye*							
Gourmet), 2.6 oz.	45	2.0	9.0	0	0	15	1.0

Food and Measure	cal.	prot. (gms)	carbo. (gms)	fat (gms)	chol. (mgs)	sod. (mgs)	fiber (gms)
fried or french-fried:							
(*Cascadian Farm* Oven French Fries)	130	2.0	24.0	4.0	0	10	2.0
(*Crispy Classics* Crinkle Cut/French Fries)	170	2.0	25.0	7.0	0	230	3.0
(*Crispy Classics* Colossal Crinkles)	170	2.0	25.0	7.0	0	290	3.0
(*Inland Valley* Crinkle Cut 32 oz.)	150	2.0	22.0	5.0	0	330	2.0
(*Inland Valley* Crinkle Cut 64 oz.)	130	2.0	22.0	4.0	5	25	2.0
(*Inland Valley* Crinkle Cut 80 oz.)	140	2.0	22.0	5.0	5	330	2.0
(*Inland Valley* French Fries)	130	2.0	21.0	4.0	0	310	2.0
(*Inland Valley* Steak Fries)	110	2.0	18.0	3.0	0	310	2.0
(*Inland Valley* Criss-Cut Fries)	160	2.0	22.0	7.0	0	300	2.0
(*Inland Valley* Curly QQQ's), 1⅓ cups	180	2.0	25.0	8.0	0	340	2.0
(*Inland Valley* Fajita Fries)	170	5.0	24.0	8.0	0	400	2.0
(*Inland Valley* Long Branch Fries) ...	160	2.0	21.0	7.0	0	390	2.0
(*Inland Valley* Tasty QQQ's), 1⅓ cups	190	2.0	25.0	9.0	0	360	2.0
(*Inland Valley* Tater-Babies)	130	2.0	19.0	5.0	0	310	2.0
(*Ore-Ida* Country-French Fries) ...	120	2.0	19.0	4.0	0	240	1.0
(*Ore-Ida* Deep Fries)	140	2.0	23.0	4.5	0	260	2.0
(*Ore-Ida* Shoestrings)	150	2.0	22.0	6.0	0	360	1.0
(*Ore-Ida* Steak Fries)	110	2.0	19.0	3.0	0	360	2.0
(*Ore-Ida* Crispers!)	210	2.0	23.0	12.0	0	420	2.0
(*Ore-Ida* Crispy Crunchies!)	160	2.0	20.0	8.0	0	240	2.0
(*Ore-Ida* Fast Food Fries)	160	2.0	22.0	7.0	0	260	2.0
(*Ore-Ida* Golden Fries)	120	2.0	20.0	3.5	0	360	2.0
(*Ore-Ida* Pixie Crinkles)	130	2.0	20.0	5.0	0	360	2.0

Food and Measure	cal.	prot. (gms)	carbo. (gms)	fat (gms)	chol. (mgs)	sod. (mgs)	fiber (gms)
Potato, frozen, french or french-fried *(cont.)*							
(*Ore-Ida Zesties*) . .	150	2.0	20.0	7.0	0	340	1.0
(*Pacific Valley* Crinkle Cut)	70	2.0	15.0	0	0	5	1.0
(*Tree of Life* Organic)	110	2.0	19.0	3.0	0	75	1.0
seasoned (*Inland Valley CrissCut Fries*)	190	2.0	21.0	11.0	0	540	2.0
hash brown:							
(*Cascadian Farm*), 1 cup	70	2.0	15.0	0	0	20	2.0
(*Inland Valley Home Browns*), 1 patty	130	2.0	15.0	7.0	0	200	2.0
(*Inland Valley Simply Shreds*), 1 cup	70	2.0	15.0	0	0	260	2.0
(*Mr. Dell's* Country Chunks), ¾ cup	70	2.0	14.0	0	0	0	2.0
(*Mr. Dell's* Original Shreds), 1 cup . .	60	2.0	12.0	0	0	0	1.0
(*Ore-Ida* Toaster), 2 pcs., 3.6 oz. . .	220	2.0	25.0	12.0	0	500	2.0
(*Ore-Ida Golden Patties*), 2.2-oz. pc.	130	1.0	14.0	8.0	0	120	1.0
shredded (*Pacific Valley*), 1 cup . .	60	2.0	15.0	0	0	5	1.0
Southern style (*Inland Valley*), ⅔ cup	70	2.0	16.0	0	0	15	2.0
Southern style (*Mr. Dell's* Big Cut), 1 cup	60	2.0	14.0	0	0	0	2.0
mashed:							
(*Inland Valley*), ⅔ cup	160	3.0	22.0	6.0	5	440	3.0
(*Inland Valley* Portionable), 8 pcs.	150	3.0	21.0	6.0	10	420	2.0
(*Ore-Ida*), ⅔ cup and ⅓ cup 2% milk	160	1.0	16.0	2.0	<5	150	1.0

Food and Measure	cal.	prot. (gms)	carbo. (gms)	fat (gms)	chol. (mgs)	sod. (mgs)	fiber (gms)
garlic, roasted (*Inland Valley*), ⅔ cup	150	3.0	24.0	5.0	5	530	2.0
O'Brien (*Inland Valley Simply Shreds O'Brien*), 1 cup ...	60	2.0	10.0	0	0	220	2.0
and onions, in sauce (*Birds Eye Simply Grillin'*), 4.5 oz. ..	180	3.0	25.0	7.0	5	580	3.0
w/peppers and onions (*Cascadian Farm* Country Style), ¾ cup	60	2.0	13.0	0	0	20	2.0
puffs:							
(*Cascadian Farm Seasoned Spud Puppies*)	150	2.0	19.0	8.0	0	400	2.0
(*Cascadian Farm Spud Puppies*) ..	150	2.0	19.0	8.0	0	320	2.0
(*Inland Valley Tater Puffs*)	160	2.0	20.0	7.0	0	380	2.0
(*Tater Tots*), 9 pcs., 3 oz.	170	4.0	21.0	8.0	0	440	2.0
mini (*Tater Tots*), 19 pcs., 3 oz. ..	180	1.0	18.0	10.0	0	440	2.0
onion (*Tater Tots*), 9 pcs., 3 oz. ...	150	1.0	21.0	7.0	0	360	2.0
roasted:							
and broccoli (*Birds Eye*), ⅔ cup	100	3.0	15.0	3.5	5	470	1.0
red (*Cascadian Farm*), 1¼ cups	110	2.0	22.0	1.5	0	170	2.0
wedges (*Pacific Valley*)	120	4.0	25.0	0	0	10	2.0
sticks (*Inland Valley Stix*)	170	2.0	19.0	10.0	0	360	2.0

Potato, mix, see "Potato dish, mix"

Potato, sweet, see "Sweet potato"

Potato chips/crisps (see also "Sweet potato chips"), 1 oz., except as noted:

Food and Measure	cal.	prot. (gms)	carbo. (gms)	fat (gms)	chol. (mgs)	sod. (mgs)	fiber (gms)
Potato chips/crisps *(cont.)*							
(*Bachman*)	160	2.0	15.0	10.0	0	150	1.0
(*Bachman* Wavy)	150	2.0	16.0	8.0	0	95	1.0
(*Barbara's* No Salt) ..	150	2.0	15.0	10.0	0	20	1.0
(*Barbara's* Regular/ Ripple)	150	2.0	15.0	10.0	0	180	1.0
(*Grandma Utz's*)	140	2.0	14.0	8.0	5	120	1.0
(*Hain* Baked Crisps) ..	110	1.0	23.0	1.5	0	150	1.0
(*Herr's/Herr's* Ripple) .	140	2.0	16.0	8.0	0	180	1.0
(*Kettle* Chips Lightly Salted)	150	2.0	15.0	9.0	0	110	1.0
(*Kettle* Crisps Lightly Salted)	110	3.0	22.0	1.5	0	135	2.0
(*Lay's* Baked)	110	2.0	23.0	1.5	0	150	2.0
(*Lay's* Classic/Wavy)	150	2.0	15.0	10.0	0	180	1.0
(*Lay's* Homestyle Classic)	150	2.0	16.0	8.0	0	190	1.0
(*Lay's* Limon)	150	2.0	15.0	10.0	0	370	1.0
(*Lay's* WOW)	75	2.0	18.0	0	0	200	1.0
(*Little Bear* Big Bag) .	160	2.0	15.0	10.0	0	100	0
(*Munchos*)	160	1.0	16.0	10.0	0	230	1.0
(*Ruffles*)	160	2.0	14.0	10.0	0	180	1.0
(*Ruffles* Baked)	120	2.0	21.0	3.0	0	200	2.0
(*Ruffles* Reduced Fat)	130	2.0	18.0	6.7	0	160	1.0
(*Ruffles* The Works!)	160	2.0	14.0	11.0	0	210	1.0
(*Ruffles* WOW)	75	2.0	17.0	0	0	200	1.0
(*Snyder's*)	140	2.0	19.0	6.0	0	90	n.a.
(*Snyder's* Ripple)	140	2.0	18.0	6.0	0	100	n.a.
(*Snyder's* Unsalted) ..	140	2.0	19.0	6.0	0	0	n.a.
(*Tastee* Yukon Gold)	130	3.0	19.0	5.0	0	160	1.0
(*Terra* Potpourri)	150	2.0	17.0	7.0	0	110	4.0
(*Terra* Yukon Gold) ..	130	2.0	19.0	5.0	0	80	0
(*Terra* Blues)	140	3.0	17.0	6.0	0	115	1.0
(*Terra Red Bliss*)	140	2.0	18.0	7.0	0	110	2.0
(*Utz*)	150	2.0	14.0	9.0	0	95	1.0
(*Utz* Homestyle)	140	2.0	14.0	8.0	0	120	1.0
(*Utz* Kettle Classics/ Wavy)	150	2.0	14.0	9.0	0	95	1.0
(*Utz* No Salt)	150	2.0	14.0	9.0	0	5	1.0
(*Utz* Ripple)	150	2.0	14.0	10.0	0	95	1.0
(*Westbrae Natural* No Salt)	160	2.0	15.0	10.0	0	10	0
(*Westbrae Natural* Ripple)	160	2.0	15.0	10.0	0	100	0

Food and Measure	cal.	prot. (gms)	carbo. (gms)	fat (gms)	chol. (mgs)	sod. (mgs)	fiber (gms)
barbecue:							
(*Bachman*)	150	2.0	13.0	10.0	0	270	1.0
(*Grandma Utz's*) . .	150	2.0	15.0	9.0	5	240	1.0
(*Hain* Baked Crisps Louisiana)	110	1.0	23.0	1.5	0	160	1.0
(*Lay's* Wavy)	150	2.0	16.0	9.0	0	210	<1.0
(*Lay's* KC Masterpiece)	150	2.0 ·	15.0	10.0	0	200	1.0
(*Lay's* KC Masterpiece Baked) . . .	120	2.0	22.0	3.0	0	210	2.0
(*Ruffles* KC Masterpiece)	150	1.0	16.0	10.0	0	190	1.0
(*Snyder's*)	150	2.0	21.0	6.0	0	230	n.a.
(*Snyder's* Rib)	140	2.0	17.0	7.0	0	290	n.a.
(*Terra* Yukon Gold)	130	3.0	19.0	5.0	0	90	2.0
(*Utz* Carolina)	150	2.0	14.0	9.0	0	270	1.0
(*Utz* Homestyle) . . .	140	2.0	15.0	8.0	0	240	1.0
(*Utz* Kettle Classics)	150	2.0	14.0	9.0	0	200	1.0
applewood, smoked cheddar (*Lay's* Bistro Gourmet)	150	2.0	14.0	10.0	0	330	1.0
hickory (*Kettle* Crisps)	110	3.0	22.0	1.5	0	160	2.0
spicy (*Lay's*)	150	2.0	15.0	9.0	0	210	1.0
barbecue, mesquite:							
(*Lay's* Homestyle) .	140	2.0	16.0	8.0	0	210	<1.0
(*Lay's* WOW)	75	2.0	17.0	0	0	250	0
(*Ruffles* KC Masterpiece)	150	1.0	15.0	10.0	0	190	1.0
barbecue cheddar (*Ruffles* Flavor Rush)	160	2.0	15.0	10.0	0	320	1.0
Buffalo style (*Ruffles*)	160	2.0	16.0	10.0	0	230	1.0
cheddar:							
(*Lay's* Cracker Barrel)	150	2.0	16.0	9.0	0	210	1.0
w/herbs (*Kettle* Chips New York)	150	2.0	15.0	9.0	0	190	1.0
sharp, and jalapeño (*Lay's* Bistro Gourmet)	150	2.0	14.0	10.0	0	350	1.0
cheddar/salsa (*Ruffles* Flavor Rush Ultimate)	160	2.0	14.0	10.0	0	320	<1.0

Food and Measure	cal.	prot. (gms)	carbo. (gms)	fat (gms)	chol. (mgs)	sod. (mgs)	fiber (gms)
Potato chips/crisps *(cont.)*							
cheddar/sour cream:							
(*Ruffles*)	160	2.0	14.0	10.0	0	190	1.0
(*Ruffles* Baked) ...	120	2.0	22.0	3.0	0	220	2.0
(*Ruffles WOW*) ...	75	3.0	16.0	0	0	230	1.0
(*Utz*)	160	2.0	14.0	10.0	0	200	1.0
chili, green, and lime							
(*Snyder's*)	150	2.0	20.0	6.0	0	300	n.a.
chili, habanero (*Kettle*							
Chips)	140	2.0	8.0	0	0	185	<1.0
crab:							
(*Utz*)	150	2.0	14.0	9.0	0	300	1.0
spicy (*Snyder's*							
Chesapeake Bay)	140	2.0	20.0	6.0	0	280	0
crème fraîche and dill							
(*Terra Blues*)	140	2.0	17.0	6.0	0	110	1.0
dill, kosher (*Snyder's*)	140	2.0	20.0	6.0	0	360	n.a.
garlic, roasted, and							
herb (*Lay's* Bistro							
Gourmet)	150	2.0	15.0	9.0	0	350	1.0
grilled steak and onion							
(*Snyder's*) ... .,	140	2.0	20.0	6.0	0	140	n.a.
honey Dijon (*Kettle*							
Chips)	150	2.0	16.0	8.0	0	150	1.0
hot:							
(*Bachman*)	150	2.0	15.0	9.0	0	230	1.0
(*Lay's* Flamin')	150	2.0	15.0	9.0	0	200	1.0
(*Utz* Red Hot)	150	2.0	14.0	9.0	0	220	1.0
Buffalo (*Snyder's*)	150	2.0	20.0	7.0	0	330	n.a.
jalapeño (*Snyder's*) ..	150	2.0	20.0	6.0	0	330	n.a.
ketchup (*Herr's Heinz*)	150	2.0	15.0	10.0	0	300	1.0
malt vinegar (*Terra*							
Frites)	150	2.0	18.0	8.0	0	200	3.0
mustard and honey							
(*Kettle* Crisps)	110	3.0	22.0	1.5	0	160	2.0
olive oil and:							
fine herbs (*Terra*							
Red Bliss)	140	2.0	18.0	7.0	0	70	3.0
roasted garlic,							
Parmesan (*Terra*							
Red Bliss)	140	2.0	16.0	7.0	0	115	2.0
sun-dried tomato,							
balsamic vinegar							
(*Terra Red Bliss*)	140	2.0	18.0	7.0	0	85	3.0

Food and Measure	cal.	prot. (gms)	carbo. (gms)	fat (gms)	chol. (mgs)	sod. (mgs)	fiber (gms)
onion, French (*Kettle* Crisps)	110	3.0	22.0	1.5	0	190	2.0
onion and garlic:							
(*Herr's*)	150	2.0	14.0	10.0	0	300	1.0
(*Terra* Yukon Gold)	130	2.0	19.0	5.0	0	65	1.0
ranch (*Lay's* Wavy) . .	150	2.0	15.0	10.0	0	200	1.0
salsa w/mesquite (*Kettle* Chips)	140	2.0	15.0	8.0	0	160	1.0
salt and pepper (*Terra* Yukon Gold)	130	2.0	19.0	5.0	0	120	1.0
salt and vinegar:							
(*Herr's*)	150	2.0	15.0	10.0	0	340	1.0
(*Lay's*)	150	2.0	15.0	10.0	0	380	1.0
(*Snyder's*)	140	2.0	19.0	6.0	0	250	n.a.
(*Terra* Yukon Gold)	130	2.0	20.0	5.0	0	110	2.0
(*Utz*)	150	2.0	14.0	9.0	0	270	1.0
sea (*Kettle* Chips)	150	2.0	15.0	8.0	0	180	1.0
sour cream/onion:							
(*Bachman*)	150	2.0	15.0	9.0	0	190	1.0
(*Lay's*)	160	2.0	12.0	11.0	<5	200	1.0
(*Lay's* Baked)	120	2.0	21.0	3.0	0	210	2.0
(*Lay's WOW*)	80	2.0	17.0	0	0	230	1.0
(*Ruffles* Flavor Rush)	150	2.0	15.0	10.0	0	260	1.0
(*Snyder's*)	150	2.0	19.0	7.0	0	150	n.a.
(*Utz*)	160	2.0	14.0	10.0	0	140	1.0
sticks:							
(*Butterfield*), ²⁄₃ cup, 1 oz. . . .	150	2.0	16.0	9.0	0	90	2.0
(*Butterfield* 1.7 oz.), 1 cup	250	3.0	26.0	15.0	1	150	3.0
(*French's*), 1 cup . .	250	3.0	23.0	16.0	0	270	1.0
hot (*Chester's* Fries Flamin')	150	2.0	17.0	8.0	0	270	<1.0
taco (*Snyder's* Fiesta)	150	2.0	20.0	7.0	0	270	n.a.
vinegar (*Bachman*) . .	150	2.0	15.0	9.0	0	260	1.0
yogurt-green onion:							
(*Barbara's*)	150	2.0	15.0	9.0	0	240	1.0
(*Kettle* Chips)	150	2.0	15.0	8.0	0	170	1.0
(*Terra* Yukon Gold)	130	2.0	19.0	5.0	0	75	1.0
Potato chips/dip kit, 1 pkg.:							
onion dip (*Ruffles*) . .	460	7.0	32.0	34.0	5	1070	3.0
ranch dip (*Ruffles*) . .	470	7.0	33.0	35.0	5	1080	3.0

Food and Measure	cal.	prot. (gms)	carbo. (gms)	fat (gms)	chol. (mgs)	sod. (mgs)	fiber (gms)
Potato dish, can or pkg., 1 cont.:							
au gratin w/ham (*Dinty Moore American Classics/Cure 81*) ..	290	12.0	29.0	14.0	35	980	1.0
butter and herb (*Bowl Appétit!*)	210	4.0	40.0	5.0	5	890	3.0
mashed:							
cheesy (*Bowl Appétit!*)	270	5.0	46.0	8.0	5	900	3.0
cheesy broccoli (*Bowl Appétit!*) .	260	5.0	43.0	9.0	0	930	3.0
sour cream/chive (*Bowl Appétit!*) .	210	4.0	41.0	4.0	5	870	3.0
scalloped w/ham (*Hormel* Microcup)	240	7.0	20.0	14.0	35	920	2.0
Potato dish, dried, 1 serving:							
and beef (*Mountain House*)	290	13.0	43.0	7.0	30	750	7.0
and cheddar, w/chives (*AlpineAire*)	350	7.0	39.0	4.5	n.a.	350	3.0
and cheese (*Mountain House*)	330	16.0	40.0	11.0	40	1020	4.0
Potato dish, frozen:							
au gratin:							
(*Cascadian Farm*), ⅔ cup	110	5.0	15.0	4.0	0	290	1.0
(*Stouffer's* Side Dish), ½ cup ...	130	4.0	15.0	6.0	15	590	1.0
ham and broccoli (*Banquet* Family), ⅔ cup	210	7.0	16.0	13.0	30	970	2.0
baked, twice, butter flavor (*Ore-Ida*), 1 pc.	160	3.0	24.0	6.0	0	330	3.0
cheddar (*Lean Cuisine Everyday Favorites* Deluxe), 10⅜ oz.	260	13.0	37.0	7.0	20	630	5.0
cheddar broccoli:							
(*Healthy Choice* Solos), 10.5-oz. pkg. ..	280	13.0	41.0	7.0	25	550	6.0
(*Michelina's*), 9.5 oz.	380	17.0	35.0	19.0	40	1120	2.0

Food and Measure	cal.	prot. (gms)	carbo. (gms)	fat (gms)	chol. (mgs)	sod. (mgs	fiber (gms)
mashed, w/gravy:							
beef gravy (*Larry's*), 4.5-oz. tray	160	3.0	21.0	7.0	0	410	<1.0
chicken gravy (*Larry's*), 4.5-oz. tray	170	4.0	21.0	8.0	0	430	<1.0
pancake, see "Potato pancake"							
pot pie, cheesy and broccoli w/ham (*Banquet*), 7 oz.	410	9.0	40.0	23.0	25	1220	2.0
roasted:							
w/broccoli (*Lean Cuisine Everyday Favorites*), 10.25-oz. pkg.	240	11.0	37.0	5.0	20	690	5.0
w/broccoli, cheese sauce (*Green Giant*), ¾ cup ..	120	4.0	19.0	3.5	5	520	2.0
w/garlic and herbs (*Green Giant*), 1¼ cups	270	3.0	33.0	14.0	0	760	4.0
w/ham (*Healthy Choice* Bowl), 8.5-oz. pkg. ...	210	17.0	26.0	4.0	30	600	6.0
scalloped:							
(*Stouffer's Family Style Favorites* 40 oz.), ½ cup ..	140	4.0	19.0	5.0	3	560	2.0
(*Stouffer's Side Dish*), ½ cup ...	170	4.0	18.0	9.0	15	540	1.0
skins (*Inland Valley Munch Skins Meals*), ⅔ cup, 5 oz.	150	3.0	24.0	5.0	5	530	2.0
stuffed, 1 pc.:							
bacon and cheese (*Larry's*)	200	4.0	24.0	10.0	5	570	1.0
bacon and cheese (*Oh Boy!*)	130	3.0	23.0	3.0	5	250	2.0
broccoli and cheese (*Larry's*)	190	4.0	23.0	9.0	5	560	1.0
cheddar cheese (*Oh Boy!*)	130	3.0	22.0	4.0	<5	270	2.0

Food and Measure	cal.	prot. (gms)	carbo. (gms)	fat (gms)	chol. (mgs)	sod. (mgs)	fiber (gms)
Potato dish, frozen, stuffed *(cont.)*							
sour cream and							
chive (*Oh Boy!*)	110	2.0	22.0	2.0	<5	260	2.0
Potato dish, mix:							
Alfredo (*Knorr* Skillet							
Potatoes), ½ cup ..	110	3.0	20.0	3.0	<5	1170	1.0
au gratin:							
(*Betty Crocker*):							
½ cup*	150	3.0	22.0	6.0	5	590	1.0
low fat, ½ cup*	110	3.0	22.0	1.5	0	560	1.0
(*Betty Crocker* 9 oz.):							
½ cup*	150	3.0	23.0	6.0	<5	620	1.0
low fat, ½ cup*	110	3.0	23.0	1.5	0	590	1.0
(*Hungry Jack*),							
½ cup	110	2.0	22.0	1.0	0	570	1.0
(*!dahoan*), ⅔ cup	110	3.0	20.0	1.5	0	690	2.0
bacon and cheddar,							
twice baked (*Betty*							
Crocker):							
⅔ cup*	210	6.0	22.0	11.0	85	580	1.0
low fat, ⅔ cup* ...	130	6.0	22.0	2.0	0	540	1.0
bacon and cheese							
(*Knorr* Skillet							
Potatoes), ½ cup ..	110	3.0	18.0	2.0	10	590	2.0
broccoli au gratin							
(*Betty Crocker*):							
½ cup*	150	3.0	21.0	6.0	<5	540	2.0
low fat, ½ cup* ...	120	3.0	21.0	2.5	0	520	2.0
cheddar, white (*Nile*							
Spice Cup), 1.5 oz.	170	5.0	29.0	4.0	10	730	3.0
cheddar and bacon:							
(*Betty Crocker*):							
½ cup*	150	3.0	21.0	6.0	<5	650	1.0
low fat, ½ cup*	120	3.0	21.0	3.0	0	620	1.0
(*Hungry Jack*),							
½ cup	110	2.0	22.0	1.0	0	500	2.0
cheddar, cheesy (*Knorr*							
Skillet Potatoes),							
½ cup	130	4.0	19.0	4.0	10	850	2.0
cheese, three (*Betty*							
Crocker):							
½ cup*	150	3.0	23.0	6.0	<5	600	2.0
low fat, ½ cup* ...	130	3.0	23.0	3.0	0	580	2.0

Food and Measure	cal.	prot. (gms)	carbo. (gms)	fat (gms)	chol. (mgs)	sod. (mgs)	fiber (gms)
chicken/vegetable (*Betty Crocker*):							
⅔ cup*	160	4.0	24.0	6.0	<5	560	2.0
low fat, ⅔ cup* . . .	120	4.0	24.0	2.5	<5	510	2.0
garlic, roasted: (*Knorr* Skillet Potatoes), ⅔ cup . . .	120	3.0	23.0	1.0	0	570	3.0
hash browns: (*Betty Crocker*), ½ cup*	190	3.0	30.0	8.0	0	620	3.0
(*Idahoan*), ⅓ cup . .	90	2.0	18.0	.5	0	110	1.0
cheesy (*Knorr* Skillet Potatoes), ⅓ cup	120	3.0	22.0	3.0	<5	990	1.0
oniony (*Knorr* Skillet Potatoes), ⅓ cup	100	2.0	20.0	.5	0	620	2.0
julienne (*Betty Crocker*):							
½ cup*	150	3.0	21.0	6.0	<5	620	1.0
low fat, ½ cup* . . .	110	3.0	21.0	2.5	0	600	1.0
kugel (*Manischewitz*), 2½ tbsp.	70	2.0	15.0	1.5	0	420	2.0
mashed:							
(*Barbara's*), ⅓ cup .	70	2.0	17.0	0	0	10	1.0
(*Betty Crocker* Potato Buds):							
⅔ cup*	160	3.0	19.0	8.0	<5	460	1.0
low fat, ⅔ cup* .	120	3.0	19.0	4.0	0	420	1.0
(*Hungry Jack* Flakes), ⅓ cup flakes . . .	80	2.0	18.0	0	0	25	1.0
(*Idahoan* Complete), ½ cup*	110	2.0	20.0	2.0	0	270	2.0
(*Idahoan* Original), ⅓ cup	80	2.0	18.0	0	0	15	2.0
(*Idahoan* Premium), ¼ cup	80	2.0	17.0	1.0	0	270	1.0
butter, creamy (*Betty Crocker*):							
½ cup*	160	3.0	20.0	8.0	<5	430	1.0
low fat, ½ cup*	130	3.0	20.0	4.5	<5	410	1.0
butter and herb: (*Betty Crocker*):							
½ cup*	160	3.0	20.0	8.0	5	470	1.0
lower fat, ½ cup*	130	3.0	20.0	4.5	<5	450	1.0
(*Idahoan*), ½ cup*	110	2.0	20.0	2.5	0	560	1.0

Food and Measure	cal.	prot. (gms)	carbo. (gms)	fat (gms)	chol. (mgs)	sod. (mgs)	fiber (gms)
Potato dish, mix, mashed *(cont.)*							
cheddar, creamy white (*Near East* Meal Cup), 1 pkg.	160	5.0	49.0	4.0	10	730	3.0
cheddar and bacon (*Betty Crocker*) ½ cup*	150	3.0	20.0	7.0	5	390	1.0
cheese, four: (*Betty Crocker*):							
½ cup*	150	3.0	20.0	7.0	<5	540	1.0
lower fat, ½ cup*	120	3.0	20.0	4.0	0	520	1.0
cheese, four (*Idahoan*), ½ cup*	100	2.0	19.0	2.5	0	550	1.0
chicken and herb (*Betty Crocker*):							
½ cup*	150	3.0	21.0	7.0	0	520	1.0
lower fat, ½ cup*	120	3.0	21.0	3.5	0	500	1.0
garlic, roasted (*Betty Crocker*):							
½ cup*	150	3.0	19.0	8.0	<5	400	2.0
lower fat, ½ cup*	130	3.0	19.0	4.5	0	380	2.0
garlic, roasted (*Idahoan*), ½ cup*	110	2.0	20.0	2.5	0	600	1.0
garlic, roasted, and rosemary (*Near East* Meal Cup), 1 pkg.	170	2.0	34.0	3.5	10	510	3.0
garlic, roasted, and rosemary (*Nile Spice* Cup), 1.6-oz. pkg. . . .	180	5.0	32.0	4.0	10	530	3.0
sour cream/chive: (*Betty Crocker*):							
½ cup*	150	3.0	21.0	7.0	5	440	1.0
lower fat, ½ cup*	120	3.0	21.0	3.5	<5	420	1.0
mashed, and gravy: beef, hearty (*Betty Crocker*), ¾ cup*	170	3.0	24.0	7.0	0	760	2.0
chicken, roasted (*Betty Crocker*), ¾ cup*	170	3.0	25.0	7.0	5	670	1.0

Food and Measure	cal.	prot. (gms)	carbo. (gms)	fat (gms)	chol. (mgs)	sod. (mgs	fiber (gms)
pancake, see "Potato pancake mix"							
ranch (*Betty Crocker*):							
½ cup*	160	3.0	25.0	6.0	<5	610	2.0
low fat, ½ cup* . . .	120	3.0	25.0	2.0	<5	580	2.0
scalloped:							
(*Betty Crocker*):							
½ cup*	160	3.0	23.0	6.0	<5	600	1.0
low fat, ⅔ cup*	110	3.0	23.0	1.0	0	570	1.0
(*Betty Crocker* 8.25 oz.):							
½ cup*	150	3.0	23.0	6.0	<5	620	1.0
low fat, ⅔ cup*	110	3.0	23.0	1.0	0	580	1.0
(*Idahoan*), ⅔ cup mix	100	2.0	21.0	1.5	0	610	1.0
scalloped, cheesy:							
(*Betty Crocker*):							
½ cup*	150	3.0	20.0	6.0	<5	540	1.0
low fat, ½ cup*	120	3.0	20.0	3.0	0	520	1.0
(*Hungry Jack*), ½ cup	110	2.0	22.0	1.5	0	520	1.0
scalloped, cheese and bacon (*Knorr Skillet Potatoes*), ½ cup	110	3.0	18.0	2.0	10	590	2.0
scalloped, creamy (*Hungry Jack*), ½ cup	110	2.0	22.0	1.5	0	420	2.0
sour cream/chive:							
(*Betty Crocker*), ½ cup*	160	3.0	22.0	7.0	5	600	2.0
(*Hungry Jack*), ½ cup	110	2.0	22.0	2.0	<5	460	1.0
Southwestern (*Knorr Skillet Potatoes*), ½ cup	140	3.0	25.0	2.5	0	750	3.0
Potato entree, see "Potato dish"							
Potato flour, 1 cup . .	571	11.0	132.9	.5	0	88	9.4
Potato knish, 1 pc.:							
frozen (*Cohen's*)	220	5.0	40.0	4.5	5	550	2.0
refrigerated (*Joshua's Coney Island*)	380	7.0	59.0	12.0	0	660	3.0

Food and Measure	cal.	prot. (gms)	carbo. (gms)	fat (gms)	chol. (mgs)	sod. (mgs)	fiber (gms)
Potato pancake, frozen:							
(*Dr. Praeger's*),							
1.5-oz. cake	80	2.0	10.0	3.0	15	150	1.0
(*Empire* Kosher),							
2-oz. cake	80	1.0	15.0	2.0	0	200	8.0
(*Empire* Kosher Mini),							
12 cakes, 3 oz. . . .	150	2.0	19.0	7.0	0	200	2.0
(*Inland Valley*),							
2-oz. cake	120	2.0	12.0	8.0	20	310	2.0
(*Kineret* Latkas),							
1.5-oz. cake	80	1.0	11.0	3.5	0	250	3.0
(*Kineret* Latkas Mini),							
10 pcs., 3 oz.	220	2.5	28.0	10.0	0	350	2.5
(*King Kold*), 2 cakes,							
2 oz.	190	4.0	28.0	8.0	0	340	<1.0
(*Ratner's*), 1.5-oz. cake	110	3.0	12.0	7.0	30	160	1.0
(*Tofutti*), 1.3-oz. cake	71	2.0	10.0	3.0	0	187	1.0
Potato pancake mix:							
(*Carmel*), 3 tbsp. . . .	80	2.0	18.0	1.0	0	500	2.0
(*Manischewitz*),							
3 tbsp.	80	2.0	18.0	1.0	0	500	2.0
(*Mrs. Manischewitz* Homestyle Latka),							
2 tbsp.	80	2.0	18.0	1.0	0	600	2.0
Potato salad:							
(*Black Bear* Northwestern), ¾ cup . .	360	5.0	18.0	30.0	30	680	3.0
(*Blue Ridge Farms*),							
½ cup	180	2.0	22.0	10.0	10	550	1.0
(*Chef's Express*), 4 oz.	260	2.0	16.0	21.0	5	450	1.0
red skin (*Blue Ridge Farms*), 4 oz., about							
½ cup	190	2.0	25.0	9.0	10	470	2.0
Potato salad seasoning (*Watkins*),							
¼ tsp.	0	0	0	0	0	135	0
Potato seasoning mix, ⅛ pkt., except as noted:							
Cheddar (*Shake 'n Bake Perfect Potatoes Zesty Cheddar*)	25	1.0	3.0	1.0	<5	410	0
french fries (*Shake 'n Bake Perfect Potatoes*)	15	0	3.0	0	0	460	0

Food and Measure	cal.	prot. (gms)	carbo. (gms)	fat (gms)	chol. (mgs)	sod. (mgs)	fiber (gms)
fries, oven (McCormick Produce Partners), ⅕ pkt. .	30	0	3.0	1.0	0	660	0
herb garlic (Shake 'n Bake Perfect Potatoes)	20	0	5.0	0	0	340	0
roasted:							
cheddar (McCormick Produce Partners)	35	0	2.0	1.5	0	420	0
Italian herb (McCormick Produce Partners)	30	0	2.0	1.5	0	430	0
onion (McCormick Produce Partners)	30	0	2.0	1.0	0	500	0
Potato starch (Manischewitz), 1 tbsp.	30	0	8.0	0	0	0	0
Potato sticks, see "Potato chips/crisps"							
Poultry seasoning, 1 tsp.	5	.1	1.0	.1	0	tr.	.2
Pout, ocean, meat only:							
raw, 4 oz.	90	18.9	0	1.0	59	69	0
baked, broiled, or microwaved, 4 oz.	116	24.2	0	1.3	76	88	0
Praline sauce (Trader Vic's), 2 tbsp.	120	1.0	21.0	5.0	0	50	0
Pretzels, 1 oz., except as noted:							
(Air Crisps)	110	3.0	22.0	1.0	0	530	<1.0
(Estee Unsalted), 23 pcs., 1.1 oz. . . .	120	3.0	25.0	1.0	0	30	1.0
(Goldfish), 43 pcs., 1.1 oz.	120	3.0	22.0	2.5	0	430	<1.0
(Snyder's Homestyle)	120	3.0	25.0	1.0	0	230	n.a.
(Snyder's Olde Tyme)	120	3.0	24.0	1.0	0	120	n.a.
(Snyder's Olde Tyme Organic Unsalted) .	120	3.0	24.0	1.0	0	75	n.a.
(Snyder's Specials) . .	120	3.0	23.0	1.0	0	450	n.a.
cheese:							
cheddar (Combos) 1.8-oz. bag	240	5.0	35.0	8.0	0	550	1.0
cheddar (Rold Gold Tiny Twists)	110	3.0	22.0	1.0	0	440	1.0
mini (Snyder's) . . .	140	3.0	19.0	5.0	0	410	n.a.

Food and Measure	cal.	prot. (gms)	carbo. (gms)	fat (gms)	chol. (mgs)	sod. (mgs)	fiber (gms)
Pretzels, cheese *(cont.)*							
nacho *(Combos),* 1.8-oz. bag	240	5.0	34.0	8.0	0	580	1.0
Dutch *(Estee),* 2 pcs., 1.1 oz.	130	3.0	26.0	1.0	0	40	1.0
hard:							
(Snyder's Unsalted)	100	3.0	22.0	0	0	90	n.a.
plain	108	2.6	22.5	1.0	0	486	.8
pumpernickel and onion *(Snyder's)*	100	3.0	21.0	1.0	0	350	n.a.
honey *(Bachman Kidzels)*	110	3.0	21.0	1.5	0	420	<1.0
honey mustard *(Rold Gold* Tiny Twists) ..	110	3.0	22.0	1.0	0	370	1.0
mini:							
(Bachman Petite) ..	100	3.0	22.0	1.0	0	800	1.0
(Snyder's)	110	3.0	25.0	0	0	250	n.a.
(Snyder's Organic) .	110	3.0	25.0	0	0	250	n.a.
(Snyder's Unsalted)	110	3.0	25.0	0	0	75	n.a.
nibblers:							
(Snyder's No Salt/ Fat Free)	120	3.0	25.0	0	0	50	n.a.
garlic bread *(Snyder's)*	130	2.0	24.0	3.0	0	180	n.a.
honey mustard onion *(Snyder's)*	130	3.0	23.0	3.0	0	95	n.a.
savory *(Snyder's)*	130	3.0	23.0	3.0	0	200	n.a.
sourdough *(Snyder's* Fat Free)	120	3.0	25.0	3.0	0	200	n.a.
pieces:							
buttermilk ranch *(Snyder's)*	130	3.0	19.0	5.0	0	250	<1.0
caramel, creamy *(Snyder's)*	130	2.0	19.0	5.0	0	150	<1.0
cheddar *(Snyder's)*	130	2.0	18.0	6.0	0	260	<1.0
honey BBQ *(Snyder's)*	130	4.0	17.0	5.0	0	150	<1.0
honey mustard onion *(Snyder's)*	140	2.0	18.0	7.0	0	240	<1.0
jalapeño *(Snyder's)*	140	2.0	20.0	5.0	0	370	<1.0
pizza flavor:							
(Combos Pizzaria)	130	3.0	19.0	4.5	0	290	1.0

Food and Measure	cal.	prot. (gms)	carbo. (gms)	fat (gms)	chol. (mgs)	sod. (mgs)	fiber (gms)
(*Combos* Pizzaria), 1.8-oz. bag	230	4.0	35.0	8.0	0	560	1.0
pepperoni (*Combo*)	140	2.0	18.0	6.0	0	290	0
pepperoni (*Combos*), 1.7-oz. bag	240	4.0	31.0	11.0	0	470	1.0
rods:							
(*Bachman*), 1.1 oz.	110	3.0	24.0	.5	0	260	1.0
(*Rold Gold*)	110	3.0	22.0	1.0	0	610	1.0
(*Snyder's*)	120	3.0	24.0	1.0	0	400	n.a.
snaps:							
(*Snyder's*)	120	3.0	25.0	1.0	0	390	n.a.
butter (*Snyder's*) ..	120	3.0	25.0	1.0	0	270	n.a.
sourdough:							
(*Bachman*)	110	3.0	22.0	1.0	0	240	1.0
(*Rold Gold* Specials)	110	3.0	23.0	0	0	470	1.0
bites (*Bachman*) ..	110	3.0	22.0	1.0	0	240	1.0
hard (*Herr's*)	100	3.0	23.0	0	0	450	2.0
hard (*Rold Gold*) ..	100	2.0	21.0	.5	0	500	1.0
hard (*Snyder's*) ...	100	3.0	22.0	0	0	240	n.a.
hard (*Wege* Original), .9-oz. pc.	120	2.0	25.0	1.0	0	470	<1.0
hard, honey wheat (*Wege*), .8-oz. pc.	120	2.0	24.0	1.5	0	20	1.0
spelt (*VitaSpelt*)	110	3.0	23.0	.5	0	350	3.0
sticks:							
(*Bachman* Stix) ...	100	2.0	20.0	1.0	0	520	1.0
(*Rold Gold*)	100	2.0	23.0	0	0	680	1.0
(*Snyder's* Dipping) .	100	3.0	22.0	0	0	330	n.a.
(*Snyder's* Olde Tyme)	110	3.0	23.0	1.0	0	300	n.a.
butter, tiny (*Snyder's*)	120	3.0	25.0	0	0	360	n.a.
honey wheat (*Snyder's* Organic)	130	3.0	24.0	2.0	0	210	n.a.
oat bran (*Snyder's* Organic)	120	3.0	25.0	0	0	320	n.a.
thins:							
(*Bachman* Thin 'n Right), 1.1 oz. ...	120	3.0	23.0	1.0	0	650	1.0
(*Rold Gold* Fat Free)	100	3.0	23.0	0	0	510	1.0
(*Snyder's*)	110	3.0	23.0	0	0	330	n.a.
twists:							
(*Bachman*)	100	3.0	22.0	1.0	0	650	1.0

Food and Measure	cal.	prot. (gms)	carbo. (gms)	fat (gms)	chol. (mgs)	sod. (mgs)	fiber (gms)
Pretzels *(cont.)*							
(*Rold Gold* Thin) ..	110	2.0	23.0	1.0	0	560	1.0
(*Rold Gold* Tiny) ..	110	2.0	23.0	1.0	0	580	1.0
(*Rold Gold* Tiny Fat Free)	100	3.0	23.0	0	0	420	1.0
Pretzels, soft:							
(*SuperPretzel*), 2.25-oz. pc.	180	6.0	36.0	1.0	0	140	2.0
bites (*SuperPretzel*), 5 pcs., 1.9 oz.	140	3.0	32.0	.5	0	115	1.0
cheese-filled (*Super-Pretzel Softstix*), 2 pcs., 1.8 oz.	140	5.0	24.0	2.5	10	250	1.0
Pretzel dip, honey-mustard:							
(*Nance's*), 2 tbsp.	90	1.0	18.0	2.0	0	600	0
(*Snyder's*), 1 oz.	70	1.0	15.0	1.0	0	240	0
Prickly pear:							
(*Andy Boy D'Arrigo*), 5-oz. pear	60	1.0	13.0	.5	0	5	5.0
(*Frieda's* Cactus Pear), 5 oz.	60	1.0	13.0	.5	0	5	5.0
4.8-oz. fruit, 3.6 oz. trimmed	42	.8	9.9	.5	0	5	3.7
1 cup	61	1.1	14.3	.8	0	7	5.4
Prosciutto, 1 oz., except as noted:							
(*Black Bear* di Parma)	80	7.0	0	6.0	25	640	0
(*Citterio/Citterio Fresco*), 2 slices, 1.1 oz.	70	8.0	0	4.5	20	730	0
(*Boar's Head* Bone-less/Skinless)	60	10.0	0	3.0	20	890	0
(*Boar's Head* Panino)	80	6.0	1.0	6.0	20	200	0
(*Boar's Head* Piccolo)	60	7.0	0	3.5	15	450	0
(*Boar's Head* Riserva Stradolce)	60	8.0	0	3.0	15	770	0
(*Primissimo*), 2 oz.	120	15.0	0	7.0	50	1080	0
Prosciutto-mozzarella roll (*Boar's Head* Prosciutto Panino), 1 oz.	80	6.0	1.0	6.0	20	200	0

Food and Measure	cal.	prot. (gms)	carbo. (gms)	fat (gms)	chol. (mgs)	sod. (mgs)	fiber (gms)
Prune, see "Plum, dried"							
Prune juice, 8 fl. oz.:							
(*Langers*)	180	0	41.0	0	0	10	1.0
(*R. W. Knudsen* Organic) . . . . . : . . .	170	1.0	45.0	0	0	20	3.0
(*Sunsweet*)	170	1.0	42.0	0	0	35	3.0
canned	182	1.6	44.7	.1	0	10	2.6
Pudding (see also specific listings), 4-oz. cont., except as noted:							
banana:							
(*Kozy Shack*)	130	3.0	22.0	3.0	15	150	0
(*Kraft Handi-Snacks*), 3.5 oz.	120	<1.0	20.0	4.0	0	130	0
butterscotch:							
(*Kraft Handi-Snacks*), 3.5 oz.	110	1.0	21.0	3.0	0	140	0
(*Swiss Miss*)	160	3.0	24.0	6.0	0	180	0
caramel sundae (*Jell-O* Fat Free)	100	2.0	23.0	0	0	230	0
chocolate:							
(*Jell-O*)	140	2.0	27.0	4.0	0	180	1.0
(*Jell-O* Fat Free) . .	100	2.0	23.0	0	0	180	<1.0
(*Kozy Shack*)	140	4.0	24.0	3.5	15	140	<1.0
(*Kraft Handi-Snacks*), 3.5 oz.	110	1.0	21.0	3.5	0	150	<1.0
(*Swiss Miss*)	160	3.0	25.0	5.0	0	180	0
(*Swiss Miss* Fat Free)	90	2.0	20.0	0	0	135	0
chocolate caramel (*Jell-O*)	140	2.0	26.0	4.0	0	170	<1.0
chocolate cream pie (*Swiss Miss*)	170	3.0	24.0	7.0	0	180	0
chocolate fudge:							
(*Kraft Handi-Snacks*), 3.5 oz.	110	1.0	21.0	3.5	0	160	<1.0
sundae (*Jell-O* Fat Free)	100	2.0	24.0	0	0	220	0
chocolate fudge caramel sundae (*Jell-O* Fat Free)	100	2.0	24.0	0	0	230	0
chocolate-vanilla swirl:							
(*Jello-O*)	140	2.0	26.0	4.0	0	170	<1.0

Food and Measure	cal.	prot. (gms)	carbo. (gms)	fat (gms)	chol. (mgs)	sod. (mgs)	fiber (gms)
Pudding *(cont.)*							
(*Swiss Miss*)	160	2.0	26.0	6.0	0	160	0
lemon meringue pie							
(*Swiss Miss*)	150	0	30.0	3.0	0	60	0
rocky road (*Kraft Handi-Snacks*),							
3.5 oz.	120	<1.0	23.0	3.5	0	110	<1.0
tapioca:							
(*Jell-O*)	130	1.0	25.0	3.0	0	150	0
(*Jell-O* Fat Free) . . .	100	2.0	23.0	0	0	230	0
(*Kozy Shack*)	130	3.0	23.0	3.0	15	140	0
(*Kraft Handi-Snacks*),							
3.5 oz.	120	1.0	20.0	3.5	0	115	0
(*Swiss Miss*)	140	2.0	24.0	3.5	0	170	0
vanilla:							
(*Jell-O*)	130	1.0	24.0	3.5	0	160	0
(*Jell-O* Fat Free) . . .	100	2.0	23.0	0	0	240	0
(*Kozy Shack*)	130	3.0	22.0	3.0	15	150	0
(*Kraft Handi-Snacks*),							
3.5 oz.	100	<1.0	20.0	3.5	0	130	0
(*Swiss Miss*)	160	2.0	24.0	6.0	0	190	0
Pudding, nondairy, 1 cont.:							
banana (*Imagine*) . . .	140	1.0	28.0	3.0	0	40	0
butterscotch (*Imagine*)	140	1.0	28.0	3.0	0	55	<1.0
chocolate (*Imagine*)	160	1.0	34.0	3.0	0	85	<1.0
lemon (*Imagine*)	140	1.0	31.0	3.0	0	55	<1.0
tofu, almond or vanilla (*Azumaya Spoonables/Nasoya Temptations*)	120	5.0	19.0	2.5	0	15	<1.0
tofu, chocolate (*Azumaya Spoonables/Nasoya Temptations*)	170	6.0	28.0	3.5	0	85	1.0
Pudding and pie filling mix, ½ cup*, except as noted:							
banana (*Watkins*), 1 tbsp.	40	0	10.0	0	0	170	0
banana cream:							
(*Jell-O*)	140	4.0	26.0	2.5	10	240	0
(*Jell-O* Instant) . . .	150	4.0	29.0	2.5	10	420	0

Food and Measure	cal.	prot. (gms)	carbo. (gms)	fat (gms)	chol. (mgs)	sod. (mgs)	fiber (gms)
(*Jell-O* Instand Fat/ Sugar Free)	70	4.0	12.0	0	<5	400	0
butterscotch:							
(*Jell-O*)	160	4.0	30.0	2.5	10	190	0
(*Jell-O* Instant)	150	4.0	29.0	2.5	10	460	0
(*Jell-O* Instant Fat/ Sugar Free)	70	4.0	12.0	0	<5	400	0
(*Watkins*), 1 tbsp.	40	0	9.0	0	0	260	0
cheesecake (*Jell-O* Instant)	160	4.0	30.0	2.5	10	420	0
chocolate:							
(*Jell-O*)	150	5.0	28.0	2.5	10	170	<1.0
(*Jell-O* Instant) ...	160	4.0	31.0	2.5	10	480	<1.0
(*Jell-O* Instant Fat/ Sugar Free)	80	5.0	14.0	0	<5	380	<1.0
(*Jell-O* Sugar Free)	90	5.0	13.0	2.5	10	170	<1.0
(*Watkins*), 1 tbsp.	30	0	6.0	0	0	110	0
milk (*Jell-O*)	150	5.0	28.0	3.0	10	190	0
white (*Jell-O* Instant)	150	4.0	29.0	2.5	10	410	0
white (*Jell-O* Instant Fat/Sugar Free)	70	4.0	12.0	0	<5	390	0
chocolate fudge:							
(*Jell-O*)	150	5.0	28.0	2.5	10	170	1.0
(*Jell-O* Instant) ...	160	5.0	31.0	3.0	10	440	<1.0
(*Jell-O* Instant Fat/ Sugar Free)	80	5.0	14.0	0	<5	380	<1.0
coconut (*Watkins*), 1 tbsp.	35	0	10.0	1.0	0	170	0
coconut cream:							
(*Jell-O*)	150	4.0	24.0	5.0	10	210	<1.0
(*Jell-O* Instant) ...	160	4.0	27.0	5.0	10	330	<1.0
custard (*Jello-O Americana*)	140	5.0	25.0	2.5	10	190	0
devil's food (*Jell-O* Instant)	160	4.0	31.0	2.5	10	500	<1.0
flan:							
(*Goya* Spanish style custard), ¼ oz. dry	60	0	13.0	.5	0	110	<1.0
(*Jell-O*)	140	4.0	26.0	2.5	10	65	0
lemon:							
(*Jell-O*)	140	4.0	25.0	2.5	10	170	0
(*Jell-O* Instant) ...	150	4.0	29.0	2.5	10	370	0

Food and Measure	cal.	prot. (gms)	carbo. (gms)	fat (gms)	chol. (mgs)	sod. (mgs)	fiber (gms)
Pudding and pie filling mix, lemon *(cont.)*							
(*Watkins*), 1 tbsp.	40	0	10.0	0	0	110	0
pistachio:							
(*Jell-O* Instant) ...	160	4.0	29.0	3.0	10	420	0
(*Jell-O* Instant Fat/							
Sugar Free)	70	4.0	12.0	.5	<5	380	0
rice, see "Rice pudding mix"							
tapioca:							
(*Jell-O Americana*)	130	4.0	28.0	0	<5	180	0
(*Minute*), 1½ tbsp.	20	0	5.0	0	0	0	0
(*Watkins*), 2½ tbsp.	35	0	9.0	0	0	150	0
vanilla:							
(*Jell-O*)	140	4.0	26.0	2.5	10	200	0
(*Jell-O* Instant) ...	150	4.0	29.0	2.5	10	410	0
(*Jell-O* Instant Fat/							
Sugar Free)	70	4.0	12.0	0	<5	390	0
(*Jell-O* Sugar Free)	80	4.0	11.0	2.5	10	170	0
(*Watkins*), 1 tbsp.	40	0	9.0	0	0	140	0
French (*Jell-O* Instant)	150	4.0	29.0	2.5	10	410	0
Pudding, plum (*Crosse & Blackwell*), ⅓ pkg.	410	4.0	91.0	4.0	10	290	4.0
Puff pastry, see "Pastry shell"							
Pummelo:							
(*Frieda's*), 5 oz.	50	1.0	13.0	0	0	0	1.0
1-lb.-3-oz. fruit w/out rind	231	4.6	58.6	.2	0	6	6.1
sections, 1 cup	72	1.4	18.3	.1	0	2	1.9
Pumpkin, fresh:							
(*Frieda's* Mini), ¾ cup, 3 oz.	20	1.0	6.0	0	0	0	2.0
pulp, ½ cup:							
raw, 1" cubes	15	.6	3.8	.1	0	1	1.0
boiled, drained, mashed	24	.9	6.0	.1	0	2	1.0
Pumpkin, canned, ½ cup:							
(*Libby's* Solid Pack) ..	40	2.0	9.0	.5	0	5	5.0
w/ or w/out winter squash	41	1.3	9.9	.3	0	6	3.4

Food and Measure	cal.	prot. (gms)	carbo. (gms)	fat (gms)	chol. (mgs)	sod. (mgs)	fiber (gms)
Pumpkin butter (*Lost Acres*), 1 tbsp. . . .	45	0	11.0	0	0	25	0
Pumpkin flower:							
raw, ½ cup	3	.2	.5	<.1	0	1	<1.0
boiled, drained, ½ cup	10	.7	2.2	.1	0	4	.6
Pumpkin leaf:							
raw, ½ cup	4	.6	.5	.1	0	2	<1.0
boiled, drained, ½ cup	7	1.0	1.2	.1	0	3	.9
Pumpkin pie spice, 1 tsp.	6	.1	1.2	.2	0	1	.3
Pumpkin seeds:							
roasted, in shell:							
1 oz. or 85 seeds . .	127	5.3	15.3	5.5	0	5	n.a.
1 cup	285	11.9	34.4	12.4	0	12	n.a.
salted, 1 oz.	127	5.3	15.3	5.5	0	163	n.a.
roasted, shelled:							
1 oz.	148	9.4	3.8	12.0	0	5	1.8
salted, 1 oz.	148	9.4	3.8	12.0	0	163	1.8
dried, shelled, 1 oz. or 142 kernels	154	7.0	5.1	13.0	0	5	n.a.
Purslane, ½ cup:							
raw	4	.3	.7	<.1	0	10	<1.0
boiled, drained	10	.9	2.1	.1	0	26	<1.0

Q

Food and Measure	cal.	prot. (gms)	carbo. (gms)	fat (gms)	chol. (mgs)	sod. (mgs)	fiber (gms)
Quail, raw:							
meat w/skin:							
1 quail, 3.8 oz.							
(4.3 oz. w/bone)	210	21.4	0	13.1	83	58	0
1 oz.	54	5.6	0	3.4	22	15	0
meat only:							
1 quail, 3.2 oz.							
(4.3 oz. w/bone							
and skin)	123	20.0	0	4.2	64	47	0
1 oz.	38	6.2	0	1.3	20	14	0
breast meat only:							
1 breast, 2 oz. . . .	69	12.7	0	1.8	32	31	0
1 oz.	35	6.4	0	.8	16	16	0
Quesadilla, frozen							
(*Cedarlane*),							
3 pcs.	250	10.0	27.0	11.0	25	420	0
Quince:							
(*Frieda's*), 5 oz.	80	1.0	21.0	0	0	5	3.0
1 medium, 5.3 oz. . .	53	.4	14.1	.1	0	4	1.7
peeled, seeded,							
1 oz.	16	.1	4.3	<.1	0	1	.5
Quinoa, dry:							
(*Eden*), ¼ cup	170	7.0	31.0	2.5	0	0	3.0
(*Frieda's*), ⅓ cup	170	6.0	31.0	2.5	0	10	3.0
Quinoa dish mix,							
cilantro, zesty							
(*Seeds of*							
Change), ½ pkg. . .	280	7.0	58.0	3.0	0	840	3.0
Quinoa seeds							
(*Arrowhead Mills*),							
¼ cup	140	5.0	25.0	2.0	0	0	4.0

R

Food and Measure	cal.	prot. (gms)	carbo. (gms)	fat (gms)	chol. (mgs)	sod. (mgs)	fiber (gms)
Rabbit, domesticated, meat only:							
roasted, 4 oz.	223	33.0	0	9.1	93	53	0
stewed, 4 oz.	234	34.5	0	9.6	98	42	0
stewed, diced, 1 cup	288	42.5	0	11.8	120	52	0
Rabbit, wild, meat only, stewed:							
4 oz.	196	37.4	0	4.0	139	51	0
diced, 1 cup	242	46.2	0	4.9	172	63	0
Raccoon, meat only, roasted, 4 oz.	289	33.1	0	16.4	109	90	0
Radiatore dish, frozen, w/vegetables (*Birds Eye*), 1 cup	200	6.0	27.0	8.0	5	430	1.0
Radiatore dish mix:							
Alfredo primavera (*Land O Lakes*), 2.5 oz.	280	11.0	45.0	7.0	5	760	2.0
w/beans (*Marrakesh Express*), 1 cup* . .	200	9.0	41.0	1.0	<5	650	3.0
cheddar, mild (*Lipton Pasta & Sauce*), ½ pkg.	210	8.0	38.0	3.0	5	830	1.0
tomato and herb (*Near East*), 1 cup*	240	8.0	41.0	6.0	5	380	3.0
Radicchio, fresh:							
(*Frieda's*), 2 cups, 3 oz.	20	1.0	4.0	0	0	20	0
trimmed, 1 oz.	7	.4	1.3	.1	0	6	0
1 medium leaf, .3 oz.	2	.1	.4	<.1	0	2	0
shredded, ½ cup	5	.3	.9	.1	0	4	0
Radish:							
(*Dole*), 7 pcs., 3 oz.	15	1.0	3.0	0	0	25	0

Food and Measure	cal.	prot. (gms)	carbo. (gms)	fat (gms)	chol. (mgs)	sod. (mgs)	fiber (gms)
Radish (*cont.*)							
10 medium, ¾"–1"	7	.3	1.6	.2	0	11	.7
sliced, ½ cup	12	.4	2.1	.3	0	14	.9
Radish, black							
(*Frieda's*), ¾ cup,							
3 oz.	15	1.0	3.0	0	0	20	1.0
Radish, Oriental:							
(*Frieda's* Daikon),							
½ cup, 1.1 oz.	15	1.0	1.0	1.0	0	0	0
(*Frieda's* Korean),							
⅔ cup, 3 oz.	15	1.0	3.0	0	0	20	1.0
(*Frieda's* Lo Bok),							
⅔ cup, 3 oz.	25	1.0	5.0	0	0	55	2.0
7" pc., 11.9 oz.	61	2.0	12.8	.3	0	71	5.4
sliced, ½ cup	8	.3	1.8	<.1	0	9	.7
boiled, drained, sliced,							
½ cup	12	.5	2.5	.2	0	10	1.2
Radish, Oriental,							
dried, ½ cup, .5 oz.	157	4.6	36.8	.8	0	161	4.8
Radish, white-icicle:							
1 medium, .6 oz.	2	.2	.5	<.1	0	3	.2
sliced, ½ cup	7	.6	1.3	.1	0	8	.7
Radish sprouts (*Jona-*							
than's), 1 cup	57	3.0	3.0	2.0	0	5	2.0
Raisin sauce:							
(*Chelten House*),							
2 tbsp.	60	0	15.0	0	0	15	0
(*Reese*), ¼ cup	150	0	36.0	0	0	55	0
Raisins, ¼ cup:							
seeded, not packed	107	.9	28.5	.2	0	11	2.5
seedless:							
(*Dole* California)	130	1.0	31.0	0	0	10	2.0
(*Dole* Cinnaraisins)	130	1.0	32.0	.5	0	5	2.0
(*Sun•Maid*)	130	1.0	31.0	0	0	10	2.0
golden (*Dole*)	130	1.0	31.0	0	0	10	2.0
golden, not packed	110	1.3	28.9	.2	0	5	1.5
Monukka/Thompson							
(*Sonoma*)	130	1.0	31.0	0	0	10	2.0
not packed	109	1.2	28.7	.2	0	5	1.5
chocolate coated, see							
"Candy"							
Raisins, baking,							
chocolate coated							
(*Nestlé*), 1⅓ tbsp.	70	<1.0	11.0	3.0	0	0	<1.0

Food and Measure	cal.	prot. (gms)	carbo. (gms)	fat (gms)	chol. (mgs)	sod. (mgs)	fiber (gms)
Raisins and cherries, dried (*Sun•Maid Fast Fruit*), ¼ cup	130	1.0	31.0	0	0	10	2.0
Rambuten, canned, in syrup, ½ cup	62	.5	15.7	.2	0	17	1.4
Ranch dip, 2 tbsp:							
(*Marie's*)	150	1.0	3.0	15.0	15	140	0
(*Marzetti* Veggie Dip)	130	1.0	2.0	13.0	25	220	0
(*Marzetti* Veggie Dip Fat Free)	35	1.0	6.0	0	0	320	0
(*Marzetti* Veggie Dip Light)	80	0	6.0	6	4	400	0
bacon (*Marie's*)	150	1.0	3.0	16.0	15	200	0
bacon (*Marzetti* Veggie Dip)	120	1.0	2.0	12.0	25	150	0
creamy (*Kraft Dips*) . .	60	1.0	3.0	4.5	0	200	0
roasted garlic (*Marzetti* Veggie Dip)	140	1.0	2.0	14.0	25	240	0
Southwestern: (*Marzetti* Veggie Dip)	140	1.0	2.0	14.0	25	170	0
(*Marzetti* Veggie Dip Fat Free)	30	1.0	6.0	0	0	380	0
Ranch dip mix: 2 tbsp.*							
(*McCormick*), 2 tbsp.*	35	0	2.0	5.0	0	340	0
(*Ruffles*), 2 tbsp.*	70	1.0	3.0	6.0	10	190	<1.0
pepper (*Watkins*), 1 tsp.	10	0	3.0	0	0	120	0
pepper, cracked (*Knorr*), ½ tsp. . .	5	0	<1.0	0	0	100	0
Rapini, see "Broccoli rabe"							
Raspberry, fresh:							
(*Dole*), 1 cup	50	1.0	17.0	0	0	0	8.0
½ cup	31	.6	7.1	.3	0	<1	4.2
Raspberry, canned, in heavy syrup (*Oregon*), ½ cup	120	1.0	30.0	0	0	10	5.0
Raspberry, frozen:							
(*Big Valley*), ⅔ cup . .	60	1.0	12.0	0	0	0	2.0
(*Birds Eye*), 5 oz. . . .	90	1.0	22.0	0	0	5	5.0
(*Cascadian Farm*), 1 cup	60	1.0	15.0	.5	0	0	7.0
(*Tree of Life*), ⅔ cup .	50	1.0	12.0	0	0	0	2.0

Food and Measure	cal.	prot. (gms)	carbo. (gms)	fat (gms)	chol. (mgs)	sod. (mgs)	fiber (gms)
Raspberry, frozen (*cont.*)							
in syrup (*Big Valley* Tub), ⅔ cup	150	<1.0	40.0	0	0	0	2.0
sweetened, ½ cup ...	129	.9	32.7	.2	0	1	5.5
Raspberry drink blends, 8 fl. oz.:							
(*R. W. Knudsen* Hibiscus)	90	<1.0	23.0	0	0	40	0
blue (*Tropicana Twister* Rush)	120	<1.0	28.0	0	0	5	0
cherry:							
(*R. W. Knudsen* Razzleberry) ...	130	<1.0	33.0	0	0	35	0
(*R. W. Knudsen* Razzleberry Aseptic)	110	1.0	29.0	0	0	25	0
Raspberry juice blends, 8 fl. oz.:							
(*Dole* Country)	140	1.0	34.0	0	0	30	0
(*Santa Cruz Organic* Nectar)	120	<1.0	30.0	0	0	25	0
kiwi (*Dole*)	140	0	35.0	0	0	35	0
peach (*R. W. Knudsen*)	150	<1.0	31.0	0	0	25	0
Raspberry syrup, ¼ cup:							
(*Knott's Berry Farm*)	210	0	52.0	0	0	50	0
red (*Smucker's*)	210	0	52.0	0	0	0	0
Raspberry topping (*Smucker's Plate Scrapers*), 2 tbsp.	100	0	25.0	0	0	5	0
Raspberry-tamarind sauce, dipping (*Helen's Tropical Exotics*), 2 tbsp. ...	50	0	11.0	1.0	0	0	1.0
Ravioli, frozen or refrigerated (see also "Ravioli entree"):							
artichoke (*Cafferata*), 10 pcs., 4.5 oz.	210	8.0	43.0	1.0	0	410	2.0
butternut squash (*Cafferata* Agnolotti), 4.5 oz.	255	11.0	47.0	5.0	26	493	4.0

Food and Measure	cal.	prot. (gms)	carbo. (gms)	fat (gms)	chol. (mgs)	sod. (mgs)	fiber (gms)
cheese:							
(*Celentano*), 4 pcs., 4.3 oz.	260	12.0	40.0	6.0	45	230	2.0
(*Celentano* Low Fat), 4.2 oz.	280	12.0	46.0	3.5	40	200	2.0
(*Mount Rose*), 11 pcs., 4.3 oz.	320	12.0	52.0	7.0	15	380	4.0
four (*Buitoni*), 1⅓ cups	380	17.0	49.0	13.0	85	500	3.0
four (*Buitoni* Light), 1 cup	230	12.0	37.0	4.0	35	390	2.0
three, mini (*Buitoni*), 1 cup	260	12.0	41.0	5.0	30	260	3.0
large (*Italian Village*), 4 pcs., 4.5 oz. ...	220	9.0	39.0	3.5	35	400	1.0
mini (*Celentano*), 12 pcs., 4 oz. ...	260	11.0	41.0	6.0	35	180	2.0
mini (*Italian Village*), 13 pcs., 3.9 oz.	210	8.0	38.0	3.0	30	280	1.0
chicken:							
Parmesan (*Buitoni*), 1¼ cups	310	14.0	44.0	9.0	55	590	3.0
roast, and garlic (*Buitoni*), 1¼ cups	330	12.0	45.0	11.0	50	400	3.0
Gorgonzola:							
(*Buitoni*), 1¼ cups	360	15.0	47.0	12.0	60	400	3.0
walnut (*Cafferata* Agnolotti), 4.5 oz.	330	15.0	36.0	14.0	70	460	<1.0
meat (*Celentano*), 4 pcs., 4.3 oz.	270	11.0	44.0	5.0	35	530	2.0
vegetable, garden (*Buitoni*), 1 cup ...	250	11.0	39.0	5.0	40	500	2.0
Ravioli entree, can or pkg., 1 cup, except as noted:							
beef:							
(*Chef Boyardee*) ...	230	9.0	37.0	5.0	20	1150	4.0
(*Chef Boyardee*), 7-oz. can	170	7.0	27.0	4.0	15	960	2.0
(*Chef Boyardee* Micro Cup), 7.5 oz.	190	6.0	29.0	5.0	15	980	2.0

Food and Measure	cal.	prot. (gms)	carbo. (gms)	fat (gms)	chol. (mgs)	sod. (mgs)	fiber (gms)
Ravioli entree, can or pkg., beef (*cont.*)							
(*Chef Boyardee* Overstuffed)	280	12.0	48.0	4.5	20	1190	4.0
(*Chef Boyardee* 99% Fat Free)	210	7.0	44.0	.5	<5	860	4.0
(*Chef Boyardee Junior* Micro Cup), 1 cont.	210	8.0	37.0	4.0	15	800	4.0
(*Dinty Moore American Classics*), 1 bowl	300	20.0	34.0	9.0	55	810	3.0
mini (*Chef Boyardee*)	240	8.0	37.0	6.0	20	1180	3.0
cheese (*Chef Boyardee* 99% Fat Free)	210	9.0	41.0	1.0	15	1150	3.0
w/tomato sauce (*Hormel* Microcup)	220	8.0	35.0	6.0	10	890	2.0
Ravioli entree, frozen, 1 pkg., except as noted:							
(*Amy's*), 8 oz.	340	15.0	44.0	12.0	20	580	6.0
cheese:							
(*Healthy Choice Solos*), 9 oz.	260	11.0	44.0	5.0	30	340	4.0
(*Lean Cuisine Everyday Favorites*), 8.5 oz.	260	12.0	38.0	7.0	35	590	4.0
(*Michelina's* Jumbo), 11 oz.	400	17.0	53.0	13.0	60	1080	4.0
(*Stouffer's*), 10⅝ oz.	230	10.0	38.0	4.5	60	790	2.0
Alfredo, and broccoli (*Michelina's*), 8 oz.	390	17.0	42.0	18.0	80	820	2.0
four (*Wolfgang Puck's*), 13 oz.	330	18.0	16.0	20.0	55	610	2.0
three (*Marie Callender's*), 16 oz.	610	27.0	92.0	15.0	40	1600	10.0
and tomato sauce (*Freezer Queen Deluxe Family*), 1 cup	280	12.0	47.0	5.0	20	1220	4.0

Food and Measure	cal.	prot. (gms)	carbo. (gms)	fat (gms)	chol. (mgs)	sod. (mgs)	fiber (gms)
and tomato sauce (*Freezer Queen* Meal), 7.75 oz.	350	5.0	57.0	11.0	45	720	6.0
meat, pomodoro sauce (*Michelina's*), 8 oz.	310	13.0	41.0	10.0	40	810	3.0
mushroom and spinach (*Wolfgang Puck's*), 13 oz. ...	260	7.0	15.0	18.0	45	1280	3.0
sweet potato (*Wolfgang Puck's*), 13 oz.	360	11.0	35.0	21.0	65	2060	4.0
Ravioli entree mix, frozen, and vegetables (*Tree of Life Easy-Meal*), 1 pkg.*							
w/tofu, oil	380	15.0	44.0	14.0	0	790	3.0
Recaito (*Goya*), 1 tsp.	0	0	0	0	0	35	0
Red bean (see also "Kidney beans"), canned, ½ cup:							
(*Allens*)	100	6.0	19.0	.5	0	310	9.0
(*Bush's Best*)	110	6.0	19.0	.5	0	460	6.0
(*S&W Louisiana*)	80	6.0	20.0	0	0	510	5.0
(*Westbrae Natural*) . .	90	6.0	16.0	0	0	140	5.0
small (*Eden*)	100	6.0	17.0	.5	0	65	5.0
small (*Goya*)	90	7.0	18.0	.5	0	360	6.0
Red kuri squash (*Frieda's*), ¾ cup, 3 oz.	30	1.0	7.0	0	0	0	1.0
Red snapper, see "Snapper"							
Redfish, see "Ocean perch"							
Refried beans, canned, ½ cup:							
(*Allens*)	150	7.0	24.0	2.5	0	360	11.0
(*Bearitos* Fat Free) . . .	110	7.0	20.0	0	0	530	8.0
(*Chi-Chi's* Fat Free) . .	120	7.0	20.0	0	0	460	4.0
(*Chi-Chi's* Fiesta)	130	6.0	20.0	3.0	0	520	4.0
(*Goya*)	150	9.0	25.0	1.5	0	510	7.0
(*Greene's Farm*)	100	6.0	20.0	0	0	520	8.0
(*Old El Paso*)	100	6.0	17.0	.5	0	570	6.0
(*Ortega*)	150	8.0	25.0	2.5	0	570	9.0
(*Rosarita* Traditional) .	100	6.0	18.0	2.0	0	510	5.0

Food and Measure	cal.	prot. (gms)	carbo. (gms)	fat (gms)	chol. (mgs)	sod. (mgs)	fiber (gms)
Refried beans (*cont.*)							
black bean:							
(*Bearitos*)	130	8.0	22.0	1.0	0	530	5.0
(*Bearitos* Fat Free) .	110	7.0	20.0	0	0	530	5.0
(*Greene's Farm*) . . .	110	7.0	19.0	0	0	520	5.0
(*Hain*)	110	6.0	18.0	.5	0	370	6.0
(*Knorr*)	140	8.0	22.0	2.5	0	480	6.0
(*La Costeña*)	180	6.0	20.0	11.0	<5	440	7.0
spicy (*Greene's Farm*)	80	6.0	17.0	0	0	510	4.0
w/cheese (*Old El Paso*)	130	7.0	18.0	3.5	5	500	6.0
w/green chilies (*Bearitos* Fat Free)	100	6.0	19.0	0	0	540	7.0
pinto bean:							
(*Bearitos*)	140	7.0	23.0	2.5	0	530	9.0
(*Bearitos* No Salt)	140	7.0	23.0	2.5	0	5	9.0
(*La Costeña*)	160	6.0	20.0	9.0	<5	410	9.0
(*La Sierra*)	150	6.0	19.0	6.0	0	400	7.0
w/sausage (*Old El Paso*)	200	7.0	14.0	13.0	10	360	4.0
spicy:							
(*Greene's Farm*) . . .	100	6.0	19.0	0	0	510	7.0
(*Old El Paso* Fat Free)	100	6.0	18.0	0	0	720	6.0
jalapeño (*Rosarita*)	100	6.0	18.0	2.0	0	630	6.0
vegetable (*Chi-Chi's*)	100	5.0	18.0	1.0	0	580	4.0
vegetarian:							
(*Hain*)	90	6.0	16.0	0	0	370	6.0
(*Hain* Canola Oil) . .	90	5.0	17.0	.5	0	370	6.0
(*Old El Paso*)	100	6.0	17.0	1.0	0	490	6.0
Refried beans, dried, w/cheese (*Alpine-Aire*), 2.25 oz.	240	15.0	27.0	8.0	10	450	11.0
Refried beans, mix, dry, ½ cup:							
black bean (*Taste Adventure*)	130	8.0	24.0	0	0	380	6.0
green chili and lime (*Taste Adventure*)	140	8.0	27.0	.5	0	410	9.0
jalapeño (*Taste Adventure*)	140	8.0	27.0	0	0	410	9.0
pinto bean (*Taste Adventure*)	130	8.0	25.0	0	0	390	9.0

Food and Measure	cal.	prot. (gms)	carbo. (gms)	fat (gms)	chol. (mgs)	sod. (mgs)	fiber (gms)
Relish, see "Pickle relish" and specific listings							
Relish, mixed, hot, Indian (*Patak's*), 1 tbsp.	40	<1.0	<1.0	4.0	0	410	0
Rémoulade sauce, in jars (*Zatarain's*), ¼ cup	80	2.0	9.0	8.0	0	780	1.0
Rennet (*Junket*), 1 tablet	1	0	0	0	0	165	0
Rhubarb, fresh:							
(*Frieda's*), ⅔ cup, 3 oz.	20	1.0	4.0	0	0	0	2.0
1 stalk	11	.5	2.3	.1	0	2	.9
diced, ½ cup	13	.6	2.8	.1	0	2	1.1
Rhubarb, canned, in extra heavy syrup (*Oregon*), ½ cup . .	180	<1.0	44.0	0	0	15	3.0
Rhubard, frozen, sweetend, cooked, ½ cup	139	.5	37.4	.1	0	2	2.4
Rice (see also "Wild rice"), dry, ¼ cup, except as noted:							
Arborio, white:							
(*Frieda's* Risotto) . .	160	3.0	36.0	0	0	0	1.0
(*Lundberg Nutra-Farmed*)	160	4.0	35.0	1.0	0	0	1.0
(*Rice Select* Risotto)	150	3.0	37.0	0	0	0	0
basmati, brown:							
(*Arrowhead Mills*)	150	3.0	33.0	1.0	0	0	2.0
(*Lundberg* Organic)	160	4.0	34.0	1.5	0	0	2.0
(*Lundberg Nutra-Farmed*/Royal) . .	170	4.0	38.0	2.0	0	0	2.0
(*Texmati*)	170	4.0	35.0	1.0	0	0	2.0
light (*Texmati*)	170	4.0	33.0	1.0	0	0	1.0
basmati, white:							
(*Lundberg* Organic)	180	4.0	38.0	.5	0	0	1.0
(*Lundberg Nutra-Farmed*)	180	4.0	41.0	.5	0	0	0
(*Texmati*)	150	3.0	34.0	.5	0	0	0
long grain (*Arrowhead Mills*)	150	4.0	34.0	0	0	0	1.0

Food and Measure	cal.	prot. (gms)	carbo. (gms)	fat (gms)	chol. (mgs)	sod. (mgs)	fiber (gms)
Rice (*cont.*)							
blends:							
(*Lundberg Black Japonica*)	170	5.0	38.0	2.0	0	0	3.0
(*Lundberg Country- wild*)	150	3.0	35.0	1.5	0	0	3.0
(*Lundberg Jubilee*)	170	4.0	39.0	1.5	0	0	3.0
(*Lundberg Wild Blend*)	150	4.0	35.0	1.5	0	0	3.0
(*Texmati Royal Blend*), ⅓ cup . .	160	4.0	34.0	.5	0	0	0
(*Watkins* Heartland)	160	4.0	35.0	0	0	0	2.0
brown/wild (*Lund- berg* Organic) . .	150	4.0	34.0	1.5	0	0	2.0
brown/wild (*Gourmet House*)	160	7.0	34.0	.5	0	0	1.0
brown/wild (*Watkins* Medley)	170	4.0	35.0	0	0	0	2.0
white/wild (*Gourmet House*)	170	4.0	35.0	0	0	0	1.0
wild/rice (*Gourmet House* Garden) . .	190	5.0	40.0	.5	0	15	1.0
brown:							
(*Lundberg Christmas*)	170	4.0	37.0	1.5	0	0	<3.0
(*Lundberg Wehani*)	170	3.0	38.0	1.5	0	0	3.0
(*River*)	150	3.0	32.0	1.0	0	0	1.0
(*Success*), ½ cup	150	4.0	33.0	1.0	0	5	2.0
(*S&W*)	150	3.0	32.0	1.0	0	0	1.0
(*Uncle Ben's* Original)	170	5.0	35.0	1.5	0	0	2.0
instant (*Uncle Ben's*), ½ cup, 1 cup* . .	190	4.0	42.0	.5	0	20	2.0
whole grain, instant (*Minute*), ½ cup, ⅔ cup*	160	3.0	32.0	1.5	0	0	1.0
brown, long grain:							
(*Arrowhead Mills*)	150	3.0	33.0	1.0	0	0	2.0
(*Carolina*)	150	3.0	32.0	1.0	0	0	1.0
(*Lundberg* Organic)	170	4.0	38.0	1.5	0	0	3.0
(*Lundberg Nutra- Farmed*)	170	3.0	37.0	2.0	0	0	3.0
(*Mahatma*)	150	3.0	32.0	0	0	0	1.0

Food and Measure	cal.	prot. (gms)	carbo. (gms)	fat (gms)	chol. (mgs)	sod. (mgs)	fiber (gms)
brown, medium grain (*Lundberg* Organic Golden Rose) ...	160	3.0	34.0	1.0	0	0	1.0
brown, short grain:							
(*Arrowhead Mills*)	170	4.0	36.0	1.0	0	0	2.0
(*Lundberg* Nutra-Farmed/Organic)	170	3.0	40.0	1.5	0	0	3.0
cracked (*Gourmet House*)	170	6.0	35.0	0	0	0	2.0
gold, parboiled (*Carolina/Mahatma*)	160	3.0	37.0	0	0	0	<1.0
glutinous or sweet ...	171	3.2	37.8	.3	0	3	1.3
Indian style (*Texmati Kasmati*)	150	3.0	34.0	.5	0	0	0
jasmine:							
(*A Taste of Thai* Soft)	160	3.0	36.0	0	0	0	0
(*Texmati Jasmati*)	150	3.0	34.0	0	0	0	0
white (*Lundberg* Nutra-Farmed/ Organic)	160	3.0	36.0	.5	0	0	n.a.
white (*Mahatma* Thai)	160	3.0	36.0	0	0	0	2.0
sushi:							
(*Lundberg* Organic)	160	3.0	36.0	0	0	0	1.0
(*Rice Select Sushi*)	190	3.0	45.0	0	0	0	0
white, long grain:							
(*Carolina*)	150	3.0	35.0	1.0	0	0	1.0
(*Mahatma*)	150	3.0	35.0	0	0	0	0
(*River/Water Maid*)	160	3.0	37.0	0	0	0	<1.0
(*Success*), ½ cup	190	4.0	44.0	0	0	5	<1.0
(*S&W*)	150	3.0	35.0	0	0	0	0
instant (*Carolina*) ..	160	4.0	36.0	0	0	0	1.0
instant (*Mahatma*)	160	4.0	36.0	0	0	5	1.0
instant (*Minute*), ½ cup, ¾ cup*	160	3.0	36.0	0	0	5	<1.0
instant (*Uncle Ben's*), ½ cup, 1 cup* ..	190	3.0	43.0	.5	0	15	1.0
instant (*Uncle Ben's Boil-in-Bag*), ⅓ cup, 1 cup* ..	190	4.0	44.0	.5	0	0	1.0
parboiled (*Uncle Ben's Converted Original*), ⅓ cup*	170	4.0	38.0	0	0	0	0

Food and Measure	cal.	prot. (gms)	carbo. (gms)	fat (gms)	chol. (mgs)	sod. (mgs)	fiber (gms)
Rice (*cont.*)							
white, short grain:							
(*Goya* Valencia) ...	150	3.0	33.0	0	0	0	0
(*Mahatma* Valencia)	160	3.0	36.0	0	0	0	<1.0
Rice and beans, see "Rice dishes, mix"							
Rice beverage, 8 fl. oz.:							
(*Hain* Supreme)	100	3.0	16.0	3.0	0	60	<1.0
(*Harmony Farms*) ...	90	13.0	21.0	0	0	100	0
(*Rice Dream*)	120	1.0	25.0	2.0	0	90	0
(*Westbrae Natural*) ..	100	1.0	18.0	2.5	0	60	0
(*Westbrae Natural* ½ gallon)	100	1.0	18.0	3.0	0	70	0
carob (*Rice Dream*) ..	150	1.0	32.0	2.5	0	100	0
chocolate (*Rice Dream*)	170	1.0	36.0	3.0	0	115	0
cinnamon (*Hain* Supreme)	130	4.0	22.0	3.0	0	60	<1.0
and soy (*EdenBlend*)	120	7.0	18.0	3.0	0	85	0
vanilla:							
(*Rice Dream*)	130	1.0	28.0	2.0	0	90	0
(*Westbrae Natural*)	120	1.0	22.0	2.5	0	65	0
(*Westbrae Natural* ½ gallon)	120	1.0	22.0	3.0	0	70	0
Rice bran, crude, 1 cup	262	11.1	41.2	17.3	0	4	18.0
Rice cake (see also "Popcorn cake"):							
plain (*Hain* Mini), 8 pcs.	60	1.0	13.0	0	0	20	0
all varieties, baked (*Hain* Ringers), 37 pcs., 1 oz.	110	2.0	21.0	2.0	0	270	1.0
apple, Granny Smith (*Estee* Mini), 5 pcs.	60	1.0	13.0	0	0	5	0
apple cinnamon:							
(*Hain*), 1 pc.	50	1.0	11.0	0	0	10	0
(*Hain* Mini), 6 pcs.	60	1.0	13.0	0	0	10	0
(*Lundberg Nutra-Farmed*), 1 pc.	80	2.0	18.0	.5	0	0	<1.0
(*Quaker* Crispy Mini's), 8 pcs. ...	60	1.0	15.0	0	0	50	0

Food and Measure	cal.	prot. (gms)	carbo. (gms)	fat (gms)	chol. (mgs)	sod. (mgs)	fiber (gms)
banana nut:							
(*Estee* Mini), 5 pcs.	60	1.0	14.0	.5	.0	30	0
(*Mother's*), 1 pc. . .	50	1.0	11.0	0	0	40	0
(*Quaker* Crispy							
Mini's), 8 pcs. . .	65	1.0	14.0	0	0	85	0
barbecue flavor							
(*Quaker* Crispy							
Mini's), 10 pcs. . . .	70	1.0	12.0	2.0	0	145	0
berry, mixed (*Estee*							
Mini), 5 pcs.	60	1.0	14.0	0	0	20	0
brown, 1 pc.:							
(*Lundberg Nutra-*							
Farmed/Organic)	70	1.0	15.0	0	0	55	0
(*Lundberg Nutra-*							
Farmed/Organic							
No Salt)	70	1.0	16.0	0	0	0	0
butter flavor, corn							
grain (*Mother's*							
Unsalted), 1 pc. . .	35	1.0	7.5	0	0	0	0
buttery caramel							
(*Lundberg Nutra-*							
Farmed), 1 pc. . . .	80	2.0	18.0	.5	0	0	<1.0
caramel corn (*Quaker*							
Crispy Mini's), 7 pcs.	60	1.0	13.0	0	0	145	0
cheese:							
cheddar (*Quaker*							
Crispy Mini's),							
9 pcs.	70	1.0	10.0	3.0	0	210	0
nacho (*Quaker*							
Crispy Mini's),							
9 pcs.	70	1.0	10.0	2.5	0	215	0
chocolate (*Quaker*							
Crispy Mini's), 7 pcs.	60	1.0	13.0	1.0	0	45	0
chocolate chip (*Estee*							
Crunchie Bar)	50	1.0	15.0	0	0	40	<1.0
cinnamon spice (*Estee*							
Mini), 5 pcs.	60	1.0	14.0	0	0	5	0
devil's food (*Hain* Mini							
Munchies), 5 pcs.	60	1.0	12.0	.5	0	20	0
honey nut:							
(*Hain*), 1 pc.	50	1.0	11.0	0	0	25	0
(*Hain* Mini), 6 pcs.	60	1.0	13.0	0	0	45	0
(*Lundberg Nutra-*							
Farmed), 1 pc.	80	2.0	18.0	.5	0	0	<1.0

Food and Measure	cal.	prot. (gms)	carbo. (gms)	fat (gms)	chol. (mgs)	sod. (mgs)	fiber (gms)
Rice cake, honey nut (*cont.*)							
(*Quaker* Crispy Mini's), 8 pcs. . . .	60	1.0	15.0	0	0	90	0
koku, 1 pc.:							
seaweed (*Lundberg* Organic)	80	2.0	17.0	0	0	95	1.0
sesame (*Lundberg* Organic)	80	2.0	17.0	0	0	35	2.0
mochi (*Lundberg Nutra-Farmed/* Organic), 1 pc. . . .	70	1.0	15.0	0	0	55	0
multigrain, w/seeds (*Lundberg* Organic), 1 pc.	80	1.0	15.0	0	0	65	<1.0
peanut butter:							
(*Estee* Crunch Mini), 5 pcs.	60	1.0	13.0	1.0	0	80	<1.0
crunch (*Hain* Mini Munchies), 5 pcs. .	50	1.0	11.0	1.0	0	60	0
popcorn (*Lundberg* Organic), 1 pc. . . .	70	1.0	16.0	0	0	55	0
ranch:							
(*Hain* Mini), 6 pcs.	70	1.0	9.0	3.5	0	190	0
(*Quaker* Crispy Mini's), 10 pcs.	75	1.0	12.0	2.5	0	195	0
sesame, 1 pc.:							
toasted (*Lundberg Nutra-Farmed*) . .	70	2.0	15.0	0	0	65	1.0
tamari (*Lundberg Nutra-Farmed/* Organic)	70	2.0	16.0	.5	0	120	2.0
sour cream/onion (*Quaker* Crispy Mini's), 10 pcs.	70	1.0	12.0	2.5	0	165	0
strawberry cheesecake (*Hain* Mini Munchies), 5 pcs.	60	1.0	12.0	0	0	15	0
tamari seaweed (*Lundberg* Organic), 1 pc.	70	1.0	15.0	0	0	125	0
vanilla (*Estee* Crunchie Bar), 1 pc.	60	1.0	14.0	0	0	35	0
wild rice (*Lundberg Nutra-Farmed/* Organic), 1 pc. . . .	70	1.0	15.0	0	0	55	0

Food and Measure	cal.	prot. (gms)	carbo. (gms)	fat (gms)	chol. (mgs)	sod. (mgs)	fiber (gms)
Rice chips, brown (*Eden*), 50 pcs., 1.1 oz.	150	2.0	19.0	7.0	0	100	0
Rice dish, canned, 1 cup:							
fried (*La Choy*)	290	7.0	64.0	2.0	0	1300	3.0
Spanish (*Old El Paso*)	140	3.0	30.0	1.0	0	860	1.0
Rice dish, frozen, 1 pkg., except as noted:							
and beans:							
Santa Fe (*Lean Cuisine Everyday Favorites*), 10⅜ oz.	300	10.0	54.0	5.0	15	650	6.0
Southwest (*Healthy Choice* Solo), 10 oz.	250	12.0	45.0	3.0	0	600	5.0
Spanish, w/chicken (*Ortega*), 10.25 oz.	400	17.0	44.0	17.0	45	1400	4.0
broccoli, cheese sauce: (*Birds Eye*), 10 oz.	290	8.0	15.0	9.0	15	1110	2.0
onion and pasta (*Freezer Queen* Family Side Dish), 1 cup	190	5.0	38.0	2.5	<5	550	3.0
cheesy, and chicken (*Healthy Choice* Solo), 9 oz.	230	15.0	34.0	4.0	30	600	5.0
risotto, cheese and mushroom (*Wolf-gang Puck's*), 11 oz.	520	20.0	68.0	18.0	30	810	4.0
Spanish, and chicken (*Michelina's*), 8 oz.	290	11.0	38.0	11.0	30	1010	2.0
Szechuan (*Cascadian Farm Veggie Bowl*), 9 oz.	210	7.0	45.0	1.5	0	630	3.0
teriyaki (*Cascadian Farm Veggie Bowl*), 9 oz.	270	9.0	44.0	7.0	0	530	2.0
w/vegetables: stir-fry (*Budget Gourmet*), 8 oz.	350	7.0	45.0	16.0	15	670	3.0

Food and Measure	cal.	prot. (gms)	carbo. (gms)	fat (gms)	chol. (mgs)	sod. (mgs)	fiber (gms)
Rice dish, frozen, w/vegetables (cont.)							
teriyaki stir-fry (*Amy's* Skillet Meals), 1 cup . . .	320	9.0	64.0	2.5	0	590	4.0
Thai stir-fry (*Amy's*), 9.5 oz.	270	7.0	36.0	11.0	0	420	2.0
wild rice pilaf (*Budget Gourmet*), 8 oz.	340	6.0	44.0	13.0	10	700	2.0
Rice dish, mix (see also "Grains, mixed, dish"), 1 cup*, except as noted:							
Alfredo broccoli (*Lipton* Rice & Sauce)	320	9.0	46.0	12.0	15	990	1.0
almond, toasted, pilaf (*Near East*)	220	5.0	41.0	5.0	10	840	2.0
and beans, black:							
(*Carolina/Mahatma*)	200	7.0	39.0	1.5	0	930	5.0
(*Goya*), ¼ cup	160	5.0	34.0	0	0	570	3.0
(*Taste Adventure* Quick Cuisine Santa Fe), ⅓ cup	160	5.0	31.0	.5	0	340	5.0
Mediterranean, pilaf (*Near East*)	260	8.0	52.0	3.5	10	890	6.0
and beans, red:							
(*Carolina/Mahatma*)	190	7.0	40.0	1.0	0	790	6.0
(*Goya*), ¼ cup	160	5.0	35.0	0	0	610	3.0
(*Success*)	240	8.0	51.0	1.0	0	920	8.0
(*Watkins*), ⅙ pkg.	140	4.0	30.0	0	0	0	2.0
jambalaya (*Taste Adventure* Quick Cuisine Louisiana), ⅓ cup	160	6.0	31.0	1.0	0	340	4.0
and beans, smoky (*Chef's Originals* Cowboy), ¼ cup . .	180	5.0	37.0	1.0	0	340	4.0
beef/beef flavor:							
(*Lipton* Rice & Sauce)	270	6.0	47.0	7.7	0	1010	1.0
(*Mahatma*)	200	4.0	41.0	2.0	0	950	<1.0
(*Rice-A-Roni*)	310	7.0	51.0	9.0	0	1130	2.0
(*Rice-A-Roni* ⅓ Less Salt)	280	7.0	53.0	5.0	0	720	2.0

Food and Measure	cal.	prot. (gms)	carbo. (gms)	fat (gms)	chol. (mgs)	sod. (mgs)	fiber (gms)
(*Success*)	190	5.0	43.0	.5	0	920	2.0
and mushroom							
(*Rice-A-Roni*) . .	290	8.0	50.0	7.0	0	1150	2.0
biryani (*Neera's*)	132	3.0	29.0	1.0	0	4	1.0
broccoli (*Rice-A-Roni*)	270	5.0	41.0	10.0	5	900	1.0
broccoli au gratin:							
(*Rice-A-Roni*)	370	8.0	46.0	17.0	5	1000	2.0
(*Rice-A-Roni* ⅓							
Less Salt)	320	7.0	49.0	11.0	5	580	2.0
(*Uncle Ben's*							
Country Inn),							
2 oz.	200	5.0	41.0	2.0	5	790	1.0
risotto (*Knorr*) . . .	260	6.0	54.0	2.5	10	880	<1.0
broccoli and cheese:							
(*Mahatma*)	200	5.0	41.0	1.5	5	620	2.0
(*Success*)	210	5.0	40.0	4.5	5	840	1.0
brown:							
hearty (*Lundberg*							
Quick), ⅓ cup . .	140	3.0	27.0	1.0	0	15	3.0
picante Spanish							
fiesta (*Lundberg*							
Quick), ½ pkg.	260	6.0	53.0	2.5	0	670	5.0
roasted garlic pesto							
(*Lundberg* Quick),							
½ pkg.	260	6.0	52.0	3.5	0	830	5.0
vegetarian chicken,							
savory (*Lundberg*							
Quick), ½ pkg.	260	6.0	53.0	2.5	0	910	5.0
and wild (*Success*)	190	6.0	41.0	1.0	0	790	3.0
wild and mushroom							
(*Lundberg* Exotic							
Quick), ½ pkg.	260	6.0	53.0	3.0	0	800	4.0
Cajun style:							
(*Lipton* Rice &							
Sauce)	270	7.0	46.0	7.0	0	910	1.0
w/beans (*Lipton*							
Rice & Sauce) . .	310	10.0	52.0	7.5	0	530	7.0
Cantonese (*Health*							
Valley), ½ cup	140	7.0	27.0	1.0	0	180	2.0
cheddar, white, and							
herbs (*Rice-A-Roni*)	340	7.0	49.0	14.0	5	940	1.0
cheddar broccoli							
(*Lipton* Rice &							
Sauce)	280	7.0	46.0	9.0	5	1010	1.0

Food and Measure	cal.	prot. (gms)	carbo. (gms)	fat (gms)	chol. (mgs)	sod. (mgs)	fiber (gms)
Rice dish, mix (*cont.*)							
cheese:							
four (*Rice-A-Roni*)	280	6.0	37.0	12.0	5	800	1.0
nacho (*Mahatma*)	250	6.0	49.0	3.0	5	1260	<1.0
three, risotto (*Marrakesh Express*) ..	200	5.0	44.0	1.5	5	410	0
chicken/chicken flavor:							
(*Carolina/Mahatma*)	190	5.0	42.0	0	0	970	<1.0
(*Health Valley*), ½ cup	140	7.0	26.0	1.0	0	290	3.0
(*Lipton* Rice & Sauce)	280	6.0	46.0	8.5	5	960	1.0
(*Rice-A-Roni*)	310	7.0	52.0	9.0	0	1130	2.0
(*Rice-A-Roni* Low Fat)	210	5.0	41.0	3.0	0	820	1.0
(*Rice-A-Roni* ⅓ Less Salt)	280	7.0	52.0	5.0	0	710	2.0
(*Success* Classic) .	150	4.0	32.0	1.0	0	720	1.0
(*Uncle Ben's Country Inn*), 2 oz.	200	5.0	42.0	1.0	0	940	1.0
broccoli (*Lipton* Rice & Sauce)	280	7.0	46.0	8.5	0	910	2.0
broccoli (*Rice-A-Roni*)	230	6.0	41.0	5.0	0	990	2.0
broccoli (*Uncle Ben's Country Inn*), 2 oz.	190	4.0	43.0	1.0	0	870	1.0
Cajun (*Rice-A-Roni*)	250	6.0	41.0	8.0	0	1010	2.0
creamy (*Lipton* Rice & Sauce)	290	6.0	45.0	11.0	0	830	1.0
fried rice (*Lipton* Rice & Sauce), ½ pkg.	240	7.0	49.0	2.0	0	940	2.0
garlic (*Rice-A-Roni*)	260	6.0	42.0	8.0	0	830	1.0
grilled (*Success*) ..	190	6.0	42.0	1.0	0	860	1.0
and herb (*Uncle Ben's Natural Select*)	200	5.0	42.0	1.0	0	680	1.0
herb roasted (*Rice-A-Roni*)	260	6.0	41.0	8.0	0	890	1.0
herb vegetable (*Bowl Appétit!*), 1 bowl	260	7.0	50.0	5.0	15	750	2.0

Food and Measure	cal.	prot. (gms)	carbo. (gms)	fat (gms)	chol. (mgs)	sod. (mgs)	fiber (gms)
w/mushrooms (Rice-A-Roni) ..	360	8.0	52.0	14.0	5	1400	2.0
Parmesan risotto (Lipton Rice & Sauce)	270	6.0	43.0	8.5	0	830	1.0
pilaf (Near East) ..	210	5.0	42.0	3.5	10	960	1.0
pilaf, and wild rice (Near East Mediterranean)	210	5.0	44.0	3.0	10	950	2.0
rice pilaf (Knorr), ⅓ cup	210	5.0	45.0	1.0	0	1000	1.0
roasted (Lipton Rice & Sauce)	260	5.0	46.0	7.5	0	880	1.0
roasted, and garlic pilaf (Near East)	210	5.0	44.0	3.0	5	590	1.0
Southwestern (Lipton Rice & Sauce)	260	5.0	47.0	7.5	0	840	1.0
teriyaki (Rice-A-Roni)	260	6.0	41.0	8.0	0	840	1.0
and vegetables (Rice-A-Roni) ..	290	7.0	51.0	7.0	0	1380	2.0
and vegetables (Uncle Ben's Country Inn), 2 oz.	190	5.0	42.0	1.5	5	580	1.0
and vegetables, savory (Rice-A-Roni Low Fat) ..	210	6.0	41.0	2.5	0	780	2.0
chili (Lundberg One-Step)	180	6.0	42.0	1.0	0	420	5.0
coconut ginger (A Taste of Thai), ¾ cup*	190	5.0	42.0	0	0	430	2.0
curry: (Lundberg One-Step)	160	5.0	38.0	1.0	0	400	5.0
pilaf (Near East) ..	210	5.0	42.0	3.0	10	680	1.0
dirty rice, Jamaican style (Neera's)	175	3.0	28.0	6.0	0	5	2.0
fried: (Rice-A-Roni)	320	7.0	50.0	11.0	0	1530	2.0
(Rice-A-Roni ⅓ Less Salt)	260	7.0	51.0	3.5	0	950	2.0

Food and Measure	cal.	prot. (gms)	carbo. (gms)	fat (gms)	chol. (mgs)	sod. (mgs)	fiber (gms)
Rice dish, mix, fried (*cont.*)							
teriyaki (*Chef's Originals*), ¼ cup	160	4.0	34.0	.5	0	330	0
garlic, roasted (*Uncle Ben's*), 2 oz.	190	6.0	41.0	1.0	0	610	1.0
garlic basil:							
(*Lundberg One-Step*)	160	6.0	37.0	1.0	0	480	5.0
(*A Taste of Thai*), ¾ cup*	160	5.0	35.0	0	0	370	0
garlic and butter (*Uncle Ben's Natural Select*), 2 oz., 1 cup*	200	5.0	43.0	.5	0	590	1.0
garlic and herb:							
(*Near East*)	220	5.0	44.0	3.5	0	680	1.0
pilaf, long grain and wild (*Near East*)	220	5.0	43.0	4.0	10	720	2.0
ginger pesto (*Chef's Originals*), ¼ cup	160	3.0	35.0	.5	0	340	0
golden (*A Taste of Thai*), ¾ cup*	180	3.0	38.0	1.5	0	390	0
herb and butter:							
(*Lipton Rice & Sauce*)	280	6.0	43.0	10.5	10	880	1.0
(*Rice-A-Roni*)	320	6.0	53.0	9.0	5	1160	1.0
jambalaya (*Mahatma*)	190	5.0	42.0	.5	0	1120	1.0
lemon herb pilaf, w/jasmine rice (*Knorr*), ⅓ cup	260	6.0	55.0	2.0	0	790	<1.0
long grain and wild:							
(*Carolina/Mahatma*)	190	5.0	41.0	.5	0	710	2.0
(*Minute*), ⅓ box	220	6.0	49.0	.5	0	880	1.0
(*Rice-A-Roni*)	240	5.0	42.0	6.0	0	930	2.0
(*Success*)	190	5.0	42.0	0	0	890	1.0
(*Uncle Ben's*), 2 oz.	190	6.0	41.0	.5	0	620	1.0
medley (*Lipton Rice & Sauce*)	270	7.0	44.0	8.5	5	870	1.0
Mexican:							
(*Chef's Originals Sonoran*), ¼ cup	180	4.0	38.0	1.0	0	440	1.0
(*Goya*), ¼ cup	160	3.0	37.0	0	0	520	0
(*Rice-A-Roni*)	250	6.0	41.0	8.0	0	780	2.0

Food and Measure	cal.	prot. (gms)	carbo. (gms)	fat (gms)	chol. (mgs)	sod. (mgs)	fiber (gms)
mushroom:							
(*Lipton* Rice & Sauce)	270	6.0	45.0	7.5	0	960	1.0
risotto (*Knorr* Italian), ⅓ cup	280	6.0	62.0	1.0	0	1280	<1.0
shiitake (*Chef's Originals*), ¼ cup ..	160	3.0	35.0	.5	0	370	0
wild, and herb pilaf (*Near East*)	220	5.0	44.0	3.5	10	560	2.0
Opelousas, and gravy (*Chef's Originals*), ¼ cup	180	4.0	40.0	1.0	0	410	1.0
Oriental:							
stir-fry (*Lipton* Rice & Sauce)	270	5.0	47.0	7.5	0	860	1.0
stir-fry (*Rice-A-Roni*)	290	6.0	54.0	6.0	0	1240	2.0
pilaf (see also specific listings):							
(*Carolina/Mahatma* Classic)	190	5.0	43.0	0	0	810	1.0
(*Casbah*), ¾ cup ..	210	6.0	38.0	.5	0	390	.5
(*Knorr*), ⅓ cup ...	210	5.0	46.0	.5	0	900	<1.0
(*Lipton* Rice & Sauce)	260	6.0	44.0	7.5	0	930	1.0
(*Lundberg* Olde World), ½ cup ..	340	11.0	73.0	3.0	0	5	10.0
(*Near East*)	210	6.0	42.0	3.0	10	890	1.0
(*Rice-A-Roni*)	310	6.0	52.0	9.0	0	1180	1.0
(*Success*)	200	5.0	44.0	0	0	630	2.0
brown rice (*Near East*)	220	6.0	41.0	4.0	10	730	2.0
long grain and wild (*Near East*)	210	6.0	42.0	3.0	10	830	2.0
long grain and wild (*Rice-A-Roni*) ..	240	5.0	43.0	6.0	0	950	2.0
primavera (*Nile Spice*), 2.2-oz. pkg. ...	240	6.0	50.0	1.5	5	620	2.0
pilau (*Neera's* Shahi)	286	6.0	48.0	8.0	0	6	2.0
primavera:							
(*Goya*), ¼ cup	160	5.0	35.0	0	0	570	1.0
(*Health Valley*), ½ cup	140	7.0	26.0	1.0	0	280	2.0

Food and Measure	cal.	prot. (gms)	carbo. (gms)	fat (gms)	chol. (mgs)	sod. (mgs)	fiber (gms)
Rice dish, mix (*cont.*)							
risotto (see also specific listings):							
fine herb (*Uncle Ben's Chef's Recipe*), 2 oz. . .	200	4.0	44.0	.5	0	470	0
garlic and herb (*Chef's Originals*), ¼ cup	130	2.0	30.0	0	0	10	0
garlic primavera (*Lundberg*), ¼ box	140	4.0	29.0	1.0	0	520	1.0
garlic Parmesan (*Lipton* Rice & Sauce), ½ pkg. .	250	8.0	45.0	5.0	10	960	1.0
garlic primavera (*Marrakesh Express*)	210	5.0	46.0	.5	0	610	1.0
Italian herb (*Lundberg*), ¼ box . . .	140	4.0	28.0	1.0	0	530	1.0
Milanese (*Alessi*), ⅓ cup	190	4.0	42.0	0	0	710	1.0
Milanese (*Knorr* Italian), ⅓ cup . .	260	4.0	59.0	1.0	0	880	1.0
Milanese, w/saffron (*Marrakesh Express*)	220	4.0	50.0	0	0	590	0
onion herb (*Knorr* Italian), ⅓ cup . .	300	6.0	66.0	1.5	0	1390	1.0
Parmesan (*Chef's Originals*), ¼ cup	130	3.0	29.0	0	0	5	0
Parmesan, creamy (*Lundberg*), ¼ box	140	5.0	27.0	1.5	0	490	1.0
porcini mushroom (*Alessi*), ⅓ cup .	190	3.0	44.0	0	0	810	1.0
portobello (*Chef's Originals*), ¼ cup	140	3.0	30.0	0	0	25	0
tomato basil (*Lundberg*), ¼ box . . .	140	4.0	30.0	1.0	0	630	1.0
sun-dried tomato (*Alessi*), ⅓ cup .	190	4.0	42.0	0	0	600	1.0

Food and Measure	cal.	prot. (gms)	carbo. (gms)	fat (gms)	chol. (mgs)	sod. (mgs)	fiber (gms)
sun-dried tomato (*Marrakesh Express*)	200	5.0	45.0	.5	0	520	1.0
vegetable (*Near East Meal Cup*), 1 pkg.	230	6.0	50.0	1.5	5	600	2.0
vegetable primavera (*Knorr*), ⅓ cup .	280	6.0	61.0	1.0	<5	1250	1.0
saffron, see "yellow," below							
salsa style (*Lipton Rice & Sauce*)	220	4.0	37.0	7.0	0	540	2.0
savory (*Chef's Originals* Louisiana), ¼ cup	180	4.0	40.0	1.0	0	330	1.0
scampi style (*Lipton Rice & Sauce*)	270	6.0	44.0	8.5	5	900	1.0
Southwestern (*Bowl Appétit!*), 1 bowl ..	260	8.0	52.0	3.0	5	920	3.0
Spanish:							
(*Carolina/Mahatma*)	180	4.0	42.0	.5	0	760	2.0
(*Lipton* Rice & Sauce)	270	6.0	47.0	7.5	0	900	2.0
(*Rice-A-Roni*)	300	8.0	51.0	8.0	0	1460	3.0
(*Success*)	190	5.0	43.0	.5	0	780	1.0
pilaf (*Casbah*), ¾ cup	200	4.0	40.0	.5	0	430	1.0
pilaf (*Near East*) ..	290	5.0	55.0	6.0	20	1130	2.0
spicy, w/beans (*Near East* Meal Cup), 1 pkg.	240	9.0	49.0	3.0	5	620	6.0
Stroganoff (*Rice-A-Roni*)	360	8.0	49.0	15.0	5	1000	1.0
teriyaki (*Lipton* Rice & Sauce)	270	5.0	45.0	8.0	0	910	1.0
Thai (*Health Valley*), ½ cup	140	7.0	27.0	1.0	0	280	2.0
tomato:							
(*Chef's Originals* French Quarter), ¼ cup	180	4.0	34.0	1.0	0	390	.5
(*Nile Spice* Meal Cup), 1 pkg. ...	140	5.0	27.0	2.5	5	540	2.0
vegetable: garden (*Rice-A-Roni*)	240	6.0	41.0	6.0	0	860	2.0

Food and Measure	cal.	prot. (gms)	carbo. (gms)	fat (gms)	chol. (mgs)	sod. (mgs)	fiber (gms)
Rice dish, mix, vegetable (*cont.*)							
roasted, and chicken pilaf (*Near East*)	220	5.0	43.0	3.5	10	800	2.0
shiitake (*Health Valley*), ½ cup . .	140	7.0	26.0	1.5	0	280	2.0
wild rice (*Lipton Rice & Sauce*)	280	7.0	48.0	7.5	0	940	2.0
yellow:							
(*Goya*), 2 oz.	180	4.0	40.0	.5	0	560	n.a.
(*Success*)	150	3.0	33.0	0	0	670	<1.0
saffron (*Carolina/ Mahatma*)	190	4.0	43.0	0	0	970	<1.0
saffron, spicy (*Mahatma*)	180	4.0	41.0	.5	0	1150	<1.0
Spanish style (*Goya*), ¼ cup	170	4.0	37.0	0	0	640	1.0
Rice dish, pkg., cheddar broccoli (*Bowl Appétit!*), 1 bowl	290	8.0	51.0	7.0	10	930	2.0
Rice entree, dried, 1 serving:							
black beans and (*AlpineAire*)	340	11.0	69.0	1.5	0	770	10.0
Mexican, w/cheese (*AlpineAire*)	240	8.0	39.0	5.0	n.a.	530	2.0
mushroom pilaf, w/vegetables (*Alpine-Aire*)	330	13.0	66.0	1.5	0	840	4.0
wild rice pilaf:							
(*AlpineAire*)	310	10.0	53.0	7.0	0	1030	8.0
mushroom (*Mountain House*)	300	9.0	55.0	5.0	10	850	3.0
Rice entree, frozen, see "Rice dish, frozen"							
Rice flour, ¼ cup, except as noted:							
brown:							
(*Arrowhead Mills*)	120	3.0	27.0	1.0	0	0	2.0
(*Hodgson Mill*), scant ¼ cup	110	3.0	23.0	1.0	0	0	1.0
(*Lundberg* Organic)	110	2.0	22.0	1.5	0	0	2.0

Food and Measure	cal.	prot. (gms)	carbo. (gms)	fat (gms)	chol. (mgs)	sod. (mgs)	fiber (gms)
(*Lundberg Nutra-Farmed*)	120	3.0	26.0	1.5	0	0	1.0
1 cup	574	11.4	120.8	4.4	0	12	7.3
white:							
(*Arrowhead Mills*) .	130	2.0	28.0	.5	0	0	1.0
1 cup	578	9.4	126.6	2.2	0	1	3.9
Rice pasta, see "Pasta"							
Rice pudding, ready-to-eat (*Kozy Shack*), ½ cup	140	4.0	22.0	3.0	20	135	0
Rice pudding mix:							
(*Jell-O Americana* Fat Free), ½ cup*	140	5.0	29.0	0	<5	160	0
(*Minute*), ¼ pkg. ...	90	<1.0	23.0	0	0	100	0
(*Watkins*), 1½ tbsp.	50	1.0	12.0	0	0	190	0
cinnamon raisin (*Uncle Ben's*), ½ cup*	160	2.0	37.0	.5	0	150	1.0
cinnamon raisin (*Lundberg* Elegant), ½ cup	70	0	16.0	0	0	0	1.0
coconut (*Lundberg* Elegant), ½ cup ...	70	0	13.0	2.0	0	0	1.0
honey almond (*Lundberg* Elegant), ½ cup	70	2.0	15.0	.5	0	0	1.0
Rice puffs (*Eden* Arare), 30 pcs., 1.1 oz.	110	3.0	24.0	0	0	160	2.0
Rice seasoning:							
Mexican (*Lawry's*), 1½ tbsp.	40	<1.0	9.0	0	0	840	0
Spanish (*Bearitos*), 1 tsp.	10	0	1.0	0	0	580	0
Rice syrup, brown (*Lundberg Sweet Dreams Nutra-Farmed*), ¼ cup ..	170	0	42.0	0	0	5	0
Rigatoni pasta, stuffed, w/cheese, frozen (*Italian Village*), 5.25 oz.	320	16.0	53.0	7.0	60	190	4.0

Food and Measure	cal.	prot. (gms)	carbo. (gms)	fat (gms)	chol. (mgs)	sod. (mgs)	fiber (gms)
Rigatoni pasta dish, mix, 1 cup*:							
cheddar, white, and broccoli sauce (*Pasta Roni*)	320	9.0	40.0	14.0	5	770	2.0
herb and butter (*Pasta Roni*)	350	9.0	42.0	16.0	5	880	2.0
Rigatoni pasta entree, frozen, 1 pkg.:							
w/broccoli and chicken (*Healthy Choice Medley*), 9 oz.	280	19.0	34.0	7.0	30	600	3.0
cheese, stuffed (*Michelina's*), 8.5 oz.	300	12.0	41.0	8.0	45	760	3.0
in cream sauce, w/broccoli, chicken (*Budget Gourmet*), 8 oz.	260	9.0	40.0	6.0	15	480	2.0
jumbo, w/meatballs (*Lean Cuisine Hearty Portions*), 15⅜ oz.	440	25.0	64.0	9.0	35	820	7.0
pomodoro (*Michelina's*), 8 oz.	220	8.0	40.0	2.5	0	410	3.0
risotto Parmigiano (*Michelina's*), 8 oz.	450	15.0	50.0	21.0	50	650	1.0
Risotto, see "Rice dish"							
Rock candy syrup (*Trader Vic's*), 1 fl. oz.	90	0	23.0	0	0	15	0
Rockfish, meat only:							
raw, 4 oz.	107	21.3	0	1.8	39	68	0
baked, broiled, or microwaved, 4 oz.	137	27.3	0	2.3	50	87	0
Roe (see also "Caviar"), mixed species:							
raw, 1 oz., 2 tbsp. ...	40	6.3	.4	1.8	106	26	0
baked, broiled, or microwaved, 1 oz.	58	8.1	.5	2.3	135	33	0
Roletti pasta dish, frozen, and vegetables (*Birds Eye*), 1 cup	190	5.0	11.0	8.0	5	350	1.0

Food and Measure	cal.	prot. (gms)	carbo. (gms)	fat (gms)	chol. (mgs)	sod. (mgs)	fiber (gms)
Roll (see also "Biscuit" and "Bun, sweet"), 1 roll, except as noted:							
(*Rhodes* Fat Free) ...	85	3.0	17.0	0	0	136	1.0
deli (*Wonder*)	180	6.0	33.0	2.5	0	360	2.0
dinner:							
(*Wonder*)	100	3.0	17.0	1.5	0	160	0
all varieties (*Awrey's*), 2 rolls, 1.6 oz.	120	4.0	22.0	1.5	0	240	<1.0
brown and serve (*Stroehmann*) ..	80	3.0	16.0	1.0	0	170	<1.0
brown and serve or plain, 2 oz.	170	4.8	28.6	4.1	<1	295	1.7
egg, 2 oz.	174	5.4	29.5	3.6	28	309	2.1
oat bran, 2 oz. ...	134	5.4	22.8	2.6	0	234	2.3
parker house (*Pepperidge Farm*), 3 rolls	150	7.0	20.0	4.5	5	230	1.0
rye, 2 oz.	162	5.8	30.1	1.9	0	506	2.8
soft (*Pepperidge Farm*)	90	4.0	15.0	1.5	0	160	<1.0
wheat, 2 oz.	155	4.9	26.1	3.8	0	193	2.2
wheat, sweet, soft (*Pepperidge Farm*)	100	3.0	17.0	1.5	0	140	<1.0
wheat, whole, 2 oz.	151	4.9	29.0	2.7	0	271	4.3
egg, twist (*Levy* Old Country)	170	5.0	30.0	4.0	5	240	1.0
French:							
(*Francisco*)	110	4.0	19.0	1.5	0	210	<1.0
2 oz.	157	4.9	28.5	2.4	0	345	1.8
hamburger:							
(*Arnold*)	140	4.0	24.0	2.5	0	270	1.0
(*Martin's Sliced*) ..	100	4.0	15.0	1.5	0	140	<1.0
(*Pepperidge Farm*)	120	5.0	21.0	2.5	0	220	1.0
(*Wonder*)	110	3.0	21.0	1.5	0	220	0
hamburger or hot dog:							
2 oz.	162	4.8	28.5	2.9	0	318	1.5
mixed grain, 2 oz. .	149	5.4	25.3	3.4	0	260	2.2
hoagie (see also "sub," below):							
(*Awrey's*)	230	8.0	46.0	1.0	0	460	2.0
(*Martin's Seeded*) .	270	11.0	2.0	4.5	0	440	2.0

Food and Measure	cal.	prot. (gms)	carbo. (gms)	fat (gms)	chol. (mgs)	sod. (mgs)	fiber (gms)
Roll, hoagie (*cont.*)							
(*Martin's* Unseeded)	260	9.0	40.0	3.0	0	460	2.0
hot dog/frankfurter:							
(*Arnold*)	120	4.0	21.0	2.0	0	240	<1.0
potato (*Arnold*) ...	130	5.0	24.0	1.5	0	200	<1.0
potato (*Martin's* Long Roll)	150	7.0	22.0	2.0	0	180	1.0
kaiser or hard:							
(*Awrey's*)	190	5.0	37.0	2.0	0	340	1.0
(*Levy* Old Country)	170	5.0	34.0	2.0	0	270	1.0
2 oz.	166	5.6	29.9	2.4	0	308	1.3
onion (*Levy* Old Country)	160	5.0	31.0	3.0	5	210	3.0
potato (*Martin's*)	100	4.0	15.0	1.0	0	130	<1.0
sandwich roll/bun:							
(*Martin's*)	150	6.0	22.0	2.0	0	210	1.0
(*Pepperidge Farm* Hearty)	210	8.0	35.0	4.5	0	390	<1.0
potato, golden (*Pepperidge Farm*) ..	220	8.0	36.0	4.5	0	360	<1.0
potato, sesame (*Arnold*) ...	170	7.0	29.0	3.0	0	250	1.0
sesame (*Arnold*) ..	140	5.0	23.0	3.0	0	230	1.0
sesame (*Marty's* Large)	190	8.0	25.0	3.5	0	290	2.0
sesame (*Pepperidge Farm*)	130	5.0	22.0	3.0	0	220	1.0
wheat, country (*Pepperidge Farm*) ..	210	8.0	36.0	4.0	0	370	1.0
sub (*Levy's* Old Country)	140	5.0	30.0	1.5	0	250	1.0
wheat:							
(*Rhodes*)	140	5.0	27.0	2.5	0	190	4.0
cracked (*Rhodes*) .	140	6.0	24.0	3.0	0	20	3.0
white (*Rhodes*)	95	3.0	17.0	2.0	0	140	0
Roll, mix, hot (*Pillsbury* Specialty), ¼ cup mix	110	3.0	21.0	1.5	0	200	<1.0
Roll, refrigerated (see also "Biscuit, refrigerated"), 1 pc.:							
crescent:							
(*Grands!* Quick), 2.5 oz.	270	5.0	29.0	15.0	0	510	<1.0

Food and Measure	cal.	prot. (gms)	carbo. (gms)	fat (gms)	chol. (mgs)	sod. (mgs)	fiber (gms)
(*Pillsbury*), 1 oz.	110	2.0	11.0	6.0	0	220	0
(*Pillsbury* Reduced Fat), 1 oz.	100	2.0	12.0	4.5	0	230	0
dinner, 1.4 oz.:							
(*Pillsbury* Traditional Tube)	110	4.0	18.0	2.0	0	270	<1.0
crusty French (*Pillsbury Home Baked Classics*)	110	4.0	19.0	1.5	0	220	0
Roll, sweet, see "Bun, sweet"							
Romaine, see "Lettuce" and "Salad blend"							
Roseapple, 1 oz.	7	.2	1.6	.1	0	<1	<1.0
Roselle, 1 oz., ½ cup	14	.3	3.2	.2	0	2	<1.0
Rosemary, dried, 1 tsp.	4	.1	.8	.2	0	1	.2
Rotini dish, mix:							
cheese, three (*Lipton Pasta & Sauce*), ½ pkg.	240	9.0	41.0	5.0	10	870	<1.0
cheese w/broccoli (*Kraft Velveeta*), 4.5 oz.	400	16.0	48.0	16.0	30	1230	2.0
w/cheese sauce, four (*Near East* Meal Cup), 1 pkg.	200	10.0	21.0	3.0	10	600	1.0
chicken and broccoli:							
(*Near East* Meal Cup), 1 pkg.	190	7.0	34.0	3.5	15	630	2.0
(*Nile Spice* Cup), 1.8-oz. pkg.	190	7.0	33.0	3.5	15	640	2.0
w/mushroom sauce (*Knorr* Side Dish), ⅔ cup	260	10.0	50.0	1.5	0	710	1.0
four cheese (*Knorr* Side Dish), ⅓ cup	130	5.0	21.0	3.5	<5	470	1.0
Rotini dish, pkg., three cheese (*Bowl Appétit!*), 1 bowl	360	13.0	56.0	10.0	15	980	2.0
Roughy, orange, meat only:							
raw, 4 oz.	78	16.7	0	.8	23	72	0
baked, broiled, or microwaved, 4 oz.	101	21.4	0	1.0	29	92	0

Food and Measure	cal.	prot. (gms)	carbo. (gms)	fat (gms)	chol. (mgs)	sod (mgs)	fiber (gms)
Rutabaga, fresh:							
1 large, 1.7 lbs.	278	9.3	62.8	1.5	0	154	19.3
cubed, ½ cup:							
raw	25	.8	5.7	.1	0	14	1.8
boiled, drained	33	1.1	7.4	.2	0	17	1.5
boiled, drained,							
mashed, ½ cup ...	47	1.6	10.5	.3	0	25	2.2
Rye, whole-grain:							
(*Arrowhead Mills*),							
¼ cup	160	6.0	34.0	1.0	0	0	6.0
1 cup	567	25.0	117.9	4.2	0	10	24.7
Rye flakes, rolled							
(*Arrowhead Mills*),							
⅓ cup	110	4.0	24.0	.5	0	0	4.0
Rye flour:							
(*Arrowhead Mills*),							
½ cup	100	5.0	20.0	1.0	0	0	4.0
(*Hodgson Mill* Organic/							
Whole Grain),							
¼ cup	90	3.0	22.0	1.0	0	0	5.0
dark, 1 cup	415	18.0	88.0	3.4	0	2	28.9
light, 1 cup	374	8.6	81.8	1.4	0	2	14.9
medium (*Pillsbury*),							
¼ cup	100	3.0	22.0	0	0	0	2.0
medium, 1 cup	361	9.9	79.0	1.8	0	3	14.9
Rye malt, see "Malt							
syrup"							

S

Food and Measure	cal.	prot. (gms)	carbo. (gms)	fat (gms)	chol. (mgs)	sod. (mgs)	fiber (gms)
Sablefish, meat only:							
raw, 4 oz.	222	15.2	0	17.4	56	64	0
baked, broiled, or							
microwaved, 4 oz.	284	19.5	0	22.2	71	82	0
smoked, 4 oz.	291	20.0	0	22.8	73	836	0
Safflower kernels,							
dried, 1 oz.	147	4.6	9.7	10.9	0	<1	1.0
Safflower meal,							
partially defatted,							
1 oz.	97	10.1	13.8	.7	0	n.a.	<3.0
Saffron, 1 tsp.	2	.1	.5	<.1	0	1	0
Sage, ground, 1 tsp.	2	.1	.4	.1	0	<1	0
Salad blend (see also							
"Lettuce" and "Salad							
kit"), fresh, 3 oz.,							
except as noted:							
(*Dole* Very Veggie) ...	20	1.0	4.0	0	0	20	1.0
(*Fresh Express* Royal							
Blend)	20	1.0	5.0	0	0	30	2.0
(*Fresh Express* Fancy							
Field Greens)	15	1.0	3.0	0	0	15	2.0
(*Fresh Express* Greener							
European)	15	1.0	3.0	0	0	10	1.0
(*Fresh Express* Riviera)	10	1.0	2.0	0	0	5	1.0
(*Fresh Express* Veggie							
Lover's)	20	1.0	4.0	0	0	15	1.0
(*Ready Pac* Classic							
Crisp/Hearty Green							
Salad)	10	<1.0	2.0	0	0	5	<1.0
(*Ready Pac* Organic							
Country Garden) ..	15	<1.0	2.0	0	0	10	<1.0
(*Ready Pac* Organic							
Harvest Crisp)	10	<1.0	2.0	0	0	5	<1.0

Food and Measure	cal.	prot. (gms)	carbo. (gms)	fat (gms)	chol. (mgs)	sod. (mgs)	fiber (gms)
Salad blend (*cont.*)							
(*Ready Pac* Spring Mix)	35	3.0	7.0	0	0	40	3.0
(*Ready Pac* All American)	15	1.0	3.0	0	0	10	1.0
(*Ready Pac Lafayette*)	10	0	3.0	0	0	5	<1.0
American:							
(*Dole*)	15	1.0	3.0	0	0	10	1.0
(*Fresh Express More Carrots*) ..	15	1.0	3.0	0	0	10	1.0
Aspen (*Ready Pac* Organic), 4.5-oz. pkg.	25	3.0	3.0	0	0	20	<1.0
Bordeaux (*Ready Pac*), 5-oz. pkg.	35	3.0	5.0	0	0	20	2.0
Caesar:							
(*Ready Pac*)	15	1.0	2.0	0	0	5	1.0
(*Ready Pac* Organic)	15	<0	2.0	0	0	10	<1.0
coleslaw:							
(*Dole* Classic)	25	1.0	5.0	0	0	25	2.0
(*Fresh Express* Angel Hair)	20	1.0	5.0	0	0	15	2.0
(*Fresh Express* Old Fashioned)	25	1.0	5.0	0	0	15	2.0
w/broccoli (*Mann's*), 4 oz.	35	1.0	6.0	0	0	65	3.0
w/carrots (*Fresh Express* 3-Color)	20	1.0	5.0	0	0	15	2.0
European (*Dole*)	15	1.0	3.0	0	0	15	1.0
French (*Dole*)	15	1.0	4.0	0	0	20	2.0
iceberg, carrots, red cabbage:							
(*Fresh Express* Iceberg Garden) ...	15	1.0	3.0	0	0	10	1.0
romaine (*Fresh Express*)	15	1.0	3.0	0	0	10	1.0
(*Fresh Express* Green & Crisp), 2 cups	15	1.0	3.0	0	0	10	1.0
romaine, double carrots (*Fresh Express* Green & Crisp)	15	1.0	4.0	0	0	15	1.0

Food and Measure	cal.	prot. (gms)	carbo. (gms)	fat (gms)	chol. (mgs)	sod. (mgs)	fiber (gms)
Italian:							
(*Dole*)	15	1.0	3.0	0	0	10	1.0
(*Fresh Express*) ...	15	1.0	2.0	0	0	10	1.0
Mediterranean (*Dole*) .	15	1.0	3.0	0	0	20	2.0
mesclun (*Ready Pac*), 4.5-oz. pkg.	35	3.0	7.0	0	0	40	3.0
Milano (*Ready Pac*) ..	15	1.0	3.0	0	0	15	2.0
Monterey (*Ready Pac* Organic)	15	1.0	3.0	0	0	10	2.0
Parisian (*Ready Pac*) .	20	1.0	4.0	0	0	20	1.0
Portofino (*Ready Pac*)	25	3.0	4.0	0	0	125	2.0
Santa Barbara (*Ready Pac*)	15	1.0	3.0	0	0	20	<1.0
Tuscany (*Dole*)	20	1.0	4.0	0	0	15	2.0
Verona (*Dole*)	10	1.0	2.0	0	0	5	1.0
Salad kit, w/dressing, fresh, 3.5 oz.:							
(*Dole* All American Toss)	50	4.0	7.0	1.0	<5	160	2.0
Caesar:							
(*Dole*)	170	3.0	7.0	15.0	10	380	2.0
(*Dole* Family)	170	3.0	8.0	15.0	10	440	2.0
(*Fresh Express*) ...	160	3.0	9.0	14.0	10	410	1.0
(*Fresh Express* Light)	100	2.0	14.0	0	0	410	1.0
(*Fresh Express* Supreme)	150	3.0	8.0	13.0	10	390	1.0
creamy garlic (*Dole*)	170	3.0	8.0	15.0	5	390	1.0
w/light dressing (*Dole*)	100	3.0	8.0	7.0	10	370	1.0
cheese, triple (*Dole* Toss)	80	5.0	4.0	5.0	15	120	1.0
coleslaw (*Fresh Express*)	120	1.0	12.0	8.0	5	135	2.0
Greek marinade (*Dole* Classic)	100	2.0	5.0	8.0	<5	340	1.0
Mediterranean marinade (*Dole*)	90	1.0	5.0	8.0	0	180	1.0
Oriental (*Fresh Express*)	140	2.0	13.0	9.0	0	350	2.0
ranch:							
(*Fresh Express*) ...	140	2.0	8.0	11.0	5	280	1.0
(*Fresh Express* Light)	100	2.0	11.0	0	0	280	1.0

Food and Measure	cal.	prot. (gms)	carbo. (gms)	fat (gms)	chol. (mgs)	sod. (mgs)	fiber (gms)
Salad kit (*cont.*)							
Romano (*Dole*)	150	2.0	8.0	13.0	0	510	2.0
sunflower ranch (*Dole*)	170	2.0	5.0	16.0	5	220	2.0
taco (*Fresh Express Taco Fiesta*)	110	3.0	7.0	8.0	10	230	1.0
Salad dressing, 2 tbsp., except as noted:							
bacon and tomato:							
(*Henri's*)	130	0	10.0	10.0	0	310	0
(*Kraft*)	140	<1.0	2.0	14.0	<5	280	0
(*Kraft ⅓ Less Fat Reduced Calorie*)	60	<1.0	3.0	5.0	<5	300	0
tangy (*Kraft Special Collection*)	130	<1.0	8.0	10.0	0	410	0
balsamic vinaigrette:							
(*Cardini's*)	150	0	2.0	16.0	0	210	0
(*Girard's Fat Free*)	25	0	6.0	0	0	400	0
(*Henri's Fat Free*) . .	15	0	4.0	0	0	300	0
(*Kraft Special Collection*)	120	0	4.0	12.0	0	290	0
(*Marzetti*)	100	0	4.0	9.0	0	330	0
(*Marzetti Light*) . . .	50	0	4.0	4.0	0	340	0
(*Newman's Own*) . .	90	0	3.0	9.0	0	350	0
(*Pfeiffer*)	100	0	4.0	9.0	0	330	0
(*Wish-Bone*)	60	0	3.0	5.0	0	280	0
roasted tomato (*Hellmann's/Best Foods*)	100	0	3.0	10.0	0	260	0
roasted tomato garlic (*Hellmann's/ Best Foods* Fat Free)	20	0	4.0	0	0	350	0
berry vinaigrette (*Wish-Bone*)	50	0	2.0	4.5	0	130	0
blue cheese:							
(*Kraft*)	160	1.0	2.0	16.0	20	320	0
(*Kraft Crumbles*) . .	160	<1.0	2.0	17.0	20	320	0
(*Kraft Light Done Right Roka*)	70	<1.0	3.0	6.0	<5	290	0
(*Kraft Roka*)	120	<1.0	1.0	13.0	<5	300	0
(*Marie's Super*) . . .	160	2.0	0	18.0	20	200	0
(*Marzetti Light*) . . .	90	1.0	5.0	8.0	15	340	1.0
(*Marzetti Low Fat*)	45	1.0	7.0	2.0	0	440	1.0
(*Ott's Fat Free*)	35	0	9.0	0	0	310	0

Food and Measure	cal.	prot. (gms)	carbo. (gms)	fat (gms)	chol. (mgs)	sod. (mgs)	fiber (gms)
(*Ott's* Original)	80	0	9.0	6.0	0	210	0
(*Ott's* Reduced Calorie)	60	0	8.0	3.0	0	210	0
(*Pfeiffer*)	170	1.0	1.0	18.0	15	280	0
(*Wish-Bone Just 2 Good!*)	45	1.0	6.0	2.0	0	320	0
chunky (*Hellmann's/ Best Foods*)	130	1.0	2.0	13.0	15	160	0
chunky (*Kraft* Reduced Calorie) ..	60	<1.0	4.0	4.0	<5	550	0
chunky (*Marie's*) ..	170	1.0	0	19.0	15	170	0
chunky (*Marzetti* Refrigerated) ...	150	1.0	1.0	16.0	20	310	0
chunky (*Wish-Bone*)	170	1.0	3.0	17.0	0	290	0
chunky (*Wish-Bone* Fat Free)	35	0	7.0	0	0	290	0
honey French (*Marzetti*)	160	1.0	11.0	13.0	0	270	0
sour cream (*Marzetti's* Dip & Dressing)	170	1.0	1.0	18.0	25	190	0
blue cheese vinaigrette:							
(*Girard's*)	100	1.0	3.0	10.0	5	500	0
(*Marie's*)	120	2.0	4.0	12.0	10	210	0
(*Marzetti* Refrigerated)	120	1.0	4.0	11.0	5	480	0
Caesar:							
(*Cardini's* Fat Free)	40	0	9.0	0	0	500	0
(*Cardini's* Light) ...	80	1.0	5.0	7.0	35	270	0
(*Cardini's* Natural) .	150	1.0	1.0	17.0	35	230	0
(*Cardini's* "The Original Caesar Dressing")	160	1.0	1.0	17.0	35	240	0
(*Girard's*)	150	1.0	1.0	15.0	10	370	0
(*Girard's* Fat Free) .	40	0	9.0	0	0	500	0
(*Girard's* Light) ...	80	1.0	5.0	7.0	10	370	0
(*Hellmann's/Best Foods* Fat Free) .	30	<1.0	8.0	0	0	420	0
(*Kraft* Classic)	140	<1.0	<1.0	15.0	5	290	0
(*Kraft* ⅓ Less Fat Reduced Calorie)	60	<1.0	2.0	6.0	<5	560	0
(*Kraft Free* Classic)	50	<1.0	11.0	0	0	350	0
(*Kraft Light Done Right* Classic) ..	70	<1.0	3.0	6.0	10	330	0

Food and Measure	cal.	prot. (gms)	carbo. (gms)	fat (gms)	chol. (mgs)	sod. (mgs)	fiber (gms)
Salad dressing, Caesar (*cont.*)							
(*Marzetti*)	120	1.0	1.0	13.0	0	360	0
(*Marzetti* Fat Free) .	40	0	9.0	0	0	500	0
(*Marzetti* Light 16 fl. oz.)	70	1.0	2.0	6.0	2	690	0
(*Marzetti* Light 12 fl. oz.)	70	1.0	2.0	6.0	3	640	0
(*Newman's Own*) . .	150	1.0	1.0	16.0	<5	450	0
(*Pfeiffer*)	120	1.0	1.0	13.0	2	350	0
(*Randall's* Nondairy)	130	1.0	1.0	11.0	30	120	0
(*Randall's* Real) . . .	130	1.0	1.0	11.0	35	120	0
(*Wish-Bone* Classic)	110	1.0	2.0	10.0	5	300	0
(*Wish-Bone* Just 2 Good!* Classic) . .	40	1.0	5.0	2.0	5	310	0
w/bacon (*Kraft*) . . .	150	1.0	1.0	15.0	15	320	0
cilantro (*El Torito* Pepita)	130	0	2.0	14.0	15	260	0
Italian (*Kraft*)	100	<1.0	2.0	10.0	0	470	0
Italian (*Kraft* Free)	25	<1.0	4.0	0	0	470	0
Parmesan vinai- grette (*Kraft*) . . .	60	1.0	1.0	5.0	<5	450	0
ranch (*Kraft*)	140	<1.0	<1.0	15.0	5	290	0
ranch (*Henri's*)	140	0	2.0	15.0	0	250	0
Caesar, creamy:							
(*Hellmann's/Best Foods*)	160	1.0	1.0	17.0	30	330	0
(*Henri's* Fat Free) . .	50	0	12.0	0	0	300	0
(*Marzetti* 16 fl. oz.)	150	1.0	1.0	15.0	10	370	0
(*Marzetti* 15 fl. oz.)	160	1.0	1.0	17.0	35	240	0
(*Newman's Own*) . .	150	1.0	1.0	16.0	<5	450	0
(*Ott's*)	110	1.0	2.0	11.0	20	290	0
(*Wish-Bone*)	180	1.0	1.0	18.0	10	290	0
(*Wish-Bone* Just 2 Good!*)	40	0	7.0	2.0	10	310	0
carrot ginger, sesame (*Randall's*)	45	0	2.0	4.5	0	60	0
Champagne:							
(*Girard's*)	150	0	2.0	16.0	0	490	0
(*Girard's* Light) . . .	60	0	2.0	5.0	0	480	0
coleslaw, see "slaw," below							
cucumber:							
(*Henri's* Fat Free) . .	60	0	14.0	0	0	480	0
creamy (*Henri's*) . .	90	0	9.0	6.0	5	390	0

Food and Measure	cal.	prot. (gms)	carbo. (gms)	fat (gms)	chol. (mgs)	sod. (mgs)	fiber (gms)
Dijon creamy vinaigrette (*Hain*)	130	0	3.0	13.0	0	280	0
Dijon lime (*Newman's Own* Parisienne) ..	120	0	0	13.0	0	220	0
dill, creamy (*Nasoya Vegi-Dressing*)	70	0	2.0	7.0	0	135	0
feta, Greek, vinaigrette (*Girard's*)	100	0	1.0	11.0	0	320	0
French:							
(*Girard's* Original)	120	0	0	13.0	0	400	0
(*Henri's* Original) ..	120	0	6.0	11.0	0	200	0
(*Kraft* ⅓ Less Fat Reduced Calorie)	50	0	6.0	3.0	0	270	0
(*Kraft* Catalina) ...	140	0	8.0	12.0	0	410	0
(*Kraft* Free Catalina)	50	0	11.0	0	0	350	0
(*Kraft* Light Done Right Catalina) ..	60	0	11.0	2.0	0	410	0
(*Marzetti* California)	160	0	11.0	12.0	0	250	0
(*Marzetti* California Fat Free)	40	0	10.0	0	0	290	0
(*Marzetti* California Light)	90	0	8.0	6.0	0	370	0
(*Marzetti* Country) .	160	0	7.0	15.0	10	180	0
(*Pfeiffer*)	150	0	7.0	13.0	10	220	0
(*Pfeiffer* California)	140	0	9.0	12.0	0	300	0
(*Pfeiffer* California Fat Free)	40	0	10.0	0	0	290	0
(*Trader Vic's*)	130	0	0	14.0	0	200	0
(*Wish-Bone* Deluxe)	120	0	5.0	11.0	0	170	0
creamy (*Estee*) ...	10	0	2.0	0	0	80	0
creamy (*Henri's*) ..	120	0	5.0	12.0	0	410	0
creamy (*Kraft*)	140	0	5.0	13.0	0	270	0
honey (*Kraft* Catalina)	130	0	7.0	11.0	0	320	0
honey (*Marzetti*) ..	170	0	10.0	14.0	0	240	0
honey (*Marzetti* Fat Free)	35	0	9.0	0	0	200	0
honey (*Marzetti* Light)	80	0	12.0	4.0	0	250	0
savory (*Hellmann's/ Best Foods*)	130	0	7.0	11.0	0	390	0
spicy (*Cardini's* Natural)	130	0	6.0	11.0	0	300	0

Food and Measure	cal.	prot. (gms)	carbo. (gms)	fat (gms)	chol. (mgs)	sod. (mgs)	fiber (gms)
Salad dressing, French (*cont.*)							
sweet/spicy (*Wish-Bone*)	140	0	6.0	12.0	0	330	0
sweet/spicy (*Wish-Bone Just 2 Good!*)	50	0	9.0	2.0	0	240	0
French style:							
(*Hellmann's/Best Foods Fat Free*)	45	0	11.0	0	0	260	0
(*Henri's Fat Free*)	40	0	11.0	0	0	230	0
(*Henri's Light*)	70	0	13.0	2.0	0	280	0
(*Kraft Free*)	45	0	11.0	0	0	290	0
(*Wish-Bone/Wish-Bone Just 2 Good!* Deluxe)	45	0	7.0	2.0	0	230	0
(*Hellmann's Light Savory*)	70	0	8.0	4.0	0	390	0
bacon tomato flavor (*Henri's*)	140	0	8.0	12.0	0	280	0
creamy (*Kraft Light Done Right*)	90	<1.0	8.0	6.0	0	280	0
garlic, creamy (*Kraft*)	110	0	2.0	11.0	0	360	0
garlic, roasted:							
(*Cardini's*)	130	0	1.0	14.0	4	310	0
(*Marzetti*)	150	1.0	2.0	15.0	15	290	0
vinaigrette (*Kraft*)	60	0	3.0	4.5	0	270	0
vinaigrette (*Randall's Lite*)	40	0	1.0	4.0	0	60	0
vinaigrette (*Pfeiffer*)	130	0	8.0	10.0	0	340	0
vinaigrette (*Wish-Bone*)	60	0	3.0	5.0	0	290	0
garlic cilantro lime (*Randall's*)	80	0	2.0	8.0	0	75	0
grape vinaigrette (*El Torito* Serrano)	25	0	7.0	0	0	290	0
Greek:							
w/feta (*Athenos Mediterranean*)	110	0	2.0	11.0	0	320	0
vinaigrette (*Kraft Special Collection*)	110	0	2.0	11.0	0	340	0
vinaigrette, w/olives and feta (*Kraft*)	120	0	2.0	12.0	0	330	0
green goddess (*Kraft*)	130	0	2.0	13.0	0	260	0
(*Henri's* Tas-Tee)	110	0	8.0	9.0	0	200	0

Food and Measure	cal.	prot. (gms)	carbo. (gms)	fat (gms)	chol. (mgs)	sod. (mgs)	fiber (gms)
(*Henri's* Tas-Tee Light)	60	0	11.0	2.0	0	220	0
herb:							
garden (*Nasoya Vegi-Dressing*) ..	70	0	2.0	7.0	0	140	0
poppy seed (*Cardini's*)	35	0	7.0	1.0	0	300	0
honey Dijon:							
(*Hellmann's/Best Foods* Fat Free)	50	0	12.0	0	0	180	0
(*Hellmann's/Best Foods* Light) ...	80	0	11.0	4.0	5	290	0
(*Kraft*)	100	0	6.0	8.0	0	180	0
(*Kraft* House)	90	0	11.0	5.0	<5	260	0
(*Kraft* Free)	50	0	12.0	0	0	330	0
(*Marzetti*)	140	0	6.0	12.0	15	180	0
(*Marzetti* Fat Free)	50	0	12.0	0	0	290	0
(*Pfeiffer*)	140	0	6.0	12.0	15	180	0
(*Wish-Bone Just 2 Good!*)	50	0	8.0	2.0	0	250	0
peppercorn (*Girard's*)	140	0	7.0	13.0	15	250	1.0
ranch (*Hellmann's*)	240	1.0	12.0	21.0	20	460	0
honey mustard:							
(*Cardini's* Summer)	150	0	5.0	14.0	0	210	0
(*Henri's*)	100	0	10.0	6.0	0	230	0
(*Henri's* Fat Free) ..	50	0	12.0	0	0	200	0
(*Marzetti's* Dip & Dressing)	130	0	6.0	12.0	15	170	0
(*Ott's*)	100	0	8.0	8.0	0	280	0
(*Randall's* Fat Free)	35	1.0	8.0	0	0	95	<1.0
jalapeño (*Randall's*)	30	1.0	7.0	0	0	130	0
Italian:							
(*Cardini's* Dressing/ Marinade)	120	0	1.0	13.0	0	220	0
(*Girard's* Olde Venice)	130	0	2.0	13.0	0	500	0
(*Hellmann's/Best Foods*)	110	0	3.0	11.0	0	460	0
(*Hellmann's/Best Foods* Fat Free)	15	0	4.0	0	0	330	0
(*Hellmann's/Best Foods* Light) ...	60	0	6.0	4.0	0	400	0
(*Henri's* Fat Free) ..	15	0	4.0	0	0	330	0
(*Henri's* Low Fat) ..	15	0	2.0	.5	0	460	0

Food and Measure	cal.	prot. (gms)	carbo. (gms)	fat (gms)	chol. (mgs)	sod. (mgs)	fiber (gms)
Salad dressing, Italian (*cont.*)							
(*Henri's* Renaissance/ Traditional)	100	0	2.0	10.0	0	490	0
(*Kraft* Golden)	70	0	2.0	7.0	0	310	0
(*Kraft* House)	110	0	2.0	11.0	<5	230	0
(*Kraft* Zesty)	80	0	2.0	8.0	0	550	0
(*Kraft* Free)	20	0	4.0	0	0	430	0
(*Kraft Free* Zesty) ..	15	0	2.0	0	0	480	0
(*Kraft* House)	70	0	3.0	6.0	<5	310	0
(*Kraft Light Done Right*)	40	0	3.0	3.0	0	270	0
(*Marzetti*)	100	0	3.0	10.0	0	580	0
(*Marzetti Fat Free 16 fl. oz.*)	20	0	4.0	0	0	290	0
(*Marzetti Fat Free 12 fl. oz.*)	15	0	4.0	0	0	280	0
(*Marzetti Light*) ...	60	0	3.0	5.0	0	600	0
(*Newman's Own* Family Recipe) ..	120	1.0	1.0	12.0	0	400	0
(*Newman's Own* Light)	45	0	3.0	4.0	0	370	0
(*Ott's*)	100	0	2.0	10.0	0	290	0
(*Pfeiffer*)	100	0	3.0	10.0	0	580	0
(*Pfeiffer* Fat Free) ..	20	0	4.0	0	0	290	0
(*Pfeiffer* Light)	50	0	3.0	4.0	0	300	0
(*Seven Seas Viva*)	90	0	2.0	9.0	0	370	0
(*Seven Seas Viva* ⅓ Less Fat)	45	0	2.0	4.0	0	310	0
(*Seven Seas Viva* Free*)	15	0	2.0	0	0	480	0
(*S&W* Light)	35	0	8.0	0	0	460	0
(*Trader Vic's*)	80	0	<1.0	9.0	0	490	0
(*Wish-Bone*)	80	0	3.0	8.0	0	490	0
(*Wish-Bone* Fat Free)	10	0	2.0	0	0	280	0
(*Wish-Bone* House)	110	0	3.0	10.0	<5	280	0
(*Wish-Bone Just 2 Good!*)	35	0	5.0	2.0	0	480	0
(*Wish-Bone Robusto*)	90	0	4.0	8.0	0	550	0
w/blue cheese crumbles (*Cardini's*)	130	1.0	2.0	13.0	5	480	0

Food and Measure	cal.	prot. (gms)	carbo. (gms)	fat (gms)	chol. (mgs)	sod. (mgs)	fiber (gms)
cheese, 3 (*Di Giorno*)	130	<1.0	<1.0	14.0	0	310	0
creamy (*Hain*)	180	0	8.0	16.0	0	210	0
creamy (*Henri's Fat Free*)	45	0	12.0	0	0	380	0
creamy (*Henri's Low Fat*)	50	0	9.0	2.0	0	420	0
creamy (*Kraft*)	100	0	2.0	11.0	0	240	0
creamy (*Kraft Free*)	60	0	13.0	0	0	320	0
creamy (*Marzetti*)	160	0	1.0	17.0	15	240	0
creamy (*Nasoya Vegi-Dressing*) ..	60	0	2.0	6.0	0	180	0
creamy (*Ott's*)	90	0	1.0	10.0	0	210	0
creamy (*Pfeiffer*) ./	160	0	1.0	17.0	15	240	0
creamy (*Seven Seas*)	90	0	2.0	9.0	0	500	0
creamy (*Seven Seas Free*)	60	0	13.0	0	0	320	0
creamy (*Wish-Bone*)	110	1.0	4.0	10.0	0	240	0
garlic, creamy (*Henri's*)	110	0	6.0	9.0	0	290	0
garlic, zesty (*Pfeiffer*)	100	0	3.0	10.0	0	590	0
golden (*Hellmann's/ Best Foods*)	90	0	3.0	9.0	0	320	0
golden (*Henri's*) ...	140	0	2.0	15.0	0	610	0
herb (*Wish-Bone Just 2 Good! Country*)	30	0	3.0	2.0	0	290	0
olive oil/oil blend (*Seven Seas* ⅓ Less Fat*)	45	0	2.0	4.0	0	460	0
Parmesan w/basil (*Kraft Special Collection*)	90	<1.0	2.0	9.0	5	360	0
Romano (*Cardini's Natural*)	130	1.0	1.0	13.0	3	280	0
Romano (*Girard's*)	130	1.0	2.0	13.0	0	510	0
Romano (*Marzetti*)	150	0	1.0	16.0	0	420	0
sweet (*Marzetti*) ...	150	0	7.0	14.0	0	250	0
Italian vinaigrette: (*Kraft* Classic)	60	.0	4.0	4.5	0	420	0
(*Kraft Special Collection* Classic) .	50	0	4.0	4.0	0	420	0

Food and Measure	cal.	prot. (gms)	carbo. (gms)	fat (gms)	chol. (mgs)	sod. (mgs)	fiber (gms)
Salad dressing, Italian vinaigrette (*cont.*)							
blue cheese (*Marzetti*)	100	1.0	3.0	9.0	0	490	0
pesto (*Kraft Special Collection*)	70	<1.0	5.0	5.0	0	270	0
roasted garlic (*Marzetti*)	130	0	8.0	10.0	0	340	0
roasted garlic (*Marzetti* House)	120	0	2.0	13.0	0	520	0
Javanese (*Trader Vic's*)	150	1.0	1.0	16.0	1	390	0
lemon herb (*Cardini's* Dressing/Marinade)	130	0	1.0	13.0	0	240	0
lime dill (*Cardini's* Dressing/Marinade)	130	0	1.0	14.0	0	240	0
mango lime vinaigrette (*Chi-Chi's*)	120	0	7.0	10.0	0	280	0
mayonnaise type, see "Mayonnaise dressing"							
mustard vinaigrette (*Henri's*)	90	0	5.0	8.0	0	300	0
oil and vinegar (*Newman's Own*)	150	0	1.0	16.0	0	150	0
olive oil vinaigrette (*Wish-Bone*)	60	0	4.0	5.0	0	290	0
Oriental:							
(*Girard's*)	120	0	6.0	11.0	0	360	0
(*Kraft* House)	60	<1.0	9.0	2.0	0	410	0
(*Wish-Bone*)	35	0	7.0	1.0	0	490	0
Parmesan:							
basil (*Wish-Bone Just 2 Good!*) ..	40	1.0	5.0	2.0	5	320	0
peppercorn (*Girard's*)	160	0	1.0	17.0	10	270	0
peppercorn (*Marzetti*)	160	0	1.0	17.0	10	260	0
roasted garlic (*Newman's Own*)	110	0	2.0	11.0	0	250	0
Romano, creamy (*Kraft Special Collection*)	140	<1.0	1.0	14.0	10	310	0
pepper, red, roasted (*Randall's* Italiana)	60	0	2.0	6.0	0	35	0

Food and Measure	cal.	prot. (gms)	carbo. (gms)	fat (gms)	chol. (mgs)	sod. (mgs)	fiber (gms)
peppercorn, cracked							
(*Marzetti*)	150	1.0	1.0	16.0	25	290	0
poppy seed:							
(*Hain* Rancher's) ..	120	<1.0	3.0	14.0	5	250	0
(*Marzetti* 16 fl. oz.)	160	0	11.0	13.0	15	310	0
(*Marzetti* 15 fl. oz.)	140	0	10	11.0	10	230	0
(*Marzetti* Fat Free							
16 fl. oz.)	60	0	14.0	0	0	190	0
(*Marzetti* Fat Free							
12 fl. oz.)	60	0	14.0	0	0	180	0
(*Ott's*)	90	0	9.0	7.0	0	210	0
(*Ott's* Fat Free)	45	0	12.0	0	0	210	0
potato salad (*Marzetti*)	150	0	5.0	15.0	25	300	0
ranch:							
(*Chi-Chi's* Serrano)	140	0	2.0	14.0	15	330	0
(*El Torito* Serrano) .	140	0	2.0	14.0	15	330	0
(*Hellmann's/Best*							
Foods Light) ...	80	0	6.0	6.0	<5	350	0
(*Hellmann's/Best*							
Foods Light							
Refrigerated) ...	80	0	4.0	7.0	15	340	0
(*Henri's* Chef's							
Recipe)	150	0	3.0	16.0	0	280	0
(*Henri's* Chef's							
Recipe Light) ...	60	0	12.0	2.0	5	290	0
(*Henri's* Fat Free) ..	45	0	11.0	0	0	380	0
(*Hidden Valley*) ...	140	1.0	1.0	14.0	10	260	0
(*Kraft*)	150	0	1.0	16.0	10	280	0
(*Kraft* Free)	50	0	11.0	0	0	350	0
(*Kraft* Light Done							
Right)	70	0	7.0	4.5	10	370	0
(*Marzetti*)	150	1.0	1.0	16.0	10	210	0
(*Marzetti* Fat Free) .	25	0	7.0	0	0	380	1.0
(*Marzetti* Low Fat) .	50	0	10.0	1.5	3	400	1.0
(*Newman's Own*) ..	140	0	2.0	15.0	10	250	0
(*Ott's*)	156	1.0	2.0	16.0	9	269	0
(*Pfeiffer*)	150	1.0	1.0	16.0	10	210	0
(*Pfeiffer* Fat Free) ..	25	0	7.0	0	0	380	1.0
(*Pfeiffer* Light)	80	0	5.0	7.0	4	370	1.0
(*Seven Seas* 1/3							
Less Fat)	100	0	5.0	9.0	0	320	0
(*Wish-Bone*)	160	0	1.0	17.0	10	200	0

Food and Measure	cal.	prot. (gms)	carbo. (gms)	fat (gms)	chol. (mgs)	sod. (mgs)	fiber (gms)
Salad dressing, ranch (*cont.*)							
(*Wish-Bone* Fat Free)	40	0	9.0	0	0	280	<1.0
(*Wish-Bone Just 2 Good!*)	40	0	5.0	2.0	0	270	0
w/bacon (*Hidden Valley*)	140	1.0	1.0	14.0	10	230	0
w/bacon (*Kraft*)	150	0	1.0	16.0	10	240	0
buttermilk (*Hellmann's/Best Foods*)	140	2.0	3.0	13.0	20	300	0
buttermilk (*Kraft*)	160	1.0	2.0	16.0	10	280	0
buttermilk (*Kraft* No MSG)	160	1.0	2.0	16.0	10	270	0
buttermilk (*Marzetti*)	180	0	1.0	20.0	3	250	0
buttermilk (*Marzetti* Light 15 fl. oz.*)	90	0	3.0	9.0	10	280	0
buttermilk (*Marzetti* Light 16 fl. oz.*)	80	0	5.0	7.0	4	370	1.0
buttermilk (*Seven Seas*)	150	0	2.0	16.0	10	280	0
buttermilk, and bacon (*Marzetti* Refrigerated)	160	1.0	1.0	17.0	10	250	0
cheese, three (*Kraft*)	170	<1.0	1.0	18.0	10	280	0
cheese, three (*Kraft Light Done Right*)	80	<1.0	2.0	7.0	10	420	0
creamy (*Hellmann's/Best Foods* Fat Free)	45	0	11.0	0	0	380	0
cucumber (*Kraft*)	140	0	3.0	15.0	0	210	0
cucumber (*Kraft Light Done Right*)	60	<1.0	2.0	5.0	<5	480	0
garden (*Marzetti*)	160	0	1.0	17.0	10	210	0
garden (*Pfeiffer*)	160	0	1.0	17.0	10	210	0
garlic (*Hellmann's/Best Foods*)	140	0	2.0	15.0	0	320	0
garlic (*Kraft*)	150	0	1.0	16.0	10	280	0
garlic (*Kraft Free*)	45	0	11.0	0	0	310	0
Italian herb (*Hellmann's/Best Foods*)	130	0	1.0	14.0	0	310	0
Parmesan (*Cardini's* Aged)	150	1.0	2.0	15.0	10	290	0

Food and Measure	cal.	prot. (gms)	carbo. (gms)	fat (gms)	chol. (mgs)	sod. (mgs)	fiber (gms)
Parmesan (*Cardini's* Lowfat)	45	1.0	7.0	2.0	0	350	0
Parmesan (*Cardini's* Natural)	150	1.0	1.0	15.0	10	240	0
Parmesan (*Henri's* Fat Free)	40	0	10.0	0	0	330	0
Parmesan (*Marie's*)	180	<1.0	<1.0	19.0	20	170	0
peppercorn (*Henri's*)	150	0	3.0	16.0	0	280	0
peppercorn (*Kraft*)	170	<1.0	1.0	18.0	10	270	0
peppercorn (*Kraft Free*)	50	0	11.0	0	0	350	0
peppercorn (*Marzetti*)	180	1.0	2.0	19.0	10	230	0
peppercorn (*Marzetti* Fat Free)	30	0	7.0	0	0	420	1.0
peppercorn (*Pfeiffer*)	180	1.0	2.0	19.0	10	230	0
sour cream and onion (*Kraft*) ...	150	0	2.0	16.0	10	280	0
Southwest (*Henri's*)	100	0	5.0	10.0	0	370	0
spring onion (*Hellmann's/Best Foods*)	130	0	2.0	14.0	0	300	0
raspberry:							
(*Girard's*)	120	0	9.0	10.0	0	65	0
(*Girard's* Fat Free) .	50	0	13.0	0	0	220	0
blush (*S&W* Light) .	40	0	10.0	0	0	410	0
raspberry vinaigrette:							
(*Hellmann's/Best Foods* Fat Free) .	35	0	9.0	0	0	140	0
(*Henri's* Fat Free) ..	35	0	10.0	0	0	130	0
(*Kraft Free*)	30	0	7.0	0	0	290	0
(*Kraft Light Done Right*)	60	0	7.0	4.0	0	270	0
(*Kraft Signature*) ..	60	0	7.0	4.0	0	210	0
(*Marzetti* House) ..	110	0	3.0	11.0	0	90	0
(*Seven Seas Free*)	30	0	7.0	0	0	290	0
red pepper, roasted (*Cardini's* Natural)	110	0	3.0	11.0	3	350	0
red wine:							
(*S&W* Light)	40	0	10.0	0	0	440	0
vinegar (*Kraft Free*)	15	0	3.0	0	0	390	0
vinegar and oil (*Marzetti*)	90	0	3.0	8.0	0	440	0

Food and Measure	cal.	prot. (gms)	carbo. (gms)	fat (gms)	chol. (mgs)	sod. (mgs)	fiber (gms)
Salad dressing (cont.)							
red wine vinaigrette:							
(Girard's Fat Free)	20	0	5.0	0	0	590	0
(Henri's Fat Free) ..	15	0	3.0	0	0	320	0
(Kraft Light Done							
Right)	50	0	3.0	4.5	0	300	0
(Marzetti Light) ...	30	0	3.0	1.5	0	460	0
(Pfeiffer)	90	0	3.0	9.0	0	450	0
(Seven Seas)	90	0	2.0	9.0	0	470	0
(Seven Seas 1/3							
Less Fat)	45	0	3.0	4.0	0	310	0
(Seven Seas Free)	15	0	3.0	0	0	390	0
(Wish-Bone)	90	0	9.0	5.0	0	230	0
(Wish-Bone Fat							
Free)	35	0	7.0	0	0	230	0
Russian:							
(Kraft)	120	0	10.0	9.0	0	300	0
(Pfeiffer)	140	0	4.0	14.0	15	240	0
(Seven Seas)	140	0	3.0	14.0	0	250	0
(Wish-Bone)	110	0	15.0	6.0	0	350	0
creamy (Kraft)	110	0	5.0	10.0	5	300	0
salsa vinaigrette							
(Chi-Chi's)	110	0	4.0	10.0	0	190	0
sesame cilantro (Annie							
Chun's Noodle/							
Salad), 1 tbsp. ...	60	0	4.0	4.0	0	400	0
sesame garlic (Nasoya							
Vegi-Dressing)	60	0	2.0	6.0	0	130	0
sesame soy:							
(Sushi Chef)	60	0	9.0	2.5	0	450	0
(Trader Vic's)	110	<1.0	3.0	11.0	0	200	0
slaw:							
(Kraft)	120	0	7.0	10.0	10	240	0
(Kraft Coleslaw) ...	110	0	7.0	9.0	10	220	0
(Henri's Fat Free) ..	50	0	13.0	0	10	270	0
(Marzetti Light) ...	100	0	10.0	7.0	25	380	0
(Marzetti Low Fat							
16 fl. oz.)	60	0	11.0	1.5	20	370	0
(Marzetti Low Fat							
12 fl. oz.)	60	0	12.0	1.5	20	370	0
(Marzetti Original)	170	0	6.0	16.0	25	390	0
(Marzetti Reduced							
Fat)	100	0	10.0	7.0	25	380	0

Food and Measure	cal.	prot. (gms)	carbo. (gms)	fat (gms)	chol. (mgs)	sod. (mgs)	fiber (gms)
(*Marzetti* Refrigerated)	170	0	6.0	16.0	25	370	0
(*Marzetti* Southern Recipe)	150	0	14.0	11.0	15	210	0
(*Pfeiffer* Coleslaw)	170	0	6.0	16.0	25	390	0
spinach salad:							
(*Girard's*)	80	0	14.0	2.0	0	250	0
(*Marzetti*)	80	0	14.0	2.0	0	250	0
sweet and saucy							
(*Marzetti*)	140	0	9.0	12.0	0	300	0
sweet and sour:							
(*Henri's*)	110	0	8.0	9.0	0	200	0
(*Marzetti*)	160	0	10.0	13.0	0	220	0
(*Marzetti* Fat Free)	50	0	13.0	0	0	300	0
(*Marzetti* Light)	100	0	11.0	6.0	0	260	0
(*Pfeiffer*)	160	0	10.0	13.0	0	220	0
tamari:							
mustard (*San-J*)	25	1.0	5.0	0	0	240	0
peanut (*San-J*)	60	3.0	9.0	2.0	0	230	1.0
sesame (*San-J*)	40	1.0	8.0	.5	0	490	0
vinaigrette (*San-J*)	60	2.0	7.0	3.0	0	740	0
teriyaki ginger (*Henri's*)	80	0	4.0	7.0	0	530	0
Thousand Island:							
(*Hain*)	110	0	6.0	9.0	<5	180	0
(*Hellmann's/Best Foods*)	130	0	5.0	12.0	10	230	0
(*Henri's*)	100	0	5.0	9.0	5	260	0
(*Henri's* Fat Free)	35	0	9.0	0	0	250	0
(*Henri's* Light)	50	1.0	8.0	2.0	20	310	0
(*Kraft*)	90	0	6.0	8.0	10	310	0
(*Kraft Free*)	40	0	9.0	0	0	280	0
(*Kraft Light Done Right*)	60	0	9.0	2.0	10	330	0
(*Marzetti*)	140	0	4.0	14.0	15	250	0
(*Marzetti* Fat Free)	45	0	11.0	0	0	290	0
(*Marzetti* Refrigerated)	150	0	5.0	15.0	25	230	0
(*Ott's*)	100	0	6.0	8.0	10	190	0
(*Pfeiffer*)	140	0	4.0	14.0	15	240	0
(*Pfeiffer* Fat Free)	45	0	11.0	0	0	370	0
(*Pfeiffer* Light)	70	0	6.0	5.0	15	360	0
(*Nasoya Vegi-Dressing*)	70	0	3.0	6.0	0	115	0

Food and Measure	cal.	prot. (gms)	carbo. (gms)	fat (gms)	chol. (mgs)	sod. (mgs)	fiber (gms)
Salad dressing, Thousand Island (*cont.*)							
(*Wish-Bone*)	140	0	7.0	12.0	10	340	0
(*Wish-Bone Just 2 Good!*)	60	0	9.0	2.0	5	300	0
w/bacon (*Kraft*) . . .	130	0	5.0	11.0	0	200	0
creamy (*Hellmann's/ Best Foods*)	130	0	4.0	13.0	0	270	0
creamy (*Kraft*), 1-oz. pouch	120	0	5.0	11.0	10	300	0
tomato, roasted, vinai- grette (*Henri's*) . . .	90	0	3.0	9.0	0	390	0
tomato, sun-dried:							
basil (*Randall's* Fat Free)	10	0	2.0	0	0	70	0
and oregano (*Kraft*)	90	0	3.0	9.0	0	320	0
vinaigrette (*Kraft Special Collection*)	60	0	4.0	5.0	0	340	0
vinaigrette (*Marzetti*)	130	0	6.0	11.0	0	330	0
vinaigrette (*Wish- Bone*)	50	0	2.0	5.0	0	280	0
white wine:							
(*S&W* Light)	40	0	10.0	0	0	450	0
vinaigrette (*Wish- Bone*)	60	0	4.0	4.5	0	260	0
Salad dressing mix*, 2 tbsp.:							
Caesar, gourmet (*Good Seasons*)	150	0	3.0	16.0	0	300	0
cheese garlic (*Good Seasons*)	140	0	1.0	16.0	0	330	0
garlic, roasted (*Good Seasons*)	150	0	2.0	15.0	0	340	0
garlic and herbs (*Good Seasons*)	140	0	1.0	15.0	0	340	0
herb, zesty (*Good Seasons* Fat Free)	10	0	2.0	0	0	260	0
honey French:							
(*Good Seasons*) . . .	160	0	5.0	15.0	0	250	0
(*Good Seasons* Fat Free)	20	0	5.0	0	0	250	0
honey mustard:							
(*Good Seasons*) . . .	150	0	3.0	15.0	0	240	0
(*Good Seasons* Fat Free)	20	0	5.0	0	0	280	0

Food and Measure	cal.	prot. (gms)	carbo. (gms)	fat (gms)	chol. (mgs)	sod. (mgs)	fiber (gms)
Italian:							
(*Good Seasons*) . . .	140	0	1.0	15.0	0	320	0
(*Good Seasons* Fat Free)	10	0	3.0	0	0	290	0
(*Good Seasons* Reduced Calorie)	50	0	2.0	5.0	0	280	0
mild (*Good Seasons*)	150	0	2.0	15.0	0	370	0
zesty (*Good Seasons*)	140	0	1.0	15.0	0	220	0
zesty (*Good Seasons* Reduced Calorie)	50	0	2.0	5.0	0	260	0
Mexican spice (*Good Seasons*)	140	0	2.0	15.0	0	310	0
Parmesan, gourmet (*Good Seasons*) . . .	150	0	2.0	16.0	0	330	0
Oriental sesame (*Good Seasons*)	150	0	3.0	16.0	0	360	0
peanut (*A Taste of Thai*)	40	1.0	5.0	1.5	0	340	1.0
Salad seasoning (*McCormick Salad Supreme*), ¼ tsp.	0	0	0	0	0	60	0
Salad toppers (see also "Croutons"), 1⅓ tbsp.:							
crunchy and flavorful (*McCormick Salad Toppins*)	35	1.0	2.0	1.5	0	90	0
garden vegetable (*McCormick Salad Toppins*)	35	<1.0	3.0	2.0	0	60	0
Salami:							
(*Boar's Head* Salame Panino), 1 oz.	80	6.0	1.0	6.0	20	160	0
(*Citterio* Milano), 6 slices, 1.1 oz. . .	110	8.0	0	8.0	35	480	0
beef, 2 oz.:							
(*Boar's Head*)	120	10.0	0	9.0	25	470	0
(*Hebrew National*)	150	8.0	0	13.0	35	420	0
(*Hebrew National* Chub)	170	8.0	0	14.0	40	420	0

Food and Measure	cal.	prot. (gms)	carbo. (gms)	fat (gms)	chol. (mgs)	sod. (mgs)	fiber (gms)
Salami, beef (*cont.*)							
(*Hebrew National Lean*)	90	9.0	1.0	5.0	25	480	0
cooked (*Boar's Head*), 2 oz.	130	8.0	0	11.0	40	550	0
cotto:							
(*Louis Rich*), 1-oz. slice	45	4.0	0	3.0	20	280	0
(*Louis Rich*), 3 slices, 3 oz. ..	130	13.0	<1.0	8.0	65	850	0
(*Oscar Mayer*), 1-oz. slice	70	4.0	<1.0	6.0	25	280	0
(*Oscar Mayer*), 2 slices, 1.7 oz.	120	6.0	1.0	10.0	45	470	0
beef (*Oscar Mayer*), 1-oz. slice	60	4.0	<1.0	4.5	20	360	0
beef (*Oscar Mayer*), 2 slices, 1.7 oz.	100	7.0	<1.0	7.0	40	610	0
dry or hard:							
(*Black Bear*), 1 oz.	110	6.0	1.0	9.0	25	500	0
(*Boar's Head*), 1 oz.	110	6.0	<1.0	9.0	25	490	0
(*Homeland*), 1 oz.	110	5.0	0	10.0	35	450	0
(*Oscar Mayer*), 1 oz.	100	7.0	<1.0	8.0	25	510	0
(*Sara Lee*), 4 slices, 1.1 oz.	160	5.0	0	15.0	40	520	0
(*Sara Lee* Deli), 4 slices, .9 oz.	130	5.0	0	10.0	35	410	0
Genoa:							
(*Boar's Head*), 2 oz.	180	12.0	1.0	14.0	55	970	0
(*Boar's Head Salame*), 1 oz. ..	90	8.0	<1.0	7.0	23	500	0
(*Citterio*), 3 slices, 1.1 oz.	100	7.0	0	8.0	30	510	0
(*Di Lusso*), 2 oz. ..	210	12.0	0	18.0	50	940	0
(*Hormel Pillow Pack*), 5 slices, 1 oz.	120	5.0	0	11.0	35	430	0
(*Oscar Mayer*), 1 oz.	100	6.0	0	9.0	30	490	0
(*San Remo Brand*), 1 oz.	120	6.0	0	9.0	30	470	0
(*Sara Lee*), 4 slices, 1.1 oz.	160	6.0	0	15.0	65	460	0
(*Sara Lee* Deli), 4 slices, .9 oz. .	130	5.0	0	11.0	50	300	0

Food and Measure	cal.	prot. (gms)	carbo. (gms)	fat (gms)	chol. (mgs)	sod. (mgs)	fiber (gms)
"Salami," vegetarian, frozen:							
(*Worthington*), 3 slices, 3 oz.	130	12.0	2.0	8.0	0	800	2.0
(*Yves* Deli Slices), 2.2 oz.	90	17.0	5.0	0	0	390	1.0
Salisbury steak, see "Beef dinner" and "Beef entree"							
Salmon, meat only:							
Atlantic, farmed, 4 oz.:							
raw	207	22.6	0	12.3	67	66	0
baked, broiled, or microwaved	234	25.0	0	14.0	71	69	0
Atlantic, wild, 4 oz.							
raw	161	22.5	0	7.2	62	50	0
baked, broiled, or microwaved	206	28.8	0	9.2	81	64	0
Chinook, 4 oz.							
raw	204	22.8	0	11.9	75	53	0
baked, broiled, or microwaved	262	29.2	0	15.2	96	68	0
chum, 4 oz.:							
raw	136	22.8	0	4.3	84	112	0
baked, broiled, or microwaved	175	29.3	0	5.5	108	73	0
coho, farmed, 4 oz.:							
raw	182	24.1	0	8.7	58	53	0
baked, broiled, or microwaved	202	27.6	0	9.3	71	59	0
coho, wild, 4 oz.							
raw	165	25.0	0	6.7	51	53	0
baked, broiled, or microwaved	158	26.6	0	4.9	62	66	0
boiled, poached, or steamed	209	31.0	0	8.5	65	60	0
pink, 4 oz.:							
raw	132	22.6	0	3.9	59	76	0
baked, broiled, or microwaved	169	29.0	0	5.0	76	98	0
sockeye, 4 oz.:							
raw	191	24.2	0	9.7	70	53	0
baked, broiled, or microwaved	245	31.0	0	12.4	99	75	0

Food and Measure	cal.	prot. (gms)	carbo. (gms)	fat (gms)	chol. (mgs)	sod. (mgs)	fiber (gms)
Salmon, canned, ¼ cup, except as noted:							
chum, drained, 4 oz. . .	160	24.3	0	6.2	44	552	0
pink:							
(*Bumble Bee*), 2.2 oz.	90	12.0	0	5.0	40	270	0
(*Chicken of the Sea Traditional*), 2 oz.	90	12.0	0	5.0	40	270	0
(*Crown Prince Natural*)	90	12.0	0	5.0	40	60	0
(*Libby's*), 2.2 oz. . . .	90	12.0	0	5.0	40	270	0
skinless/boneless (*Crown Prince*), ⅓ cup	90	12.0	0	5.0	40	270	0
skinless/boneless, in water (*Chicken of the Sea*), 2 oz. . . .	60	10.0	0	2.0	20	280	0
red:							
(*Chicken of the Sea*), 2 oz.	110	13.0	0	7.0	40	270	0
(*Crown Prince*), ⅓ cup	120	13.0	0	7.0	40	270	0
blueback (*Rubinstein's*)	110	13.0	0	7.0	40	270	0
sockeye (*Bumble Bee*), 2.2 oz. . . .	110	13.0	0	7.0	40	270	0
sockeye (*Icy Point*)	110	13.0	0	7.0	40	270	0
sockeye, drained, w/bone, 4 oz. . .	174	23.2	0	8.3	50	611	0
Salmon, marinated (*Spence & Co. Gravlax*), 2 oz. . . .	120	13.0	<1.0	7.0	30	910	<1.0
Salmon, smoked, 2 oz.:							
(*Ocean Beauty*) . . .	86	14.0	<1.0	4.0	28	1154	0
Atlantic:							
(*Ducktrap River Kendall Brook*) . .	130	11.0	0	9.0	10	690	0
(*Ducktrap River Spruce Point*) . .	110	12.0	0	7.0	35	680	0
(*Ducktrap River Winter Harbor*) . .	130	11.0	0	9.0	10	690	0

Food and Measure	cal.	prot. (gms)	carbo. (gms)	fat (gms)	chol. (mgs)	sod. (mgs)	fiber (gms)
plain or cracked pepper and garlic (*Louis Kemp*) . . .	90	13.0	0	4.5	20	350	0
Chinook.	66	10.4	0	2.4	13	445	0
lox (*Vita*)	50	11.0	<1.0	1.0	20	800	0
Norwegian (*Frionor*)	93	12.0	0	5.0	39	484	0
Nova (*Vita*)	50	11.0	<1.0	1.0	20	580	0
pastrami style (*Ducktrap River Spruce Point*)	130	11.0	0	9.0	10	690	0
roasted (*Ducktrap River*)	100	13.0	0	6.0	10	430	0
sockeye (*Lascco Copper River*)	70	15.0	0	1.0	30	400	0
Salmon, smoked, pâté:							
(*Ducktrap River*), ¼ cup	150	7.0	1.0	14.0	35	410	0
(*Trois Petits Cochons*), 2 oz.	90	6.0	2.0	7.0	65	370	0
Salmon, smoked, spread:							
(*Vita*), ¼ cup	180	5.0	29.0	5.0	35	440	0
(*Sabra Salads* Lox), 1 oz.	104	.9	.9	10.7	9	158	0
Salmon burger, frozen, 1 pc.:							
(*Ocean Beauty*), 3.2 oz.	80	18.0	1.0	.5	35	380	1.0
(*Omega Foods*), 3.2 oz.	100	18.0	3.0	2.0	20	150	0
veggie (*Dr. Praeger's*), 2.8 oz.	100	7.5	11.0	3.0	7	200	3.0
Salmon entree, frozen:							
croquette (*Dr. Praeger's*), 2.2-oz. pc.	120	10.0	12.0	5.0	25	170	1.0
grilled, fillet, 1 pc.:							
creamy dill (*Mrs. Paul's*)	90	17.0	1.0	2.5	30	200	0
honey mustard (*Mrs. Paul's*) . . .	90	16.0	3.0	2.0	30	320	0
Salmon oil, see "Oil"							

Food and Measure	cal.	prot. (gms)	carbo. (gms)	fat (gms)	chol. (mgs)	sod. (mgs)	fiber (gms)
Salmon seasoning							
(*Old Bay* Classic),							
⅕ pkg.	40	1.0	3.0	1.5	0	115	0
Salsa, 2 tbsp., except							
as noted:							
(*Buckaroo* Greenhorn							
Salsa/Dip)	10	0	1.0	0	0	230	0
(*Chi-Chi's* Garden) ...	15	0	3.0	0	0	130	0
(*D. L. Jardine's* Bobos)	15	1.0	4.0	0	0	230	1.0
(*Embasa* Mexican) ...	5	0	1.0	0	0	170	<1.0
(*Embasa* Verde)	5	0	1.0	0	0	200	1.0
(*Featherweight*)	15	0	3.0	0	0	100	1.0
(*Herdez* Casera)	10	0	1.0	0	0	240	0
(*Herdez* Ranchera) ...	15	0	1.0	0	0	220	0
(*Herdez* Verde)	10	0	1.0	0	0	310	0
(*La Victoria* Ranchera)	10	0	2.0	0	0	125	0
(*La Victoria* Verde) ...	10	0	1.0	0	0	190	0
(*La Victoria* Victoria)	10	0	2.0	0	0	115	0
(*Ortega* Thick &							
Chunky)	10	0	2.0	0	0	210	<1.0
(*Pace* Chunky)	10	0	3.0	0	0	220	0
(*Sonoma*)	15	1.0	3.0	0	0	160	1.0
(*Sonoma* Coasteña) ..	20	0	5.0	0	0	65	0
(*Tostitos* Restaurant),							
4 tbsp.	30	<2.0	6.0	0	0	420	<2.0
(*Watkins JR's* Thick &							
Chunky)	10	0	2.0	0	0	218	0
all styles:							
(*Chi-Chi's*)	10	0	2.0	0	0	150	0
(*El Torito* Original							
Restaurant)	10	0	2.0	0	0	180	0
(*Old El Paso*)	10	0	2.0	0	0	230	0
(*Old El Paso* Thick							
n' Chunky)	10	0	3.0	0	0	230	0
(*Red Gold*)	10	0	2.0	0	0	120	1.0
(*Tostitos*), 4 tbsp.	30	2.0	6.0	0	0	520	2.0
except black bean							
corn (*Muir Glen*)	10	0	2.0	0	0	125	0
and beef (*Ortega*) ...	50	3.0	5.0	2.0	5	170	1.0
black bean:							
(*Buckaroo*)	15	1.0	3.0	0	0	260	0
(*Buckaroo* Whistle-							
Berries)	35	2.0	6.0	0	0	95	2.0

Food and Measure	cal.	prot. (gms)	carbo. (gms)	fat (gms)	chol. (mgs)	sod. (mgs)	fiber (gms)
(*D. L. Jardine's* Buckshot)	15	1.0	3.0	0	0	260	0
(*Mrs. Renfro's*) . . .	15	1.0	3.0	0	0	230	0
corn (*Buckaroo*) . .	20	1.0	4.0	0	0	290	<1.0
corn (*Muir Glen*) . .	15	1.0	3.0	0	0	125	<1.0
corn (*Walnut Acres*)	15	1.0	3.0	0	0	125	<1.0
cheese, see "Cheese dip"							
cherry (*Buckaroo* Wild & Wooly)	20	0	5.0	0	0	160	0
chipotle:							
(*Embasa*)	5	0	1.0	.5	0	190	<1.0
(*Pace*)	10	0	3.0	0	0	210	<1.0
corn (*Mrs. Renfro's*)	15	0	3.0	0	0	230	0
cilantro:							
(*Pace*)	10	0	3.0	0	0	220	0
(*Walnut Acres*) . . .	10	0	2.0	0	0	135	0
fire-roasted tomato:							
(*Pace*)	10	0	2.0	0	0	200	0
(*Tostitos*), 4 tbsp.	30	<2.0	4.0	0	0	560	2.0
mild or medium (*El Torito*)	10	0	2.0	0	0	170	0
garlic (*Pace* Grande)	10	0	3.0	0	0	220	0
garlic, roasted:							
(*Buckaroo*)	10	0	2.0	0	0	110	0
(*Mrs. Renfro's*) . . .	10	0	2.0	0	0	190	0
(*Newman's Own*) . .	10	1.0	2.0	0	0	150	1.0
(*Ortega*)	10	0	2.0	0	0	240	0
green, hot (*Mrs. Renfro's*)	10	0	2.0	0	0	390	0
green chili:							
(*Buckaroo*)	10	0	1.0	0	0	230	0
(*La Victoria*)	10	0	2.0	0	0	170	0
habanero:							
(*D. L. Jardine's* XXX Hot)	10	0	2.0	0	0	220	0
(*Mrs. Renfro's*) . . .	15	0	3.0	0	0	310	0
(*Shotgun Willie's* Hotter'n Hell) . . .	10	0	2.0	0	0	220	0
hot:							
(*El Paso* Chili Fresco)	5	0	1.0	0	0	135	<1.0
(*La Victoria* Thick 'N Chunky)	10	0	2.0	0	0	110	<1.0

Food and Measure	cal.	prot. (gms)	carbo. (gms)	fat (gms)	chol. (mgs)	sod. (mgs)	fiber (gms)
Salsa, hot (*cont.*)							
(*Mrs. Renfro's*) ...	15	0	3.0	0	0	310	0
(*Newman's Own*) ..	10	0	2.0	0	0	150	<1.0
jalapeño:							
(*El Pato*)	10	0	2.0	0	0	30	<1.0
(*Shotgun Willie's* Hotter'n Hell) ...	10	0	2.0	0	0	390	0
green or red (*La Victoria* Jalapeña)	10	0	2.0	0	0	150	0
lime/garlic (*Pace*) ...	15	0	3.0	0	0	210	0
medium:							
(*D. L. Jardine's* Texacante)	10	0	2.0	0	0	130	0
(*La Victoria* Suprema)	10	0	1.0	0	0	135	0
(*La Victoria* Thick 'N Chunky)	10	0	2.0	0	0	125	0
(*Mrs. Renfro's*) ...	15	0	3.0	0	0	280	0
(*Ortega* Homestyle)	10	<1.0	2.0	0	0	220	<1.0
mild:							
(*La Victoria* Suprema)	10	0	2.0	0	0	105	0
(*La Victoria* Thick 'N Chunky)	10	0	2.0	0	0	130	0
(*Mrs. Renfro's*) ...	10	0	2.0	0	0	240	0
(*Ortega* Mexican) ..	15	1.0	3.0	0	0	180	1.0
(*Snyder's*)	10	0	2.0	0	0	220	0
mild or medium (*Newman's Own*)	10	0	2.0	0	0	105	<1.0
peach:							
(*Buckaroo* Twenty-Four Kick)	10	0	3.0	0	0	120	0
(*D. L. Jardine's*) ...	20	0	4.0	0	0	90	0
(*Mrs. Renfro's*) ...	10	0	3.0	0	0	170	0
(*Newman's Own*) ..	25	0	6.0	0	0	90	1.0
(*Walnut Acres*) ...	20	0	5.0	0	0	85	0
picante (see also "Picante sauce"):							
medium (*La Victoria*)	10	0	1.0	0	0	150	0
mild (*La Victoria*) ..	10	0	1.0	0	0	180	0
pineapple (*Newman's Own*)	15	0	3.0	0	0	90	1.0

Food and Measure	cal.	prot. (gms)	carbo. (gms)	fat (gms)	chol. (mgs)	sod. (mgs)	fiber (gms)
pinto bean, spicy (*Buckaroo* Cowboy Thunder)	15	1.0	3.0	0	0	105	0
raspberry (*D. L. Jardine's*)	15	0	4.0	0	0	90	0
red pepper, roasted:							
(*Guiltless Gourmet*)	10	0	2.0	0	0	120	0
and garlic (*Pace*) ..	10	0	3.0	0	0	220	<1.0
roasted (*Mrs. Renfro's*)	10	0	2.0	0	0	220	0
roasted tomato (*Chi-Chi's*)	10	0	2.0	0	0	180	0
Southwestern grill (*Guiltless Gourmet*)	10	0	2.0	0	0	150	0
taco, see "Taco sauce"							
tomatillo (*D. L. Jardine's* Verde) ...	10	0	2.0	.5	0	180	0
tropical (*Watkins*) ...	50	0	12.0	0	0	400	0
Salsa seasoning, ½ tsp.:							
(*Bearitos*)	5	0	1.0	0	0	80	0
(*Lawry's*)	5	0	1.0	0	0	90	0
mild (*McCormick Produce Partners*) .	5	0	0	0	0	120	0
spicy (*McCormick Produce Partners*) .	5	0	0	0	0	130	0
Salsa–sour cream dip mix (*Watkins*), 1 tsp.	10	0	2.0	0	0	160	0
Salsify:							
raw:							
(*Frieda's*), ¾ cup, 3 oz.	70	3.0	16.0	0	0	15	3.0
untrimmed, 1 lb. ..	325	13.0	73.4	.8	0	79	13.0
sliced, ½ cup	55	2.2	12.5	.1	0	13	2.2
boiled, drained, sliced, ½ cup	46	1.9	10.5	.1	0	11	2.1
Salt (see also specific listings), ¼ tsp.:							
(*Morton*)	0	0	0	0	0	590	0
sea (*Hain*)	0	0	0	0	0	590	0
Salt, seasoned (see also specific listings), ¼ tsp.:							
(*Lawry's*)	0	0	0	0	0	380	0

Food and Measure	cal.	prot. (gms)	carbo. (gms)	fat (gms)	chol. (mgs)	sod. (mgs)	fiber (gms)
Salt, seasoned (*cont.*)							
(*McCormick* Salt 'n Spice)	0	0	0	0	0	250	0
(*McCormick Season-All*), ¼ tsp.	0	0	0	0	0	350	0
(*Watkins* Seasoning)	0	0	0	0	0	270	0
spicy (*McCormick Season-All*)	0	0	0	0	0	250	0
Salt, substitute, ¼ tsp., except as noted:							
(*Estee* Salt-It)	0	0	0	0	0	0	0
seasoned (*Lawry's* Salt Free 17)	0	0	0	0	0	0	0
Salt pork, raw, 1 oz. .	212	1.4	0	22.8	25	404	0
Sandwich, see specific listings							
Sandwich sauce, ¼ cup, except as noted:							
(*Kraft* Burger), 2 tbsp.	150	0	4.0	15.0	15	210	0
Sloppy Joe:							
(*Del Monte* Original)	50	1.0	16.0	0	0	600	0
(*Heinz*), ½ cup . . .	70	3.0	14.0	.5	0	770	2.0
(*Hormel* Not-So-Sloppy Joe)	60	1.0	13.0	0	0	640	1.0
(*Libby's*), ⅓ cup . .	50	1.0	12.0	0	0	430	1.0
(*Manwich* Original)	30	1.0	6.0	0	0	380	1.0
hickory flavor (*Del Monte*)	70	1.0	18.0	0	0	700	0
Sandwich sauce seasoning mix, see "Sloppy Joe seasoning mix"							
Sandwich spread (see also "Meat spread," and specific listings):							
(*Hellmann's/Best Foods*), 1 tbsp. . . .	50	0	2.0	5.0	<5	180	0
(*Kraft*), 1 tbsp.	50	0	3.0	4.0	<5	105	0
(*Kraft* Reduced Fat), 1 tbsp.	35	0	3.0	2.5	0	130	0
(*Loma Linda*), ¼ cup	80	4.0	7.0	4.5	0	260	3.0

Food and Measure	cal.	prot. (gms)	carbo. (gms)	fat (gms)	chol. (mgs)	sod. (mgs)	fiber (gms)
Sapodilla:							
(*Frieda's*), 3-oz. fruit	70	0	17.0	1.0	0	10	5.0
1 medium, 3" x 2½"	140	.7	33.9	1.9	0	20	9.0
½ cup	100	.5	24.1	1.3	0	15	6.4
Sapote:							
(*Frieda's*), 5 oz.	190	3.0	47.0	1.0	0	15	4.0
11.2-oz. fruit, 7.9 oz.							
trimmed	301	4.8	76.0	1.4	0	23	5.9
trimmed, 1 oz.	38	.6	9.6	.2	0	3	.7
Sardine, fresh, see							
"Herring"							
Sardine, canned:							
Atlantic, in oil:							
drained, 2 oz.	118	14.8	0	6.5	81	286	0
2 medium, 3" long	50	5.9	0	2.8	34	121	0
in hot sauce (*Chicken*							
of the Sea Brisling),							
3.75-oz. can	220	16.0	2.0	16.0	145	560	1.0
in lemon sauce:							
(*Bela*), ¼ cup	130	12.0	0	9.0	20	115	0
(*Goya*), ¼ cup	120	10.0	0	9.0	20	300	0
in hot sauce (*Bela*),							
¼ cup	110	13.0	0	7.0	20	120	0
in mustard:							
(*Chicken of the Sea*							
Brisling), 3.75 oz.	260	15.0	6.0	20.0	95	820	0
(*Crown Prince*),							
⅓ cup	90	10.0	1.0	5.0	35	280	1.0
(*Crown Prince*							
Brisling), 1 can	210	14.0	<1.0	16.0	45	710	<1.0
(*Underwood*), 1 can	180	17.0	2.0	12.0	105	820	1.0
in oil (*Chicken of the*							
Sea Brisling), 2.9 oz.	220	18.0	1.0	16.0	100	400	0
in olive oil, drained:							
(*Bela*), ¼ cup	120	13.0	0	7.0	20	130	0
(*Crown Prince*),							
2.9-oz. can	210	16.0	1.0	16.0	65	420	1.0
(*Crown Prince* Cross-							
pack), 2.9-oz. can	210	16.0	1.0	15.0	65	500	<1.0
(*Crown Prince*							
Natural Brisling							
2-Layer),							
3-oz. can	290	17.0	0	24.0	75	320	<1.0
(*Goya*), ¼ cup	130	13.0	0	9.0	20	20	0

Food and Measure	cal.	prot. (gms)	carbo. (gms)	fat (gms)	chol. (mgs)	sod. (mgs)	fiber (gms)
Sardine, canned, in olive oil (*cont.*)							
skinless/boneless (*Crown Prince*), 6 pcs.	230	24.0	0	15.0	40	300	<1.0
skinless/boneless (*Granadaisa*), ¼ cup	120	13.0	0	7.0	24	280	0
in soy oil, drained:							
(*Crown Prince*), 1 can	210	15.0	0	17.0	50	320	0
(*Crown Prince* No Salt), 2.9-oz. can	230	17.0	0	18.0	45	125	0
spiced (*Goya*), ¼ cup	120	12.0	0	9.0	20	280	0
in tomato sauce:							
(*Chicken of the Sea* Oval), 5 oz.	110	24.0	1.0	1.5	50	760	0
(*Crown Prince* Brisling), 3.75-oz. can	210	16.0	0	16.0	50	600	<1.0
(*Crown Prince* Oval), ⅓ cup	80	10.0	1.0	4.0	36	170	1.0
(*Goya*), ¼ cup	130	12.0	1.0	9.0	20	300	0
Pacific, 2 oz.	101	9.3	n.a.	6.8	35	235	<1.0
in water:							
(*Chicken of the Sea* Brisling), 2.9 oz.	150	14.0	0	10.0	55	75	0
(*Chicken of the Sea* Tall), 2 oz.	80	13.0	1.0	1.5	55	320	0
(*Crown Prince*), ⅓ cup	70	12.0	0	2.0	40	180	0
(*Crown Prince Natural* Brisling), 3-oz. can	290	17.0	<1.0	24.0	120	70	<1.0
skinless/boneless (*Crown Prince Natural*), 3.2-oz. can	130	22.0	0	5.0	35	360	0
Sardine oil, see "Oil"							
Satsuma, see "Tangerine"							
Sauce (see also specific sauce listings), all purpose:							
(*Aunt Nellie's* Old Style), 1 tbsp.	70	0	3.0	6.0	10	260	0

Food and Measure	cal.	prot. (gms)	carbo. (gms)	fat (gms)	chol. (mgs)	sod. (mgs)	fiber (gms)
(*Silver Dollar City*), 2 tbsp.	30	0	8.0	0	0	180	0
Sauerbraten seasoning mix (*Knorr Recipe Classics*), 1 tbsp.	35	<1.0	6.0	1.0	0	440	0
Sauerkraut, 2 tbsp., except as noted:							
(*Boar's Head*)	5	0	1.0	0	0	180	<1.0
(*Bush's Best*)	5	0	1.0	0	0	180	1.0
(*Cascadian Farm* Old World)	5	0	<1.0	0	0	250	<1.0
(*Cascadian Farm* Low Sodium)	5	0	1.0	0	0	120	<1.0
(*Claussen*), ¼ cup ...	5	0	1.0	0	0	220	1.0
(*Del Monte*)	0	0	<1.0	0	0	180	<1.0
(*Eden*), ½ cup	25	2.0	4.0	0	0	580	3.0
(*Hebrew National*) ...	5	0	1.0	0	0	180	1.0
(*Libby's*)	5	0	1.0	0	0	200	<1.0
(*Silver Floss*)	5	0	1.0	0	0	180	1.0
(*S&W*)	5	0	1.0	0	0	220	0
Bavarian:							
(*Bush's Best*)	15	0	3.0	0	0	105	1.0
(*Del Monte*)	15	0	4.0	0	0	180	0
red cabbage (*S&W*) .	15	0	3.0	0	0	160	0
Sauerkraut juice (*Bush's Best*), 1 cup	15	2.0	1.0	0	0	1670	0
Sausage (see also specific listings), cooked, except as noted:							
(*Jones Dairy Farm* Golden Brown), 1 patty	150	5.0	1.0	14.0	30	240	0
(*Jones Dairy Farm* Gold Brown Light), 2 links	100	7.0	1.0	8.0	25	230	0
(*Jones Dairy Farm* Golden Brown Mild), 2 links	190	6.0	1.0	18.0	35	300	0
apple cinnamon: (*Johnsonville* Breakfast), 3 links ...	190	10.0	1.0	16.0	40	610	0

Food and Measure	cal.	prot. (gms)	carbo. (gms)	fat (gms)	chol. (mgs)	sod. (mgs)	fiber (gms)
Sausage, apple cinnamon (*cont.*)							
(*Jones Dairy Farm* Golden Brown), 2 links	170	5.0	2.0	16.0	35	310	0
beef:							
(*Jones Dairy Farm* Golden Brown), 2 links	170	7.0	1.0	15.0	40	410	0
hot (*Johnsonville* Hot Links), 2.7 oz.	230	9.0	2.0	20.0	40	620	0
smoked (*Healthy Choice*), 2 oz. ..	80	8.0	6.0	2.5	20	480	0
smoked (*Thorn Apple Valley*), 3.2-oz. link	290	11.0	4.0	25.0	55	710	0
brown and serve:							
(*Little Sizzlers*), 3 links	230	8.0	1.0	22.0	45	670	0
(*Little Sizzlers*), 2 patties	190	7.0	1.0	18.0	40	560	0
(*Swift Premium Brown 'N Servo Original*), 3 links	210	7.0	2.0	19.0	45	410	0
(*Swift Premium Brown 'N Serve Original*), 2 patties	170	6.0	2.0	16.0	40	370	0
cheese, smoked:							
(*Johnsonville Beddar with Cheddar*), 2.7-oz. link	240	9.0	2.0	21.0	60	640	0
(*Johnsonville Beddar with Cheddar Light*), 2.3-oz. link	140	10.0	3.0	9.0	35	640	0
(*Oscar Mayer* Little Smokies), 6 links	180	7.0	1.0	16.0	40	590	0
(*Oscar Mayer* Smokies), 1 link .	130	6.0	1.0	12.0	30	450	0
(*Thorn Apple Valley*), 3.2-oz. link	290	11.0	4.0	25.0	55	740	0
chicken, 2-oz. link, except as noted:							
Andouille, Cajun-style (*Bilinski's*) .	80	9.0	1.0	4.0	60	300	0

Food and Measure	cal.	prot. (gms)	carbo. (gms)	fat (gms)	chol. (mgs)	sod. (mgs)	fiber (gms)
apple, fresh, raw (*Aidell's*)	100	8.0	1.0	7.0	40	300	0
apple, smoked (*Aidell's*), 3.5-oz. link	210	16.0	1.0	16.0	90	730	0
apple, smoked, cocktail (*Aidell's*), 6 links, 2 oz.	100	8.0	1.0	8.0	50	370	0
apple and Chardonnay (*Bilinski's*) ..	70	10.0	2.5	5.5	60	350	0
cilantro (*Bilinski's*) .	70	9.0	1.0	3.5	40	270	1.0
jalapeño (*Bilinski's*)	70	9.0	0	4.0	55	270	0
lemon, smoked (*Aidell's*), 3.5-oz. link	210	15.0	1.0	16.0	90	700	0
pesto (*Bilinski's*) ..	90	10.0	0	5.0	40	320	0
spinach (*Bilinski's*)	70	9.0	1.0	3.5	40	270	1.0
sun-dried tomato (*Bilinski's*)	70	10.0	2.0	3.5	40	280	0
teriyaki, fresh, raw (*Aidell's*), 3.5-oz. link	210	15.0	6.0	15.0	85	590	0
chicken/turkey, 3.5-oz. link, except as noted:							
artichoke, smoked (*Aidell's*)	180	14.0	2.0	14.0	75	610	0
curry, smoked (*Aidell's* Burmese)	220	18.0	3.0	15.0	95	730	0
habanero (*Aidell's*), 3.2-oz link	160	15.0	2.0	10.0	55	540	0
pesto, smoked (*Aidell's*)	220	18.0	1.0	16.0	75	780	0
smoked (*Aidell's* New Mexico) ...	210	15.0	2.0	16.0	80	600	0
w/sun-dried tomatoes and basil, fresh, raw (*Aidell's*)	200	15.0	1.0	15.0	85	550	0
Thai, fresh, raw (*Aidell's*)	200	15.0	1.0	16.0	75	600	0
chorizo: (*Fiorucci* Cantimpalo), 1 oz.	110	5.0	1.0	10.0	25	490	0

Food and Measure	cal.	prot. (gms)	carbo. (gms)	fat (gms)	chol. (mgs)	sod. (mgs)	fiber (gms)
Sausage, chorizo (*cont.*)							
beef, raw (*Aidell's*), 3.5-oz. link	400	13.0	3.0	37.0	70	550	0
pork, spicy (*Battisoni*), 1 oz. ...	80	4.0	0	7.0	20	180	0
dinner (*Jones Dairy Farm*), 1 link	150	8.0	1.0	14.0	35	310	0
duck/turkey, smoked (*Aidell's*), 3.5-oz. link	220	17.0	1.0	16.0	60	700	0
French, garlic (*Trois Petits Cochons Saucisson a l'Ail*), 2 oz.	80	11.0	1.0	3.5	35	430	0
garlic (*Johnsonville Irish O' Garlic*), 3-oz. link	290	14.0	1.0	25.0	65	800	0
Italian, chicken, w/peppers, onions, 2 oz.:							
mild (*Bilinski's*) ...	70	9.0	1.0	3.5	60	270	0
hot (*Bilinski's*)	70	9.0	1.0	4.2	60	270	0
Italian, dry (*Boar's Head*), 1 oz.	100	9.0	<1.0	7.0	22	510	0
Italian, pork, 1 link:							
raw (*Aidell's*), 3.5-oz. link	230	16.0	0	18.0	40	550	0
grilled (*Johnsonville Fresh*), 3 oz. ...	290	14.0	1.0	25.0	65	800	0
mild (*Johnsonville Cooked*), 2.7 oz.	240	9.0	2.0	22.0	50	760	0
Italian, turkey, 1 link:							
hot, raw (*Perdue*), 3.2 oz.	150	16.0	1.0	9.0	60	500	0
hot, cooked (*Perdue*), 2.8 oz.	150	16.0	1.0	9.0	60	470	0
hot, raw (*Shady Brook Farms*) ...	90	12.0	1.0	4.0	45	450	0
sweet, raw (*Perdue*), 2.7 oz.	150	16.0	1.0	9.0	60	510	0
sweet, cooked (*Perdue*), 2.4 oz.	150	16.0	1.0	9.0	60	490	0
sweet, raw (*Shady Brook Farms*) ...	90	12.0	1.0	4.0	40	420	0

Food and Measure	cal.	prot. (gms)	carbo. (gms)	fat (gms)	chol. (mgs)	sod. (mgs)	fiber (gms)
Italian style, ground:							
burger, grilled (*Johnsonville*), 2.5 oz.	240	11.0	1.0	21.0	50	580	0
mild or hot (*Johnsonville*), 2.5 oz.	210	10.0	0	18.0	45	500	0
w/pepper and onions (*Wampler*), 1 cup	210	17.0	14.0	11.0	70	1120	3.0
lamb/beef, w/rosemary, fresh, raw (*Aidell's*), 3.5-oz. link	220	16.0	2.0	16.0	65	600	<1.0
maple flavor:							
(*Johnsonville* Vermont Breakfast), 3 links ...	200	10.0	1.0	18.0	40	600	0
(*Jones Dairy Farm* Golden Brown), 2 links	190	5.0	1.0	18.0	35	260	0
pickled, smoked, or hot (*Hormel*), 6 links	140	8.0	1.0	11.0	40	380	0
pork, fresh:							
link, raw, 1 oz. ...	118	3.3	.3	11.4	19	189	0
link, cooked, .5 oz. (1 oz. raw)	105	5.6	.3	8.8	24	367	0
patty, raw, 2 oz. ..	286	6.6	.6	22.8	39	378	0
pork, link:							
(*Johnsonville* Original Breakfast), 3 links ...	190	10.0	1.0	16.0	40	610	0
(*Jones Dairy Farm* All Natural Light), 2 links	130	8.0	1.0	11.0	20	420	0
(*Jones Dairy Farm* All Natural Little), 3 links	190	8.0	1.0	17.0	45	420	0
(*Little Sizzlers*), 3 links	230	8.0	0	22.0	45	610	0
(*Oscar Mayer Little Friers*), 2 links ..	180	9.0	1.0	16.0	45	450	0
(*Perri* Breakfast), 3 links	190	10.0	1.0	16.0	40	610	0
brown sugar/honey (*Johnsonville* Breakfast), 3 links	190	7.0	5.0	15.0	35	460	0

Food and Measure	cal.	prot. (gms)	carbo. (gms)	fat (gms)	chol. (mgs)	sod. (mgs)	fiber (gms)
Sausage (cont.)							
pork, ground, seasoned, raw (*Johnsonville*), 2.5 oz. ..	210	10.0	0	18.0	45	500	0
pork, patty:							
(*Johnsonville Original/Vermont Maple Breakfast*), 2 pcs, ...	180	11.0	1.0	15.0	40	580	0
(*Jones Dairy Farm All Natural*), 1 pc.	130	5.0	0	12.0	30	250	0
(*Little Sizzlers*), 2 pcs.	230	8.0	0	22.0	45	610	0
pork, roll, original or hot (*Jones Dairy Farm All Natural*), 2 oz.	230	9.0	1.0	21.0	50	430	0
pork, smoked:							
Andouille (*Aidell's Cajun Brand*), 3.5-oz. link	220	16.0	1.0	17.0	55	770	<1.0
whiskey fennel (*Aidell's*), 3.5-oz. link	220	17.0	1.0	17.0	60	520	<1.0
pork/bacon (*Jones Dairy Farm* Golden Brown), 2 links ...	170	6.0	1.0	16.0	30	370	0
pork/beef, fresh, .5-oz. link	112	3.9	.8	10.3	20	228	0
pork/turkey (*Healthy Choice*), 2 links or 1 patty ..	50	7.0	3.0	1.5	20	340	0
pork/veal, smoked, (*Aidell's Bier*), 3.5-oz. link	240	17.0	0	19.0	35	720	0
sandwich patty (*Jones Dairy Farm*), 1 pc.	170	5.0	1.0	16.0	30	280	0
smoked:							
(*Boar's Head*), 4.6-oz. link	360	17.0	2.0	31.0	75	1050	0
(*Healthy Choice*), 2 oz.	80	7.0	6.0	2.5	25	480	0
(*Johnsonville*), 2.7-oz. link	240	9.0	2.0	21.0	60	640	0

Food and Measure	cal.	prot. (gms)	carbo. (gms)	fat (gms)	chol. (mgs)	sod. (mgs)	fiber (gms)
(*Johnsonville Little Smokies*), 6 links, 2 oz. . . .	180	6.0	1.0	16.0	35	480	0
(*Thorn Apple Valley*), 3.2-oz. link	280	11.0	4.0	25.0	55	700	0
hot (*Boar's Head* Skinless), 3.2 oz.	250	12.0	1.0	22.0	55	740	0
turkey (*Jennie-O*), 2 oz.	70	9.0	0	3.0	55	510	0
spicy (*Jones Dairy Farm* Golden Brown), 2 links	190	6.0	1.0	18.0	35	300	0
turkey, raw, except as noted:							
(*Jennie-O Breakfast Lover's*), 1 link . .	130	9.0	0	11.0	45	330	0
(*Jennie-O Breakfast Lover's* Patties), 2 oz.	130	9.0	0	11.0	45	330	0
(*Louis Rich*), 2.5-oz. link	110	12.0	1.0	6.0	55	430	0
(*Shady Brook Farms* Breakfast), 2 links	80	10.0	1.0	4.0	35	480	0
(*Shady Brook Farms* Dinner), 1 link . .	190	12.0	1.0	4.0	45	450	0
(*Wampler* Breakfast), 4 oz.	230	17.0	1.0	17.0	100	880	0
cranberry, smoked (*Aidell's*), 3.5-oz. link	210	16.0	1.0	16.0	85	730	<1.0
Italian, see "Italian," above							
maple (*Shady Brook Farms* Breakfast), 1 link	100	11.0	3.0	4.0	45	290	0
w/scallions and herbs, fresh (*Aidell's*), 3.5-oz. link	200	15.0	1.0	12.0	70	700	<1.0
turkey/chicken, see "chicken/turkey," above							

Food and Measure	cal.	prot. (gms)	carbo. (gms)	fat (gms)	chol. (mgs)	sod. (mgs)	fiber (gms)
Sausage, canned:							
pickled, regular, or hot (*Hormel*), 6 links, 2 oz.	140	8.0	1.0	11.0	40	380	0
Polish (*Maxwell Street*), 2 oz.	170	7.0	2.0	14.0	35	640	0
smoked (*Vienna*), 2 oz.	150	7.0	1.0	13.0	30	560	0
Vienna:							
(*Armour*), 3 links .	150	5.0	0	14.0	50	430	0
(*Goya*), 3 links	130	5.0	1.0	12.0	50	320	0
(*Hormel*), 2 oz. . . .	150	5.0	0	14.0	45	420	0
(*Libby's*), 3 links . .	150	6.0	<1.0	14.0	45	460	0
chicken (*Hormel*), 2 oz.	110	6.0	1.0	9.0	55	400	0
chicken (*Libby's*), 3 links	100	6.0	0	8.0	50	450	0
Sausage, dried, pork, patties (*Mountain House*), 1 patty . . .	110	12.0	1.0	6.0	45	530	0
Sausage, frozen, Italian (*Rosina Bites*), 4 pcs., 2 oz.	180	11.0	<1.0	15.0	40	430	1.0
"Sausage," vegetarian (see also specific listings):							
.9-oz. link	64	4.6	2.5	4.5	0	222	.7
1.3-oz. patty	97	7.0	3.7	6.9	0	337	1.1
canned:							
(*Loma Linda* Little Links), 2 links . .	90	8.0	2.0	6.0	0	230	2.0
(*Worthington Saucettes*), 1 link	90	6.0	1.0	6.0	0	200	1.0
frozen:							
(*Boca* Breakfast), 2 links	100	10.0	6.0	4.0	0	330	5.0
(*Boca* Breakfast), 1 patty	60	8.0	6.0	4.0	0	260	3.0
(*Morningstar Farms* Breakfast), 2 links	80	9.0	3.0	3.0	0	320	2.0
(*Morningstar Farms* Breakfast), 1 patty	80	10.0	3.0	3.0	0	270	2.0
(*Worthington Prosage* Links), 2 links	80	9.0	3.0	3.0	0	320	2.0

Food and Measure	cal.	prot. (gms)	carbo. (gms)	fat (gms)	chol. (mgs)	sod. (mgs)	fiber (gms)
(*Worthington Prosage* Patties), 1 patty	80	9.0	3.0	3.0	0	300	2.0
(*Yves* Breakfast Links), 1.75 oz.	60	11.0	3.0	0	0	390	2.0
(*Yves* Breakfast Patties), 2 oz. . .	70	11.0	4.0	2.0	0	350	2.0
bits (*Morningstar Farms* Sausage Style Crumbles), ⅔ cup	90	11.0	5.0	3.0	0	370	2.0
Italian (*Boca*), 1 link	120	11.0	6.0	6.0	0	990	5.0
roll (*Worthington Prosage*), ⅝" slice	140	10.0	2.0	10.0	0	390	2.0
smoked (*Boca*), 1 link	130	12.0	7.0	5.0	0	890	2.0
refrigerated (*Morningstar Farms* Breakfast), 2 patties	120	15.0	5.0	5.0	0	380	3.0
Sausage, wrapped, frozen, cocktail, smoked (*Master Choice* Piggies in a Blanket), 3 pcs. . .	300	7.0	21.0	21.0	30	400	<1.0
Sausage hash, canned (*Mary Kitchen*), 1 cup	410	20.0	23.0	27.0	85	1020	2.0
Sausage, peppers, onions, refrigerated (*DeLuca*), 2 pcs., ¼ cup sauce	250	11.0	4.0	22.0	75	600	1.0
Sausage seasoning, (*Tone's*), 1 tsp. . . .	12	.4	2.7	.3	0	1	.7
Sausage stick, 1 pc., except as noted: (*Johnsonville* Snack Stix), 1 oz.	120	5.0	0	11.0	25	400	0
beef/beef jerky:							
(*Rustler's*), .16 oz.	20	2.0	<1.0	1.5	5	105	<1.0
(*Rustler's*), .17 oz.	20	2.0	<1.0	1.5	5	115	<1.0
(*Rustler's*), .22 oz.	30	2.0	1.0	2.0	10	140	<1.0
(*Rustler's*), .32 oz.	40	3.0	1.0	2.5	10	210	<1.0

Food and Measure	cal.	prot. (gms)	carbo. (gms)	fat (gms)	chol. (mgs)	sod. (mgs)	fiber (gms)
Sausage stick, beef/beef jerky(cont.)							
hickory smoked (*Pemmican*), 1 oz.	70	12.0	4.0	1.0	35	610	<1.0
peppered or teriyaki (*Pemmican*), 1 oz.	70	13.0	3.0	1.0	35	670	1.0
sweet and hot (*Pemmican*), 1 oz.	80	11.0	6.0	.5	30	470	1.0
sweet mesquite (*Pemmican*), 1 oz.	70	12.0	3.0	2.0	25	560	0
hot:							
(*Rustler's Flamin' Hot*), .26 oz. . . .	40	2.0	<1.0	3.0	5	130	<1.0
(*Rustler's Flamin' Hot*), .28 oz. . . .	40	2.0	<1.0	3.0	10	140	<1.0
smoked (*Rustler's Steak Strip*), .8 oz.	60	8.0	1.0	2.0	20	580	0
spicy:							
(*Rustler's*), .3 oz.	50	2.0	<1.0	4.0	10	140	<1.0
(*Rustler's*), .5 oz.	70	3.0	1.0	6.0	20	250	<1.0
turkey:							
peppered (*Pemmican*), 1 oz	60	10.0	4.0	.5	20	670	0
sweet smoked (*Pemmican*), 1 oz.	70	9.0	5.0	1.0	25	700	0
Sausage biscuit, see "Breakfast sandwich"							
Savory, ground, 1 tsp.	4	.1	1.0	.1	0	<1	<1.0
Scallion, see "Onion, green"							
Scallop, meat only:							
raw, 4 oz.	100	19.0	2.7	.9	38	183	0
raw, 2 large or 5 small, 1.1 oz.	26	5.0	.7	.2	10	48	0
Scallop, frozen (*Contessa*), 4 oz., 1 cup	80	17.0	3.0	0	35	180	0
"Scallop," imitation:							
bay style (*Louis Kemp Scallop Delights*), ½ cup, 3 oz.	80	9.0	12.0	0	10	385	0
from surimi, 4 oz. . . .	112	14.5	12.1	.5	25	902	0

Food and Measure	cal.	prot. (gms)	carbo. (gms)	fat (gms)	chol. (mgs)	sod. (mgs)	fiber (gms)
Scallop, smoked							
(*Ducktrap River*),							
¼ cup	60	10.0	0	1.0	60	260	0
"Scallop," vegetarian,							
canned:							
(*Loma Linda Tender*							
Bits), 6 pcs.	110	11.0	7.0	4.5	0	440	3.0
(*Worthington Vege-*							
table Skallops),							
½ cup	90	15.0	3.0	1.5	0	410	3.0
Scallop entree, frozen:							
fried (*Mrs. Paul's*),							
13 pcs., 3.75 oz. ...	220	11.0	27.0	7.0	25	440	1.0
stuffed w/seafood							
(*Ocean's Cuisine*),							
3.5 oz.	200	10.0	13.0	13.0	45	490	1.0
Scallop squash,							
½ cup:							
raw, sliced	12	.8	2.5	.1	0	1	1.2
boiled, drained, sliced	14	.9	3.0	.2	0	1	1.1
boiled, drained,							
mashed	19	1.2	4.0	.2	0	1	1.4
Scampi sauce							
(*Zatarain's*), 1 tbsp.	5	0	0	0	0	200	0
***Schlotzsky's Deli*,**							
1 serving:							
sandwich, on sour-							
dough, except as							
noted:							
BLT:							
large	1141	41.0	140.0	46.0	80	3066	6.0
regular	578	21.0	70.0	24.0	41	1548	3.0
small	379	13.0	47.0	15.0	26	1010	2.0
cheese, original:							
large	1857	87.0	159.0	98.0	180	4365	8.0
regular	854	38.0	79.0	44.0	72	2107	4.0
small	596	27.0	53.0	31.0	54	1432	3.0
chicken, Dijon:							
large	972	74.0	150.0	10.0	137	3981	8.0
regular, on wheat	497	38.0	74.0	6.0	68	2091	6.0
small, on wheat	330	25.0	50.0	4.0	46	1373	4.0
chicken, pesto:							
large	999	73.0	145.0	15.0	141	3799	7.0
regular	512	37.0	73.0	9.0	71	1927	4.0

Food and Measure	cal.	prot. (gms)	carbo. (gms)	fat (gms)	chol. (mgs)	sod. (mgs)	fiber (gms)
***Schlotzsky's Deli,* sandwich, chicken, pesto** (*cont.*)							
small	346	25.0	49.0	6.0	48	1297	2.0
chicken, Santa Fe:							
large	1182	82.0	155.0	29.0	185	4232	9.0
regular, jalapeño							
cheese bun ..	642	43.0	77.0	19.0	106	2302	4.0
small, jalapeño							
cheese bun ..	431	29.0	52.0	13.0	72	1547	3.0
chicken breast:							
large	1008	72.0	158.0	15.0	155	4522	6.0
regular	535	37.0	81.0	10.0	85	2365	3.0
small	363	25.0	55.0	7.0	58	1596	2.0
chicken club:							
large	1351	88.0	149.0	45.0	209	4678	8.0
regular	686	44.0	75.0	23.0	106	2403	4.0
small	458	29.0	50.0	15.0	71	1591	3.0
corned beef:							
large	1134	81.0	139.0	25.0	167	4751	6.0
regular, dark rye .	587	40.0	70.0	15.0	84	2488	4.0
small, dark rye ..	388	27.0	47.0	10.0	56	1625	3.0
Deluxe Original:							
large	1986	111.0	167.0	97.0	273	8478	8.0
regular	970	53.0	84.0	47.0	128	4264	4.0
small	717	39.0	57.0	37.0	103	3130	3.0
ham/cheese, original:							
large	1625	93.0	163.0	67.0	183	6807	8.0
regular	789	44.0	82.0	32.0	83	3428	4.0
small	537	30.0	55.0	22.0	58	2298	3.0
The Original:							
large	1591	74.0	157	75.0	157	5019	8.0
regular	778	34.0	79.0	36.0	75	2528	4.0
small	550	24.0	53.0	27.0	55	1755	3.0
pastrami/Swiss:							
large	1681	114.0	148.0	69.9	304	7211	6.0
regular, dark rye .	861	57.0	74.0	37.0	152	3718	4.0
small, dark rye ..	570	38.0	49.0	24.0	101	2445	3.0
The Philly:							
large	1709	121.0	157.0	66.0	244	4477	7.0
regular	824	57.0	78.0	32.0	113	2189	4.0
small	559	39.0	52.0	22.0	78	1467	2.0
Reuben, corned beef:							
large	1594	102.0	147.0	62.0	262	6944	7.0
regular, dark rye	833	51.0	74.0	35.0	132	3514	4.0
small, dark rye ..	528	32.0	50.0	21.0	80	2269	3.0

Food and Measure	cal.	prot. (gms)	carbo. (gms)	fat (gms)	chol. (mgs)	sod. (mgs)	fiber (gms)
Reuben, pastrami:							
large	1777	113.0	152.0	77.0	308	7765	7.0
regular, dark rye	924	56.0	77.0	43.0	155	3924	4.0
small, dark rye ..	619	38.0	51.0	29.0	103	2679	3.0
Reuben, turkey:							
large	1656	101.0	159.0	69.0	247	7704	7.0
regular, dark rye	863	50.0	80.0	39.0	124	3893	4.0
small, dark rye ..	579	33.0	54.0	26.0	83	2659	3.0
roast beef:							
large	1185	87.0	145.0	28.0	164	3362	6.0
regular	617	43.0	73.0	17.0	83	1733	3.0
small	413	29.0	49.0	11.0	55	1162	2.0
roast beef/cheese:							
large	1749	120.0	163.0	70.0	255	4987	8.0
regular	848	57.0	82.0	34.0	119	2451	4.0
small	580	39.0	55.0	24.0	83	1666	3.0
Texas Schlotsky's:							
large	1544	84.0	155.0	65.0	184	6446	6.0
regular, jalapeño	816	43.0	76.0	37.0	98	3357	3.0
cheese bun	561	30.0	51.0	26.0	69	2263	2.0
small, jalapeño							
cheese bun ..	537	30.0	51.0	23.0	69	2288	2.0
tuna, albacore:							
large	1000	59.0	147.0	26.0	122	3099	6.0
regular	533	31.0	74.0	16.0	69	1655	4.0
small	361	21.0	50.0	11.0	47	1122	3.0
tuna melt:							
large	1631	93.0	158.0	77.0	214	4474	7.0
regular, wheat ..	818	45.0	79.0	40.0	106	2293	5.0
small, wheat	562	31.0	53.0	28.0	74	1552	3.0
turkey, original:							
large	1772	108.0	162.0	77.0	241	6235	8.0
regular	862	51.0	81.0	37.0	112	3095	4.0
small	607	36.0	54.0	28.0	83	2136	3.0
turkey, smoked:							
large	988	68.0	150.0	13.0	118	4229	6.0
regular	498	34.0	75.0	7.0	60	2123	3.0
small	335	23.0	50.0	5.0	40	1426	2.0
turkey/bacon club:							
large	1790	108.0	161.0	80.0	240	6086	7.0
regular, on wheat	874	52.0	79.0	40.0	113	3009	5.0
small, on wheat	596	35.0	53.0	27.0	78	2012	3.0
turkey guacamole:							
large	1317	73.0	166.0	42.0	118	5255	6.0

Food and Measure	cal.	prot. (gms)	carbo. (gms)	fat (gms)	chol. (mgs)	sod. (mgs)	fiber (gms)
Schlotzsky's Deli, sandwich, turkey guacamole (cont.)							
regular	683	36.0	84.0	24.0	60	2680	3.0
small	448	24.0	56.0	15.0	40	1764	2.0
vegetable club:							
large	1112	39.0	151.0	41.0	46	2716	9.0
regular	584	19.0	76.0	24.0	24	1435	5.0
small	393	13.0	50.0	16.0	16	962	3.0
vegetarian:							
large	966	34.0	150.0	26.0	48	2398	8.0
regular	519	18.0	75.0	17.0	32	1329	5.0
small	351	12.0	51.0	11.0	22	889	4.0
Western vegetarian:							
large	1261	35.0	150.0	61.0	125	2235	8.0
regular	651	18.0	75.0	33.0	62	1161	4.0
small	449	12.0	51.0	23.0	47	790	3.0
soup, 8-oz. cup:							
bean, 7, medley ...	145	7.0	24.0	2.0	0	1260	8.0
beef and black bean	150	10.0	25.0	1.0	5	1060	7.0
broccoli cheese ...	252	7.0	23.0	17.0	17	1104	1.0
cheese, Wisconsin	319	4.0	26.0	25.0	22	1104	1.0
chicken noodle ...	122	8.0	18.0	2.0	39	1104	1.0
chicken gumbo ...	110	4.0	13.0	5.0	20	1114	2.0
chicken tortilla	167	10.0	24.0	3.0	22	1026	3.0
chicken w/wild rice	378	10.0	24.0	28.0	78	1201	1.0
chili, Timberline ...	210	14.0	24.0	7.0	32	814	7.0
clam bisque, Tuscan	219	5.0	19.0	16.0	15	950	1.0
clam chowder,							
Boston	233	5.0	24.0	15.0	10	1062	1.0
corn chowder	284	2.0	38.0	17.0	6	1010	1.0
minestrone	89	3.0	17.0	1.0	0	1048	3.0
potato, cream of,							
w/bacon	226	2.0	31.0	13.0	5	1209	2.0
ravioli tomato	111	6.0	21.0	2.0	17	1115	1.0
red beans and rice	167	8.0	32.0	1.0	0	934	4.0
tomato Milano	89	4.0	17.0	0	0	437	2.0
tortellini	122	6.0	19.0	3.0	22	1360	1.0
vegetable:							
beef barley	100	6.0	12.0	3.0	11	1160	2.0
cheese	289	6.0	24.0	19.0	28	1338	2.0
Santa Fe	120	5.0	20.0	2.0	5	680	5.0
Schlotzsky's	220	10.0	44.0	2.0	0	2200	6.0
vegetarian	138	3.0	20.0	6.0	6	1536	6.0
salad, deli, 5 oz.:							
coleslaw	188	1.0	24.0	10.0	6	275	3.0

Food and Measure	cal.	prot. (gms)	carbo. (gms)	fat (gms)	chol. (mgs)	sod. (mgs)	fiber (gms)
macaroni	275	4.0	23.0	19.0	13	642	2.0
pasta, California . . .	58	0	10.0	3.0	0	250	1.0
potato	288	4.0	35.0	15.0	13	600	4.0
potato, mustard . . .	250	4.0	31.0	13.0	6	1050	4.0
salad, leaf, plain:							
Caesar	152	11.0	11.0	8.0	15	505	4.0
chef's:							
ham/turkey	248	23.0	15.0	11.0	51	1442	3.0
smoked turkey . .	243	24.0	15.0	10.0	53	1275	3.0
chicken, Caesar . . .	254	28.0	13.0	10.0	63	935	4.0
chicken, Chinese . .	150	20.0	11.0	3.0	47	448	3.0
garden	61	3.0	8.0	1.0	0	119	3.0
garden, small	25	1.0	3.0	1.0	0	55	1.0
Greek	180	10.0	13.0	10.0	23	654	4.0
dressings, 1 pkt.:							
balsamic vinaigrette,							
Greek	170	0	2.0	17.0	0	330	0
Caesar	260	2.0	1.0	27.0	25	250	0
Italian, light	90	0	3.0	8.0	0	690	0
ranch	270	0	1.0	29.0	5	370	0
ranch, spicy	230	1.0	2.0	25.0	15	310	0
ranch, spicy, light	140	1.0	9.0	11.0	15	350	0
sesame ginger							
vinaigrette	170	1.0	8.0	15.0	0	370	0
Thousand Island . .	220	0	6.0	21.0	30	360	0
salad extras, 1 pkt.:							
chow mein noodles	74	2.0	1.0	4.0	0	111	1.0
garlic cheese							
croutons	46	1.0	5.0	2.0	0	142	0
pizza, 8" sourdough:							
bacon, tomato, and							
mushroom	635	27.0	78.0	24.0	38	1891	4.0
cheese, double . . .	603	26.0	77.0	21.0	34	1772	4.0
cheese, double, and							
pepperoni	744	32.0	77.0	34.0	62	2206	4.0
chicken, barbecue .	653	38.0	78.0	20.0	74	2103	3.0
chicken, Thai	681	40.0	88.0	19.0	72	2303	5.0
chicken and pesto	649	40.0	78.0	19.0	74	2187	4.0
combination, the							
original	648	26.0	79.0	25.0	41	1994	5.0
Mediterranean	524	21.0	72.0	18.0	32	1879	3.0
New Orleans	666	40.0	79.0	20.0	74	2493	4.0
smoked turkey and							
jalapeño	647	38.0	81.0	19.0	62	2591	4.0

Food and Measure	cal.	prot. (gms)	carbo. (gms)	fat (gms)	chol. (mgs)	sod. (mgs)	fiber (gms)
Schlotzsky's Deli, pizza (cont.)							
Southwestern	635	38.0	76.0	19.0	71	2015	4.0
tomato and pesto ..	539	23.0	76.0	16.0	27.0	1670	4.0
vegetarian special .	551	24.0	76.0	17.0	27	1757	4.0
breads/buns:							
dark rye, regular ..	327	10.0	68.0	2.0	0	819	3.0
dark rye, small	218	7.0	45.0	1.0	0	546	2.0
jalapeño cheese:							
regular	353	12.0	66.0	4.0	6	945	2.0
small	235	8.0	44.0	3.0	4	630	2.0
sourdough:							
large	667	22.0	136.0	4.0	0	1725	5.0
regular	333	11.0	68.0	2.0	0	863	2.0
small	225	7.0	46.0	1.0	0	582	2.0
wheat, regular	336	12.0	66.0	3.0	0	864	4.0
wheat, small	226	8.0	45.0	2.0	0	583	2.0
desserts, 1 pc.:							
cheesecake:							
cookies & creme	330	6.0	36.0	18.0	35	320	1.0
New York	310	7.0	31.0	18.0	60	230	0
strawberry swirl .	300	6.0	30.0	17.0	55	230	0
cookie:							
chocolate chip ..	160	2.0	23.0	7.0	10	150	0
fudge chocolate							
chip	170	2.0	22.0	8.0	10	170	1.0
oatmeal raisin ..	150	1.0	24.0	5.0	10	140	1.0
peanut butter ...	170	2.0	21.0	8.0	10	190	1.0
sugar	160	2.0	23.0	6.0	15	180	0
white chocolate							
macadamia ..	170	2.0	22.0	8.0	10	140	0
fudge brownie cake	410	5.0	46.0	25.0	35	135	3.0
Scone, all fruit varieties (Health Valley Fat Free), 2.1-oz. pc.	180	4.0	43.0	0	0	190	5.0
Scorpion drink mixer (Trader Vic's), 4 fl. oz.	80	0	21.0	0	0	20	0
Scrapple, 2 oz.:							
(Dietz & Watson)	150	5.0	7.0	9.0	35	300	0
(Jones Dairy Farm) ..	120	5.0	7.0	8.0	30	280	0
Scrod, fresh, see "Cod, Atlantic"							
Scup, meat only:							
raw, 4 oz.	119	21.4	0	3.1	n.a.	48	0

Food and Measure	cal.	prot. (gms)	carbo. (gms)	fat (gms)	chol. (mgs)	sod. (mgs)	fiber (gms)
baked, broiled, or microwaved, 4 oz.	153	27.5	0	4.0	n.a.	61	0
Sea bass, meat only:							
raw, 4 oz.	110	20.9	0	2.3	47	77	0
baked, broiled, or microwaved, 4 oz.	141	26.8	0	2.9	60	99	0
Sea breeze drink mixer (*Mr & Mrs T*), 4 fl. oz.	80	0	19.0	0	0	45	0
Sea trout, meat only:							
raw, 4 oz.	118	19.0	0	4.1	94	66	0
baked, broiled, or microwaved, 4 oz.	151	24.3	0	5.3	120	84	0
Seafood, see specific listings							
Seafood sauce (see also specific listings), cocktail, ¼ cup, except as noted:							
(*Crosse & Blackwell*)	100	1.0	23.0	0	0	710	0
(*Del Monte*)	100	1.0	24.0	0	0	910	0
(*Golden Dipt*)	100	0	18.0	0	0	1280	0
(*Kraft* Cocktail)	60	1.0	13.0	.5	0	800	1.0
(*Kraft* Cocktail), .75 oz.	25	0	5.0	0	0	270	0
(*Old Bay*)	110	0	18.0	.5	0	960	0
(*Red Gold*)	70	0	17.0	0	0	480	1.0
(*S&W*), 1 tbsp.	20	0	5.0	0	0	220	0
hot, extra (*Golden Dipt*)	100	0	18.0	0	0	1300	0
Seafood seasoning (see also "Fish seasoning and coating mix" and specific listings):							
(*McCormick* Chesapeake Style), ¼ tsp.	0	0	0	0	0	350	0
(*Old Bay*), ¼ tsp. ...	0	0	0	0	0	160	0
Seafood stuffing, frozen (*Massachusetts Bay Clam Co.*), 1 oz.	80	2.0	7.0	5.0	2	230	.5

Food and Measure	cal.	prot. (gms)	carbo. (gms)	fat (gms)	chol. (mgs)	sod. (mgs)	fiber (gms)
Seasoning (see also specific listings), ¼ tsp., except as noted:							
(*Ac'cent*), ⅛ tsp. . . .	0	0	0	0	0	160	0
(*Sazon Goya* con Achiote)	0	0	0	0	0	160	0
(*Sazon Goya* con Azafran)	0	0	0	0	0	150	0
(*Sa-son* con Culantro)	0	0	0	0	0	170	0
(*Sa-son Ac'cent*)	0	0	0	0	0	150	0
Key West (*McCormick Spice Blends*)	0	0	0	0	0	100	0
Monterey (*McCormick Spice Blends*)	0	0	0	0	0	80	0
Santa Fe (*McCormick Spice Blends*)	0	0	0	0	0	70	0
Seasoning and coating mix (see also "Batter mix" and specific listings), country mild (*Shake 'n Bake*), ⅛ pkg. . .	35	0	5.0	2.0	0	240	0
Seasoning sauce, see specific listings							
Seaweed:							
agar:							
raw, 2 tbsp.	3	.5	.7	0	0	1	<.1
dried, 1 oz.	87	1.8	22.9	.1	0	29	2.2
flakes/bar (*Eden*), 1 tbsp.	10	0	2.0	0	0	10	2.0
arame (*Eden*), ½ cup .	30	1.0	7.0	0	0	120	7.0
hiziki (*Eden*), ½ cup .	30	0	6.0	0	0	160	6.0
Irish moss, raw, 1 oz.	14	.4	3.5	<.1	0	19	.4
kelp, raw, 1 oz.	12	.5	2.7	.2	0	66	.4
kombu (*Eden*), ½ of 7" pc.	10	0	2.0	0	0	90	1.0
laver, raw, 1 oz. . . .	10	1.6	1.4	.1	0	1	4.1
nori, 1 sheet:							
(*Eden/Eden* Sushi)	10	1.0	1.0	0	0	5	1.0
(*Sushi Chef*)	10	1.0	2.0	0	0	20	1.0
spirulina, 1 oz.:							
raw	8	1.7	.7	.1	0	28	n.a.
dried	82	16.3	6.8	2.2	0	297	1.0

Food and Measure	cal.	prot. (gms)	carbo. (gms)	fat (gms)	chol. (mgs)	sod. (mgs)	fiber (gms)
wakame:							
raw, 1 oz.	13	.9	2.6	.2	0	247	.1
(*Eden*), ½ cup	25	2.0	4.0	0	0	660	4.0
flakes (*Eden*), 1 tsp.	3	0	0	0	0	72	2.0
Semolina, whole-grain, 1 cup	601	21.2	121.6	1.8	0	2	6.5
Semolina flour:							
(*Hodgson Mill*), scant ¼ cup	110	4.0	22.0	.5	0	0	2.0
(*La Rinascente*), 2 oz.	200	7.0	41.0	1.0	0	0	2.0
mix (*Arrowhead Mills*), ½ cup	240	9.0	50.0	1.0	0	0	4.0
Sesame flour, 1 oz.:							
high fat	149	8.7	7.6	10.5	0	12	1.8
partially defatted	108	11.4	10.0	3.4	0	12	1.7
low fat	95	14.2	10.1	.5	0	11	1.4
Sesame meal, partially defatted, 1 oz. . . .	161	4.8	7.4	13.6	0	11	1.1
Sesame oil, 1 tsp.:							
(*Sun Luck*)	45	0	0	5.0	0	0	0
pure or hot (*House of Tsang*)	45	0	0	5.0	0	0	0
Sesame paste (see also "Tahini"), from whole seeds, 1 tbsp.	95	2.9	4.1	8.1	0	2	.9
Sesame seasoning (*Eden* Shake), ½ tsp.	10	0	0	.5	0	40	<1.0
Sesame seeds:							
whole:							
brown (*Arrowhead Mills*), ¼ cup . . .	200	7.0	8.0	20.0	0	20	5.0
dried, 1 tbsp.	52	1.6	2.1	4.5	0	1	1.1
roasted, toasted, 1 oz.	160	4.8	7.3	13.6	0	3	4.0
kernels:							
(*Arrowhead Mills*), ¼ cup	210	7.0	5.0	20.0	0	0	5.0
dried, 1 tsp.	16	.7	.3	1.5	0	1	<1.0
toasted, 1 oz.	161	4.8	7.4	13.6	0	11	4.8
Sesame spread (*Oskri*), 1.1 oz. . . .	170	2.0	26.0	8.0	0	40	1.0
Sesbania flower:							
raw, 1 cup	5	.3	1.4	<.1	0	3	n.a.
steamed, ½ cup	11	.6	2.7	<.1	0	6	n.a.

Food and Measure	cal.	prot. (gms)	carbo. (gms)	fat (gms)	chol. (mgs)	sod. (mgs)	fiber (gms)
Shad, meat only:							
raw, 4 oz.	223	19.2	0	15.6	85	58	0
baked, broiled, or							
microwaved, 4 oz.	286	24.6	0	20.0	109	74	0
Shallot, fresh:							
(*Frieda's*), 1 oz.	20	1.0	5.0	0	0	0	0
peeled, 1 oz.	20	.7	4.8	<.1	0	3	<1.0
chopped, 1 tbsp. . . .	7	.3	1.7	<.1	0	1	<1.0
Shallot, freeze-dried,							
1 tbsp.	3	.1	.7	tr.	0	1	<1.0
Shark, meat only, raw,							
4 oz.	148	23.8	0	5.1	58	90	0
Sheepshead, meat							
only:							
raw, 4 oz.	123	22.9	0	2.7	56	81	0
baked, broiled, or							
microwaved, 4 oz.	143	29.5	0	1.8	73	83	0
Shellie beans, canned							
w/liquid, ½ cup . . .	37	2.1	7.6	.2	0	408	4.1
Shells, pasta, mix,							
and cheese:							
(*Kraft Velveeta* Origi-							
nal), 4 oz.	360	14.0	45.0	13.0	25	1030	2.0
(*Velveeta* Light), 4 oz.	310	17.0	49.0	6.0	20	1090	3.0
creamy (*Land O Lakes*),							
3.5 oz.	350	13.0	40.0	14.0	25	800	2.0
white cheddar (*Pasta*							
Roni), 1 cup*	310	9.0	40.0	13.0	5	730	2.0
Shells, pasta, entree,							
frozen, 1 pkg.,							
except as noted:							
and American cheese							
(*Stouffer's*), ½ of							
12-oz. pkg.	280	12.0	36.0	10.0	20	810	1.0
and cheese w/jalapeño							
(*Michelina's*), 8 oz.	350	14.0	46.0	11.0	25	500	2.0
and cheese sauce							
(*Freezer Queen*							
Meal), 8.5 oz.	270	6.0	43.0	9.0	15	700	6.0
stuffed, broccoli							
(*Celentano*), 10 oz.	230	10.0	32.0	4.5	20	510	4.0
stuffed, cheese:							
(*Celentano*), 10 oz.	320	12.0	31.0	15.0	40	810	3.0

Food and Measure	cal.	prot. (gms)	carbo. (gms)	fat (gms)	chol. (mgs)	sod. (mgs)	fiber (gms)
(*Celentano* Low Fat), 10 oz.	250	11.0	32.0	6.0	25	630	3.0
(*Healthy Choice*), 10.35 oz.	370	18.0	60.0	6.0	20	570	5.0
no sauce (*Celentano*), 4 pcs., ½ of 12.5-oz. pkg.	320	16.0	36.0	12.0	70	470	2.0
Sherbet (see also "Sorbet"), ½ cup, except as noted:							
berry rainbow (*Dreyer's/Edy's*) ...	130	1.0	29.0	1.0	5	35	0
cherry chip (*Darigold*)	130	1.0	28.0	2.0	5	35	<1.0
cherry lemonade or citrus swirl (*Blue Bell*) ....:..	130	2.0	29.0	1.0	<5	35	0
lemon bar (*Dreyer's/ Edy's*)	150	1.0	30.0	2.5	10	50	0
lemon or lime (*Blue Bell*)	130	2.0	29.0	1.0	<5	35	0
orange:							
(*Blue Bell*)	130	1.0	29.0	1.0	<5	30	0
(*Breyers*)	130	1.0	27.0	1.5	5	40	0
(*Darigold*)	120	1.0	26.0	1.0	5	35	0
(*Turkey Hill* Grove)	120	1.0	26.0	1.0	5	20	0
cherry (*Dreyer's/ Edy's Starburst*)	150	1.0	33.0	2.0	5	40	0
Swiss (*Dreyer's/ Edy's*)	150	1.0	30.0	3.0	5	40	0
orange, and vanilla ice cream:							
(*Baldwin*)	140	2.0	21.0	6.0	20	40	0
(*Breyers* Take Two)	130	2.0	20.0	5.0	15	30	0
(*Darigold* Float) ...	120	2.0	21.0	4.0	15	40	0
swirl (*Dreyer's/ Edy's*)	120	2.0	23.0	2.0	10	40	0
swirl (*Turkey Hill*)	140	2.0	19.0	6.0	20	25	0
pineapple (*Blue Bell*)	120	1.0	28.0	1.0	<5	30	0
rainbow:							
(*Baldwin*)	110	1.0	42.0	1.0	5	35	0
(*Blue Bell*), 3-oz. cup	110	1.0	25.0	1.0	<5	30	0
(*Blue Bell* Pint) ...	130	1.0	28.0	1.0	<5	30	0
(*Blue Bell* Quart) ..	130	1.0	29.0	1.0	<5	30	0

Food and Measure	cal.	prot. (gms)	carbo. (gms)	fat (gms)	chol. (mgs)	sod. (mgs)	fiber (gms)
Sherbet, rainbow (*cont.*)							
(*Breyers*)	130	1.0	27.0	1.5	5	40	0
(*Darigold*)	120	1.0	26.0	1.0	5	30	0
fruit (*Turkey Hill*) . .	120	1.0	26.0	1.0	5	20	0
tropical (*Dreyer's/ Edy's*)	130	1.0	29.0	1.0	5	35	0
raspberry:							
(*Darigold*)	120	1.0	26.0	1.0	5	30	0
chocolate swirl (*Dreyer's/Edy's*)	130	2.0	28.0	1.5	5	40	0
strawberry (*Dreyer's/ Edy's Starburst*) . .	160	1.0	33.0	2.5	5	40	0
Sherbet bar (see also "Iced confection bar"), 1 bar:							
(*Popsicle* Cyclone) . . .	50	1.0	11.0	.5	<5	15	0
all flavors (*Creamsicle* No Sugar)	25	0	5.0	0	0	10	0
orange:							
(*Blue Bell* Pop Up)	90	<1.0	20.0	1.0	<5	20	0
(*Good Humor* Pop-Ups)	80	<1.0	19.0	1.0	<5	15	0
orange lemon (*Pop-sicle* Smile!)	90	0	20.0	.5	<5	10	0
w/vanilla ice cream:							
orange (*Creamsicle* Single)	120	1.0	21.0	3.0	10	30	0
orange raspberry (*Creamsicle*), 2.75 fl. oz.	110	1.0	19.0	3.0	10	25	0
orange raspberry (*Creamsicle* Pop), 1.75 fl. oz.	80	<1.0	14.0	2.0	5	20	0
rainbow (*Good Humor* Pop-Ups)	90	<1.0	19.0	1.0	<5	15	0
Shortening, 1 tbsp.:							
(*Jewel/Swiftning*)	110	0	0	12.0	1	10	0
(*Wesson*)	110	0	0	12.0	0	0	0
soy and cottonseed . .	113	0	0	12.8	0	0	0
vegetable:							
(*Smart Balance*) . . .	110	0	0	12.0	0	0	0
(*Snowdrift*)	110	0	0	12.0	1	0	0
regular/butter flavor (*Crisco*)	110	0	0	12.0	0	0	0

Food and Measure	cal.	prot. (gms)	carbo. (gms)	fat (gms)	chol. (mgs)	sod. (mgs)	fiber (gms)
Shrimp, meat only:							
raw, 4 oz.	120	23.0	1.0	2.0	173	168	0
raw, 4 large, 1 oz. . . .	30	5.7	.3	.5	43	42	0
boiled or steamed:							
4 oz.	112	23.7	0	1.2	221	254	0
4 large, .8 oz.	22	4.6	0	.2	43	49	0
Shrimp, canned,							
2 oz., except as							
noted:							
(*Crown Prince*							
Natural), ½ can,							
2.1 oz.	120	26.0	2.0	.5	250	810	1.0
medium (*Bumble Bee*)	45	10.0	0	1.0	115	650	0
medium or small							
(*Chicken of the Sea*)	45	10.0	1.0	.5	145	650	0
small (*Crown Prince*),							
½ can, 2.1 oz. . . .	120	26.0	2.0	.5	250	310	1.0
tiny:							
(*Chicken of the Sea*)	45	10.0	1.0	.5	145	650	0
(*Orleans* Cocktail)	44	10.0	0	0	113	650	0
(*3 Diamonds*)	55	11.0	1.0	.5	185	260	0
tiny or broken (*Crown Prince*), ½ can,							
2.1 oz.	60	13.0	<1.0	.5	145	360	0
drained, 1 cup	154	29.6	1.3	2.5	222	216	0
Shrimp, freeze-dried							
(*AlpineAire*), 1 oz.	110	23.0	2.0	1.0	0	170	0
Shrimp, frozen:							
raw (*Contessa*), 4 oz.	70	17.0	1.0	0	135	550	0
cooked (*Contessa*),							
4 oz.	60	13.0	0	0	130	360	0
cooked, w/sauce							
(*Contessa Party Platter*), 3.75 oz. . . .	80	14.0	6.0	0	105	750	0
"Shrimp," imitation,							
from surimi, 4 oz.	115	14.1	10.4	1.7	41	800	0
Shrimp, smoked							
(*Ducktrap River*),							
¼ cup	60	10.0	0	2.0	120	440	0
Shrimp entree, freeze-dried, 1 serving:							
Alfredo (*AlpineAire*) . .	320	17.0	44.0	9.0	25	710	1.0
Newburg (*AlpineAire*)	300	14.0	49.0	6.0	15	510	1.0

Food and Measure	cal.	prot. (gms)	carbo. (gms)	fat (gms)	chol. (mgs)	sod. (mgs)	fiber (gms)
Shrimp entree, frozen, 1 pkg., except as noted:							
Alfredo:							
(*Mrs. Paul's* Bowl), 11-oz. cont. ...	410	21.0	40.0	19.0	110	880	5.0
w/fettuccine (*Michelina's*), 8 oz.	310	16.0	31.0	12.0	100	530	2.0
w/penne (*Gorton's* Bowl), 10.5 oz.	290	13.0	49.0	5.0	45	980	2.0
and angel hair pasta (*Lean Cuisine Cafe Classics*), 10 oz. ..	280	15.0	44.0	5.0	60	690	3.0
Buffalo (*Mrs. Paul's/ Van de Kamps*), 20 pcs., 4 oz.	320	11.0	35.0	15.0	90	970	0
butterfly, 7 pcs.:							
(*Mrs. Paul's*)	270	10.0	27.0	14.0	80	530	<1.0
(*Van de Kamp's*) ..	300	10.0	30.0	15.0	80	610	3.0
Cajun, w/out sauce (*Mrs. Paul's*), about 21 pcs., 4 oz.	70	13.0	2.0	.5	155	1120	0
Cajun sauce (*Contessa Shrimp on the Bar-B*), ¼ of 24-oz. pkg.	140	22.0	3.0	4.5	190	880	0
fantail, breaded (*Mrs. Friday's*), 4 oz., about 7 pcs.	300	12.0	28.0	15.0	90	500	4.0
fried rice (*Yu Sing*), 8 oz.	350	9.0	64.0	5.0	40	780	2.0
herb sauce, Italian (*Contessa Shrimp on the Bar-B*), ¼ of 24-oz. pkg.	150	21.0	6.0	4.5	190	960	0
garlic butter, w/fettucine (*Gorton's* Bowl), 10.5 oz. ...	280	13.0	46.0	5.0	40	680	3.0
w/linguine:							
(*Contessa Mediterranean*), 1⅓ cups	170	9.0	26.0	3.0	60	840	2.0
(*Mrs. Paul's*), 1½ cups	180	14.0	30.0	1.0	40	550	4.0

Food and Measure	cal.	prot. (gms)	carbo. (gms)	fat (gms)	chol. (mgs)	sod. (mgs)	fiber (gms)
lo mein (*Yu Sing*), 8 oz.	210	9.0	38.0	1.0	30	1030	3.0
peanut, Thai style (*Mrs. Paul's* Bowl), 11-oz. cont.	390	16.0	61.0	9.0	65	590	4.0
popcorn:							
(*Gorton's*), 3.6 oz., about 22 pcs. . .	250	10.0	27.0	12.0	90	840	0
(*Mrs. Paul's*), 20 pcs.	290	10.0	31.0	13.0	75	680	<1.0
(*Van de Kamp's*), 20 pcs.	270	10.0	30.0	12.0	80	850	2.0
garlic and herb (*Gorton's*), 3.2 oz., about 20 pcs. . .	240	7.0	26.0	12.0	65	810	0
scampi (*Contessa*), ¾ of 12-oz. pkg.	340	10.0	5.0	30.0	85	790	0
stir-fry:							
(*Contessa*), 1¾ cups	140	9.0	26.0	.5	55	1250	4.0
(*Mrs. Paul's* Bowl), 11-oz. cont.	390	14.0	80.0	1.0	65	1740	3.0
(*Mrs. Paul's/Van de Kamp's*), 1⅔ cups	260	10.0	54.0	.5	40	920	3.0
stuffed (*Van de Kamp's*), 3 pcs., 4.5 oz.	290	12.0	32.0	13.0	70	720	<1.0
sweet and sour (*Contessa*), 1½ cups	180	9.0	40.0	0	50	430	3.0
teriyaki, w/rice (*Gorton's* Bowl), 10.5 oz.	320	10.0	57.0	6.0	35	1250	2.0
w/vegetables (*Healthy Choice*), 11.8 oz.	270	15.0	39.0	6.0	50	580	6.0
Shrimp sauce (*Crosse & Blackwell*), ¼ cup	110	1.0	25.0	0	0	790	0
Sloppy Joe sauce, see "Sandwich sauce"							
Sloppy Joe seasoning:							
(*Bearitos*), 2 tsp. . . .	25	0	6.0	0	0	320	0
(*Lawry's*), 2 tsp.	20	0	5.0	0	0	530	0

Food and Measure	cal.	prot. (gms)	carbo. (gms)	fat (gms)	chol. (mgs)	sod. (mgs)	fiber (gms)
Sloppy Joe seasoning (*cont.*)							
(*Manwich*), ¼ oz. . . .	20	0	5.0	0	0	355	0
(*McCormick*),							
⅛ pkg.	15	0	3.0	0	0	360	0
(*Tempo*), 1⅓ tbsp. . .	45	1.0	11.0	0	0	680	0
Smelt, rainbow,							
meat only:							
raw, 4 oz.	110	20.0	0	2.8	80	68	0
baked, broiled, or							
microwaved, 4 oz.	141	25.6	0	3.5	102	87	0
Smoothie mix,							
⅓ pkt.:							
all flavors, except							
chocolate-banana							
and strawberry							
frost (*McCormick*							
Produce Partners)	80	0	18.0	0	0	0	0
chocolate-banana							
frost (*McCormick*							
Produce Partners)	80	0	18.0	0	0	10	0
strawberry frost							
(*McCormick*							
Produce Partners)	80	0	19.0	0	0	0	0
Smoothie mix,							
frozen, ⅔ cup:							
banana-raspberry-							
strawberry or							
strawberry-							
banana (*Tree of*							
Life)	90	1.0	23.0	0	0	0	3.0
mango-strawberry-							
raspberry (*Tree*							
of Life)	70	1.0	18.0	0	0	0	4.0
strawberry-banana-							
blueberry (*Tree*							
of Life)	90	1.0	22.0	0	0	0	3.0
Snack chips (see							
also "Snack mix"							
and specific list-							
ings), 1 oz.,							
except as noted:							
multigrain:							
(*Garden of Eatin'*							
Garden Grains) .	150	2.0	18.0	7.0	0	100	1.0

Food and Measure	cal.	prot. (gms)	carbo. (gms)	fat (gms)	chol. (mgs)	sod. (mgs)	fiber (gms)
(Sunchips)	140	2.0	19.0	6.0	0	115	2.0
cheddar (Sunchips Harvest)	140	2.0	19.0	6.0	0	190	2.0
onion, French (Sunchips)	140	2.0	18.0	7.0	0	160	2.0
onion flavor:							
(Funyons)	140	2.0	18.0	7.0	0	270	<1.0
rings (Utz)	140	1.0	18.0	7.0	0	340	0
Snack mix, ½ cup, except as noted:							
(Boston's)	125	3.0	20.0	3.5	0	320	2.0
(Buckaroo Saddle-bag Hunter's Mix), 1 oz.	170	6.0	6.0	14.0	0	200	<4.0
(Cheez-It)	130	3.0	21.0	4.5	0	330	2.0
(Cheez-It Big Crunch), ¾ cup ...	110	3.0	20.0	6.0	0	360	<1.0
(Cheez-It Blitz Mix/ Hoops Edition)	130	3.0	21.0	4.5	0	330	2.0
(Cheez-It Get Nutty) ..	150	4.0	17.0	8.0	0	280	1.0
(Cheez-It Party Mix) ..	140	4.0	19.0	5.0	0	270	1.0
(Chex Bold Party Blend)	140	3.0	20.0	6.0	0	390	2.0
(Chex Bold Party Blend), 1.6-oz. pkg.	220	4.0	33.0	9.0	0	640	4.0
(Chex Traditional), ⅔ cup	130	2.0	22.0	4.0	0	410	1.0
(Chex Traditional), 1.6-oz. pkg.	210	4.0	36.0	7.0	0	670	2.0
(Doo Dads)	150	3.0	20.0	7.0	0	410	2.0
(Gardetto's Snak•ens)	160	3.0	18.0	8.0	0	330	1.0
(Gardetto's Snak•ens), 1.6-oz. pkg.	240	4.0	28.0	13.0	0	510	1.0
(Gardetto's Snak•ens Reduced Fat)	130	3.0	19.0	5.0	0	330	<1.0
(Gardetto's Snak•ens Reduced Fat), 1.6-oz. pkg.	220	4.0	31.0	8.0	0	510	1.0
(Ritz)	150	2.0	21.0	7.0	0	430	1.0

Food and Measure	cal.	prot. (gms)	carbo. (gms)	fat (gms)	chol. (mgs)	sod. (mgs)	fiber (gms)
Snack mix (cont.)							
(Ritz), 1.5-oz. pkg. . . .	200	3.0	27.0	9.0	0	650	2.0
(Rold Gold), ¾ cup . .	160	3.0	18.0	8.0	0	380	1.0
(Snack 'Ums Big Boomin' Pops), 1 cup	120	2.0	27.0	0	0	135	0
(Snack 'Ums Big Rollin' Froot Loops), 1¼ cups . .	120	2.0	28.0	1.0	0	150	1.0
(Snack 'Ums Rice Krispies Treats Krunch), 1 cup . . .	130	2.0	26.0	1.5	0	10	0
cheddar:							
(Chex)	140	3.0	21.0	5.0	0	330	2.0
(Chex), 1.6-oz. pkg.	220	5.0	34.0	9.0	0	530	3.0
(Ritz)	150	2.0	20.0	7.0	0	490	1.0
cheese:							
(Cheez-It), ¾ cup .	110	3.0	19.0	5.0	0	450	<1.0
Italian blend (Gardetto's)	140	3.0	20.0	5.0	0	350	<1.0
Italian blend (Gardetto's), 1.6-oz. pkg. . . .	200	5.0	30.0	7.0	0	530	1.0
honey, toasted (Wheatables)	130	3.0	20.0	5.0	0	350	2.0
honey nut:							
(Chex)	130	2.0	22.0	4.0	0	270	1.0
(Chex), 1.6-oz. pkg.	210	3.0	37.0	6.0	0	450	2.0
hot and spicy:							
(Chex), ⅔ cup . . .	130	2.0	21.0	4.5	0	390	2.0
(Chex), 1.6-oz. pkg.	210	4.0	35.0	7.0	0	640	3.0
Italian recipe:							
(Gardetto's)	150	3.0	20.0	6.0	0	290	1.0
(Gardetto's), 1.6-oz. pkg. . . .	220	5.0	30.0	9.0	0	440	2.0
nacho fiesta:							
(Chex), ⅔ cup . . .	120	2.0	22.0	3.5	0	350	1.0
(Chex), 1.6-oz. pkg.	200	4.0	36.0	6.0	0	570	2.0
peanut lovers:							
(Chex)	140	3.0	19.0	6.0	0	370	1.0
(Chex), 1.6-oz. pkg.	210	5.0	30.0	9.0	0	550	2.0
peanut butter crunch (Wheatables)	160	4.0	21.0	7.0	0	430	1.0

Food and Measure	cal.	prot. (gms)	carbo. (gms)	fat (gms)	chol. (mgs)	sod. (mgs)	fiber (gms)
pretzel, mustard:							
(*Gardetto's*)	130	3.0	24.0	2.0	0	220	1.0
(*Gardetto's*),							
1.6-oz. pkg. ...	190	5.0	36.0	3.0	0	340	2.0
Snail, sea, see "Whelk"							
Snap beans (see also "Green beans"), all varieties (*Frieda's*), ²⁄₃ cup, 3 oz.	25	2.0	0	0	0	5	3.0
Snapper, meat only:							
raw, 4 oz.	113	23.3	0	1.5	42	73	0
baked, broiled, or microwaved, 4 oz.	145	30.0	0	2.0	53	65	0
Snow pea, see "Peas, edible-podded"							
Snow pea sprouts (*Jonathan's*), 1 cup	40	3.0	8.0	0	0	0	3.0
Soft drinks, carbonated, 8 fl. oz., except as noted:							
apple, spiced (*Natural Brew*), 12 fl. oz. ...	170	0	42.0	0	0	18	0
apple raspberry (*Fruitworks*)	100	0	28.0	0	0	70	0
berry (*After the Fall Berrymeister Spritzer*), 12 fl. oz.	170	<1.0	42.0	0	0	25	0
birch beer (*Pennsylvania Dutch*)	110	0	28.0	0	0	30	0
blackberry (*Clearly Canadian*)	100	0	24.0	0	0	11	0
boysenberry, 12 fl. oz.:							
(*R. W. Knudsen Spritzer*)	160	<1.0	40.0	0	0	25	0
(*R. W. Knudsen Spritzer Light*) ..	110	0	28.0	0	0	15	0
cherry:							
(*Clearly Canadian*) .	80	0	23.0	0	0	11	0
(*Crush*)	120	0	34.0	0	0	30	0
(*7-Up*)	100	0	26.0	0	0	35	0
(*Sundrop*)	120	0	31.0	0	0	20	0
cream (*Stewart's*), 12 fl. oz.	190	0	48.0	0	0	30	0

Food and Measure	cal.	prot. (gms)	carbo. (gms)	fat (gms)	chol. (mgs)	sod. (mgs)	fiber (gms)
Soft drinks, cherry (*cont.*)							
lime (*Slice*), 12 fl. oz.	160	0	43.0	0	0	50	0
spice (*Slice*), 12 fl. oz.	150	0	40.0	0	0	35	0
cherry, black:							
(*IBC*)	120	0	32.0	0	0	40	0
(*Koala*)	90	0	23.0	0	0	25	0
(*Koala*), 11 fl. oz.	130	0	32.0	0	0	30	0
(*After the Fall Spritzer*), 12 fl. oz.	180	<1.0	45.0	0	0	20	0
(*R. W. Knudsen Spritzer*), 12 fl. oz.	170	<1.0	42.0	0	0	25	0
cherry amaretto (*Natural Brew*), 12 fl. oz.	160	0	40.0	0	0	20	0
cherry ginger brew (*Reed's*), 12 fl. oz.	150	0	38.5	0	0	5	0
chocolate (*Hershey's*)	120	0	25.0	0	0	170	0
citrus (*Citra*)	90	0	25.0	0	0	40	0
club soda:							
(*Canada Dry*)	0	0	0	0	0	60	0
(*Schweppes*)	0	0	0	0	0	45	0
coconut (*Goya*), 12 fl. oz.	200	0	45.0	0	0	65	0
cola:							
(*Coca-Cola* Classic/ Caffeine Free) . .	100	0	27.0	0	0	35	0
(*Pepsi/Pepsi* Caffeine Free) . .	100	0	27.0	0	0	25	0
(*Santa Cruz Organic*), 12 fl. oz.	140	0	36.0	0	0	0	0
(*Slice*), 12 fl. oz. . .	160	0	43.0	0	0	35	0
(*Vanilla Coke*)	100	0	28	0	0	25	0
berry (*Pepsi Blue*)	100	0	28	0	0	25	0
champagne (*Goya*), 12 fl. oz.	200	0	47.0	0	0	60	0
ginseng (*Natural Brew*), 12 fl. oz.	170	0	42.0	0	0	20	0
lemon (*Pepsi* Twist)	100	0	27.0	0	0	25	0
cola, cherry:							
(*Coca-Cola*)	100	0	28.0	0	0	30	0
(*R. W. Knudsen Spritzer*), 12 fl. oz.	170	<1.0	42.0	0	0	20	0

Food and Measure	cal.	prot. (gms)	carbo. (gms)	fat (gms)	chol. (mgs)	sod. (mgs)	fiber (gms)
wild (*Pepsi*)	110	0	29.0	0	0	25	0
Collins mixer:							
(*Canada Dry*)	100	0	21.0	0	0	15	0
(*Schweppes*)	100	0	21.0	0	0	15	0
cranberry (*R. W. Knudsen Spritzer*), 12 fl. oz.	190	1.0	45.0	0	0	65	0
cranberry raspberry:							
(*Koala*)	90	0	21.0	0	0	25	0
(*Koala*), 11 fl. oz.	120	0	29.0	0	0	35	0
cream/creme:							
(*A&W*)	120	0	31.0	0	0	30	0
(*Barq's*)	110	0	30.0	0	0	45	0
(*Hires*)	120	0	32.0	0	0	30	0
(*IBC*)	120	0	32.0	0	0	50	0
(*Mug*)	120	0	32.0	0	0	45	0
creme, vanilla, 12 fl. oz.:							
(*After the Fall Spritzer*)	170	1.0	42.0	0	0	25	0
(*Natural Brew*)	170	0	42.0	0	0	18	0
(*R. W. Knudsen Spritzer*).......	160	<1.0	35.0	0	0	20	0
(*Dr Pepper*)	100	0	27.0	0	0	35	0
(*Dr. Slice*), 12 fl. oz. ...	140	0	39.0	0	0	35	0
fruit punch/blend:							
(*Goya*), 12 fl. oz. ...	190	0	45.0	0	0	40	0
(*Hawaiian Punch Fruit Juicy Red*)	130	0	33.0	0	0	90	0
(*Slice*), 12 fl. oz. ..	190	0	50.0	0	0	55	0
(*Tahitian Treat*) ...	110	0	30.0	0	0	25	0
ginger ale:							
(*After the Fall Spritzer* Nantucket), 12 fl. oz.	160	1.0	40.0	0	0	25	0
(*Canada Dry*)	90	0	24.0	0	0	15	0
(*Natural Brew* Outrageous), 12 fl. oz.	170	0	42.0	0	0	18	0
(*R. W. Knudsen Spritzer*), 12 fl. oz.	160	1.0	40.0	0	0	25	0
(*Schweppes*)	80	0	22.0	0	0	25	0
(*Vernors*), 12 fl. oz.	150	0	39.0	0	0	25	0
cranberry (*Canada Dry*)	90	0	25.0	0	0	15	0

Food and Measure	cal.	prot. (gms)	carbo. (gms)	fat (gms)	chol. (mgs)	sod. (mgs)	fiber (gms)
Soft drinks, ginger ale (*cont.*)							
cranberry or strawberry (*After the Fall Spritzer*), 12 fl. oz.	150	0	37.0	0	0	15	0
raspberry (*After the Fall Spritzer*), 12 fl. oz.	140	0	35.0	0	0	15	0
ginger beer:							
(*Goya*), 12 fl. oz. ..	190	0	47.0	0	0	30	0
(*Reed's* Extra Ginger Brew), 12 fl. oz.	145	0	37.4	0	0	5	0
(*Stewart's*), 12 fl. oz.	200	0	50.0	0	0	30	0
grape:							
(*Crush*)	130	0	35.0	0	0	30	0
(*Goya*), 12 fl. oz. ..	230	0	57.0	0	0	5	0
(*Minute Maid*)	130	0	34.0	0	0	45	0
(*R. W. Knudsen Spritzer*), 12 fl. oz.	170	1.0	41.0	0	0	30	0
(*Slice*), 12 fl. oz. ..	190	0	51.0	0	0	70	0
(*Welch's*)	130	0	34.0	0	0	40	0
Concord (*After the Fall Spritzer*), 12 fl. oz.	180	<1.0	43.0	0	0	30	0
white (*Clearly Canadian*)	90	0	21.0	0	0	11	0
grapefruit (*Natural Brew*), 12 fl. oz. ..	160	0	40.0	0	0	0	0
grapefruit kiwi lime:							
(*Koala*)	90	0	22.0	0	0	25	0
(*Koala*), 12 fl. oz.	130	0	32.0	0	0	35	0
guava berry (*Fruitworks*), 12 fl. oz. ..	170	0	46.0	0	0	80	0
kiwi lime (*R. W. Knudsen Spritzer*), 10 fl. oz.	130	1.0	32.0	0	0	25	0
kiwi-strawberry (*After the Fall Spritzer*), 12 fl. oz.	150	0	38.0	0	0	15	0
lemon, bitter (*Schweppes*)	110	0	28.0	0	0	20	0
lemon-ginger (*tré limone*)	90	0	22.0	0	0	30	0

Food and Measure	cal.	prot. (gms)	carbo. (gms)	fat (gms)	chol. (mgs)	sod. (mgs)	fiber (gms)
lemonade (see also "Lemonade"):							
(*Country Time*) ...	90	0	23.0	0	0	90	0
Jamaican (*R. W. Knudsen Spritzer*), 12 fl. oz.	170	<1.0	41.0	0	0	25	0
pink (*Fruitworks*) ..	110	0	30.0	0	0	50	0
lemon-lime (*R. W. Knudsen Spritzer*), 12 fl. oz.	170	1.0	42.0	0	0	25	0
lime, 12 fl. oz.:							
Caribbean (*After the Fall Spritzer*)	170	<1.0	41.0	0	0	20	0
mandarin (*R. W. Knudsen Spritzer*)	170	1.0	42.0	0	0	25	0
malt beverage (*Goya*), 12 fl. oz.	230	1.0	56.0	0	0	80	0
mango, 12 fl. oz.:							
(*R. W. Knudsen Spritzer Fandango*)	190	1.0	45.0	0	0	30	0
(*R. W. Knudsen Spritzer Light*) ..	110	0	28.0	0	0	10	0
ginger (*After the Fall Spritzer*)	150	0	36.0	0	0	10	0
Hawaiian (*After the Fall Spritzer*) ...	190	<1.0	45.0	0	0	30	0
(*Mountain Dew*)	110	0	31.0	0	0	50	0
(*Mountain Dew Code Red*)	110	0	31.0	0	0	70	0
orange:							
(*After the Fall Spritzer Mimosa*), 12 fl. oz.	170	<1.0	39.0	0	0	35	0
(*Crush*)	120	0	34.0	0	0	30	0
(*Minute Maid*)	120	0	32.0	0	0	25	0
(*Natural Brew*), 12 fl. oz.	150	0	38.0	0	0	30	0
(*Orangina*)	90	0	23.0	0	0	25	0
(*Orangina*), 10 fl. oz.	120	<1.0	28.0	0	0	115	0
(*Slice*), 12 fl. oz. ..	190	0	51.0	0	0	50	0
(*Sunkist*)	130	0	35.0	0	0	30	0
cream (*Stewart's*), 12 fl. oz.	190	0	48.0	0	0	40	0

Food and Measure	cal.	prot. (gms)	carbo. (gms)	fat (gms)	chol. (mgs)	sod. (mgs)	fiber (gms)
Soft drinks (*cont.*)							
orange-mango:							
(*Koala*)	80	0	20.0	0	0	25	0
(*Koala*), 12 fl. oz.	120	0	30.0	0	0	40	0
orange–passion fruit:							
(*Fruitworks*),							
12 fl. oz.	160	0	43.0	0	0	110	0
(*Koala*)	90	0	21.0	0	0	25	0
(*R. W. Knudsen*							
Spritzer), 12 fl. oz.	160	1.0	40.0	0	0	25	0
peach:							
(*Crush*)	120	0	33.0	0	0	25	0
(*R. W. Knudsen*							
Spritzer), 12 fl. oz.	160	2.0	37.0	0	0	35	0
Georgia (*After the*							
Fall Spritzer),							
12 fl. oz.	150	<1.0	37.0	0	0	35	0
peach-papaya (*Fruit-*							
works)	110	0	30.0	0	0	70	0
pineapple:							
(*After the Fall*							
Spritzer Mandarin),							
12 fl. oz.	160	<1.0	38.0	0	0	20	0
(*Goya*), 12 fl. oz. ..	170	0	43.0	0	0	40	0
(*Slice*), 12 fl. oz. ..	190	0	51.0	0	0	70	0
pineapple-passion							
fruit, tropical							
(*After the Fall*							
Spritzer), 12 fl. oz.	170	<1.0	42.0	0	0	20	0
raspberry:							
(*After the Fall*							
Spritzer), 12 fl. oz.	170	<1.0	42.0	0	0	25	0
(*R. W. Knudsen*							
Spritzer), 12 fl. oz.	170	0	38.0	0	0	25	0
(*R. W. Knudsen*							
Spritzer Light),							
12 fl. oz.	110	0	28.0	0	0	15	0
cream (*Clearly*							
Canadian)	75	0	19.0	0	0	11	0
raspberry-guava:							
(*Koala*)	90	0	21.0	0	0	25	0
(*Koala*), 12 fl. oz.	130	0	32.0	0	0	35	0
root beer:							
(*A&W*)	120	0	31.0	0	0	30	0

Food and Measure	cal.	prot. (gms)	carbo. (gms)	fat (gms)	chol. (mgs)	sod. (mgs)	fiber (gms)
(Barq's)	100	0	30.0	0	0	50	0
(Hires)	120	0	31.0	0	0	45	0
(IBC)	110	0	29.0	0	0	40	0
(Mug)	110	0	29.0	0	0	45	0
(Santa Cruz Organic), 12 fl. oz.	140	0	36.0	0	0	0	0
(Stewart's), 12 fl. oz.	160	0	40.0	0	0	30	0
seltzer, plain or flavored	0	0	0	0	0	0	0
(7-Up)	100	0	26.0	0	0	50	0
(Sierra Mist), 12 fl. oz.	150	0	39.0	0	0	35	0
(Slice Red), 12 fl. oz.	190	0	51.0	0	0	55	0
(Sprite)	100	0	26.0	0	0	45	0
(Squirt)	100	0	27.0	0	0	15	0
(Squirt Ruby Red)	120	0	31.0	0	0	15	0
strawberry:							
(Crush)	110	0	30.0	0	0	30	0
(R. W. Knudsen Spritzer), 12 fl. oz.	170	<1.0	42.0	0	0	25	0
(Slice), 12 fl.oz.	170	0	47.0	0	0	55	0
strawberry-kiwi (R. W. Knudsen Spritzer Light), 12 fl. oz.	110	0	28.0	0	0	15	0
strawberry-kiwi-peach (Koala)	90	0	22.0	0	0	25	0
strawberry-melon:							
(Clearly Canadian)	80	0	20.0	0	0	11	0
(Fruitworks)	110	0	30.0	0	0	70	0
summer brew (Natural Brew), 12 fl. oz.	160	0	40.0	0	0	0	0
(Sundrop)	130	0	34.0	0	0	20	0
tangerine, 12 fl. oz.:							
(After the Fall Spritzer)	180	<1.0	44.0	0	0	35	0
(R. W. Knudsen Spritzer)	170	2.0	40.0	0	0	35	0
(R. W. Knudsen Spritzer Light)	110	2.0	28.0	0	0	15	0
tangerine citrus (Fruitworks)	100	0	28.0	0	0	50	0
tonic:							
(Canada Dry)	100	0	24.0	0	0	15	0
(Schweppes)	80	0	23.0	0	0	20	0

Food and Measure	cal.	prot. (gms)	carbo. (gms)	fat (gms)	chol. (mgs)	sod. (mgs)	fiber (gms)
Soft drinks (*cont.*)							
(*Vernor's*)	100	0	26.0	0	0	15	0
(*Wink*)	110	0	29.0	0	0	25	0
winter brew (*Natural Brew*), 12 fl. oz. ...	180	0	44.0	0	0	20	0
Sofrito (*Goya* Jar), 1 tsp.	0	0	0	0	0	45	0
Sole, see "Flatfish"							
Sole entree, frozen, 5-oz. pc., except as noted:							
au gratin (*Oven Poppers*)	220	24.0	5.0	11.0	75	450	<1.0
w/shrimp and lobster in Newburg sauce (*Oven Poppers*) ...	130	19.0	3.0	5.0	90	440	<1.0
stuffed:							
w/broccoli, cheese (*Oven Poppers*)	150	20.0	4.0	6.0	55	330	1.0
w/crab (*Oven Poppers*)	250	17.0	15.0	13.0	70	400	1.0
w/crab, miniatures (*Oven Poppers*), 2-oz. pc.	120	6.0	8.0	7.0	25	140	0
w/garlic, shrimp, almonds (*Oven Poppers*)	250	19.0	15.0	13.0	80	430	2.0
w/shrimp, lobster (*Oven Poppers*)	150	20.0	7.0	5.0	80	430	1.0
Sonic, 1 serving:							
burgers:							
bacon cheeseburger	727	23.0	44.0	49.0	67	1433	2.0
No. 1	577	14.0	43.0	36.0	37	753	2.0
No. 2	481	14.0	43.0	25.0	29	761	2.0
No. 1 cheeseburger	647	18.0	44.0	42.0	52	1103	2.0
No. 2 cheeseburger	551	18.0	44.0	31.0	44	1111	2.0
Super Sonic No. 1	929	28.0	45.0	66.0	96	1476	2.0
Super Sonic No. 2	839	28.0	46.0	55.0	88	1571	3.0
toaster sandwiches:							
bacon cheddar burger	675	26.0	60.0	38.0	59	1786	4.0
BLT	581	19.0	42.0	41.0	47	1307	3.0
chicken club	675	39.0	75.0	29.0	85	1458	3.0
grilled cheese	282	12.0	39.0	12.0	15	830	2.0

Food and Measure	cal.	prot. (gms)	carbo. (gms)	fat (gms)	chol. (mgs)	sod. (mgs)	fiber (gms)
sandwiches:							
chicken, breaded . .	582	28.0	66.0	23.0	53	427	2.0
chicken, grilled . . .	343	27.0	31.0	13.0	70	829	2.0
steak, country fried	748	24.0	56.0	47.0	60	804	2.0
chicken strip:							
dinner	749	32.0	86.0	32.0	47	1973	5.0
snack	272	19.0	22.0	13.0	35	760	0
coney, regular:							
plain	262	8.0	22.0	16.0	30	657	1.0
cheese	366	13.0	24.0	24.0	52	962	1.0
coney, extra long: . . .							
plain	483	14.0	44.0	27.0	50	1162	1.0
cheese	666	23.0	47.0	42.0	87	1648	2.0
corn dog	262	6.0	23.0	17.0	15	480	1.0
kids' meal:							
chicken strips, 2 . .	184	13.0	15.0	9.0	23	507	0
corn dog	262	6.0	23.0	17.0	15	480	1.0
grilled cheese	282	12.0	39.0	12.0	15	830	2.0
hot dog, plain	262	8.0	22.0	16.0	30	657	1.0
Jr. burger	353	14.0	27.0	21.0	45	1294	1.0
regular fries	195	2.0	22.0	11.0	0	648	4.0
regular tots	259	0	27.0	16.0	0	1046	3.0
"Faves & Craves":							
Ched 'R Peppers . .	256	8.0	29.0	12.0	28	1056	4.0
fries:							
large	252	3.0	30.0	13.0	0	758	5.0
large cheese . . .	322	7.0	31.0	19.0	15	1108	5.0
large chili cheese	357	8.0	32.0	22.0	22	1062	5.0
regular	195	2.0	22.0	11.0	0	648	4.0
regular cheese . .	265	6.0	23.0	17.0	15	998	4.0
regular chili							
cheese	299	8.0	24.0	19.0	22	952	4.0
Super Sonic	358	5.0	44.0	18.0	0	963	7.0
Fritos chili pie	611	18.0	36.0	44.0	53	816	3.0
mozzarella sticks . .	382	20.0	35.0	19.0	50	1300	0
onion rings:							
large	507	12.0	102.0	7.0	0	486	10.0
regular	331	8.0	66.0	5.0	0	311	7.0
Super Sonic	706	16.0	141.0	10.0	1	788	11.0
tater tots:							
large	365	0	40.0	21.0	0	1358	4.0
large cheese . . .	435	4.0	41.0	27.0	15	1708	4.0
large chili cheese	547	9.0	43.0	36.0	37	1844	5.0
regular	259	0	27.0	16.0	0	1046	3.0

Food and Measure	cal.	prot. (gms)	carbo. (gms)	fat (gms)	chol. (mgs)	sod. (mgs)	fiber (gms)
Sonic, "Fave & Craves," tater tots (*cont.*)							
regular cheese ..	329	4.0	28.0	22.0	15	1396	3.0
regular chili cheese	363	5.0	28.0	25.0	22	1350	3.0
add-ons, 1 oz., except as noted:							
bacon, .5 oz.	80	5.0	0	7.0	15	330	0
cheddar, shredded	104	6.0	1.0	9.0	28	491	0
cheese, .67 oz. ...	70	4.0	1.0	6.0	15	350	0
honey mustard dressing, 1.1 oz.	110	0	9.0	9.0	10	300	0
marinara sauce ...	15	0	3.0	0	0	260	0
ranch dressing	147	0	2.0	16.0	5	215	0
slaw, .9 oz.	45	0	4.0	3.0	0	45	1.0
Sonic chili	52	2.0	1.0	4.0	8	59	0
Sonic green chilies	10	0	3.0	0	0	24	0
Sonic hickory barbe-cue sauce	41	0	10.0	0	0	429	0
Thousand Island dressing	150	0	3.0	15.0	10	170	0
Sopressata, 1 oz., except as noted:							
(*Boar's Head* Cala-brese)	100	9.0	0	7.0	15	510	0
(*Boar's Head* Grande)	100	8.0	<1.0	8.0	15	540	0
(*Boar's Head* Veneta)	100	9.0	0	7.0	20	600	0
(*Citterio* Salame), 6 slices, 1.1 oz. ..	110	7.0	0	8.0	35	320	0
(*Citterio Fresco*), 3 slices, 1.1 oz. ..	110	7.0	0	8.0	35	320	0
hot (*Beretta*), 2 oz. ..	230	15.0	<1.0	19.0	25	1240	0
w/wine (*Fiorucci*)	80	7.0	0	6.0	25	450	0
Sorbet (see also "Sherbert"), ½ cup, except as noted:							
berry, mixed (*Sharon's Sorbet*)	90	0	23.0	0	0	11	1.0
blackberry (*Cascadian Farm*)	80	1.0	20.0	0	0	5	2.0
boysenberry (*Dreyer's/ Edy's Whole Fruit*)	150	0	37.0	0	0	20	0
chocolate:							
(*Cascadian Farm*) ..	100	1.0	27.0	1.0	0	70	2.0
(*Häagen-Dazs*)	120	2.0	28.0	0	0	70	2.0

Food and Measure	cal.	prot. (gms)	carbo. (gms)	fat (gms)	chol. (mgs)	sod. (mgs)	fiber (gms)
(*Sharon's Sorbet*)	130	1.0	22.0	5.0	0	5	1.0
coconut (*Sharon's Sorbet*)	160	1.0	22.0	8.0	0	8	1.0
and ice cream:							
blackberry (*Cascadian Farm* Sorbet & Cream)	110	2.0	21.0	3.0	8	30	1.0
lemon (*Cascadian Farm* Sorbet & Cream)	110	2.0	22.0	3.0	11	45	0
orange (*Cascadian Farm* Sorbet & Cream)	120	2.0	29.0	3.0	10	30	<1.0
orange swirl (*Dreyer's/Edy's 50/50 Bar*)	100	2.0	18.0	2.5	15	35	0
peach (*Cascadian Farm* Sorbet & Cream)	110	2.0	21.0	3.0	10	45	<1.0
raspberry (*Cascadian Farm* Sorbet & Cream)	110	2.0	22.0	3.0	10	30	1.0
lemon:							
(*Cascadian Farm Luscious Lemon*)	90	0	23.0	0	0	5	<1.0
(*Dreyer's/Edy's Whole Fruit*) ...	140	0	35.0	0	0	20	0
(*Häagen-Dazs Zesty Lemon*) ..	120	0	31.0	0	0	0	<1.0
(*Sharon's Sorbet*) .	75	0	19.0	0	0	8	0
mango:							
(*Cascadian Farm Mango Magic*) ..	90	0	23.0	0	0	5	1.0
(*Dreyer's Whole Fruit*)	130	0	33.0	0	0	0	0
(*Häagen-Dazs*)	120	0	31.0	0	0	0	<1.0
(*Sharon's Sorbet*)	80	0	20.0	0	0	0	1.0
orange (*Edy's Whole Fruit*)	130	0	33.0	0	0	0	0
orange (*Häagen-Dazs*)	120	0	30.0	0	0	0	<1.0
passion fruit (*Sharon's Sorbet*)	80	1.0	20.0	0	0	8	0
peach:							
(*Cascadian Farm*) ..	90	0	23.0	0	0	0	1.0

Food and Measure	cal.	prot. (gms)	carbo. (gms)	fat (gms)	chol. (mgs)	sod. (mgs)	fiber (gms)
Sorbet, peach (cont.)							
(Edy's Whole Fruit)	130	0	32.0	0	0	10	0
(Häagen-Dazs Orchard)	130	0	33.0	0	0	0	<1.0
raspberry:							
(Cascadian Farm) . .	80	1.0	20.0	0	0	5	2.0
(Dreyer's/Edy's Whole Fruit) . . .	130	0	33.0	0	0	15	0
(Häagen-Dazs)	120	0	30.0	0	0	0	2.0
(Sharon's Sorbet)	80	0	20.0	0	0	8	2.0
strawberry:							
(Cascadian Farm) . .	80	1.0	20.0	0	0	0	1.0
(Dreyer's Whole Fruit)	130	0	32.0	0	0	10	0
(Edy's Whole Fruit)	120	0	31.0	0	0	10	0
(Häagen-Dazs)	120	0	30.0	0	0	0	1.0
tropical (Häagen-Dazs)	120	0	31.0	0	0	0	<1.0
Sorbet bar (see also "Fruit bar"), 1 bar:							
marshmallow swirl (Cool Cotton Candy)	100	1.0	20.0	2.0	10	20	0
orange/vanilla and cream (Häagen-Dazs)	120	2.0	16.0	5.0	35	20	0
raspberry/vanilla and yogurt (Häagen-Dazs)	90	2.0	21.0	0	0	15	<1.0
tangerine (Dreyer's/ Edy's Whole Fruit)	80	0	20.0	0	0	0	0
Sorghum, whole-grain, 1 cup.	650	21.7	143.3	6.3	0	12	n.a.
Sorghum syrup:							
(Arrowhead Mills), 1 tbsp.	60	0	16.0	0	0	0	0
½ cup	479	0	123.7	0	0	13	0
1 tbsp.	61	0	15.7	0	0	2	0
Sorrel, see "Dock"							
Soup, ready-to-serve, 1 cup, except as noted:							
asparagus, cream of (Baxter's)	130	2.0	13.0	7.0	5	880	6.0

Food and Measure	cal.	prot. (gms)	carbo. (gms)	fat (gms)	chol. (mgs)	sod. (mgs)	fiber (gms)
bean:							
(*Dominique's* U.S. Senate)	170	11.0	29.0	1.5	0	800	9.0
3 (*Coco Pazzo*) . . .	240	13.0	25.0	6.0	0	710	12.0
4, chili (*Walnut Acres*)	150	6.0	28.0	1.5	0	640	4.0
5 (*Coco Pazzo*) . . .	220	11.0	31.0	6.0	0	830	10.0
5, vegetable (*Health Valley*)	140	10.0	32.0	0	0	250	10.0
w/bacon (*Campbell's* Classic)	170	8.0	25.0	4.0	<5	870	<8.0
Italian, and pasta (*Healthy Choice*)	100	6.0	17.0	1.5	0	480	3.0
navy (*Sylvia's*)	170	11.0	29.0	1.5	0	800	9.0
and pasta (*Baxter's* Healthy Reward Italian/Pasta Fagioli)	110	4.0	14.0	1.5	0	460	4.0
w/pasta (*Healthy Choice* Mediterranean)	120	8.0	22.0	1.5	0	480	4.0
white, escarole (*Coco Pazzo* Tuscan)	210	10.0	31.0	6.0	0	700	8.0
bean, black (*Greene's Farm*), ½ of 15-oz. can	160	10.0	32.0	1.5	0	510	9.0
(*Hain* Healthy)	90	4.0	18.0	0	0	480	4.0
(*Health Valley*) . . .	130	7.0	25.0	1.0	0	380	5.0
(*Health Valley* No Salt)	130	7.0	25.0	1.0	0	25	5.0
(*Progresso* Hearty)	170	8.0	30.0	1.5	<5	730	10.0
vegetable (*Amy's*)	110	6.0	22.0	1.0	0	580	5.0
vegetable (*Health Valley* Fat Free)	110	11.0	24.0	0	0	280	9.0
bean and ham:							
(*Campbell's* Select)	180	9.0	31.0	2.0	5	700	8.0
(*Campbell's* Chunky)	180	11.0	30.0	2.0	10	800	8.0
(*Healthy Choice*) . .	160	12.0	29.0	1.5	5	480	5.0
beef:							
barley (*Progresso*)	130	10.0	13.0	4.0	25	780	3.0
barley (*Progresso* 99% Fat Free) . .	130	9.0	20.0	2.0	10	710	4.0

Food and Measure	cal.	prot. (gms)	carbo. (gms)	fat (gms)	chol. (mgs)	sod. (mgs)	fiber (gms)
Soup, beef (*cont.*)							
mushroom (*Progresso*)	100	9.0	12.0	2.0	19	1200	1.0
pasta (*Campbell's Chunky*)	100	9.0	16.0	3.0	20	800	2.0
and potato (*Healthy Choice*)	110	7.0	21.0	1.0	5	480	2.0
w/white and wild rice (*Campbell's Chunky*)	150	10.0	23.0	2.5	15	960	2.0
beef broth:							
(*College Inn*)	20	4.0	0	0	0	620	0
(*Health Valley*) ...	15	3.0	0	0	0	380	0
(*Health Valley* No Salt)	15	3.0	0	0	0	150	0
(*Health Valley* Quart)	10	0	2.0	0	0	360	0
(*Swanson*)	10	2.0	0	0	0	890	0
(*Swanson* Lower Sodium)	10	2.0	0	0	0	440	0
w/onion (*College Inn* French Onion)	35	5.0	4.0	0	0	920	0
w/onion (*Swanson*)	20	2.0	2.0	0	0	890	0
beef vegetable:							
(*Progresso*)	120	10.0	13.0	3.0	20	880	2.0
(*Progresso* 99% Fat Free)	160	11.0	24.0	2.0	10	870	3.0
country (*Campbell's Chunky*)	180	13.0	20.0	5.0	30	950	4.0
borscht:							
(*Manischewitz* Clear)	80	<1.0	21.0	0	0	680	2.0
(*Manischewitz* Reduced Sodium)	80	<1.0	21.0	0	0	350	0
w/shredded beets (*Manischewitz*)	90	1.0	21.0	0	0	540	3.0
broccoli:							
(*Walnut Acres* Home-style)	110	4.0	17.0	3.0	10	650	2.0
carotene (*Health Valley* Fat Free)	70	6.0	16.0	0	0	240	7.0
creamy (*Imagine*)	70	3.0	10.0	1.5	0	370	2.0
butternut squash, creamy (*Imagine*)	120	2.0	23.0	2.0	0	370	2.0
broth (*Imagine* No Chicken)	20	1.0	4.0	.5	0	460	<1.0

Food and Measure	cal.	prot. (gms)	carbo. (gms)	fat (gms)	chol. (mgs)	sod. (mgs)	fiber (gms)
chicken:							
(*Healthy Choice* Fiesta)	90	6.0	16.0	1.0	5	480	2.0
(*Progresso* Home-style)	90	7.0	11.0	1.5	15	900	<1.0
hearty (*Healthy Choice*)	130	8.0	21.0	2.0	10	480	3.0
chicken, grilled:							
w/sun-dried tomato (*Campbell's* Select)	100	7.0	17.0	2.0	10	780	2.0
and vegetables w/pasta (*Campbell's* Chunky) . .	110	6.0	17.0	2.0	10	860	2.0
chicken, roasted:							
w/vegetables (*Progresso* Garden)	70	6.0	9.0	1.5	15	920	<1.0
w/vegetables (*Progresso* 99% Fat Free)	90	7.0	12.0	1.5	10	660	1.0
w/white wild rice (*Campbell's* Select)	110	7.0	17.0	1.0	10	920	2.0
w/wild rice (*Progresso* 99% Fat Free)	90	6.0	12.0	1.5	10	700	<1.0
chicken barley (*Progresso*)	110	8.0	16.0	1.5	15	850	3.0
chicken broccoli:							
creamy (*Progresso* 99% Fat Free) . .	90	6.0	13.0	2.0	15	550	1.0
cheese, potato (*Campbell's* Chunky)	190	7.0	14.0	12.0	20	960	1.0
chicken broth:							
(*Boston Market*) . .	15	1.0	1.0	1.0	0	1090	0
(*Butterball* Reduced Sodium)	10	1.0	2.0	0	0	620	0
(*College Inn*)	10	1.0	0	1.0	0	880	0
(*Hain* Home Style)	25	1.0	3.0	2.0	20	630	0
(*Hain* Home Style No Salt)	25	1.0	3.0	2.0	20	340	0
(*Health Valley*) . . .	40	6.0	0	1.5	25	90	0

Food and Measure	cal.	prot. (gms)	carbo (gms)	fat (gms)	chol. (mgs)	sod. (mgs)	fiber (gms)
Soup, chicken broth (*cont.*)							
(*Health Valley* Fat Free)	25	6.0	0	0	0	390	0
(*Health Valley* Fat Free No Salt) ...	40	6.0	0	1.5	25	150	0
(*Health Valley* Fat Free Quart)	30	5.0	2.0	0	0	390	0
(*Imagine* Free Range)	20	1.0	2.0	.5	5	570	<1.0
(*Manischewitz*), ½ cup	15	<1.0	2.0	.5	0	740	2.0
(*Swanson*)	15	1.0	1.0	0	<5	980	0
(*Swanson Natural Goodness*)	15	2.0	1.0	0	0	570	0
w/Italian herbs or roasted garlic (*Swanson*)	20	1.0	3.0	0	<5	950	0
chicken consommé (*Rokeach*)	50	4.0	0	4.0	0	1350	2.0
chicken corn chowder:							
(*Campbell's Chunky*)	240	8.0	19.0	15.0	25	800	2.0
(*Healthy Choice*) ..	150	7.0	29.0	2.5	10	480	4.0
chicken, w/meatballs (*Progresso* Chickarina)	130	8.0	12.0	5.0	20	1010	<1.0
chicken mushroom chowder (*Campbell's Chunky*)	230	7.0	14.0	17.0	15	910	2.0
chicken noodle:							
(*Campbell's* Classic)	80	3.0	11.0	2.0	15	890	<1.0
(*Campbell's Chunky* Classic)	130	8.0	15.0	3.5	20	880	1.0
(*Campbell's Healthy Request*)	100	6.0	13.0	3.0	15	360	1.0
(*Campbell's Simply Home*)	90	6.0	13.0	1.0	10	850	1.0
(*Campbell's Soup to Go*), 1 cont. ...	100	7.0	16.0	2.0	15	900	1.0
(*Hain* Home Style)	150	8.0	24.0	3.0	45	480	1.0
(*Hain* Home Style No Salt)	110	9.0	13.0	2.0	25	80	1.0
(*Health Valley* 99% Fat Free)	130	9.0	20.0	2.0	15	390	2.0

Food and Measure	cal.	prot. (gms)	carbo. (gms)	fat (gms)	chol. (mgs)	sod. (mgs)	fiber (gms)
(*Healthy Choice* Old Fashioned)	120	6.0	27.0	.5	0	480	5.0
(*Progresso*)	90	9.0	9.0	2.0	25	950	<1.0
(*Progresso* 99% Fat Free)	90	7.0	13.0	1.5	20	950	1.0
egg (*Campbell's Select*)	90	6.0	13.0	2.0	15	880	1.0
egg (*Wolfgang Puck's*)	150	8.0	16.0	5.0	30	610	1.0
vegetable (*Rokeach*)	90	4.0	14.0	1.5	10	1290	2.0
chicken pasta:							
(*Campbell's Simply Home*)	90	6.0	15.0	2.0	10	780	2.0
(*Healthy Choice*) . .	110	6.0	19.0	2.5	5	480	2.0
and mushroom (*Campbell's Chunky*)	120	8.0	16.0	4.0	15	930	1.0
w/roasted garlic (*Campbell's Select*)	110	6.0	17.0	2.0	10	800	1.0
chicken rice:							
(*Campbell's* Classic)	80	2.0	14.0	2.0	<5	850	<1.0
(*Campbell's* Select)	100	4.0	19.0	1.0	10	900	2.0
(*Campbell's Healthy Request* Hearty)	100	5.0	16.0	2.0	15	360	1.0
(*Campbell's Soup to Go*), 1 cont. . . .	140	6.0	25.0	2.0	10	990	1.0
(*Health Valley* 99% Fat Free)	130	8.0	21.0	2.0	15	390	2.0
(*Healthy Choice*) . .	100	5.0	16.0	2.0	5	480	3.0
(*Rienzi*)	110	6.0	17.0	2.5	5	930	2.0
savory, white and wild (*Campbell's Chunky*)	140	9.0	18.0	3.0	25	840	2.0
w/vegetables (*Progresso*)	90	6.0	12.0	2.0	10	890	1.0
white/wild (*Campbell's Simply Home*)	100	5.0	19.0	2.0	10	830	2.0
wild (*Progresso*) . .	100	7.0	15.0	1.5	15	850	1.0
chicken and rotini:							
(*Progresso* Hearty)	90	8.0	12.0	1.5	15	970	<1.0
roasted (*Progresso*)	80	6.0	11.0	1.5	15	970	<1.0

Food and Measure	cal.	prot. (gms)	carbo. (gms)	fat (gms)	chol (mgs)	sod. (mgs)	fiber (gms)
Soup (*cont.*)							
chicken vegetable:							
(*Campbell's* Select)	100	5.0	17.0	2.0	10	880	2.0
(*Campbell's Chunky* Hearty)	90	6.0	12.0	2.0	10	800	2.0
(*Campbell's Healthy Request*)	110	6.0	18.0	2.0	15	360	2.0
Italian style (*Campbell's* Select) ...	130	8.0	20.0	2.0	15	880	3.0
w/pasta (*Wolfgang Puck's*)	140	8.0	17.0	5.0	15	620	2.0
spicy (*Campbell's Chunky*)	110	7.0	15.0	2.0	15	760	3.0
white meat (*Progresso*)	90	7.0	13.0	1.5	15	820	2.0
chili beef:							
(*Campbell's Chunky*), 10¾-oz. can ...	300	21.0	38.0	7.0	20	1080	9.0
(*Healthy Choice*)	190	16.0	34.0	2.0	5	480	8.0
chili pepper (*A Taste of Thai*)	45	1.0	5.0	2.5	5	460	2.0
clam chowder, Manhattan (*Campbell's Chunky*)	140	6.0	20.0	3.5	5	880	2.0
clam chowder, New England:							
(*Campbell's* Select)	190	5.0	14.0	13.0	10	960	1.0
(*Campbell's* Select 98% Fat Free) ..	110	4.0	17.0	3.0	10	780	2.0
(*Campbell's Chunky*)	240	7.0	23.0	13.0	15	890	2.0
(*Campbell's Healthy Request*)	110	5.0	18.0	2.0	10	360	2.0
(*Dominique's*)	200	7.0	13.0	14.0	15	970	4.0
(*Healthy Choice*) ..	120	7.0	22.0	1.0	5	480	4.0
(*Progresso*)	190	5.0	21.0	10.0	15	830	1.0
(*Snow's*)	170	6.0	14.0	11.0	20	960	1.0
coconut ginger (*A Taste of Thai*)	100	2.0	11.0	5.0	0	570	2.0
consommé, madrilene:							
clear (*Dominique's*)	30	8.0	<1.0	0	0	890	0
red (*Dominique's*)	35	7.0	2.0	0	0	900	<1.0
corn:							
creamy (*Imagine*)	100	5.0	15.0	3.0	0	340	1.0
tortilla (*Buckaroo*)	130	3.0	22.0	4.0	0	560	2.0

Food and Measure	cal.	prot. (gms)	carbo. (gms)	fat (gms)	chol. (mgs)	sod. (mgs)	fiber (gms)
vegetable (*Health Valley* Fat Free)	70	5.0	17.0	0	0	135	7.0
corn chowder:							
(*Greene's Farm*), ½ of 15-oz. can ...	120	3.0	26.0	2.0	5	520	3.0
(*Walnut Acres*) ...	150	4.0	28.0	3.0	10	690	2.0
escarole, in chicken broth (*Progresso*)	25	1.0	3.0	1.0	<5	930	1.0
garlic, roasted, and lentil (*Progresso*) ..	120	7.0	20.0	1.5	0	960	5.0
gazpacho (*Dominique's*)	60	2.0	12.0	.5	0	570	2.0
ginger carrot (*Walnut Acres*)	100	2.0	22.0	1.0	0	550	3.0
gumbo (*Healthy Choice* Zesty)	100	6.0	15.0	2.0	10	480	3.0
hot and sour (*Rice Road*)	90	3.0	15.0	3.0	0	1340	2.0
leek, Scotch (*Baxter's*)	80	6.0	8.0	2.5	0	980	3.0
lemon grass (*A Taste of Thai*)	35	2.0	6.0	.5	0	850	2.0
lentil:							
(*Amy's*)	130	8.0	19.0	4.0	0	590	9.0
(*Coco Pazzo*)	220	15.0	30.0	6.0	0	610	16.0
(*Health Valley*) ...	80	3.0	18.0	0	0	380	4.0
(*Health Valley* No Salt)	100	8.0	21.0	1.0	0	25	8.0
(*Progresso*)	140	9.0	22.0	2.0	0	750	7.0
(*Progresso* 99% Fat Free)	130	8.0	20.0	1.5	0	440	6.0
(*Rienzi*)	130	7.0	22.0	2.0	0	800	6.0
and carrot (*Health Valley* Fat Free)	100	10.0	25.0	0	0	220	10.0
sausage (*Dominique's*)	200	12.0	25.0	6.0	10	880	6.0
savory (*Campbell's Select*)	130	8.0	23.0	1.0	0	770	4.0
vegetarian (*Hain Healthy*)	170	12.0	30.0	.5	0	480	11.0
lobster bisque (*Baxter's*)	120	6.0	11.0	6.0	70	990	0
macaroni and bean:							
(*Progresso*)	160	7.0	23.0	4.0	<5	800	6.0
(*Rienzi*)	150	7.0	26.0	2.5	0	910	6.0

Food and Measure	cal.	prot. (gms)	carbo. (gms)	fat (gms)	chol. (mgs)	sod. (mgs)	fiber (gms)
Soup (cont.)							
matzo ball (Manische-							
witz)	110	3.0	13.0	5.0	35	710	0
menudo:							
(Juanita's Menudito)	170	15.0	12.0	7.0	90	1150	3.0
(Pico Pica)	200	14.0	12.0	9.0	90	1250	2.0
hot and spicy							
(Juanita's)	170	15.0	12.0	7.0	90	1200	3.0
minestrone:							
(Amy's)	90	3.0	17.0	1.5	0	540	3.0
(Baxter's Healthy							
Reward)	110	4.0	21.0	1.0	0	425	4.0
(Campbell's Classic)	90	4.0	16.0	2.0	<5	960	<3.0
(Campbell's Plus!							
Hearty)	130	5.0	26.0	1.0	0	670	4.0
(Campbell's Select							
Old World)	120	4.0	21.0	2.0	5	950	2.0
(Campbell's Simply							
Home)	140	5.0	27.0	1.0	5	840	3.0
(Campbell's Soup to							
Go), 1 cont. . . .	140	6.0	27.0	1.0	0	1040	4.0
(Hain Home Style)	110	5.0	20.0	2.0	0	480	4.0
(Health Valley Fat							
Free)	90	8.0	21.0	0	0	210	8.0
(Health Valley) . . .	70	3.0	17.0	0	0	380	4.0
(Health Valley No							
Salt)	70	3.0	17.0	0	0	45	3.0
(Progresso)	120	5.0	21.0	2.0	0	960	5.0
(Progresso 99% Fat							
Free)	110	5.0	19.0	1.0	0	630	4.0
(Rienzi)	130	5.0	21.0	2.5	0	700	4.0
(Rokeach)	170	8.0	32.0	1.0	0	740	5.0
(Walnut Acres							
Classic)	100	3.0	22.0	0	0	650	3.0
herb and shells							
(Progresso)	120	5.0	22.0	1.5	0	1050	4.0
Tuscany style							
(Campbell's							
Select)	160	5.0	23.0	5.0	5	890	7.0
mulligatawny, hot							
(Patak's Sabzi)	100	4.0	20.0	1.0	0	1540	3.0
mushroom, cream of:							
(Amy's), ¾ cup . . .	120	2.0	10.0	9.0	5	590	2.0

Food and Measure	cal.	prot. (gms)	carbo. (gms)	fat (gms)	chol. (mgs)	sod. (mgs)	fiber (gms)
(*Campbell's* Select 98% Fat Free) ..	80	1.0	15.0	2.0	5	810	1.0
(*Hain* Home Style)	150	4.0	28.0	2.5	10	480	2.0
(*Rokeach*)	120	2.0	13.0	7.0	5	770	2.0
mushroom barley:							
(*Hain* Healthy)	130	5.0	26.0	1.5	15	480	5.0
(*Health Valley*) ...	70	2.0	17.0	0	0	380	3.0
(*Health Valley* No Salt)	70	2.0	17.0	0	0	25	3.0
mushroom broth (*Health Valley* Fat Free)	10	0	2.0	0	0	380	0
mushroom rice (*Campbell's* Select)	80	3.0	16.0	1.0	0	810	1.0
noodle:							
(*Amy's* No Chicken)	90	5.0	12.0	3.0	0	480	2.0
Oriental, w/vegetables (*Campbell's* Select)	100	4.0	18.0	1.0	5	890	3.0
onion, French:							
(*Baxter's* Healthy Reward)	90	2.0	18.0	1.5	0	480	1.0
(*Progresso*)	50	<1.0	9.0	1.5	<5	900	1.0
(*Rokeach*)	80	1.0	12.0	3.0	0	620	2.0
(*Wolfgang Puck's* Country)	140	6.0	16.0	5.0	10	960	1.0
pasta:							
Bolognese or cacciatore (*Health Valley* Fat Free)	100	4.0	20.0	0	0	290	4.0
fagioli (*Health Valley* Fat Free)	120	6.0	25.0	0	0	290	4.0
primavera (*Health Valley* Fat Free)	110	3.0	23.0	0	0	290	3.0
Romano or rotini (*Health Valley* Fat Free)	100	4.0	20.0	0	0	290	4.0
and vegetables (*Campbell's* Plus!)	110	4.0	20.0	1.5	<5	660	4.0
pea, split:							
(*Amy's*)	100	7.0	19.0	0	0	570	4.0
(*Health Valley* Organic)	110	10.0	23.0	0	0	160	8.0

Food and Measure	cal.	prot. (gms)	carbo. (gms)	fat (gms)	chol. (mgs)	sod. (mgs)	fiber (gms)
Soup, pea, split (*cont.*)							
(*Health Valley* Organic No Salt)	110	10.0	23.0	0	0	115	8.0
(*Progresso* 99% Fat Free)	170	10.0	29.0	1.5	0	620	5.0
and carrot (*Health Valley* Fat Free)	110	8.0	17.0	0	0	230	4.0
green (*Progresso*)	170	10.0	25.0	3.0	5	870	5.0
vegetarian (*Hain Healthy*)	110	7.0	20.0	.5	0	15	7.0
pea, split, w/ham:							
(*Campbell's* Select)	170	10.0	30.0	2.0	10	860	6.0
(*Campbell's Chunky*)	180	11.0	27.0	3.5	10	860	4.0
(*Campbell's Healthy Request*)	170	10.0	29.0	2.0	10	360	4.0
(*Healthy Choice*) ..	170	13.0	28.0	2.0	5	480	5.0
penne in chicken broth (*Progresso* Hearty)	80	4.0	14.0	1.0	0	1020	<1.0
pepper steak (*Campbell's Chunky*)	140	11.0	17.0	3.0	20	810	3.0
portobello, creamy (*Imagine*)	80	4.0	10.0	3.0	0	310	2.0
potato (*Rokeach*)	115	2.0	21.0	2.5	0	560	2.0
potato, baked:							
w/bacon, chives (*Healthy Choice*)	140	7.0	25.0	2.0	10	480	4.0
w/bacon bits and chives (*Campbell's Chunky*) ..	150	4.0	22.0	5.0	5	890	2.0
w/cheddar and bacon bits (*Campbell's Chunky*) ..	180	5.0	23.0	8.0	10	840	2.0
w/steak and cheese (*Campbell's Chunky*)	200	10.0	21.0	9.0	20	970	2.0
potato, w/broccoli, cheese (*Progresso*)	160	5.0	21.0	6.0	<5	960	1.0
potato, w/roasted garlic:							
creamy (*Campbell's* Select)	180	3.0	20.0	9.0	10	770	2.0
creamy (*Campbell's Healthy Request*)	110	2.0	20.0	2.0	5	360	3.0

Food and Measure	cal.	prot. (gms)	carbo. (gms)	fat (gms)	chol. (mgs)	sod. (mgs)	fiber (gms)
potato, white cheddar (*Progresso* 99% Fat Free)	100	2.0	20.0	1.5	<5	680	2.0
potato and ham (*Healthy Choice*) ..	140	6.0	25.0	2.5	10	480	3.0
potato ham chowder (*Campbell's Chunky* Old Fashioned) ...	210	5.0	17.0	13.0	15	800	2.0
potato leek:							
(*Baxter's* Healthy Reward)	80	2.0	16.0	1.0	0	420	3.0
(*Health Valley*) ...	70	2.0	15.0	0	0	230	3.0
(*Health Valley* No Salt)	70	4.0	15.0	0	0	35	3.0
(*Imagine* Organic) .	90	3.0	14.0	2.5	0	380	2.0
pozole (*Juanita's*) ...	170	8.0	22.0	5.0	25	1000	5.0
pumpkin (*Walnut Acres* Autumn Harvest)	100	3.0	19.0	2.0	5	620	2.0
ravioli, tomato:							
cheese w/vegetables (*Campbell's Chunky*)	150	4.0	27.0	3.5	5	930	4.0
w/vegetables (*Campbell's Healthy Request*)	150	4.0	26.0	2.0	5	360	3.0
rotini, vegetable (*Health Valley* Fat Free)	100	4.0	20.0	0	0	290	4.0
sirloin burger (*Campbell's Chunky*)	180	10.0	17.0	8.0	25	910	3.0
sirloin steak, grilled, w/hearty vegetables (*Campbell's Chunky*)	120	9.0	20.0	2.0	20	950	2.0
steak and potato (*Campbell's Chunky*)	160	13.0	19.0	4.0	25	910	3.0
tomato:							
(*Campbell's*)	120	2.0	27.0	0	0	760	1.0
(*Campbell's* Classic)	120	.2.0	27.0	0	0	760	<1.0
(*Health Valley*) ...	80	3.0	18.0	0	0	380	1.0
(*Health Valley* No Salt)	80	3.0	18.0	0	0	35	1.0
(*Walnut Acres* Savory)	120	4.0	23.0	2.0	5	580	2.0

Food and Measure	cal.	prot. (gms)	carbo (gms)	fat (gms)	chol. (mgs)	sod. (mgs)	fiber (gms)
Soup, tomato (*cont.*)							
(*Walnut Acres* Zesty)	80	3.0	19.0	.5	0	590	2.0
cream of (*Amy's*) . .	100	2.0	17.0	2.0	10	690	4.0
creamy (*Campbell's*)	140	2.0	32.0	0	5	760	2.0
creamy (*Campbell's* Classic)	140	3.0	25.0	4.0	<10	730	<2.0
creamy (*Imagine*)	90	2.0	17.0	1.5	0	520	2.0
basil (*Progresso*) . .	160	3.0	29.0	3.0	0	1060	2.0
chunky (*Hain* Home Style)	120	3.0	27.0	1.0	0	480	2.0
garden (*Campbell's* Select)	100	3.0	22.0	0	10	750	3.0
lentil, mild Indian (*Patak's*)	120	6.0	21.0	2.0	0	1020	2.0
w/roasted garlic, herbs (*Campbell's*)	150	2.0	34.0	0	0	770	2.0
rotini (*Progresso*)	140	4.0	30.0	.5	0	1000	2.0
tomato vegetable:							
(*Health Valley* Fat Free)	80	6.0	17.0	0	0	240	5.0
(*Wolfgang Puck's* Country)	150	2.0	18.0	8.0	20	850	2.0
garden (*Progresso* 99% Fat Free) . .	100	3.0	19.0	1.5	0	660	2.0
tortellini, cheese:							
w/chicken and vege- tables (*Campbell's Chunky*) . .	110	5.0	18.0	2.0	15	860	2.0
and herb (*Progresso*)	140	4.0	23.0	3.0	<5	700	2.0
turkey broth (*College Inn*)	10	0	1.0	0	0	1010	0
turkey noodle (*Progresso*)	90	7.0	11.0	1.5	20	1060	<1.0
turkey rice:							
white and wild (*Healthy Choice*)	100	6.0	17.0	1.5	5	480	3.0
wild (*Greene's Farm*), ½ of 15-oz. can	110	6.0	19.0	1.5	10	770	2.0
vegetable:							
(*Campbell's* Select)	110	3.0	20.0	1.0	0	760	3.0

Food and Measure	cal.	prot. (gms)	carbo. (gms)	fat (gms)	chol. (mgs)	sod. (mgs)	fiber (gms)
(*Campbell's* Select Fiesta)	120	4.0	24.0	0	0	810	3.0
(*Campbell's* Chunky)	130	3.0	22.0	3.5	0	870	4.0
(*Campbell's* Healthy Request) Hearty) .	100	3.0	20.0	1.0	0	360	3.0
(*Health Valley*) . . .	80	3.0	18.0	0	0	380	4.0
(*Health Valley* No Salt)	80	3.0	18.0	0	0	40	4.0
(*Progresso*)	90	3.0	17.0	1.0	0	930	2.0
(*Progresso* Vegetarian)	100	4.0	20.0	.5	0	990	4.0
(*Rokeach*)	110	3.0	22.0	1.5	0	790	3.0
barley (*Health Valley* Fat Free)	90	6.0	19.0	0	0	210	4.0
w/beef stock (*Campbell's* Classic) . . .	80	3.0	17.0	0	0	790	<2.0
clam (*Healthy Choice*)	80	4.0	17.0	.5	0	480	2.0
country (*Campbell's Healthy Request*)	110	2.0	23.0	1.0	<5	360	3.0
country (*Campbell's Simply Home*) . .	110	3.0	23.0	0	0	700	3.0
country (*Healthy Choice*)	100	5.0	22.0	.5	0	450	5.0
garden (*Baxter's* Healthy Reward)	70	<1.0	15.0	1.0	0	370	2.0
garden (*Campbell's Simply Home*) . .	110	4.0	22.0	0	5	720	2.0
garden (*Campbell's Soup to Go*), 1 cont.	130	6.0	25.0	1.0	5	870	3.0
garden (*Healthy Choice*)	120	6.0	27.0	.5	0	480	5.0
garden, 14 (*Health Valley* Fat Free)	80	6.0	17.0	0	0	250	4.0
w/pasta (*Campbell's Chunky* Hearty)	140	4.0	24.0	3.0	5	920	3.0
w/pasta (*Rienzi*) . . .	100	3.0	20.0	5.0	0	870	3.0
roasted, w/barley and wild rice (*Campbell's* Plus!)	130	3.0	25.0	1.0	<5	680	5.0
thick (*Wolfgang Puck's* Country)	180	4.0	25.0	7.0	15	760	7.0

Food and Measure	cal.	prot. (gms)	carbo. (gms)	fat (gms)	chol. (mgs)	sod. (mgs)	fiber (gms)
Soup (*cont.*)							
vegetable beef:							
(*Campbell's* Select)	100	6.0	16.0	2.0	5	930	2.0
(*Campbell's Chunky* Old Fashioned) ..	160	12.0	16.0	5.0	25	900	3.0
(*Campbell's Healthy* Request Hearty)	130	9.0	19.0	2.0	20	360	3.0
(*Healthy Choice*) ..	120	10.0	20.0	1.0	5	480	3.0
w/pasta (*Campbell's Soup to Go*), 1 cont.	130	8.0	22.0	2.0	10	980	2.0
vegetable broth:							
(*Hain* Healthy)	30	1.0	8.0	0	0	480	<1.0
(*Hain* Healthy No Salt)	30	1.0	8.0	0	0	20	<1.0
(*Health Valley* Fat Free)	20	0	5.0	0	0	210	0
(*Health Valley* Fat Free Quart)	15	0	3.0	0	0	360	0
(*Imagine*)	30	1.0	5.0	.5	0	480	1.0
(*Swanson*) ...	20	0	3.0	0	0	970	0
vichyssoise (*Dominique's*)	130	3.0	17.0	6.0	10	860	2.0
wild rice (*Hain*)	80	3.0	15.0	1.5	0	480	1.0
Soup, condensed, undiluted, ½ cup, except as noted:							
asparagus, cream of (*Campbell's*)	110	2.0	9.0	7.0	<5	870	1.0
barley and:							
bean (*Rokeach*) ...	120	5.0	22.0	1.5	0	840	6.0
mushroom (*Manischewitz*)	100	3.0	16.0	2.5	0	1040	4.0
bean:							
black (*Campbell's*)	110	5.0	19.0	2.0	0	900	5.0
bacon (*Campbell's*)	170	8.0	25.0	4.0	<5	870	8.0
ham and bacon (*Campbell's Healthy Request*)	150	7.0	24.0	3.0	5	430	7.0
navy (*Walnut Acres*)	110	7.0	19.0	1.0	0	460	7.0
beef w/vegetables and barley (*Campbell's*)	80	5.0	11.0	2.0	10	910	1.0
broccoli, cream of:							
(*Campbell's*)	90	2.0	9.0	5.0	<5	770	1.0

Food and Measure	cal.	prot. (gms)	carbo. (gms)	fat (gms)	chol. (mgs)	sod. (mgs)	fiber (gms)
(*Campbell's 98% Fat Free*)	70	2.0	11.0	2.0	5	720	1.0
(*Campbell's Healthy Request*)	60	2.0	9.0	2.0	5	420	1.0
(*Walnut Acres*), ⅔ cup	90	4.0	11.0	3.0	10	360	2.0
cheese (*Campbell's*)	110	2.0	10.0	6.0	5	820	1.0
cheese (*Campbell's 98% Fat Free*) . .	60	1.0	11.0	2.0	<5	810	<1.0
carrot, cream of (*Walnut Acres*), ⅔ cup	150	2.0	11.0	11.0	15	510	1.0
celery, cream of:							
(*Campbell's*)	100	2.0	9.0	7.0	<5	900	1.0
(*Campbell's 98% Fat Free*)	60	1.0	8.0	3.0	<5	780	1.0
(*Campbell's Healthy Request*)	70	1.0	11.0	2.0	5	430	1.0
cheese:							
cheddar (*Campbell's*)	130	3.0	11.0	8.0	15	950	1.0
nacho (*Campbell's Fiesta*)	130	4.0	10.0	8.0	15	790	1.0
chicken:							
alphabet, w/vegetables (*Campbell's*)	80	4.0	11.0	2.0	10	880	1.0
clear (*Manischewitz*)	15	<1.0	2.0	.5	0	740	2.0
clear (*Rokeach*) . . .	20	1.0	2.0	1.5	0	720	0
cream of (*Campbell's*)	120	3.0	10.0	8.0	10	880	1.0
cream of (*Campbell's 98% Fat Free*)	80	3.0	9.0	3.0	10	910	<1.0
cream of (*Campbell's Healthy Request*)	70	2.0	12.0	2.0	10	430	1.0
cream of, and broccoli (*Campbell's*)	120	3.0	9.0	8.0	15	860	2.0
cream of, and broccoli (*Campbell's Healthy Request*)	80	3.0	10.0	3.0	10	450	1.0

Food and Measure	cal.	prot. (gms)	carbo. (gms)	fat (gms)	chol. (mgs)	sod. (mgs)	fiber (gms)
Soup, condensed, chicken (cont.)							
cream of, Dijon (*Campbell's*) ...	130	3.0	12.0	8.0	10	840	1.0
cream of, w/herbs (*Campbell's*) ...	80	3.0	9.0	4.0	10	890	1.0
cream of, mushroom (*Campbell's*) ...	120	3.0	9.0	8.0	10	980	1.0
and dumplings (*Campbell's*) ...	80	4.0	10.0	3.0	15	960	1.0
gumbo (*Campbell's*)	60	2.0	9.0	2.0	5	970	1.0
w/kreplach (*Manischewitz*)	35	2.0	5.0	1.0	0	880	3.0
w/matzo balls (*Manischewitz*)	80	3.0	9.0	4.0	25	880	2.0
rice (*Campbell's*) ..	70	2.0	10.0	2.0	<5	850	<1.0
rice (*Campbell's Healthy Request*)	60	2.0	8.0	2.0	10	420	1.0
rice, wild and white (*Campbell's*) ...	60	2.0	10.0	2.0	5	810	<1.0
and stars (*Campbell's*)	70	3.0	10.0	2.0	10	940	<1.0
chicken noodle:							
(*Campbell's*)	60	3.0	8.0	2.0	10	890	<1.0
(*Campbell's* Homestyle)	70	3.0	8.0	2.0	15	960	<1.0
(*Campbell's Healthy Request*)	60	2.0	8.0	2.0	10	450	1.0
(*Campbell's Noodle O's*)	80	3.0	11.0	2.0	15	950	1.0
(*Manischewitz*) ...	35	2.0	6.0	.5	0	830	1.0
creamy (*Campbell's*)	130	4.0	12.0	7.0	15	880	1.0
curly (*Campbell's*)	80	3.0	12.0	2.0	15	840	1.0
chicken vegetable:							
(*Campbell's*)	80	3.0	12.0	2.0	10	910	2.0
(*Campbell's Healthy Request*)	80	3.0	12.0	2.0	5	440	2.0
Southwestern (*Campbell's*) ...	110	5.0	20.0	1.0	<5	830	4.0
chili beef w/beans (*Campbell's* Fiesta)	170	7.0	24.0	5.0	10	880	6.0
clam bisque (*Chincoteague* Premium) ..	100	8.0	13.0	2.0	15	990	1.0

Food and Measure	cal.	prot. (gms)	carbo. (gms)	fat (gms)	chol. (mgs)	sod. (mgs)	fiber (gms)
clam chowder, Manhattan:							
(*Campbell's*)	70	2.0	12.0	2.0	<5	890	1.0
(*Chincoteague*) ...	100	8.0	13.0	2.0	15	990	1.0
clam chowder, New England:							
(*Campbell's*)	90	4.0	13.0	2.0	<5	960	1.0
(*Campbell's* 98% Fat Free)	80	3.0	13.0	2.0	<5	940	1.0
(*Chincoteague*) ...	80	5.0	10.0	2.5	10	590	<1.0
(*Olde Cape Cod* All Natural)	80	5.0	11.0	2.0	10	600	<1.0
corn chowder:							
(*Chincoteague* Premium)	100	2.0	16.0	3.5	0	890	1.0
(*Olde Cape Cod* Old Fashioned)	110	4.0	18.0	2.0	10	600	1.0
(*Walnut Acres*) ...	80	2.0	15.0	2.5	0	370	1.0
crab:							
cream of (*Chincoteague* Chesapeake Bay)	200	11.0	23.0	6.0	35	830	0
red, vegetable (*Chincoteague*)	90	5.0	12.0	2.5	15	880	2.0
crab and cheddar (*Chincoteague* Chesapeake Bay) ..	90	4.0	10.0	3.5	20	590	0
lentil (*Manischewitz*)	140	7.0	24.0	2.0	0	1310	4.0
lobster bisque:							
(*Chincoteague* Premium)	90	4.0	10.0	4.0	15	650	0
(*Olde Cape* All Natural Gourmet)	60	1.0	8.0	2.0	5	770	0
minestrone:							
(*Campbell's*)	90	4.0	15.0	2.0	<5	960	3.0
(*Campbell's Healthy Request*)	80	3.0	15.0	1.0	5	460	3.0
(*Manischewitz*) ...	90	3.0	16.0	1.5	0	760	2.0
(*Walnut Acres*) ...	120	5.0	21.0	3.0	0	340	5.0
mushroom:							
(*Rokeach*)	80	<1.0	13.0	3.0	0	750	1.0
beefy (*Campbell's*)	70	4.0	6.0	3.0	10	900	1.0
golden (Campbell's)	80	2.0	10.0	3.0	<5	920	1.0

Soup, condensed, mushroom, cream of *(cont.)*

Food and Measure	cal.	prot. (gms)	carbo. (gms)	fat (gms)	chol. (mgs)	sod. (mgs)	fiber (gms)
mushroom, cream of:							
(*Campbell's*)	100	1.0	9.0	7.0	<5	870	1.0
(*Campbell's 98% Fat Free*)	70	1.0	9.0	3.0	<5	900	<1.0
(*Campbell's Healthy Request*)	70	1.0	10.0	2.0	5	460	1.0
w/roasted garlic (*Campbell's*) . . .	70	1.0	10.0	2.0	<5	790	<1.0
noodle:							
double, in chicken broth (*Campbell's*)	100	4.0	15.0	2.0	15	830	1.0
and ground beef (*Campbell's*) . . .	100	5.0	11.0	4.0	20	890	1.0
mega, in chicken broth (*Campbell's*)	60	2.0	10.0	2.0	<5	880	<1.0
onion:							
cream of (*Campbell's*)	110	2.0	12.0	6.0	15	880	1.0
French (*Campbell's*)	45	2.0	6.0	2.0	<5	900	1.0
oyster:							
chowder (*Olde Cape Cod*)	70	2.0	11.0	2.5	10	680	0
stew (*Campbell's*)	80	2.0	5.0	6.0	20	910	0
pasta w/chicken (*Campbell's Fun Shapes*)	60	2.0	10.0	2.0	5	880	1.0
pea:							
green (*Campbell's*) .	180	9.0	29.0	3.0	5	870	5.0
split, and egg barley (*Rokeach*)	150	7.0	24.0	3.0	5	670	2.0
split, and barley (*Walnut Acres*) . .	150	10.0	28.0	.5	0	340	10.0
split, w/ham (*Campbell's*)	180	9.0	28.0	3.0	<5	850	5.0
pepperpot (*Campbell's*)	90	4.0	9.0	4.0	20	940	1.0
potato, cream of (*Campbell's*)	90	2.0	14.0	3.0	10	880	1.0
potato kale (*Walnut Acres*), ⅔ cup	90	2.0	16.0	2.5	0	300	2.0
Scotch broth (*Campbell's*)	70	3.0	9.0	2.0	<5	880	2.0
shrimp, cream of (*Campbell's*)	90	2.0	8.0	6.0	15	880	1.0

Food and Measure	cal.	prot. (gms)	carbo. (gms)	fat (gms)	chol. (mgs)	sod. (mgs)	fiber (gms)
shrimp bisque (*Chinco-teague* Premium) ..	80	2.0	10.0	3.0	20	590	0
shrimp and tomato bisque, garlic (*Olde Cape Cod*)	60	4.0	8.0	1.0	25	690	<1.0
sweet potato chowder (*Walnut Acres*), ⅔ cup	130	3.0	25.0	3.0	0	420	3.0
tomato:							
(*Campbell's*)	80	2.0	19.0	0	0	710	1.0
(*Campbell's Healthy Request*)	90	1.0	18.0	2.0	0	450	1.0
(*Rokeach*)	60	1.0	13.0	1.0	0	740	1.0
(*Walnut Acres*) ...	70	2.0	13.0	1.0	5	380	1.0
bisque (*Campbell's*)	130	2.0	23.0	3.0	<5	880	1.0
Italian, w/basil, ore-gano (*Campbell's*)	100	1.0	23.0	0	<5	800	2.0
noodle (*Campbell's*)	120	3.0	25.0	1.0	5	720	1.0
rice (*Campbell's* Old Fashioned)	110	1.0	23.0	2.0	<5	770	1.0
rice (*Rokeach*)	110	2.0	26.0	0	0	660	2.0
w/roasted garlic and herbs (*Campbell's*)	100	1.0	23.0	0	0	850	1.0
turkey:							
noodle (*Campbell's*)	70	3.0	9.0	2.0	10	970	<1.0
vegetable (*Camp-bell's*)	70	3.0	11.0	2.0	5	840	2.0
vegetable:							
(*Campbell's*)	80	3.0	16.0	0	0	790	2.0
(*Campbell's* Old Fashioned)	70	2.0	10.0	2.0	<5	940	1.0
(*Campbell's Healthy Request*)	90	3.0	16.0	1.0	5	440	2.0
(*Rokeach*)	80	2.0	18.0	0	0	610	3.0
beef (*Campbell's*) ..	70	5.0	12.0	0	5	810	2.0
beef (*Campbell's Healthy Request*)	75	4.0	11.0	2.0	5	450	2.0
California style (*Campbell's*) ...	60	2.0	11.0	1.0	<5	790	2.0
pasta (*Campbell's* Hearty)	80	2.0	17.0	0	<5	800	2.0
pasta (*Campbell's Healthy Request* Hearty)	90	2.0	17.0	1.0	5	460	2.0

Food and Measure	cal.	prot. (gms)	carbo. (gms)	fat (gms)	chol. (mgs)	sod. (mgs)	fiber (gms)
Soup, condensed, vegetable (*cont.*)							
vegetarian							
(*Campbell's*) ...	80	2.0	15.0	1.0	0	860	2.0
won ton (*Campbell's*) .	45	3.0	5.0	1.0	10	920	<1.0
Soup, semicondensed,							
undiluted, ⅔ cup,							
except as noted:							
black bean (*Pepperidge*							
Farm)	120	5.0	19.0	2.5	0	1050	4.0
chicken curry							
(*Pepperidge Farm*) .	170	9.0	16.0	8.0	25	1030	2.0
chicken w/wild rice							
(*Pepperidge Farm*) .	80	5.0	8.0	3.5	15	960	1.0
clam chowder:							
Manhattan (*Book-*							
binder's), ½ cup	80	6.0	12.0	.5	0	1140	2.0
New England (*Pep-*							
peridge Farm) ..	160	8.0	13.0	8.0	20	1160	1.0
consommé,							
madrilene (*Pep-*							
peridge Farm)	50	5.0	6.0	.5	0	910	0
corn chowder (*Pep-*							
peridge Farm)	70	3.0	14.0	8.0	10	1050	2.0
crab bisque (*Book-*							
binder's), ½ cup ..	120	5.0	10.0	7.0	25	920	1.0
gazpacho (*Pepper-*							
idge Farm)	70	1.0	12.0	2.0	0	1050	2.0
lobster bisque:							
(*Bookbinder's*),							
½ cup	90	4.0	10.0	4.0	25	710	<1.0
(*Pepperidge Farm*) .	160	4.0	12.0	11.0	40	1090	1.0
mushroom, shiitake							
(*Pepperidge Farm*) .	80	3.0	10.0	3.0	<5	1100	2.0
onion, French (*Pepper-*							
idge Farm)	50	3.0	7.0	1.0	<5	1080	1.0
pepperpot (*Book-*							
binder's), ½ cup ..	110	7.0	16.0	2.0	20	1260	2.0
vichyssoise (*Pepper-*							
idge Farm)	70	2.0	11.0	8.0	15	950	2.0
watercress (*Pepper-*							
idge Farm)	80	1.0	11.0	3.5	<5	930	2.0
Soup, frozen, 7.5 oz.,							
except as noted							

Food and Measure	cal.	prot. (gms)	carbo. (gms)	fat (gms)	chol. (mgs)	sod. (mgs)	fiber (gms)
barley mushroom (*Tabatchnick*)	70	2.0	13.0	0	0	540	3.0
bean (*Tabatchnick Yankee*)	160	10.0	27.0	1.5	0	570	11.0
beef noodle (*Reames*), 3.3 oz.	140	8.0	21.0	2.0	40	920	1.0
broccoli, cream of (*Tabatchnick*)	90	3.0	12.0	4.0	5	740	3.0
cabbage (*Tabatchnick*)	60	1.0	14.0	0	0	160	2.0
chicken:							
(*Tabatchnick* New York)	35	2.0	6.0	0	0	850	0
w/dumplings (*Tabatchnick*) ..	70	1.0	13.0	2.0	20	830	1.0
noodle (*Reames* Hearty Home- style), 3 oz.	130	7.0	21.0	2.0	40	1030	1.0
corn chowder (*Tabatchnick*)	150	3.0	22.0	6.0	5	650	1.0
lentil (*Tabatchnick*) ..	140	8.0	25.0	0	0	460	7.0
minestrone (*Tabatchnick*)	150	9.0	27.0	1.0	0	550	10.0
mushroom:							
(*Tabatchnick* No Salt)	70	2.0	13.0	0	0	98	3.0
cream of (*Tabatchnick*)	110	3.0	12.0	6.0	10	430	<1.0
onion (*Tabatchnick*) .	50	2.0	11.0	0	0	600	1.0
pea:							
(*Tabatchnick*)	180	12.0	31.0	1.5	0	520	11.0
(*Tabatchnick* No Salt)	180	12.0	31.0	1.5	0	79	11.0
potato:							
(*Tabatchnick* New England)	150	4.0	21.0	6.0	9	540	2.0
(*Tabatchnick* Old Fashioned)	70	2.0	16.0	0	0	540	2.0
spinach, cream of (*Tabatchnick*)	90	3.0	11.0	4.0	5	630	2.0
tomato rice (*Tabatchnick*)	60	2.0	11.0	1.5	0	260	1.0
vegetable:							
(*Tabatchnick*)	110	5.0	20.0	1.0	0	580	4.0

Food and Measure	cal.	prot. (gms)	carbo. (gms)	fat (gms)	chol. (mgs)	sod. (mgs)	fiber (gms)
Soup, semicondensed, vegetable (*cont.*)							
(*Tabatchnick* No Salt)	110	5.0	20.0	1.0	0	77	4.0
wild rice (*Tabatchnick*)	120	3.0	24.0	1.0	0	610	1.0
Soup, mix (see also "Soup base mix"), 1 pkg. or cont., except as noted:							
bean:							
(*Hodgson Mill Choice*), ¼ cup .	150	9.0	27.0	0	0	5	11.0
black (*Knorr Taste-Breaks* Cup) . . .	190	9.0	36.0	1.0	0	660	10.0
black (*Mrs. Manischewitz*)	200	11.0	37.0	1.0	0	320	5.0
black (*Near East*) . .	190	13.0	40.0	1.5	0	650	13.0
black (*Nile Spice*) . .	170	11.0	35.0	1.5	0	600	11.0
black (*Taste Adventure*), ¾ cup	210	13.0	38.0	1.0	0	530	9.0
black, spicy, w/cous-cous (*Health Valley* Fat Free), ⅓ cup	130	6.0	29.0	0	0	290	5.0
black, zesty, w/rice (*Health Valley* Fat Free), ⅓ cup . . .	100	5.0	22.0	0	0	240	4.0
lima, w/barley (*Manischewitz*), ⅙ pkg.	80	4.0	19.0	.5	0	670	3.0
multi (*AlpineAire*), 1.75 oz.	170	10.0	28.0	2.5	0	570	8.0
navy (*Knorr Taste-Breaks*)	130	6.0	25.0	.5	0	820	7.0
navy (*Nile Spice* Home Style)	200	7.0	37.0	2.5	0	490	2.0
navy (*Taste Adventure*), ¾ cup . . .	160	10.0	30.0	0	0	390	9.0
and rice, see "rice and beans," below							
seven, and barley, all varieties							

Food and Measure	cal.	prot. (gms)	carbo. (gms)	fat (gms)	chol. (mgs)	sod. (mgs)	fiber (gms)
(*Arrowhead Mills*), ¼ cup ...	170	12.0	35.0	0	0	0	7.0
bean and ham (*Hormel Micro Cup*)	190	9.0	29.0	4.0	15	680	7.0
beef noodle:							
(*House of Tsang*) ..	120	5.0	23.0	1.0	5	1100	1.0
vegetable (*Herb-Ox*)	130	5.0	23.0	1.5	25	820	1.0
beef vegetable (*Hormel Micro Cup*)	90	6.0	15.0	1.0	10	790	1.0
broccoli, cream of:							
(*AlpineAire*), 1.2 oz.	130	5.0	21.0	3.0	15	1090	2.0
(*Knorr Recipe Classics*), 3 tbsp.	70	2.0	10.0	2.5	0	730	1.0
broccoli cheese w/ham (*Hormel* Micro Cup)	170	4.0	10.0	13.0	30	710	1.0
cheddar broccoli (*Nile Spice* Home Style) .	110	4.0	19.0	3.0	10	570	3.0
chicken:							
broth (*Cup-a-Soup*)	45	2.0	8.0	0	0	440	0
cream of (*Cup-a-Soup*)	70	1.0	12.0	2.0	0	660	0
noodle (*Cup-a-Soup*)	50	2.0	8.0	1.0	10	560	0
noodle (*Herb-Ox*) .	110	6.0	19.0	1.5	30	750	0
noodle (*Hormel* Micro Cup)	110	8.0	13.0	2.5	35	790	0
noodle (*House of Tsang*)	130	5.0	25.0	1.0	5	700	1.0
noodle (*Mrs. Mani-schewitz*)	140	3.0	26.0	2.0	15	840	0
noodle (*Nile Spice*)	90	3.0	16.0	1.0	15	690	1.0
noodle, hearty (*Cup-a-Soup*)	60	3.0	10.0	1.0	15	600	0
rice (*Hormel* Micro Cup)	110	5.0	17.0	3.0	15	950	1.0
rice (*Mrs. Mani-schewitz*)	130	3.0	28.0	1.0	0	840	1.0
rice (*Mrs. Grass*), ¼ pkg.	80	2.0	15.0	1.0	0	1130	0
rice, creamy (*Knorr Savory*), 3 tbsp.	90	3.0	14.0	2.5	<5	860	0
roasted, rotini (*Near East*)	100	4.0	21.0	1.0	5	500	2.0

Food and Measure	cal.	prot. (gms)	carbo. (gms)	fat (gms)	chol. (mgs)	sod. (mgs)	fiber (gms)
Soup mix, chicken (*cont.*)							
vegetable (*Cup-a-Soup*)	50	2.0	8.0	1.0	10	500	0
vegetable (*Nile Spice* Home Style)	110	4.0	21.0	1.5	5	650	2.0
chili:							
(*Herb-Ox*)	200	9.0	37.0	1.5	0	930	4.0
no beans (*Herb-Ox*)	210	16.0	17.0	9.0	35	970	3.0
clam chowder, New England (*Hormel Micro Cup*)	130	5.0	17.0	5.0	25	820	1.0
coconut ginger (*A Taste of Thai*), 2 tsp.	15	0	2.0	1.0	0	620	0
corn:							
(*House of Tsang* Velvet)	170	5.0	34.0	1.0	5	1230	1.0
sweet (*Nile Spice* Home Style)	110	3.0	22.0	2.0	5	400	3.0
corn chowder:							
(*AlpineAire* Kernel's), 2 oz.	200	13.0	35.0	1.5	0	15	11.0
(*Knorr TasteBreaks* Cup)	140	3.0	26.0	3.0	10	700	2.0
roasted (*Near East*)	140	4.0	28.0	2.5	5	620	3.0
sweet (*Taste Adventure*), ¾ cup ...	190	13.0	35.0	1.0	0	470	5.0
w/tomatoes (*Health Valley* Fat Free), ¼ cup	100	5.0	21.0	0	0	270	3.0
garlic, roasted, herb (*Knorr Recipe Classics*), 3 tbsp.	80	2.0	13.0	1.5	0	860	0
garlic mushroom (*Lipton Recipe Secrets*), 1 cup* ..	20	0	4.0	0	0	530	0
gazpacho (*Nile Spice*)	100	2.0	23.0	.5	0	570	2.0
herb:							
fiesta, w/red pepper (*Lipton Recipe Secrets*), 1 cup*	30	1.0	6.0	0	0	560	0
savory, w/garlic (*Lipton Recipe Secrets*), 1 cup*	30	1.0	6.0	0	0	480	0

Food and Measure	cal.	prot. (gms)	carbo. (gms)	fat (gms)	chol. (mgs)	sod. (mgs)	fiber (gms)
hot and sour (*Knorr Recipe Classics*), 2 tbsp.	45	0	8.0	1.5	0	880	0
leek (*Knorr Recipe Classics*), 2 tbsp.	70	2.0	9.0	2.5	<5	810	0
lentil:							
(*Herb-Ox*)	140	9.0	35.0	.5	0	790	2.0
(*Nile Spice* Home Style)	170	11.0	34.0	1.5	0	540	11.0
curry (*Taste Adventure*), ¾ cup	210	17.0	36.0	1.0	0	620	19.0
hearty (*Mrs. Manischewitz*)	140	6.0	26.0	1.0	0	1090	2.0
w/couscous (*Health Valley* Fat Free), ⅓ cup	130	7.0	28.0	0	0	270	5.0
matzo ball (*Mrs. Manischewitz*)	40	1.0	9.0	1.5	14	800	1.0
minestrone:							
(*AlpineAire* Alpine), 1.75 oz.	170	7.0	33.0	1.0	0	510	7.0
(*Manischewitz*), ¼ pkg.	150	9.0	27.0	0	0	700	3.0
(*Mrs. Manischewitz*)	210	9.0	39.0	1.5	0	760	6.0
(*Near East*)	140	7.0	27.0	2.0	5	540	5.0
(*Nile Spice*)	140	8.0	30.0	1.0	0	590	8.0
(*Taste Adventure*), ¾ cup	140	9.0	27.0	.5	0	210	8.0
Mediterranean (*Knorr* Savory), 3 tbsp.	100	2.0	18.0	2.0	0	810	3.0
miso:							
dark (*San-J*)	40	3.5	4.0	1.5	0	1190	1.0
mild (*San-J*)	50	3.0	6.0	1.5	0	1250	1.0
mushroom:							
beefy (*Lipton Recipe Secrets*), 1 cup*	35	<1.0	7.0	0	0	640	0
country (*Nile Spice* Home Style)	140	4.0	26.0	2.5	5	590	1.0
cream of (*Cup-a-Soup*)	60	1.0	10.0	2.0	0	610	0

Food and Measure	cal.	prot. (gms)	carbo (gms)	fat (gms)	chol. (mgs)	sod. (mgs)	fiber (gms)
Soup mix, mushroom (*cont.*)							
and noodle (*House of Tsang*)	120	5.0	23.0	1.0	5	1050	1.0
noodle:							
buckwheat (*West-brae Natural Ramen*), ½ pkg.	140	5.0	30.0	1.0	0	750	2.0
rice, brown (*West-brae Natural Ramen*), ½ pkg.	140	5.0	30.0	1.0	0	750	2.0
ring noodle (*Cup-a-Soup*)	50	2.0	9.0	1.0	15	560	0
noodle, beef:							
(*Nissin Cup Noodles*)	300	6.0	38.0	14.0	0	1080	2.0
(*Nissin Cup Noodles Twin*), ½ pkg.	150	3.0	20.0	6.0	0	720	1.0
(*Nissin Top Ramen*), ½ pkg.	190	4.0	28.0	7.0	0	700	<1.0
hot sauce (*Nissin Cup Noodles*) . . .	290	6.0	35.0	14.0	0	1090	2.0
picante (*Nissin Top Ramen*), ½ pkg.	180	4.0	26.0	7.0	0	830	1.0
noodle, chicken:							
(*Mrs. Grass* Home-style), ¼ pkg. . .	70	3.0	10.0	1.5	10	840	1.0
(*Nissin Cup Noodles*)	300	6.0	36.0	14.0	<5	1170	2.0
(*Nissin Cup Noodles Twin*), ½ pkg. . .	150	3.0	20.0	7.0	0	710	<1.0
(*Nissin Top Ramen*), ½ pkg.	180	4.0	26.0	7.0	0	800	<1.0
w/broth, real (*Mrs. Grass*), ¼ pkg. .	60	2.0	10.0	1.5	20	960	0
Cajun (*Nissin Cup Noodles*)	300	7.0	37.0	14.0	0	1240	2.0
Cajun (*Nissin Top Ramen*), ½ pkg.	180	4.0	26.0	7.0	0	890	<1.0
creamy (*Nissin Cup Noodles*)	300	7.0	39.0	13.0	5	1240	2.0
creamy (*Nissin Top Ramen*), ½ pkg.	190	5.0	26.0	7.0	<5	710	1.0
flavor, hearty (*Knorr TasteBreaks*) . . .	120	4.0	20.0	2.0	20	910	1.0

Food and Measure	cal.	prot. (gms)	carbo. (gms)	fat (gms)	chol. (mgs)	sod. (mgs)	fiber (gms)
flavor (*Knorr* Savory), 3 tbsp.	70	3.0	11.0	1.5	10	650	1.0
hot sauce (*Nissin Cup Noodles*) ...	300	6.0	37.0	13.0	<5	1130	2.0
mushroom (*Nissin Cup Noodles*) ...	300	5.0	38.0	14.0	0	1140	2.0
mushroom (*Nissin Top Ramen*), ½ pkg.	190	4.0	27.0	7.0	0	720	1.0
sesame (*Nissin Top Ramen*), ½ pkg.	190	4.0	27.0	7.0	0	900	1.0
spicy (*Nissin Cup Noodles*)	300	6.0	38.0	14.0	0	1120	3.0
teriyaki (*Nissin Cup Noodles*)	300	7.0	37.0	14.0	0	1030	2.0
teriyaki (*Nissin Top Ramen*), ½ pkg.	190	4.0	28.0	7.0	0	600	1.0
vegetable (*Nissin Cup Noodles*) ...	300	7.0	37.0	14.0	0	1120	2.0
vegetable (*Nissin Cup Noodles Twin*), ½ pkg. ..	160	3.0	21.0	7.0	0	720	<1.0
vegetable (*Nissin Top Ramen*), ½ pkg.	190	4.0	27.0	7.0	0	790	1.0
w/vegetables (*Health Valley* Fat Free), ⅓ cup ...	110	5.0	24.0	0	0	270	3.0
noodle, chili (*Nissin Top Ramen*), ½ pkg.	190	4.0	26.0	8.0	0	690	<1.0
noodle, mushroom (*Westbrae Natural Ramen*), ½ pkg. ..	140	5.0	30.0	.5	0	710	3.0
noodle, onion, French (*Nissin Cup Noodles*)	300	7.0	40.0	12.0	5	1170	2.0
noodle, Oriental (*Nissin Top Ramen*), ½ pkg.	190	4.0	26.0	7.0	0	830	1.0
noodle, pork: (*Nissin Cup Noodles*)	300	6.0	36.0	14.0	0	1130	2.0

Food and Measure	cal.	prot. (gms)	carbo. (gms)	fat (gms)	chol. (mgs)	sod. (mgs)	fiber (gms)
Soup mix, noodle, pork (*cont.*)							
(*Nissin Top Ramen*), ½ pkg.	180	4.0	26.0	7.0	0	760	<1.0
noodle, seafood (*Nissin Cup Noodles*)	300	7.0	36.0	14.0	0	1240	2.0
noodle, seaweed (*Westbrae Natural* Ramen), ½ pkg. . .	140	5.0	30.0	.5	0	690	3.0
noodle, shrimp:							
(*Nissin Cup Noodles*)	300	6.0	38.0	14.0	10	1070	2.0
(*Nissin Cup Noodles* Twin), ½ pkg. . .	150	3.0	21.0	6.0	<5	730	<1.0
(*Nissin Top Ramen*), ½ pkg.	190	4.0	27.0	7.0	0	800	1.0
hot sauce (*Nissin Cup Noodles*) . . .	300	7.0	38.0	13.0	10	1210	2.0
picante (*Nissin Cup Noodles*)	310	6.0	37.0	15.0	5	980	2.0
onion:							
(*Lipton Recipe Secrets*), 1 cup*	20	0	4.0	0	0	610	0
(*Mrs. Grass* Soup/ Dip), ¼ pkg. . . .	30	1.0	6.0	0	0	890	0
(*Mrs. Grass* Soup/ Dip Reduced Sodium), ¼ pkg.	30	1.0	7.0	0	0	440	0
beefy (*Lipton Recipe Secrets*), 1 cup*	25	0	5.0	.5	0	610	0
French (*Knorr Recipe Classics*), 2 tbsp.	35	1.0	6.0	1.0	0	790	0
golden (*Lipton Recipe Secrets*), 1 cup*	50	1.0	10.0	1.5	0	640	0
onion mushroom:							
(*Lipton Recipe Secrets*), 1 cup*	30	<1.0	6.0	1.0	0	630	0
(*Mrs. Grass* Soup/ Dip), ¼ pkg. . . .	50	1.0	10.0	.5	0	1090	0
oxtail, tomato beef flavor (*Knorr Recipe Classics*), 2 tbsp. .	60	2.0	9.0	2.0	<5	1030	0

Food and Measure	cal.	prot. (gms)	carbo. (gms)	fat (gms)	chol. (mgs)	sod. (mgs)	fiber (gms)
pasta:							
Italiano (*Health Valley* Fat Free), ½ cup	140	5.0	31.0	0	0	270	3.0
marinara, Mediterranean, or Parmesan (*Health Valley* Fat Free), ½ cup	100	5.0	20.0	0	0	290	1.0
pea, golden (*Taste Adventure*), ¾ cup	220	15.0	39.0	1.0	0	500	5.0
pea, green (*Cup-a-Soup*)	80	4.0	12.0	1.0	0	520	3.0
pea, split:							
(*AlpineAire* Soup-er), 2 oz.	200	14.0	34.0	1.5	0	380	9.0
(*Knorr TasteBreaks*)	150	8.0	28.0	1.0	0	730	4.0
(*Near East/Nile Spice*)	200	13.0	35.0	1.0	0	600	8.0
(*Taste Adventure*), ¾ cup	220	16.0	40.0	1.0	0	500	16.0
w/barley (*Manischewitz*), ⅛ pkg.	110	7.0	21.0	0	0	780	3.0
garden, w/carrots (*Health Valley* Fat Free), ½ cup ...	110	7.0	22.0	0	0	270	2.0
potato, creamy:							
broccoli (*Health Valley* Fat Free), ⅓ cup	80	4.0	17.0	0	0	290	3.0
cheddar (*AlpineAire*), 2 oz.	210	7.0	36.0	4.0	20	1290	3.0
potato cheese, w/ham (*Hormel* Micro Cup)	190	4.0	15.0	13.0	50	750	1.0
potato leek:							
(*Herb-Ox*)	140	3.0	24.0	3.5	15	840	2.0
(*Knorr TasteBreaks*)	130	4.0	22.0	2.5	10	920	1.0
(*Nile Spice* Home Style)	110	4.0	19.0	3.0	10	570	3.0
rice, Spanish (*Herb-Ox*)	250	6.0	54.0	.5	0	1240	1.0
rice and beans:							
black (*Uncle Ben's* Hearty), 1.5 oz.	150	7.0	28.0	1.5	0	720	7.0
red (*Near East*) ...	190	11.0	40.0	1.5	0	540	10.0

Food and Measure	cal.	prot. (gms)	carbo. (gms)	fat (gms)	chol. (mgs)	sod. (mgs)	fiber (gms)
Soup mix (*cont.*)							
seafood chowder (*Mountain House*), ½ pouch	250	15.0	44.0	6.0	65	1050	1.0
spinach, cream of (*Knorr Recipe Classics*), 2 tbsp.	70	2.0	10.0	2.5	0	760	<1.0
tomato:							
(*Cup-a-Soup*)	90	2.0	19.0	1.0	5	540	<1.0
basil (*Knorr Recipe Classics*), 3 tbsp.	80	2.0	13.0	2.5	0	920	0
herb (*Nile Spice*) ..	90	2.0	20.0	1.0	5	590	2.0
vegetable:							
(*Knorr Recipe Classics*), 2 tbsp. ..	60	1.0	10.0	1.5	0	880	2.0
(*Lipton Recipe Secrets*), 1 cup*	30	<1.0	7.0	0	0	600	1.0
(*Mrs. Grass* Homestyle Soup/Dip), ¼ pkt.	35	1.0	7.0	0	0	860	1.0
chicken flavor (*Knorr Taste-Breaks*)	120	4.0	21.0	1.5	<5	860	1.0
cream of (*Knorr Savory*), 3 tbsp.	100	2.0	12.0	4.5	0	870	1.0
herb (*Arrowhead Mills*), ⅓ cup ...	150	4.0	30.0	1.0	0	160	3.0
w/mushrooms (*Manischewitz*), ⅕ pkg.	120	7.0	22.0	0	0	700	3.0
and noodle (*House of Tsang*)	120	4.0	25.0	1.0	5	980	1.0
spring (*Knorr Recipe Classics*), 2 tbsp.	25	1.0	5.0	0	0	610	1.0
vegetarian (*Knorr TasteBreaks*) ...	160	6.0	32.0	1.0	0	870	3.0
vichyssoise (*Nile Spice*)	100	3.0	18.0	3.0	10	590	1.0
wild rice:							
(*Herb-Ox*)	230	7.0	33.0	7.0	25	1190	3.0
herb (*Arrowhead Mills*), ⅓ cup ...	140	4.0	28.0	1.0	0	220	3.0

Food and Measure	cal.	prot. (gms)	carbo. (gms)	fat (gms)	chol. (mgs)	sod. (mgs)	fiber (gms)
Soup base mix:							
beef:							
(*Watkins* Soup/ Gravy), 2 tsp.	15	<1.0	2.0	1.0	0	710	0
stew, hearty (*Wyler's Stew Starter*), ⅛ pkg.	70	1.0	16.0	0	0	700	2.0
vegetable (*Wyler's Soup Starter*), ⅛ pkg.	100	3.0	21.0	.5	0	950	2.0
broccoli, cream of (*McCormick Produce Partners*), ⅓ pkt.	35	0	4.0	0	0	700	0
cheddar cheese broccoli (*McCormick Produce Partners*), ⅓ pkt.	70	1.0	5.0	3.0	0	720	0
cheese (*Watkins* Soup/ Gravy), 2½ tbsp.	80	1.0	14.0	2.0	5	440	0
chicken:							
(*Watkins* Soup/ Gravy), 2 tsp.	15	<1.0	3.0	.5	0	580	0
noodle (*Watkins* Soup/Gravy), 1 tbsp.	30	1.0	5.0	0	5	470	0
noodle (*Wyler's Soup Starter*), ⅛ pkg.	80	2.0	15.0	1.0	5	780	1.0
vegetable, hearty (*Wyler's Soup Starter*), ⅐ pkg.	70	2.0	14.0	.5	0	700	2.0
w/white and wild rice (*Wyler's Soup Starter*), ⅛ pkg.	70	2.0	15.0	.5	0	1040	1.0
chili, three bean (*Wyler's Soup Starter*), ⅙ pkg.	150	7.0	28.0	1.0	0	970	8.0
cream (*Watkins* Soup/ Gravy), 2½ tbsp.	90	1.0	4.0	8.0	15	1150	0
mushroom (*Watkins* Soup/Gravy), 2 tbsp.	60	2.0	9.0	2.0	0	540	0

Food and Measure	cal.	prot. (gms)	carbo. (gms)	fat (gms)	chol. (mgs)	sod (mgs)	fiber (gms)
Soup base mix (*cont.*) onion:							
(*Watkins* Soup/ Gravy), 2 tsp. . . .	20	<1.0	3.0	.5	0	400	0
French (*McCormick Produce Partners*), ⅓ pkt.	40	0	5.0	0	0	1150	0
potato: cream of (*Mc-Cormick Produce Partners*), ¼ pkt.	25	0	3.0	0	0	710	0
garlic and chives (*Wyler's Soup Starter*), ⅙ pkg.	130	2.0	23.0	3.5	0	840	2.0
vegetable, garden (*Mc-Cormick Produce Partners*), ⅓ pkt.	40	1.0	5.0	0	0	930	0
Sour cream, see "Cream, sour"							
Sour cream–onion salt (*Watkins*), ¼ tsp.	0	0	0	0	0	300	0
Soursop, ½ cup	75	1.1	18.9	.3	0	16	3.7
Soy bean, see "Soybean"							
Soy beverage, 8 fl. oz., except as noted:							
(*Edensoy/Edensoy* Extra)	130	10.0	13.0	4.0	0	105	0
(*Edensoy* Light)	93	5.0	14.0	2.0	0	84	0
(*Hain* Supreme)	80	6.0	9.0	3.0	0	90	<2.0
(*Harmony Farms*) . . .	90	13.0	21.0	0	0	100	0
(*NutraBlend*)	120	7.0	9.0	6.0	0	150	<1.0
(*Silk*)	100	7.0	8.0	4.0	0	75	0
(*Soy Dream* Original)	130	7.0	17.0	4.0	0	140	0
(*Vitasoy* Creamy Original)	110	9.0	9.0	5.0	0	150	1.0
(*Vitasoy* Creamy Original Refrigerated) . .	110	7.0	12.0	4.0	0	140	1.0
(*Vitasoy* Creamy Unsweetened)	80	6.0	5.0	4.0	0	150	0
(*Vitasoy* Enriched Original)	90	6.0	9.0	4.0	0	140	1.0
(*Vitasoy* Light Original)	60	4.0	7.0	2.0	0	115	0

Food and Measure	cal.	prot. (gms)	carbo. (gms)	fat (gms)	chol. (mgs)	sod. (mgs)	fiber (gms)
(*WestSoy* Drink)	90	4.0	14.0	1.5	0	90	2.0
(*WestSoy* Drink Nonfat)	80	3.0	15.0	0	0	85	1.0
(*WestSoy* Lite)	100	3.0	15.0	2.0	0	120	0
(*WestSoy* Original) . .	140	7.0	18.0	4.5	0	125	3.0
(*WestSoy* Plus)	130	7.0	18.0	3.5	0	130	3.0
(*WestSoy* Unsweetened)	90	9.0	30.0	4.5	0	30	4.0
apple (*NutraBlend*) . .	110	1.0	25.0	1.0	0	65	<1.0
apple splash (*WestSoy* Singles Juice Bar), 6.3 fl. oz.	90	2.0	18.0	1.0	0	15	2.0
berry splash (*WestSoy* Singles Juice Bar), 6.3 fl. oz.	100	2.0	19.0	1.0	0	15	2.0
carob:							
(*Soy Dream*)	210	7.0	36.0	4.0	0	160	0
(*Vitasoy* Supreme)	150	8.0	20.0	4.5	0	180	<1.0
chai:							
(*Silk*)	130	6.5	20.0	3.0	0	125	1.0
(*Power Dream* Sky High), 11 fl. oz.	250	10.0	42.0	5.0	0	70	<1.0
(*WestSoy* Singles), 6.3 fl. oz.	110	1.0	20.0	2.0	0	45	<1.0
chocolate:							
(*Power Dream* X-Treme), 11 fl. oz.	260	10.0	48.0	5.0	0	180	2.0
(*Silk*)	140	5.0	23.0	3.5	0	75	0
(*Soy Dream*)	210	7.0	37.0	3.5	0	160	1.0
(*Vitasoy* Rich)	160	7.0	24.0	4.0	0	180	1.0
creamy (*WestSoy* Vigor-aid)	240	10.0	38.0	6.0	0	100	7.0
cocoa:							
(*Vitasoy* Light)	110	5.0	18.0	2.5	0	120	<1.0
(*Vitasoy* Rich)	150	8.0	21.0	4.5	0	180	1.0
(*WestSoy* Lite)	150	3.0	28.0	2.5	0	140	0
(*WestSoy* Plus) . . .	180	7.0	29.0	3.5	0	30	4.0
coffee:							
(*Café Westbrae*) . . .	130	2.0	25.0	2.5	0	85	0
(*Power Dream* Java Jolt), 11 fl. oz.	240	1.0	42.0	4.5	0	70	2.0
vanilla, French (*Café Westbrae*)	130	2.0	23.0	2.5	0	40	0

Food and Measure	cal.	prot (gms)	carbo (gms)	fat (gms)	chol. (mgs)	sod. (mgs)	fiber (gms)
Soy beverage, coffee (*cont.*)							
vanilla, French (*West-Soy* Lite Singles),							
6.3 fl. oz.	100	1.0	18.0	2.0	0	35	<1.0
green tea (*Vitasoy*) ..	130	7.0	16.0	4.0	0	180	1.0
mango (*Power Dream*							
Passion), 11 fl. oz.	320	8.0	65.0	4.5	0	100	1.0
mocha:							
(*Café Westbrae*) ...	120	2.0	24.0	2.5	0	65	0
(*Silk*)	130	6.5	20.0	3.0	0	125	1.0
(*WestSoy* Lite							
Singles),							
6.3 fl. oz.	100	1.0	18.0	2.0	0	50	<1.0
orange:							
(*NutraBlend*)	100	1.0	24.0	1.0	0	60	<1.0
twist (*WestSoy*							
Singles Juice Bar),							
6.3 fl. oz.	90	2.0	16.0	1.0	0	15	2.0
rice/soy blend, see							
"Rice beverage"							
vanilla:							
(*Edensoy/Edensoy*							
Extra)	150	6.0	23.0	3.0	0	90	0
(*Edensoy* Light) ...	120	3.0	21.0	2.0	0	87	0
(*Hain* Supreme) ...	100	6.0	12.0	3.0	0	90	2.0
(*NutraBlend*)	140	7.0	15.0	6.0	0	160	<1.0
(*Power Dream*							
Blast), 11 fl. oz.	240	10.0	39.0	5.0	0	170	2.0
(*Silk*)	100	6.0	10.0	3.5	0	95	0
(*Soy Dream*)	150	7.0	22.0	4.0	0	140	0
(*Vitasoy* Delight) ..	120	7.0	14.0	4.0	0	115	0
(*Vitasoy* Light)	90	4.0	14.0	2.0	0	110	0
(*Vitasoy* Light							
Enriched)	90	4.0	13.0	2.0	0	105	0
(*Vitasoy* Lowfat) ..	90	4.0	13.0	2.0	0	120	0
(*WestSoy* Drink) ..	120	4.0	22.0	2.0	0	120	0
(*WestSoy* Drink							
Nonfat)	90	3.0	17.0	0	0	85	1.0
(*WestSoy* Lite)	120	3.0	21.0	2.5	0	120	0
(*WestSoy* Plus) ...	140	7.0	19.0	3.5	0	130	3.0
French (*WestSoy*							
Vigor-aid)	260	10.0	44.0	6.0	0	120	7.0
Soy beverage mix:							
(*SoyNilla*), 5 tbsp. ..	130	13.5	18.0	0	0	160	3.0

Food and Measure	cal.	prot. (gms)	carbo. (gms)	fat (gms)	chol. (mgs)	sod. (mgs)	fiber (gms)
all purpose (*Loma Linda Soyagen*), ¼ cup	130	6.0	12.0	6.0	0	150	3.0
carob (*Loma Linda Soyagen*), ¼ cup ..	130	6.0	13.0	6.0	0	170	2.0
malted, 1 pkg.:							
almond (*WestSoy*)	240	6.0	27.0	11.0	0	140	0
almond (*WestSoy* Lite)	160	6.0	26.0	4.0	0	140	0
carob (*WestSoy*) ..	270	7.0	33.0	12.0	0	140	0
cocoa-mint (*West-Soy*)	270	7.0	32.0	12.0	0	140	0
cocoa-mint (*West-Soy* Lite)	160	6.0	26.0	4.0	0	140	0
vanilla (*WestSoy*) .	240	6.0	28.0	12.0	0	140	0
vanilla royale (*West-Soy*)	160	6.0	26.0	6.0	0	140	0
Soy butter, see "Soy spread"							
Soy flour:							
(*Arrowhead Mills*), ½ cup	200	16.0	16.0	9.0	0	0	8.0
(*Hodgson Mill*), scant ¼ cup	80	15.0	9.0	0	0	10	6.0
(*Hodgson Mill* Organic), ¼ cup	110	9.0	9.0	5.0	0	0	5.0
stirred, 1 cup:							
full fat, raw	371	29.4	29.9	17.6	0	11	8.2
defatted	329	47.0	38.4	1.2	0	20	17.5
low fat	287	40.9	33.4	2.4	0	16	9.0
Soy meal, defatted, raw, 1 cup	414	54.8	49.0	2.9	0	3	14.0
Soy milk, see "Soy beverage"							
Soy nuts, roasted:							
(*Frieda's* Salted), ⅓ cup, 1.1 oz. ...	140	11.0	9.0	7.0	0	50	1.0
(*Frieda's* Unsalted), ⅓ cup, 1.1 oz. ...	140	11.0	9.0	7.0	0	0	1.0
(*Skee's Soy Nutz* Salted), 1 oz.	150	12.0	9.0	7.0	0	80	3.0
all varieties (*Tofutti*), 1 oz.	130	10.0	8.0	6.0	0	125	2.0

Food and Measure	cal.	prot. (gms)	carbo. (gms)	fat (gms)	chol. (mgs)	sod. (mgs)	fiber (gms)
Soy nuts (*cont.*)							
barbecue, honey, hot/ spicy, or wasabi (*Frieda's*), ¼ cup ..	140	10.0	11.0	7.0	0	110	5.0
chocolate dipped, see "Candy"							
honey (*Skee's Soy Nutz*), 1 oz.	140	12.0	10.0	6.0	0	170	5.0
onion-garlic (*Skee's Soy Nutz*), 1 oz. ..	150	13.0	7.0	8.0	0	260	4.0
toasted (*AlpineAire*), 2.5 oz.	350	29.0	19.0	18.0	0	1390	19.0
Soy protein, concentrate, 1 oz.:							
w/alcohol	94	16.5	8.8	.1	0	1	<2.0
acid/water wash	94	16.5	8.8	.1	0	255	<2.0
Soy sauce, 1 tbsp., except as noted:							
(*House of Tsang* Dark)	10	0	1.0	0	0	920	0
(*House of Tsang* Light)	5	0	0	0	0	930	0
(*House of Tsang* Low Sodium)	5	0	0	0	0	300	0
(*Kikkoman*)	10	2.0	0	0	0	920	0
(*Kikkoman* Lite)	10	1.0	1.0	0	0	575	0
(*La Choy*)	10	1.5	1.0	0	0	1225	0
(*La Choy* Lite)	15	1.5	2.0	0	0	530	0
(*Sushi Chef* Dark) ...	10	2.0	1.0	0	0	990	0
(*Sushi Chef* Reduced Sodium)	20	0	3.0	0	0	510	0
(*Westbrae Natural* Organic)	10	<1.0	2.0	0	0	700	0
garlic, spicy (*Watkins*)	10	1.0	1.0	0	0	910	0
ginger flavor:							
(*House of Tsang*) ..	20	1.0	4.0	0	0	760	0
(*House of Tsang* Low Sodium) ...	10	0	2.0	0	0	320	0
hot, honey (*Watkins*)	20	1.0	5.0	0	0	650	0
mild (*Westbrae Natural*)	10	<1.0	2.0	0	0	430	0
shoyu:							
(*Eden* Imported Organic)	15	2.0	2.0	0	0	1040	0
(*Eden* Imported Traditional)	15	2.0	2.0	0	0	1010	0

Food and Measure	cal.	prot. (gms)	carbo. (gms)	fat (gms)	chol. (mgs)	sod. (mgs)	fiber (gms)
(*Eden* Reduced Sodium)	10	2.0	2.0	0	0	500	0
(*San-J* Organic) ...	15	2.0	1.0	0	0	960	0
or gai (*Westbrae Natural* Traditional)	10	<1.0	2.0	0	0	830	0
tamari:							
(*Eden* Domestic) ..	15	2.0	2.0	0	0	860	0
(*Eden* Imported) ..	10	2.0	2.0	0	0	990	0
(*San-J*)	15	2.0	1.0	0	0	960	0
(*San-J* Reduced Sodium)	20	2.0	1.0	0	0	700	0
tamari, wheat free:							
(*San-J* Organic) ...	15	2.0	1.0	0	0	940	0
(*San-J* Organic Reduced Sodium)	20	2.0	2.0	0	0	700	0
(*Westbrae Natural*)	10	2.0	<1.0	0	0	760	0
Soy spread, 2 tbsp.:							
(*Soy Wonder*)	170	8.0	10.0	11.0	0	170	1.0
butter, roasted (*Natural Touch*)	170	6.0	10.0	11.0	0	170	1.0
Soybean (see also "Edamame"), ½ cup:							
raw, shelled	188	16.6	14.1	8.7	0	19	5.4
boiled, drained	127	11.1	10.0	5.8	0	13	3.8
Soybean, canned, ½ cup:							
(*Westbrae Natural* High Protein)	150	13.0	11.0	7.0	0	140	3.0
black (*Eden* Organic) .	120	11.0	8.0	6.0	0	30	7.0
Soybean, dried (see also "Soy nuts"):							
raw (*Arrowhead Mills*), ¼ cup	170	15.0	14.0	8.0	0	0	10.0
boiled, ½ cup	149	14.3	8.5	7.7	0	1	5.2
dry-roasted, ½ cup ..	387	34.0	28.1	18.6	0	2	7.0
roasted, ½ cup	405	30.3	28.9	21.8	0	140	7.0
Soybean curd or cake, see "Tofu"							
Soybean kernels, roasted, toasted:							
1 oz. or 95 kernels ...	129	10.5	8.7	6.8	0	1	1.0
whole, 1 cup	490	40.0	33.0	25.9	0	4	3.9

Food and Measure	cal.	prot. (gms)	carbo. (gms)	fat (gms)	chol. (mgs)	sod. (mgs)	fiber (gms)
Soybean spread/dip, 2 tbsp.:							
cucumber-dill or garden vegetable (*Maxbean*)	45	3.0	n.a.	2.0	0	n.a.	1.0
garlic, roasted (*Maxbean*)	45	3.0	n.a.	2.5	0	n.a.	1.0
horseradish (*Maxbean*)	40	3.0	n.a.	2.0	0	n.a.	1.0
ranch (*Maxbean*)	45	4.0	n.a.	2.0	0	n.a.	1.0
roasted red pepper (*Maxbean*)	40	3.0	n.a.	2.5	0	n.a.	1.0
Soybean sprouts, (*Jonathan's*), 1 cup . .	100	11.0	8.0	6.0	0	10	2.0
steamed, ½ cup	38	4.0	3.1	2.1	0	5	.4
Spaghetti, see "Pasta"							
Spaghetti dish, mix:							
Italian, tangy (*Kraft Dinner*), 2 oz.	200	8.0	38.0	1.5	0	600	1.0
w/meat sauce (*Kraft Dinner*), 5.5 oz. . . .	330	11.0	47.0	10.0	15	810	3.0
w/tomato sauce: (*Classico It's Pasta Anytime*), 15.25 oz.	490	15.0	93.0	6.0	0	940	10.0
beef flavor (*Classico It's Pasta Anytime*), 15.25 oz.	490	15.0	93.0	6.0	<5	930	11.0
Spaghetti entree, can or pkg., 1 cup, except as noted: (*Franco-American SpaghettiOs w/Calcium*)	190	2.0	37.0	1.0	<5	650	3.0
w/franks: (*Franco-American SpaghettiOs*) . . .	240	9.0	30.0	10.0	15	1190	5.0
rings (*Kid's Kitchen*)	240	9.0	32.0	9.0	30	810	1.0
marinara, w/roasted vegetables (*Cascadian Farm*), 10 oz.	230	11.0	38.0	4.0	10	600	4.0
w/meatballs: (*Chef Boyardee*) . . .	250	9.0	32.0	10.0	25	950	3.0
(*Chef Boyardee Micro Cup*), 7.5 oz.	210	7.0	25.0	9.0	20	870	1.0

Food and Measure	cal.	prot. (gms)	carbo. (gms)	fat (gms)	chol. (mgs)	sod. (mgs)	fiber (gms)
(*Dinty Moore American Classics*), 1 bowl	290	13.0	44.0	7.0	20	1020	3.0
(*Franco-American SpaghettiOs*) ...	240	11.0	32.0	8.0	20	1070	3.0
(*Kid's Kitchen*)	220	11.0	28.0	7.0	25	950	1.0
rings (*Kid's Kitchen*)	230	11.0	31.0	7.0	25	1190	1.0
in tomato cheese sauce (*Franco-American Spa-ghettiOs*)	180	6.0	37.0	1.0	10	870	3.0
Spaghetti entree, dried, 1 serving: marinara, w/mush-rooms (*AlpineAire*)	320	17.0	53.0	4.0	n.a.	550	5.0
w/meat and sauce: (*Mountain House Double /Four*) ..	270	14.0	37.0	8.0	20	790	2.0
(*Mountain House Single*)	340	17.0	46.0	10.0	25	990	3.0
and meatballs (*Alpine-Aire*)	320	19.0	37.0	12.0	n.a.	1140	5.0
Spaghetti entree, frozen, 1 pkg., except as noted: (*Kid Cuisine* Bowl Silly), 8 oz.	250	9.0	38.0	7.0	15	1190	3.0
Bolognese (*Michel-ina's*), 8.5 oz.	280	12.0	47.0	4.0	10	770	3.0
cheesy, bake: (*Stouffer's*), 12 oz.	460	21.0	47.0	21.0	130	1320	4.0
(*Stouffer's Family Favorites*), ¼ of 40-oz. pkg.	370	16.0	37.0	17.0	85	1210	3.0
marinara: (*Budget Gourmet*), 8 oz.	270	8.0	45.0	6.0	5	680	3.0
(*Michelina's*), 8 oz.	260	9.0	49.0	2.0	0	400	3.0
w/meat sauce: (*Healthy Choice Solo*), 10 oz. ...	290	14.0	40.0	8.0	20	600	7.0
(*Lean Cuisine Every-day Favorites*), 11.5 oz.	300	13.0	51.0	5.0	15	580	6.0

Food and Measure	cal.	prot. (gms)	carbo. (gms)	fat (gms)	chol. (mgs)	sod. (mgs)	fiber (gms)
Spaghetti entree, frozen, w/meat sauce (*cont.*)							
(*Stouffer's*), 12 oz.	440	20.0	56.0	15.0	35	770	5.0
and garlic bread (*Marie Callender's*), 17 oz.	670	27.0	85.0	25.0	35	1160	9.0
w/meatballs:							
(*Lean Cuisine Everyday Favorites*), 9.5 oz.	270	18.0	37.0	6.0	20	690	4.0
(*Michelina's*), 9 oz.	300	14.0	43.0	8.0	20	860	3.0
(*Stouffer's*), 12⅝ oz.	390	19.0	49.0	13.0	30	850	5.0
w/tomato basil sauce (*Michelina's*), 8 oz.	260	9.0	48.0	3.0	5	470	3.0
Spaghetti sauce, see "Pasta sauce"							
Spaghetti squash:							
raw (*Frieda's*), ¾ cup, 3 oz.	30	1.0	6.0	0	0	15	1.0
baked or boiled, drained, ½ cup . . .	23	.5	5.0	.2	0	14	1.1
Spareribs, see "Pork"							
Spelt chips (*VitaSpelt* Flatchips), 1 oz. . . .	70	2.0	15.0	.5	0	110	.5
Spelt flakes, see "Cereal, ready-to-eat"							
Spelt flour, ¼ cup:							
(*Arrowhead Mills*) . . .	100	4.0	24.0	.5	0	0	5.0
(*Hodgson Mill* Organic)	115	4.0	22.0	1.0	0	0	2.0
Spelt kernels (*Purity Foods* Berries), ¼ cup	130	7.0	32.0	1.0	0	0	8.0
Spinach, fresh:							
raw:							
(*Mann's* Salad Spinach), 3 oz.	40	2.0	10.0	0	0	160	5.0
baby (*Dole* Organic Blend), 3 oz. . . .	35	2.0	9.0	0	0	135	4.0
baby (*Fresh Express*), 1½ cups, 3 oz.	20	2.0	3.0	0	0	65	2.0
baby (*Ready Pac*), 4 cups, 3 oz. . . .	40	2.0	10.0	0	0	160	5.0
chopped, ½ cup . .	6	.8	1.0	.1	0	22	.8

Food and Measure	cal.	prot. (gms)	carbo. (gms)	fat (gms)	chol. (mgs)	sod. (mgs)	fiber (gms)
shredded (*Dole*), 1½ cups, 3 oz.	40	2.0	10.0	0	0	160	5.0
boiled, drained, ½ cup	21	2.7	3.4	.2	0	63	2.2
cooked (*Ready Pac* Microwave), ½ cup, 3 oz.	20	2.0	3.0	0	0	60	<1.0
Spinach, canned:							
leaf, ½ cup:							
(*Popeye*)	30	3.0	4.0	0	0	190	2.0
(*Popeye* Low Sodium)	30	3.0	4.0	0	0	35	2.0
(*Bush's Best*)	30	3.0	4.0	0	0	390	2.0
(*Del Monte*)	30	2.0	4.0	0	0	360	2.0
(*Del Monte* No Salt)	30	2.0	4.0	0	0	85	2.0
(*S&W*)	30	3.0	4.0	0	0	440	2.0
chopped, ½ cup							
(*Del Monte*)	30	2.0	4.0	0	0	360	2.0
(*Popeye/Sunshine*)	30	3.0	4.0	0	0	190	2.0
drained, ½ cup	25	3.0	3.6	.5	0	29	2.6
Spinach, frozen (see also "Spinach dish"):							
(*Tree of Life* Organic), 1 cup	20	2.0	2.0	0	0	110	2.0
leaf:							
blocks (*Bonduelle*), 3-oz. block	25	2.0	4.0	0	0	0	3.0
cut (*Birds Eye*), 1 cup	20	2.0	2.0	0	0	110	2.0
cut (*Green Giant*), ¾ cup	15	2.0	2.0	0	0	100	2.0
leaf or chopped:							
(*Seabrook Farms*), ⅓ cup	20	2.0	2.0	0	0	115	2.0
drained, ½ cup ...	27	3.0	5.1	.2	0	82	2.6
chopped (*Birds Eye*), ⅓ cup	20	3.0	3.0	0	0	80	2.0
Spinach, malabar, cooked, 1 cup	10	1.3	1.2	.4	0	24	.9
Spinach, New Zealand, chopped:							
raw, 1 oz. or ½ cup ..	4	.4	.7	.1	0	37	n.a.

Food and Measure	cal.	prot. (gms)	carbo. (gms)	fat (gms)	chol. (mgs)	sod. (mgs)	fiber (gms)
Spinach, New Zealand (*cont.*)							
boiled, drained,							
½ cup	11	1.2	2.0	.2	0	97	n.a.
Spinach, water							
(*Frieda's* Ong Choy),							
2 cups, 3 oz.	20	2.0	3.0	0	0	65	2.0
Spinach dip, 2 tbsp.:							
(*Marie's*)	140	0	3.0	14.0	10	200	0
(*Marzetti* Veggie Dip)	140	1.0	1.0	14.0	25	240	0
Spinach dip mix							
(*McCormick*),							
2 tbsp.*	40	0	2.0	5.0	0	140	0
Spinach dish, frozen:							
creamed:							
(*Birds Eye*), ½ cup	100	3.0	7.0	7.0	35	660	1.0
(*Boston Market*),							
½ cup	190	6.0	9.0	14.0	25	580	2.0
(*Seabrook*), ½ cup	120	4.0	10.0	6.0	15	450	3.0
(*Stouffer's* Side							
Dish), ½ of							
9-oz. pkg.	230	4.0	8.0	20.0	35	560	2.0
(*Tabatchnick*),							
7.5 oz.	60	2.0	8.0	2.0	5	270	2.0
pancake (*Dr. Praeger's*)							
1.3-oz. cake	70	2.0	8.5	3.0	15	155	1.0
soufflé (*Stouffer's*),							
⅓ of 12-oz. pkg. ..	140	6.0	10.0	8.0	90	480	1.0
Spinach entree, pack-							
aged, w/rice, 1 pkg.:							
w/cheese (*Tamarind*							
Tree Palak Paneer) .	380	14.0	46.0	15.0	35	640	6.0
w/garbanzos (*Tama-*							
rind Tree Saag							
Chole)	370	14.0	55.0	10.0	0	800	13.0
Spinach-feta pocket,							
frozen (*Amy's*),							
4½-oz. pc.	250	11.0	34.0	9.0	20	590	3.0
Spinach-feta appetizer,							
frozen (*Apollo/*							
Athens), 5 pcs.,							
5 oz.	390	12.0	34.0	23.0	70	730	2.0
Spinach-feta snack							
(*Amy's*), 5–6 pcs. .	170	7.0	24.0	6.0	15	430	2.0

Food and Measure	cal.	prot. (gms)	carbo. (gms)	fat (gms)	chol. (mgs)	sod. (mgs)	fiber (gms)
Spiny lobster, meat only:							
raw, 4 oz.	127	23.4	2.8	1.7	80	201	0
boiled or steamed:							
2 lbs. in shell	233	43.1	5.1	3.2	146	370	0
4 oz.	138	29.9	3.5	2.2	102	257	0
Spiral pasta entree, frozen, w/spicy tomato sauce (*Michelina's*),							
8 oz.	210	8.0	41.0	1.5	0	570	3.0
Spleen, braised:							
beef, 4 oz.	164	28.5	0	4.8	394	65	0
lamb, 4 oz.	177	30.0	0	5.4	437	66	0
pork, 4 oz.	169	32.0	0	3.6	572	121	0
veal, 4 oz.	146	27.3	0	3.3	507	66	0
Split peas:							
dry, ¼ cup:							
green (*Arrowhead Mills*)	170	12.0	31.0	.5	0	20	7.0
green (*Goya*)	110	11.0	27.0	0	0	25	11.0
green (*Jack Rabbit*)	110	11.0	27.0	0	0	25	11.0
yellow (*Goya*)	110	10.0	28.0	0	0	20	12.0
yellow (*Jack Rabbit*)	110	10.0	28.0	0	0	20	12.0
boiled, ½ cup	116	8.2	20.7	.4	0	2	8.1
Sports drink, 8 fl. oz.:							
all flavors (*Gatorade*)	50	0	14.0	0	0	110	0
lemon-lime (*AriZona*)	60	0	16.0	0	0	100	0
Spot, meat only:							
raw, 4 oz.	140	21.0	0	5.6	68	33	0
baked, broiled, or microwaved, 4 oz.	179	26.9	0	7.1	87	42	0
Sprouts, see "Bean sprouts" and specific listings							
Sprouts, mixed, 1 cup:							
(*Jonathan's*)	100	7.0	21.0	0	0	10	4.0
(*Jonathan's* Gourmet)	20	3.0	3.0	0	0	10	2.0
hot and spicy (*Jonathan's*)	25	3.0	4.0	0	0	15	2.0
salad (*Jonathan's*) ...	80	4.0	10.0	0	0	15	4.0
Squab, fresh, raw:							
meat w/skin, 4 oz. ..	333	20.9	0	27.0	108	61	0
breast meat only, 4 oz.	161	19.8	0	8.5	102	62	0

Food and Measure	cal.	prot. (gms)	carbo. (gms)	fat (gms)	chol. (mgs)	sod. (mgs)	fiber (gms)
Squash (see also specific squash listings), frozen, cooked (*Birds Eye*), ½ cup	50	1.0	12.0	0	0	0	4.0
Squid, fresh, meat only, raw, 4 oz. . . .	104	17.7	3.5	1.6	265	50	0
Squid, frozen, tubes, tentacles (*Soundings*), 4 oz.	110	17.0	3.0	2.0	260	50	0
Squirrel, meat only, roasted, 4 oz.	196	34.9	0	5.3	137	135	0
Star fruit, see "Carambola"							
Steak marinade, see "Marinade"							
Steak sauce, 1 tbsp., except as noted:							
(*A1*)	15	0	3.0	0	0	280	0
(*A1* Bold/Spicy)	20	0	5.0	0	0	260	0
(*A1* Sweet/Tangy) . . .	30	0	8.0	0	0	200	0
(*A1* Thick/Hearty) . . .	25	0	6.0	0	0	290	0
(*Crosse & Blackwell*)	30	0	7.0	0	0	95	0
(*Heinz 57*)	20	0	4.0	0	0	190	0
(*HP*)	15	0	3.0	0	0	150	0
(*Lea & Perrins* Sweet & Spicy)	25	0	6.0	0	0	140	0
(*Lea & Perrins* Traditional)	25	0	5.0	0	0	390	0
(*Newman's Own*)	20	0	4.0	.5	0	85	0
(*Peter Luger*)	30	0	7.0	0	0	125	0
(*Texas Best*)	15	0	4.0	0	0	200	0
(*Watkins*)	20	0	4.0	0	0	220	0
peppercorn (*Lawry's* Weekday Gourmet), 2 tbsp.	40	<1.0	3.0	3.0	0	370	0
Steak seasoning, ¼ tsp.:							
broiled (*McCormick*)	0	0	0	0	0	20	0
Montreal (*McCormick Grill Mates*)	0	0	0	0	0	170	0
Montreal, spicy (*McCormick Grill Mates*)	0	0	0	0	0	150	0

Food and Measure	cal.	prot. (gms)	carbo. (gms)	fat (gms)	chol. (mgs)	sod. (mgs)	fiber (gms)
Stir-fry sauce (see also "Marinade," and specific listings), 1 tbsp., except as noted:							
(*House of Tsang Bangkok Padang*)	45	1.0	4.0	2.5	0	250	0
(*House of Tsang Classic*)	25	0	4.0	.5	0	570	0
(*House of Tsang Saigon Sizzle*)	45	0	8.0	1.0	0	380	0
(*Kikkoman*)	20	<1.0	4.0	0	0	520	0
garlic and ginger (*Rice Road*)	25	0	3.0	1.0	0	310	0
herb and roasted garlic (*Lawry's* Seasoning)	5	0	1.0	0	0	210	0
lemon (*Rice Road*) . .	15	0	4.0	0	0	310	0
lemon basil (*Lawry's* Seasoning)	10	0	3.0	0	0	260	0
sesame ginger (*Lawry's* Seasoning)	15	0	3.0	0	0	280	0
spicy, Szechuan (*House of Tsang*) . .	20	0	4.0	.5	0	520	0
sweet and sour (*House of Tsang*) . .	35	0	8.0	0	0	50	0
sweet and spicy (*Lawry's* Seasoning)	20	0	4.0	0	0	320	0
teriyaki (*House of Tsang Korean*)	30	0	6.0	.5	0	460	0
Stir-fry seasoning mix (*McCormick Produce Partners*), ⅕ pkg.	20	0	4.0	0	0	520	0
Stomach, pork, raw, 1 oz.	44	4.7	0	2.7	55	15	0
Strawberry, fresh:							
(*Dole*), 8 medium, 5.2 oz.	45	1.0	12.0	0	0	0	4.0
halves, ½ cup	23	.5	5.3	.3	0	1	1.8
pureed, ½ cup	35	.7	8.1	.4	0	1	2.7
Strawberry, canned, ½ cup:							
in light syrup (*Oregon*)	100	1.0	23.0	0	0	5	2.0
in heavy syrup	117	.7	29.9	.3	0	5	2.2

Food and Measure	cal.	prot. (gms)	carbo. (gms)	fat (gms)	chol. (mgs)	sod. (mgs)	fiber (gms)
Strawberry, dried:							
(*Frieda's*), ½ cup, 1.4 oz.	150	1.0	34.0	0	0	0	3.0
freeze-dried, whole (*AlpineAire*), .5 oz.	50	1.0	12.0	0	0	0	2.0
Strawberry, frozen:							
(*Big Valley*), ⅔ cup . .	50	<1.0	12.0	0	0	0	2.0
(*Cascadian Farm*), 1 cup	90	1.0	20.0	0	0	0	6.0
(*Tree of Life* Organic), ¾ cup	50	<1.0	13.0	0	0	0	2.0
whole:							
(*Birds Eye*), ½ cup .	100	<1.0	25.0	0	0	0	1.0
(*Sun-Vale* No Sugar), 1 cup	40	0	9.0	0	0	0	2.0
sliced:							
in sugar (*Big Valley* Tub), ⅔ cup . . .	150	<1.0	38.0	0	0	0	2.0
sweetened (*Sun-Vale*), ⅔ cup . . .	150	1.0	36.0	1.0	0	0	4.0
in light syrup (*Birds Eye* Lite), 10 oz. . .	120	1.0	31.0	0	0	0	1.0
in syrup (*Birds Eye*), 4.75 oz.	120	1.0	31.0	0	0	0	1.0
unsweetened, ½ cup	39	.5	10.1	.1	0	2	2.3
Strawberry drink:							
(*Capri Sun All Natural Strawberry Cooler*), 6.75 fl. oz.	90	0	25.0	0	0	20	0
(*Hawaiian Punch Surfin'*), 8 fl. oz. . .	120	0	31.0	0	0	100	0
Strawberry drink blends, 8 fl. oz., except as noted:							
banana:							
(*AriZona*)	140	0	34.0	.5	0	25	0
(*Libby's* Nectar), 11.5-fl.-oz. can	220	<1.0	52.0	0	0	10	0
(*WipperSnapple*), 10 fl. oz.	160	0	40.0	0	0	60	0
guava (*Santa Cruz* Organic)	100	<1.0	24.0	0	0	25	0

Food and Measure	cal.	prot. (gms)	carbo. (gms)	fat (gms)	chol. (mgs)	sod. (mgs)	fiber (gms)
kiwi:							
(*Capri Sun All Natural*), 6.75 fl. oz.	100	0	26.0	0	0	20	0
(*Dole*)	130	0	33.0	0	0	20	0
(*Dole*), 11.5 fl. oz.	180	0	46.0	0	0	30	0
(*Kool-Aid Bursts*), 6.75 fl. oz.	100	0	24.0	0	0	30	0
(*Libby's* Nectar), 11.5-fl.-oz. can	200	0	49.0	0	0	10	0
(*Tropicana Twister*)	130	0	33.0	0	0	20	0
sparkling cider (*R. W. Knudsen*)	110	<1.0	28.0	0	0	15	0
Strawberry drink mix*, 8 fl. oz., except as noted:							
(*Kool-Aid* Sugar Sweetened)	60	0	16.0	0	0	0	0
kiwi (*Kool-Aid Slammin'*)	70	0	17.0	0	0	15	0
star fruit (*Kool-Aid* Sugar Sweetened)	70	0	17.0	0	0	0	0
Strawberry milk, see "Milk, flavored"							
Strawberry milk drink mix (*Nesquik*), 2 tbsp.	90	0	22.0	0	0	0	0
Strawberry pie glaze (*Smucker's*), 2 oz.	80	0	21.0	0	0	0	0
Strawberry syrup, ¼ cup, except as noted:							
(*Hershey's*), 2 tbsp.	100	0	26.0	0	0	10	0
(*Knott's Berry Farm*)	210	0	52.0	0	0	50	0
(*Maple Grove Farms*)	210	0	53.0	0	0	0	0
(*Nesquik*), 2 tbsp. ..	110	0	27.0	0	0	0	0
(*Smucker's*)	210	0	52.0	0	0	0	0
(*Smucker's* Sundae Syrup), 2 tbsp.	100	1.0	25.0	0	0	110	0
Strawberry topping, 2 tbsp.:							
(*Kraft*)	110	0	29.0	0	0	15	0
(*Mrs. Richardson's*) ..	70	0	18.0	0	0	5	0
(*Smucker's*)	100	0	26.0	0	0	0	0

Food and Measure	cal.	prot. (gms)	carbo. (gms)	fat (gms)	chol. (mgs)	sod. (mgs)	fiber (gms)
String bean, see "Green bean"							
Stroganoff mix, vegetarian (*Natural Touch*), 4 tbsp. . . .	90	5.0	10.0	3.5	10	610	3.0
Stroganoff sauce, beef (*Lawry's*), 1 tbsp. .	20	0	5.0	0	0	500	0
Strudel, see "Apple pastry"							
Stuffing, ¾ cup:							
corn bread (*Pepperidge Farm*)	170	4.0	33.0	2.0	0	480	2.0
herb seasoned:							
(*Chatham Village* Traditional)	150	5.0	30.0	.5	0	760	1.0
(*Pepperidge Farm*) .	170	5.0	33.0	1.5	0	600	3.0
Stuffing mix, dry, ⅙ pkg., except as noted:							
(*Bell's*), ½ cup	130	5.0	25.0	1.5	0	510	1.0
(*Kellogg's Croutettes*), 1 cup	120	5.0	25.0	0	0	460	0
apple raisin (*Pepperidge Farm Farmhouse*), ½ cup	70	1.0	10.0	3.0	10	230	<1.0
for beef (*Stove Top*) . .	110	4.0	22.0	1.0	0	490	<1.0
chicken flavor:							
(*Pepperidge Farm One Step*), ½ cup	140	4.0	24.0	4.0	<5	440	<1.0
(*Pepperidge Farm Farmhouse*), ½ cup	110	2.0	12.0	6.0	<5	300	<1.0
(*Stove Top* Flexible Serve), 1 oz. . . .	120	3.0	19.0	3.0	0	460	<1.0
(*Stove Top* Lower Sodium)	110	4.0	21.0	1.0	0	260	<1.0
cornbread:							
(*Stove Top*)	110	3.0	21.0	1.0	0	490	1.0
(*Stove Top* Flexible Serve), 1 oz. . . .	110	3.0	20.0	2.5	0	490	1.0
Southwestern (*Pepperidge Farm One Step*), ½ cup . . .	150	4.0	23.0	5.0	0	440	1.0

Food and Measure	cal.	prot. (gms)	carbo. (gms)	fat (gms)	chol. (mgs)	sod. (mgs)	fiber (gms)
cranberry:							
(*Stove Top*)	110	3.0	20.0	1.0	0	400	<1.0
and herb (*Chatham Village*), 1 cup . .	130	4.0	28.0	0	0	530	2.0
herb:							
(*Chatham Village* Traditional), 1 cup	150	4.0	32.0	0	0	520	2.0
(*Stove Top* Flexible Serve Homestyle), 1 oz.	110	3.0	19.0	2.5	0	440	<1.0
pork flavor (*Stove Top*)	110	3.0	20.0	1.0	0	450	<1.0
San Francisco style (*Stove Top*)	110	4.0	20.0	1.0	0	460	1.0
turkey (*Pepperidge Farm Farmhouse*), ½ cup	90	3.0	14.0	3.0	<5	350	<1.0
Sturgeon, meat only:							
raw, 4 oz.	120	18.3	0	4.6	68	61	0
baked, broiled, or microwaved, 4 oz.	153	23.5	0	5.9	87	78	0
smoked, 4 oz.	196	35.4	0	5.0	91	838	0
Subway, 1 serving:							
breakfast sandwich:							
bacon & egg	305	13.0	29.0	15.0	184	500	1.0
cheese & egg	302	13.0	29.0	15.0	187	520	1.0
ham & egg	291	15.0	30.0	12.0	189	700	1.0
western egg	285	13.0	31.0	12.0	182	510	2.0
6" Classic sub:							
Cold Cut Trio	415	19.0	40.0	20.0	57	1670	3.0
Italian BMT	453	21.0	40.0	24.0	56	1740	3.0
meatball	501	23.0	46.0	25.0	56	1350	4.0
Seafood & Crab, w/light mayo . . .	378	14.0	46.0	16.0	24	1270	3.0
steak & cheese . . .	362	23.0	41.0	13.0	37	1190	4.0
Subway Melt	380	23.0	41.0	15.0	41	1690	3.0
tuna, w/light mayo .	419	18.0	39.0	21.0	42	1180	3.0
6" Select sub:							
asiago Caesar chicken	391	22.0	41.0	15	46	1000	3.0
honey mustard melt	373	23.0	47.0	11.0	41	1570	3.0
roast beef, horse- radish	401	18.0	42.0	17.0	28	880	3.0

Food and Measure	cal.	prot. (gms)	carbo. (gms)	fat (gms)	chol. (mgs)	sod. (mgs)	fiber (gms)
Subway, 6" Select sub (*cont.*)							
steak & cheese,							
Southwest	412	23.0	42.0	18.0	44	1120	4.0
deli style sandwich:							
ham	194	10.0	30.0	3.5	12	750	2.0
roast beef	206	12.0	31.0	4.0	13	600	2.0
turkey breast	200	12.0	31.0	3.5	10	700	2.0
tuna w/light mayo	309	12.0	31.0	15.0	26	810	2.0
7 Under 6 sub:							
ham	261	17.0	39.0	4.5	25	1260	3.0
roast beef	264	18.0	39.0	4.5	20	850	3.0
roast chicken breast	311	25.0	40.0	6.0	48	880	3.0
Subway Club	294	22.0	40.0	5.0	29	1250	3.0
turkey breast	254	16.0	39.0	3.5	15	1000	3.0
turkey breast & ham	267	18.0	40.0	4.5	23	1210	3.0
Veggie Delite	200	7.0	37.0	2.5	0	500	3.0
wraps:							
asiago Caesar							
chicken	413	22.0	47.0	15.0	46	1320	2.0
steak & cheese ...	353	22.0	46.0	9.0	37	1400	3.0
turkey breast &							
bacon	321	18.0	45.0	7.0	23	1510	2.0
condiments/extras:							
bacon, 2 slices ...	45	2.0	0	4.0	8	180	0
cheese, 2 triangles	41	2.0	0	3.5	10	200	0
mayo, 1 tbsp.	111	0	0	12.0	9	80	0
mayo, light, 1 tbsp.	46	0	0	5.0	6	100	0
mustard, 2 tsp. ...	8	1.0	0	0	0	115	0
oil blend, 1 tsp. ..	45	0	0	5.0	0	0	0
vinegar, 1 tsp.	1	0	0	0	0	0	0
Classic salad, w/out							
dressing:							
Cold Cut Trio	234	14.0	11.0	15.0	57	1370	3.0
Italian BMT	273	16.0	11.0	19.0	56	1440	3.0
meatball	320	18.0	18.0	20.0	56	1050	4.0
steak & cheese ...	182	17.0	12.0	8.0	37	890	4.0
Seafood & Crab,							
w/light mayo ...	198	9.0	17.0	11.0	24	970	4.0
Subway Melt	203	17.0	12.0	10.0	41	1410	3.0
tuna, w/light mayo	238	13.0	11.0	16.0	42	880	3.0
7 Under 6 salad, w/out							
dressing:							
ham	112	11.0	11.0	3.0	25	1070	3.0
roast beef	114	12.0	11.0	3.0	20	660	3.0

Food and Measure	cal.	prot. (gms)	carbo. (gms)	fat (gms)	chol. (mgs)	sod. (mgs)	fiber (gms)
roast chicken breast	137	16.0	12.0	3.0	36	730	3.0
Subway Club	145	17.0	12.0	3.5	30	1070	3.0
turkey breast	105	11.0	11.0	2.0	15	820	3.0
turkey breast & ham	117	13.0	11.0	3.0	23	1030	3.0
Veggie Delite	50	2.0	9.0	1.0	0	310	3.0
dressing, 2 oz.:							
French, fat free . . .	70	0	17.0	0	0	390	0
Italian, fat free	20	0	4.0	0	0	610	0
ranch, fat free	60	0	14.0	0	0	530	0
cookie:							
chocolate chip	209	3.0	29.0	10.0	12	135	1.0
chocolate chunk . .	210	2.0	30.0	10.0	12	150	1.0
M&M's	210	2.0	29.0	10.0	13	135	1.0
macadamia nut . . .	221	2.0	27.0	12.0	13	140	1.0
oatmeal raisin	197	3.0	29.0	8.0	14	180	1.0
peanut butter	220	3.0	26.0	12.0	0	200	1.0
sugar	222	2.0	28.0	12.0	18	170	0
Succotash, canned,							
½ cup:							
kernel (*Libby's*)	90	2.0	19.0	0	0	280	3.0
cream style (*Blue Boy*)	90	2.0	19.0	0	0	280	3.0
cream-style	103	3.5	23.4	.7	0	325	4.0
Succotash, frozen:							
(*John Cope's*), ⅔ cup	80	6.0	17.0	0	0	50	2.0
boiled, drained,							
½ cup	79	3.7	17.0	.8	0	38	4.6
Sucker, white meat							
only:							
raw, 4 oz.	105	19.0	0	2.6	47	45	0
baked, broiled, or							
microwaved, 4 oz.	135	24.4	0	3.4	60	58	0
Sugar, beet or cane:							
brown:							
1 oz.	107	0	27.6	0	0	11	0
1 cup, not packed	546	0	141.0	0	0	57	0
1 cup, packed	828	0	214.0	0	0	86	0
granulated:							
1 oz.	110	0	28.3	0	0	<1	0
1 cup	773	0	199.8	0	0	<1	0
1 tbsp.	46	0	12.0	0	0	<1	0
1 tsp.	15	0	4.0	0	0	<1	0
powdered or confec-							
tioners':							
1 cup, sifted	389	0	99.5	0	0	1	0

Food and Measure	cal.	prot. (gms)	carbo. (gms)	fat (gms)	chol. (mgs)	sod. (mgs)	fiber (gms)
Sugar, beet or cane, powdered or confectioners' (*cont.*)							
1 tbsp., unsifted ..	31	0	8.0	0	0	<1	0
Sugar, maple, 1 oz.	99	0	25.5	0	0	4	0
Sugar, substitute (see also "Fructose"):							
(*Equal*), 1 pkt.	4	0	<1.0	0	0	0	0
(*NutraSweet*), 1 tsp.	2	0	<1.0	0	0	0	0
(*Sweet 'n Low*), 1 pkt.	4	0	1.0	0	0	0	0
(*Weight Watchers*) ...	5	0	1.0	0	0	30	0
Sugar, turbinado (*Hain*), 1 tsp.	15	0	4.0	0	0	0	0
Sugar apple:							
1 medium, 9.9 oz. ..	146	3.2	36.6	.5	0	15	6.8
½ cup	118	2.6	29.6	.4	0	12	5.5
Sugar loaf squash (*Frieda's*), ¾ cup, 3 oz.	30	1.0	7.0	0	0	0	1.0
Sugar snap peas, see "Peas, edible-podded"							
Summer sausage:							
(*Johnsonville* Chub Original/Beef/Garlic), 2 oz.	180	10.0	1.0	15.0	40	680	0
beef (*Oscar Mayer*), 2 slices, 1.7 oz. ..	140	7.0	<1.0	12.0	40	670	0
smoked (*Old Smokehouse*), 2 oz.	200	2.0	2.0	18.0	55	970	0
Summer squash (see also specific listings), all varieties, 1 cup:							
raw, sliced	23	1.3	4.9	.2	0	2	2.2
boiled, drained, sliced	36	1.6	7.8	.6	0	2	2.5
Sunburst squash, baby (*Frieda's*), ⅔ cup, 3 oz.	15	1.0	3.0	0	0	0	1.0
Sunchoke, see "Jerusalem artichoke"							
Sunfish, pumpkinseed, meat only:							
raw, 4 oz.	101	22.0	0	.8	76	91	0
baked, broiled, or microwaved, 4 oz.	129	28.2	0	1.0	98	117	0

Food and Measure	cal.	prot. (gms)	carbo. (gms)	fat (gms)	chol. (mgs)	sod. (mgs)	fiber (gms)
Sunflower butter:							
(*Kettle Roaster Fresh*),							
1 oz.	168	5.0	6.0	15.0	0	3	0
1 tbsp.	93	3.2	4.4	7.6	0	1	.8
Sunflower seed, 1 oz.							
kernels, except as							
noted:							
(*Frito-Lay*)	180	7.0	5.0	15.0	0	150	2.0
(*House of Bazzini*							
Salted), ¼ cup	200	8.0	6.0	17.0	0	180	4.0
(*Planters*), ¼ cup . . .	200	7.0	6.0	17.0	0	180	4.0
(*Planters*), 3-oz. pkg.	280	10.0	8.0	23.0	0	180	4.0
in shell, roasted							
(*Planters*), ¾ cup . .	180	7.0	5.0	15.0	0	120	2.0
raw, ¼ cup:							
(*Blue Diamond*) . . .	190	7.0	6.0	17.0	0	0	3.0
(*House of Bazzini*)	180	8.0	5.0	15.0	0	10	2.0
dried (*Arrowhead*							
Mills), ¼ cup	180	8.0	6.0	15.0	0	10	2.0
dry-roasted, unsalted	165	5.5	6.8	14.1	0	1	3.2
oil-roasted:							
(*Blue Diamond*),							
¼ cup	210	7.0	5.0	20.0	0	210	2.0
unsalted	174	6.1	4.2	16.3	0	1	4.2
toasted, unsalted	176	4.9	5.8	16.1	0	1	3.3
barbecue (*Frito-Lay*) .	200	7.0	6.0	15.0	0	200	2.0
hot (*Frito-Lay* Flamin')	180	7.0	5.0	15.0	0	380	2.0
Sunflower seed flour,							
partially defatted,							
1 cup	261	38.5	28.7	1.3	0	2	4.2
Sunflower sprouts,							
(*Jonathan's*), 1 cup	45	2.0	2.0	4.0	0	0	1.0
Surimi, pollock, 4 oz.	112	17.2	7.8	1.0	34	162	0
Swamp cabbage:							
raw, .6-oz. shoot	2	.3	.4	<.1	0	15	.3
boiled, drained,							
chopped, ½ cup . .	10	1.0	1.8	.1	0	60	.9
Sweet dumpling							
squash (*Frieda's*),							
¾ cup, 3 oz.	30	1.0	7.0	0	0	0	1.0
Sweet peas, see							
"Peas, green"							
Sweet potato:							
raw, 5" x 2" potato . . .	136	2.1	31.6	.4	0	17	3.9

Food and Measure	cal.	prot. (gms)	carbo. (gms)	fat (gms)	chol. (mgs)	sod. (mgs)	fiber (gms)
Sweet potato (*cont.*)							
baked in skin:							
5" x 2" potato	118	2.0	27.7	.1	0	12	3.4
mashed, ½ cup . . .	103	1.7	24.3	.1	0	10	3.0
boiled w/out skin:							
4 oz.	119	1.9	27.5	.3	0	15	2.8
mashed, ½ cup . . .	172	2.7	39.8	.5	0	21	4.1
Sweet potato, canned, ½ cup, except as noted:							
whole (*Royal Prince/ Trappey's*), 3 pcs., 6.1 oz.	200	1.0	48.0	0	0	40	4.0
cut:							
(*Allens/Princella/ Sugary Sam*), ⅔ cup	160	0	40.0	.5	0	35	3.0
(*Glory Foods*)	120	0	30.0	0	0	30	2.0
candied (*S&W Yams*)	170	2.0	46.0	0	0	360	4.0
mashed (*Princella/ Sugary Sam*), ⅔ cup	120	1.0	28.0	.5	0	30	3.0
candied (*Royal Prince*)	210	1.0	50.0	0	0	30	2.0
orange-pineapple (*Royal Prince*)	210	1.0	50.0	0	0	30	3.0
in syrup:							
(*Sylvia's Yams*) . . .	120	0	30.0	0	0	30	2.0
w/liquid	101	1.1	23.9	.2	0	50	2.8
drained	106	1.3	24.9	.3	0	38	2.9
Sweet potato, frozen:							
baked, cubed, ½ cup	88	1.5	20.6	.1	0	7	2.6
candied:							
(*Green Giant*), ¾ cup	240	2.0	41.0	7.0	0	430	3.0
(*Mrs. Paul's*), 5 oz.	300	1.0	73.0	1.0	0	130	3.0
w/apple (*Mrs. Paul's*), 1¼ cups	270	0	66.0	0	0	90	3.0
Sweet potato chips, 1 oz.:							
(*Tastee*)	140	2.0	17.0	7.0	0	90	2.0
(*Terra* No Salt)	140	1.0	18.0	7.0	0	10	1.0
barbecue, mesquite (*Terra*)	140	1.0	18.0	7.0	0	65	1.0

Food and Measure	cal.	prot. (gms)	carbo. (gms)	fat (gms)	chol. (mgs)	sod. (mgs)	fiber (gms)
cinnamon nutmeg							
(*Tastee*)	140	2.0	17.0	7.0	0	90	2.0
nacho cheese (*Terra*)	140	1.0	18.0	7.0	0	70	1.0
jalapeño (*Terra*)	140	1.0	20.0	7.0	0	70	2.0
salsa (*Terra*)	140	0	20.0	7.0	0	75	2.0
spiced:							
(*Terra*)	140	1.0	16.0	7.0	0	105	3.0
cinnamon (*Terra*) . .	140	1.0	17.0	7.0	0	70	2.0
Sweet potato leaf:							
raw, chopped, ½ cup	6	.7	1.1	.1	0	2	<1.0
steamed, ½ cup	11	.7	2.3	.1	0	4	.6
Sweet and sour drink							
mixer (*Mr & Mrs T*),							
4 fl. oz.	150	0	34.0	0	0	115	0
Sweet and sour sauce,							
2 tbsp., except as							
noted:							
(*Contadina*)	40	0	8.0	1.0	0	115	0
(*Kikkoman*)	35	0	9.0	0	0	190	0
(*Kraft*)	60	0	13.0	0	0	125	0
(*San-J*)	50	<1.0	13.0	0	0	320	0
duck sauce:							
(*Ka•Me*)	60	0	15.0	0	0	180	0
(*Ty Ling*)	70	0	19.0	0	0	260	0
w/ginger (*Ka•Me*) . . .	50	0	13.0	0	0	60	0
Hawaiian style (*World*							
Harbors)	60	0	14.0	0	0	250	0
tangerine (*Heaven and*							
Earth), 1 tbsp. . . .	25	<1.0	6.0	0	0	5	0
Sweetbreads, see							
"Pancreas" and							
"Thymus"							
Swiss chard, fresh:							
raw:							
(*Frieda's*), 1 cup,							
3 oz.	15	2.0	3.0	0	0	180	1.0
chopped, ½ cup . .	3	.3	.7	<.1	0	38	.3
boiled, drained,							
chopped, ½ cup . .	18	1.7	3.6	.1	0	158	1.8
Swisswurst (*Johnson-*							
ville), 2.7-oz. link . .	240	9.0	2.0	21.0	60	640	0
Swordfish, fresh,							
meat only:							
raw, 4 oz.	137	22.5	0	4.6	45	102	0

Food and Measure	cal.	prot. (gms)	carbo. (gms)	fat (gms)	chol (mgs)	sod (mgs)	fiber (gms)
Swordfish (*cont.*)							
baked, broiled, or microwaved, 4 oz.	176	28.8	0	5.8	57	130	0
Syrup, see specific syrup listings							
Szechuan sauce (see also "Stir-fry sauce"):							
(*Ka•Me*), 1 tbsp.	25	1.0	2.0	1.5	0	390	0
(*San-J*), 1 tsp.	5	0	1.0	0	0	180	0

T

Food and Measure	cal.	prot. (gms)	carbo. (gms)	fat (gms)	chol. (mgs)	sod. (mgs)	fiber (gms)
Tabouli (*Frieda's*), ½ cup	160	5.0	30.0	4.0	0	210	5.0
Tabouli salad mix:							
(*Casbah*), 1.25 oz. . .	120	3.0	24.0	.5	0	410	1.0
(*Cedar's*), 2 tbsp. . . .	30	1.0	3.0	1.0	0	63	1.0
(*Near East*), ⅔ cup*	110	4.0	23.0	3.0	0	270	5.0
(*Yorgo*), 2 tbsp.	25	1.0	3.0	1.0	0	55	1.0
Taco, frozen, 1 pc.:							
beef/cheese, soft:							
(*El Monterey Family Classics*), 5.5 oz.	440	19.0	42.0	23.0	40	880	3.0
spicy (*El Monterey Family Classics*), 5 oz.	380	17.0	37.0	19.0	35	710	2.0
spicy (*El Monterey Family Classics*), 5.5 oz.	420	19.0	40.0	21.0	40	790	2.0
beef/pork, soft (*El Monterey Family Classics*), 4 oz. . . .	230	12.0	29.0	8.0	25	480	1.0
Taco Bell, 1 serving:							
burrito:							
bean	370	13.0	54.0	12.0	10	1080	12.0
chili cheese	330	13.0	40.0	13.0	25	900	4.0
fiesta, beef	380	14.0	49.0	15.0	30	1100	4.0
fiesta, chicken	370	17.0	48.0	12.0	35	1000	3.0
fiesta, steak	370	18.0	47.0	12.0	25	1020	3.0
grilled *Stuft*, beef . .	730	27.0	75.0	35.0	65	2090	11.0
grilled *Stuft*, chicken	690	33.0	73.0	29.0	70	1900.	8.0
grilled *Stuft*, steak	690	30.0	72.0	30.0	60	1970	8.0
7-layer	520	16.0	65.0	22.0	25	1270	13.0
burrito *Supreme:*							
beef	430	17.0	50.0	18.0	40	1210	9.0
chicken	410	20.0	49.0	16.0	45	1120	8.0

Food and Measure	cal	prot. (gms)	carbo. (gms)	fat (gms)	chol. (mgs)	sod. (mgs)	fiber (gms)
Taco Bell, **burrito** *Supreme* (*cont.*)							
steak	420	21.0	48.0	16.0	35	1140	8.0
double, beef	510	23.0	52.0	23.0	60	1500	11.0
double, chicken	460	27.0	50.0	17.0	70	1200	3.0
double, steak	470	28.0	48.0	18.0	55	1230	3.0
chalupa *Baja*:							
beef	420	14.0	30.0	27.0	35	760	3.0
chicken	400	17.0	28.0	24.0	40	660	2.0
steak	400	17.0	27.0	24.0	30	680	2.0
chalupa nacho cheese:							
beef	370	13.0	30.0	22.0	25	740	3.0
chicken	350	16.0	29.0	19.0	25	640	2.0
steak	350	16.0	28.0	30.0	20	660	1.0
chalupa *Supreme*:							
beef	380	14.0	29.0	23.0	40	580	3.0
chicken	360	17.0	28.0	20.0	45	490	2.0
steak	360	17.0	27.0	20.0	35	500	2.0
cheesy gordita crunch	560	21.0	44.0	33.0	60	980	6.0
cheesy gordita crunch *Supreme*	610	22.0	47.0	37.0	70	990	6.0
gordita *Baja*:							
beef	360	13.0	29.0	21.0	35	810	4.0
chicken	340	16.0	28.0	18.0	40	710	3.0
steak	340	17.0	27.0	18.0	30	730	3.0
gordita nacho cheese:							
beef	310	13.0	30.0	15.0	25	780	4.0
chicken	290	15.0	29.0	13.0	25	690	3.0
steak	290	16.0	28.0	13.0	20	700	2.0
gordita *Supreme*:							
beef or steak	300	17.0	27.0	14.0	35	550	3.0
chicken	300	16.0	28.0	13.0	45	530	3.0
taco:							
Double Decker	380	15.0	43.0	17.0	30	740	9.0
regular	170	9.0	12.0	10.0	30	330	4.0
soft, beef	210	11.0	20.0	10.0	30	570	3.0
soft, chicken	190	13.0	19.0	7.0	35	480	2.0
soft, steak	280	12.0	20.0	17.0	35	630	2.0
taco *Supreme*:							
Double Decker	420	15.0	45.0	21.0	40	760	10.0
regular	260	10.0	20.0	16.0	40	350	4.0
specialties:							
Enchirito, beef	370	18.0	33.0	19.0	50	1300	9.0
Enchirito, chicken	350	21.0	32.0	16.0	55	1210	7.0
Enchirito, steak	350	22.0	31.0	16.0	45	1220	7.0

Food and Measure	cal.	prot. (gms)	carbo. (gms)	fat (gms)	chol. (mgs)	sod. (mgs)	fiber (gms)
Mexican pizza	390	18.0	28.0	25.0	45	930	8.0
MexiMelt	290	15.0	22.0	15.0	45	830	4.0
taco salad, w/salsa	850	30.0	69.0	52.0	70	2250	16.0
taco salad, w/salsa, w/out shell	400	24.0	31.0	22.0	70	1510	15.0
tostada	250	10.0	27.0	12.0	15	640	11.0
quesadilla, cheese	350	16.0	31.0	18.0	50	860	3.0
quesadilla, chicken	400	25.0	33.0	19.0	75	1050	3.0
nachos and sides:							
Mexican rice	190	5.0	23.0	9.0	15	750	<1.0
nachos	320	5.0	34.0	18.0	<5	560	3.0
nachos BellGrande	760	20.0	83.0	39.0	35	1300	17.0
nachos, mucho grande	1320	31.0	116.0	82.0	75	2670	18.0
nachos Supreme ..	440	14.0	44.0	24.0	35	800	9.0
Pintos'n Cheese ...	180	9.0	18.0	8.0	15	640	10.0
twists, cinnamon ..	150	1.0	27.0	4.5	0	190	<1.0
Taco entree, frozen, 1 pkg.:							
beef:							
mini (Swanson Fun Feast), 7.2 oz. .	400	12.0	53.0	15.0	30	680	4.0
w/salsa, rice (Michelina's), 8 oz.	380	14.0	50.0	14.0	30	670	2.0
roll-ups (Kid Cuisine), 7.35 oz. .	420	9.0	55.0	18.0	25	740	4.0
Taco entree kit, pkg.:							
(Old El Paso):							
2 pcs. w/beef*	300	17.0	19.0	17.0	55	840	2.0
2 pcs. w/chicken*	240	20.0	19.0	9.0	50	840	2.0
(Ortega 12 Pack), 2 tsp. seasoning, 1 tbsp. sauce, 2 shells	150	3.0	24.0	5.0	0	700	3.0
(Ortega 18 Pack), 2 tsp. seasoning, 1 tbsp. sauce, 2 shells	150	3.0	25.0	5.0	0	740	3.0
soft (Chi-Chi's), seasoning, 2 shells	300	6.0	54.0	7.0	0	1360	2.0
soft (Old El Paso):							
2 pcs. w/beef*	390	22.0	33.0	19.0	65	1270	2.0
2 pcs. w/chicken* .	330	26.0	33.0	10.0	60	1270	2.0

Food and Measure	cal.	prot. (gms)	carbo. (gms)	fat (gms)	chol. (mgs)	sod. (mgs)	fiber (gms)
Taco filling, frozen:							
beef (*Ortega*), ⅓ cup	100	7.0	4.0	6.0	20	290	1.0
chicken (*Tyson*),							
¼ cup	90	9.0	4.0	4.0	35	330	0
Taco John's,							
1 serving:							
burritos:							
bean	380	15.0	53.0	11.0	15	820	12.0
beefy	440	22.0	44.0	20.0	55	860	6.0
chicken and potato	450	15.0	56.0	18.0	20	1310	9.0
meat and potato ..	500	15.0	58.0	23.0	25	1200	8.0
super	450	19.0	51.0	19.0	35	910	10.0
platters:							
beef/bean chimi ...	740	26.0	82.0	35.0	40	1780	10.0
beef enchilada	830	34.0	79.0	41.0	70	2190	11.0
chicken enchilada .	690	27.0	71.0	32.0	50	2220	10.0
smothered burrito .	880	35.0	101.0	36.0	55	1930	17.0
specialties:							
chicken festiva:							
burrito	550	17.0	56.0	28.0	40	1150	9.0
salad	690	22.0	39.0	50.0	75	1450	5.0
salad, no dres-							
sing	370	21.0	27.0	20.0	55	680	5.0
chicken super							
nachos	810	26.0	57.0	54.0	55	1550	7.0
Potato Olés Bravo .	570	9.0	55.0	35.0	10	1750	6.0
Sierra chicken sand-							
wich	480	25.0	37.0	27.0	65	880	2.0
super nachos	900	23.0	68.0	60.0	45	1350	10.0
Super Potato Olés .	970	22.0	82.0	61.0	45	2920	10.0
taco salad	770	24.0	55.0	50.0	55	1890	3.0
taco salad, no							
dressing	600	24.0	50.0	33.0	55	970	3.0
tacos:							
crispy	190	9.0	13.0	12.0	25	250	0
Sierra, beef	500	18.0	39.0	30.0	45	530	2.0
Sierra, chicken	430	18.0	37.0	24.0	40	670	3.0
softshell	230	11.0	23.0	10.0	25	500	0
softshell, chicken ..	170	11.0	21.0	5.0	20	610	4.0
Taco Bravo	360	15.0	40.0	15.0	25	660	6.0
taco burger	280	14.0	29.0	11.0	35	580	1.0
sides:							
chili, Texas style ..	380	21.0	23.0	22.0	55	950	4.0
Mexican rice	250	6.0	44.0	5.0	0	860	0

Food and Measure	cal.	prot. (gms)	carbo. (gms)	fat (gms)	chol. (mgs)	sod. (mgs)	fiber (gms)
nachos	440	7.0	35.0	30.0	10	740	4.0
Potato Olés	410	4.0	45.0	24.0	n.a.	1190	4.0
Potato Olés, large ..	540	5.0	59.0	32.0	n.a.	1570	6.0
Potato Olés, small .	310	3.0	33.0	18.0	n.a.	880	3.0
refried beans	360	18.0	45.0	11.0	15	1020	15.0
side salad	290	3.0	15.0	25.0	20	560	2.0
desserts:							
apple grande	258	5.0	40.0	9.0	7	240	1.0
churro	158	2.0	13.0	11.0	10	115	1.0
choco taco	311	3.0	37.0	17.0	20	100	1.0
cinnamon mint							
swirl, 1	60	0	14.0	0	0	5	0
cookies, 1 bag	130	1.0	20.0	5.0	0	70	0
local favorites:							
burrito:							
chicken fajita ...	320	18.0	41.0	10.0	35	890	7.0
combination	410	18.0	49.0	15.0	35	840	9.0
El Grande	730	33.0	69.0	36.0	85	1630	8.0
El Grande,							
chicken	630	33.0	66.0	26.0	75	1850	3.0
ranch, beef	440	16.0	43.0	22.0	45	830	1.0
ranch, chicken ..	380	16.0	41.0	17.0	40	940	2.0
smothered	540	25.0	57.0	24.0	50	1120	11.0
cheese crisp	220	10.0	9.0	16.0	35	250	0
chilto	440	21.0	41.0	22.0	60	1060	7.0
enchilada, double ..	780	38.0	58.0	43.0	100	1950	8.0
Mexi Rolls	670	28.0	53.0	40.0	65	1470	2.0
Mexican pizza	560	23.0	47.0	31.0	50	720	4.0
Potato Olés w/nacho							
cheese	530	7.0	50.0	34.0	10	1930	4.0
quesadilla	460	18.0	41.0	24.0	45	860	7.0
quesadilla, chicken	430	20.0	42.0	20.0	45	990	7.0
taco, El Grande ...	480	24.0	30.0	29.0	65	760	1.0
taco, El Grande,							
chicken	330	17.0	24.0	18.0	40	740	1.0
tostada	200	9.0	13.0	12.0	25.0	250	0
tostada, bean	160	6.0	17.0	7.0	5	230	3.0
Taco mix, vegetarian (Natural Touch), 3 tbsp.	10	8.0	5.0	1.0	0	590	3.0
Taco pizza kit (Old El Paso), 1 crust, w/beef*	350	19.0	17.0	23.0	70	660	1.0

Food and Measure	cal.	prot. (gms)	carbo. (gms)	fat (gms)	chol. (mgs)	sod. (mgs)	fiber (gms)
Taco sauce, 1 tbsp., except as noted:							
(*Chi-Chi's*)	10	0	1.0	0	0	75	0
green:							
medium (*La Victoria*)	0	0	<1.0	0	0	75	0
mild (*La Victoria*) . .	0	0	<1.0	0	0	70	0
hot (*Mrs. Renfro's*), 2 tbsp.	10	0	2.0	0	0	210	0
medium (*Ortega*)	10	0	2.0	0	0	125	0
medium or hot (*Old El Paso*)	5	0	1.0	0	0	90	0
mild:							
(*Mrs. Renfro's*), 2 tbsp.	10	0	3.0	0	0	240	0
(*Old El Paso*)	5	0	1.0	0	0	85	0
mild or hot (*Ortega*) . .	10	0	2.0	0	0	120	0
red:							
medium (*La Victoria*)	5	0	1.0	0	0	75	0
mild (*La Victoria*) . .	5	0	1.0	0	0	90	0
Taco seasoning mix:							
(*Bearitos*), 2¼ tsp. . .	20	1.0	4.0	0	0	510	0
(*Chi-Chi's* Fiesta), ⅕ pkg.	25	0	4.0	0	0	400	1.0
(*El Torito*), ⅕ pkt. . . .	25	0	5.0	0	0	430	0
(*Hain*), 2 tsp.	20	1.0	4.0	0	0	230	<1.0
(*Lawry's*), 2 tsp.	15	0	3.0	0	0	300	0
(*McCormick* Original), ⅙ pkg.	20	0	3.0	0	0	430	0
(*McCormick* 30% Less Sodium), ⅙ pkg. . .	20	0	3.0	0	0	300	0
(*Old El Paso*), 2 tsp. .	15	0	4.0	0	0	560	0
(*Ortega*), 2 tsp.	20	0	4.0	0	0	430	0
chicken:							
(*Lawry's*), 2 tsp. . . .	20	0	5.0	0	0	450	0
(*McCormick*), ¼ pkg.	25	0	4.0	0	0	450	0
hot (*McCormick*), ⅙ pkg.	20	0	3.0	0	0	430	0
mild (*McCormick*), ⅙ pkg.	20	1.0	4.0	0	0	460	0
salad (*Lawry's*), 1 tsp.	15	0	3.0	0	0	200	0

Food and Measure	cal.	prot. (gms)	carbo. (gms)	fat (gms)	chol. (mgs)	sod. (mgs)	fiber (gms)
Taco shell:							
(*Old El Paso*), 3 pcs.	150	2.0	19.0	7.0	0	135	2.0
soft, see "Tortilla"							
tostada:							
(*Los Pericos*), 1 pc.	90	1.0	10.0	5.0	0	105	0
(*Old El Paso*), 3 pcs.	150	2.0	19.0	7.0	0	135	2.0
white/yellow corn (*Chi-Chi's*), 2 pcs.	170	2.0	22.0	8.0	0	330	2.0
TacoTime, 1 serving:							
burrito:							
bean, soft, double	506	23.0	77.0	12.0	22	860	19.0
bean, soft, value, single	380	16.0	58.0	10.0	15	715	13.0
Casita Burrito	647	40.0	54.0	31.0	89	1233	16.0
combination, soft, double	617	39.0	66.0	23.0	63	1343	18.0
crisp, bean	427	15.0	53.0	18.0	12	453	9.0
crisp, chicken	422	17.0	32.0	25.0	54	795	2.0
crisp, meat	552	34.0	39.0	30.0	58	1000	7.0
meat, soft, double	726	57.0	55.0	33.0	99	1809	17.0
meat, soft, value, single	491	31.0	48.0	21.0	56	1197	12.0
veggie	491	21.0	70.0	16.0	24	643	10.0
taco:							
beef, shredded, soft, super	368	12.0	38.0	11.0	22	556	7.0
cheeseburger	633	31.0	48.0	36.0	66	1291	7.0
chicken, soft	387	21.0	41.0	16.0	48	933	7.0
crisp	295	22.0	16.0	17.0	48	609	5.0
flour, soft, rolled	512	33.0	46.0	23.0	63	1111	12.0
meat, natural, super	627	41.0	60.0	27.0	82	915	14.0
soft, value	316	24.0	23.0	15.0	48	599	5.0
salads, no dressing:							
taco, chicken	370	19.0	27.0	21.0	48	861	3.0
taco, regular	479	30.0	30.0	28.0	63	895	7.0
Tostada Delight, meat	628	36.0	48.0	33.0	82	1004	13.0
nachos/sides:							
Mexi Fries:							
large	532	6.0	54.0	34.0	0	1598	n.a.
regular	266	3.0	27.0	17.0	0	799	n.a.
nachos	680	26.0	61.0	38.0	78	1250	11.0
nachos deluxe	1048	46.0	91.0	57.0	109	2252	17.0
quesadilla, cheese	205	11.0	17.0	11.0	30	255	1.0

Food and Measure	cal.	prot. (gms)	carbo. (gms)	fat (gms)	chol. (mgs)	sod. (mgs)	fiber (gms)
***TacoTime*, nachos/sides** (*cont.*)							
refritos	326	18.0	44.0	10.0	22	525	13.0
rice, Mexican	159	3.0	30.0	2.0	0	530	1.0
sauces/shells:							
chips, 2 oz.	266	4.0	35.0	12.0	0	461	3.0
dressing, 1 oz.:							
sour cream	137	1.0	2.0	14.0	8	207	0
Thousand Island	160	0	4.0	16.0	10	220	0
enchilada sauce,							
1 oz.	12	0	3.0	0	0	133	1.0
guacamole, 1 oz.	29	0	2.0	2.0	0	94	1.0
hot sauce, 1 oz. . .	10	0	2.0	0	0	120	0
salsa, ranchero,							
2 oz.	21	1.0	3.0	1.0	0	192	1.0
sour cream, 1 oz. .	55	1.0	1.0	5.0	19	11	0
taco shell, 6"	110	2.0	14.0	6.0	0	48	2.0
tortilla:							
flour, 7"	88	4.0	16.0	1.0	0	42	1.0
flour, 8"	107	5.0	16.0	3.0	0	33	2.0
flour, 10"	213	6.0	31.0	4.0	0	393	6.0
flour, fried, 8"	205	4.0	24.0	11.0	0	203	1.0
flour, fried, 10" . . .	318	6.0	37.0	16.0	0	315	2.0
wheat, 11"	175	8.0	33.0	3.0	0	84	2.0
dessert:							
cherry empanada . .	250	5.0	37.0	9.0	0	46	n.a.
Crustos . . . . , ...	373	9.0	47.0	15.0	0	86	n.a.
Tahini:							
(*Arrowhead Mills*).							
2 tbsp.	190	6.0	5.0	19.0	0	5	3.0
(*Joyva*), 2 tbsp.	200	5.0	3.0	18.0	0	75	1.0
(*Telma* Tehina),							
½ cup	230	7.0	7.0	19.0	0	250	3.0
Tahini sauce mix							
(*Casbah*), ¼ pkg.	200	4.0	10.0	13.0	0	160	.5
Tahini spread/dip							
(*Sabra Salads*),							
1 oz.	80	2.6	1.3	7.0	0	67	.8
Tamale, canned,							
2 pcs., except as							
noted:							
(*Wolf*)	210	6.0	23.0	12.0	20	450	4.0
beef:							
(*Hormel*), 7.5 oz. .	200	6.0	22.0	10.0	25	1060	3.0

Food and Measure	cal.	prot. (gms)	carbo. (gms)	fat (gms)	chol. (mgs)	sod. (mgs)	fiber (gms)
(*Hormel/Hormel* Hot/Spicy)	140	4.0	15.0	7.0	15	710	2.0
jumbo (*Hormel*) ..	190	6.0	21.0	10.0	25	980	3.0
chicken (*Hormel*) ...	130	3.0	15.0	7.0	30	660	1.0
Tamale, frozen, 1 pc.:							
(*Goya*)	240	6.0	31.0	10.0	15	390	2.0
beef, 4.5 oz.:							
(*El Monterey*)	300	9.0	24.0	19.0	30	640	3.0
(*El Monterey Family Classics*)	230	11.0	26.0	10.0	20	700	2.0
chicken (*El Monterey/ El Monterey Family Classics*), 4.5 oz.	250	9.0	27.0	11.0	20	750	2.0
Tamale dinner, frozen, beef, 1 pkg.:							
(*Patio*), 12 oz.	440	12.0	51.0	21.0	35	2460	8.0
and enchilada (*Patio*), 12.25 oz.	480	12.0	54.0	24.0	35	2040	9.0
Tamale pocket, frozen (*Amy's*), 4.5 oz. ..	250	8.0	39.0	7.0	10	580	3.0
Tamale pot pie, frozen, Mexican (*Amy's*), 8 oz.	220	10.0	41.0	3.0	0	480	11.0
Tamari, see "Soy sauce"							
Tamarillo, fresh (*Frieda's*), 2 pcs., 4.2 oz.	40	2.0	9.0	0	0	0	4.0
Tamarind:							
(*Frieda's*), 1.1-oz. pod	70	1.0	19.0	0	0	10	2.0
1 fruit, 3" x 1"	5	.1	1.3	<.1	0	1	.1
pulp, ½ cup	144	1.7	37.5	.4	0	17	3.1
Tamarind nectar (*Goya*), 12 fl. oz. ..	240	1.0	59.0	0	0	20	1.0
Tandoori paste, (*Patak's*), 2 tbsp.	30	<1.0	3.0	1.0	0	1440	2.0
Tangerine, fresh:							
(*Dole*), 1 medium, 3.8 oz.	50	1.0	15.0	.5	0	0	3.0
(*Frieda's* Delite/Pixie Mandarin/Satsuma), 1 cup, 5 oz.	60	0	16.0	0	0	0	3.0
(*Frieda's* Page Mandarin), 1 cup, 5 oz.	60	0	12.0	0	0	0	3.0

Food and Measure	cal.	prot. (gms)	carbo. (gms)	fat (gms)	chol. (mgs)	sod. (mgs)	fiber (gms)
Tangerine (*cont.*)							
1 large 2½" diam.,							
3.5 oz.	43	.6	11.0	.2	0	1	2.3
sections, 1 cup	86	1.2	21.8	.4	0	2	4.5
Tangerine, canned:							
in juice, ½ cup	46	.8	11.9	<1	0	6	.9
in light syrup:							
(*Del Monte*),							
½ cup	80	0	19.0	0	0	10	<1.0
(*Del Monte* Snack							
Cup), ½ cup ...	70	0	17.0	0	0	10	<1.0
(*Dole*), ½ cup	80	0	19.0	0	0	10	<1.0
(*Garden Treat* Man-							
darin), ⅔ cup ..	100	<1.0	23.0	0	0	15	<1.0
½ cup	77	.6	20.4	.1	0	8	.9
Tangerine drink, ruby							
red:							
(*Tropicana Twister*),							
8 fl. oz.	130	0	32.0	0		20	0
(*Tropicana Twister*),							
11.5 fl. oz.	190	0	46.0	0		30	0
Tangerine juice,							
8 fl. oz.:							
(*Noble* Express)	125	1.0	30.0	0	0	0	0
fresh	106	1.2	25.0	1.2	0	2	.5
canned, sweetened ..	125	1.3	29.9	.5	0	2	.5
frozen*	111	1.0	26.7	.3	0	2	.5
Tannier, see "Malanga"							
Tapenade, see							
"Tomato tapenade"							
Tapioca, see							
"Pudding" and							
"Pudding and							
pie filling mix"							
Taquito, frozen,							
4.5-oz. pc.:							
beef/cheese (*El*							
Monterey Family							
Classics)	330	12.0	36.0	15.0	30	430	1.0
chicken/cheese (*El*							
Monterey Family							
Classics)	310	11.0	36.0	13.0	20	540	1.0
Taquito, breakfast,							
frozen: egg, bacon,							

Food and Measure	cal.	prot. (gms)	carbo. (gms)	fat (gms)	chol. (mgs)	sod. (mgs)	fiber (gms)
cheese, salsa (*El Monterey Family Classics*), 4.5 oz.	290	12.0	38.0	11.0	110	740	1.0
Taramosalata (*Krinos*), 1 tbsp.	90	1.0	0	10.0	15	115	0
Taro, fresh, ½ cup:							
raw, sliced	56	.8	13.8	.1	0	6	2.1
cooked, sliced	94	.3	22.8	.1	0	10	3.4
Tahitian:							
raw, sliced	25	1.7	4.3	.6	0	31	n.a.
cooked, sliced	30	2.8	4.7	.5	0	37	n.a.
Taro chips:							
(*Terra*), 1 oz.	140	1.0	19.0	6.0	0	110	4.0
1 oz.	141	.7	19.3	7.1	0	97	n.a.
½ cup	57	.3	8.1	3.1	0	44	n.a.
spiced (*Terra*), 1 oz.	130	1.0	20.0	5.0	0	170	2.0
Taro leaf:							
raw, ½ cup	6	.7	.9	.1	0	1	.5
steamed, ½ cup	17	2.0	2.9	.3	0	1	1.5
Taro root (*Frieda's*), ⅔ cup, 3 oz.	90	1.0	22.0	0	0	10	3.0
Taro shoots, ½ cup:							
raw, sliced	5	.4	1.0	<.1	0	<1	n.a.
cooked, sliced	10	.5	2.2	.1	0	1	n.a.
Tarragon, ground, 1 tsp.	5	.4	.8	.1	0	1	.1
Tart shell, see "Pastry shell"							
Tartar sauce, 2 tbsp.:							
(*Golden Dipt*)	160	0	3.0	15.0	0	220	0
(*Golden Dipt* Fat Free)	35	0	6.0	0	0	210	0
(*Hellmann's/Best Foods*)	80	0	3.0	7.0	10	300	0
(*Hellmann's/Best Foods* Low Fat)	40	0	7.0	1.5	0	360	0
(*Kraft*)	150	0	1.0	16.0	15	460	0
(*Kraft Free* Nonfat)	25	0	5.0	0	0	200	0
(*Maille* Dipping)	140	0	3.0	14.0	<5	300	0
(*Marzetti* Sauce Shoppe)	120	0	4.0	11.0	20	290	0
(*Old Bay*)	130	0	3.0	12.0	0	170	0
lemon and herb flavor (*Kraft*)	150	0	<1.0	16.0	15	170	0

Food and Measure	cal.	prot. (gms)	carbo. (gms)	fat (gms)	chol. (mgs)	sod. (mgs)	fiber (gms)
TCBY, all flavors, ½ cup:							
ice cream:							
low fat	120	3.0	22.0	2.5	5	75	0
low fat, no sugar ..	100	3.0	20.0	2.5	10	55	0
sorbet, soft serve ...	100	0	24.0	0	0	30	0
yogurt, soft serve:							
96% fat free	130	4.0	23.0	3.0	15	60	0
nonfat	110	4.0	23.0	0	<5	60	0
nonfat, no sugar ..	80	4.0	20.0	0	<5	35	0
Tea (see also "Tea, iced"), plain, regular, or instant, all varieties, 1 bag or tsp.	0	0	0	0	0	0	0
Tea, iced, 8 fl. oz.:							
(*AriZona*)	90	0	25.0	0	0	20	0
(*AriZona Rx Health*) ..	70	0	19.0	0	0	20	0
(*AriZona Rx Energy*)	120	0	31.0	0	0	25	0
(*AriZona Rx Memory*)	80	0	20.0	0	0	20	0
(*AriZona Rx Stress*) ..	70	0	18.0	0	0	20	0
(*Crystal Light*)	5	0	0	0	0	15	0
(*R. W. Knudsen/Santa Cruz Organic Hibiscus Cooler*)	90	<1.0	23.0	0	0	40	0
(*Turkey Hill*)	90	0	22.0	0	0	15	0
(*Turkey Hill* Decaf) ...	80	0	20.0	0	0	15	0
cherry (*Snapple* Very)	100	0	25.0	0	0	10	0
cranberry twist (*Snapple*)	100	0	26.0	0	0	10	0
ginseng (*AriZona* Extract)	60	0	15.0	0	0	20	0
green tea:							
w/ginseng (*After the Fall Green Tea Express*)	90	0	23.0	0	0	10	0
w/ginseng (*AriZona*)	70	0	18.0	0	0	20	0
w/ginseng and honey (*Turkey Hill*)	70	0	17.0	0	0	20	0
lime (*Snapple*)	100	0	25.0	0	0	10	0
plum (*AriZona* Asia)	70	0	18.0	0	0	20	0
mandarin orange (*AriZona*)	70	0	19.0	0	0	20	0

Food and Measure	cal.	prot. (gms)	carbo. (gms)	fat (gms)	chol. (mgs)	sod. (mgs)	fiber (gms)
lemon:							
(*AriZona*)	90	0	25.0	0	0	20	0
(*AriZona* Thermal) .	90	0	23.0	0	0	20	0
(*Nestea*)	80	0	21.0	0	0	25	0
(*Snapple*)	100	0	25.0	0	0	10	0
(*Turkey Hill* Cooler)	100	0	24.0	0	0	10	0
lemonade:							
(*Minute Maid*)	110	0	29.0	0	0	25	0
(*Snapple*)	110	0	28.0	0	0	10	0
frozen* (*Minute Maid*)	100	0	28.0	0	0	0	0
mint (*Snapple*)	110	0	27.0	0	0	10	0
mint w/chamomile (*Turkey Hill* Cooler)	90	0	21.0	0	0	10	0
oolong, blueberry (*Turkey Hill*)	100	0	24.0	0	0	10	0
oolong w/ginkgo, gin- seng (*Turkey Hill*)	100	0	25.0	0	0	10	0
orange (*Turkey Hill* Cooler)	100	0	25.0	0	0	10	0
peach:							
(*AriZona*)	90	0	25.0	0	0	20	0
(*Crystal Light*)	5	0	0	0	0	15	0
(*Snapple*)	100	0	26.0	0	0	10	0
peach or raspberry (*Turkey Hill* Cooler)	110	0	28.0	0	0	10	0
raspberry:							
(*AriZona*)	90	0	25.0	0	0	20	0
(*Snapple*)	100	0	26.0	0	0	10	0
sweet (*Snapple*)	120	0	31.0	0	0	10	0
Tea, iced, mix:							
(*Country Time* Classic), 8 fl. oz.*	90	0	22.0	0	0	10	0
(*Crystal Light*), 8 fl. oz.*	5	0	0	0	0	0	0
(*Nestea* 100%/Sun Tea), 2 tsp.	0	0	<1.0	0	0	0	0
(*Nestea* Sugar Free), 2 tsp.	5	0	1.0	0	0	0	0
herb, lemon, or orange spice (*Nestea*), 1 tbsp.	15	0	3.0	0	0	0	0
lemon:							
(*Nestea*), 2 tsp. . . .	5	0	1.0	0	0	0	0

Food and Measure	cal.	prot. (gms)	carbo. (gms)	fat (gms)	chol. (mgs)	sod. (mgs)	fiber (gms)
Tea, iced, mix, lemon (*cont.*)							
and sugar (*Nestea*), 2 tbsp.	80	0	19.0	0	0	0	0
lemonade (*Nestea*), 2 tbsp.	80	0	19.0	0	0	0	0
peach or raspberry:							
(*Country Time*), 8 fl. oz.*	90	0	22.0	0	0	10	0
(*Crystal Light*), 8 fl. oz.*	5	0	0	0	0	0	0
peach, raspberry, or tangerine (*Watkins*), 4 tsp.	80	0	21.0	0	0	0	0
Teff seeds or flour (*Arrowhead Mills*), 2 oz.	200	7.0	41.0	1.0	0	6	7.7
Tempeh:							
1 oz.	55	5.3	2.7	3.1	0	3	n.a.
½ cup	160	15.4	7.8	9.0	0	7	n.a.
Tempura batter mix (*Golden Dipt* Fry Easy), ¼ cup	100	1.0	20.0	0	0	150	0
Tenderizer, see "Meat tenderizer"							
Teriyaki entree, frozen (*Lean Cuisine* Every-day Favorites), 10-oz. pkg.	290	18.0	45.0	4.0	20	590	4.0
Teriyaki sauce (see also "Marinade"):							
(*Kikkoman* Baste & Glaze), 2 tbsp. ...	50	1.0	11.0	0	0	810	0
(*San-J*), 1 tbsp.	10	1.0	3.0	0	0	450	0
(*Sun Luck* Honey Mirin), 1 tbsp. ...	30	<1.0	6.0	0	0	320	0
(*Sushi Chef*), 1 tbsp.	35	0	9.0	0	0	590	0
(*S&W* Cooking Sauce), 1 tbsp.	25	1.0	5.0	0	0	220	0
(*Watkins* Tangy), 1 tbsp.	15	1.0	2.0	0	0	620	0
chicken (*Lawry's* Week-day Gourmet), 2 tbsp.	40	0	10.0	0	0	630	0

Food and Measure	cal.	prot. (gms)	carbo. (gms)	fat (gms)	chol. (mgs)	sod. (mgs)	fiber (gms)
Hawaiian style, and marinade (*World Harbors*), 2 tbsp.	70	0	17.0	0	0	270	0
w/honey, pineapple (*Kikkoman* Baste & Glaze), 2 tbsp.	80	1.0	18.0	0	0	770	0
hot, tropical style (*World Harbors Maui Mountain*), 2 tbsp.	70	0	17.0	0	0	300	0
Polynesian (*Trader Vic's*), 1 tbsp.	15	0	3.0	0	0	430	0
sesame garlic (*Rice Road*), 1 tbsp.	15	0	4.0	0	0	300	0
Texas toast, see "Bread, frozen"							
Thai sauce (see also "Peanut sauce" and specific listings):							
chili, 1 tsp.:							
garlic pepper (*A Taste of Thai*)	10	0	2.0	0	0	230	0
pepper paste (*A Taste of Thai*)	20	0	2.0	1.0	0	572	0
sweet green or red (*A Taste of Thai*)	10	0	2.0	0	0	40	0
curry, 1 tbsp.:							
green (*Ka•Me*)	10	0	2.0	0	0	440	0
red (*Ka•Me*)	15	0	4.0	0	0	250	0
curry base, see "Curry sauce base"							
and marinade, East Asian style (*World Harbors*), 2 tbsp.	40	0	8.0	0	0	350	0
pad Thai (*A Taste of Thai*), 2 tbsp.	90	1.0	20.0	1.0	0	790	1.0
seasoning (*A Taste of Thai*), 1 tbsp.	15	2.0	1.0	0	0	1730	0
Thyme, ground:							
(*Watkins*), ¼ tsp.	0	0	0	0	0	0	0
1 tsp.	4	.1	.9	.1	0	1	.3
Thymus, 4 oz.:							
beef, braised	362	24.8	0	28.3	333	132	0
veal, braised	197	35.8	0	4.9	532	75	0

Food and Measure	cal.	prot. (gms)	carbo. (gms)	fat (gms)	chol. (mgs)	sod. (mgs)	fiber (gms)
Tikka sauce, see "Curry sauce"							
Tilefish, meat only:							
raw, 4 oz.	109	19.9	0	2.6	57	60	0
baked, broiled, or microwaved, 4 oz.	167	27.8	0	5.3	73	67	0
Tiramisu, see "Cake, frozen"							
Toaster bagel, muffin, and pastry, 1 pc.:							
all fruits (*Weight Watchers*)	190	2.0	38.0	3.0	0	180	2.0
apple (*Toaster Strudel*)	190	3.0	26.0	8.0	5	190	<1.0
apple cinnamon:							
(*Pop-Tarts*)	210	2.0	37.0	6.0	0	180	1.0
(*Pop-Tarts Pastry Swirls*)	250	2.0	37.0	11.0	0	180	<1.0
bagel, cream cheese:							
(*Toaster Bagel Shoppe*)	130	4.0	24.0	2.0	<5	230	<1.0
w/blueberry or strawberry (*Toaster Bagel Shoppe*) ..	130	4.0	24.0	1.5	0	190	<1.0
cinnamon raisin (*Toaster Bagel Shoppe*)	130	3.0	25.0	2.5	0	180	<1.0
berry, frosted:							
(*Pop-Tarts Snack-Stix*)	190	2.0	37.0	4.5	0	250	1.0
wild (*Pop-Tarts*) ...	210	2.0	39.0	5.0	0	170	1.0
blueberry:							
(*Eggo Toaster Delights*)	130	3.0	21.0	4.0	15	270	<1.0
(*Pop-Tarts*)	200	2.0	36.0	5.0	0	190	1.0
(*Thomas' Toast-r-Cakes*)	90	1.0	15.0	3.0	5	160	<1.0
(*Toaster Strudel*) ..	190	3.0	26.0	8.0	5	190	<1.0
frosted (*Pop-Tarts*)	200	2.0	37.0	5.0	0	170	1.0
brown sugar–cinnamon:							
(*Pop-Tarts*)	210	3.0	35.0	6.0	0	190	1.0
(*Toaster Strudel*) ..	190	3.0	26.0	8.0	5	230	<1.0
frosted (*Pop-Tarts*)	210	3.0	35.0	6.0	0	190	1.0
frosted (*Pop-Tarts Low Fat*)	190	2.0	39.0	3.0	0	230	1.0

Food and Measure	cal.	prot. (gms)	carbo. (gms)	fat (gms)	chol. (mgs)	sod. (mgs)	fiber (gms)
frosted (*Toastettes KoolStuf*)	190	2.0	34.0	5.0	0	170	<1.0
caramel apple (*Toaster Strudel*)	190	3.0	26.0	8.0	5	210	<1.0
cheese:							
(*Pop-Tarts Pastry Swirls*)	260	3.0	36.0	11.0	0	180	0
cherry (*Pop-Tarts Pastry Swirls*) ..	250	2.0	37.0	11.0	0	200	<1.0
cherry:							
(*Toaster Strudel*) ..	190	3.0	26.0	8.0	5	200	<1.0
(*Toastettes KoolStuf Burst*)	190	2.0	35.0	5.0	0	160	<1.0
frosted (*Pop-Tarts*)	200	2.0	38.0	5.0	0	170	1.0
chocolate:							
(*Toaster Strudel*) ..	190	3.0	25.0	9.0	5	180	<1.0
chip (*Pop-Tarts*) ...	200	3.0	35.0	6.0	0	230	<1.0
fudge, frosted (*Pop-Tarts*)	200	3.0	37.0	5.0	0	220	1.0
fudge, frosted (*Pop-Tarts Low Fat*) ..	190	3.0	39.0	3.0	0	270	2.0
chocolate-vanilla creme, frosted (*Pop-Tarts*)	200	3.0	37.0	5.0	0	220	1.0
cinnamon:							
(*Eggo Toaster Delights*)	130	3.0	20.0	4.5	15	270	0
creme (*Pop-Tarts Pastry Swirls*) ..	260	2.0	36.0	12.0	0	230	<1.0
cookies and creme (*Pop-Tarts Snack-Stix*)	200	3.0	35	6.0	0	280	<1.0
corn (*Thomas' Toast-r-Cakes*)	100	1.0	17.0	3.5	5	180	<1.0
cream cheese:							
(*Toaster Strudel Danish Style*) ...	200	3.0	23.0	11.0	15	230	<1.0
cherry, raspberry, or strawberry (*Toaster Strudel*)	200	3.0	24.0	10.0	10	220	0
eggs, w/cheese:							
(*Toaster Scrambles*)	180	4.0	14.0	12.0	25	400	0
and bacon (*Toaster Scrambles*)	180	4.0	14.0	12.0	25	380	0

Toaster bagel, muffin, and pastry, eggs, w/cheese (*cont.*)

Food and Measure	cal.	prot. (gms)	carbo. (gms)	fat (gms)	chol. (mgs)	sod. (mgs)	fiber (gms)
bacon and sausage combo (*Toaster Scrambles*)	180	4.0	14.0	12.0	25	370	0
ham or sausage (*Toaster Scrambles*)	180	4.0	14.0	12.0	25	370	0
Western (*Toaster Scrambles*)	170	4.0	14.0	11.0	25	340	0
frosted (*Pop-Tarts Wild Magicburst*) ..	200	2.0	37.0	6.0	0	180	1.0
fudge, frosted (*Toastettes KoolStuf Super Blast*)	180	2.0	32.0	5.0	0	220	<1.0
grape, frosted (*Pop-Tarts*)	200	2.0	38.0	5.0	0	170	<1.0
raisin bran (*Thomas' Toast-r-Cake*)	90	2.0	15.0	3.0	10	190	<1.0
raspberry:							
(*Toaster Strudel*) ..	190	3.0	26.0	8.0	5	200	0
frosted (*Pop-Tarts*)	210	3.0	37.0	5.0	0	170	<1.0
s'mores:							
(*KoolStuf Honey Maid*)	190	3.0	36.0	4.0	0	190	<1.0
frosted (*Pop-Tarts*)	200	3.0	36.0	6.0	0	200	1.0
strawberry:							
(*Eggo Toaster Delights*)	130	3.0	20.0	4.5	15	260	0
(*Pop-Tarts*)	200	2.0	37.0	5.0	0	190	1.0
(*Pop Tarts Pastry Swirls*)	260	2.0	38.0	11.0	0	170	<1.0
(*Toaster Strudel*) ..	190	3.0	26.0	8.0	5	190	<1.0
frosted (*Pop-Tarts*)	200	2.0	38.0	5.0	0	170	1.0
frosted (*Pop-Tarts Low Fat*)	190	2.0	39.0	3.0	0	210	1.0
frosted (*Pop-Tarts Snack-Stix*)	190	2.0	37.0	4.5	0	240	1.0
waffle:							
apple cinnamon or maple (*Eggo Waf-Fulls*)	150	2.0	25.0	5.0	10	310	<1.0
blueberry or strawberry (*Eggo Waf-Fulls*)	150	2.0	25.0	5.0	10	300	<1.0

Food and Measure	cal.	prot. (gms)	carbo. (gms)	fat (gms)	chol. (mgs)	sod. (mgs)	fiber (gms)
wildberry (*Toaster Strudel*)	190	3.0	25.0	9.0	5	190	<1.0
Toffee baking bits (*Skor*), 1 tbsp. ...	70	0	7.0	4.5	10	60	0
Toffee topping (*Heath* Shell), 2 tbsp.	230	<1.0	17.0	17.0	0	40	<1.0
Tofu:							
fresh, ½ cup	94	10.0	2.3	5.9	0	9	1.5
fresh, extra firm:							
(*Azumaya*), 2.8 oz.	70	8.0	<1.0	4.0	0	0	0
(*Azumaya* Lite), 2.8 oz.	60	9.0	3.0	2.0	0	80	2.0
(*Nasoya*), 3 oz. ...	90	8.0	3.0	5.0	0	0	0
fresh, firm:							
(*Azumaya*), 2.8 oz.	70	7.0	2.0	4.0	0	0	0
(*Frieda's*), 3 oz. ...	60	6.0	2.0	3.0	0	10	0
(*Nasoya*), 3 oz. ...	70	7.0	2.0	3.5	0	0	<1.0
(*Tree of Life* Organic/ Vacuum Pack), ⅕ block	100	9.0	2.0	5.0	0	5	0
(*Tree of Life* 30% Reduced Fat), ⅕ block	90	10.0	4.0	4.0	0	5	2.0
1 oz.	41	4.5	1.2	2.5	0	4	.7
½ cup	183	19.9	5.4	11.0	0	17	2.9
enriched (*Nasoya*), 3 oz.	45	7.0	0	1.0	0	30	0
fresh, silken:							
(*Azumaya*), 3.2 oz.	50	7.0	1.0	2.0	0	0	0
(*Azumaya* Lite), 3.2 oz.	40	7.0	1.0	1.0	0	70	1.0
(*Nasoya*), 3.2 oz.	45	4.0	2.0	2.5	0	5	0
enriched (*Nasoya*), ⅕ of 1-lb. block	40	7.0	1.0	1.0	0	65	0
fresh, soft (*Nasoya*), 3 oz.	60	7.0	1.0	3.5	0	0	0
fresh, flavored, 3 oz.:							
5-spice (*Nasoya*)	70	7.0	0	4.0	0	220	0
garlic onion (*Nasoya*)	70	7.0	1.0	4.0	0	250	0
baked, 2 pcs., except as noted:							
(*Tree of Life* Organic), ⅓ block	150	16.0	5.0	8.0	0	310	0

Food and Measure	cal.	prot. (gms)	carbo. (gms)	fat (gms)	chol. (mgs)	sod. (mgs)	fiber (gms)
Tofu, baked (*cont.*)							
chili picante							
(*Azumaya*)	200	20.0	9.0	10.0	0	320	2.0
mesquite (*Azumaya*)	190	20.0	6.0	10.0	0	480	2.0
mesquite smoke							
(*Nasoya*)	220	21.0	17.0	9.0	0	560	2.0
Oriental (*Tree of Life* Organic),							
⅓ block	130	15.0	5.0	7.0	0	330	0
savory or island spice (*Tree of Life* Organic),							
⅓ block	140	15.0	4.0	7.0	0	320	0
teriyaki (*Azumaya*)	200	20.0	9.0	10.0	0	730	2.0
teriyaki (*Nasoya*) ..	230	20.0	21.0	9.0	0	700	3.0
Tex-Mex (*Nasoya*)	230	21.0	21.0	9.0	0	360	4.0
Thai peanut							
(*Nasoya*)	240	21.0	19.0	10.0	0	540	3.0
Thai peanut, spicy							
(*Azumaya*)	190	20.0	6.0	10.0	0	500	2.0
salted and fermented							
(fuyu), 1 oz.	33	2.3	1.5	2.3	0	814	<1.0
smoked (*Tree of Life* Original), ½ block .	120	18.0	3.0	4.0	0	120	0
Tofu, ground (*Tree of Life Ready Ground*),							
3 oz.	60	7.0	2.0	4.0	0	10	0
Tofu pudding, see "Pudding, nondairy"							
Tofu sauce (*Westbrae Natural*), 1 tsp.	5	0	1.0	0	0	210	0
Tofu seasoning mix (*TofuMate*), ¼ pkg.:							
breakfast scramble ..	15	1.0	3.0	0	0	330	0
eggless salad	15	0	4.0	0	0	310	0
mandarin stir-fry	30	1.0	6.0	0	0	310	0
Mediterranean herb ..	15	1.0	3.0	0	0	330	0
Szechuan stir-fry	25	1.0	4.0	0	0	280	0
Texas taco	15	1.0	3.0	0	0	360	0
Tom and Jerry drink batter (*Trader Vic's*),							
1 tbsp.	116	2.0	23.0	2.0	35	240	0

Food and Measure	cal.	prot. (gms)	carbo. (gms)	fat (gms)	chol. (mgs)	sod. (mgs)	fiber (gms)
Tomatillo, fresh:							
(*Frieda's*), ⅔ cup,							
3 oz.	25	1.0	5.0	1.0	0	0	2.0
1 medium, 1⅝" diam.	11	.3	2.0	.4	0	tr.	.6
chopped, ½ cup	21	.6	3.8	.7	0	1	1.3
Tomatillo, canned:							
whole:							
(*Embasa*), 3 pcs.,							
2.1 oz.	15	0	3.0	0	0	15	2.0
(*La Costeña*), 4 pcs.,							
4.3 oz.	40	1.0	4.0	2.5	0	260	4.0
(*La Victoria* Entero),							
5 pcs., 4.5 oz. . .	40	1.0	7.0	1.0	0	410	5.0
crushed:							
(*Embasa*), ¼ cup . .	10	0	2.0	0	0	290	2.0
(*La Victoria*), 4.5 oz.	45	2.0	8.0	.5	0	400	7.0
Tomato, fresh, ripe:							
raw:							
(*Frieda's* Baby							
Roma/Teardrop),							
⅔ cup, 3 oz. . . .	20	1.0	4.0	0	0	10	1.0
2⅗" tomato	26	1.0	5.7	.4	0	11	1.4
chopped, 1 cup . . .	38	1.5	8.4	.6	0	16	2.0
boiled:							
2 medium, 8.8 oz. .	66	2.6	14.3	1.0	0	27	2.5
1 cup	65	2.6	14.0	1.0	0	27	2.4
dried, see "Tomato,							
dried"							
orange:							
3.9-oz. tomato	18	1.3	3.5	.2	0	47	1.0
chopped, 1 cup . . .	25	1.8	5.0	.3	0	66	1.4
yellow:							
7.8-oz. tomato	32	2.1	6.3	.6	0	49	1.5
chopped, 1 cup . . .	21	1.4	4.1	.4	0	32	1.0
Tomato, canned (see							
also "Tomato paste,"							
"Tomato puree," and							
"Tomato sauce")							
½ cup, except as							
noted:							
(*S&W Italian Recipe*) .	35	1.0	7.0	0	0	270	2.0
whole, peeled:							
(*Del Monte*)	25	1.0	6.0	0	0	250	2.0
(*Hunt's*)	20	<1.0	4.0	0	0	210	<1.0

Food and Measure	cal.	prot. (gms)	carbo. (gms)	fat (gms)	chol. (mgs)	sod. (mgs)	fiber (gms)
Tomato, canned, whole, peeled (*cont.*)							
(*Hunt's* No Salt) . . .	20	1.0	4.0	0	0	25	1.0
(*Progresso*)	25	1.0	5.0	0	0	220	1.0
(*Progresso* Italian) .	20	1.0	4.0	0	0	220	1.0
(*Red Gold*)	25	1.0	5.0	0	0	220	1.0
(*S&W*)	25	1.0	4.0	0	0	220	1.0
(*S&W* No Salt)	20	2.0	4.0	0	0	20	1.0
plain or basil (*Muir Glen*)	30	1.0	5.0	0	0	260	1.0
chunky:							
chili (*Del Monte*) . .	30	1.0	8.0	0	0	670	2.0
pasta (*Del Monte*) .	45	1.0	11.0	0	0	560	2.0
crushed:							
(*Contadina*), ¼ cup	20	<1.0	4.0	0	0	150	1.0
(*Del Monte* Original/ Italian)	45	2.0	9.0	0	0	390	1.0
(*Eden*)	20	1.0	3.0	0	0	0	1.0
(*Hunt's*)	30	2.0	6.0	0	0	340	1.0
(*Progresso*), ¼ cup	20	<1.0	3.0	0	0	95	1.0
(*S&W* Italian Style), ¼ cup	20	1.0	4.0	0	0	95	1.0
fire roasted (*Muir Glen*), ¼ cup . . .	20	1.0	5.0	0	0	160	1.0
w/garlic (*Del Monte*)	50	2.0	11.0	0	0	510	1.0
garlic, roasted (*Contadina*), ¼ cup	20	<1.0	3.0	0	0	150	1.0
heavy puree (*S&W*), ¼ cup	20	0	4.0	0	0	120	1.0
Italian herbs (*Contadina*), ¼ cup . . .	20	<1.0	3.0	0	0	150	<1.0
diced:							
(*Contadina*)	30	<1.0	6.0	0	0	200	1.0
(*Del Monte*)	25	1.0	6.0	0	0	250	2.0
(*Del Monte* No Salt)	25	1.0	6.0	0	0	50	2.0
(*Eden*)	30	1.0	6.0	0	0	5	2.0
(*Red Gold* Chili Ready)	35	1.0	8.0	0	0	220	1.0
(*Muir Glen*)	25	1.0	4.0	0	0	290	1.0
(*Muir Glen* No Salt)	25	1.0	4.0	0	0	45	1.0
(*Red Gold*)	25	1.0	5.0	0	0	220	1.0
(*S&W Ready Cut*)	25	1.0	4.0	0	0	190	1.0

Food and Measure	cal.	prot. (gms)	carbo. (gms)	fat (gms)	chol. (mgs)	sod. (mgs)	fiber (gms)
(S&W Ready Cut Pasta Sauce) ...	35	2.0	9.0	0	0	470	2.0
(S&W/S&W Ready Cut No Salt)	25	1.0	4.0	0	0	30	1.0
basil, garlic, oregano (Del Monte)	50	2.0	11.0	0	0	650	<1.0
basil, garlic, oregano (Hunt's)	25	<1.0	6.0	0	0	520	1.0
basil/garlic, garlic/ onion, green chili, or herb (Muir Glen)	25	1.0	4.0	0	0	290	1.0
fire roasted (Muir Glen), ¼ cup ...	30	1.0	6.0	0	0	290	1.0
garlic (S&W)	30	2.0	5.0	1.0	0	240	1.0
garlic, roasted (Contadina)	45	1.0	10.0	0	0	560	<1.0
garlic and onion (Del Monte)	40	2.0	8.0	.5	0	610	<1.0
green chili (Chi-Chi's), ¼ cup ...	20	0	4.0	0	0	290	0
green chili (Del Monte)	30	1.0	6.0	0	0	550	1.0
green chili (Eden) .	30	2.0	5.0	0	0	35	2.0
green chili (Red Gold)	25	1.0	5.0	0	0	340	1.0
green pepper, onion (Del Monte)	40	1.0	9.0	0	0	480	<2.0
Italian (Red Gold)	50	1.0	7.0	2.0	0	270	1.0
Italian (S&W)	25	1.0	4.0	0	0	190	1.0
Italian herb (Contadina)	45	1.0	10.0	0	0	470	<1.0
jalapeño (Del Monte)	30	1.0	6.0	0	0	540	1.0
jalapeño (S&W) ..	25	2.0	5.0	0	0	290	<1.0
onion (S&W)	35	2.0	6.0	0	0	310	1.0
onion, sauteed (Contadina)	40	1.0	9.0	0	0	300	<1.0
diced, in puree: (S&W Ready Cut)	30	2.0	6.0	0	0	410	2.0
medium (S&W) ...	30	2.0	6.0	0	0	410	2.0
ground, peeled (Muir Glen), ¼ cup	10	<1.0	2.0	0	0	100	2.0

Food and Measure	cal.	prot. (gms)	carbo. (gms)	fat (gms)	chol. (mgs)	sod. (mgs)	fiber (gms)
Tomato, canned (*cont.*)							
stewed:							
(*Contadina*)	35	1.0	9.0	.0	0	220	1.0
(*Del Monte*)	35	1.0	9.0	0	0	360	2.0
(*Del Monte* No Salt)	35	1.0	9.0	0	0	50	2.0
(*Hunt's*)	30	<1.0	7.0	0	0	370	1.0
(*Muir Glen*)	30	1.0	7.0	0	0	290	<1.0
(*S&W*)	35	1.0	7.0	0	0	270	2.0
(*S&W* No Salt)	35	1.0	7.0	0	0	15	2.0
Cajun (*Del Monte*)	35	1.0	9.0	0	0	460	2.0
Cajun, Italian, or							
Mexican (*S&W*)	35	1.0	7.0	0	0	270	2.0
Italian (*Contadina*)	35	1.0	8.0	0	0	260	1.0
Italian (*Del Monte*)	30	1.0	8.0	0	0	420	2.0
Mexican (*Del*							
Monte)	35	1.0	9.0	0	0	400	2.0
wedges (*Del Monte*)	35	1.0	9.0	0	0	380	2.0
Tomato, dried:							
(*Roland* Sun-dried),							
2 pcs.	45	2.0	8.0	0	0	45	2.0
1 oz.	73	4.0	15.8	.8	0	594	3.5
1 pc., 32 pcs. per cup	5	.3	1.1	.1	0	42	.3
½ cup	70	3.8	15.3	.8	0	500	3.3
bits (*Sonoma*), 2 tsp.	15	1.0	3.0	0	0	5	1.0
halves (*Sonoma*),							
2 pcs.	15	1.0	2.0	0	0	5	1.0
halves or chopped							
(*Frieda's*), ⅓ cup,							
1.1 oz.	100	2.0	19.0	1.0	0	10	2.0
marinated, in oil:							
(*Frieda's* Julienne							
Marinated),							
1 tbsp.	35	1.0	4.0	2.0	0	60	1.0
(*Hogue Farms*),							
3 pcs.	40	1.0	3.0	2.5	0	5	1.0
(*Norpaco*), 1 tbsp.	60	2.0	6.0	3.0	0	20	2.0
(*Sonoma*),							
2–3 halves	35	1.0	3.0	2.5	0	5	1.0
drained, ½ cup . . .	117	2.8	12.8	7.7	0	146	3.2
julienne (*Sonoma*),							
8 strips	35	1.0	3.0	2.5	0	5	1.0
and roasted garlic							
(*Sonoma*),							
8 strips	40	1.0	4.0	3.0	0	40	1.0

Food and Measure	cal.	prot. (gms)	carbo. (gms)	fat (gms)	chol. (mgs)	sod. (mgs)	fiber (gms)
yellow, halves or chopped (*Frieda's*), ½ cup, 3 oz.	220	12.0	47.0	2.5	0	1780	10.0
Tomato, dried, blend: (*Frieda's* Tomato Toss), ½ cup, 1.1 oz. ...	100	6.0	19.0	0	0	105	4.0
(*Sonoma Toss-Ta*), ½ cup	70	4.0	13.0	0	0	75	3.0
(*Sonoma Toss-Ta* Ranchero), 3 tsp.	15	1.0	3.0	0	0	80	1.0
in oil (*Sonoma* Spice Medley), drained, 1 tbsp.	50	1.0	3.0	4.0	0	200	1.0
Tomato, dried, seasoning (*Sonoma* Season It), 2 tsp.	20	1.0	3.0	0	0	25	1.0
Tomato, green, raw, 1 large, 6.4 oz. ...	44	2.2	9.3	.4	0	24	2.0
Tomato, pickled: (*Ba-Tampte*), ½ pc., 1.5 oz.	5	0	1.0	0	0	310	0
(*Claussen*). 1 oz. ...	5	0	1.0	0	0	320	<1.0
Tomato, sun-dried, see "Tomato, dried"							
Tomato dip mix, 1 tsp.:							
bacon (*Watkins*)	10	1.0	2.0	0	0	170	0
horseradish (*Watkins*)	10	0	2.0	0	0	100	0
Tomato juice, 8 fl. oz.:							
(*Campbell's*)	50	1.0	10.0	0	0	750	1.0
(*Del Monte*)	50	2.0	10.0	0	0	760	1.0
(*Del Monte* Not from Concentrate)	40	3.0	7.0	0	0	550	0
(*Eden*)	35	1.0	6.0	1.0	0	560	1.0
(*Muir Glen*)	40	3.0	7.0	0	0	620	1.0
(*R. W. Knudsen*)	60	2.0	14.0	0	0	390	0
(*Red Gold*)	45	1.0	10.0	0	0	750	2.0
(*Red Gold* No Salt) ..	45	1.0	10.0	0	0	25	2.0
(*Sacramento*)	40	3.0	8.0	0	0	550	2.0
(*Welch's*)	50	2.0	10.0	0	0	730	2.0
Tomato flakes (*Alpine-Aire*), .5 oz.	50	2.0	10.0	0	0	20	1.0
Tomato paste, 2 tbsp.:							
(*Contadina*)	30	2.0	6.0	0	0	20	1.0
(*Del Monte*)	30	1.0	7.0	0	0	25	2.0

Food and Measure	cal.	prot. (gms)	carbo. (gms)	fat (gms)	chol. (mgs)	sod. (mgs)	fiber (gms)
Tomato paste (*cont.*)							
(*Hunt's*)	25	1.0	6.0	0	0	85	2.0
(*Muir Glen*)	30	2.0	6.0	0	0	20	1.0
(*Progresso*)	30	2.0	6.0	0	0	20	1.0
(*Red Gold*)	30	2.0	6.0	0	0	20	1.0
Italian seasoning (*Contadina*)	35	1.0	7.0	.5	0	290	1.0
garlic, roasted (*Contadina*)	35	1.0	6.0	.5	0	300	1.0
pesto (*Contadina*) . . .	35	1.0	5.0	.5	0	300	<1.0
Tomato pesto, see "Pesto sauce"							
Tomato powder (*AlpineAire*), .67 oz.	70	3.0	13.0	.5	0	25	0
Tomato puree, ¼ cup:							
(*Contadina*)	20	<1.0	4.0	0	0	15	<1.0
(*Muir Glen*)	20	1.0	5.0	0	0	20	1.0
(*Progresso*)	25	1.0	5.0	0	0	15	1.0
(*Red Gold*)	25	1.0	5.0	0	0	10	1.0
thick (*Progresso*)	20	<1.0	5.0	0	0	15	1.0
Tomato relish, 1 tbsp., except as noted:							
(*Country Sides* Garden Style), ¼ cup	50	<1.0	11.0	0	0	170	1.0
(*Heinz* Piccalilli)	15	0	4.0	0	0	75	0
hot (*Mrs. Renfro's*) . .	10	0	3.0	0	0	40	0
medium, Indian (*Patak's*)	10	0	2.0	.5	0	70	0
mild (*Mrs. Renfro's*)	10	0	3.0	0	0	45	0
Tomato sauce, can or jar (see also "Pasta sauce" and "Tomato, canned"), ¼ cup:							
(*Contadina*)	15	<1.0	3.0	0	0	280	<1.0
(*Contadina* Extra Thick & Zesty)	20	1.0	3.0	0	0	340	1.0
(*Del Monte*)	20	<1.0	4.0	0	0	340	<1.0
(*Del Monte* No Salt) . .	20	<1.0	4.0	0	0	20	<1.0
(*Goya*)	20	1.0	4.0	0	0	280	1.0
(*Hunt's*)	15	1.0	3.0	0	0	380	<1.0
(*Hunt's* for Chili)	25	1.0	5.0	0	0	460	1.0
(*Hunt's* for Lasagna) .	40	2.0	8.0	.5	0	430	1.0
(*Hunt's* for Meat Loaf)	30	1.0	7.0	0	0	410	2.0
(*Hunt's* No Salt)	15	1.0	3.0	0	0	15	<1.0

Food and Measure	cal.	prot. (gms)	carbo. (gms)	fat (gms)	chol. (mgs)	sod. (mgs)	fiber (gms)
(*Hunt's* for Pasta) ...	50	2.0	11.0	1.0	0	810	2.0
(*Hunt's* for Tacos) ...	15	<1.0	4.0	0	0	470	<1.0
(*Muir Glen*)	20	<1.0	4.0	0	0	310	1.0
(*Muir Glen* Chunky) ..	20	<1.0	4.0	0	0	160	1.0
(*Muir Glen* No Salt) ..	20	<1.0	5.0	0	0	30	1.0
(*Progresso*)	20	1.0	4.0	0	0	260	1.0
(*Red Gold*)	20	0	5.0	0	0	280	1.0
(*S&W*)	20	1.0	4.0	0	0	260	1.0
w/garlic and onion (*Contadina's*)	20	<1.0	4.0	0	0	270	<1.0
w/herbs and cheese ..	36	1.3	6.2	1.2	0	331	1.3
Italian style (*Contadina*)	15	<1.0	4.0	0	0	320	<1.0
w/onions	26	1.0	6.1	.1	0	338	1.1
w/onions, green pepper, and celery	26	.6	5.5	.5	0	341	.9
w/tomato tidbits, no salt	20	.8	4.3	.1	0	9	.9
Tomato tapenade, sun-dried:							
(*Sonoma*), 1 tbsp. ...	70	1.0	4.0	6.0	0	5	1.0
(*Susan Elaine's* Tuscan), 2 tbsp.	33	0	6.0	1.0	0	92	1.0
Tomato-beef drink (*Beefamato*), 8 fl. oz.	50	0	11.0	0	0	830	0
Tomato-chili cocktail (*Snap-E-Tom*):							
6 fl. oz.	40	2.0	8.0	0	0	500	1.0
10 fl. oz.	60	3.0	13.0	0	0	840	2.0
Tomato-clam drink, 8 fl. oz.:							
(*Clamato*)	60	1.0	11.0	0	0	880	1.0
(*Clamato* Bloody Caesar)	50	1.0	12.0	0	0	860	0
(*Clamato* Picante) ...	60	1.0	13.0	0	0	930	0
Tomato-olive relish (*Sonoma* Muffaletta), drained, 2 tbsp. ..	70	1.0	3.0	6.0	0	140	1.0
Tongue, braised:							
beef, 4 oz.	321	25.1	.4	23.5	121	68	0
lamb, 4 oz.	312	24.5	0	23.0	214	76	0
pork, 4 oz.	307	27.3	0	21.1	166	124	0
veal (calves), 4 oz. ...	229	29.3	0	11.5	n.a.	73	0

Food and Measure	cal.	prot. (gms)	carbo. (gms)	fat (gms)	chol. (mgs)	sod. (mgs)	fiber (gms)
Tongue lunch meat, beef, 2 oz.:							
and bloodwurst (*Boar's Head*)	170	10.0	1.0	14.0	90	380	0
corned (*Hebrew National*)	120	10.0	0	9.0	50	330	0
Tortellini (see also "Tortelloni"), refrigerated:							
cheese, 1 cup:							
(*Celentano*)	420	18.0	68.0	8.0	26	520	3.0
three (*Buitoni*)	290	13.0	49.0	5.0	30	510	3.0
chicken and herb (*Buitoni*), ¾ cup ..	260	10.0	40.0	7.0	35	250	2.0
meat (*Celentano*), 1 cup	340	21.0	55.0	4.0	35	200	3.0
spinach cheese (*Buitoni*), ¾ cup ..	260	12.0	40.0	6.0	40	370	3.0
Tortellini entree, canned, meat (*Chef Boyardee*), 7.5 oz.	260	12.0	48.0	3.5	30	810	4.0
Tortellini entree, frozen, 1 pkg.:							
cheese:							
(*Healthy Choice* Bowl), 10.35 oz.	320	14.0	50.0	7.0	60	600	4.0
(*Wolfgang Puck's*), 12 oz.	360	13.0	49.0	13.0	40	420	13.0
chicken, spicy (*Wolfgang Puck's*), 12 oz.	490	16.0	51.0	24.0	90	910	6.0
mushroom (*Wolfgang Puck's*), 12 oz. ...	430	14.0	54.0	18.0	40	660	6.0
Tortelloni (see also "Tortellini"), refrigerated, 1 cup:							
cheese and roasted garlic (*Buitoni*) ...	270	12.0	38.0	8.0	30	260	2.0
chicken, lemon (*Di Giorno*)	270	11.0	42.0	7.0	35	380	1.0
chicken and prosciutto (*Buitoni*)	360	15.0	45.0	13.0	60	400	1.0
mozzarella and cheese (*Buitoni*)	320	15.0	45.0	9.0	50	360	2.0

Food and Measure	cal.	prot. (gms)	carbo. (gms)	fat (gms)	chol. (mgs)	sod. (mgs)	fiber (gms)
mozzarella, garlic (*Di Giorno*)	300	15.0	42.0	8.0	45	400	1.0
pesto (*Di Giorno*)	320	16.0	49.0	7.0	45	410	3.0
sausage, Italian, and tomato (*Di Giorno*)	350	14.0	51.0	9.0	40	450	3.0
Tortilla (see also "Wraps"):							
corn (*Azteca*), 2 pcs., 1.2 oz.	90	2.0	18.0	1.0	0	15	2.0
flour, 1 pc., except as noted:							
(*Azteca*), 2 pcs., 1.7 oz.	150	4.0	27.0	3.0	0	320	2.0
(*Azteca*), 1.4-oz. pc.	130	4.0	23.0	2.5	0	270	2.0
(*Azteca* Burrito Size), 1.75 oz.	160	4.0	28.0	3.0	0	330	3.0
(*Azteca* Fat Free), 1.4-oz. pc.	110	3.0	24.0	0	0	340	1.0
(*Old El Paso*), 2 pcs.	160	3.0	26.0	4.5	0	370	0
soft taco (*Old El Paso*), 2 pcs.	160	3.0	26.0	4.5	0	350	0
Tortilla chips, see "Corn chips/crisps"							
Tortilla entree, frozen (*Michelina's* Sunset), 8-oz. pkg.	310	11.0	43.0	9.0	25	730	2.0
Tostado shell, see "Taco shell"							
Trail mix, 3 tbsp., except as noted:							
(*AlpineAire* Bear Ate My Food), 4 oz. ..	550	9.0	67.0	27.0	0	20	6.0
(*AlpineAire* Bits of Hawaii), 4 oz. ...	380	0	84.0	5.0	0	75	5.0
(*AlpineAire* Call Me Tamari), 4 oz.	640	22.0	26.0	50.0	0	530	7.0
(*AlpineAire* Can't Get Out of the Tent), 4 oz.	540	14.0	53.0	30.0	0	15	15.0
(*AlpineAire* Nanners on the Trail), 2.5 oz. ..	340	1.0	45.0	18.0	0	0	0
(*AlpineAire* No Fish in the Lake), 4 oz. ...	530	11.0	68.0	24.0	0	35	6.0

Food and Measure	cal	prot. (gms)	carbo. (gms)	fat (gms)	chol. (mgs)	sod. (mgs)	fiber (gms)
Trail mix (*cont.*)							
(*AlpineAire* Over the Top), 4 oz.	560	9.0	60.0	32.0	0	10	9.0
(*AlpineAire* Stumbling Down the Trail), 4 oz.	550	13.0	60.0	29.0	0	50	7.0
(*AlpineAire* Trail Blazer), 4 oz.	620	19.0	38.0	44.0	0	15	11.0
(*Estee* Fruit & Nuts), ¼ cup	210	6.0	19.0	12.0	<5	45	2.0
(*Sonoma*), ¼ cup, 1.4 oz.	160	3.0	24.0	7.0	0	5	2.0
apple cranberry crunch (*Planters*) . .	140	0	10.0	11.0	0	50	2.0
Cajun crunch (*Planters*), ⅓ cup .	130	1.0	20.0	5.0	0	310	2.0
caramel nut crunch (*Planters*)	140	2.0	15.0	8.0	0	100	1.0
Caribbean crunch (*Planters*)	140	2.0	12.0	10.0	0	75	2.0
fruit and nuts:							
(*Planters* 6 oz.) . . .	130	3.0	14.0	7.0	0	10	1.0
(*Planters* 10 oz.) . .	120	2.0	14.0	7.0	0	10	2.0
nuts and chocolate (*Planters*)	170	2.0	16.0	11.0	0	20	2.0
nuts and raisins (*Planters*)	160	4.0	11.0	12.0	0	15	3.0
Tree fern, cooked, chopped, ½ cup . .	28	.2	7.8	.1	0	3	2.6
Triticale, whole-grain, 1 cup	646	25.1	138.5	4.0	0	10	34.8
Triticale flour, whole-grain, 1 cup	440	17.1	95.1	2.4	0	3	19.0
Tropical punch, see "Fruit punch"							
Trout, meat only:							
mixed species:							
raw, 4 oz.	168	23.6	0	7.5	66	59	0
baked, broiled, or microwaved, 4 oz.	215	30.2	0	9.6	84	76	0
rainbow, farmed:							
raw, 4 oz.	156	23.7	0	6.1	67	40	0
baked, broiled, or microwaved, 4 oz.	192	27.5	0	8.2	77	48	0

Food and Measure	cal.	prot. (gms)	carbo. (gms)	fat (gms)	chol. (mgs)	sod. (mgs)	fiber (gms)
rainbow, wild:							
raw, 4 oz.	135	23.2	0	3.9	67	35	0
baked, broiled, or							
microwaved, 4 oz.	170	26.0	0	6.6	78	64	0
sea, see "Sea trout"							
Trout, smoked, 2 oz.:							
(*Ducktrap River*)	110	14.0	0	6.0	15	590	
peppered, rainbow							
(*Spence & Co.*) . . .	100	14.0	0	5.0	30	430	0
Trout, smoked, canned,							
golden (*Reese*),							
3.75-oz. can drained	110	20.0	0	12.0	65	430	0
Trout, smoked, pâté,							
¼ cup:							
(*Ducktrap River*)	130	9.0	1.0	10.0	25	380	0
(*Ducktrap River*							
Lowfat)	70	10.0	1.0	3.0	5	280	0
Tuna, meat only:							
bluefin:							
raw, 4 oz.	163	26.5	0	5.6	43	44	0
baked, broiled, or							
microwaved, 4 oz.	209	33.9	0	7.1	56	57	0
skipjack:							
raw, 4 oz.	117	25.0	0	1.2	53	42	0
baked, broiled, or							
microwaved, 4 oz.	150	32.0	0	1.5	68	53	0
yellowfin:							
raw, 4 oz.	123	26.5	0	1.1	51	42	0
baked, broiled, or							
microwaved, 4 oz.	158	34.0	0	1.4	66	53	0
Tuna, canned, drained,							
2 oz. or ¼ cup,							
except as noted:							
chunk light, in oil:							
(*Bumble Bee*)	110	13.0	0	6.0	30	250	0
(*Chicken of the Sea*)	110	13.0	0	6.0	30	250	0
(*Star-Kist*)	110	13.0	0	6.0	30	250	0
(*Star-Kist* Pouch) . .	110	11.5	0	6.0	30	250	0
chunk light, in water:							
(*Bumble Bee*)	60	13.0	0	.5	30	250	0
(*Bumble Bee*), 3 oz.	70	15.0	0	1.0	40	350	0
(*Chicken of the Sea*)	60	13.0	0	.5	30	250	0
(*Chicken of the Sea*							
50% Less Salt) .	60	13.0	0	.5	30	125	0

Food and Measure	cal.	prot. (gms)	carbo. (gms)	fat (gms)	chol. (mgs)	sod. (mgs)	fiber (gms)
Tuna, canned, chunk light, in water (*cont.*)							
(*Chicken of the Sea Low Sodium*) . . .	60	13.0	0	.5	30	90	0
(*Crown Prince Natural* Tongol)	60	14.0	0	0	35	140	0
(*Crown Prince Natural* Tongol Low Sodium) . . .	60	14.0	0	0	35	50	0
(*Star-Kist*)	60	13.0	0	.5	30	250	0
chunk white, in water:							
(*Chicken of the Sea*)	60	13.0	0	1.0	25	250	0
(*Chicken of the Sea* Very Low Sodium)	60	14.0	0	.5	25	35	0
(*Star-Kist*)	60	13.0	0	1.0	25	250	0
solid, in olive oil:							
(*Chicken of the Sea Genova*)	130	14.0	0	8.0	30	250	0
(*Progresso*)	160	13.0	0	12.0	30	250	0
solid white, in oil:							
(*Bumble Bee*)	90	14.0	0	3.0	25	250	0
(*Bumble Bee*), 3 oz.	130	19.0	0	5.0	35	350	0
(*Chicken of the Sea*)	90	14.0	0	3.0	25	250	0
(*Star-Kist*)	90	15.0	0	3.0	25	250	0
solid white, in water:							
(*Bumble Bee*)	70	15.0	0	1.0	25	250	0
(*Bumble Bee*), 3 oz.	90	20.0	0	1.0	35	350	0
(*Chicken of the Sea*)	70	15.0	0	1.0	25	250	0
(*Crown Prince Natural* Albacore)	65	15.0	0	.5	30	150	0
(*Crown Prince Natural* Albacore Low Sodium) . . .	65	15.0	0	0	0	80	0
Tuna, freeze-dried, Albacore (*Alpine-Aire*), 1 oz.	110	26.0	0	.5	0	0	0
"Tuna," vegetarian, drained:							
canned, ⅓ cup:							
(*Natural Touch Tuno*)	60	7.0	2.0	2.0	0	360	1.0
(*Worthington Tuno*)	80	7.0	4.0	4.0	0	380	1.0

Food and Measure	cal.	prot. (gms)	carbo. (gms)	fat (gms)	chol. (mgs)	sod. (mgs)	fiber (gms)
frozen:							
(*Worthington Tuno*),							
½ cup	80	6.0	2.0	6.0	0	290	1.0
(*Veggie Master*							
Vege Fillet),							
¼ pkg.	104	6.7	3.8	6.3	0	219	7.0
Tuna burger, frozen,							
3.2-oz. pc.:							
(*Ocean Beauty*)	90	17.0	3.0	1.0	40	350	0
(*Omega Foods*)	90	19.0	3.0	.5	5	183	0
Tuna entree, dried,							
w/noodles, cheese							
(*AlpineAire*),							
1½ cups	310	17.0	40.0	9.0	20	840	2.0
Tuna entree, frozen,							
1 pkg.:							
(*Healthy Choice* Solo							
Casserole), 9 oz. ...	240	15.0	30.0	7.0	25	580	4.0
and noodle:							
(*Marie Callender's*							
Homestyle),							
10 oz.	430	14.0	34.0	27.0	60	1260	5.0
(*Stouffer's* Cas-							
serole), 10 oz. ...	360	18.0	36.0	16.0	30	1060	2.0
Tuna entree mix (*Tuna*							
Helper), 1 cup*:							
au gratin	310	13.0	38.0	12.0	20	920	1.0
au gratin, less fat	250	13.0	38.0	6.0	15	880	1.0
broccoli:							
cheesy	270	12.0	31.0	11.0	20	870	<1.0
cheesy, less fat ...	220	12.0	31.0	5.0	15	820	<1.0
creamy	290	12.0	33.0	13.0	15	830	1.0
creamy, less fat ...	230	12.0	33.0	5.0	15	780	1.0
cheddar, garden	290	13.0	36.0	11.0	20	990	1.0
cheddar, garden,							
less fat	240	13.0	36.0	5.0	15	950	1.0
fettuccine Alfredo ...	310	14.0	32.0	14.0	15	950	1.0
fettuccine Alfredo,							
less fat	240	14.0	32.0	6.0	15	870	1.0
pasta,:							
cheesy	270	12.0	31.0	11.0	20	870	<1.0
cheesy, less fat ...	220	12.0	31.0	5.0	15	820	<1.0
creamy	290	12.0	32.0	13.0	15	880	2.0
creamy, less fat ...	230	12.0	32.0	6.0	15	830	2.0

Food and Measure	cal.	prot. (gms)	carbo. (gms)	fat (gms)	chol. (mgs)	sod. (mgs)	fiber (gms)
Tuna entree mix (*cont.*)							
tetrazzini	300	14.0	34.0	12.0	20	970	1.0
tetrazzini, less fat	240	14.0	34.0	5.0	15	910	1.0
tuna melt	300	12.0	34.0	13.0	20	920	0
tuna melt, less fat . . .	240	12.0	34.0	6.0	15	870	0
Tuna salad:							
(*Sabra Salads*), 1 oz.	85	3.0	3.4	6.7	9	169	1.0
(*Wampler*), ⅓ cup . .	180	7.0	9.0	12.0	20	450	1.0
chunky (*Wampler*), ⅓ cup	180	4.0	8.0	13.0	20	380	1.0
Tuna salad kit:							
(*Bumble Bee*), 3.5 oz.	190	8.0	6.0	15.0	15	270	1.0
(*Bumble Bee* Fat Free), 3.5 oz.	90	7.0	10.0	0	15	380	0
w/crackers (*Bumble Bee*), 3.8 oz.	250	17.0	15.0	13.0	45	550	0
Tuna seasoning (*Old Bay Classic*), ⅕ pkg.	30	0	2.0	1.0	0	120	0
Turban squash (*Frieda's*), ¾ cup, 3 oz.	30	1.0	7.0	0	0	0	1.0
Turbot, European, meat only:							
raw, 4 oz.	108	18.2	0	3.4	54	170	0
baked, broiled, or microwaved, 4 oz.	138	23.3	0	4.3	70	218	0
Turkey (see also "Turkey, frozen and refrigerated"), fresh, all classes, roasted:							
meat w/skin, 4 oz. . .	236	31.9	0	11.0	93	77	0
meat only:							
4 oz.	193	3.2	0	5.6	86	79	0
diced, 1 cup	238	41.0	0	7.0	107	99	0
skin only, 1 oz.	125	5.6	0	11.2	32	15	0
dark meat:							
w/skin, 4 oz.	251	31.2	0	13.1	101	86	0
meat only, 4 oz. . .	212	32.4	0	8.2	96	90	0
meat only, diced, 1 cup	262	40.0	0	10.1	119	110	0
light meat:							
w/skin, 4 oz.	223	32.4	0	9.4	86	71	0
meat only, 4 oz. . .	178	33.9	0	3.7	78	73	0

Food and Measure	cal.	prot. (gms)	carbo. (gms)	fat (gms)	chol. (mgs)	sod. (mgs)	fiber (gms)
meat only, diced, 1 cup	219	41.9	0	4.5	97	89	0
breast, meat w/skin:							
½ breast, 1.9 lbs., (4.2 lbs. raw w/bone)........	1637	248.1	0	64.1	643	541	0
4 oz.	214	32.6	0	8.4	84	71	0
ground, see "Turkey ground"							
leg, meat w/skin:							
1.2 lbs. (1.5 lbs. raw w/bone)	1133	152.2	0	53.6	466	420	0
4 oz.	236	31.6	0	11.1	96	87	0
wing, meat w/skin:							
6.6 oz. (9.9 oz. raw w/bone)	426	50.9	0	23.1	150	114	0
4 oz.	260	31.0	0	14.1	92	69	0
Turkey, canned, chunk, 2 oz.:							
(*Hormel*)	70	11.0	0	3.0	35	340	0
white (*Hormel*)	60	13.0	0	1.0	25	330	0
Turkey, cured, dark (*Wampler*), 2 oz. .	80	8.0	2.0	4.5	30	600	0
Turkey, freeze-dried, diced (*AlpineAire*), .5 oz.	60	12.0	0	1.5	45	25	0
Turkey, frozen or re- frigerated, raw, 4 oz., except as noted:							
whole:							
(*Jennie-O*)	170	22.0	0	8.0	85	120	0
(*Norbest* Gold Label Hen)	195	22.0	0	12.0	65	95	0
(*Norbest* Tender- Times Hen)	170	22.0	0	8.0	75	190	0
(*Norbest* Tender- Times Tom)	180	21.0	0	10.0	65	180	0
whole, young:							
(*Norbest* Family Tradition Tom) ..	170	23.0	0	8.5	80	80	0
(*Norbest* Family Traditions/Free Range Hen)	190	23.0	0	10.0	70	70	0

Food and Measure	cal.	prot. (gms)	carbo. (gms)	fat (gms)	chol. (mgs)	sod. (mgs)	fiber (gms)
Turkey, frozen or refrigerated, raw, whole, young (*cont.*)							
(*Norbest* Free Range Tom)	170	23.0	0	9.0	80	80	0
(*Shady Brook Farms* Prime)	180	23.0	0	9.0	85	75	0
basted (*Jennie-O* Young Frozen) . .	160	21.0	0	8.0	80	260	0
boneless:							
(*Jennie-O* Young) . .	170	21.0	0	8.0	70	160	0
(*Jennie-O* Frozen)	140	21.0	0	6.0	60	930	0
roast (*Norbest*) . . .	135	18.0	0	7.0	65	490	0
breast:							
(*Empire* Kosher Hen)	160	24.0	0	6.0	70	180	0
(*Jennie-O*)	170	23.0	0	8.0	70	105	0
(*Norbest* Tender-Timed)	170	22.0	0	9.0	60	270	0
(*Shady Brook Farms* Hotel Style)	180	24.0	0	9.0	85	65	0
(*Shady Brook Farms* Prime Young) . .	180	24.0	0	9.0	70	60	0
basted (*Jennie-O*)	170	21.0	0	7.0	60	740	0
split (*Shady Brook Farms*)	190	24.0	0	9.0	70	60	0
split, rotisserie (*Shady Brook Farms*)	180	23.0	0	9.0	65	400	0
split, honey roast (*Shady Brook Farms*)	190	24.0	4.0	9.0	65	170	0
breast, boneless:							
(*Jennie-O* Young) . .	170	22.0	0	8.0	65	150	0
(*Jennie-O* Young Frozen)	130	22.0	0	2.5	50	990	0
chops (*Shady Brook Farms*)	160	23.0	0	7.0	70	260	0
cutlet (*Shady Brook Farms*)	130	28.0	0	.5	70	55	0
cutlet, thin (*Perdue Fit 'n Easy*), 3.3 oz.	100	23.0	0	1.0	50	45	0
fillet (*Perdue*)	120	27.0	0	1.0	60	55	0

Food and Measure	cal.	prot. (gms)	carbo. (gms)	fat (gms)	chol. (mgs)	sod. (mgs)	fiber (gms)
London broil (*Perdue Fit 'n Easy*)	120	27.0	0	1.0	60	55	0
London broil (*Shady Brook Farms*)	130	28.0	0	.5	70	55	0
slices (*Jennie-O*) ..	90	22.0	0	.5	40	55	0
tenders (*Empire* Kosher)	120	26.0	0	1.5	70	70	0
breast half, marinated rotisserie (*Perdue*) .	170	20.0	2.0	9.0	55	390	0
drums (*Empire* Kosher)	110	19.0	0	4.0	85	110	0
drumstick (*Shady Brook Farms*)	140	18.0	0	7.0	55	50	0
ground, see "Turkey, ground"							
hindquarter (*Jennie-O*)	180	21.0	0	12.0	80	80	0
leg quarter (*Shady Brook Farms*)	170	22.0	0	9.0	70	80	0
pan roast, 5 oz.:							
(*Jennie-O* Extra Lean)	120	20.0	0	3.0	55	780	0
(*Jennie-O* Fat Free)	100	20.0	0	0	40	720	0
combo (*Jennie-O*)	150	20.0	0	7.0	60	750	0
white (*Jennie-O*) ..	150	20.0	0	7.0	55	760	0
tenderloin:							
(*Jennie-O*)	120	28.0	0	.5	50	70	0
(*Perdue Fit 'n Easy*)	120	27.0	0	1.0	60	55	0
(*Shady Brook Farms*)	130	28.0	0	.5	70	55	0
butter garlic (*Perdue*)	110	24.0	2.0	1.0	55	740	0
cracked black pepper (*Perdue*) .	110	2.0	1.0	1.0	50	810	0
thigh (*Shady Brook Farms*)	145	20.0	0	7.0	75	80	0
wing:							
(*Shady Brook Farms*)	220	23.0	0	14.0	80	60	0
portion (*Shady Brook Farms*) ...	240	23.0	0	16.0	75	60	0

Food and Measure	cal.	prot. (gms)	carbo. (gms)	fat (gms)	chol. (mgs)	sod. (mgs)	fiber (gms)
Turkey, frozen or re-frigerated, cooked, 3 oz., except as noted:							
(*Boar's Head Deli Dinners Ovengold*)	90	18.0	1.0	2.0	55	540	0
whole:							
dark (*Perdue* Hen)	180	20.0	0	11.0	85	65	0
dark (*Perdue* Tom)	160	21.0	0	9.0	90	55	0
white (*Perdue* Hen)	150	22.0	0	7.0	65	45	0
white (*Perdue* Tom)	140	23.0	0	5.0	65	50	0
barbecued (*Empire* Kosher), 5 oz. . . .	250	35.0	0	12.0	100	320	0
oven-roasted (*Shady Brook Farm*)	130	17.0	1.0	6.0	50	540	0
smoked (*Norbest*)	145	16.0	0	9.0	50	720	0
smoked (*Shady Brook Farms*) . . .	150	24.0	3.0	4.0	60	660	0
breast:							
(*Perdue* Whole) . .	150	22.0	0	7.0	60	40	0
(*Perdue* Half) . . .	150	23.0	0	7.0	75	40	0
cutlet, thin sliced (*Perdue Fit 'n Easy*), 2.4 oz. . .	90	20.0	0	.5	45	30	0
fillet, London broil, or tenderloin (*Perdue Fit 'n Easy*)	110	26.0	0	.5	60	40	0
oven-roasted (*Jennie-O*), 2 oz.	70	11.0	0	2.0	25	450	0
oven-roasted (*Shady Brook Farms*)	60	13.0	1.0	0	35	520	0
breast, flavored:							
garlic peppered (*Jennie-O*), 2 oz.	50	11.0	0	0	20	400	0
honey cured (*Jennie-O*), 2 oz.	80	10.0	0	2.5	30	690	0
honey roast (*Shady Brook Farms*) . . .	70	13.0	4.0	0	30	510	0
rotisserie (*Jennie-O*), 2 oz.	60	12.0	0	0	25	580	0

Food and Measure	cal.	prot. (gms)	carbo. (gms)	fat (gms)	chol. (mgs)	sod. (mgs)	fiber (gms)
breast, smoked:							
(*Shady Brook Farms*)	130	17.0	2.0	6.0	50	760	0
hickory (*Jennie-O*), 2 oz.	70	11.0	0	2.0	25	450	0
hickory (*Shady Brook Farms*) ...	60	13.0	1.0	0	35	560	0
breast half, marinated rotisserie (*Perdue*)	130	18.0	1.0	6.0	55	320	0
drumstick, smoked (*Shady Brook Farms*)	180	22.0	3.0	8.0	70	620	0
nuggets (*Louis Rich*), 4 pcs., 3.25 oz. ...	260	13.0	15.0	16.0	35	640	0
tenderloin, seasoned:							
cracked pepper (*Perdue*)	90	20.0	1.0	1.0	45	690	0
butter garlic (*Perdue*)	100	20.0	2.0	1.0	45	830	0
thigh, smoked (*Shady Brook Farms*)	160	14.0	2.0	10.0	55	700	0
wing (*Perdue*)	160	22.0	0	8.0	90	65	0
wing, smoked (*Shady Brook Farms*)	200	22.0	3.0	10.0	65	680	0
wing drumettes (*Perdue*), 3.3-oz. pc.	180	24.0	0	9.0	95	70	0
Turkey, ground, 4 oz., except as noted:							
raw:							
(*Jennie-O*)	130	22.0	0	5.0	75	75	0
(*Jennie-O* Frozen)	170	19.0	0	13.0	110	80	0
(*Norbest*)	170	21.0	0	10.0	75	75	0
(*Perdue Fit 'n Easy*)	170	21.0	0	9.0	90	120	0
(*Wampler*)	210	18.0	0	15.0	100	30	0
raw, breast:							
(*Jennie-O* Frozen)	140	20.0	0	7.0	95	75	0
(*Perdue Fit 'n Easy*)	120	27.0	0	1.5	65	60	0
(*Shady Brook Farms* Only One)	120	28.0	0	.5	70	55	0
(*Shady Brook Farms* 85% Fat Free) ..	220	21.0	0	15.0	75	75	0
(*Shady Brook Farms* 93% Fat Free) ..	170	22.0	0	8.0	80	85	0

Food and Measure	cal.	prot. (gms)	carbo. (gms)	fat (gms)	chol. (mgs)	sod. (mgs)	fiber (gms)
Turkey, ground (*cont.*)							
raw, burger:							
(*Empire* Kosher) ..	150	2.0	0	7.0	90	130	0
(*Jennie-O*)	160	19.0	0	9.0	120	85	0
(*Perdue Fit 'n Easy*)	170	21.0	0	9.0	90	120	0
(*Shady Brook Farms*)	170	20.0	0	9.0	95	90	0
(*Wampler*)	210	18.0	0	15.0	100	30	0
barbecue (*Wampler*)	220	18.0	3.0	15.0	100	250	0
specially seasoned (*Wampler*)	180	21.0	1.0	11.0	75	400	0
cooked, 3 oz.:							
(*Perdue Fit 'n Easy*)	160	20.0	0	9.0	85	85	0
breast (*Perdue Fit 'n Easy*)	110	25.0	0	1.0	50	40	0
"Turkey," vegetarian:							
canned (*Worthington* Turkee), 3 slices ..	170	13.0	3.0	12.0	0	580	2.0
frozen:							
(*Yves* Deli Slices), 2.2 oz.	85	18.0	4.0	0	0	480	1.0
smoked, roll (*Worthington* Meatless), ⅜" slice	140	10.0	3.0	10.0	0	600	2.0
smoked, sliced (*Worthington* Meatless), 3 slices	140	10.0	3.0	10.0	0	620	2.0
Turkey bacon, 1 slice:							
(*Briar Street Market*)	25	2.0	0	2.0	10	150	0
(*Butterball*)	30	2.0	0	2.5	10	170	0
(*Butterball* Thin & Crispy)	20	1.0	0	2.0	5	115	0
(*Jennie-O* Extra Lean)	20	3.0	0	.8	10	140	0
(*Jennie-O* Fat Free) ..	20	3.0	0	0	10	140	0
(*Louis Rich*)	35	2.0	0	2.5	15	180	0
Turkey bologna, 2 oz., except as noted:							
(*Healthy Deli*)	70	8.0	3.0	2.5	15	460	0
(*Louis Rich*), 1-oz. slice	50	3.0	1.0	4.0	20	270	0
(*Louis Rich*), 3 slices, 3 oz.	160	10.0	4.0	12.0	55	810	0

Food and Measure	cal.	prot. (gms)	carbo. (gms)	fat (gms)	chol. (mgs)	sod. (mgs)	fiber (gms)
(*Norbest*)	130	7.0	0	11.0	45	640	0
(*Wampler*)	100	8.0	1.0	8.0	40	340	0
(*Wampler* Family Size Chunk)	130	8.0	1.0	11.0	50	550	0
Turkey burger, see "Turkey, ground"							
Turkey dinner, frozen, 1 pkg.:							
breast:							
(*Healthy Choice* Traditional), 10.5 oz.	320	20.0	49.0	5.0	30	600	5.0
(*Swanson Traditional Favorites*), 11.75 oz.	330	18.0	50.0	6.0	40	1290	4.0
grilled (*Healthy Choice*), 10 oz.	260	21.0	33.0	5.0	30	600	5.0
roast (*Stouffer's* HomeStyle), 16 oz.	460	24.0	55.0	16.0	60	1620	7.0
and gravy w/dressing (*Banquet Extra Helping*), 17 oz. ..	620	28.0	54.0	32.0	80	2250	10.0
w/stuffing, baked (*Swanson Traditional Favorites*), 13.5 oz.	450	20.0	59.0	15.0	25	1080	5.0
white meat, mostly (*Swanson Hungry-Man*), 16.75 oz. ..	500	30.0	61.0	15.0	50	1550	7.0
Turkey entree, can or pkg.:							
and dressing (*Dinty Moore American Classics*), 1 bowl ..	290	22.0	32.0	8.0	45	1120	3.0
stew, 1 cup:							
(*Dinty Moore* Can)	140	10.0	19.0	3.0	20	910	2.0
(*Dinty Moore* Microwave Cup)	130	9.0	16.0	2.5	10	760	2.0
Turkey entree, dried, 1 serving:							
(*AlpineAire* Wild Thyme)	370	21.0	47.0	11.0	55	610	7.0

Food and Measure	cal.	prot. (gms)	carbo. (gms)	fat (gms)	chol. (mgs)	sod. (mgs)	fiber (gms)
Turkey entree, dried (*cont.*)							
mashed potato and gravy w/ (*Alpine-Aire*)	300	13.0	56.0	2.0	35	640	4.0
Romanoff (*AlpineAire*)	330	24.0	35.0	11.0	70	670	1.0
teriyaki (*AlpineAire*) ..	290	17.0	50.0	2.5	40	590	1.0
tetrazzini:							
(*Mountain House Double*)	280	16.0	27.0	12.0	40	910	2.0
(*Mountain House Single*)	350	20.0	35.0	15.0	50	1070	3.0
Turkey entree, frozen, 1 pkg., except as noted:							
breast medallions:							
and stuffing (*Marie Callender's* Bowl), 11 oz.	320	26.0	33.0	10.0	50	1210	5.0
grilled (*Marie Callender's*), 9.5 oz.	290	24.0	31.0	8.0	30	780	3.0
chili, see "Chili entree"							
croquettes, gravy and (*Freezer Queen Family*), 1 patty w/gravy, ⅙ pkg. ..	140	8.0	14.0	6.0	20	600	2.0
divan (*Healthy Choice* Bowl), 11 oz.	270	21.0	30.0	7.0	40	600	4.0
glazed, tenderloins (*Lean Cuisine Cafe Classics*), 9 oz. ...	260	14.0	41.0	4.5	25	640	4.0
and gravy, w/dressing: (*Freezer Queen* Meal), 9.25 oz.	230	14.0	31.0	5.0	55	1060	3.0
rolls (*Freezer Queen Deluxe Family*), 1 roll	170	12.0	33.0	4.0	35	820	3.0
and whipped potato (*Freezer Queen Homestyle*), 9 oz.	210	10.0	31.0	5.0	20	620	3.0
w/gravy and stuffing (*Marie Callender's*), 14 oz.	420	31.0	36.0	17.0	65	1500	5.0
gravy and, w/dressing (*Morton*), 9 oz. ...	240	10.0	27.0	10.0	40	1200	4.0

Food and Measure	cal.	prot. (gms)	carbo. (gms)	fat (gms)	chol. (mgs)	sod. (mgs)	fiber (gms)
home style:							
(*Lean Cuisine Everyday Favorites*), 9⅜ oz.	250	21.0	28.0	6.0	40	610	3.0
w/potato (*Birds Eye Turkey Voila!*), 1 cup cooked . . .	200	12.0	24.0	6.0	10	830	3.0
meat loaf, marinara, green beans, potato (*Mamma Rita's*), ½ of 18-oz. pkg. . .	300	27.0	22.0	12.0	90	230	3.0
pie/pot pie:							
(*Banquet*), 7 oz. . .	370	10.0	38.0	20.0	45	850	3.0
(*Marie Callender's*), 9.5 oz.	660	13.0	56.0	43.0	20	1100	3.0
(*Marie Callender's* 16.5 oz.), 1 cup	540	12.0	45.0	35.0	15	1060	1.0
(*Stouffer's*), 10 oz.	750	26.0	62.0	44.0	80	1010	3.0
(*Stouffer's*), ½ of 16-oz. pkg.	590	17.0	53.0	34.0	55	890	2.0
(*Swanson*), 7 oz.	400	10.0	42.0	21.0	25	700	3.0
(*Swanson Potato-Topped*), 12 oz.	350	17.0	33.0	17.0	50	1080	6.0
white meat, deep dish (*Swanson Hungry-Man*), 1 cup	520	13.0	53.0	29.0	40	940	3.0
roast:							
(*Lean Cuisine Skillet Sensations*), ½ of 24-oz. pkg.	220	14.0	37.0	2.0	25	790	6.0
breast (*Healthy Choice* Medley), 8.5 oz.	220	18.0	26.0	5.0	25	600	5.0
breast (*Lean Cuisine Cafe Classics*), 9.75 oz.	270	13.0	49.0	2.0	25	590	3.0
breast (*Lean Cuisine Hearty Portions*), 14 oz.	320	11.0	43.0	6.0	30	840	6.0
breast (*Stouffer's* HomeStyle), 9⅝ oz.	310	19.0	27.0	14.0	35	1020	3.0

Food and Measure	cal.	prot. (gms)	carbo. (gms)	fat (gms)	chol. (mgs)	sod. (mgs)	fiber (gms)
Turkey entree, frozen, roast (*cont.*)							
white meat (*Banquet*), 9 oz. . . .	230	14.0	30.0	6.0	25	1070	5.0
roasted, slow, breast, and mashed potato (*Healthy Choice Duo*), 8.5 oz.	200	20.0	19.0	5.0	40	600	4.0
sliced, gravy and:							
(*Banquet* Family), 2 slices w/gravy	140	7.0	5.0	10.0	40	600	1.0
(*Banquet* Hot Sandwich Toppers), 5-oz. bag	140	8.0	3.0	11.0	30	670	0
(*Freezer Queen* Cook-in-Pouch), 5 oz.	70	7.0	6.0	2.0	15	750	1.0
(*Freezer Queen* Family), 4.5 oz., ⅙ pkg.	60	5.0	6.0	2.0	15	550	<1.0
white meat (*Freezer Queen Family Buffet*), ¼ pkg.	290	14.0	39.0	8.0	40	1510	3.0
tetrazzini (*Stouffer's*), 10 oz.	400	20.0	36.0	19.0	60	1010	2.0
white meat, mostly (*Banquet*), 9.25 oz.	270	14.0	30.0	11.0	55	1060	3.0
Turkey fat, 1 tbsp. . . .	115	0	0	12.8	13	0	0
Turkey frankfurter, see "Frankfurter"							
Turkey giblets:							
simmered, 4 oz.	189	30.1	2.4	5.8	474	67	0
simmered, diced, 1 cup	243	38.5	3.0	7.4	606	85	0
Turkey gravy, can or jar, ¼ cup:							
(*Boston Market*)	25	1.0	3.0	1.0	5	370	0
(*Franco-American*) . . .	25	1.0	3.0	1.0	<5	290	0
(*Franco-American Slow Roast*)	25	1.0	4.0	.5	<5	320	0
(*Heinz* Home Style) . .	25	1.0	3.0	1.0	0	340	0
(*Heinz* Home Style Fat Free)	10	1.0	2.0	0	0	320	0
Turkey gravy mix:							
(*Lawry's*), 1 tbsp. . . .	25	0	4.0	1.0	0	310	0

Food and Measure	cal.	prot. (gms)	carbo. (gms)	fat (gms)	chol. (mgs)	sod. (mgs)	fiber (gms)
(*McCormick*), ¼ cup*	20	0	3.0	0	0	350	0
roasted (*Knorr*), 1 tbsp.	25	2.0	4.0	.5	<5	300	0
Turkey ham, 2 oz., except as noted:							
(*Carl Buddig*), 2.5-oz. pkg.	100	13.0	1.0	5.0	40	1020	0
(*Healthy Deli*)	70	10.0	2.0	2.5	30	470	0
(*Jennie-O*), 1 oz. ...	60	9.0	0	3.0	40	600	0
(*Norbest*), 3 oz.	100	14.0	0	4.0	45	920	0
(*The Turkey Store*) ...	70	9.0	2.0	3.0	40	620	0
(*The Turkey Store Premium*)	70	9.0	2.0	3.0	35	660	0
(*Wampler* Family Size Chunk)	60	8.0	1.0	2.0	30	630	0
(*Wampler* 12% Water)	60	10.0	0	2.5	40	590	0
(*Wampler* 20% Water)	50	8.0	1.0	2.0	30	530	0
Black Forest:							
(*Shady Brook Farms*)	70	10.0	3.0	2.5	30	470	0
(*The Turkey Store*)	70	9.0	2.0	3.0	35	660	0
(*Wampler/Wampler Deli Roast Collection*)	60	10.0	2.0	1.5	25	650	0
honey:							
(*Jennie-O*), 1 oz. .	70	9.0	0	3.0	35	660	0
roasted (*Sara Lee*)	70	5.0	2.0	3.0	40	700	0
Turkey ham salad (*Wampler*), ⅓ cup	150	7.0	9.0	10.0	30	500	1.0
Turkey kielbasa, see "Kielbasa"							
Turkey liver, see "Liver"							
Turkey lunch meat (see also "Turkey ham," etc.), breast, 2 oz., except as noted:							
(*Alpine Lace* Fat Free)	45	10.0	0	0	25	350	0
(*Boar's Head* Lower Sodium)	60	12.0	0	1.5	25	320	0
(*Boar's Head* Lower Sodium Skinless) ..	60	12.0	0	.5	20	340	0
(*Boar's Head Salsalito*)	60	13.0	1.0	.5	25	460	0
(*Briar Street Market*)	50	10.0	2.0	0	15	500	<1.0

Food and Measure	cal.	prot. (gms)	carbo. (gms)	fat (gms)	chol. (mgs)	sod. (mgs)	fiber (gms)
Turkey lunch meat (*cont.*)							
(*Briar Street Market* Reduced Sodium) .	50	10.0	1.0	0	15	340	0
(*Carl Buddig*), 2.5-oz. pkg.	110	12.0	1.0	7.0	40	780	0
(*Light & Lean 97*), 1-oz. slice	30	5.0	0	1.0	15	380	0
(*Jennie-O*)	50	11.0	0	.5	20	460	0
(*Jennie-O Skinless*) . .	50	11.0	0	0	20	460	0
(*Jennie-O Skinless Petite*)	50	11.0	0	.5	20	480	0
(*Norbest* Gold Label Golden Browned) . .	60	10.0	0	.5	30	500	0
(*Shady Brook Farms* No Salt)	70	16.0	0	0	40	30	0
(*The Turkey Store* . . . Golden Roast), 3 oz.	100	19.0	2.0	2.5	35	740	0
(*Wampler* 5 Diamond)	50	13.0	0	0	30	240	0
(*Wampler* 5 Diamond Skin On)	70	12.0	0	2.5	35	240	0
(*Wampler* 4 Diamond Skinless)	60	11.0	0	1.5	20	400	0
(*Wampler* 4 Diamond Skinless No Salt) . .	80	12.0	0	0	30	25	0
Black Forest (*Healthy Deli*)	60	11.0	1.0	.5	20	480	0
browned:							
(*Briar Street Market*)	50	10.0	2.0	0	15	500	<1.0
(*Healthy Choice*) . .	50	10.0	1.0	1.0	20	400	0
Cajun:							
(*Perdue Carving*) . .	50	9.0	1.0	1.0	20	800	0
(*The Turkey Store*)	50	12.0	1.0	0	20	460	0
cured (*Norbest* Gourmet)	70	7.0	0	4.5	35	620	0
flame seared (*Healthy Choice*)	60	12.0	2.0	.5	20	470	0
garlic, roasted, herb:							
(*Louis Rich*), 3 slices, 1.9 oz.	50	10.0	1.0	.5	25	750	0
(*Louis Rich Carving Board*), 3 slices, 1.9 oz.	60	11.0	2.0	1.0	25	640	0

Food and Measure	cal.	prot. (gms)	carbo. (gms)	fat (gms)	chol. (mgs)	sod. (mgs)	fiber (gms)
garlic pesto or honey Dijon (*The Turkey Store*)	50	12.0	1.0	0	20	460	0
honey roasted:							
(*Carl Buddig* 6 oz.)	85	9.0	2.0	5.0	30	600	0
(*Carl Buddig* Premium), 2.5-oz. pkg. . . .	70	12.0	4.0	1.0	30	770	0
(*Healthy Deli*)	60	10.0	3.0	.5	20	480	0
(*Perdue Carving*) . .	50	10.0	1.0	1.0	20	390	0
(*Sara Lee*)	60	12.0	1.0	.5	20	550	0
(*Sara Lee*), 2 slices, 1.6 oz.	50	10.0	1.0	.5	20	450	0
(*Shady Brook Farms*)	60	11.0	3.0	.5	30	400	0
(*The Turkey Store* Golden Roast) . .	60	12.0	2.0	.5	20	500	0
cracked pepper (*Shady Brook Farms*)	60	11.0	4.0	0	25	470	0
cured (*Louis Rich*)	60	10.0	2.0	1.0	25	600	0
cured (*Louis Rich*), 3 slices, 2.2 oz.	70	11.0	2.0	1.0	30	670	0
Italian style (*Healthy Choice*), 1-oz. slice	25	5.0	1.0	0	10	240	0
lemon pepper (*The Turkey Store*)	50	12.0	1.0	0	20	460	0
maple glazed:							
(*Boar's Head Honey Coat*)	70	14.0	2.0	.5	30	440	0
baby (*Boar's Head Honey Coat*) . . .	70	14.0	2.0	.5	30	480	0
oil browned:							
(*Wampler 5 Diamond*)	45	9.0	1.0	.5	20	530	0
(*Wampler 5 Diamond Skin On*)	70	11.0	3.0	1.0	15	390	0
(*Wampler 4 Diamond*)	60	10.0	1.0	1.5	25	490	0
(*Wampler 3 Diamond*)	50	12.0	1.0	1.5	20	360	0
(*Wampler 3 Diamond Fat Free*)	45	9.0	1.0	0	20	440	0

Food and Measure	cal.	prot. (gms)	carbo. (gms)	fat (gms)	chol. (mgs)	sod. (mgs)	fiber (gms)
Turkey lunch meat, oil browned (*cont.*)							
(*Wampler* 3 Diamond Skinless)	45	9.0	1.0	.5	20	530	0
oven browned							
(*Wampler* 4 Diamond)	50	9.0	0	1.0	20	540	0
oven roasted:							
(*Boar's Head* Golden Oven)	60	11.0	0	2.0	25	370	0
(*Boar's Head* Golden Oven Skinless)	60	12.0	<1.0	1.0	25	350	0
(*Boar's Head* Ovengold)	60	12.0	1.0	1.5	35	360	0
(*Boar's Head* Ovengold Skinless)	60	13.0	0	1.0	20	350	0
(*Briar Street Market*)	45	8.0	2.0	1.0	15	560	1.0
(*Briar Street Market* Lower Sodium)	50	10.0	1.0	0	15	320	0
(*Briar Street Market* No Salt)	70	13.0	0	2.0	25	30	0
(*Briar Street Market* Skinless)	50	10.0	2.0	0	15	500	<1.0
(*Carl Buddig* Premium), 2.5-oz. pkg.	60	12.0	1.0	1.0	30	770	0
(*Healthy Choice*), 1-oz. slice	30	5.0	1.0	1.0	15	240	0
(*Healthy Choice* Deli), 1-oz. slice	25	5.0	1.0	0	10	240	0
(*Healthy Choice Deli Traditions* 6 oz.), 6 slices, 1.9 oz.	60	9.0	2.0	1.5	20	470	0
(*Healthy Choice Deli Traditions* 9 oz.), 5 slices, 1.9 oz.	60	9.0	2.0	1.5	25	450	0
(*Healthy Choice* Skinless)	50	10.0	1.0	1.0	20	430	0
(*Healthy Deli* Gourmet)	60	11.0	1.0	.5	20	440	0
(*Healthy Deli* Less Sodium)	60	10	1.0	.5	20	310	0
(*Healthy Deli* Natural Shape)	60	11.0	1.0	.5	20	480	0

Food and Measure	cal.	prot. (gms)	carbo. (gms)	fat (gms)	chol. (mgs)	sod. (mgs)	fiber (gms)
(*Hebrew National* Thin Sliced) ...	50	11.0	1.0	.5	20	430	0
(*Louis Rich*), 3 slices, 1.9 oz.	50	9.0	2.0	1.0	20	590	0
(*Louis Rich*), 3 slices, 2.3 oz.	70	11.0	3.0	1.5	25	730	0
(*Louis Rich*), 4 slices, 2 oz. ..	60	9.0	2.0	1.0	20	620	0
(*Louis Rich* Fat Free)	50	11.0	1.0	0	20	660	0
(*Louis Rich* Fat Free), 1-oz. slice	25	4.0	1.0	0	10	340	0
(*Louis Rich* Fat Free), 2 slices, 1.8 oz.	45	8.0	2.0	0	15	600	0
(*Louis Rich* Carving Board*), 6 slices, 2.1 oz.	60	12.0	1.0	.5	25	720	0
(*Norbest* Bronze Label)	60	7.0	2.0	2.0	20	560	0
(*Norbest* Gold Label)	60	10.0	0	1.5	25	500	0
(*Norbest* Silver Label)	60	8.0	2.0	2.0	25	500	0
(*Oscar Mayer*), 1 oz.	30	4.0	1.0	1.0	10	300	0
(*Perdue*)	50	10.0	1.0	1.0	20	420	0
(*Perdue Carving*) ..	70	12.0	1.0	2.0	25	510	0
(*Perdue Health-sense*)	60	10.0	3.0	0	20	290	0
(*Sara Lee*)	60	12.0	0	1.5	25	480	0
(*Sara Lee*), 2 slices, 1.6 oz.	45	8.0	2.0	.5	20	470	0
(*Shady Brook Farms*)	60	12.0	1.0	0	20	400	0
(*The Turkey Store*)	50	11.0	1.0	.5	20	500	0
(*The Turkey Store* Homestyle)	50	12.0	0	.5	25	480	0
(*The Turkey Store* Presliced)	50	11.0	1.0	.5	25	660	0
(*Wampler* Family Size Chunk)	45	7.0	2.0	1.0	15	660	0
(*Wampler* 3 Diamond)	50	9.0	1.0	1.0	15	390	0
(*Wampler* 2 Diamond)	50	8.0	1.0	1.5	10	430	0
(*Wampler* 1 Diamond)	50	7.0	1.0	2.0	20	490	0

Turkey lunch meat, oven roasted (*cont.*)

Food and Measure	cal.	prot. (gms)	carbo. (gms)	fat (gms)	chol. (mgs)	sod. (mgs)	fiber (gms)
cured (*Carl Buddig*), 2.5-oz. pkg. ...	110	12.0	1.0	7.0	40	780	0
glazed (*Healthy Deli Gourmet*)	60	11.0	1.0	.5	20	440	0
Italian (*Healthy Deli*)	70	10.0	4.0	.5	20	480	0
rotisserie flavor (*Sara Lee*)	70	11.0	1.0	2.0	25	450	0
pan roasted:							
(*Perdue Carving Classics*)	70	14.0	0	2.0	30	390	0
(*Perdue Carving Classics* Skinless)	60	13.0	0	.5	30	390	0
(*Wampler Deli Roast Collection*)	60	10.0	2.0	1.5	25	650	0
(*Wampler Deli Roast Collection* All-Natural)	50	10.0	2.0	1.0	25	650	0
braised (*Perdue Carving Classics* Homestyle)	70	13.0	1.0	2.0	45	360	0
cracked pepper (*Perdue Carving Classics*)	50	10.0	2.0	0	20	470	0
hickory smoked (*Perdue Carving Classics*)	70	12.0	1.0	2.5	30	540	0
peppered:							
(*Healthy Choice*), 1-oz. slice	25	5.0	1.0	0	10	240	0
(*Healthy Deli* Tutta Bella)	60	11.0	2.0	0	20	480	0
(*Wampler Deli Roast Collection*)	40	8.0	1.0	0	20	520	0
(*Sara Lee*)	50	10.0	2.0	0	20	420	0
cracked (*Sara Lee*)	60	11.0	2.0	.5	20	400	0
cracked (*Sara Lee*), 3 slices, 2 oz. ..	60	11.0	2.0	.5	20	480	0
cracked (*The Turkey Store*)	50	12.0	1.0	0	20	460	0
hot red (*Jennie-O* Rio Grande)	60	12.0	0	0	25	630	0

Food and Measure	cal.	prot. (gms)	carbo. (gms)	fat (gms)	chol. (mgs)	sod. (mgs)	fiber (gms)
garlic (*Jennie-O* Mediterranean)	60	13.0	0	.5	25	630	0
smoked (*Jennie-O* Smoky Mountain)	60	17.0	0	.5	35	440	0
roasted, 1-oz. slice:							
(*Louis Rich*)	25	4.0	<1.0	.5	10	400	0
breast and white (*Louis Rich*)	30	5.0	<1.0	.5	10	310	0
rotisserie seasoned:							
(*Healthy Choice Deli Traditions*), 6 slices, 1.9 oz.	60	9.0	2.0	1.5	20	470	0
(*Louis Rich*), 2 slices, 1.6 oz.	45	9.0	<1.0	0	20	480	0
(*Louis Rich*), 3 slices, 2.3 oz.	70	11.0	3.0	1.5	25	730	0
(*Wampler Deli Roast Collection*)	50	9.0	1.0	1.5	20	500	0
salsa-roasted (*Shady Brook Farms*)	50	11.0	1.0	0	25	530	0
slow roasted (*Shady Brook Farms*)	60	11.0	1.0	0	20	400	0
smoked:							
(*Boar's Head Cracked Pepper Mill*)	60	13.0	0	.5	30	460	0
(*Carl Buddig* 6 oz.) .	80	9.0	1.0	5.0	30	600	0
(*Carl Buddig*), 2.5-oz. pkg. ...	110	12.0	1.0	7.0	40	780	0
(*Carl Buddig* Premium), 2.5-oz. pkg. ...	60	12.0	1.0	1.0	30	680	0
(*Healthy Choice*), 1-oz. slice	30	5.0	2.0	1.0	15	240	0
(*Healthy Choice Deli Traditions* 9 oz.), 5 slices, 1.9 oz.	60	9.0	30	1.5	25	450	0
(*Healthy Choice Deli Traditions* 6 oz.), 6 slices, 1.9 oz. .	60	9.0	30	1.5	25	470	0
(*Healthy Choice Skinless*)	50	10.0	1.0	1.0	20	430	0
(*Healthy Deli* Brick Oven)	60	11.0	1.0	0	20	470	0

Food and Measure	cal.	prot. (gms)	carbo. (gms)	fat (gms)	chol. (mgs)	sod. (mgs)	fiber (gms)
Turkey lunch meat, smoked (cont.)							
(*Louis Rich*), 1 oz.	35	5.0	<1.0	1.5	15	280	0
(*Louis Rich*), 2 slices, 1.6 oz.	45	9.0	<1.0	0	20	540	0
(*Louis Rich* Fat Free), 1 oz.	25	4.0	1.0	0	10	310	0
(*Louis Rich Carving Board*)	60	9.0	2.0	1.0	20	620	0
(*Louis Rich Carving Board*), 3 slices, 1.9 oz.	50	9.0	2.0	1.0	20	590	0
(*Louis Rich Carving Board*), 4 slices, 2.3 oz.	70	11.0	3.0	1.5	25	730	0
(*Norbest* Bronze Label)	60	7.0	2.0	2.5	20	540	0
(*Norbest* Gold Label)	60	10.0	0	1.5	30	510	0
(*Norbest* Silver Label)	60	8.0	2.0	1.5	25	540	0
(*Oscar Mayer*), 1 oz.	30	4.0	<1.0	1.0	10	320	0
(*Oscar Mayer Free*), 4 slices, 1.8 oz.	40	8.0	2.0	0	15	570	0
(*Wampler* Family Size Chunk)	50	8.0	2.0	1.0	20	720	0
(*Wampler* 5 Diamond Skin On)	70	12.0	0	2.5	20	420	0
(*Wampler* 4 Diamond)	60	11.0	2.0	2.0	20	490	0
(*Wampler* 3 Diamond)	45	8.0	1.0	1.0	15	430	0
(*Wampler* 2 Diamond)	60	8.0	2.0	2.5	20	380	0
(*Wampler* 1 Diamond)	50	8.0	1.0	1.5	20	520	0
Cajun style (*Boar's Head*)	60	13.0	<1.0	.5	25	390	0
cured, hickory or mesquite (*Jennie-O*)	50	11.0	0	.5	25	590	0
hardwood (*Sara Lee*)	60	12.0	1.0	.5	20	550	0

Food and Measure	cal.	prot. (gms)	carbo. (gms)	fat (gms)	chol. (mgs)	sod. (mgs)	fiber (gms)
hardwood (*Sara Lee*), 2 slices, 1.6 oz.	45	9.0	1.0	.5	20	450	0
hickory (*Jennie-O*)	60	12.0	0	1.0	25	430	0
hickory (*Perdue*) ..	60	9.0	1.0	2.5	40	770	0
hickory (*Shady Brook Farms*) ...	50	12.0	1.0	0	25	470	0
hickory (*The Turkey Store*)	60	11.0	1.0	1.0	20	560	0
hickory, Black Forest (*Boar's Head* Lower Sodium)	60	13.0	0	.5	25	360	0
hickory, honey cured (*The Turkey Store*)	60	11.0	2.0	1.0	20	500	0
honey (*Healthy Choice*)	60	10.0	2.0	1.0	20	360	0
honey (*Perdue Carving*)	50	10.0	2.0	0	20	510	0
honey cured (*The Turkey Store*) ...	60	11.0	2.0	1.0	20	500	0
honey cured (*Wampler* 4 Diamond)	70	9.0	4.0	2.0	25	560	0
honey cured (*Wampler* 4 Diamond Petite)	50	9.0	4.0	0	25	380	0
honey cured, hickory or mesquite (*Jennie-O*)	50	11.0	0	.5	25	530	0
mesquite (*Boars Head Mesquite Wood Smoked*)	60	13.0	1.0	.5	25	440	0
mesquite (*Healthy Choice*), 1 oz. ..	25	5.0	1.0	0	10	210	0
mesquite (*Louis Rich*), 3 slices, 1.9 oz.	50	11.0	<1.0	.5	25	810	0
mesquite (*Louis Rich Carving Board*)	60	10.0	2.0	1.0	25	670	0

Food and Measure	cal.	prot. (gms)	carbo. (gms)	fat (gms)	chol. (mgs)	sod. (mgs)	fiber (gms)
Turkey lunch meat, smoked (*cont.*)							
mesquite (*Louis Rich Carving Board*), 3 slices, 1.9 oz.	50	9.0	2.0	1.0	25	640	0
mesquite (*Healthy Choice Savory Selections*), 6 slices, 1.9 oz.	60	9.0	3.0	1.5	25	470	0
mesquite (*Healthy Deli*)	60	11.0	1.0	.5	20	480	0
mesquite (*Light & Lean* 97), 1 oz.	30	5.0	0	1.0	15	380	0
mesquite (*Louis Rich Carving Board*), 3 slices, 1.9 oz.	50	11.0	1.0	.5	25	810	0
mesquite (*Norbest* Gold Label)	50	10.0	3.0	0	25	490	0
mesquite (*Perdue Carving*)	50	10.0	0	1.0	25	510	0
mocquite (*Sara Lee*)	60	12.0	1.0	.5	20	560	0
mesquite (*The Turkey Store*) ...	60	11.0	1.0	1.0	20	500	0
mesquite, honey cured (*Wampler 4 Diamond*)	50	9.0	4.0	0	25	380	0
picnic cured, dark (*Wampler* Family Size Chunk)	80	8.0	2.0	4.5	30	600	0
white (*Norbest*) ...	70	7.0	2.0	3.0	25	540	0
Southwest grill: (*Healthy Choice*) ..	60	11.0	2.0	1.0	20	400	0
(*Healthy Choice*), 1 oz.	25	5.0	1.0	0	10	240	0
spiced (*Wampler Deli Roast Collection Classic*)	70	16.0	1.0	.5	25	380	0
sun-dried tomato (*The Turkey Store*)	50	12.0	1.0	0	20	460	0
Tex-Mex (*Black Bear*)	60	12.0	1.0	.5	20	460	0
Turkey meatballs, see "Meatballs"							

Food and Measure	cal.	prot. (gms)	carbo. (gms)	fat (gms)	chol. (mgs)	sod. (mgs)	fiber (gms)
Turkey pastrami, 2 oz.:							
(*Boar's Head*)	60	13.0	1.0	.5	25	440	0
(*Boar's Head* Round)	60	14.0	0	.5	30	390	0
(*Healthy Deli*)	70	10.0	2.0	2.5	30	480	0
(*Jennie-O*)	70	11.0	0	2.5	40	640	0
(*Norbest*)	70	10.0	0	3.0	30	570	0
(*Shady Brook Farms*)	60	10.0	1.0	2.0	35	470	0
(*The Turkey Store*) ...	70	10.0	1.0	3.0	40	670	0
(*Wampler*)	80	11.0	1.0	4.0	40	290	0
hickory smoked							
(*Perdue*)	70	9.0	2.0	3.0	40	670	0
Turkey pepperoni							
(*Hormel Pillow Pack*), 17 slices, 1.1 oz.	80	9.0	0	4.0	40	550	0
Turkey pie, see "Turkey entree"							
Turkey pocket, frozen, 4.5-oz. pc.:							
broccoli and cheese							
(*Lean Pockets*) ...	230	10.0	30.0	7.0	35	480	2.0
ham and cheese:							
(*Croissant Pockets*)	320	12.0	39.0	13.0	40	600	2.0
(*Hot Pockets*)	310	12.0	43.0	10.0	40	730	2.0
(*Lean Pockets*) ...	290	13.0	42.0	7.0	30	600	2.0
Turkish salad (*Sabra Salads*), 1 oz.	13	.5	2.5	0	0	150	.7
Turkey salami:							
(*Norbest*), 2 oz.	85	9.0	2.0	5.0	30	510	0
(*Wampler*), 2 oz. ...	90	9.0	1.0	6.0	55	560	0
cooked, 1 oz.	56	4.6	.2	3.9	23	285	0
Turkey sausage, see "Sausage"							
Turmeric, 1 tsp.	8	.2	1.4	.2	0	1	.5
Turnip, ½ cup, except as noted:							
raw:							
1 large 6.5 oz. ...	49	1.7	11.4	.2	0	123	11.4
cubed	18	.6	4.1	.1	0	44	1.2
boiled, drained:							
cubed	16	.6	3.8	.6	0	39	1.6
mashed	24	.8	5.6	.9	0	58	2.3
Turnip, frozen, boiled, drained, ½ cup ...	18	1.2	3.4	.2	0	28	1.6

Food and Measure	cal	prot. (gms)	carbo. (gms)	fat (gms)	chol. (mgs)	sod. (mgs)	fiber (gms)
Turnip greens, fresh:							
raw:							
untrimmed, 1 lb. . .	85	4.8	18.2	1.0	0	126	7.6
chopped, ½ cup . .	7	.4	1.6	.1	0	11	.7
boiled, chopped,							
½ cup	15	.8	3.1	.2	0	21	2.2
Turnip greens, canned,							
½ cup:							
(*Allens/Sunshine*) . . .	25	2.0	3.0	.5	0	15	2.0
(*Stubb's*)	25	2.0	3.0	.5	0	15	2.0
chopped:							
(*Bush's Best*)	25	2.0	3.0	0	0	300	2.0
w/diced turnip							
(*Allens/Sunshine*)	30	1.0	5.0	.5	0	20	3.0
w/diced turnip							
(*Bush's Best*) . . .	30	1.0	5.0	0	0	380	2.0
w/liquid	17	1.6	2.8	.4	0	325	1.5
seasoned:							
(*Glory Foods*)	45	3.0	6.0	.5	0	630	2.0
(*Sylvia's*)	40	1.0	8.0	0	0	490	3.0
Turnip greens, frozen,							
1 cup:							
chopped (*Birds Eye*)	30	2.0	2.0	0	0	20	2.0
w/diced turnip:							
(*Birds Eye*)	25	2.0	2.0	0	0	20	2.0
boiled, drained	28	3.4	4.7	.3	0	24	2.9
Turnover, frozen or							
refrigerated, 1 pc.:							
apple (*Pillsbury*)	170	2.0	23.0	8.0	0	310	<1.0
blueberry (*Pepperidge*							
Farm)	280	4.0	33.0	15.0	0	230	1.0
cherry (*Pillsbury*) . . .	170	2.0	23.0	8.0	0	310	0
raspberry (*Pepperidge*							
Farm)	290	4.0	33.0	15.0	0	230	2.0

U-V

Food and Measure	cal.	prot. (gms)	carbo. (gms)	fat (gms)	chol. (mgs)	sod. (mgs)	fiber (gms)
Uzbek melon (*Frieda's*),							
1 cup, 5 oz.	35	1.0	9.0	0	0	15	1.0
Vanilla extract,							
imitation, 1 tbsp.:							
w/alcohol	31	0	.3	0	0	<1	0
w/out alcohol	7	0	1.8	0	0	<1	0
Vanilla syrup (*Ferrara*),							
2 oz.	130	0	32.0	0	0	12	0
Veal, meat only, 4 oz.:							
cubed, lean only,							
braised or stewed	213	39.6	0	4.9	164	105	0
ground, broiled	195	27.6	0	8.6	117	94	0
leg:							
braised, lean w/fat	239	41.0	0	7.2	152	76	0
braised, lean only	230	41.6	0	5.8	159	76	0
roasted, lean w/fat	181	31.4	0	5.3	117	77	0
roasted, lean only	170	31.8	0	3.8	117	77	0
loin:							
braised, lean w/fat	322	34.2	0	19.5	134	91	0
braised, lean only	256	38.1	0	10.4	142	95	0
roasted, lean w/fat	246	28.1	0	14.0	117	105	0
roasted, lean only	198	29.8	0	7.9	120	109	0
rib:							
braised, lean w/fat	285	36.8	0	14.2	158	108	0
braised, lean only	247	39.1	0	8.9	163	112	0
roasted, lean w/fat	259	27.2	0	15.8	125	104	0
roasted, lean only	201	29.2	0	8.4	130	110	0
shank, braised:							
lean w/fat	217	35.8	0	7.0	141	105	0
lean only	201	35.4	0	4.9	143	107	0
shoulder, whole:							
braised, lean w/fat	259	36.4	0	11.5	143	108	0
braised, lean only	226	38.2	0	6.9	147	110	0

Food and Measure	cal.	prot. (gms)	carbo. (gms)	fat (gms)	chol. (mgs)	sod. (mgs)	fiber (gms)
veal, shoulder, whole (*cont.*)							
roasted, lean w/fat	209	28.7	0	9.5	128	109	0
roasted, lean only	193	29.3	0	7.5	129	110	0
shoulder, arm:							
braised, lean w/fat	268	38.1	0	11.6	168	99	0
braised, lean only	228	40.5	0	6.0	176	102	0
roasted, lean w/fat	208	28.9	0	9.4	122	102	0
roasted, lean only	186	29.6	0	6.6	124	103	0
shoulder, blade:							
braised, lean w/fat	255	35.4	0	11.4	174	111	0
braised, lean only	224	37.0	0	7.3	179	115	0
roasted, lean w/fat	211	28.5	0	9.8	133	113	0
roasted, lean only	194	29.1	0	7.8	135	116	0
sirloin:							
braised, lean w/fat	286	35.4	0	14.9	122	90	0
braised, lean only	231	38.5	0	7.4	128	92	0
roasted, lean w/fat	229	28.5	0	11.9	116	94	0
roasted, lean only	191	29.8	0	7.1	118	96	0
Veal dinner, frozen, parmigiana, 1 pkg.:							
(*Stouffer's* HomeStyle), 17.5 oz.	530	27.0	66.0	17.0	60	1130	7.0
(*Swanson Traditional Favorites*), 11.25 oz.	390	19.0	40.0	18.0	85	1060	5.0
Veal entree, frozen, parmigiana, 1 pkg.:							
(*Banquet*), 8.75 oz.	330	12.0	34.0	16.0	20	1240	3.0
(*Freezer Queen* Meal), 9 oz.	330	20.0	37.0	11.0	80	660	5.0
(*Stouffer's* HomeStyle), 11⅝ oz.	410	18.0	48.0	16.0	60	1270	4.0
Vegetable batter mix (*McCormick Produce Partners*), ¼ cup	120	2.0	16.0	.5	0	500	0
Vegetable burger, see "Burger, vegetarian"							
Vegetable chips (see also specific listings):							
(*Eden*), 1.1 oz.	130	<1.0	24.0	4.0	0	260	0
(*Snyder's Eat Smart* Crisps), 1 oz.	160	2.0	18.0	8.0	0	290	n.a.
(*Terra Chips*), 1 oz. . .	140	1.0	18.0	7.0	0	70	3.0

Food and Measure	cal.	prot. (gms)	carbo. (gms)	fat (gms)	chol. (mgs)	sod. (mgs)	fiber (gms)
(*Terra Chips*), .75-oz. bag	110	1.0	14.0	6.0	0	55	2.0
(*Terra Stix*), 1 oz. ...	150	1.0	16.0	9.0	0	110	3.0
sea (*Eden*), 1.1 oz. ..	140	<1.0	23.0	5.0	0	220	0
Vegetable dinner, frozen, 1 pkg.:							
(*Amy's* Country), 11 oz.	380	11.0	60.0	12.0	15	570	9.0
loaf (*Amy's* Veggie), 10 oz.	260	8.0	47.0	5.0	0	690	7.0
Vegetable dip mix, garden:							
(*McCormick*), 2 tbsp.*	35	0	2.0	5.0	0	170	0
(*Watkins*), 1 tsp, ...	10	0	2.0	0	0	100	0
Vegetable dish, can or jar, ½ cup, except as noted:							
curry, 1½ cups:							
(*Patak's* Aloo Mattar Sabzi)	240	5.0	25.0	14.0	0	770	3.0
(*Patak's* Tikka Masala)	190	5.0	27.0	5.0	0	690	3.0
hot/spicy (*House of Tsang* Szechuan) ..	70	1.0	14.0	1.0	0	1130	1.0
sweet/sour (*House of Tsang* Hong Kong)	160	0	40.0	0	0	580	0
teriyaki (*House of Tsang* Tokyo)	100	1.0	23.0	0	0	1240	1.0
Vegetable dish, frozen (see also "Vegetable entree, frozen," "Vegetables, mixed, frozen," and specific listings):							
Bavarian (*Birds Eye*), ½ of 9-oz. pkg.	150	5.0	15.0	8.0	30	460	3.0
California (*Birds Eye*), ½ cup	100	3.0	9.0	5.0	10	240	3.0
French country (*Birds Eye*), ⅔ cup	110	2.0	10.0	6.0	10	290	2.0
Italian, w/bowties (*Birds Eye*), 1 cup	150	3.0	13.0	9.0	10	380	2.0
Oriental style (*Birds Eye*), ½ cup	60	2.0	4.0	4.0	10	260	2.0

Food and Measure	cal.	prot. (gms)	carbo. (gms)	fat (gms)	chol. (mgs)	sod. (mgs)	fiber (gms)
Vegetable dish, frozen (*cont.*)							
pasta and, see "Pasta dish, frozen"							
New England, and pasta shells (*Birds Eye*), 9-oz. pkg. ..	260	6.0	29.0	14.0	15	480	3.0
pancake (*King Kold*), 2 cakes, 2 oz.	120	2.0	11.0	8.0	0	260	2.0
stir-fry (*Birds Eye*), ½ cup	60	2.0	5.0	4.0	10	270	1.0
Vegetable entree, frozen (see also "Vegetable entree mix, frozen" and "Vegetarian entree"), 1 pkg.:							
au gratin (*Cascadian Farm Veggie Bowl Cascade*), 9 oz. ...	170	9.0	24.0	6.0	10	630	4.0
Caribbean, and rice (*Cascadian Farm Veggie Bowl*), 9 oz.	280	7.0	52.0	5.0	0	500	3.0
casserole, fiesta (*Cascadian Farm Veggie Bowl*), 9 oz.	340	12.0	52.0	11.0	15	330	7.0
Chinese style, and white chicken w/rice (*Budget Gourmet*), 8 oz.	250	6.0	40.0	6.0	10	670	3.0
Italian style, w/white chicken and rice (*Budget Gourmet*), 8 oz.	250	7.0	39.0	6.0	15	540	2.0
pie/pot pie:							
(*Amy's*), 7.5 oz. ..	420	9.0	54.0	19.0	50	590	4.0
(*Amy's* Country), 7.5 oz.	370	12.0	47.0	16.0	40	580	4.0
(*Amy's* Nondairy), 7.5 oz.	320	7.0	50.0	9.0	0	590	4.0
(*Cedarlane* Less Fat), 7.4 oz.	390	12.0	60.0	8.0	20	250	4.0
w/beef (*Morton*), 7 oz.	190	5.0	33.0	21.0	20	1380	2.0

Food and Measure	cal.	prot. (gms)	carbo. (gms)	fat (gms)	chol. (mgs)	sod. (mgs)	fiber (gms)
w/chicken (*Morton*), 7 oz.	320	8.0	32.0	18.0	25	1040	2.0
Mediterranean (*Cedarlane*), 7.5 oz.	490	13.0	43.0	29.0	20	590	4.0
Sante Fe (*Cedarlane*), 7.5 oz.	490	13.0	50.0	26.0	15	660	5.0
w/turkey (*Morton*), 7 oz.	310	8.0	29.0	18.0	25	1060	2.0
shepherd's pie (*Amy's*), 8 oz.	160	5.0	27.0	4.0	0	490	5.0
spicy Szechuan style, and white chicken w/pasta (*Budget Gourmet*), 8 oz. . .	280	9.0	41.0	9.0	10	880	3.0
stir-fry, w/rice (*Michelina's*), 8 oz.	240	5.0	44.0	4.0	0	1040	3.0
wraps, see "Vegetarian entree, frozen"							
Vegetable entree mix, frozen:							
basil herb primavera (*Birds Eye Easy Recipe Creations*), 2¼ cups	260	9.0	31.0	11.0	25	750	3.0
beef broccoli stir-fry (*Green Giant Create a Meal!*), 1⅓ cups* w/beef or chicken	290	27.0	15.0	13.0	60	1150	4.0
beefy noodle (*Green Giant Create a Meal!*), 1¼ cups* w/hamburger	350	26.0	31.0	14.0	70	1130	3.0
cheesy pasta-vegetable (*Green Giant Create a Meal!*), 1¼ cups* w/hamburger	420	29.0	29.0	21.0	95	1350	2.0
chicken Alfredo (*Green Giant Create a Meal!*), 1¼ cups* w/chicken	400	35.0	36.0	13.0	75	1100	3.0

Food and Measure	cal.	prot. (gms)	carbo. (gms)	fat (gms)	chol. (mgs)	sod. (mgs)	fiber (gms)
Vegetable entree mix, frozen (*cont.*)							
curry, South Indian (*Cascadian Farm Quickstart*), 2¼ cups* w/tofu ..	300	11.0	35.0	13.0	0	620	3.0
garlic ginger stir-fry (*Green Giant Create a Meal!*), 1½ cups* w/chicken or beef	270	27.0	25.0	7.0	55	1130	4.0
garlic herb (*Green Giant Create a Meal!*), 1¾ cups* w/chicken	350	31.0	35.0	9.0	70	760	5.0
garlic herb pasta (*Green Giant Create a Meal!*), 1¼ cups* w/chicken	380	32.0	30.0	15.0	80	870	3.0
lemon pepper chicken (*Green Giant Create a Meal!*), 1⅔ cups* w/chicken	310	29.0	30.0	8.0	65	1400	5.0
lo mein stir-fry (*Green Giant Create a Meal!*), 1¼ cups* w/chicken or beef	320	30.0	33.0	7.0	60	920	3.0
Oriental lo mein (*Birds Eye Easy Recipe Creations*), 2¼ cups	230	8.0	40.0	3.5	5	1200	2.0
Parmesan herb (*Green Giant Create a Meal!*), 1¾ cups* w/chicken	340	31.0	29.0	11.0	70	1050	5.0
sesame ginger teriyaki (*Birds Eye Easy Recipe Creations*), 2¼ cups	140	6.0	24.0	1.5	0	1230	4.0
Southwest skillet (*Cascadian Farm Quickstart*), 2¼ cups* w/tofu	290	13.0	42.0	10.0	0	640	5.0
stew, home-style (*Green Giant Create a Meal!*), 1 cup* w/hamburger	340	24.0	24.0	16.0	70	1370	3.0

Food and Measure	cal.	prot. (gms)	carbo. (gms)	fat (gms)	chol. (mgs)	sod. (mgs)	fiber (gms)
sweet and sour:							
w/pineapple (*Birds Eye Easy Recipe* Creations),							
1⅔ cups	200	2.0	45.0	.5	0	330	3.0
stir-fry (*Green Giant Create a Meal!*), 1¼ cups*							
w/chicken or beef	340	25.0	43.0	7.0	60	620	3.0
Szechuan:							
spicy, w/cashews (*Birds Eye Easy Recipe* Creations),							
2¼ cups	180	6.0	29.0	4.5	0	1410	4.0
stir-fry (*Green Giant Create a Meal!*), 1¼ cups*							
w/chicken or beef	310	26.0	20.0	14.0	60	1390	4.0
teriyaki stir-fry:							
(*Green Giant Create a Meal!*), 1¼ cups*							
w/chicken or beef	230	27.0	18.0	6.0	55	920	4.0
(*Tree of Life Easy/Meal*), 1 pkg.*							
w/tofu, oil	270	13.0	24.0	14.0	0	560	6.0
teriyaki veggies/rice (*Cascadian Farm Quickstart*),							
2¼ cups* w/tofu ..	330	11.0	40.0	18.0	0	650	4.0
Thai stir-fry (*Tree of Life EasyMeal*),							
1 pkg.* w/tofu, oil	270	14.0	21.0	14.0	0	230	5.0
Thai veggies/rice (*Cascadian Farm Quickstart*),							
2¼ cups* w/tofu ..	310	12.0	41.0	12.0	0	470	3.0
tortellini parmigiana (*Birds Eye Easy Recipe* Creations),							
2¼ cups	240	9.0	25.0	12.0	25	870	4.0

Food and Measure	cal.	prot. (gms)	carbo. (gms)	fat (gms)	chol. (mgs)	sod. (mgs)	fiber (gms)
Vegetable juice, 8 fl. oz., except as noted:							
(*Muir Glen* Original), 5.5 fl. oz.	50	1.0	10.0	0	0	420	2.0
(*R. W. Knudsen Very Veggie* Original/ Organic/Spicy)	50	3.0	10.0	1.0	0	960	0
(*R. W. Knudsen Very Veggie* Low Sodium)	50	1.0	11.0	.5	0	35	0
(*Red Gold*)	50	1.0	11.0	0	0	650	2.0
(*V8*)	50	2.0	10.0	0	0	600	2.0
(*V8* Calcium)	60	2.0	12.0	0	0	660	3.0
(*V8* Low Sodium) ...	50	0	13.0	0	0	140	2.0
(*V8* A•C•E Vitamin Rich)	50	1.0	11.0	0	0	440	2.0
cocktail	46	1.5	11.0	.2	0	653	1.9
spicy hot (*V8*)	50	1.0	10.0	0	0	740	1.0
Vegetable oyster, see "Salsify"							
Vegetable pie, see "Vegetable entree, frozen"							
Vegetable pocket/ sandwich (see also specific listings), 1 pc.:							
Mediterranean (*Amy's*), 4.5 oz.	220	9.0	33.0	7.0	15	540	3.0
pie (*Amy's*), 5 oz. ...	300	8.0	45.0	9.0	0	490	3.0
roasted vegetables (*Amy's*), 4.5 oz. ..	220	6.0	35.0	8.0	0	480	4.0
Vegetable protein (*AlpineAire*), 2 oz.	200	30.0	17.0	1.5	0	10	10.0
Vegetables, see specific listings							
Vegetables, mixed, fresh:							
(*Mann's* Medley), 4 oz.	35	3.0	8.0	0	0	35	3.0
Oriental stir-fry (*Frieda's*), 3 oz. ...	15	1.0	3.0	0	0	35	1.0

Food and Measure	cal.	prot. (gms)	carbo. (gms)	fat (gms)	chol. (mgs)	sod. (mgs)	fiber (gms)
Vegetables, mixed, can or jar, ½ cup, except as noted:							
(*Del Monte*)	40	2.0	8.0	0	0	360	2.0
(*Del Monte* No Salt) . .	40	2.0	8.0	0	0	25	2.0
(*Libby's*)	45	1.0	9.0	0	0	340	2.0
(*S&W*)	35	1.0	7.0	0	0	370	2.0
(*Veg-All* Original)	40	1.0	8.0	0	0	290	2.0
(*Veg-All* Original No Salt)	40	1.0	8.0	0	0	25	2.0
(*Veg-All* Homestyle Large Cut)	40	1.0	8.0	0	0	350	2.0
Cajun (*Veg-All*)	50	2.0	10.0	0	0	410	3.0
Chinese, mixed (*La Choy*)	10	1.0	1.0	0	0	30	<1.0
chop suey (*La Choy*), ⅔ cup	15	1.0	3.0	0	0	320	1.0
drained	38	2.1	7.6	.2	0	121	2.5
hot/spicy (*Veg-All*) . .	40	1.0	8.0	0	0	370	2.0
stir-fry (*La Choy*) . . .	15	<1.0	4.5	0	0	200	3.0
Vegetables, mixed, dried, ½ cup:							
(*AlpineAire*)	70	2.0	14.0	0	0	75	2.0
garden (*AlpineAire*) . .	80	3.0	15.0	.5	0	55	3.0
Vegetables, mixed, frozen (see also "Vegetable dishes, frozen"), ⅔ cup, except as noted:							
(*Birds Eye*), ⅓ cup . .	50	2.0	12.0	0	0	35	3.0
(*Green Giant*), ¾ cup	50	2.0	10.0	0	0	40	2.0
(*John Cope's* 5-Way)	60	3.0	12.0	0	0	55	3.0
(*John Cope's* 4-Way)	60	2.0	10.0	.5	0	50	2.0
(*Seabrook Farms*) . . .	70	3.0	13.0	.5	0	55	2.0
(*Tree of Life*), ½ cup	65	3.0	13.0	0	0	60	3.0
Alfredo (*Green Giant*), ¾ cup	70	4.0	9.0	2.5	5	440	3.0
boiled, drained	54	2.6	11.9	.1	0	32	4.0
California blend:							
(*Cascadian Farm*) . .	20	1.0	4.0	0	0	20	0
(*John Cope's*), ¾ cup	30	2.0	5.0	0	0	35	2.0
in cheddar sauce (*Cascadian Farm* Medley)	80	4.0	11.0	2.5	5	260	2.0

Food and Measure	cal.	prot. (gms)	carbo. (gms)	fat (gms)	chol. (mgs)	sod. (mgs)	fiber (gms)
Vegetables, mixed, frozen (*cont.*)							
Chinese stir-fry (*Cascadian Farm*), 1 cup	25	2.0	6.0	0	0	15	2.0
gumbo blend:							
(*Birds Eye*), ¾ cup .	40	2.0	10.0	0	0	30	2.0
(*McKenzie's*)	35	1.0	8.0	0	0	30	2.0
Santa Fe (*Cascadian Farm*), 3 oz.	60	3.0	12.0	.5	0	65	3.0
seasoning blend:							
(*Birds Eye*), ¾ cup	20	1.0	5.0	0	0	25	1.0
(*McKenzie's*), 1.1 oz.	10	1.0	2.0	0	0	10	0
soup mix:							
(*Birds Eye*)	45	1.0	9.0	0	0	45	2.0
(*McKenzie's*) . . . . :	40	2.0	9.0	0	0	40	2.0
stew mix (*Birds Eye* Southern)	40	1.0	9.0	0	0	40	1.0
teriyaki (*Green Giant*), 1¼ cup	80	2.0	6.0	5.0	0	490	2.0
Thai stir-fry (*Cascadian Farm*), ¾ cup	25	2.0	6.0	0	0	15	2.0
winter blend (*John Cope's*), 1 cup	25	2.0	4.0	0	0	20	2.0
Vegetables, mixed, pickled:							
(*Krinos*), 3 oz.	0	0	0	0	0	900	2.0
(*Zorba*), ½ cup	20	<1.0	2.0	1.0	0	850	0
Vegetarian dish (see also "Vegetarian entree" and specific listings):							
canned:							
(*Loma Linda* Swiss Steak), 3.25-oz. pc. . . .	120	9.0	8.0	6.0	0	430	4.0
(*Loma Linda* Tender Bits), 6 pcs., 3 oz.	110	11.0	7.0	4.5	0	440	3.0
(*Loma Linda* Nuteena), ⅜" slice	160	6.0	6.0	13.0	0	120	2.0
(*Worthington* Prime Stakes), 3.2-oz. pc.	120	10.0	4.0	7.0	0	440	4.0

Food and Measure	cal.	prot. (gms)	carbo. (gms)	fat (gms)	chol. (mgs)	sod. (mgs)	fiber (gms)
(*Worthington Savory Slices*), 3 slices, 3 oz. ..	150	10.0	6.0	9.0	0	540	3.0
(*Worthington Vegetable Steaks*), 2 slices, 2.5 oz.	80	15.0	3.0	1.5	0	300	3.0
(*Worthington Choplets*), 2 slices	90	17.0	3.0	1.5	0	500	2.0
(*Worthington Multigrain Cutlets 20 oz.*), 2 slices, 3.2 oz.	100	15.0	5.0	2.0	0	390	4.0
(*Worthington Multigrain Cutlets 50 oz.*), 1 slice, 2.5 oz.	80	12.0	4.0	1.5	0	300	3.0
(*Worthington Numete*), ⅜" slice	130	6.0	5.0	10.0	0	270	3.0
(*Worthington Protose*), ⅜" slice ..	130	13.0	5.0	7.0	0	280	3.0
cutlets (*Loma Linda Dinner Cuts*), 2 pcs.	90	17.0	3.0	1.5	0	500	2.0
cutlets (*Worthington*), 2.2-oz. slice	70	11.0	3.0	1.0	0	340	2.0
stew, country (*Worthington*), 1 cup	210	13.0	20.0	9.0	0	830	5.0
frozen:							
(*Natural Touch Dinner Entree*), 3-oz. patty	220	19.0	2.0	15.0	0	380	2.0
(*Worthington Dinner Roast*), ¾" slice, 3 oz.	180	12.0	5.0	12.0	<5	580	3.0
(*Worthington FriPats*), 1 patty	130	14.0	4.0	6.0	0	320	3.0
black pepper steak (*Veggie Master Vege*), ¼ pkg. ..	97	7.1	6.8	4.6	0	247	4.8

Food and Measure	cal.	prot. (gms)	carbo. (gms)	fat (gms)	chol. (mgs)	sod. (mgs)	fiber (gms)
Vegetarian dish, frozen (*cont.*)							
croquettes (*Worthington* Golden), 4 pcs.	210	14.0	14.0	10.0	0	600	3.0
ground, original or Italian (*Yves* Ground Round), ⅓ cup	60	10.0	4.0	0	0	270	3.0
patty (*Worthington* Stakelets), 2.5 oz. pc.	140	12.0	6.0	8.0	0	480	2.0
mix, dry:							
loaf (*Natural Touch*), 4 tbsp.	100	14.0	10.0	.5	0	700	7.0
loaf, savory (*Loma Linda*), ⅓ cup . .	90	14.0	7.0	1.5	0	560	5.0
patty (*Loma Linda*), ⅓ cup	90	14.0	7.0	1.0	0	480	5.0
Vegetarian entree, frozen (see also "Vegetable entree, frozen," "Vegetarian dish," and specific listings):							
Aztec (*Cascadian Farm Meals for a Small Planet*), 3½ cups . .	290	12.0	53.0	4.0	0	560	8.0
Cajun (*Cascadian Farm Meals for a Small Planet*), 3½ cups . .	290	10.0	56.0	3.0	0	500	8.0
Indian (*Cascadian Farm Meals for a Small Planet*), 3½ cups	340	12.0	62.0	5.0	0	610	9.0
Mediterranean (*Cascadian Farm Meals for a Small Planet*), 3¼ cups	230	9.0	36.0	7.0	0	440	5.0
Moroccan (*Cascadian Farm Meals for a Small Planet*), 3½ cups	310	13.0	50.0	5.0	0	410	13.0
pot pie, see "Vegetable entree, frozen"							

Food and Measure	cal.	prot. (gms)	carbo. (gms)	fat (gms)	chol. (mgs)	sod. (mgs)	fiber (gms)
sandwich, burger and cheese stuffed (*Morningstar Farms* Meat-Free), 4.5-oz. pc.	290	14.0	40.0	8.0	10	400	2.0
stew, w/"meatballs" (*Yves*), 10.5 oz. . .	170	17.0	24.0	0	0	1020	7.0
Szechuan:							
(*Cascadian Farm Meals for a Small Planet*), 3½ cups	340	14.0	56.0	9.0	0	690	8.0
(*Cedarlane* Veggie Chick'n), ½ of 10-oz. pkg.	220	7.0	40.0	3.0	0	510	2.0
teriyaki (*Cedarlane* Veggie Chick'n), ½ of 10-oz. pkg. . .	220	7.0	43.0	3.0	0	580	2.0
wrap, vegetable, 6 oz.:							
w/couscous (*Cedarlane*)	220	14.0	36.0	3.0	0	580	3.0
w/rice, teriyaki (*Cedarlane*)	280	9.0	56.0	3.0	0	480	2.0
vegetarian pizza (*Cedarlane*)	220	17.0	32.0	3.0	0	520	2.0
Vegetarian entree mix, pkg. (see also specific listings), 1 pkg.:							
curried garbanzos and potatoes (*Tamarind Tree* Alu Chole) . . .	350	12.0	63.0	6.0	0	620	9.0
peas and mushrooms (*Tamarind Tree* Dhingri Mutter) . . .	290	8.0	53.0	5.0	0	680	7.0
vegetables, creamy, w/nuts (*Tamarind Tree* Navratan Korma)	430	12.0	60.0	16.0	5	700	7.0
vegetables, spicy (*Tamarind Tree* Jalfrazi)	310	8.0	57.0	6.0	0	600	7.0
Venison, meat only, roasted, 4 oz.	179	34.3	0	3.6	127	61	0

Food and Measure	cal.	prot. (gms)	carbo. (gms)	fat (gms)	chol. (mgs)	sod. (mgs)	fiber (gms)
Vermicelli dish, mix, roasted garlic and olive oil, 1 cup*:							
(*Near East*)	310	10.0	48.0	9.0	<5	510	3.0
(*Pasta Roni*)	360	9.0	49.0	15.0	0	1030	2.0
Vienna sausage, see "Sausage, canned"							
Vine spinach, raw, untrimmed, 1 lb. . .	86	8.2	15.4	1.4	0	109	4.0
Vinegar, 1 tbsp.:							
all varieties, except balsamic (*Progresso*)	0	0	0	0	0	0	0
apple cider or red wine (*Eden* Organic) . . .	0	0	0	0	0	0	0
balsamic:							
(*Pompeian*)	5	0	2.0	0	0	0	0
(*Progresso*)	10	0	1.0	0	0	0	0
(*Regina*)	5	0	2.0	0	0	5	0
cider (*Sterling True*) . .	0	0	0	0	0	0	0
plum or brown rice (*Eden* Organic) . . .	2	0	0	0	0	0	0
red wine:							
(*Pompeian*)	2	0	0	0	0	0	0
(*Regina*)	0	0	<1.0	0	0	0	0
sushi (*Sushi Chef*) . .	20	0	6.0	0	0	570	0
white wine (*Regina*) . .	0	0	<1.0	0	0	0	0

W

Food and Measure	cal.	prot. (gms)	carbo. (gms)	fat (gms)	chol. (mgs)	sod. (mgs)	fiber (gms)
Waffle, 1 pc.:							
(*Thomas'* Homestyle)	140	3.0	19.0	5.0	0	390	<1.0
blueberry (*Thomas'*)	140	2.0	20.0	5.0	0	400	<1.0
buttermilk (*Thomas'*)	130	3.0	18.0	4.5	0	470	<1.0
Waffle, frozen, 2 pcs., except as noted:							
(*Aunt Jemima* Homestyle)	200	5.0	32.0	6.0	<5	440	1.0
(*Aunt Jemima* Lowfat)	170	4.0	32.0	2.5	0	380	1.0
(*Belgian Chef*)	180	3.0	34.0	2.0	0	420	0
(*Eggo* Homestyle)	190	5.0	29.0	7.0	20	440	2.0
(*Eggo* Homestyle Low Fat)	160	5.0	31.0	2.5	15	300	1.0
(*Eggo Minis* Homestyle), 3 sets of 4 pcs.	260	7.0	38.0	9.0	25	600	2.0
(*Eggo Nutri-Grain*)	170	5.0	28.0	5.0	0	420	3.0
(*Eggo Nutri-Grain* Low Fat)	140	5.0	28.0	2.5	0	430	3.0
(*Eggo Special K*)	120	6.0	26.0	0	0	280	1.0
(*Hungry Jack* Homestyle)	180	3.0	29.0	6.0	0	540	<1.0
(*Hungry Jack* Homestyle Low Fat)	170	4.0	34.0	2.0	0	350	1.0
apple cinnamon:							
(*Eggo*)	200	5.0	30.0	7.0	20	400	2.0
(*Hungry Jack*)	200	4.0	33.0	6.0	0	540	<1.0
banana bread (*Eggo*)	190	5.0	30.0	6.0	0	280	2.0
blueberry:							
(*Aunt Jemima*)	210	5.0	34.0	6.0	<5	470	1.0
(*Eggo*)	200	4.0	30.0	7.0	20	410	1.0
(*Eggo Nutri-Grain* Low Fat)	150	5.0	30.0	2.5	0	420	3.0
(*Hungry Jack*)	210	3.0	33.0	7.0	0	540	<1.0

Food and Measure	cal.	prot. (gms)	carbo. (gms)	fat (gms)	chol. (mgs)	sod. (mgs)	fiber (gms)
Waffle, frozen (*cont.*)							
buttermilk:							
(*Aunt Jemima*)	200	5.0	33.0	6.0	<5	550	1.0
(*Eggo*)	190	5.0	28.0	7.0	20	420	2.0
(*Hungry Jack*)	190	4.0	29.0	6.0	0	530	<1.0
chocolate chip (*Eggo*)	200	4.0	32.0	7.0	15	380	1.0
cinnamon toast, 3 sets of 4:							
(*Eggo*)	290	5.0	46.0	10.0	25	480	1.0
(*Hungry Jack*)	270	4.0	45.0	9.0	0	600	<1.0
multibran (*Eggo Nutri-Grain*)	160	5.0	29.0	5.0	0	390	5.0
nut and honey (*Eggo*)	220	6.0	30.0	9.0	20	390	2.0
oat, golden (*Eggo*) . . .	140	5.0	26.0	2.5	0	270	3.0
strawberry (*Eggo*) . . .	200	5.0	30.0	7.0	20	420	2.0
wildberry (*Hungry Jack*)	200	3.0	33.0	6.0	0	540	<1.0
Waffle, toaster, see "Toaster bagel, muffin, and pastry"							
Waffle mix, see "Pancake mix"							
Waffle sticks, frozen, 3 pcs.:							
(*Aunt Jemima Home-style*)	310	6.0	48.0	10.0	10	680	3.0
chocolate chip (*Aunt Jemima*)	330	6.0	47.0	13.0	10	640	3.0
cinnamon sugar (*Aunt Jemima*)	320	6.0	52.0	10.0	10	610	3.0
Walnut, dried:							
(*Bazzini's Nut Club*), ¼ cup	210	5.0	3.0	20.0	0	0	3.0
(*Blue Diamond* Halves and Pieces), ⅓ cup	210	5.0	6.0	20.0	0	0	3.0
(*Fisher*), 1 oz.	200	5.0	3.0	20.0	0	0	3.0
black:							
shelled, 1 oz.	172	6.9	3.4	16.1	0	<1	1.4
chopped, 1 cup . . .	759	30.4	15.1	70.7	0	2	6.3
English or Persian:							
shelled, 1 oz.	182	4.1	5.2	17.6	0	3	1.4
pcs., 1 cup	770	17.2	22.0	74.2	0	12	5.8
halves, 1 cup	642	14.3	18.3	61.9	0	10	4.8

Food and Measure	cal.	prot. (gms)	carbo. (gms)	fat (gms)	chol. (mgs)	sod. (mgs)	fiber (gms)
sesame glazed							
(*Diamond*), ¼ cup	190	3.0	15.0	13.0	0	160	2.0
Walnut topping,							
(*Smucker's*),							
2 tbsp.	170	2.0	20.0	9.0	0	0	0
Wasabi root, fresh,							
sliced, ½ cup	71	3.1	15.3	.4	0	11	5.0
Wasabi sauce:							
(*S&B* Tube), 1 tsp. . .	15	0	3.0	.5	0	100	0
(*Sushi Chef*), 1 tbsp.	90	0	0	10.0	5	75	0
w/ginger (*Gold's*),							
1 tsp.	15	0	1.0	1.5	5	15	0
Water chestnut, fresh:							
(*Frieda's*), 1.1 oz. . . .	30	0	7.0	0	0	0	1.0
4 medium, 1.3 oz. . .	35	.5	8.6	< .1	0	5	1.1
sliced, ½ cup	60	.9	14.8	.1	0	9	1.9
Water chestnut, can							
or jar:							
whole, 4 pcs., 1 oz.	14	.3	3.5	< .1	0	2	.7
sliced, ½ cup:							
(*La Choy*)	25	1.0	5.0	0	0	10	1.0
w/liquid	35	.5	8.7	< .1	0	6	1.8
Watercress:							
(*Frieda's*), 1 cup,							
3 oz.	10	2.0	1.0	0	0	35	2.0
10 sprigs, 11¼"	3	.6	.3	< .1	0	10	.6
chopped, ½ cup	2	.4	.2	< .1	0	7	.4
Watermelon, fresh:							
1" slice, 10" diam. . . .	152	3.0	34.6	2.0	0	10	2.4
diced, ½ cup	25	.5	5.7	.3	0	2	.4
yellow, seedless							
(*Frieda's*), ½ cup,							
3 oz.	25	1.0	6.0	0	0	0	0
Watermelon drink							
(*R. W. Knudsen*							
Cooler), 8 fl. oz. . .	120	<1.0	29.0	0	0	10	0
Watermelon rind,							
pickled, sweetened							
(*Reese*), 2 cubes . .	70	0	17.0	0	0	40	0
Watermelon seeds,							
dried, 1 oz.	158	8.1	4.4	13.5	0	28	n.a.
Wax beans, fresh,							
see "Green bean"							

Food and Measure	cal.	prot. (gms)	carbo. (gms)	fat (gms)	chol. (mgs)	sod. (mgs)	fiber (gms)
Wax beans, can or jar, ½ cup:							
cut:							
(*Del Monte* Golden)	20	1.0	4.0	0	0	360	2.0
(*Libby's*)	25	<1.0	4.0	0	0	380	2.0
(*S&W*)	20	1.0	4.0	0	0	360	2.0
cut or French sliced							
(*Blue Boy*)	25	<1.0	4.0	0	0	380	2.0
green and cut (*S&W*)	20	1.0	4.0	0	0	390	2.0
Wax gourd, 1 cup:							
raw, cubed	17	.5	4.0	.3	0	147	3.8
boiled, drained, cubed	23	.7	5.3	.4	0	187	1.8
Welsh rarebit, frozen							
(*Stouffer's*), ¼ cup	120	5.0	5.0	9.0	20	280	0
Wendy's, 1 serving:							
burgers:							
Big Bacon Classic	570	34.0	46.0	29.0	100	1460	3.0
cheeseburger:							
Jr.	310	17.0	34.0	12.0	45	820	2.0
Jr., bacon	380	20.0	34.0	18.0	55	890	2.0
Jr., deluxe	350	17.0	37.0	16.0	45	890	2.0
Kid's Meal	310	17.0	34.0	12.0	45	820	2.0
Classic Single							
w/everything ...	410	24.0	37.0	19.0	70	890	2.0
hamburger Jr.	270	14.0	34.0	9.0	30	600	2.0
hamburger Kid's							
Meal	270	14.0	33.0	9.0	30	600	2.0
chicken sandwich:							
breaded fillet	430	27.0	46.0	16.0	55	750	2.0
club	470	30.0	47.0	19.0	65	920	2.0
grilled	300	24.0	36.0	7.0	55	740	2.0
spicy	430	27.0	47.0	15.0	60	1240	3.0
condiments:							
American cheese ..	70	3.0	1.0	5.0	15	320	0
American cheese Jr.	45	2.0	0	3.5	10	220	0
bacon, 1 slice	20	1.0	0	1.5	5	80	0
honey mustard,							
reduced cal., 1 tsp.	25	0	2.0	1.5	0	40	0
ketchup, 1 tsp. ...	10	0	2.0	0	0	75	0
mayonnaise,							
1½ tsp.	30	0	1.0	3.0	5	60	0
mustard, ½ tsp. ..	5	0	0	0	0	50	0
onion, 4 rings	5	0	1.0	0	0	0	0
pickles, 4 slices ...	0	0	0	0	0	105	0

Food and Measure	cal.	prot. (gms)	carbo. (gms)	fat (gms)	chol. (mgs)	sod. (mgs)	fiber (gms)
tomato, 1 slice	5	0	1.0	0	0	0	0
salads, *Garden Sensations*, no croutons/ dressing:							
Caesar side	70	7.0	2.0	4.0	15	250	1.0
chicken BLT	310	33.0	10.0	16.0	60	1100	4.0
Mandarin Chicken .	150	20.0	17.0	1.5	10	650	3.0
almonds	130	4.0	4.0	12.0	0	70	2.0
noodles	60	1.0	10.0	2.0	0	180	0
side salad	35	2.0	7.0	0	0	20	3.0
spring mix ......:	180	11.0	12.0	11.0	30	230	5.0
taco supremo	360	27.0	29.0	17.0	65	1090	8.0
chips ....:....	220	3.0	25.0	11.0	0	150	2.0
salsa	30	1.0	6.0	0	0	440	0
sour cream ...	60	1.0	1.0	6.0	15	40	0
salad croutons, garlic, 1 pkt.	70	1.0	9.0	2.5	0	120	1.0
dressings, 1 pkt.:							
blue cheese	290	2.0	3.0	30.0	45	870	0
Caesar	150	1.0	1.0	16.0	20	240	0
French style, fat free	90	0	21.0	0	0	240	1.0
honey mustard ...	310	1.0	12.0	29.0	25	410	0
honey mustard, low fat	120	0	23.0	3.5	0	370	0
Oriental sesame ...	280	2.0	21.0	21.0	0	620	0
ranch, creamy	250	0	5.0	25.0	15	640	0
ranch, creamy, reduced fat	80	1.0	7.0	9.0	15	610	1.0
vinagrette	220	0	9.0	20.0	0	830	0
Crispy Chicken Nuggets:							
5 pcs.	220	11.0	13.0	14.0	35	480	0
4 pc. Kid's Meal ...	180	9.0	10.0	11.0	25	380	0
nuggets sauce, 1 pkt.:							
barbecue	40	1.0	10.0	0	0	160	0
honey mustard ...	130	0	6.0	12.0	10	210	0
sweet and sour ...	45	0	12.0	0	0	115	0
chili:							
large, 12 oz.	300	25.0	31.0	9.0	50	1310	7.0
small, 8 oz. ......:	200	15.0	21.0	6.0	35	870	5.0
cheddar, shredded, 2 tbsp.	70	4.0	1.0	6.0	15	110	0
hot chili, 1 pkt. ...	5	0	2.0	0	0	280	0
saltines, 2	25	1.0	4.0	.5	0	80	0

Food and Measure	cal.	prot. (gms)	carbo. (gms)	fat (gms)	chol. (mgs)	sod. (mgs)	fiber (gms)
Wendy's (cont.)							
baked potato:							
plain, 10 oz.	310	7.0	72.0	0	0	25	7.0
bacon cheese	580	18.0	79.0	22.0	40	950	7.0
broccoli cheese . . .	480	9.0	81.0	14.0	5	510	9.0
sour cream chive . .	370	7.0	73.0	6.0	15	40	7.0
sour cream pkt. . . .	60	1.0	2.0	5.0	20	55	0
whipped margarine pkt.	60	0	0	7.0	0	115	0
french fries:							
Biggie	440	5.0	63.0	19.0	0	380	7.0
Great Biggie	530	6.0	75.0	23.0	0	450	8.0
Kid's Meal	250	3.0	36.0	11.0	0	220	4.0
medium	390	4.0	56.0	17.0	0	340	6.0
Frosty:							
junior	170	4.0	28.0	4.0	20	100	0
medium	440	11.0	73.0	11.0	50	260	0
small	330	8.0	56.0	8.0	35	200	0
Whataburger, 1 serving:							
breakfast:							
bacon, 2 slices . . .	75	6.0	1.0	5.0	7	311	0
biscuit, plain	290	5.0	33.0	15.0	0	720	n.a.
w/bacon, egg, cheese	491	21.0	35.0	29.0	244	1370	n.a.
w/egg, cheese . .	416	14.0	34.0	24.0	237	1060	n.a.
w/sausage	503	16.0	34.0	34.0	39	1054	n.a.
w/sausage, gravy	479	8.0	48.0	32.0	16	1567	n.a.
w/sausage, egg, cheese	629	25.0	34.0	43.0	275	1394	n.a.
Breakfast-on-a-Bun, bacon	322	18.0	29.0	16.0	223	814	n.a.
Breakfast-on-a-Bun, sausage	460	23.0	29.0	30.0	354	838	n.a.
cinnamon roll	430	6.0	63.0	6.0	25	160	n.a.
eggs, scrambled, 2	162	13.0	2.0	11.0	454	134	n.a.
hash brown stick, 4 pcs.	140	0	16.0	8.0	0	440	n.a.
omelet sandwich w/cheese	292	15.0	15.0	28.0	255	724	n.a.
pancakes, 3 cakes:							
plain	300	9.0	57.0	3.0	0	1080	n.a.
w/bacon	375	16.0	58.0	8.0	8	1391	n.a.
w/sausage	513	20.0	57.0	22.0	9	1414	n.a.

Food and Measure	cal.	prot. (gms)	carbo. (gms)	fat (gms)	chol. (mgs)	sod. (mgs)	fiber (gms)
sausage	212	11.0	0	18.0	38	334	0
sausage and egg . .	382	22.0	17.0	28.0	355	727	n.a.
taquito:							
bacon and egg . .	377	20.0	28.0	20.0	348	881	n.a.
potato and egg . .	372	14.0	35.0	19.0	340	791	n.a.
burgers:							
Justaburger	295	16.0	27.0	12.0	35	682	n.a.
Whataburger	596	31.0	53.0	29.0	75	1166	n.a.
Whataburger, small							
bun, no oil	424	27.0	31.0	21.0	75	876	n.a.
Whataburger,							
double meat	836	51.0	53.0	46.0	150	1304	n.a.
Whataburger Jr. . .	305	17.0	29.0	15.0	35	688	n.a.
chicken sandwich:							
grilled	453	31.0	49.0	18.0	84	1164	n.a.
grilled, no dressing	397	31.0	47.0	12.0	75	1075	n.a.
grilled, no dressing,							
no oil	370	31.0	47.0	9.0	75	1075	n.a.
grilled, small bun,							
w/mustard, no							
dressing/oil	335	29.0	30.0	8.0	75	1125	n.a.
Whatachick'N	580	28.0	56.0	30.0	64	1096	n.a.
chicken strips, 2	380	18.0	22.0	24.0	30	700	n.a.
salads:							
garden	56	3.0	11.0	0	0	32	n.a.
garden w/cheddar .	225	13.0	11.0	15.0	43	234	n.a.
grilled chicken	216	25.0	19.0	5.0	75	632	n.a.
grilled chicken							
w/cheddar	385	35.0	19.0	19.0	118	834	n.a.
dressing, 2 oz.:							
ranch	310	10.0	3.0	33.0	20	470	0
ranch, lowfat	70	2.0	10.0	4.0	20	640	0
Thousand Island . .	160	0	12.0	12.0	15	490	0
vinaigrette, lowfat	35	0	6.0	2.0	0	890	0
sides:							
fries, Jr. . . . . :	240	3.0	37.0	14.0	0	206	n.a.
fries, large	560	7.0	69.0	29.0	0	411	n.a.
fries, regular	420	5.0	51.0	21.0	0	309	n.a.
onion rings, large .	464	6.0	54.0	26.0	0	608	n.a.
onion rings, regular	307	4.0	36.0	17.0	0	403	n.a.
peppered gravy,							
3 oz.	53	0	8.0	5.0	0	345	n.a.
Texas toast slice . .	137	4.0	21.0	5.0	0	270	n.a.

Food and Measure	cal.	prot. (gms)	carbo. (gms)	fat (gms)	chol. (mgs)	sod. (mgs)	fiber (gms)
Whataburger (*cont.*)							
desserts/shakes:							
cookie, 2 oz.:							
chocolate chunk	140	3.0	35.0	8.0	25	10	n.a.
white chocolate							
macadamia ..	240	3.0	31.0	12.0	25	20	n.a.
hot apple pie	250	2.0	34.0	12.0	0	181	n.a.
shake, medium:							
chocolate	905	19.5	145.7	24.8	90	479	0
strawberry	782	18.1	114.3	24.1	90	421	0
vanilla	834	19.3	121.9	25.7	96	449	0
shake, small:							
chocolate	616	13.1	100.2	16.7	60	325	0
strawberry	620	12.1	101.0	16.1	60	296	0
vanilla	559	12.9	81.7	17.2	64	301	0
Wheat, whole-grain:							
durum, 1 cup	651	26.3	136.6	4.7	0	3	n.a.
hard red:							
spring, 1 cup	632	29.6	130.6	3.7	0	4	24.2
winter, 1 cup	628	24.2	136.7	3.0	0	4	24.2
winter (*Arrowhead*							
Mills), ¼ cup ...	160	6.0	34.0	1.0	0	0	7.0
hard white, 1 cup ...	657	21.7	145.7	3.3	0	4	n.a.
soft red winter, 1 cup	556	17.4	124.7	2.6	0	4	21.0
soft white, 1 cup	571	18.0	126.6	3.3	0	3	21.3
Wheat, parboiled, see "Bulgur"							
Wheat, sprouted,							
1 cup	214	8.1	45.9	1.4	0	18	1.2
Wheat bran (see also "Cereal"):							
(*Arrowhead Mills*),							
¼ cup	35	2.0	10.0	1.0	0	0	6.0
crude, 2 tbsp.	15	1.1	4.5	.3	0	<1	3.0
toasted (*Kretschmer*),							
¼ cup	30	3.0	10.0	1.0	0	0	7.0
unprocessed (*Quaker*),							
⅓ cup	30	3.0	11.0	0	0	0	8.0
untoasted (*Hodgson Mill*), 2 tbsp.	55	4.0	7.0	1.0	0	0	4.0
Wheat flakes, rolled (*Arrowhead Mills*),							
⅓ cup	110	4.0	24.0	.5	0	0	5.0

Food and Measure	cal.	prot. (gms)	carbo. (gms)	fat (gms)	chol. (mgs)	sod. (mgs)	fiber (gms)
Wheat flour, ¼ cup, except as noted:							
(*All Trump*)	100	4.0	22.0	0	0	0	<1.0
(*Hodgson Mill* 50/50 Wheat)	100	4.0	21.0	1.0	0	0	2.0
(*La Piña*)	100	2.0	23.0	0	0	0	<1.0
all-purpose, white:							
(*Gold Medal/Gold Medal* Organic) .	100	3.0	22.0	0	0	0	<1.0
(*Red Band*)	100	2.0	23.0	0	0	0	<1.0
(*Robin Hood*)	100	3.0	22.0	0	0	0	<1.0
1 cup	455	12.9	95.4	1.2	0	2	3.4
all purpose, unbleached:							
(*Arrowhead Mills*), ⅓ cup	160	5.0	33.0	.5	0	0	0
(*Gold Medal/Robin Hood*)	100	3.0	22.0	0	0	0	<1.0
(*Hodgson Mill*) . . .	100	3.0	23.0	0	0	0	1.0
(*Pillsbury*)	100	3.0	21.0	0	0	0	<1.0
bread:							
(*Eagle Mills* Bread Machine)	100	3.0	22.0	0	0	0	<1.0
(*Gold Medal* Better for Bread)	100	4.0	22.0	0	0	0	<1.0
(*Hodgson Mill* Best for Bread)	100	4.0	22.0	0	0	5	1.0
(*Red Band*)	100	4.0	22.0	0	0	0	<1.0
wheat blend (*Gold Medal* Better for Bread)	100	4.0	21.0	.5	0	0	1.0
cake:							
(*Betty Crocker Softasilk*)	100	2.0	23.0	0	0	0	<1.0
(*Swan's Down*) . . .	100	2.0	22.0	0	0	0	0
1 cup	395	8.9	85.1	.9	0	2	1.8
gluten, see "Wheat gluten"							
mix, self-rising (*Aunt Jemima*), 3 tbsp.	90	3.0	20.0	0	0	310	1.0
pasta, see "Semolina flour"							
pastry:							
(*Arrowhead Mills*) .	110	4.0	23.0	.5	0	0	3.0

Food and Measure	cal.	prot. (gms)	carbo. (gms)	fat (gms)	chol. (mgs)	sod. (mgs)	fiber (gms)
Wheat flour, pastry (cont.)							
whole wheat (*Hodgson Mill*)	110	3.0	22.0	.5	0	0	3.0
presifted:							
(*Pillsbury* Shake & Blend)	100	3.0	23.0	0	0	0	<1.0
(*Wondra*)	100	3.0	23.0	0	0	0	<1.0
seasoned (*Kentucky Kernel*)	90	3.0	20.0	0	0	1360	0
self-rising:							
(*Gold Medal/Robin Hood*)	100	3.0	22.0	0	0	400	<1.0
(*Pillsbury*)	100	3.0	22.0	0	0	360	<1.0
(*Red Band*)	100	2.0	22.0	0	0	400	<1.0
1 cup	442	12.4	92.8	1.2	0	1587	4.0
tortilla mix, 1 cup	449	10.7	74.5	11.8	0	751	n.a.
whole grain, 1 cup	407	16.4	87.1	2.2	0	1	15.1
whole wheat:							
(*Gold Medal*)	90	4.0	21.0	.5	0	0	3.0
graham (*Hodgson Mill*)	100	3.0	22.0	1.0	0	0	3.0
white (*Hodgson Mill*)	100	3.0	21.0	.5	0	0	3.0
stone-ground (*Arrowhead Mills*)	130	5.0	25.0	.5	0	0	4.0
Wheat germ:							
(*Kretschmer*), 2 tbsp.	50	4.0	6.0	1.0	0	0	2.0
crude, 1 oz.	102	6.6	14.7	2.8	0	3	3.7
honey crunch (*Kretschmer*), 1⅔ tbsp.	50	4.0	8.0	1.0	0	0	1.0
raw (*Arrowhead Mills*), 3 tbsp.	50	4.0	10.0	1.5	0	0	2.0
toasted, 1 oz.	108	8.3	14.1	3.0	0	1	3.7
Wheat gluten:							
(*Arrowhead Mills*), 3 tbsp.	35	5.0	3.0	0	0	0	0
(*General Mills* Supreme Hygluten), ¼ cup	100	4.0	22.0	0	0	0	<1.0
(*Hodgson Mill* Vital), 1 tbsp.	30	6.0	2.0	0	0	0	1.0
Wheat kernels (*Purity Foods* Berries), ¼ cup	160	6.0	34.0	1.0	0	0	7.0

Food and Measure	cal.	prot. (gms)	carbo. (gms)	fat (gms)	chol. (mgs)	sod. (mgs)	fiber (gms)
Wheat malt syrup, see "Malt syrup"							
Wheat pilaf mix (see also "Grains, mixed, dish"):							
(*Near East*), 2 oz. ...	180	6.0	42.0	.5	0	650	5.0
(*Near East*), 1 cup* ..	210	6.0	42.0	3.5	10	710	5.0
bulgur (*Casbah*), ¾ cup	240	10.0	36.0	1.0	0	460	4.0
Whelk, meat only, raw, 4 oz.	156	27.0	8.8	.5	74	234	0
Whey, fluid:							
acid, 1 cup	59	1.9	12.6	.2	0	118	0
sweet, 1 cup	66	2.1	12.6	.9	5	132	0
Whipped topping, see "Cream topping"							
Whiskey, see "Liquor"							
Whiskey sour drink mixer (*Mr & Mrs T*), 4 fl. oz.	100	0	23.0	0	0	50	0
White bean, mature:							
boiled, ½ cup	125	8.6	22.6	.3	0	6	5.7
small:							
dry (*Jack Rabbit*), ¼ cup	70	8.0	22.0	0	0	15	14.0
boiled, ½ cup	124	8.7	22.5	.3	0	5	5.6
White bean, canned:							
w/liquid, ½ cup	153	9.5	28.7	.4	0	595	6.3
small (*S&W*), ½ cup	80	7.0	19.0	1.0	0	440	6.0
Spanish style (*Goya*), 7.5 oz.	130	13.0	29.0	1.0	0	990	12.0
White Castle:							
sandwiches, 1 pc.:							
breakfast	340	14.0	17.0	25.0	130	900	0
cheeseburger	160	7.0	11.0	9.0	15	250	2.0
cheeseburger, bacon	200	10.0	12.0	13.0	25	400	3.0
cheeseburger, double	290	14.0	16.0	18.0	30	430	5.0
chicken ring	200	5.0	15.0	14.0	20	1370	1.0
fish	180	7.0	27.0	7.0	10	390	1.0
hamburger	140	6.0	11.0	7.0	10	135	2.0
hamburger, double	240	11.0	16.0	14.0	20	200	4.0
chicken rings, 6 pcs.	210	16.0	10.0	14.0	50	420	0

Food and Measure	cal	prot. (gms)	carbo. (gms)	fat (gms)	chol. (mgs)	sod. (mgs)	fiber (gms)
White Castle (cont.)							
sides:							
cheese sticks, 5 pcs.	420	17.0	37.0	23.0	40	1240	3.0
french fries, small	115	0	15.0	6.0	0	15	2.0
onion rings, 8 pcs.	290	3.0	38.0	13.0	1	300	4.0
shakes, 16 oz.:							
chocolate	250	9.0	37.0	8.0	30	160	0
vanilla	260	9.0	40.0	8.0	30	170	0
White sauce mix							
(*Knorr*), 2 tsp. . . .	25	0	4.0	1.0	0	220	0
Whitefish, meat only:							
raw, 4 oz.	153	21.7	0	6.7	68	58	0
baked, broiled, or microwaved,							
4 oz.	195	27.7	0	8.5	87	74	0
Whitefish, smoked:							
(*Ducktrap River*),							
2 oz.	70	12.0	0	2.0	5	730	0
4 oz.	122	26.5	0	1.1	37	1156	0
Whitefish salad,							
smoked (*Rite Brand*),							
2 tbsp.	100	8.0	<1.0	10.0	15	180	0
Whiting, meat only:							
raw, 4 oz.	102	20.8	0	1.5	76	82	0
baked, broiled, or microwaved,							
4 oz.	130	26.6	0	1.9	95	150	0
Wiener, see "Frank-furter"							
Wild rice:							
raw, ¼ cup:							
(*Gourmet House*) . .	170	6.0	35.0	0	0	0	2.0
(*Gourmet House* Quick)	170	6.0	25.0	0	0	0	2.0
(*Lundberg* Organic)	160	6.0	34.0	.5	0	0	3.0
cooked, 1 cup	166	6.5	35.0	.6	0	6	1.5
dried, instant (*Alpine-Aire*), 1 oz.	110	4.0	22.0	0	0	0	1.0
Wild rice blends, see "Rice"							
Wild rice dishes, see "Rice dishes"							
Wine, 3.5 fl.oz.:							
dessert or apertif[1] . . .	158	.2	12.2	0	0	9	0

Food and Measure	cal.	prot. (gms)	carbo. (gms)	fat (gms)	chol. (mgs)	sod. (mgs)	fiber (gms)
dry or table[2]:							
red	74	.2	1.8	0	0	5	0
rose	73	.2	1.4	0	0	5	0
white	70	.1	.8	0	0	5	0
Wine, cooking, 2 tbsp., except as noted:							
Burgundy (*Regina*) ..	25	0	3.0	0	0	190	0
Marsala (*Holland House*)	45	0	4.0	0	0	190	0
red (*Holland House*) .	20	0	1.0	0	0	190	0
rice (*Sun Luck* Mirin), 1 tbsp.	20	0	5.0	0	0	55	0
Sauterne (*Regina*) ...	20	0	3.0	0	0	190	0
sherry:							
(*Holland House*) ..	45	0	5.0	0	0	190	0
(*Regina*)	35	0	5.0	0	0	190	0
white, plain or w/lemon (*Holland House*)	20	0	0	0	0	190	0
Winged bean, fresh:							
raw, sliced, ½ cup ...	11	1.5	1.0	.2	0	1	n.a.
boiled, drained, ½ cup	12	1.6	1.0	.2	0	1	n.a.
Winged bean, mature:							
dry, ½ cup	372	27.0	38.0	14.9	0	35	14.1
boiled, ½ cup	126	9.1	12.8	5.0	0	11	n.a.
Winged bean leaves, trimmed, 1 oz. ...	21	1.7	4.0	.3	0	n.a.	n.a.
Winged bean tuber, trimmed, 1 oz. ...	45	3.3	8.0	.3	0	n.a.	n.a.
Winter squash (see also specific listings), all varieties, 1 cup:							
raw, cubed	43	1.7	10.2	.3	0	5	1.7
boiled, drained, cubed	80	1.8	17.9	1.3	0	2	5.7
Witloof, see "Chicory, witloof"							

1. *Includes fortified wines containing more than 15% alcohol, such as port, sherry, vermouth, etc.*
2. *Includes wines containing less than 15% alcohol, such as Burgundy, Chablis, champagne, etc.*

Food and Measure	cal.	prot. (gms)	carbo. (gms)	fat (gms)	chol. (mgs)	sod. (mgs)	fiber (gms)
Wolf fish, Atlantic, meat only:							
raw, 4 oz.	109	19.9	0	2.7	52	97	0
baked, broiled, or microwaved, 4 oz.	139	25.4	0	3.5	67	124	0
Wonton wrapper (see also "Wrappers"):							
(*Frieda's*), 4 pcs.	80	3.0	17.0	0	0	160	1.0
(*Nasoya*), 8 pcs.	260	6.0	31.0	.5	20	370	1.0
Worcestershire sauce, 1 tsp.:							
(*A.1.*)	5	0	1.0	0	0	70	0
(*Heinz*)	0	0	0	0	0	60	0
(*Lea & Perrins*)	5	0	1.0	0	0	65	0
white wine (*Lea & Perrins*)	3	0	.7	0	0	50	0
Wrappers (see also "Egg roll wrapper" and "Wonton wrapper"):							
large square (*Azumaya*), 3 pcs.	170	7.0	35.0	.5	10	410	1.0
round square (*Azumaya*), 10 pcs.	160	6.0	31.0	.5	10	370	1.0
square (*Azumaya*), 8 pcs.	160	6.0	31.0	.5	10	370	1.0
Wraps (see also "Tortilla"), unfilled, 2-oz. pc., except as noted:							
plain (*Aladdin Bread*)	190	4.0	33.0	4.0	0	320	1.0
garlic pesto:							
(*Aladdin Bread*)	180	4.0	33.0	4.0	0	400	1.0
(*Cedar's*), 2.5 oz.	190	7.0	36.0	3.0	0	345	5.0
multigrain, 6 (*Cedar's Mountain Bread*)	200	7.0	35.0	4.0	0	380	4.0
jalapeño (*Aladdin Bread*)	190	4.0	33.0	4.0	0	410	1.0
Southwestern:							
(*Aladdin Bread*)	190	4.0	33.0	4.0	0	390	1.0
(*Cedar's*), 2.5 oz.	185	8.0	36.0	3.0	0	350	5.0
spinach (*Cedar's*), 2.5 oz.	180	8.0	36.0	3.0	0	300	5.0

Food and Measure	cal.	prot. (gms)	carbo. (gms)	fat (gms)	chol. (mgs)	sod. (mgs)	fiber (gms)
tomato basil (*Cedar's*), 2.5 oz.	185	8.0	36.0	3.0	0	345	5.0
wheat:							
(*Cedar's* Mountain Bread)	180	7.0	34.0	4.0	0	340	4.0
whole (Aladdin Bread)	180	4.0	33.0	4.0	0	480	1.0
white (Cedar's Mountain Bread)	180	4.0	29.0	4.0	0	310	1.0
Wraps, filled, see "Vegetarian entree, frozen" and "Pasta entree, frozen"							

Food and Measure	cal.	prot. (gms)	carbo. (gms)	fat (gms)	chol. (mgs)	sod. (mgs)	fiber (gms)
Yam, cubed, ½ cup:							
raw	89	1.2	20.9	.1	0	7	3.1
baked or boiled	79	1.0	18.8	.1	0	6	2.7
Yam, canned or frozen, see "Sweet potato"							
Yam, mountain, Hawaiian, ½ cup:							
raw, cubed	46	.9	11.1	.1	0	9	n.a.
steamed, cubed	59	1.2	14.4	.1	0	9	n.a.
Yam, name, see "Name yam"							
Yam bean, tuber:							
raw:							
(*Frieda's* Jicama), ¾ cup, 3 oz. ...	35	1.0	7.0	0	0	5	1.0
sliced, ½ cup	23	.4	5.3	.1	0	3	2.9
boiled, drained, 4 oz.	43	.8	10.0	.1	0	5	n.a.
Yard-long bean, fresh:							
raw (*Frieda's* Long Bean), ¾ cup, 3 oz.	40	2.0	7.0	0	0	0	0
boiled, drained, sliced, ½ cup	25	1.3	4.8	.1	0	2	n.a.
Yard-long bean, mature:							
dry, ½ cup	292	20.4	52.0	1.1	0	14	4.0
boiled, ½ cup	102	7.1	18.1	.4	0	4	1.4
Yeast, baker's:							
active:							
(*Hodgson Mill*), ⁵⁄₁₆ oz.	30	4.0	3.0	0	0	0	1.0
dry, 1 tbsp.	35	3.4	4.6	.6	0	6	.3
compressed, .6-oz. ..	6	<.1	1.1	0	0	2	<.1

Food and Measure	cal.	prot. (gms)	carbo. (gms)	fat (gms)	chol. (mgs)	sod. (mgs)	fiber (gms)
fast rise (*Hodgson Mill*), 5⁄16 oz.	25	3.0	4.0	0	0	0	1.0
Yellow beans, dried, boiled, ½ cup	126	8.1	22.2	1.0	0	4	n.a.
Yellow eye beans (*Frieda's*), ½ cup	120	7.0	22.0	0	0	0	9.0
Yellow squash, fresh, see "Crookneck squash"							
Yellow squash, canned (*Sunshine*), ½ cup	25	0	5.0	0	0	160	2.0
Yellow squash, frozen, sliced (*Birds Eye Southern*), 2⁄3 cup .	15	<1.0	2.0	0	0	15	1.0
Yellowtail, meat only: raw, 4 oz.	166	26.3	0	6.0	62	44	0
baked, broiled, or microwaved, 4 oz.	212	33.6	0	7.6	81	57	0
Yogurt, 8 oz., except as noted:							
plain:							
(*Colombo* Lowfat)	130	10.0	16.0	2.5	15	125	0
(*Colombo* Nonfat)	100	10.0	16.0	0	10	125	0
(*Crowley* Nonfat) . .	100	8.0	17.0	0	<5	130	0
(*Dannon* Lowfat) . .	150	12.0	18.0	4.0	20	190	0
(*Dannon* Nonfat) . .	130	12.0	19.0	0	5	190	0
(*Darigold* Lowfat) . .	160	14.0	21.0	2.5	15	190	0
(*Friendship*)	150	12.0	18.0	3.0	15	190	0
(*Stonyfield Farm*) .	180	9.0	12.0	10.0	40	125	0
(*Stonyfield Farm* Lowfat), 6 oz. . .	80	7.0	10.0	1.5	5	105	0
(*Stonyfield Farm* Lowfat)	110	9.0	14.0	2.0	10	135	0
(*Stonyfield Farm* Nonfat)	100	9.0	15.0	0	<5	150	0
(*Yoplait* Nonfat), 6 oz.	80	7.0	12.0	0	5	120	0
all flavors:							
(*Colombo* Light) . .	120	7.0	21.0	0	5	110	0
(*Dannon Sprinkl'ins*), 4.1 oz.	120	6.0	22.0	1.0	0	85	0

Food and Measure	cal.	prot. (gms)	carbo. (gms)	fat (gms)	chol. (mgs)	sod. (mgs)	fiber (gms)
Yogurt (*cont.*)							
all fruit flavors:							
(*Breyers* 1% Lowfat)	230	9.0	44.0	2.0	20	120	0
(*Breyers* Creme Savers)	230	7.0	42.0	3.0	25	230	0
(*Crowley* Swiss Style)	240	8.0	47.0	2.5	10	135	0
(*Yoplait* 99% Fat Free), 6 oz.	170	5.0	33.0	1.5	10	80	0
(*Yoplait* Custard Style), 6 oz. . . .	190	7.0	32.0	3.5	15	90	0
(*Yoplait* Custard Style), 4 oz. . . .	120	5.0	21.0	2.0	10	60	0
(*Yoplait* Exprésse), 2.25-oz. tube . . .	70	2.0	11.0	1.5	5	40	0
(*Yoplait* Go-Gurt), 2.25-oz. tube . .	70	3.0	11.0	2.0	5	40	0
(*Yoplait* Trix), 4 oz.	120	4.0	23.0	1.5	5	55	0
(*Yoplait* Yumsters), 4 oz.	120	5.0	21.0	2.0	10	60	0
except banana/straw- berry (*Colombo* Classic)	220	7.0	42.0	2.0	15	115	0
apple cinnamon:							
(*Breyers Light*) . . .	120	8.0	22.0	0	10	105	0
(*Dannon* Fruit on the Bottom)	210	9.0	39.0	2.0	10	140	1.0
apple cobbler							
(*Breyers* Smooth & Creamy*)	230	7.0	46.0	2.0	20	120	0
apricot mango:							
(*Darigold* Lowfat) . .	240	10.0	45.0	2.5	15	130	0
(*Stonyfield Farm* Nonfat)	160	8.0	31.0	0	0	125	<1.0
(*Stonyfield Farm* Nonfat), 1 cup . .	170	8.0	30.0	0	0	130	0
(*Yoplait* Light), 6 oz.	100	5.0	19.0	0	<5	85	0
banana (*Stonyfield Farm* Blended), 6 oz.	170	6.0	32.0	1.5	5	85	3.0
banana cream pie:							
(*Dannon Light 'n Fit*)	120	8.0	21.0	0	<5	130	0
(*Yoplait* Light), 6 oz.	100	6.0	19.0	0	<5	90	0

Food and Measure	cal.	prot. (gms)	carbo. (gms)	fat (gms)	chol. (mgs)	sod. (mgs)	fiber (gms)
banana/strawberry (*Colombo* Classic)	230	7.0	47.0	2.0	10	90	0
berries, mixed (*Dannon* Fruit on the Bottom)	210	9.0	39.0	2.0	10	190	0
berries and cream (*Yoplait* Light), 6 oz.	100	5.0	19.0	0	<5	85	0
blackberry pie (*Dannon Light 'n Fit*)	120	8.0	22.0	0	<5	130	0
blueberries and cream: (*Breyers Light*) . . .	120	8.0	21.0	0	10	105	<1.0
(*Breyers Smooth & Creamy*)	230	7.0	46.0	2.0	20	110	0
blueberry: (*Dannon* Fruit on the Bottom)	210	9.0	39.0	2.0	10	200	1.0
(*Dannon Light 'n Fit*)	120	8.0	23.0	0	<5	130	0
(*Darigold* Lowfat) . .	240	10.0	45.0	2.5	15	150	0
(*Stonyfield Farm* Lowfat), 6 oz. . .	130	6.0	23.0	1.5	5	90	0
(*Stonyfield Farm* Nonfat)	160	8.0	30.0	0	0	130	<1.0
(*Yoplait* Light), 6 oz.	100	5.0	19.0	0	<5	85	0
wild (*Stonyfield Farm*), 6 oz. . . .	160	5.0	22.0	5.0	20	85	0
blueberry peach (*Dannon* Fruit on the Bottom), 4 oz. . . .	100	5.0	20.0	1.0	5	100	0
blueberry vanilla cream (*Dannon Double Delights*), 6 oz.	180	7.0	36.0	1.0	5	105	0
Boston cream pie (*Yoplait* Light), 6 oz.	100	6.0	19.0	0	<5	90	0
boysenberry: (*Dannon* Fruit on the Bottom)	210	9.0	39.0	2.0	10	170	1.0
(*Darigold* Lowfat) . .	240	10.0	45.0	2.5	15	170	0
cappuccino: (*Dannon Light 'n Fit*)	120	8.0	23.0	0	<5	135	0
(*Stonyfield Farm* Nonfat)	160	9.0	31.0	0	0	135	0

Food and Measure	cal.	prot. (gms)	carbo. (gms)	fat (gms)	chol. (mgs)	sod. (mgs)	fiber (gms)
Yogurt (*cont.*)							
caramel:							
(*Stonyfield Farm Lowfat*), 6 oz. ..	170	6.0	33.0	1.5	5	135	0
(*Stonyfield Farm Nonfat*)	220	8.0	46.0	0	0	180	0
chocolate (*Stonyfield Farm*), 4 oz.	110	4.0	21.0	1.0	5	65	2.0
cheesecake, 6 oz.:							
cherry (*Dannon Double Delights*)	180	7.0	35.0	1.0	5	115	0
chocolate (*Dannon Double Delights*)	220	8.0	46.0	1.0	5	160	0
strawberry (*Dannon Double Delights*)	170	7.0	33.0	1.0	5	115	0
cherry:							
(*Dannon* Fruit on the Bottom)	210	9.0	40.0	2.0	10	150	0
(*Darigold Lowfat*) ..	240	10.0	44.0	2.5	15	150	0
(*Stonyfield Farm Nonfat*)	160	8.0	31.0	0	0	130	<1.0
(*Yoplait Light*), 6 oz.	100	5.0	19.0	0	<5	85	0
cherry, black:							
(*Breyers Light Jubilee*)	120	8.0	21.0	0	10	105	0
(*Breyers Smooth & Creamy Parfait*)	230	7.0	46.0	2.0	20	110	0
(*Breyers Smooth & Creamy Parfait*), 4 oz.	110	3.0	23.0	1.0	10	55	0
cherry vanilla:							
(*Dannon Light 'n Fit*)	120	8.0	24.0	0	<5	130	0
cream (*Breyers Light*)	120	8.0	21.0	0	10	105	0
chocolate (*Stonyfield Farm Nonfat*)	200	8.0	46.0	0	0	135	<1.0
chocolate, white:							
raspberry (*Dannon Light 'n Fit*)	120	8.0	22.0	0	<5	135	0
raspberry (*Darigold Lowfat*)	240	10.0	45.0	2.5	15	150	0
strawberry (*Yoplait Light*), 6 oz. ...	100	5.0	19.0	0	<5	85	0

Food and Measure	cal.	prot. (gms)	carbo. (gms)	fat (gms)	chol. (mgs)	sod. (mgs)	fiber (gms)
coconut cream pie:							
(*Dannon Light 'n Fit*)	120	8.0	22.0	0	<5	130	0
(*Yoplait*), 6 oz. . . .	190	5.0	34.0	3.0	10	85	0
coffee (*Dannon*)	220	11.0	37.0	4.0	15	170	0
cranberry raspberry							
(*Dannon*)	220	11.0	37.0	4.0	15	170	0
crème caramel							
(*Dannon Light 'n Fit*)	120	8.0	22.0	0	<5	130	0
dulce de leche							
(*Dannon La Crème*),							
4 oz.	140	5.0	20.0	5.0	20	80	0
lemon:							
(*Colombo* Classic) .	180	8.0	32.0	2.0	15	120	0
(*Dannon*)	220	11.0	37.0	4.0	15	170	0
(*Stonyfield Farm*							
Lotsa Nonfat) . . .	160	9.0	30.0	0	0	140	0
(*Stonyfield Farm*							
Luscious Lowfat),							
6 oz.	130	6.0	23.0	1.5	5	115	0
(*Yoplait*), 6 oz. . . .	180	5.0	36.0	1.5	10	80	0
chiffon (*Breyers*							
Light)	120	8.0	21.0	0	10	105	0
chiffon (*Dannon*							
Light 'n Fit)	120	8.0	22.0	0	<5	130	0
chiffon (*Darigold*							
Light), 6 oz. . . .	100	8.0	18.0	0	5	130	0
meringue pie							
(*Dannon Double*							
Delights), 6 oz. .	180	7.0	37.0	1.0	5	190	0
lime pie, Key:							
(*Breyers Light*) . . .	120	8.0	22.0	0	10	105	0
(*Breyers Light*),							
4 oz.	60	4.0	11.0	0	5	50	0
(*Darigold* Light),							
6 oz.	100	8.0	18.0	0	5	110	0
(*Yoplait* Light), 6 oz.	100	5.0	19.0	0	<5	85	0
maple, creamy							
(*Stonyfield Farm*),							
6 oz.	160	6.0	19.0	6.0	25	90	0
maple vanilla (*Stony-*							
field Farm Lowfat),							
6 oz.	120	6.0	19.0	1.5	5	95	0
marionberry (*Darigold*							
Light), 6 oz.	100	8.0	18.0	0	5	110	0

Food and Measure	cal.	prot. (gms)	carbo. (gms)	fat (gms)	chol. (mgs)	sod. (mgs)	fiber (gms)
Yogurt (*cont.*)							
mocha:							
(*Stonyfield Farm Mocha-ccino*), 6 oz.	170	6.0	22.0	6.0	20	95	0
latte (*Stonyfield Farm* Lowfat), 6 oz.	120	8.0	20.0	1.5	5	100	0
orange:							
(*Yoplait* Light Sunrise), 6 oz.	100	5.0	19.0	0	<5	85	0
crème (*Yoplait* Light), 6 oz.	100	5.0	19.0	0	<5	85	0
orange mango (*Dannon Light 'n Fit*)	120	8.0	21.0	0	<5	130	0
orange vanilla cream (*Breyers Smooth & Creamy*)	230	7.0	45.0	2.0	20	110	0
passion fruit banana (*Yoplait* Light), 6 oz.	100	5.0	19.0	0	<5	85	0
peach:							
(*Breyers Light 'n Lively*), 4 oz.	120	3.0	24.0	1.0	10	50	0
(*Dannon* Fruit on the Bottom)	210	9.0	40.0	2.0	10	140	0
(*Dannon La Crème*), 4 oz.	140	5.0	20.0	3.0	20	80	0
(*Dannon Light 'n Fit*)	120	8.0	23.0	0	<5	130	0
(*Darigold* Lowfat)	240	10.0	45.0	2.5	15	150	0
(*Stonyfield Farm* Blended), 6 oz.	170	5.0	33.0	1.5	5	85	3.0
(*Stonyfield Farm* Just Peachy Lowfat), 6 oz.	130	6.0	22.0	1.5	5	110	<1.0
(*Stonyfield Farm* Nonfat)	150	8.0	30.0	0	0	130	<1.0
(*Yoplait* Light), 6 oz.	100	5.0	19.0	0	<5	85	0
a la mode (*Breyers* 1.5% Lowfat)	290	8.0	59.0	2.5	15	110	0
peaches and cream:							
(*Breyers Light*)	120	8.0	21.0	0	10	105	0
(*Breyers Smooth & Creamy*)	240	7.0	48.0	2.0	20	105	0

Food and Measure	cal.	prot. (gms)	carbo. (gms)	fat (gms)	chol. (mgs)	sod. (mgs)	fiber (gms)
(*Breyers Smooth & Creamy*), 4 oz. . .	120	3.0	24.0	1.0	10	50	0
(*Darigold* Light), 6 oz.	100	8.0	18.0	0	5	110	0
piña colada (*Yoplait*), 6 oz.	170	5.0	33.0	2.0	10	95	0
strawberries and cream (*Stonyfield Farm*), 6 oz.	160	5.0	22.0	5.0	20	85	0
raspberries and cream:							
(*Breyers Light*) . . .	120	8.0	22.0	0	10	120	0
(*Breyers Smooth & Creamy*)	240	7.0	48.0	2.0	20	115	0
(*Breyers Smooth & Creamy*), 4 oz. . .	120	3.0	24.0	1.0	10	55	0
raspberry:							
(*Dannon* Fruit on the Bottom)	210	9.0	40.0	2.0	10	150	1.0
(*Dannon La Crème*), 4 oz.	140	5.0	20.0	3.0	20	85	0
(*Dannon Light 'n Fit*)	120	8.0	22.0	0	<5	190	0
(*Darigold* Light), 6 oz.	100	8.0	18.0	0	5	125	0
(*Darigold* Lowfat) . .	240	10.0	45.0	2.5	15	170	0
(*Stonyfield Farm* Lowfat), 6 oz. . .	130	6.0	23.0	1.5	5	100	1.0
(*Stonyfield Farm* Nonfat)	160	8.0	31.0	0	0	130	<1.0
(*Yoplait* Light), 6 oz.	100	5.0	19.0	0	<5	85	0
a la mode (*Breyers* 1.5% Lowfat) . . .	290	8.0	58.0	2.5	15	115	0
raspberry Bavarian creme (*Dannon Double Delights*), 6 oz.	170	7.0	34.0	1.0	5	105	0
raspberry lemon (*Darigold* Lowfat) . .	240	10.0	45.0	2.5	15	130	0
raspberry peach Melba (*Yoplait* Light), 6 oz.	100	5.0	19.0	0	<5	85	0
raspberry strawberry banana (*Dannon Danimals*), 4 oz. . .	120	5.0	21.0	2.0	5	75	0

Food and Measure	cal.	prot. (gms)	carbo. (gms)	fat (gms)	chol. (mgs)	sod. (mgs)	fiber (gms)
Yogurt (*cont.*)							
strawberry:							
(*Breyers Light Classic*)	120	8.0	21.0	0	10	105	0
(*Breyers Light Classic*), 4 oz. . .	60	4.0	11.0	0	5	50	0
(*Breyers Light 'n Lively*), 4 oz. . . .	110	3.0	23.0	1.0	10	50	0
(*Breyers Light 'n Lively* Fruit Cup), 4 oz.	120	4.0	23.0	1.0	10	55	0
(*Breyers Smooth & Creamy* Classic)	230	7.0	46.0	2.0	20	105	0
(*Breyers Smooth & Creamy* Classic), 4 oz.	110	3.0	23.0	1.0	10	50	0
(*Colombo* Lowfat) .	190	9.0	31.0	3.0	20	130	0
(*Dannon La Crème*), 4 oz.	140	5.0	20.0	3.0	20	75	0
(*Dannon* Fruit on the Bottom)	210	9.0	40.0	2.0	10	140	0
(*Dannon Light 'n Fit*)	120	8.0	23.0	0	<5	160	0
(*Darigold Light*), 6 oz.	100	8.0	18.0	0	5	110	0
(*Darigold* Lowfat) . .	240	10.0	45.0	2.5	15	150	0
(*Stonyfield Farm* Blended), 6 oz. .	170	5.0	33.0	1.5	5	85	3.0
(*Stonyfield Farm* Lowfat), 6 oz. . .	130	6.0	23.0	1.5	5	90	0
(*Stonyfield Farm* Nonfat)	160	8.0	32.0	0	0	130	<1.0
(*Yoplait* Light), 6 oz.	100	5.0	19.0	0	<5	85	0
a la mode (*Breyers* 1.5% Lowfat) . . .	290	8.0	58.0	2.5	15	110	0
strawberry banana:							
(*Breyers Light*) . . .	120	8.0	22.0	0	10	115	<1.0
(*Breyers Smooth & Creamy*)	240	7.0	49.0	2.0	20	100	0
(*Breyers Smooth & Creamy*), 4 oz. . .	120	3.0	24.0	1.0	10	50	0
(*Dannon* Fruit on the Bottom)	210	9.0	40.0	2.0	10	140	0
(*Dannon Light 'n Fit*)	120	8.0	22.0	0	<5	140	0
(*Darigold* Lowfat) . .	240	10.0	46.0	2.5	15	130	0

Food and Measure	cal.	prot. (gms)	carbo. (gms)	fat (gms)	chol. (mgs)	sod. (mgs)	fiber (gms)
(*Stonyfield Farm*), 4 oz.	100	4.0	20.0	1.0	5	70	2.0
(*Yoplait* Light), 6 oz.	100	5.0	19.0	0	<5	85	0
strawberry banana, cherry, or raspberry (*Dannon* Blended Nonfat), 4 oz.	100	5.0	21.0	0	0	75	0
strawberry blueberry (*Dannon* Blended Nonfat), 4 oz.	100	5.0	21.0	0	0	85	0
strawberry cheesecake:							
(*Breyers Light*) ...	120	8.0	22.0	0	10	115	<1.0
(*Breyers Smooth & Creamy*)	230	7.0	47.0	2.0	20	105	0
strawberry kiwi:							
(*Dannon Light 'n Fit*)	120	8.0	22.0	0	<5	140	0
(*Darigold* Lowfat) ..	240	10.0	45.0	2.5	15	150	0
strawberry mixed berries (*Dannon* Fruit on the Bottom), 4 oz.	110	5.0	20.0	1.0	5	70	0
strawberry peach (*Dannon* Blended Nonfat), 4 oz.	100	5.0	20.0	0	0	75	0
tangerine chiffon (*Dannon Light 'n Fit*)	120	8.0	22.0	0	<5	130	0
tropical w/peaches (*Dannon* Fruit on the Bottom)	240	9.0	44.0	3.0	15	150	0
tropical punch banana (*Dannon Danimals*), 4 oz.	110	5.0	20.0	2.0	5	75	0
vanilla:							
(*Breyers* 1.5% Lowfat)	220	10.0	39.0	3.0	20	135	0
(*Breyers Smooth & Creamy*)	240	7.0	47.0	2.0	20	105	0
(*Colombo* Classic)	180	8.0	32.0	2.0	15	120	0
(*Colombo* Fat Free)	160	8.0	32.0	0	5	140	0
(*Dannon*)	230	11.0	36.0	4.0	15	170	0
(*Dannon La Crème*), 4 oz.	140	5.0	20.0	3.0	20	75	0
(*Dannon Light 'n Fit*)	120	8.0	22.0	0	<5	130	0
(*Darigold* Lowfat) ..	240	10.0	45.0	2.5	15	150	0

Food and Measure	cal.	prot. (gms)	carbo. (gms)	fat (gms)	chol. (mgs)	sod. (mgs)	fiber (gms)
Yogurt, vanilla (*cont.*)							
(*Stonyfield Farm*), 1 cup	230	8.0	30.0	8.0	30	130	0
. (*Stonyfield Farm Lowfat*), 6 oz. ..	120	6.0	20.0	1.5	5	100	0
(*Stonyfield Farm Lowfat*), 1 cup ..	160	9.0	27.0	2.0	10	135	0
(*Yoplait* Custard Style), 6 oz. ...	190	8.0	32.0	3.5	15	90	0
French (*Colombo Lowfat*)	180	8.0	32.0	2.5	15	120	0
French (*Stonyfield Farm*), 6 oz. ...	170	8.0	23.0	6.0	20	95	0
French (*Stonyfield Farm* Nonfat) ...	160	9.0	30.0	0	0	135	0
truffle (*Stonyfield Farm*), 6 oz. ...	220	7.0	37.0	5.0	20	100	0
very (*Yoplait* Light), 6 oz. ....:.	100	6.0	19.0	0	<5	90	0
vanilla raspberry, French (*Dannon* Fruit on the Bottom)	240	9.0	43.0	3.0	15	150	0
vanilla strawberry (*Dannon Danimals*), 4 oz.	120	5.0	21.0	2.0	5	75	0
French (*Dannon* Fruit on the Bottom)	240	9.0	43.0	3.0	15	140	0
watermelon cherry (*Dannon Danimals*), 4 oz.	110	5.0	21.0	2.0	5	85	0
Yogurt, frozen, ½ cup:							
apple pie (*Häagen-Dazs*)	230	7.0	35.0	6.0	55	70	2.0
banana split (*Blue Bell* Nonfat)	110	4.0	24.0	0	0	75	0
(*Ben & Jerry's Phish Food*)	230	4.0	32.0	5.0	15	110	1.0
caramel w/cake (*Ben & Jerry's Ooey Gooey Cake*)	190	4.0	35.0	3.5	25	115	0

Food and Measure	cal.	prot. (gms)	carbo. (gms)	fat (gms)	chol. (mgs)	sod. (mgs)	fiber (gms)
caramel fudge (*Dreyer's/Edy's Caramel Fudge Cosmo*)	140	2.0	23.0	4.0	10	50	0
caramel praline crunch (*Dreyer's/Edy's Fat Free*)	100	3.0	23.0	0	0	60	0
cherry, black, vanilla swirl (*Dreyer's/Edy's Fat Free*)	90	3.0	20.0	0	0	45	0
cherry fudge (*Ben & Jerry's Cherry Garcia*)	170	4.0	32.0	3.0	20	80	0
chocolate:							
(*Breyers*)	130	3.0	23.0	3.0	10	45	<1.0
(*Cascadian Farm*) ..	130	4.0	25.0	3.0	9	85	1.0
(*Dreyer's/Edy's* Decadence)	120	2.0	20.0	3.5	10	45	0
(*Kemp's by Green's* Nonfat)	100	4.0	21.0	0	<5	80	<1.0
(*Stonyfield Farm*) ..	100	4.0	19.0	0	0	55	<1.0
chocolate w/almonds (*Kemp's by Green's*)	130	4.0	20.0	5.0	10	60	<1.0
chocolate cherry cordial (*Turkey Hill* Fat Free)	110	3.0	24.0	0	0	70	0
chocolate chip:							
(*Dreyer's/Edy's Chips Supreme*) .	120	2.0	19.0	4.0	10	35	0
chocolate (*Häagen-Dazs*)	230	10.0	32.0	7.0	60	55	2.0
cookie dough (*Ben & Jerry's*)	200	4.0	35.0	4.5	10	120	1.0
cookie dough (*Turkey Hill* Half Gallon)	140	3.0	23.0	4.5	10	120	0
cookie dough (*Turkey Hill* Pint)	140	3.0	24.0	4.0	10	115	0
chocolate fudge:							
(*Dreyer's/Edy's* Fat Free)	100	3.0	22.0	0	0	55	0
brownie (*Ben & Jerry's*)	190	5.0	36.0	2.5	5	105	1.0
chocolate marshmallow (*Turkey Hill* Fat Free)	130	3.0	30.0	0	0	40	0

Yogurt, frozen (cont.)

Food and Measure	cal.	prot. (gms)	carbo. (gms)	fat (gms)	chol. (mgs)	sod. (mgs)	fiber (gms)
coffee:							
(*Häagen-Dazs*)	200	8.0	31.0	4.5	65	50	0
(*Stonyfield Farm* Decaf)	90	4.0	19.0	0	<5	65	0
(*Stonyfield Farm* Soft Gourmet) ..	90	3.0	19.0	0	0	50	0
fudge sundae (*Edy's* Fat Free)	100	3.0	22.0	0	0	60	0
cookies and cream:							
(*Dreyer's/Edy's*) ...	110	2.0	19.0	3.0	10	45	0
mint (*Turkey Hill* Fat Free)	110	4.0	24.0	0	0	80	0
crème caramel (*Stonyfield Farm*)	120	4.0	23.0	1.5	<5	90	0
(*Dreyer's/Edy's Hokey Pokey*)	140	3.0	21.0	4.5	10	70	0
(*Dreyer's/Edy's* Mumbo Jumbo)	120	2.0	21.0	3.0	5	85	0
dulce de leche (*Häagen-Dazs*)	190	6.0	35.0	2.5	5	75	0
lemon chiffon (*Cascadian Farm*)	120	4.0	22.0	2.0	9	90	<1.0
mint chocolate chip (*Stonyfield Farm*) ..	130	4.0	22.0	3.0	0	50	<1.0
mocha almond (*Stonyfield Farm*)	130	5.0	23.0	2.5	0	60	1.0
mocha coffee chip (*Kemp's by Green's*)	120	3.0	20.0	3.5	10	65	0
mocha fudge (*Cascadian Farm*)	120	3.0	24.0	2.0	8	85	<1.0
Neapolitan:							
(*Kemp's by Green's* Nonfat)	100	3.0	20.0	0	0	70	0
(*Turkey Hill* Fat Free)	100	3.0	22.0	0	0	50	0
peach:							
(*Häagen-Dazs* Melba)	210	7.0	37.0	3.5	50	45	0
(*Kemp's by Green's*)	120	2.0	22.0	2.0	10	60	0
peach raspberry (*Turkey Hill*)	110	3.0	20.0	2.0	10	60	0
raspberry:							
(*Stonyfield Farm*) ..	100	3.0	21.0	0	0	55	0
(*Stonyfield Farm* Soft)	90	3.0	19.0	0	0	50	0

Food and Measure	cal.	prot. (gms)	carbo. (gms)	fat (gms)	chol. (mgs)	sod. (mgs)	fiber (gms)
black (*Turkey Hill*) .	110	3.0	20.0	2.5	10	60	0
raspberry chocolate swirl (*Cascadian Farm*)	110	3.0	21.0	2.0	7	80	<1.0
raspberry coconut (*Ben & Jerry's Raspberry Gone Coconuts*)	210	7.0	34.0	5.0	15	90	1.0
strawberry:							
(*Blue Bell* Nonfat) .	120	4.0	25.0	0	0	80	0
(*Breyers*)	120	2.0	22.0	2.5	10	35	0
(*Häagen-Dazs* Nonfat)	140	5.0	31.0	0	<5	40	0
(*Kemp's by Green's* Nonfat)	110	3.0	23.0	0	0	70	0
strawberry cheesecake (*Häagen-Dazs*)	230	7.0	36.0	6.0	65	130	<1.0
tin roof sundae:							
(*Dreyer's/Edy's*) ...	130	3.0	20.0	4.0	5	50	0
(*Turkey Hill*)	140	4.0	21.0	4.5	10	100	0
toffee crunch (*Dreyer's/ Edy's Heath*)	120	2.0	18.0	4.0	10	45	0
vanilla:							
(*Blue Bell* Country Lowfat)	120	4.0	23.0	1.5	10	90	0
(*Breyers*)	120	3.0	22.0	3.0	10	40	0
(*Cascadian Farm*) ..	130	4.0	24.0	3.0	10	100	<1.0
(*Dreyer's/Edy's*) ...	100	2.0	17.0	2.5	10	30	0
(*Dreyer's/Edy's* Fat Free) .:......	90	3.0	19.0	0	0	45	0
(*Häagen-Dazs*)	200	9.0	31.0	4.5	65	55	0
(*Kemp's by Green's*)	120	3.0	20.0	2.5	10	65	0
(*Kemp's by Green's* Nonfat)	110	3.0	22.0	0	<5	75	0
(*Stonyfield Farm*) ..	90	4.0	19.0	0	<5	65	0
bean (*Turkey Hill*) .	110	4.0	17.0	2.5	10	70	0
French or simply (*Stonyfield Farm* Soft)	90	3.0	19.0	0	0	50	0
vanilla chocolate:							
(*Turkey Hill*)	110	3.0	19.0	3.0	0	70	0
swirl (*Dreyer's/Edy's* Fat Free)	90	3.0	19.0	0	0	45	0

Food and Measure	cal.	prot. (gms)	carbo. (gms)	fat (gms)	chol. (mgs)	sod. (mgs)	fiber (gms)
Yogurt, frozen (*cont.*)							
vanilla chocolate straw-							
berry (*Breyers*) ...	120	3.0	22.0	2.5	10	40	0
vanilla fudge:							
(*Häagen-Dazs*)	220	9.0	37.0	4.0	60	115	0
(*Turkey Hill* Fat Free)	110	3.0	24.0	0	0	80	0
swirl (*Kemp's by*							
Green's Nonfat)	120	3.0	25.0	0	0	70	0
swirl (*Stonyfield*							
Farm)	110	4.0	23.0	0	0	60	0
vanilla orange sherbet							
swirl (*Turkey Hill*							
Nonfat)	100	3.0	22.0	0	0	40	0
vanilla raspberry swirl							
(*Häagen-Dazs*)	170	5.0	31.0	2.5	30	30	<1.0
"Yogurt," soy, 6 oz.,							
except as noted:							
plain (*Silk*), 8 oz. ...	150	5.0	24.0	3.5	0	40	1.0
apricot-mango (*Silk*)	170	4.0	34.0	2.0	0	20	1.0
banana-strawberry,							
blueberry, Key lime,							
or mixed berry							
(*Silk*)	170	4.0	33.0	2.0	0	20	1.0
cherry, black (*Silk*) ..	160	4.0	30.0	2.0	0	20	1.0
chocolate-vanilla or							
strawberry-peach							
(*Stonyfield Farm*							
O'Soy), 4 oz.	90	4.0	15.0	1.5	0	20	3.0
lemon (*Silk*)	170	4.0	35.0	2.0	0	20	1.0
lemon kiwi (*Silk*)	170	4.0	34.0	2.0	0	20	1.0
peach (*Silk*)	170	4.0	32.0	2.0	0	20	1.0
raspberry or straw-							
berry (*Silk*)	170	4.0	35.0	2.0	0	20	1.0
vanilla:							
(*Silk*)	110	4.0	27.0	2.5	0	30	1.0
(*Silk*), 8 oz.	150	5.0	35.0	3.5	0	40	1.0
Yogurt bar, 1 pc.:							
blackberry (*Cascadian*							
Farm)	80	3.0	14.0	1.0	5	45	<1.0
cherry fudge (*Ben &*							
Jerry's Cherry							
Garcia)	250	6.0	32.0	13.0	15	85	2.0
chocolate (*Cascadian*							
Farm)	100	3.0	18.0	1.5	5	70	0

Food and Measure	cal.	prot. (gms)	carbo. (gms)	fat (gms)	chol. (mgs)	sod. (mgs)	fiber (gms)
vanilla (*Cascadian Farm*)	100	2.0	18.0	1.5	5	70	0
Yogurt drink (see also "Kefir"):							
all flavors:							
(*Dannon Actimel*), 3.3 fl. oz.	90	3.0	16.0	2.0	10	45	0
(*Dannon Danimals Drinkable*), 3.1 fl. oz.	90	4.0	16.0	1.5	5	55	0
banana berry (*Dannon Frusion* Smoothie), 1 bottle	270	8.0	52.0	3.5	15	130	0
berries, wild (*Dannon Frusion* Smoothie), 1 bottle	270	8.0	53.0	3.5	15	170	0
peach passion fruit (*Dannon Frusion* Smoothie), 1 bottle	270	8.0	51.0	3.5	15	180	0
Youngberry juice, blend (*Ceres*), 5.25 fl. oz.	87	0	21.0	0	0	n.a.	0
Yu choy sum (*Frieda's*), 1 cup, 3 oz.	20	2.0	3.0	0	0	20	0
Yuca root (*Frieda's*), ⅔ cup, 3 oz.	100	3.0	23.0	0	0	5	1.0

Z

Food and Measure	cal.	prot. (gms)	carbo. (gms)	fat (gms)	chol. (mgs)	sod. (mgs)	fiber (gms)
Ziti entree, frozen, 1 pkg.:							
baked (*Celentano*), 9 oz., ⅛ pkg.	250	8.0	24.0	13.0	15	580	3.0
Parmesano (*Budget Gourmet*), 8 oz. . .	260	10.0	42.0	7.0	5	530	3.0
Zucchini, fresh, w/skin, ½ cup, except as noted:							
raw:							
chopped	9	.7	1.8	.1	0	2	.7
sliced	8	.7	1.6	.1	0	2	7
baby (*Frieda's*), ⅔ cup, 3 oz. . . .	20	2.0	3.0	0	0	0	0
baby, 1 large, 3⅛"	3	.4	.5	<.1	0	tr.	<.1
boiled, drained:							
sliced	14	.6	3.5	<.1	0	2	1.3
mashed	19	.8	4.7	.1	0	3	1.7
Zucchini, canned, Italian style, ½ cup:							
(*Del Monte*)	30	1.0	7.0	0	0	490	1.0
w/tomato juice	33	1.2	7.8	.1	0	424	1.0
Zucchini, frozen, w/skin, boiled, drained, 1 cup	38	2.6	7.9	.3	0	5	2.9
Zucchini, breaded, frozen (*Empire Kosher*), 7 pcs., 3 oz.	100	5.0	18.0	.5	0	280	1.0
Zucchini, marinated, sun-dried, in jars							

Food and Measure	cal.	prot. (gms)	carbo. (gms)	fat (gms)	chol. (mgs)	sod. (mgs)	fiber (gms)
(*Antica Italia*), 1 oz.	160	0	2.0	17.0	0	15	1.0
Zucchini soufflé, frozen (*Melrose*), ½ cup	90	3.0	19.0	0	0	160	3.0

Corinne T. Netzer

SHE KNOWS WHAT'S GOOD FOR YOU!

___ 22564-7 THE COMPLETE BOOK OF FOOD COUNTS / $7.50

___ 23679-7 THE CORINNE T. NETZER 2003 CALORIE COUNTER / $7.50

___ 22609-0 CORINNE T. NETZER'S BIG BOOK OF MIRACLE CURES / $6.99

___ 23682-7 THE CORINNE T. NETZER CARBOHYDRATE COUNTER / $6.99

___ 22055-6 THE CORINNE T. NETZER FAT GRAM COUNTER / $5.99

___ 61367-1 THE COMPLETE BOOK OF VITAMIN AND
               MINERAL COUNTS / $23.00

___ 50410-4 THE CORINNE T. NETZER DIETER'S DIARY / $10.95

___ 50821-5 THE DIETER'S CALORIE COUNTER / $10.95

___ 50695-6 THE CORINNE T. NETZER LOW-FAT DIARY / $9.95

___ 50852-5 THE CARBOHYDRATE DIETER'S DIARY / $8.95

___ 21665-6 THE CORINNE T. NETZER CARBOHYDRATE GRAM COUNTER / $5.99

___ 50367-1 THE CORINNE T. NETZER ENCYCLOPEDIA OF FOOD VALUES / $29.95

___ 50417-1 101 LOW CHOLESTEROL RECIPES / $15.00

Please enclose check or money order only, no cash or CODs. Shipping & handling costs: $5.50 U.S. mail, $7.50 UPS. New York and Tennessee residents must remit applicable sales tax. Canadian residents must remit applicable GST and provincial taxes. Please allow 4 – 6 weeks for delivery. All orders are subject to availability. This offer subject to change without notice. Please call 1-800-726-0600 for further information.

Bantam Dell Publishing Group, Inc.   TOTAL AMT $_____
Attn: Customer Service   SHIPPING & HANDLING $_____
400 Hahn Road   SALES TAX (NY, TN) $_____
Westminster, MD 21157

                              TOTAL ENCLOSED $_____

Name _____

Address _____

City/State/Zip _____

Daytime Phone (_____) _____